Veterinary Medical Virology

Veterinary Medical Virology

Author

Dr. C.B. PRASAD

M.V.Sc., Ph.D., FRVCS (SWEDEN)

Ex University Professor cum Chief Scientist and Chairman

Department of Veterinary Microbiolgy, Bihar Veterinary College, Patna

Rajendra Agriculture University, Pusa, Patna-800 014, Bihar

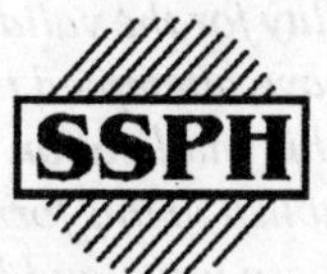

SATISH SERIAL PUBLISHING HOUSE

403, Express Tower, Commercial Complex, Azadpur, Delhi-110033 (India)

Phone : 011-27672852, Fax : 91-11-27672046

E-mail : info@satishserial.com, hkjain1975@yahoo.com

Website : www.satishserial.com

Published by :

SATISH SERIAL PUBLISHING HOUSE
403, Express Tower, Commercial Complex, Azadpur, Delhi-110033 (INDIA)
Phone : 011-27672852 Fax : 91-11-27672046
E-mail : info@satishserial.com, hkjain1975@yahoo.com

ISBN 978-93-81226-51-3

Typeset at: Harminder Kharb *for* Laxmi Art Creation # 9971212252
Printed at: Salasar Imaging Systems, Delhi-110035

*The book, veterinary medical virology is dedicated to my daughter, **MEENAKSHI KUMARI**. The completion of the book would not have been possible without her help inspite of the fact that she is suffering from fanconi syndrome and strugling for life.*

Foreword

The book, Veterinary Medical Virology compiled by Dr C. B. Prasad is based on his longstanding experience on various aspects of Veterinary Microbiology. His teaching & research experience in reputed Veterinary Colleges & Research Institutes in India & abroad, & visits to several countries related to research & training in the subject extends to about 38 years.

The present book on Veterinary Medical Virology has been divided into two parts; Basic Virology & Pathogenic Viruses. Basic Virology has been written in seven chapters (1 to 7), while Pathogenic Viruses include chapters 8 to 33. Chapter 34 covers diseases caused by prion proteins. Basic Virology is essential for the students, practising veterinarians, medicos & other readers to understand the basic concept, nature & characteristics of various families of viruses, their mode of replication, the mechanism of virus-cell interactions, & ongoing fight between host defensive mechanisms & viral strategy to thwart host protective measures. Topics on viral immunity & viral vaccines are very specific & informative; especially veterinary viral vaccines have been described in details giving the dose, mode of administration, & schedule of vaccination which are essential for controlling viral diseases especially when they are not responsive to antibiotics. All chapters are very informative, self explanatory & include latest informations for the benefit of students, practioners and teachers.

Presentation made in Table 1-3 is of utmost importance as it summarizes each virus family classification, taxonomy & serotypes & diseases caused by the member viruses in humans & animals.

As regards Pathogenic Viruses in part two, similar procedure has been adopted to present each chapter: describing characteristics of the family, viral genome, virus replication, virus classification, and in tabular form virus family classification & diseases caused by the member viruses in humans & animals. While describing each viral disease in animals, the general presentation includes summary description of each disease, etiology, occurrence, hosts susceptible, transmission, pathogenesis, clinical symptoms & lesions, diagnosis, treatment, control & vaccination.

The book covers the syllabus prescribed by the Veterinary Council of India on Veterinary Virology for both undergraduate & postgraduate students of veterinary colleges in India. The publication of Veterinary Medical Virology has fulfilled the long felt need in the discipline especially detailing vaccination policy to be adopted to control viral diseases. The book is required to be acquired by each and every Library of veterinary medical institutions as an important and latest addition in the field of virology.

I greatly appreciate the sincere effort of Dr. C.B. Prasad for his earnest desire to undertake to write the book single-handed providing latest information on Veterinary Medical Virology; I do hope that this book will greatly benefit the students, teachers, practioners & also medical profession.

Prof. Allauddin Ahmad*
Ph. D., D.Sc. (H.C.), FNAVS.
Patna, dated 10.4.2012

M. 09430487932, Tel: 06122585010
30-A, Indirapuri Colony, Patna 800014

a) Former Vice Chancellor, Jamia Hamdard (N. Delhi) and S. K. University of Agrc. Sciences & Technology (J & K).
b) Past President of Association of Indian Universities and Association of Agril. Universities in India.
c) Ex Vice Chairman, International Islamic Forum for Science and Technology & Human Resource Development (Jakarta).
d) Ex Member of the executive & General Council of the Association of Commonwealth Universities.
e) Ex Dy Director General (Education) & National Project Director (UNDP), ICAR, Govt. of India, N. Delhi.
f) Ex Member Bihar State Farmers' Commission.

Preface

The inspiration for writing the present book "Veterinary Medical Virology" is the outcome of my longstanding 38 years experience of teaching and research in various aspects of veterinary Microbiology including Virology at several colleges and Research Institutions in India & abroad. During the tenure of heading the Dept of Veterinary Microbiology while working as Assistant Professor, Associate Professor & University Professor cum Chairman of Microbiology both at College of Veterinary Science & Animal Husbandry, Kanke, Ranchi (now Birsa Agriculture University) & at Bihar Veterinary College, Patna (Rajendra Agricultural University, Bihar), Lectures on Veterinary Virology, Veterinary Immunology, Veterinary Bacteriology & Mycology were published that became very popular among the students. All these experiences & repeated requests by UG & PG students to write a book on Veterinary Medical Virology in concise & simple language with latest information on viral diseases with detail informations on vaccination policy in each case encouraged me to write the present book.

While teaching, all available multi-authors written foreign books on Virology were consulted but none satisfied the students quench, & none described vaccination policy & vaccines with detail which are the backbone of controlling viral diseases. Accordingly, it was laboured hard to present the book in a simple, concise understandable & comprehensive manner incorporating all available informations on viral diseases with viral vaccines in detail that could be beneficial to the students, the practising veterinarians, teachers in understanding the subject in simple language & adopting a suitable vaccination policy for the control of viral diseases. It is sincerely believed & hoped that this book will be worth reading & beneficial for the students of Virology, Pathology, Medicine, the practising veterinarians, medicos & students of other biological sciences.

It would be pertinent to mention that while writing this book, syllabus of Veterinary Council of India as regards to Veterinary Virology has been fully covered.

The book, Veterinary Medical Virology, has been divided into two parts; Basic Virology & Pathogenic Viruses & presented in 34 chapters. Basic Virology has been written in seven chapters from chapter 1 to 7, while Pathogenic Viruses include from chapter 8 to chapter 33. Chapter 34 describes prion diseases.

The seven chapters of Basic Medical Virology in Part-I are as follows:

Chapter 1: Historical development, general characteristics, structure & taxonomy of viruses.

Chapter 2: Propagation, purification & enumeration of viruses

Chapter 3: Viral replication, viral genetics & recombination

Chapter 4: Virus-cell interactions and viral pathogenesis

Chapter 5: Antiviral immunity

Chapter 6: Control of viral diseases, vaccines & vaccination policy

Chapter 7: Laboratory diagnosis of viral infections

Chapter 1 in Table 1-2 summarizes the characteristics of 26 important families of viruses of medical & veterinary importance, & Table 1-3 is very important as it furnishes the gist of each virus family with classification, taxonomy & diseases caused by the member viruses. It would be beneficial for the students & readers to go through these two tables first.

Chapter 2 details cultivation of viruses in cell cultures, in embryonated eggs & animals, & various methods to purify & enumerate the viruses.

Chapter 3 is important to have a concept into understanding virus replication of different groups of viruses of medical & veterinary importance.

Chapter 4 describes the virus-cell interactions, which is worth reading in understanding the ongoing mechanisms of virus-cell interactions, fight between host defensive mechanisms & viral strategy to thwart host defenses to cause disease or recover from viral diseases.

Chapter 5 describes the general principles of viral immunity, newer concept on recognition of viral components & nucleic acid to initiate immune responses, & describes mechanism of both non specific & adaptive immune responses to combat viral diseases.

Chapter 6 is very important as all available vaccines against important animal diseases have been mentioned to combat viral diseases. The chapter also describes general policy to be adopted to control viral diseases in cattle, sheep, goats, pigs, horses, dogs, cats & poultry along with choice as to which vaccine is to be used against each viral disease. It is worth reading.

Chapter 7 includes the common virological tests including modern tests & principles in vogue to diagnose viral diseases.

Pathogenic Viruses in Part-II start from chapters 8 to 34 as follows:

Chapter 8: Characteristics of and diseases caused by group I double-stranded DNA adenoviruses

Chapter 9: Characteristics of and diseases caused by group I double-stranded DNA asfarviruses

Chapter 10: Characteristics of and diseases caused by group I double-stranded DNA herpesviruses

Chapter 11: Characteristics of and diseases caused by group I double-stranded DNA poxviruses

Chapter 12: Characteristics of and diseases caused by group I double-stranded DNA papillomaviruses

Chapter 13: Characteristics of and diseases caused by group I double-stranded DNA polyomaviruses

Chapter 14: Characteristics of and diseases caused by group II single-stranded DNA parvoviruses

Chapter 15: Characteristics of and diseases caused by group II single-stranded circoviruses

Chapter 16: Characteristics of and diseases caused by group III double-stranded RNA reoviruses

Chapter 17: Characteristics of and diseases caused by group III double-stranded RNA birnaviruses

Chapter 18: Characteristics of and diseases caused by group IV single-stranded (+) RNA picornaviruses

Chapter 19: Characteristics of and diseases caused by group IV single-stranded (+) RNA caliciviruses

Chapter 20: Characteristics of and diseases caused by group IV single-stranded (+) RNA togaviruses

Chapter 21: Characteristics of and diseases caused by group IV single-stranded (+) RNA flaviviruses

Chapter 22: Characteristics of and diseases caused by group IV single-stranded (+) RNA coronaviruses

Chapter 23: Characteristics of and diseases caused by group IV single-stranded (+) RNA arteriviruses

Chapter 24: Characteristics of and diseases caused by group IV single-stranded (+) RNA astroviruses

Chapter 25: Characteristics of and diseases caused by group V single-stranded (-) RNA orthomyxoviruses

Chapter 26: Characteristics of and diseases caused by group V single-stranded (-) RNA paramyxoviruses

Chapter 27: Characteristics of and diseases caused by group V single-stranded (-) RNA rhabdoviruses

Chapter 28: Characteristics of and diseases caused by group V single-stranded (-) RNA bornaviruses

Chapter 29: Characteristics of and diseases caused by group V single-stranded (-) RNA filoviruses

Chapter 30: Characteristics of and diseases caused by group V single-stranded (-) RNA arenaviruses

Chapter 31: Characteristics of and diseases caused by group V single-stranded (-) RNA bunyaviruses

Chapter 32: Characteristics of and diseases caused by group VI double-stranded RNA-RT retroviruses

Chapter 33: Characteristics of and diseases caused by group VII double-stranded DNA-RT hepadnaviruses

Chapter 34: Characteristics of and diseases caused by prions proteins/ transmissible spongiform encephalopathies

General plan in describing pathogenic viruses from chapters 8 to 33 is: characteristics of the family, viral genome, virus replication, virus classification, & in tabular form virus family classification & diseases caused by the member virus species in humans & animals. While describing each viral disease in animals, the general presentation is: a summary description of each disease, etiology, occurrence, hosts susceptible, transmission, pathogenesis, clinical symptoms & lesions, diagnosis, treatment & control, & vaccination. In presenting each chapter most up to date informations have been incorporated after consulting internet search, recent articles & books on these topics. Recent Products of veterinary commercial companies on vaccine, type of vaccines (live, attenuated, killed, marker or recombinant vaccine preparation) with dose, schedule of vaccination including primary, booster & subsequent annual or otherwise vaccination policy in animals & poultry have been described.

As regards prion diseases, the topic includes: Characteristics of Prions, PrP^{C} & PrP^{Sc}, various hypotheses on prion diseases, transmission, sterilization & pathogenesis, Table 34-1depicting various prion diseases, prion diseases caused by various transmissible spongiform encephalopathies, clinical infections in humans, clinical infections in animals, Scrapie, Bovine spongiform encephalopathy, Transmissible mink encephalopathy, Feline spongiform encephalopathy, Chronic wasting disease & Exotic ungulate encephalopathy.

During writing this book, I came across highly informative picture presentation on virology by Swiss Molecular Biology, Swiss Institute of Bioinformatics under the heading ViralZone & some other pictures. The pictures are so informative that each veterinary medical student,clinician, teachers & other readers can understand the virus morphology easily, & hence I have included the pictures in this book. I highly acknowledge their contribution.

I would be failing in my duty if I do not mention the contribution of my crippled daughter, Meenakshi Kumari, who is unable to stand & walk; although not educated but she is master of computer application. She helped me in managing the computer writing & corrected the computer whenever it went wrong. My wife, Mrs Saroj Devi always encouraged me to continue writing & complete the book. My son, Er Avinash Kumar silently & patiently prayed for the completion of the book. The whole income if any will be spent towards treating my disabled daughter & furtherance of development of veterinary virology.

My students, whom I taught for such long period & who could not satisfy from multi-author written books on Virology always encouraged me to write in concise, simple understandable informative manner the book on Veterinary Medical Virology depicting all recent developments & especially mentioning the details of viral vaccines. I gratefully acknowledge their constant encouragement.

I take opportunity to extend my gratitude to all my respected teachers, late Dr Rubarth of Sweden, late Dr C. M. Singh, Dr P. Kumar, Dr B. S. Rajya, Dr B. S. Malik, Dr Allauddin Ahmad (ex Vice Chancellor of S. K. University of Agriculture, JK), Dr. H.R. Mishra (ex Dean & Vice Chancellor of Birsa Agriculture University), Dr R. D. Sinha, & Dr B. K. Gupta of C.D.R.I., Lucknow from whom I got great inspiration.

I am extremely thankful to my colleagues, Dr R. P. Sinha, ex Professor of Medicine, BAU, Ranchi, Dr D.P. Singh, ex Professor of Surgery & a successful veterinary practitioner, Dr S. S. Singh, ex Professor of Livestock Production & Management, B.V.C., Patna, Dr Arun Prasad, Professor & Head of Dept of Microbiology, Ranchi & Dr K. C. P. Singh, present Dean of Veterinary Faculty, College of Animal Science, Chhattisgarh, my friends Sri Ram Akbal Sinha, Advocate, Hajipur, Sri A. K. Ghosh, Dr Rajeshwar Prasad Sinha & ErAjit Kumar who always encouraged me to do something better in life.

10.4.2012

Dr. C.B. PRASAD
Ex University Professor
cum Chief Scientist and Chairman
Dept of Vet.Microbiolgy
Bihar Veterinary College, Patna
Rajendra Agriculture University, Pusa
Patna-800 014, Bihar

Residence
B-45, Indirapuri colony
Road No. 1, Patna-800 014
M.: 9430213239

Contents

Part 1 : Basic Virology

Part 2 : Pathogenic Viruses

Part 1 : Basic Virology

Chapter 1

Historical Development, General Characteristics, Structure & Taxonomy of Viruses

Contents

Historical Development of Virology

The foundation of the medical and veterinary virology dates back to period of the concept of the specificity of causation of diseases. Louis Pasteur, called the father of microbiology was the first in 1857 to discover the specificity of microbial fermentations; in 1865 he founded the concept of infectious diseases of silkworms, and between 1877 and 1895 extended the concept to human and animal diseases. Pasteur's early work centered on septic war wounds; he then turned to anthrax and other bacterial diseases, and lastly to rabies. In 1885, Pasteur gave the first rabies vaccine to a boy, Joseph Meister, bitten severely by a rabid dog, that day marked the opening of the modern era of infectious disease science aimed at disease prevention and control.

Robert Koch, called the father of Bacteriology discovered the causative agents of tuberculosis and cholera and contributed to the development of laboratory methods in bacteriology. Koch also worked on several diseases which eventually showed were caused by viruses. As a result of the work of Pasteur, Koch and others, the identification of the causative agents of many important human diseases proceeded at rapid pace around the turn of the twentieth century.

Pasteur, Koch and their colleagues, & others extended the field of the infectious disease in many ways. The **Table 1-1** presented in the last of this chapter gives in chronically order some of the discoveries and technologies that were made in the advancement of medical and veterinary virology. The table includes as many as possible of the important and interesting pathogens that are the focus of medical and veterinary virology and comparative virology research. The arboviruses proved to be a special case because of their profusion, so a selective approach was taken in order to emphasize those viruses causing major human and veterinary diseases.

In 1884 the French microbiologist Charles Chamberland invented a filter, known today as the Chamber land filter or Chamberland-Pasteur filter that has pores smaller than bacteria. Among the founders of the science of virology, the evidence for the existence of filterable, very small infectious agents was provided in 1898 by Martinus Beijerinck in Holland and Dimitri Ivanovski in Russia. They made extracts from diseased tobacco plants infected with **tobacco mosaic virus**, and passed the extracts through fine filters that retained bacteria. The filtrates contained an agent that was able to infect new plants, but no bacteria could be cultured from the filtrates. The agent remained infective through several transfers to new plants, eliminating the possibility of a toxin. Beijerinck called it a *contagium vivum fluidum* (soluble living germ) and **reintroduced the word *virus*.** Beijerinck maintained that viruses were liquid in nature, a theory later discredited by Wendell Stanley, who proved they were particulate. Beijerinck **called the agent a 'virus' which means poison in Latin,** and the term has since been retained till now. At around the same time in 1898, **Freidrich Loeffler and Paul Frosch** discovered the **first virus of vertebrates; they passed the material through a similar filter & transmitted foot and mouth disease from animal to animal in inoculum that had been highly diluted.** Other imminent founders of virology to be remembered are as follows. **Sanarelli in 1898** discovered myxoma virus. In 1990 **Walter Reed & James Carroll** discovered the first human virus, Yellow fever virus & demonstrated virus transmission through mosquitoes. M'fadyean discovered Horse sickness virus in 1900. Gentanni, Lodge & Gruber in 1901 discovered fowl plague virus. Remlinger & Riffat Bay in 1903 discovered rabies virus. De Schweinitz & Dorset discovered hog cholera virus. Arnold Theiler in 1900s discovered rinderpest, & African horse sickness. Ellermann & bang in 1908 discovered **avian leukemia virus- the first cancer causing virus.** In 1909 Landsteiner & Popper discovered poliovirus. Rous in 1911 discovered the first solid tumor virus- Ross sarcoma virus. Laidlaw & Dunkin in 1926 discovered canine distemper virus.

In 1931 Shope discovered swine influenza virus. Andrewes, Laidlaw, Smith & Burnet in 1933 isolated influenza virus. Max Theiler in 1933 discovered yellow fever vaccine. Olafson, Pritchard, Gillepsi, Baker & colleagues in 1940s-1950 discovered Bovine viral diarrhea. In 1950s Sigurdsson studied scrapie & maedi/visna in sheep & proposed that they are caused by slow growing viruses. The second half of the 20th century was the golden age of virus discovery and most of the 2,000 recognized species of animal, plant, and bacterial viruses were discovered during these years. Salk & Sabin in 1954 & 1957 developed inactivated virus & attenuated virus polio vaccines. In 1957, equine arteritis and the cause of Bovine virus diarrhea (a pestivirus) were discovered. In 1963, the hepatitis B virus was discovered by Baruch Blumberg, and in 1965, Howard Temin described the first retrovirus. Reverse transcriptase, the key enzyme that retroviruses use to translate their RNA into DNA, was first described in

1970, independently by Howard MartinTemin and David Baltimore. In 1983 Luc Montaigne's team at the Pasteur Institute in France, first isolated the retrovirus now called HIV. Charmichael, Parrish & colleagues in 1978 discovered canine parvovirus. Petersen & colleagues in 1987 discovered feline immunodeficiency virus. Stanleg B Prusiner studied the nature of prions, the causative agent of bovine spongiform encephalopathy, srapie & other transmissible spongiform encephalopathy & won Novel Prize in medicine in 1999.

In the early 20th century, the English bacteriologist Frederick Twort discovered a group of viruses that infect bacteria, now called bacteriophage or commonly *phages*, and the French-Canadian microbiologist Felix d Herelle described viruses that, when added to bacteria on agar would produce areas of dead bacteria. He accurately diluted a suspension of these viruses and discovered that the highest dilutions (lowest virus concentrations), rather than killing all the bacteria, formed discrete areas of dead organisms. Counting these areas and multiplying by the dilution factor allowed him to calculate the number of viruses in the original suspension.

By the end of the 19th century, viruses were defined in terms of their infectivity, their ability to be filtered, and their requirement for living hosts. Viruses had been grown only in plants and animals. In 1906, Ross Granville invented a method for growing tissue in lymph, and, in 1913, E. Steinhardt, C. Israeli, and R. A. Lambert used this method to grow vaccinia virus in fragments of guinea pig corneal tissue. In 1928, H. B. Maitland and M. C. Maitland grew vaccinia virus in suspensions of minced hens' kidneys. Their method was not widely adopted until the 1950s, when poliovirus was grown on a large scale for vaccine production. Another breakthrough came in 1931, when the American pathologist Ernest Willium Goodpasture grew influenza and several other viruses in fertilized chickens' eggs. In 1949, John F. Enders, Thomas Weller & Fredrick Rabbins grew polio virus in cultured human embryo cells, the first virus to be grown without using solid animal tissue or eggs. This work enabled Jonas Salk to make an effective poliovirus vaccine.

The first images of viruses were obtained upon the invention of electron microscope in 1931 by the German engineers Ernst Ruska and max Knoll. In 1935, American biochemist and virologist, Wendell Meredith Stanley examined the tobacco mosaic virus and found it was mostly made of protein. A short time later, this virus was separated into protein and RNA parts. The tobacco mosaic virus was the first to be crystallized and its structure could therefore be elucidated in detail. The first X-ray diffraction pictures of the crystallized virus were obtained by Bernal and Fankuchen in 1941. On the basis of her pictures, Rosalind Franklin discovered the full DNA structure of the virus in 1955. In the same year, Heinz Fraenkel-Conrat and Robley Williams showed that purified tobacco mosaic virus RNA and its coat protein can assemble by themselves to form functional viruses, suggesting that this simple mechanism was probably the means through which viruses were created within their host cells.

General Characteristics of Viruses

Ubiquity & origin of viruses on earth:

The ubiquitous nature of viruses has its impact throughout the living world; virus disease can be found in higher animals, birds, plants, arthropods, protozoa and bacteria. Viruses infect all cellular life forms: eukaryotes-vertebrate animals, invertebrate animals, plants & fungi, & prokaryotes-bacteria and archaea. The viruses that infect prokaryotes are called **bacteriophages** or simply phage. The presence of virus is obvious in host organisms showing signs of disease. Many healthy organisms, however, are hosts of non-pathogenic virus infections, some of which are active, while some are quiescent. Furthermore, the genomes of many organisms contain remnants of ancient virus genomes that integrated into their host genomes long ago. The viruses present within their hosts are also found in soil, air and water. Many aqueous environments contain very high concentrations of viruses that infect the host organisms that live in those environments. There is a strong correlation between how intensively a species is studied and the number of viruses found in that species. There are many viruses known that infect mankind & animals than any other species, and new human & animal viruses continue to emerge. Many viruses have been found in the intestinal bacterium, *Escherichia coli*. It is presumed that the viruses that have been discovered represent only a small fraction of the viruses on the Earth. Most of the known plants, animals, fungi, bacteria and archaea have not yet been investigated for the presence of viruses, and new potential hosts for viruses continue to be discovered.

Viruses are found wherever there is life and have probably existed since living cells first evolved. The **origin of viruses is unclear** because they do not form fossils, so molecular techniques have been the most useful means of hypothesising how they arose. However, these techniques rely on the availability of ancient viral DNA or RNA but most of the viruses that have been preserved and stored in laboratories are less than 90 years old. Molecular methods have only been successful in tracing the ancestry of viruses that evolved in the 20th century.

There are three main theories of the origins of viruses:

a. *Regressive theory:* If they are not cells and require living cells for replication, then viruses must not have been present prior to cellular evolution and could therefore have coevolved with cells. Viruses may have once been small cells that parasitized larger cells. Over time, genes not required by their parasitism were lost. The bacteria, richettsia and chlamydia are living cells that, like viruses, can reproduce only inside host cells. They lend credence to this theory, as their dependence on parasitism is likely to have caused the loss of genes that enabled them to survive outside a cell.

b. *Cellular origin theory:*Viruses were once cells but have lost all cellular functions retaining only information to replicate themselves using hosts machinery. Some viruses may have evolved from bits of DNA or RNA that "escaped" from the genes of a larger organism. The escaped DNA could have come from plasmids, pieces of DNA that can move between cells while others may have evolved from bacteria.

c. *Coevolution theory:* Viruses may have evolved from complex molecules of protein and DNA at the same time as cells first appeared on earth and would have been dependent on cellular life for many millions of years. Or viruses have evolved from plasmids (plasmids are self replicating independent DNA) or from RNA viroids. These "early" viruses did not contain genes for capsids. As viroids moved from cell to another, it picked up such genes.

Several viruses cause disease: Viruses are etiological agents of many human & animal diseases, ranging from the trivial (e.g. common colds) to the lethal rabies, HIV infection, Ebolavirus, Corona SARS in humans. Similarly Foot & mouth diseases, Rinderpest, IBR in cattle, Infectious canine hepatitis, Parvoviral canine infection, Canine distemper in dogs, & many other diseases (**Table1-3**); viruses also play roles in the development of several types of cancer. Viruses besides causing individuals to suffer, virus diseases can also affect the well-being of societies. Smallpox had a great impact in the past and AIDS is having a great impact today. Similar is the case with rinderpest & foot and mouth disease in animals that had wiped out large population of animals in the past. There is therefore a requirement to understand the nature of viruses, how they replicate and how they cause disease. This knowledge permits the development of effective means for prevention, diagnosis and treatment of virus diseases through the production of vaccines, diagnostic reagents and techniques, and antiviral drugs. These medical applications therefore constitute major aspects of the science of virology.

Veterinary virology is also very important because of the economic impact of the many viruses that cause disease in domestic animals e. g. foot and mouth disease virus in animals. Viruses can cause immense economic damage in the dairy industry, where phages can infect the lactic acid bacteria that are responsible for the fermentations that produce cheese, yogurt and other milk products.

Some viruses are useful:

Some viruses are studied because they have useful potential applications.

- *Phage typing of bacteria:* Some bacteria, such as some *Salmonella* species, are classified into strains on the basis of the spectrum of phages to which they are susceptible. Identification of the phage types of bacterial isolates can provide useful epidemiological information during outbreaks of disease caused by these bacteria.
- *Sources of enzymes:* A number of enzymes used in molecular biology are virus enzymes. Examples include reverse transcriptases from retroviruses and RNA polymerases from phages.
- *Pesticides:* Some insect pests are controlled with baculoviruses, and myxoma virus has been used to control rabbits.
- *Anti-bacterial agents:* In the mid-20th century phages were used to treat some bacterial infections of humans. Interest waned with the discovery of antibiotics, but has been renewed with the emergence of antibiotic-resistant strains of bacteria.
- *Anti-cancer agents:* Genetically modified strains of viruses, such as herpes simplex virus and vaccinia virus are being investigated for treatment of cancers. These strains have been modified so that they are able to infect and destroy specific tumor cells, but are unable to infect normal cells.
- *Gene vectors for protein production:* Viruses such as certain baculoviruses and adenoviruses are used as vectors to take genes into animal cells growing in culture. This technology can be used to insert into cells genes encoding useful proteins, such as vaccine components, and the cells can then be used for mass production of the proteins.

- *Gene vectors for treatment of genetic diseases:* Children with severe combined immunodeficiency have been successfully treated using retroviruses as vectors to introduce into their stem cells a non-mutated copy of the mutated gene responsible for the disease.

Virus studies contribute to our knowledge:

Viruses have thrown much light in our understanding of the basic knowledge of molecular biology, cell biology and cancer as enumerated below:

- Alfred Hershey and Martha Chase through their experiment published in 1952, used phage T2 and *E. coli* to provide strong evidence that genes are composed of DNA.
- The first enhancers to be characterized were in genes of simian virus 40 (SV40).
- The first transcription factor to be characterized was the transplantation (T) antigen of SV40.
- The first nuclear localization signal of a protein was identified in the T antigen of SV40.
- Introns were discovered during studies of adenovirus transcription.
- The role of the cap structure at the 5′ end of eukaryotic mRNA was discovered during studies with vaccinia virus and a reovirus.
- The first internal ribosomal entry site was discovered using the RNA of poliovirus.
- The first RNA pseudoknot was discovered in the genome of turnip yellow mosaic virus.

The nature of viruses:

Virology is concerned with study of very small particles, called virions. The units in which virions are normally measured are nanometers (1 nm = 10^{-9} m). Viruses are among the smallest infectious agents, and most of them can only be seen by electron microscopy. Most viruses cannot be seen by light microscopy, i.e., they are submicroscopic; their sizes range from 20 to 300 nm. They are so small that it would take 30,000 to 750,000 of them, side by side, to stretch to one cm. Although virions are very small, their dimensions cover a large range. There are predominantly two kinds of shapes found amongst viruses: rods or filaments, and spheres. The rod shape is due to the linear array of the nucleic acid and the protein subunits making up the capsid. The sphere shape is actually a 20-sided polygon (icosahedrons). Amongst the smallest are parvoviruses, with diameters about 20 nm, while the microbe-mimicking virus (mimivirus), **isolated from an amoeba**, is amongst the largest.

A concentrated suspension of virions might contain 10^{12} virions/ml. A single virus-infected cell might produce 10^5 virions. A person infected with HIV might produce 10^{11} virions in a day.

Virions are not cells; they are acellular. They do not contain organelles, except for the virions of the arenaviruses, which contain cell ribosomes that were packaged when the virions were assembled.

The viruses have genes: The virion contains the genome of the virus. Whereas the genomes of cells are composed of double-stranded DNA, there are 7 types of a virus genome:

- Double-stranded DNA
- Single-stranded DNA
- Double-stranded RNA
- Single-stranded positive-sense RNA.
- Single-stranded negative-sense RNA.
- RNA viruses-reverse transcribing
- DNA viruses-reverse transcribing

The genome is enclosed in a protein coat known as a **capsid**. The genome plus the capsid, plus outer envelope in some cases, and other components in many cases, constitute the **virion**. The functions of the virion are to protect the genome and to deliver it into a cell in which it can replicate. Generally, virus genomes are much smaller than cell genomes. How viruses being so small encode all their requirements in a small genome; this is achieved in a number of ways.

- Viruses use host cell proteins. The genomes of large viruses duplicate some of the functions of the host cell, but the small viruses rely heavily on functions of the host cell. There is, however, **one function that an RNA virus must encode, no matter how small its genome**. That function is an **RNA polymerase**, because cells do not encode enzymes that can replicate virus RNA. Large number of the genome of an RNA virus is taken up with the gene for an RNA polymerase.
- Viruses code efficiently. There may be overlapping genes and genes encoded within genes. The small genome of hepatitis B virus is a good example.
- Many virus proteins are multifunctional. A virus protein may have several enzyme activities.

Viruses are parasites:

A virus is a very small, acellular parasite of cells. **Virus genome is composed of either DNA or RNA but not both,** is enclosed in a protein coat, called capsid, & sometimes external envelope. **Viruses belong to biology because they possess genes, replicate, evolve, and are adapted to particular hosts, biotic habitats, and ecological niches.**Viruses differ from cells in the way in which they multiply. A new cell is always formed directly from a pre-existing cell, but a new virion is never formed directly from a pre-existing virion. New virions components are formed separately by a process of replication, which takes place inside a host cell and involves the synthesis of virus components separately followed by their assembly into virions. **Viruses are therefore parasites of cells,** and are dependent on their hosts for most of their requirements, including

- Building-blocks such as amino acids and nucleosides;
- Protein-synthesizing machinery (ribosomes);
- Energy, in the form of adenosine triphosphate.

A virus modifies the intracellular environment of its host in order to enhance the efficiency of the replication process. Modifications might include production of new membranous structures, reduced expression of cell genes or enhancement of a cell process. Some large phages encode proteins that boost photosynthesis in the cells of their photosynthetic bacterial hosts, thereby probably boosting the yields of virus from the cells.

Summing up, viruses are obligate intracellular parasites. This means that they cannot replicate on their own but instead have to rely on host cells and the cellular biosynthetic machinery for reproduction. They enter the cytosol or nucleus of a host cell, and force the cell to synthesize new virus particles according to instructions that they provide in the form of RNA or DNA. A virus particle is generally very small and structurally quite simple. In addition to proteins and sometimes also lipids, it contains as an essential component one or more molecules of DNA or RNA. These constitute the genome of the virus that carries genes necessary for the production of new viruses in the host cell. The number of genes varies from a small number to a few hundred depending on the virus. In a virus particle isolated from the extra cellular space, the genome is present in a highly condensed form and protected by a coat of proteins called viral capsid. Capsids take the form of a helix or they have an icosahedral protein shell that encloses the genome. In enveloped viruses, the capsid is further covered by a lipid bilayer membrane, the viral envelope. The membrane contains additional viral proteins that are usually glycosylated and often form spike-like projections required for cell attachment and penetration into the host cell. Virus particles serve as carriers for the viral genome and accessory proteins from the infected host cell to an uninfected cell. Importantly, the particle must also protect the genome in transit so that it can be delivered in a replication competent form. The target cell can be a neighboring cell in the same tissue and organism, or a cell in another organism. The **lifecycle** of a typical virus occurs in four stages: Entry and uncoating, replication, assembly, and release. Once infected, the new host cell produces and releases thousands of new virus particles. The cell often suffers from the infection and eventually dies. Many viruses are therefore dangerous pathogens.

To repeat, some general characteristics of viruses are:

- Viruses **possess** one type of nucleic acid: **either DNA or RNA but not both.**
- They **carry out no metabolism on their own and must replicate using the host cell's metabolic machinery**. Viruses don't grow and divide, but new viral components are synthesized separately and assembled within the infected host cell to infect a new cell. They grow & **reproduce** at a faster rate only in living host cells. They must assemble into complete viruses (virions) to go from one host cell to another.
- Viruses can **mutate.**
- They are totally dependent on a host cell for replication & are strict intracellular parasites.
- Since viruses lack metabolic machinery of their own, lack ribosomes & other factors needed for virus replication; and are totally dependent on their host cell for replication, they cannot be grown in synthetic culture media. Animal viruses are normally grown in animals, embryonated eggs, or in **cell cultures** wherein animal host cells are grown in a synthetic medium and the viruses are then grown in these cells.
- Viral genomes encode minimal information to ensure genome replication and packaging; production of viral proteins; and subvert cellular functions to allow the production of virions.
- Some viruses like phages infect prokaryotic cells, & plant viruses infect plant, while others animal viruses infect humans, animals, birds & other eukaryotic cells.
- Some viruses destroy cells, producing overt disease; others persist in the infected cells either in a latent or persistent state; and still other may cause cellular malignant transformation.
- A virus is an ultramicroscopic **obligate intracellular parasite** whose genome is made of **either DNA or RNA but not both**, and contains a

protein coat, called capsid, & often an outer covering called an envelope. The viruses do not possess metabolic system of their own & hence depend upon the machinery of the host cell for replication. They are simple, **acellular** & they contain no cytoplasm or cellular organelles. There are two phases of viruses, extracellular that possess few enzymes, if any, and do not reproduce, & intracellular where they exist mainly as replicating nucleic acids that exert control over the host cell's metabolism in the synthesis of new virus.

Are viruses living or nonliving?

Are viruses alive? There is an ongoing debate as to whether viruses are living or nonliving; the view taken depends on how life is defined. Anyone with a cold or the flu or other virus infection feels as if they are under attack by some organism. But in the scientific community it's still an open-ended question. This is why viruses do not belong to a kingdom of living things. After all, virus is not even a single-celled organism. A virus is little more than a strand of DNA or RNA covered by a protein coat or in some cases covered by an envelope. Viruses are a thousand times smaller than bacteria and come in a wide range of shapes. Some look like weird, tall spiders whereas others look like prickly porcupine like soccer balls. One thing is for sure; viruses are very much a part of life on Earth and the human experience. Viruses infect animals, plants, and even bacteria. Humans are in a constant battle with viruses. HIV (the virus that causes AIDS), the Ebola virus, and the West Nile virus continue to make headlines and take millions of lives. Other maladies, such as colds, the flu, chicken pox, measles, and hepatitis, are more common, but sometimes deadly. Similarly, several viral diseases in animals are proving obstrucles in animal production, milk production, their zoonotic potential, & are serious concern in international trade & imports. Symptoms vary depending on which kind of cell is under attack. Cold viruses attack the nose and throat, the rabies virus attacks the brain and nervous system, and the human immunodeficiency virus (HIV) attacks white blood cells in the bloodstream. Viruses can even cause some kinds of cancers and leukemia.

To determine whether a virus is alive or not, we could compare the virus's characteristics to what many biologists consider the **requirements of life**. All living things have several common characteristics. Some nonliving things may have one or more of the characteristics but not all of them. For a virus then to be classified as alive it must: **reproduce, obtain and use energy, grow, develop, and die, & respond to the environment.**

Viruses do have DNA or RNA, and DNA is the code for life. Having genetic material is an important step towards being classified as alive. DNA controls the evolution of the cell and the organism. Like living things, viruses evolve through time and thus can adapt to their environment. But unlike cells, viruses cannot use their genetic material by themselves. They need a living cell in order to function and reproduce; otherwise they are playing dead.

Because viruses are not cells, they can't divide by binary fission like bacteria. Yet they do reproduce themselves in an extraordinary way. Their structure enables viruses to attack a plant or animal cell called a **host cell**. The protein shell protecting the virus's DNA is covered with spike like protrusions/ spikes. These spikes allow the virus to attack onto the cells they infect. Once hooked on, the virus injects its genetic material into the host cell. The virus's DNA takes control of the cell once it's within the cytoplasm and begins to make the cell produce virus DNA and other parts of viruses. The host cell is forced to expend all of its energy and resources to help the virus replicate and make hundreds more viruses. The poor, weak cell usually bursts like an overinflated balloon from all the viruses and is destroyed in the process. Then, the replicated virus attaches itself to a new, unaffected host cell, and the viral infection continues.

Living things do more than just reproduce. They also must obtain food to fuel the cell's metabolic activity. Some organisms, such as animals, eat other living things for energy. Other organisms, such as plants, harness the Sun's energy to make their own food. Because viruses aren't cells and have no activity within it, it has no need for food. However, the virus-controlled host cell needs material and energy to reproduce the viruses. May be viruses can fit the requirement that life forms need to obtain and use energy. All other living things also grow or get bigger. **A virus does nothing inside its protein coat; therefore it does not grow**. But some scientists argue that a virus's growth occurs inside the host cell where parts of viruses are built during reproduction.

Plants and animals react to the environment. All living things have ways of sensing the world around them and can respond to changes in their environment. Do viruses react? Viruses cannot move themselves, but there are some differences in opinion that viruses do react to changes in the environment. The virus's DNA or RNA can evolve over time, thereby increasing its chances for survival and adapting to the environment. Like bacteria, they adapt through genetic mutations caused by rapid reproduction. That is why it is so hard to cure viral diseases. Viruses keep changing their DNA and protein coat to prolong their "life form" and keep ahead of the game.

As humans, we like to classify things because it helps us understand the physical world. Viruses must have a host cell to live and reproduce. Outside of the host cell, viruses are pieces of genetic molecules that can do nothing by themselves. **Viruses are right on the border between living and nonliving.** Some biologists currently see the virus as a nonliving infectious particle. Other biologists disagree and suggest they are alive because of what happens inside the host cell.

Viruses have genes and when they infect cells, these genes are replicated, so in this sense viruses are living. They are, however, very different to cellular life forms. When viruses are outside their host cells they exist as virus particles (virions), which are inert, and could be described as nonliving, but viable bacterial spores are inert and are not considered to be nonliving. When Beijerinck selected the word **'virus' he chose the Latin word for poison.** This term has now been in use for over a century and virology has developed into a huge subject. More recently, the term virus has acquired further meanings. Computers are threatened by **infection** with viruses that can be found **in the wild** once they have been **released** by their authors. These viruses are **specific** for certain file types. Infected files may be put on several web sites and a virus *epidemic* may ensue.

Study of viruses

- **Physical characteristics** of a virus include presence of genetic material-nucleic acid of either RNA (ssRNA, dsRNA, segmented RNA) or DNA (ssDNA, dsDNA), a protein coat (subunit structure) covering its genome, nucleoprotein, a capsid (capsomers, geometrical constraints), & some possessing an outer envelope. Genetic material is limited about 10^3 to 10^5 bases long that codes for unique proteins, **polymerases** for RNA replication, kinases, proteases, structural proteins & nonstructural accessory proteins.

- **Biological characteristics** include viral replication inside the cell, host cell tropism & lytic vs nonlytic infection. Viral replication cycles include binding/entry to a cell, its uncoating, genome replication, protein production, assembly, & budding or release to infect other susceptible cells.

- **Host cell tropism** is due to presence of appropriate receptors on host cells that results in lytic vs. non-lytic infection.

- **Characterization & study of viruses** are performed by the following methods: Structural & Morphological study is conducted by X-ray crystallography, electron microscopy; Biochemical study by gel electrophoresis, filtration, metabolic labeling; Enzymatic assays (reverse transcriptase, neuraminidase); Cell/Virus interaction: by hemagglutination, titration, focus forming, plaque assay, syncytia, in vivo labeling; Immunological: ELISA, Western blot, IFA, plaque-reduction, neutralization; Physical: Differential centrifugation, solvent resistance; Nucleic acid based: PCR, sequencing, hybridization, etc; & Host/Virus interaction: Host range, LD50, vaccination-challenge, suckling mice, & epidemiology studies.

- **Epidemiological study** is conducted by tracking prevalence of viruses in host populations from blood components and tissue samples, virus culture in vitro (tissue culture) or in vivo (susceptible animal model); by Molecular testing by PCR methods, Southern blot, ELISA, assay for antigen (viral protein) & assay for antibody directed against virus.

  The details of virus infection and replication vary greatly with host type; all viruses share 6 basic steps in their replication cycles. These include: 1) attachment; 2) penetration; 3) uncoating; 4) replication; 5) assembly; 6) release.

- *Viral pathogenesis:* Studies mechanism of disease production, virus sequential replication at various sites, targeted cells & host response to virus.

- *Manifestations of viral infections*: Include asymptomatic infection, acute viral syndrome (influenza, rhinovirus, etc), persistent viral syndrome (EBV), chronic infection (Borna disease), reactivating (HSV-1/2, VZV (chicken pox/shingles)- progressive (HBV, HCV, HIV), Cancer (EBV, HPV-16, HBV, HCV, KSHV), death (HIV) & acute death (smallpox, Ebola, SARS). The range of structural and biochemical effects that viruses have on the host cell is extensive. These are called cytopathic effects (CPE). Most virus infections eventually result in the death of the host cell. The causes of death include cell lysis (bursting), alterations to the cell's surface membrane and apoptosis (cell "suicide"). Often cell death is caused by cessation of its normal activity due to proteins produced by the virus, not all of which are components of the virus particle.

Some viruses cause no apparent changes to the infected cell. Cells in which the virus is **latent and inactive,** show few signs of infection and often function normally. This causes **persistent infections** and the virus is often dormant for many months or years. This is often the case with herpesviruses.

Viruses, such as Epstein-Barr virus often cause cells to proliferate without causing malignancy, but viruses, such as papillomaviruses are an established cause of cancer. When a cell's DNA is damaged by a virus and if the cell cannot repair, this often triggers apoptosis. One of the results of apoptosis is destruction of the damaged DNA by the cell itself. Some viruses have mechanisms to limit apoptosis so that the host cell does not die before progeny viruses have been produced. HIV, for example, does this.

Diseases: Common human diseases caused by viruses include the common cold, flu, chickenpox and cold sores. Serious diseases such as Ebola and AIDS are also caused by viruses. Many viruses cause little or no disease and are said to be "benign". The more harmful viruses are described as virulent. Viruses cause different diseases depending on the types of cell that they infect. Some viruses can cause life-long or chronic infections where the viruses continue to reproduce in the body despite the host's defense mechanisms. This is common in hepatitis B virus and hepatitis C virus infections. People chronically infected with a virus are known as carriers. They serve as important reservoirs of the virus. If there are a high proportion of carriers in a given population, a disease is said to be endemic. There are many ways in which viruses spread from host to host but each species of virus uses only one or two. Many viruses that infect plants are carried by organisms; such organisms are called vectors. Some viruses that infect animals and humans are also spread by vectors, usually blood-sucking insects. However, direct animal-to-animal, person-to-person or animal-to-person transmission is more common. Some virus infections, (norovirus and rotavirus), are spread by contaminated food and water, hands and communal objects and by intimate contact with another infected person, while others are airborne (influenza virus). Viruses such as HIV, hepatitis B and hepatitis C are often transmitted by unprotected sex or contaminated hypodermic needles. It is important to know how each different kind of virus is spread to prevent infections and epidemic.

Host resistance to virus infection

Animals & humans, have many natural defenses against viruses. Some are **non-specific** and protect against many viruses regardless of the type. This **innate immunity** is inborn & not improved by repeated exposure to viruses and does not retain a "memory" of the infection. The skin of animals, particularly its surface, which is made from dead cells, prevents many types of viruses from infecting the host. The acidity of the contents of the stomach kills many viruses that have been swallowed. When a virus overcomes these barriers and enters the host, other innate defenses prevent the spread of infection in the body. A special hormone called interferon is produced by the body when viruses are present, and this stops the viruses from reproducing by killing the infected cell and its close neighbors. Inside cells, there are enzymes that destroy the RNA of viruses. This is called RNA interference. Some blood cells engulf and destroy other virus infected cells.

Specific immunity or adaptive immunity to viruses develops over time and lymphocytes play a central role. Lymphocytes retain a "memory" of virus infections and produce many special molecules called antibodies or cellular immune response. The antibodies attach to viruses and stop the virus from infecting cells. Antibodies are highly selective and attack only one type of virus. The body makes many different antibodies, especially during the initial infection, however, after the infection subsides, some antibodies remain and continue to be produced, often giving the host life-long immunity to the virus. Cellular immune response destroys virus carrying cells.

Prevention and treatment of viral disease in humans and other animals:

Vaccines

Vaccination is a way of preventing diseases caused by viruses. Vaccines simulate a natural infection and its associated immune response, but do not cause the disease. Their use has resulted in a dramatic decline in illness and death caused by infections such as polio, measles, mumps and rubella. Vaccines are available to prevent over thirteen viral infections of humans and more are used to prevent viral infections of animals. Vaccines may consist of either live or killed viruses. Live vaccines contain weakened forms of the virus, but these vaccines can be dangerous when given to people with weak immunity. In these people, the weakened virus can cause the original disease. Biotechnology and genetic engineering techniques are used to produce "designer" vaccines that only have the capsid proteins of the virus. Hepatitis B vaccine is an example of this type of vaccine. These vaccines are safer because they can never cause the disease.

Antiviral drugs

Over the past 20 years, the development of antiviral drugs has increased rapidly, mainly driven by the AIDS pandemic. Antiviral drugs are often nucleoside analogues, which are molecules very similar, but not identical to DNA building blocks. When the replication of virus DNA begins, some of these fake building blocks are incorporated. As soon as that happens, replication stops prematurely—the fake building blocks lack the essential features that allow the addition of further building blocks. Thus, DNA production is halted, and the virus can no longer reproduce. Examples of nucleoside analogues are acyclovir for herpesvirus infections and lamividin for HIV and hepatitis B virus infections. Acyclovir is one of the oldest and most frequently prescribed antiviral drugs.

Basic Viral Structural Forms of Viruses

Viruses have the simplest structure made of a nucleic acid genome of either DNA or RNA but not both, a protein coat called capsid, and often some viruses contain an external membrane called an **envelope**.

Basic morphology of viruses exhibit **five different basic structural forms** of viruses as mentioned below.

- Naked icosahedral - adenoviruses and picornaviruses.
- Naked helical - tobacco mosaic virus; no known human or animal viruses have this structure.
- Enveloped icosahedral - togaviruses and flaviviruses.
- Enveloped helical - rhabdoviruses and paramyxoviruses.
- Complex - bacteriophages and poxviruses.

In an attempt to clarify the **terminology for virus components,** Caspar *et al.* (1962) made a number of proposals which were generally accepted. Briefly, the proposals are as follows:

1. The **capsid** denotes the protein shell that encloses the nucleic acid. It is built of structure units.
2. **Structural units** are the smallest functional building units of the capsid.
3. **Capsomers** are morphological units seen on the surface of particles and represent clusters of structure units.
4. The capsid together with its enclosed nucleic acid is called the **Nucleocapsid**.
5. The nucleocapsid may be invested in an **Envelope** which may contain material of host cell as well as viral origin.
6. The **virion** is the complete infective virus particle.

Capsid

The virus capsid protects the viral genome during its transfer from cell to cell. Capsid is a complex and highly organized entity which gives form to the virus. The capsid accounts for most of the virion mass. **The protein coat or capsid** of a **virion** is composed of multiple copies of one or more types of proteins. These proteins assemble, forming structural units called **capsomeres**. Subunits are called **protomeres** that aggregate to form capsomeres which in turn aggregate to form the capsid. Capsids consist of multiples copies of one single protein or by association of different proteins. Capsid made up of multiple copies of a single protein is economical, since a single gene can encode the unit protein required to cover the whole viral genome.

The capsid exhibit **three types of symmetry**:

Icosahedral: Naked icosahedral - adenoviruses and picornaviruses, & Enveloped icosahedral - togaviruses and flaviviruses.

Helical: Naked helical - tobacco mosaic virus; no known human or animal viruses have this structure & Enveloped helical - rhabdoviruses and paramyxoviruses.

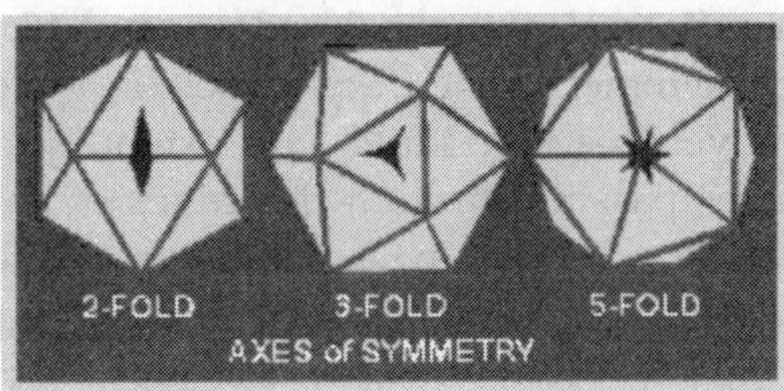

Figure 1.1 : Two-fold, three-fold, five- fold axes of symmetry

Complex symmetry: Capsid consists of several oligomeric structural subunits made of protein called protomers. The observable 3-dimensional morphological subunits, which may or may not correspond to individual proteins, are called capsomers. Once the virus has infected the cell, it will start replicating itself, using the mechanisms of the infected host cell. During replication, new capsid subunits are synthesized according to the genetic material of the virus, using the protein biosynthesis mechanism of the cell. During the assembly process, a **portal** subunit is assembled at one vertex of the capsid. Through this portal, viral DNA or RNA is transported into the capsid. The structure and assembly of the herpesvirus capsid portal protein has been imaged via cryo-electron microscopy.

In geometry, an **icosahedron** is a regular polyhedron with **20 identical equilateral triangular faces, 30 edges and 12 vertices.** It is one of the five Platonic solids.

In 1956, James Watson (1928 -) and Francis Crick (1916 -) proposed on theoretical considerations and on the basis of rather flimsy experimental evidence, principles of virus structure that have been amply confirmed and universally accepted. They formed two proposals:

1. The only reasonable way to build a protein shell with small viral nucleic acids is to use the same type of molecule over and over again, hence their **theory of identical subunits.**
2. The subunits must be packed so as to provide each with an identical environment in the protein shell or capsid; only possible in **Cubic (=icosahedral) or Helical symmetry**.

Icosahedral symmetry: A body with cubic symmetry possesses a number of axes about which it may be rotated to give a number of identical appearances. The occurrence of icosahedral features in quite unrelated viruses is not a matter of chance, but a preference. An **Icosahedron** is composed of **20 facets, each an equilateral triangle, 30 edges, and 12 vertices,** and have axes of **5:3:2** rotational symmetry. There are, in fact, six 5-fold axes of symmetry passing through the vertices, ten 3-fold axes extending through each face and fifteen 2-fold axes passing through the edges of an icosahedron. The simplest icosahedral capsids with 5:3:2 symmetry are built up by using 3 identical subunits to form each triangular face, thereby requiring 60 identical subunits to form a capsid. A few virus particles are constructed in this way, e.g. bacteriophage ØX174. Each unit would be related identically (equivalent) and asymmetrically with its neighbors, and none of the units would coincide with an axis of symmetry.

Axes of symmetry: There are, in fact, six 5-fold axes of symmetry passing through the vertices, ten 3-fold axes extending through each face and fifteen 2-fold axes passing through the edges of an icosahedron.

As soon as the first high resolution micrographs of negatively stained icosahedral viruses were obtained, it seemed that there was a **structural paradox**. The number of morphological units observed on the surface of known icosahedral viruses at that time was never 60 or multiples of 60, and was often more than 60 severely restricts the size of the genome that can be packaged, and **more than 60 subunits cannot be arranged in an equivalent fashion around an icosahedron.** Furthermore, the capsomers themselves appeared to be symmetrical and were located on symmetry axes, e.g. **herpesvirus**. There was direct evidence that capsomers of **herpesvirus were hexagonal and pentagonal** in section. It was therefore clear that the capsomers were not equivalent to the subunits of Crick and Watson (1956). An obvious solution to the problem was provided by supposing that the **symmetrical capsomers are built from a number of Asymmetrical subunits**. In this way it is possible to build a variety of complicated bodies in which 5:3:2 symmetry is preserved and in which the number of subunits is a multiple of 60 as predicted by Crick and Watson.

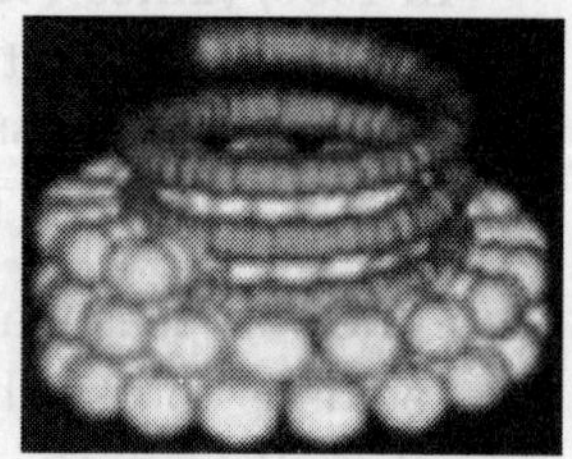

Figure 1.2 : TMV with helical symmetry

In **1962 Donald Caspar and Aaron Klug** developed two theoretical framework accounting for the structural properties of larger (> 60 units) particles with icosahedral symmetry.

1. Caspar and Klug proposed that when a capsid contains more than 60 subunits, each subunit occupies a **quasi-equivalent position**; that is, the bonding properties of subunits in different structural environments are similar (but not identical, as in the case of the simplest, 60-structure).

2. The second important idea was that of **triangulation**, the description of the triangular face of a large icosahedral structure in terms of its subdivision into smaller triangles termed facets. This process is described by the **Triangulation number,** which gives the number of structural units per face. The icosahedron itself has 20 equilateral triangular facets and therefore 20 T structure units given by the rule: T=P x f(SQR) where P can be any number of the series 1,3,7,13,19,21,31, and f is any integer. Morphological units can be clustered as 20T trimmers, 30T dimmers or separated as 60T monomers. The number of morphological units that would be produced by a clustering into hexamers and pentamers can be calculated as follows: There are 10(T-1) hexamers plus 12 (and only 12) pentamers. In adenoviruses each side of the equilateral face consists of 6 capsomers linked to each other by divalent bounds. By using special equation to calculate capsomers number which are fixed in number and genetically controlled as the following:

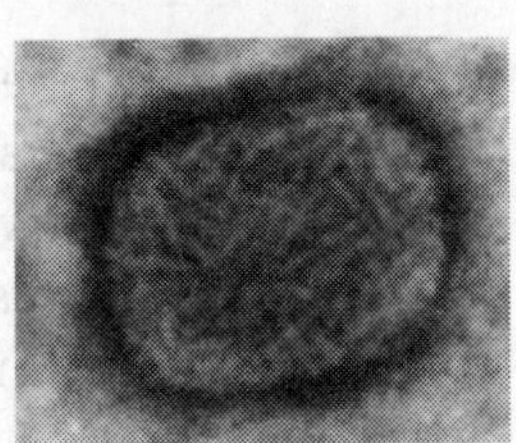

Figure 1.3 : poxviruses with complex symmetry.

Capsomers No = 10 (edge capsomers No. - 1)^2 +2

= 10 (6 – 1)^2 +2

= 10 ×25 +2 = 252

In herpes viruses where edge capsomers No are 5

= 10 (5 – 1)^2 +2

= 10 ×16 +2 = 162

But in less capsomers number, other equation used.

Capsomers No. = 30 (edge capsomers No. - 1)^2 +2

= 30 (2 – 1)^2 +2

= 30 ×1 +2 = 32

E.g. for cubical symmetry viruses: adeno and picorna which are naked, herpes and toga which are enveloped.

Helical symmetry: **Tobacco mosaic virus (TMV)** is representative of one of the two major structural classes seen in viruses of all types, those with helical symmetry. The simplest way to arrange multiple, identical protein subunits is to use rotational symmetry & to arrange the irregularly shaped proteins around the circumference of a circle to form a disc. Multiple discs can then be stacked on top of one another to form a cylinder, with the virus genome coated by the protein shell or contained in the hollow centre of the cylinder.

Closer examination of the TMV particle by X-ray crystallography reveals that the structure of the capsid actually consists of a helix rather pile of stacked disks. A helix can be defined mathematically by two parameters:

1. The **amplitude** (diameter) &
2. The **pitch** (the distance covered by each complete turn of the helix). Helices are rather simple structures formed by stacking repeated components with a constant relationship (amplitude & pitch) to one another - if this simple constraint is broken a spiral forms rather than a helix – results unsuitable for containing a virus genome.

Complex viruses structures: The majority of viruses can be fitted into one of the two structural classes outlined above, i.e. those with helical symmetry or icosahedral symmetry. However, there are many viruses whose structure is more complex. In these cases, although the general principles of symmetry already described are often used to build part of the virus shell.

The larger & more complex viruses cannot be simply defined by a mathematical equation as can a simple helix or icosahedron.

An example of such a group & the problems of complexity are shown by the members of the poxvirus family. These viruses have oval or 'brick-shaped' particles 200-400nm long. In fact, these particles are so large that they were first observed using high resolution optical microscopes in 1886 & thought at that time to be 'the spores of micrococci'

The envelope: Many viruses-e.g. herpesviruses & poxviruses among DNA viruses, & orthomyxoiruses, paramyxoviruses, rhabdoviruses, flaviviruses, togaviruses, coronaviruses & retroviruses among RNA viruses have **viral envelopes** covering their protein capsids; it is necessary for virus infectivity. A virus is **naked virus** when it lacks an envelope. The envelopes are derived from the **host cell membranes- nuclear, Golgi apparatus, endoplasmic reticulum or plasma membrane** with phospholipids and proteins, but also include some viral glycoproteins. Consequently, an envelope is composed of a lipid bilayer with virus-encoded proteins inserted on it. Functionally, viral envelopes are used to help viruses enter host cells. Spikes projecting from the envelope are the glycoprotein projections which have enzymatic or adsorption or hemagglutinating activity. These spikes arise from the envelope and are highly antigenic. Glycoproteins on the surface of the envelope serve to identify and bind to receptors sites on the host's membrane. These envelope- associated proteins perform 4 vital functions-receptor binding, membrane fusion, uncoating, & receptor destruction. Glycoproteins, in the form of dimmers or trimers assemble into virion peplomers or spikes. **Fusion proteins** are glycosylated & involve in virus entry & release. The viral envelope fuses with the host's membrane, allowing the capsid and viral genome to enter and infect the host. **Viral matrix proteins** are nonglycosylated present in orthomyxoiruses, paramyxoviruse, rhabdoviruses, flaviviruses, & retroviruses associated with the inner surface of the lipid bilayer of the viral envelope, & have been implicated in control of viral transcription and serve as the "glue" that binds the nucleocapsid to the appropriate membrane site during viral budding from the host cell

Usually, the cell from which the virus itself buds will often die or be weakened, and shed more viral particles for an extended period. The lipid bilayer envelope of these viruses is relatively sensitive to desiccation, heat, and detergents, therefore these viruses are easier to sterilize than non-enveloped viruses, have limited survival outside host environments, and typically must transfer directly from host to host. Enveloped viruses can cause persistent infection.

Envelope is an amorphous structure composed of lipid, protein and carbohydrate which lies to the outside of the capsid. It contains a mosaic of antigens from the host and the virus. The viral envelope is derived from host cell membranes. Hence bacteriophages, have complex structure having a protein tails, the instrument for attachment or penetration of viral DNA into susceptible host cells.

Viral genome: A virus genome has either DNA or RNA but not both and is called a DNA virus or a RNA virus respectively. The vast majority of viruses have RNA genomes. Plant viruses mostly have single-stranded RNA genomes and bacteriophages mostly have double-stranded DNA genomes.

- The viral DNA can be double-stranded (ds) as in case of viruses of the families *Adenoviridae, Asfarviridae, Herpesviridae, Poxviridae, Papillomaviridae, Polyomaviridae* or partially double-stranded, e.g. *Hepadnaviridae*. Double-stranded genomes consist of two complementary paired nucleic acids (±) analogous to a ladder.
- The viral DNA can be single-stranded (ss) as in case of *Parvoviridae* and *Circoviridae*.

- The viral DNA can be linear or **circular.** RNA viruses having circular DNA include papillomaviruse, polyomaviruse, circoviruses & hepadnaviruses. Some linear DNA viruses like poxviruses have their ends covalently cross linked at their termini making the molecules large single stranded circle. Linear ds DNA of many DNA viruses & RNA of retroviruses have repeat sequences at the ends permitting circularization.
- Size of the viral DNA genome varies from 1.7 kb (circovirus) to about 200 kp (herpesviruses & poxviruses) to have 2-200 genes coding for 200 proteins. But coding capacity is actually more as DNA or RNA sequences may be read in 3 different frames; either one or both DNA can be transcribed; in some case genes are overlapping resulting in various transcripts, & a single primary RNA transcript is spliced or cleaved to yield several mRNAs.
- Size of the sis viral RNA genome varies from 1.7 kb to about 27kb, which are much smaller than ds DNA viruses & hence these viruses encode lesser proteins.
- The viral RNA can be double-stranded (ds) as in case of *Reoviridae & Birnaviridae.*
- All the rest viral RNA can be single-stranded (ss) either of positive sense (called the plus-strand) as in case of viruses belonging to the families- *Picornaviridae, Togaviridae, Calciviridae, Flaviviridae, Cornaviridae, Astroviridae, & Arteriviridae.* Positive-sense viral RNA is in the same sense as viral mRNA and thus at least a part of it can be immediately translated by the host cells.
- The viral RNA can be single-stranded (ss) negative sense (called the minus-strand) as in case of viruses belonging to the families- *Orthomyxoviridae, Paramyxoviridae, Rhabdoviridae, Bornaviridae, Arenaviridae, Filoviridae & Bunyaviridae.* Negative-sense viral RNA is complementary to mRNA and thus must be converted to positive-sense RNA by an **RNA-dependent RNA polymerase** before translation.
- The *Retroviridae* have diploid linear, positive sense RNA that replicate through reverse transcriptase via DNA intermediates.
- RNA viral genomes are linear & among RNA viruses, the genome is either monopartite having a single piece of linear RNA as in case of all RNA viruses except *Reoviridae, Birnaviridae, Orthomyxoviridae & Bunyaviridae.* Oher RNA viruses are multipartite often divided up into separate parts or segments in which case it is called **segmented.** For multipartite RNA viruses, each segment often codes for only one protein

and they are usually found together in one capsid. Segmentd RNA viruses include *Reoviridae* (10, 11, 12 segments), *Birnaviridae* (two segments), *Orthomyxoviridae* (8, 7, 6 segments), *Bunyaviridae* (3 segments) & *Arenavridae* (2 segments). All ss RNA viruses are not covalently linked except circular ss RNA delta hepatitis virus. But ss RNA bunyaviruses & arenaviruses appear circular because of sticky hydrogen bonded ends. Single-stranded RNA viruses have secondary structures, base pairing regions resulting in loops & hairpins. These control virus replication, transcription, translation & packaging.

- The virus particles of *Hepadnaviridae* contain a genome consisting of circular ds DNA with a region of ss DNA, that is partially double-stranded and partially single-stranded. The particles are DNA-reverse transcribing viruses.
- DNA nomenclature for viruses with single-sense genomic ss DNA is similar to RNA nomenclature, in that the **coding strand** for the viral mRNA is complementary to it (-), and the **non-coding strand** is a copy of it (+). However, several types of ss DNA and ss RNA viruses have genomes that are **ambisense** in that transcription can occur from both strands in a double-stranded replicative intermediate. Examples are **arenaviruses**, which are ss RNA viruses of animals.
- Genome size varies greatly between species. The smallest viral genome of the ssDNA circoviruses codes for only two proteins and have a genome size of only 2 kilobases; the largest, mimiviruses have genome sizes of over 1.2 megabases and code for over one thousand proteins. RNA viruses generally have smaller genome sizes than DNA viruses because of a higher error-rate when replicating, and have a maximum upper size limit. Beyond this limit, errors in the genome when replicating render the virus useless or uncompetitive. To compensate for this, RNA viruses often have segmented genome which is split into smaller molecules, thus reducing the chance that an error in a single-component genome will incapacitate the entire genome. In contrast, DNA viruses generally have larger genomes because of the high fidelity of their replication enzymes. Single-strand DNA viruses are an exception to this rule, however, as mutation rates for these genomes can approach the extreme of the ssRNA virus case.

How antigenic shift, or reassortment, can result in novel and highly pathogenic strains of human influenza. Viruses undergo genetic change by several mechanisms. These include a process called **genetic drift** where individual bases in the DNA or RNA mutate to other bases. Most of these point mutations are "silent"; they do not change the protein that the gene encodes, but others can confer evolutionary advantages such as resistance to antiviral drugs. **Antigenic shift** occurs when there is a major change in the genome of the virus. This can be a result of recombination or reassortment. When this happens with influenza A viruses, pandemics might result. RNA viruses often exist as quasispecies or swarms of viruses of the same species but with slightly different genome nucleoside sequences. Such quasispecies are a prime target for natural selection.

- Segmented genomes confer evolutionary advantages; different strains of a virus with a segmented genome can shuffle and combine genes and produce progeny viruses or (offspring) that have unique characteristics. This is called reassortment or *viral sex*. **Genetic recombination** is the process by which a strand of DNA is broken and then joined to the end of a different DNA molecule. This can occur when viruses infect cells simultaneously and studies of viral evolution have shown that recombination has been rampant in the species studied. Recombination is common to both RNA and DNA viruses.
- The DNA genome may have their ends covalently linked to each other (circular = polyomavirus, circoviruses) or not linked (linear = adenovirus, herpesvirus, parvoviruses). The genome of poxviruses is dsDNA whose ends are covalently attached to each other. The majority of these are single-stranded and a few are double stranded (reoviruses, birnaviruses). Most RNA viruses have their genomes in a single piece (monopartite) while others have it segmented in 10 segments (reoviruses), 7 or 8 segments (orthomyxoviruses), three segments (bunyaviruses) and two segments (arenaviruses). Regarding ssRNAs, there are two major sequence possibilities:
- In some viruses (Arenavirus and Bunyaviruses) portions of the RNA genome are transcribed, generating mRNAs, which are then translated. The copy of these mRNAs (complementary, supposedly negative-sense RNAs) may also be translated. This arrangement is unique among viruses and is said to be **ambisense.**

Viral proteins

- Viral proteins are those that are found in any species of virus, and more than 490 viral proteins have been identified. Aggregated form of viral proteins can form inclusion bodies. The viral proteins encoded by different viral genomes vary & include as few as two proteins to over hundreds.
- The viral proteins are mainly divided in to **structural proteins** forming the viral envelope and capsid, & **nonstructural proteins that** are produced

inside the infected cells and play roles in different steps of viral replication. However, there are also viral regulatory & accessory proteins.

- *Viral structural proteins* are those that form part of the physical structure of the virion like capsid & envelope; the capsid packages the nucleic acid genome. In case of enveloped viruses, a protein layer lie between the capsid and the envelope called the **tegument;** these are also structural proteins. Viral matrix proteins are non glycosylated, associated with the inner surface of the lipid bilayer of the viral envelope - they are implicated in control of viral transcription and may possibly serve as the "glue" that binds the nucleocapsid to the appropriate membrane site during viral budding from the host cell. Viral matrix proteins are associated with the inner surface of the lipid bilayer of the viral envelope. These proteins have been implicated in control of viral transcription and may possibly serve as the "glue" that binds the nucleocapsid to the appropriate membrane site during viral budding from the host cell. Among the structural proteins of the capsid or envelope, some form the ligands, which interact with receptors on the surface of target cells. Viral glycoproteins are processed in the lumen of the rough endoplasmic reticulum, oligosaccharides attach to the polypeptide chain, & then sent to the Golgi apparatus, to secretary vesicles, and ultimately fuse with the plasma membrane where they are present on the surface of the infected cell. Such glycoproteins play important role in enveloped viruses; these mediate interactions between the virions and cells & in some cases constitute targets for neutralizing antibodies.

- *Viral nonstructural proteins* include proteins encoded by a viral genome that are produced in the organisms they infect, but are not packaged into the virus particles. Some of these proteins play roles within the infected cell during virus replication, transcription, translation & shut down of host cell functions or act in regulation of virus replication or virus assembly. Viral regulatory and accessory proteins include a broad range of viral proteins that play indirect roles in the biological processes and activities of viruses. Nonstructural proteins include replicases as DNA dependent RNA polymerase, & enzymes associated with viral DNA replication, proteases, & ligages, & reverse transcriptase of retroviruses & hepadnaviruses, which makes a DNA copy of a RNA template. These proteins either regulate the expression of viral genes or are involved in modifying host cell functions. Many of the proteins in this category serve multiple functions. Among virus encoded non-structural proteins, some play multiple accessory roles in the regulation of viral and cellular gene expression, regulation of different steps of the viral cycle, counteraction of host defenses, cell transformation, & others.

Lipids

- Since viruses are derived from the cellular membranes of the host cell, they are composed mainly of phospholipids (50-60%) and the remainder is cholesterol. The composition of lipid varies as per its source of origin. The lipid bilayer of the host membranes surrounding the virion of enveloped viruses also possesses viral proteins and glycoproteins, such as the characteristic spikes of some enveloped viruses. The overall lipid composition of enveloped viruses is approximately 20-35% dry weight of which 50-60% is phospholipids, & the remainder is cholesterol.

Carbohydrates

- In viruses, the carbohydrates constitute oligosaccharide side chains of glycoproteins, glycolipids, and mucopolysacharides. These carbohydrates are that of the host cell. The carbohydrates are present in the viral envelope. The glycoproteins have an N- or O- glycosidic linkage. The larger, more complex viruses contain internal glycoproteins or glycosylated capsid proteins.

Summary

1. Viruses contain either DNA or RNA as their genetic material, but not both. This nucleic acid usually has unique chemical and/or physical features which makes it distinguishable from human nucleic acid.
2. Viral nucleic acid is enclosed in a capsid made up of protein subunits called protomers.
3. Some species of viruses have a membrane, the envelope, surrounding the capsid; other species do not have an envelope, i.e., they are naked. Enveloped viruses have glycoprotein spikes arising from their envelope. These spikes have enzymatic, absorptive, hemagglutinating and/or antigenic activity.
4. The morphology of a virus is determined by the arrangement of the protomers. When protomers aggregate into units of five or six (capsomers) and then condense to form a geometric figure having 20 equal triangular faces, 30 edges and 12 apices, the virus is said to have icosahedral (cubic) morphology. When protomers aggregate to form a capped tube, they are said to have helical morphology. Any other arrangement of the protomers results in a complex morphology.
5. All viruses undergo a replication cycle in their host cell consisting of adsorption, penetration, uncoating, nucleic acid replication, maturation and release stages.

6. During the viral replication cycle, an accumulation of mature viruses, incomplete viruses and viral parts occurs within the cell. This accumulation is the inclusion body. The size, shape, location and chemical properties of the inclusion body are used by the pathologist to diagnose viral infectious diseases.
7. A virally-infected cell generally presents three signals that it is infected. The first is the production of double-stranded RNA, which induces interferon; the second is the expression of viral protein on the surface of the plasma membrane, thus causing activation of cytotoxic T cells, natural killer cells and sometimes induction of antibody synthesis. The third is the formation of an inclusion body either within the cytoplasm or the nucleus or very rarely within both the cytoplasm and nucleus.
8. In general, all DNA-containing viruses replicate in the host cell nucleus. The exceptions to the rule are the poxviruses.
9. In general, all RNA-containing viruses replicate in the host cell cytoplasm. The exceptions to the rule are the retroviruses and the orthomyxoviruses.

Taxonomy & Classification of Animal Viruses

Currently there are two main schemes used for the classification of viruses: the International Committee on the Taxonomy of Viruses (ICTV) system, and Baltimore classification system, which places viruses into one of seven groups. Accompanying this broad method of classification are specific naming conventions and further classification guidelines set out by the ICTV. ICTV is responsible for developing, refining, and maintaining universal virus taxonomy. A complete catalog of known viruses is maintained by the ICTV at ICTVdb. ICTV nomenclature is used to classify animals' viruses.

According to David Baltimore (1971), Novel Prize winner, viruses can be placed in one of the seven following groups depending on a combination of their nucleic acid (DNA or RNA), strandedness (single-stranded or double-stranded), sense, and method of replication. These groups are designated by Roman numerals and discriminate viruses depending on their mode of replication, and genome type:

I *Double-stranded (ds) DNA viruses* (Adenoviruses; Herpesviruses; Poxviruses, etc.). Most DNA viruses replicate in the nucleus e.g. adenoviruses using cellular proteins. Poxviruses replicate in the cytoplasm and make their own enzymes for nucleic acid replication.

II *Single-stranded (+)sense DNA viruses* (Parvoviruses, Circoviruses) Replication occurs in the nucleus, involving the formation of a (-) sense strand, which serves as a template for (+) strand RNA and DNA synthesis.

III **Double-stranded RNA viruses** (Reoviruses; Birnaviruses)
These viruses have segmented genomes. Each genome segment is transcribed separately to produce monocistronic mRNAs.

IV **Single-stranded (+) sense RNA viruses** (Picornaviruses; Togaviruses, etc.)

a) Polycistronic mRNA e.g. Picornaviruses; Hepatitis A. Genome RNA = mRNA. Means naked RNA is infectious & contains no virion particle associated polymerase. Translation results in the formation of a polyprotein product, which is subsequently cleaved to form the mature proteins.

b) Complex transcription e.g. togaviruses. Two or more rounds of translation are necessary to produce the genomic RNA.

V **Single-stranded (-) sense RNA viruses** (Orthomyxoviruses, Paramyxoviruses, Rhabdoviruses, etc.)
Must have a virion particle RNA directed RNA polymerase.

a) Segmented e.g. Orthomyxoviruses. First step in replication is transcription of the (-) sense RNA genome by the virion RNA-dependent RNA polymerase to produce monocistronic mRNAs, which also serve as the template for genome replication.

b) Non-segmented e.g. Rhabdoviruses. Replication occurs as above and monocistronic mRNAs are produced.

VI **Single-stranded (+) sense RNA with DNA intermediate in life-cycle** (Retroviruses)

Genome is (+) sense but unique among viruses in that it is diploid, and does not serve as mRNA, but act as a template for reverse transcription.

VII **Double-stranded DNA with RNA intermediate** (Hepadnaviruses)
This group of viruses also relies on reverse transcription, but unlike the Retroviruses, this occurs inside the virus particle on maturation. On infection of a new cell, the first event to occur is repair of the gapped genome, followed by transcription.

I dsDNA viruses;

II ssDNA (+) sense DNA, III: dsRNA viruses; IV: (+) ssRNA viruses; V: (-) ssRNA viruses; VI: ssRNA-RT with DNA intermediate in life-cycle (e.g. *Retroviridae*); & VII: dsDNA-RT viruses (e.g. Hepadnaviruses)

Animal viruses are classified into 26 families whose various properties are presented in the Table 1-2 on the basis of characteristics & criteria as mentioned above & to be enumerated below:

Table 1.2 : Various properties of 26 virus families of medical & veterinary importance.

SN/Groups/ Family	Virion size diam (nm)	E/ NE	Capsid symmetry	Capso mers no	Genome nature	Genome size (kb)	Rep lC N	Matu ration	Genome ends/ their features
I dsDNA viruses									
1. *Adenoviridae*	80-100	NE	Icosahedral	252	Linear, dsDNA	36-44	N	None	ITR at both ends, covalently bound terminal protein & the 5′ ends with the protein-primers.
2. *Asfarviridae*	175-215	E	Icosahedral	1892-2172	Linear, dsDNA	170-190	N	PM	Both ends coval ently closed, have ITR.
3. *Herpesviridae*	150-200	E	Icosahedral	162	Linear, dsDNA	120-230	N	NM	Contain Terminal & internal reiterated repeats.
4. *Poxviridae*	220-450x 140-260	E	Complex	NA	Linear, dsDNA	170-250	C	Golgi M	3′ & 5′ends covalent ly closed with invert ed terminal repeats.
5. *Papillomaviridae*	40-55	NE	Icosahedral	72	circular, supercoiled dsDNA	5-8	N	None	Transcribed as a bicistronic or poly-cistronic form containing two or more ORFs & are polyadenylated at either an early or late poly(A) site.
6. *Polyomaviridae*	45	NE	Icosahedral	72	Linear, dsDNA	5	N	None	Contain histones H2a, H2b, H3, & H4 from the host
II ssDNA viruses									
7. *Parvoviridae*	25	NE	Icosahedral	32	Linear, (-) ssDNA	5	N	None	Genome +or- sen se, palindromic sequence at the end enabling circularization during replication
8. *Circoviridae*	17-22	NE	Icosahedral	32?	Circular, (+) ssDNA	1.7-2.3	N	None	Ambisense or + sense.
III dsRNA viruses									
9. *Reoviridae*	60-80	NE	Icosahedral	92	Linear, ssRNA, 10, 11, 12 segments	16-27	C	None	L (large), M (medium) and S (small) segments, each encodes 1-3 proteins.
10. *Birnaviridae*	60	NE	Icosahedral	92	Linear, ssRNA, 2 segments	7	C	None	5′-end has a cap on both segments & genome-linked protein (VPg).
IV (+) ssRNA viruses									
11. *Picornaviridae*	28-30	NE	Icosahedral	60	Linear, (+) ssRNA	7.2-8.4	C	None	3′ end with shorter UTR with role in (-) strand synthes-is, polyA, 5′ end with VPg-primer & has Internal Ribosome Entry Site (IRES).

12. *Calciviridae*	30-38	N	Icosahedral	32	Linear, (+) ssRNA	7.4-7.7	C	None	5′ end with (VPg) & 3′end has poly A.
13. *Togaviridae*	70	E	Icosahedral	60	Linear, (+) ssRNA	9.7-11.8	C	PM	5′ end has cap & 3′ end a tail.
14. *Flaviviridae*	45-60	E	Icosahedral	60	Linear, (+) ssRNA	9.5-12.5	C	ER	5′ end has a cap or VPg but hepaciv iruses & pestiviruses are uncapped and has IRES, no poly A at 3′ end.
15. *Coronaviridae*	80-120	E	Helical	NA	Linear, (+) ssRNA	22-32	C	ER	5′ end is capped & 3′ end is polyadenylated.
16. *Arteriviridae*	50-70	• +	Helical	NA	Linear, (+) ssRNA	22	C	ER	5′ end has leader RNA, & also each subgenomic RNAs.
17. *Astroviridae*	28-3 0	N	Icosahedral	32	Linear, (+) ssRNA	7.2-7.9	C	None	5′ end has no cap & 3′ end has polyadenylated tail.
V (-) ssRNA viruses									
18. *Orthomyxoviridae*	80-120	E	Helical	NA	Linear, (-), ssRNA, 6,7,8 segments	10-13.6	N	PM	ITRs at both ends , 3 polymerase polyp eptides, PB1, PB2 & PA at each end of each segment.
19. *Paramyxoviridae*	150-350	E	Helical	NA	Linear, (-), ssRNA	15-16	C	PM	5′-end lacks a terminal protein, nor a cap & 3′ end has no poly A.
20. *Rhabdoviridae*	180x75	E	Hlical	NA	Linear, (-), ssRNA	13-16	C	PM	5′ has no cap or 3′has no polyA tail.
21. *Bornaviridae*	50-60	E	Icosahedral	?	Linear, (-) ssRNA	10-13.6	N	?	
22. *Filoviridae*	790-970 x80	E	Helical	NA	Linear, (-) ssRNA	19.1	C	PM	3′end not poly A, 5′end not capped.
23. *Arenaviridae*	100-300	E	Helical	NA	Linear, (-) ssRNA, 2 segments	10-14	C	PM	-sense or ambisense with sticky ends enable circularizaion.
24. *Bunyaviridae*	80-120	E	Helical	NA	Linear, (-) ssRNA, 3 segments	11-21	C	GM	- Sense or ambisense & sticky ends allow circularization.
VI RNA viruses-RT									
25. *Retroviridae*	80-100	E	Icosahedral	?	Linear, (++) ssRNA-RT	7-11	C+ N	PM	Diploid+ sense, each H bonded at 3′ end, with 3′ end poly A & 5′ ends capped.
VII DNA viruses-RT									
26. Hepadna*viridae*	42	NE	Icosahedral	42	Circular, dsDNA, Some part partially dsDNA	3.2	N	None	ds DNA but a region of ssDNA.

C= cytoplasm; ds= double-stranded; E= Envelope, ER= endoplasmic reticulum, GM=Golgi membrane; ITR = inverted terminal repeats; N= nucleus; NE= naked or non-enveloped; NM=nuclear membrane; PM=Plasma membrane; ss= single-stranded.

ICTV VIRAL CLASSIFICATION

It starts at the level of order and follows as thus, with the taxon suffixes given in italics:

Order (*-virales*)

Family (*-viridae*)

Subfamily (*-virinae*)

Genus (*-virus*)

Species

So far, six orders have been established by the ICTV:

1. *Caudovirales*, 2. *Herpesvirales*, 3. *Mononegavirales*, 4. *Nidovirales*, 5. *Picornavirales and* 6. *Tymovirales.*

1. *Caudovirales* are tailed dsDNA (group I) bacteriophages.
2. *Herpesvirales* contains large eukaryotic dsDNA viruses, & includes 3 families- *Alloherpesviridae, Herpesviridae* & *Malaherpesviridae,* among which ***Herpesviridae*** contains viruses of medical & veterinary importance.
3. *Mononegavirales* includes non-segmented (-) strand ssRNA (Group V) plant and animal viruses. This order includes four families; *Bornaviridae, Filoviridae, Paramyxoviridae* & *Rhabdoviridae.*
4. *Nidovirales* is composed of (+) strand ssRNA (Group IV) viruses with vertebrate hosts. It includes the following families: *Arteriviridae, Coronaviridae & Roniviridae.*
5. *Picornavirales* contains small (+) strand ssRNA viruses that infect a variety of plant, insect, and animal hosts. It contains the following families: *Calciviridae, Comoviridae, Dicistroviridae, Iflaviridae, Marnaviridae, Picornaviridae, Potyviridae, Sequiviridae, & Secoviridae.*
6. *Tymovirales* contains monopartite ssRNA viruses that infect plants.

Other variations occur between the orders, for example, Nidovirales are isolated for their differentiation in expressing structural and non-structural proteins separately. However, this system of nomenclature differs from other taxonomic codes on several points. A minor point is that names of orders and families are italicized, as in the ICBN. Most notably, species names generally take the form of *[Disease] virus.* The establishment of an order is based on the inference that the virus families contained within a single order have most likely evolved from a common ancestor. The majority of virus families, about

65 families still unassigned to an order. Currently (2009) 6 orders, 87 families, 19 subfamilies, 348 genera, and 2,288 species of virus have been defined.

Animal viruses can be classified into **26 families** (**Table** 1-2) of medical & veterinary importance as per the following characteristics:

Characteristics of viral nucleic acid

1. Nucleic acid type- DNA or RNA.
2. Nucleic acid strand; if it is circular or linear, single stranded or double strand, or segmented or monopartite.
3. Nucleic acid size & diameter
4. Nucleic acid replication site; if it replicated in the cytoplasm or nucleus of infected cells.
5. Presence of transcriptase enzyme.
6. Complete or partial nucleotide sequences of the viruses.
7. Mode of mRNA replication; whether the virus belongs to one of the I-VII Groups: I: dsDNA viruses; II: ssDNA (+) sense DNA, III: dsRNA viruses; IV: (+) ssRNA viruses; V: (-)ssRNA viruses; VI: ssRNA-RT with DNA intermediate in life-cycle (e.g. *Retroviridae*); & VII: dsDNA-RT viruses (e.g. Hepadnaviruses)

Characteristics of viral capsid

1. Shape & size of capsid.
2. Symmetry of capsid with N.A (Helical, Cubical, Binal, Complex).
3. Site of capsid assembly inside the infected cells.
4. Lipid solvent sensitivity.
5. Number of capsomers which comprise the capsid in icosahedral symmetry or helical symmetry.

Animal viruses have been broadly classified into two groups which are RNA group & DNA group as per the above characters. DNA & RNA viruses have the following 26 families of veterinary & medical importance.

DNA viruses families

Group I ds DNA virus families

1. *Adenoviridae*
2. *Asfarviridae*

3. *Herpesviridae*
4. *Poxviridae*
5. *Papillomaviridae*
6. *Polyomaviridae*

Group II ss DNA virus families

7. *Parvoviridae*
8. *Circoviridae*

RNA viruses families

Group III ds RNA virus families

9. *Reoviridae*
10. *Birnaviridae*

Group IV ss positive sense (+) RNA virus families

11. *Picornaviridae*
12. *Caliciviridae*
13. *Togaviridae*
14. *Flaviviridae*
15. *Coronaviridae*
16. *Arteriviridae*
17. *Astroviridae*

Group V negative sense (-) ss RNA virus families

18. *Orthomyxoviridae*
19. *Paramyxoviridae*
20. *Rhabdoviridae*
21. *Bornaviridae*
22. *Filoviridae*
23. *Arenaviridae*
24. *Bunyaviridae*

Group VI RNA virus-reverse transcribing families

25. *Retroviridae*

Group VII DNA virus-reverse transcribing

26. *Hepadnaviridae*

Table 1.3 : Taxonomy of viruses of veterinary & medical importance & diseases caused by the member viruses.

SN	Order/Family	Subfamily	Genus	Species/serotypes	Diseases caused
ds DNA viruses					
1	*Adenoviridae*	-	*Mastadenovirus*	TS: *Human adenovirus C*/ HAdV	*Human adenovirus C* causes respiratory disease in humans.
				Canine adenovirus/ CAdV-1	**Infectious canine hepatitis** in dogs, foxes, wolves, coyotes etc.
				Canine adenovirus/ CAdV-2	**Kennel cough** or infectious laryngotracheitis in dogs.
				Equine adenovirus A/EAdV-1	Mild **URT symptoms** in equines, severe in **Arabian foals.**
			Aviadenovirus	**TS: *Fowl adenovirus A*/ FAdV-1/CELO**	FAdV-1/CELO chicken embryo lethal orphan virus causes **Quail bronchitis.**
				Fowl adenovirus B/FAdV-5	FAdV-5 causes **inclusion body hepatitis** in young chicks
			Atadenovirus	TS: *Ovine adenovirus D* /OAdV-7	Subclinical infection
				Duck adenovirus A /EDSV	DAdV-1/EDSV causes **egg drop syndrome** in broiler chickens.
			Siadenvirus	TS: *Frog adenovirus*	Adenoviruses of frogs.
				Turkey adenovirus A/TAdV-3	**TAdV-3** causes 3 disease syndromes: **adenovirus splenomegaly** in chickens, **marble spleen disease** in pheasants **& hemorrhagic enteritis** in young turkey.
2	*Asfarviridae*		*Asfivirus*	TS: *African swine fever virus*/ASFV	**African swine fever.**
3	O. *Herpesvirale/ Herpesviridae*	*Alphaherpes virinae*	*Simplexvirus*	TS: *Human herpesvirus 1*/ HHV-1	Oral & or genital infections, cold sores, genital herpes & encephalitis.

		Bovine herpesvirus 2/BHV-2	**Bovine ulcerative mammilitis & pseudolumpy-skin disease.**
	Varicellovirus	TS: *Human herpesvirus 3/ HHV-3*	Chickenpox & Shingles.
		Bovine herpesvirus 1/BHV-1	Infectious bovine Rhinotracheitis (IBR) in cattle.
		Bovine herpesvirus 5/BHV-5	**Causes meningoencephalitis in cattle.**
		Equid herpesvirus 1/EqHV 1	**Equine abortion in horses.**
		Equid herpesvirus 3/EqHV 3	**Equine coital exanthema in horses.**
		Equid herpesvirus 4/EqHV-4	**Rhinopneumonitis in horses.**
		Canid herpesvirus 1/CaHV-1	**Severe hemorrhagic disease in puppies.**
		Felid herpesvirus 1/ FeHV-1	**Feline viral rhinotracheitis & keratitis in cats.**
		Suid herpesvirus1 SuHV-1	**Pseudorabies** disease in pigs, cattle, sheep, dogs & cats.
	Mardivirus	TS: *Gallid herpesvirus 2/* GaHV2/MDV1	**Marek's disease** in chickens.
	Iltovirus	TS: *Gallid herpesvirus 1/* GaHV 1	Infectious laryngotracheitis (ILT) in chickens & pheasants
Betaherpe svirinae	*Cytomegalovirus*	TS: *Human herpesvirus 5*	Infectious mononucleosis (IM) like syndrome, retinitis, etc.
	Muromega lovirus	TS: *Murid herpesvirus 1 1/ MuHV-1*	Infect peritoneal macrophages, DC & hepatocytes, inducing significant pathology in both the spleen & liver
	Roseolovirus	TS: *Human herpesvirus 6/* HHV-6	Roseola infantum or exanthem subitum.

		Gammaherpesvirinae	*Lymphocryptovirus*	TS: *Human herpesvirus* 4/HHV-4	IM; Burkitt's lymphoma; Hodgkin's disease; CNS lymphoma in AIDS patients; Nasopharyngeal carcinoma, HIV-associated hairy leukoplakia (PTLD).
			Rhadinovirus	TS: *Human herpesvirus 8* / HHV-8	Kaposi's sarcoma; primary effusion lymphoma; some types of multicentric Castlesman's disease.
				Alcelaphine herpesvirus 1/ AlHV1	**MCF in cattle, deer & other ruminants in Africa.**
				Alcelaphine herpes virus 2 / ALHV 2	**MCF in antelope &** hartebeest to cattle.
				Ovine herpesvirus 2- Sheep-associated MCF	**MCF in cattle, deer & other ruminants in rest of world.**
		Unassigned	Unassigned	*Anatid herpesvirus* 1/AnHV1	**Duck plague/ duck viral hepatitis** in ducks, & geese.
		Unassigned	Unassigned	*Suid herpesvirus*/ SuHV	**Inclusion body rhinitis in piglets**
4	*Poxviridae*	*Chordopoxvirinae*	*Orthopoxvirus*	TS: *Vaccinia virus*/ VACV	*Vaccinia virus* infects sheep, water buffaloes, rabbits, cattle, horses, humans, & acts as vaccine vectors.
				Buffalopox virus/ BPXV	**Buffalopox** is adisease of water buffaloes.
				Camelpox virus/ CAMV-CMS, -GRI	**Camelpox** in Asia, Africa, Middle East.
				Cowpox virus/ CPX-BR, -GRI	**Cowpox** in cattle, domestic & zoo cats, humans, zoo animals, anteaters, & rodents.
				Monkeypox virus/ MPXV-ZAI	**Monkeypox** affects monkeys & humans, is prevalent in central and West Africa.

			Parapoxvirus	TS: *Orf virus*/ ORFV-SAOO, -NZ2	**Orf or contagious pustular dermatitis in lambs & goats.**
				Bovine papular stomatitis virus/ BPSV	Bovine papular stomatitis in cattle.
				Pseudocowpox virus PCPV	**Pseudocowpox**/ milkers nodule occurs in cows.
			Capripoxvirus	TS: *Sheeppox virus*/ SPPV-A, NIS-99	**Sheeppox** endemic in Asia, Africa, SE Europe in sheep, goats.
				Goatpox virus/ GTPV-G20	**Goatpox**
				Lumpy skin disease virus/LSDV-NI, -NW	**Lumpy skin disease in cattle** also in buff, giraffes, impalas in Africa
			Suipoxvirus	TS: *Swinepox virus* /SWPV	**Swinepox** occurs in pigs worldwide.
			Avipoxvirus	TS: *Fowlpox virus* / FPV	**Fowlpox** in chickens, turkeys, grouse, quail, pheasants, canaries, pigeons, sparrow, starlings & other avian species.
			Leporipoxvirus	TS: *Myxoma virus*/ MYXV-LAU	**Myxomatosis** is endemic in wild rabbits (*Sylvilagus*) in N & S. America; *Oryctolagus* in Europe, S America, Australia.
			Molluscipoxvirus	TS: *Molluscum contagtiosum virus*/ MOCV	Molluscum contagiosum occurs in humans- in children.
				Yaba monkey tumor virus/YMTV	Yaba monkey tumor.
				Tanapox virus/ TAPV	Tanapox occurs in humans near Tana river in Kenya.
		Entomopo xvirinae			Viruses of insects
5	*Papilloma viridae*		*Alphapapill omavirus*	TS: *Human papillamavirus 32*/ HPV-32,42	Papillomatosis in humans; **HPV-16, 18: are high risk tumor producers** associated with **human uterine cancers**; induce in-vitro cell transformation.

Betapapillo mavirus	TS: *Human papillo-mavirus* 5/HPV-5	HPV-5, 9, 49 cause Epidermodysplasia verruciformis.
Gammapapill omavirus	TS: *Human papilla-mavirus* 4/HPV-4	HPV-4,65,95,48,50, 60, 88 cause lesions.
Deltapapill omavirus	TS: *European elk papillomavirus* / *EEPV*	EEPV transform C127 mouse cell line, & induce fibrosarcoma in young hamsters after SC inj.
	Bovine papillomavirus1/BPV1, 2	BPV-1 infects paragenital areas, penis, teats & udders/ BPV-2 infects skin, alimentary tract & urinary bladder. **Both produce carcinomas when grazing land is infested with braken.**
Epsilonpapill omavirus	TS: *Bovine papillamavirus* 5/BPV-5	BPV-5 causes cutaneous papillomas in cattle.
Zetapapillo mavirus	TS: *Equus caballus papillomavirus* 1/ EcPV	Causes cutaneous lesions in horses.
Etapapillo mavirus	TS: *Frinzilla coelebs papillomavirus*	Causes cutaneous lesions in avian hosts.
Thetapapillo mavirus	TS: *Psittacus erithacus timmeh papillomaviru*	Causes cutaneous lesions in avian hosts.
Iotapapilloma virus	TS: *Mastomys natalensis papillomavirus*	Causes cutaneous lesions in rodents.
Kappapapillo *mavirus*	TS: *Cottontail rabbitpapillomavirus*	Causes cutaneous & mucosal lesions in rabbits.
Lambdapapillo mavirus	TS: *Canine oral papillomavirus*/COPV	Infects cats & dogs & cause & mucosal lesions.
Mupapapilloma virus	TS: *Human papillomavirus* 1/ HPVI, 63	Cutaneous lesions in Humans- species specific I/C inclusions.
Nupapapilloma virus	TS: *Human papillomavirus* 41	Benign & malignant lesions in the hosts.
Xipapapilloma virus	*Bovine papillomavirus* 3/BPV 3, 4, 6	True papillomas on mucosal surfaces; BPV-3 infects skin, BPV-4 upper

					alimentary tract, also causes squamous cell carcinoma; BPV-6 produces udder & teat papillomas of cattle.
			Omikronpapillomavirus	TS:*Phocoena spinipinnis papillomavirus*	Causes genital warts in cetaceans.
			Pipapapilloma virus	TS: *Hamster oral papillo-mavirus*/ HaOPV	Causes mucosal lesions in hamsters.
6	*Polyomaviridae*		*Polyomavirus*	TS: *Simian virus* 40/SV40	Infects monkeys but does not cause symptoms; infection is widespread within the humans & detected in human brain tumor.
				Budgerian fledgling diseasepolyomavirus/ BFDV	Causes acute, often fatal generalized **Budgerian fledgling disease** in young budgerigars.
				JC *polyomavirus*/ JCPyV	Infects R T, kidney & brain in humans; in immunocompromized reactivated in the brain causing progressive multifocal leucoence-phalopathy (PML).
				Merkel cell polyomavirus/ MCPYV	Merkel skin carcinoma in humans.
ss DNA viruses					
7	*Parvoviridae*	*Parvovirinae*	*Parvovirus*	TS: *Murine minute virus*/MVMc	Natural infections are symptomatic; neonatal mice are susceptible to lethal renal and/or intestinal hemorrhages during experimental infection.
				Feline panleukopenia virus/FPV	**Feline panleukopenia** in domestic & wild cats.
				Canine parvovirus/ CPV-2	**CPV2 causes canine parvovirus infn,** a highly contagious disease of young dogs-severe diarrhea, vomition, leucopenia, immune-suppression & often death.

				Porcine parvovirus/ PPV-kr	**Porcine parvovirus infn** in pigs is a cause of **infectious infertility.**
			Erythrovirus	TS: *Human parvovirus 19*/B19V	Childhood rash-exanthema, erythema infectiosum or aplastic anemia.
			Dependovirus	TS: *Adeno-associated virus 2*/AAV2	Infects humans and some other primate species. AAV is not currently known to cause disease.
				Duck parvovirus/ BDPV, MDPV	**Derzy's disease/ hepatitis** in Muscovy ducks.
				Goose parvovirus/GPV	**Goose viral hepatitis**
			Amdovirus	TS: *Aleutian mink disease virus*/AMDV	**Aleutian mink disease** causes abortion & death in minks & ferrets.
			Bocavirus	TS: *Bovine parvovirus*/ BPV	Subclinical in cattle; sporadic outbreaks with **enteritis & diarrhea in calves.**
8	*Circoviridae*		*Circovirus*	TS: *Porcine circovirus 1*/PCV-1, -2	PCV-2 causes **postweaning multi-systemic wasting syndrome (PMSWD)** & other syndromes.
				Beak and feather disease virus/BFDV	Beak & Feather disease is a fatal infn in young birds, attacks the feather follicles and the beak & claws-growing cells of the bird, affect the liver, brain, and immune system.
			Gyrovirus	TS: *Chicken anemia virus/*	**Chicken anemia** affects young chicks, causes anemia, bone marrow atrophy, & immunosuppression.
		Densovirinae			Not of Veterinary importance
Ds RNA viruses					
9	*Reoviridae*		*Orthoreovirus*	TS: *Mammalian orthoreovirus*/ MRV-1, 2, 3	Mild res & enteric infection in humans & in many animal sps.

			Avianorthoreovirus/ ARV-s1133, 176, SK138a	Causes **arthritis, tendinitis, gastro enteritis, hepatitis, & myocarditis** in chickens & turkeys.
		Orbivirus	*African horse sickness virus*/ AHSV 1 to 9	**African horse sickness.**
			TS: *Bluetongue virus*/ BTV- 1 to 24	**Bluetongue,** *Culicoides* borne disease of sheep, cattle, goats, buffaloes, deer, and antelopes.
			Epizootic hemorrhagic disease virus/ EHDV	Culicoides borne- affects **white tailed mule deer, cattle, & buffaloes.**
			Equine encephalosis virus/EEV 1to 8	**Equine encephalosis** is an acute illness of horses in S Africa.
			Palyam virus/ PAV	It is culicine & *Culicoides* borne, causes **fetal lesions, abortion in cattle, & sheep.**
		Rotavirus	TS: *Rotavirus* A/RV-A	Gastroenteritis with diarrhea in young animals up to 8 weeks old.
		Coltivirus	TS: *Colorado tick fever virus*/ CTFV-56-14-03	Encephalitis, flu-like in child, it is ticks & mosquitoes-borne
		Seadornavirus	*Banna virus*/ BAV-ch	*Seadornavirus*-South East Asia dodeca RNA virus; *Banna virus* causes encephalitis in humans in Japan & Indonesia, & **isolated from pigs & cattle.**
10	*Birnaviridae*	*Birnavirus*	*Infectious bursal disease virus*/IBDV 1,2	IBDV-2 in young chickens causes IBD/ Gumboro disease with immunosuppression, mortality at 3 to 6 weeks of age.
(+) ssRNA viruses				
11	O. *Piconavirale* *Picornaviridae*	*Enterovirus*	TS: *Human enterovirus* C/ HEC-19 types:+ CV-A + PV-1,2,3	*Human enterovirus* C/ Poliovirus (PV-1, 2, 3); **poliomyelitis,** which is being controlled globally.
			E V-B5-Swine vesicular disease	Swine vesicular disease (SVD)-vesicular lesions

		on feet, coronary band, lips, tongue, snout, & lameness.
	Porcine enterovirus B /PEV-9,10	PEV-9, 10 causes **SMEDI (stillbirth, mummification, embryonic death, and infertility)**
Cardiovirus	TS: *Encephalomyocarditis virus*/EMCV-1	**Encephalomyocarditisin rodents**, the natural host & **humans, monkeys & pigs**
Aphthovirus	TS: *Foot-and-mouth disease virus*/ FMDV-O, A, C, Asia1, SAT1, SAT2, SAT3	**FMD** forms vesicles in mouth-excessive salivation, on the feet with lameness, & myocarditis & death in newborn.
	Equine rhinitis A virus/ ERAV	ERAV causes **acute respiratory disease in horses.**
Hepatovirus	TS: *Hepatitis A virus*/ HAV	Hepatitis A virus causes an acute infectious of liver in humans.
Parechovirus	TS: *Human Parechovirus* / HPeV 1 to 14	Mild res & GIT illness & also myocarditis in humans.
Erbovirus	TS: *Equine rhinitis virus*/ ERBV-1 to 3	Upper respiratory febrile disease in foals & weanlings.
Kobuvirus	TS: *Aichi virus*/AiV	Causes gastroenteritis in humans.
Teschovirus	TS: *Porcine teschovirus*/ PTV-1 to 11	Teschen disease or Talfan disease in pigs by serotype 1
Sapelovirus	TS: *Porcine sapelovirus*/PSV	PSV is causes of acute diarrhea, res distress, & **polioencephalomyelitis of pigs** in China.
Senecovirus	TS: *Seneca valley virus* / SVV-001	SVV-001 used as oncolytic agent.
Tremovirus	TS: *Avian encephalomyelitis virus*/AEV-1	**Avian encephalomyelitis** in turkeys, chickens, pheasants & Japanese quails.

		Avihepatovirus	TS: *Duck hepatitis A virus*/ DHAV 1 to 3	DHAV-1 causes acute disease of young domestic (Pekin) ducklings.
12	O. *Picornavirales Caliciviridae*	*Vesivirus*	*Vesicular exanthema of swine virus*/ VESV-13 types	Vesicular exanthema (VE) in swine, horses & dogs **resemble FMD.**
			Feline calicivirus/ FCV-many types	FCV in kittens causes **important feline respiratory disease.**
		Lagovirus	*Rabbit haemorrhagic disease virus*/RHDV	RHDV affects mononuclear cells, is acute with resp & fatal coagulative hepatic necrosis.
		Norovirus	*Norwalk virus*/NWV	Norwalk virus causes gastroenteritis in humans.
		Sappovirus	*Sapporo virus*/SV	Causes gastroenteritis in infants & children.
		Nebovirus	*Newbury-1 virus*	**Bovine enteric calicivirus,** Jena virus & Newbury agent 1
13	*Togaviridae*	*Alphavirus*	*TS: Sindbis virus*	Infects humans; cycle between birds & mosquitoes.
			Eastern equine encephalitis virus/ EEEV	**Encephalitis in horses, humans & pheasants** in N & S America
			Venezuelanequine encephalitis virus/ V EEV	**Encephalitis in horses, donkeys, humans, & small mammals in C. & S.** America; cycle between rodents & mosquitoes.
			Westernequine encephalitis virus/ *WEEV*	Mild encephalitis in horses & humans in America; virus cycle between birds & mosquitoes.
			Getah virus/GETV	**Sporadic disease in horses** in East USA, S.E Asia, Australia with fever, urticaria & edema of limbs.
		Rubivirus	*Rubella virus*/RUBV	Rubella, an exanthematous disease in humans.

14	*Flaviviridae*		*Flavivirus*	TS: *Yellow fever virus*/YFV	Yellow fever in humans is an acute hemorrhagic disease caused by female mosquitoes *Aedes aegypti.*
				Louping ill virus/ LIV, 5 types	**Louping ill** in sheep, often cattle, deer, horses, pigs, red goose, humans-ticks-fever & CNS.
				Powassan virus/ POWV	Powassan virus causes tick-borne **encephalitis in small mammals.**
				Japanese encephalitis virus/JE V	JE is mosquito-borne in Asia in **birds & bats, pigs, horses, humans.**
				Israel turkey meningitisvirus/ITV	**Israel turkey meningitis** in Israel & S. Africa in turkeys with paralysis.
				Wesselsbron virus/ WESSV	WESSV occurs in sheep, cattle, & humans in Africa, Thailand; causes hepatitis & abortion in ewes.
			Hepacivirus	*Hepatitis C virus*/ HCV	HCV causes an acute hepatitis & chronic hepatitis in humans
			Hepatitis G Virus	*Hepatitis G virus*/ HGV-C	Hepatitis G virus or GB virus C (GBV-C) infects humans.
			Pestivirus	*Border disease virus*/ BDV,2 subtypes	**Border disease** in sheep, kids & rarely in calves; pregnant ewes abort & show congenital defects.
				Bovine viral diarrhea virus1/ BVDV-1	**BVD-1** if NCP infected cattle again infected with CP biotype, acute MD results & cattle die of MD.
				Classical swine fever virus/CSFV	**Classical swine fever** occurs in S. Africa with neurological signs, abortion in pregnants, & still birth.
15	O. Nidovirales *Coronaviridae*	*Corona virinae*	*Alphacorona virus*	*Canine corona virus* /CCoV	***Canine corona us* infection** occurs in

			dogs of all ages with diarrhea, vomition, and enteritis.
		Feline corona virus (Feline infectious peritonitis virus)/ FCoV/FIPV	**Feline cornavirus infn** is mild in cats, produce mild gastroenteritis **FIPV (wet & dry forms) is a progressive debilitating disease.**
		Porcine epidermal dirrhoea virus/PEDV	PEDV produces **watery diarrhea in swine.**
		Transmissible gastro-enteritis virus/TGEV	Causes transmissible gastroenteritis (TGE) in newborn pigs with vomition, diarrhea, dehydration, acidosis & high mortality.
	Betacoronavirus	*Bovine corona virus*/ BCoV	BCoV causes **diarrhea in calves & winter dysentery in adult cattle.**
		Porcine haemagglutinating encephalomyelitis virus/ PEV	PEV/ vomition & wasting disease virus **infects young pigs in America & Europe with symptoms of vomition & wasting & acute encephalomyelitis.**
		Sars corona virus/ SARS CoV	**Severe acute respiratory syndrome** with fever, flu-like symptoms in humans worldwide.
	Gammacorona virus	TS: *Infectious bronchitis virus*/ IBV-8 serotypes	**IBV** causes infectious bronchitis in young chickens.
		Turkery corona virus/ TCoV	TCoV causes **Blue comb disease or transmissible enteritis** in turkeys.
Torovirinae	*Torovirus*	*Bovine torovirus*/ BToV-Breda	Causes **diarrhea in newborn calves** not fed colostrums.
		TS: *Equine torovirus*/ EToV-Berne	EToV-Berne virus reported from **diarrhea in horses.**
		Porcine torovirus/ PToV	**Common in swine after weaning,** virus

				shed after 4-14 days post weaning **with normal stool.**
16	O. *Nidovirales* *Arteriviridae*	*Arterivirus*	TS: *Equine arteritis virus*/ EAV	Res in **horses, donkey, & mules** with pneumonia in foals, edema in dependent limbs, **abortion, fetal death, & vascular damage.**
			Lactate dehydrogenase elevating virus/LDEV	Mice **persistently infected-Macrophages for life with a life-long viremia.**
			Porcine respiratory & reproductive syndrome virus/PRRSV	**PRRSV** cause mild & short anorexia in adults **& resp signs in newborn, abortion in pregnant sows, still-births & mummified fetuses.**
			Simian hemorrhagic fever virus/SHFV	Systemic disease, a highly pathogenic virus in monkeys causing some death.
17	*Astroviridae*	*Mamastrovirus*	*Bovine astrovirus*/ BAstV-1, 2	**Causes mild or subclinical gastroenteritis in bovine.**
			Feline astrovirus/ FAstV-1	Sick animals develop **green and watery diarrhea.**
			TS: *Human astrovirus*/ HAstV-1, 8	Watery diarrhea in children & mild gastroenteritis in adults.
			Ovine astrovirus/ OAstV-1	Causes **diarrhea in lambs & calves.**
			Porcine astrovirus/ PAstV-1	Isolated in some cases from pigs with acute diarrhea.
		Avastrovirus	*Chicken astrovirus*/ CAstV, AHV-1,2	Causes **mild gastroenteritis in chickens.**
			Duck astrovirus/ DAstV-1	Mild gastroenteritis in ducks with often acute **fatal hepatitis.**
			TS:*Turkey astrovirus*/ TAstV-1, 2	Causes **diarrhea, growth depression** in poults; type 2 is more pathogenic.

(-) ss RNA viruses

18	*Orthomyxo-viridae*	*Infuenzavirus A*		*Human influenza A virus*	H1N1, H1N2, H3N2 are influenza A virus subtypes currently circulating among humans causing epidemics & pandemics.
				Avian influenza A viruses	Avian influenza A virus subtypes are: H5N1, H7N2, H1N7, H7N3, H13N6, H5N9, H11N6, H3N8, H9N2, H5N2, H4N8, H10N7, H2N2, H8N4, H14N5, H6N5, H12N5 and others.
				Swine infuenza A viruses	H1N1, H1N2, and H3N2 are the common subtypes worldwide.
				Equine influenza A viruses	Subtypes are **H7N7** or **equine-1** commonly affects horse heart muscle, and **H3N8** or **equine-2** is usually more severe.
				Canine influenza A viruses	**H3N8** is now endemic in birds, horses and dogs.
			Infuenzavirus B	*Influenza B virus*	Infects mostly humans, is less common than *Influenzavirus A*. Also infects **seal & the ferrets.**
			Influenzavirus C	*Influenza C virus*	Infects humans, dogs & pigs, often causing severe illness and local epidemics.
			Isavirus	*Infectious salmon anemia virus*	Infects Atlantic salmon.
			Thogotovirus	*Thogoto virus*	*Thogoto virus* & *Dhori virus* infect humans.
9	O. *Mononega-virales Paramy-roviridae*	*Paramyxo virinae*	*Respirovirus*	TS: *Sendai virus*/SeV	Murine parainfluenza virus-1 causes RT infection in mice, G. pigs, rats, & occasionally pigs.
				Bovine parainfluenza virus 3/ BPIV-3	Mild respiratory infection in cattle & sheep.

	Rubulavirus	TS: *Mumps virus*/ MuV	Causes mumps in children with swelling of the parotid glands.
		Porcine rubula virus/ PoRV-2 strains	Causes **blue eye disease with encephalitis & res disease in piglets,** & reproductive failure in adult pigs, & corneal opacity.
	Morbillivirus	TS: *Measles virus*/ MeV	Causes measles in humans.
		Canine distemper virus/CDV	CDV is a pantropic disease of dogs & other carnivores with a diphasic fever, gastroenteritis & res signs, leucopenia, neurological symptoms & hard footpad.
		Rinderpest virus/RPV	RP in cattle, buffaloes & wildlife.
		Peste des petits ruminants virus/ PPRV	A disease of goats & sheep with fever, necrotic stomatitis, gastroenteritis & pneumonia.
	Henipavirus	TS: *Hendra virus*/ HeV	Res distress, neurological sign & rapid death in horses, also infects humans.
		Nipah virus/NiV	Severe res or neurological distress, & encephalitis in pigs & humans with high mortality rate.
	Avulavirus	*New castle disease virus* or *Avian parmyxovirus-1* (NDV/APMV-1)	Disease of birds affecting many domestic and wild avian sps with **severeres or nervous signs or diarrhea & high mortality.**
Pneumo-virinae	*Pneumovirus*	*Bovine respiratory syncytial virus*/BRSV	BRSV causes **severe res disease in young beef & dairy cattle** initially but mild to subclinical in subsequent infections.
		Avian metapneumo-virus /AMPV	Disease in turkeys and chickens with upper res

				disease & drops in egg prodn in layers & breeders.
20	O. *Mononega-virales* *Rhabdoviridae*	*Vesiculovirus*	TS: *Vesicular stomatitis Indiana virus*/VSIV	VSIV causes vesicular lesions like FMD in cattle, horses, pigs and humans & occasionally sheep and goats.
		Lyssavirus	*Rabies virus*/RABV	**Rabies** (RABV) is a viral disease of all warm- blooded animals.
		Ephemerovirus	TS: *Bovine ephemeral fever virus*/BEFV	**Bovine ephemeral fever** is an arthropod-borne disease of cattle with **fever, muscular shivering, stiffness, lameness, nasal & ocular discharges, & enlarged peripheral lymph nodes.**
21	O. *Mononega virales* *Bornaviridae*	*Bornavirus*	*Bornavirus disease virus*/BDV	Subacute **meningo-encephalitis in horses, sheep, cattle, rabbits & cats.**
22	O. *Mononega virales* *Filoviridae*	*Ebolavirus*	TS: *Zaire ebola virus* /ZEBOV/*Sudan ebola virus*/SEBOV	Zaire ebola virus causes ebola hemorrahagic fever (EHF) in humans.
			Côte d'Ivoire e bolavirus/ Bundibugyo ebola virus	Infects humans.
		Marburgvirus	TS: *Lake Victoria Marburg virus*/ MARV	Marburg hemorrhagic fever (MHV) occurs in humans & non-human primates.
23	*Arenaviridae*	*Arenavirus*	TS: *Lymphocytic choriomeningitis virus*/ LCMV4	LCMV-4 **infects wild rodents, mice and occasionally humans** with occasional meningitis.
			Lassa virus/LASV	Causes **Lassa fever**, is maintained in its natural rodent reservoir, the multimammate rat with high fever, myalgia, coagulo-pathy, hemorrhagic skin rash, infects humans.

24	*Bunyaviridae*		*Phlebovirus*	TS: *Rift Valley fever virus*/RVFV	Abortion, new-born mortality & hepatitis in cattle, sheep & goat.
			Nairovirus	TS: *Dugbe virus*/ Nairobi sheep disease virus/NSDV	Hemorrhagic gastroenteritis in sheep & goats.
			Ortho*bunyavirus*	*Akabane virus*/ AKAV	Congenital malformation, arthrogryposis and hydranencephaly in livestock.
				TS: *Bunyamwera virus* *Cache valley virus*/ CVV	Teratogenic effect, & congenital malformation in sheep.
				California encephalitis virus, San Angelo virus/SAV	Congenital malformation in sheep experimentally.
				Main Drain virus/ MDV	Encephalomyelitis, congenital malformation in sheep experimentally
			Hantavirus	TS: *Hantaan virus*/ *Sin Nombre virus*/ SNV, others	Hantaan Cardio-pulmonary syndrome in humans- HCPS, some develop serious kidney disease, death in 5 days due to heart and lung failure.
				Puumala virus/ PUUV	Hemorrhagic fever with renal syndrome-HFRS or Nephropathi epidemica in humans.
RNA viruss-RT					
25	*Retroviridae*	*Orthoretrovirinae*	*Alpharetrovirus*	TS: *Avian leukosis virus*/ALV	ALV-disturbed blood formation in chickens, neoplastic conditions: lymphoid, erythroid, myeloid leukosis, fibrosarcoma & nephroblastoma.
			Betaretrovirus	*Jaagsiekte sheep retrovirus*/JSSRV	Causes a contagious lung cancer in sheep called Jaagsiekte, or ovine pulmonary adenocarcinoma OPA.
				TS: *Mouse mammary tumor virus*/MMTV	Causes mammary breast cancer, which is milk transmitted.

Gammaretrovirus	TS: *Murine leukemia virus* /MLV	MLVs cause cancer in mice hosts. Some MLVs may infect other vertebrates.
	Feline leukemia virus/ FeLV	Causes **cancer of the blood cells (lymphocytes)-leukemia.**
Deltaretrovirus	TS: *Bovine leukemia virus*/ BLV	Causes **B-cell leukemia called enzootic bovine leukosis in adult cattle.**
	Human T-lymphotropic virus/ HTLV -1, 2, 3	Causes adult T cell leukemia /lymphoma in humans.
Lentivirus	*Bovine immunodeficiency virus*/ BIV	Infects cattle lymphocytes and monocytes/ macrophages.
	Equine infectious anemia virus/ EIAV	**EIA/swamp fever in horses** runs in 3 clinical forms: **acute, subacute & chronic forms.**
	Feline immunodeficiency virus/ FeIV	FeIV replicates in CD[4] helper T lymphocytes, macrophases, astroccytes, & microglial cells. The infected cats remain persistently viremic, but don't die.
	TS: *Human immunodeficiency virus*/ HIV-1	HIV-1,2 causes AIDS in humans with progressive failure of immune system favouring life-threatening opportunistic infections & cancers to develop.
	Caprine arthritis encephalitic virus/ CAEV	Causes polyarthritis in adult goats, encephalitis in kids, mastitis, hypogalactia, chronic interstitial pneumonia, progressive weight loss & a persistent, lifelong infection.

				Visna/maedi virus/ VISNA	Causes encephalitis and chronic pneumonitis in sheep or ovine progressive pneumonia.
		Spumavirinae	*Spumavirus*	TS: *Simian foamy virus*	*Bovine foamy virus, Feline foamy virus & Equine foamy virus.*
26	*Hepadnaviridae*		*Orthohepad-navirus*	TS: *Hepatitis B virus navirus*	Infects liver of humans, chimps, gibbons, wooly monkeys & causes hepatitis; chronic hepatitis leads to cirrhosis & incidence of hepatocellular carcinoma.
				Ground squirrel hepatitis virus/GSHV	Causes hepatitis or hepatocellular carcinoma in squirrels in northern California.
				Woodchuk *hepatitis virus*/WHV	Causes acute hepatitis & usually hepato-cellular carcinoma but not cirrhosis.
				Wooly monkey hepatitis B virus/ WMHBV	Asymptomatic carrier state, hepatitis, hepatocellular carcinoma.
			Avihepadnavirus	*Duck hepatitis B virus*/ DHBV	Infects Anas species ducks (not Muscovy ducks), acquired congenitally; produces chronic viremia.

ds= double-sranded; F = family; G= genus; GIT=Gastrointestinal tract; O= Order; RT= reverse transcriptase; res, RT= respiratory tract; ss= single stranded; TS= type species

Characteristics & Description of 26 Viral Families

Group1 ds DNA virus families

Family 1 : *Adenoviridae*

(G. adeno = gland)

General characteristics

1. Naked, 70-90 nm in diameter ds DNA viruses.
2. Icosahedral symmetry with 252 capsomers.
3. Genome linear-26 -45 Kbp, Early **(E) genes** & **Late (L) genes**, 3′ & 5′ ends" have inverted terminal repeats & the 5′ ends have **terminal 55**

kDa protein used as **primers** in viral replication; encodes more than 30 proteins including 10 structural proteins.

4. Fibers project from twelve vertices of capsid. Pentons & fibers determine type specific antigenicity & elicit neutralizing antibodies.

5. Replicate in nuclei forming intranuclear inclusion bodies, Early (E) phase & late (L) phase; **knob domain of the fiber** protein binds to CD46 for the group B human adenovirus serotypes, and the coxsackievirus adenovirus receptor (CAR) for all other serotypes.

6. Agglutinate rat or monkey RBCs

7. Infect birds, many mammals and man, **can undergo latent infection in lymphoid tissues & become reactivated some time later**. Several types have oncogenic potential.

8. Resist freezing, mild acid & lipid solvents, 56C for 10 min, stable to chemical or physical agents, adverse pH allowing **prolonged survival outside the body.**

Classification of *Adenoviridae*

Genus 1 *Mastadenovirus*; type species: *Human adenovirus C*; other importance species are; *Canine adenovirus-1*(CAD-1) causes **infectious canine hepatitis (ICH)** in dogs, *Canine adenovirus-2* **(CAD-2)** causes **kennel cough** or infectious laryngotracheitis in dogs.

Genus 2 *Aviadenovirus*; type species: *Fowl adenovirus A* **(FAdV-1/CELO, chicken embryo lethal orphan virus)** causes a widespread but inapparent infection; CELO virus also causes **Quail bronchitis;** *Fowl adenovirus B* **(FAdV- 5)** & many types cause **inclusion body hepatitis in young chickens.**

Genus 3 *Atadenovirus;* type species: *Ovine adenovirus D;* other species are: *Duck adenovirus A* **(DAdV-1/ EDSV) causes egg drop syndrome in chickens.**

Genus 4 *Siaadenovirus;;* type species: *Frog adenovirus;* other virus species are *Turkey adenovirus A* **(TAdV-3)**/Avian adenovirus splenomegaly virus causes **adenovirus splenomegaly in chickens;** Marble spleen disease virus **(TAdV-3)** causes **marble spleen disease in pheasants, alsò** causes **marble spleen disease in pheasants &** Turkey haemorhagic enteritis **in young turkey poults.**

Genus 5 *Ichtadenovirus;* type species: *Sturgeon adenovirus A.*

Family 2: Asfarviridae

Derived from African swine fever and related viruses

General characteristics:

1. Enveloped, 175-215 nm in diameter, dsDNA viruses.
2. Icosahedral symmetry, 1892-2172 capsomers
3. Genome linear ds DNA 170-190 kb, both ends covalently closed, have inverted terminal repeats.
4. Replicate in cytoplasm of host cells & in soft ticks.
5. Sylvatic (Warthogs, Bushpigs-reservoirs) & domestic transmission cycles, **transmitted by soft ticks**, majority causes hemadsorption
6. Stable at 4-20°C, persist for months in meat.

Classification of Asfarviridae

Group: Group I dsDNA viruses

Family: *Asfarviridae*

Genus: *Asfivirus;* Type species: *African swine fever virus* causes African swine fever.

Family 3: *Herpesviridae*

(G. herpein= to creep) meaning to the latent, recurring & lytic infections.

General characteristics

1. Enveloped spherical to pleomorphic, 120-200 nm in diameter, dsDNA viruses, **tegument** in between capsid & envelope
2. Capsid with icosahedral symmetry, 162 capsomers.
3. Genome linear dsDNA 120-230kb; contain terminal & internal reiterated sequences.
4. Replicate in nucleus with intranuclear inclusion bodies. Virion attaches via glycoprotein gB, gC & gD to the cell surface sialic acid receptors.
5. Virus assembly occurs via budding through the inner lamella of the nuclear membrane modified by the insertion of herpes glycoproteins, throughout the Golgi and finally released at the plasma membrane.
6. **Latency** is a common with herpesvirus infection with reactivation on stresses; **during latency the viral genome is maintained in the nucleus as circular episomes with limited expression of viral genes.**

7. Some cell-associated infections are oncogenic; some infections are silent or mild in natural hosts but serious in other hosts, e.g. pseudorabies.
8. This family contains more than 100 viruses causing diseases in human, birds, mammals, fish, amphibian & reptiles.

Classification of *Herpesviridae*

Group: Group I ds DNA

Order: *Herpesvirales*

Family: *Herpesviridae*

Subfamily 1: *Herpesvirinae*: Members of *Alphaherpesvirinae* are neurotropic, i.e. they infect nervous system tissues, have a short reproductive cycle of about18 hours with efficient cell destruction and variable host range, The viruses of this subfamily establish **latent infections in neural cells,** most herpesviruses of veterinary importance are found in the genus *Varicellovirus.*

G1: *Simplexvirus;* type species: *Human hepesvius 1* or Herpes simplex virus; others *Bovine herpesvirus* 2 (BHV-2) causes **bovine ulcerative mammitis.**

G2: *Varicellovirus* ; type species: *Human hepesvirus* 3 or Varicella-zoster virus; causes Infectious bovine rhinotracheitis (**BHV-1**), Bovine meningoencephalitis (BHV-5), Equine abortion (EqHV-1) & equine rhinotracheitis (EqHV-4), Equine coital exanthema (EqHV-3), Fatal haemorrhagic disease of puppies (CaHV-1), Feline rhinotracheitis (FeHV-1), Pseudorabies (SuHV-1).

G3: *Mardivirus;* type species: *Gallid herpesvirus* 2 (GaHV-2/MDV-1) *causes* **Marek's disease** in poulty

G4: *Iltovirus;* type spcies: *Gallid herpesvius 1* (GaHV-1) causes **Infectious laryngotracheitis in birds**

Subfamily 2: *Betaherpesvirinae*: Members of *Betaherpesvirinae* are lymphotropic, have a long reproductive cycle, restricted host range, the infected cells become enlarged (cytomegalo), & the viruses may become latent in secretory glands & lymphoreticular cells.

G1: *Cytomegalovirus* ; type species: *Human herpesvius 5*

G2: *Muromegalovirus;* type species: *Murid herpesvirus 1*

G3: *Roseolovirus* ; type species: *Human herpesvirus 6*

G4: *Proboscivirus;* Elephantid herpesvirus1: TS

Subfamily 3: *Gammaherpesvirinae*: Members of *Gammaherpesvirinae* are also lymphotropic and specific for either T or B lymphocytes. If lymphocytes are infected, viral expression is minimal, some replicate in the epithelial cells & fibroblasts with cell lysis, & several species can lead to neoplastic transformation of lymphocytes.

G1: *Lymphocryptovirus;* type species: *Human herpesvirus 4* or Epstein-Barr virus

G2: *Rhadinovirus;* type species: *Human herpesvirus 8; Alcelaphine herpesvirus* 1 (AlHV1) causes **Malignant catarrhal fever in cattle in Africa** & *Ovine herpesvirus* 2 (OvHV-2) causes MCF in cattle in **rest of the world.**

G3: *Macavirus*: type species: *Alcelaphine herpesvirus 1*

G4: *Percavirus;* type species: *Equid herpesvirus* 2

Unassigned

Genus: *Cercopithecine;* type species: *Cercopithecine herpesvirus 1; Anatid herpesvirus 1*(AnHV-1) causes Duck plague/duck viral hepatitis in ducks & geese.

Family 4 : *Poxviridae*

General characters

1. Enveloped, largest 220-450 nm x 140- 260 nm, ds DNA viruses.
2. Complex symmetry, brick shaped or ovoid viruses.
3. Genome; linear, dsDNA 130-375kb.
4. Contain DNA dependent RNA polymerase or RNA transcriptase that helps in uncoating the virus
5. Replicate in cytoplasm at sites called virolasm or viral factories, cytoplasmic inclusions, virus is released through cell lysis or often budding.
6. Pock or skin lesions prominent feature.
7. Genetic recombination within genera results in extensive serological cross reaction and cross-protection.
8. Virions are stable at room temperature under dry conditions, but sensitive to heat, detergents, formaldehyde and oxidizing agents.

Classificaton of *Poxviridae*

Group I dsDNA virus

Family: *Poxviridae*

Subfamily 1: *Chordopoxvirinae*

Genus 1: *Orthopoxvirus*; type species: *Vaccinia virus*; other species are: *Camelpox virus, Cowpox virus, Ectromelia virus, Monkeypox virus, Racoonpox virus, Taterapox virus, Vaccinia virus, Variola virus & Volepox virus*- causes Vaccinia virus infection, Cowpox, Buffalopox, Felinepox, Horsepox, Camelox, Monkeypox.

Genus 2: *Parapoxvirus*; type species: *Orf virus*; species: *Bovine papular stomatitis virus, Parapoxvirus of red deer in New Zealand & Pseudocowpox virus*- **Orf, Pseudocowpox, Bovine papular stomatitis**.

Genus 3: *Capripoxvirus*; type species: *Sheeppox virus*; other species are: *Goatpox virus, Lumpy skin disease virus*- **Sheep & goatpox, Lumpy skin disease**.

Genus 4: *Avipoxvirus; type species: Fowlpox virus*; other species are: *Canarypox virus, fowlpox virus, Juncopox virus, Mynapox virus, Pigeonpox virus, Psitacinepox virus, Quailpox virus, Sparrowpox virus, Starlingpox virus & Turkeypox virus* – **Fowlpox,** pigeon pox, Turkey pox.

Genus 5: *Suipoxvirus*; type species: *Swinepox virus*-**Swinepox**, the only species.

Genus 6: *Leporipoxvirus*; type species: *Myxoma virus*; other species are: *Hare fibroma virus, Myxoma virus, Rabbit fibroma virus, Squirrel fibroma virus*- **Rabbit myxomatosis**.

Genus 7: *Molluscipoxvirus*; type species: *Molluscum contagiosum virus*, the only species.

Genus 8: *Yatapoxvirus*; type species: *Yaba money tumor virus*; other species are: *Tanapoxvirus, Yaba money tumor virus.*

Genus 9: *Cervidpoxvirus*; type species: *Deerpox virus W-848-83*, the only species.

Genus *Unassigned*; species: *Squirrelpox virus.*

Subfamily 2: *Entomopxvirinae* - Viruses of insects.

Family 5 : *Papillomaviridae*

(L. papilli=pustule, oma=tumours)

General characteristics

1. Non-enveloped, circular, 40-55 nm diameter ds DNA viruses.
2. Icosahedral symmetry with 72 star-shaped capsomers (T=7).
3. Genome single molecule of circular, superoiled, ds DNA about 5.3-8 kbp long, early region & late region.
4. **L1 protein forms viral capsid & is responsible for producing neutralizing antibodies.**
5. Replications in **nucleus of basal cells of squamous surface epithelium.**
6. During assembly of the virion particles, nucleus breaks down and the virus is released.
7. Resistant to lipid- solvents, acids, 60°C for 30 minutes.

Classification of *Papillomaviridae*

Group I ds DNA

Family: *Papillomaviridae*

G 1: ***Alphapapillomavirus;* type species: *Human papillomavirus* 32**

G 2: *Betapapillomavirus*; type species: *Human papillomavirus 5*

G 3: *Gammapapillomavirus*; type species: *Human papillomavirus 4*

G 4: *Deltapapillomavirus;* type species: *European elk papillomavirus,* Others are *Bovine papillomavirus 1,2*

G 5: *Epsilonpapillomavirus;* type species: *Bovine papillomavirus 5*

G 6: *Etapapillomavirus;* type species: *Frinzilla coelebs papillomavirus*

G 7: *Iotapapillomavirus;* type species: *Mastomys natalensis papillomavirus*

G 8: *Kappapapillomavirus;* type species: *Cottontail rabbitpapillomavirus*

G 9: *Lambdapapillomavirus;* type species: *Canine oral papillomavirus*

G 10: *Mupapillomavirus;* type species: *Human papillomavirus 1*

G 11: *Nupapillomavirus;* type species: *Human papillomavirus 41*

G 12: *Omikronpapillomavirus;* type species: *Phocoena spinipinnis papillomavirus*

G 13: *Pipapapillomavirus;* type species: *Hamster oral papillomavirus*

G 14: *Thetapapillomavirus;* type species: *Psittacus erithacus timmeh papillomavirus*

G 15: *Xipapillomavirus;* type species: *Bovine papillomavirus 3*

G 16: *Zetapapillomavirus;* type species: *Equine papillomavirus 1* Cause papilloma & fibropapilloma in domestic animals.

Deltapapillomavirus (BPV1, 2), Genus: *Epsilonpapillomavirus* (BPV 5), & Genus: *Xipapapillomavirus* (BPV- 3, 4, 6) – Cause Bovine papillomatosis, Bovine alimentary tract papilloma-carcoma; Genus: *Zetapapillomavirus*(EqPV-1)-cause s Equine papillomatosis, Genus : *Xipapapillomavirus* 4 (BPV-4)-causes Equine sarcoids, Genus - *Lambdapapillomavirus* (COPV)-causes Canine oral papillomatosis.

Family 6 : *Polyomaviridae*
(G. poly= several, oma= tumor)
General characteristics

1. Naked, about 45nm in diameter, ds DNA viruses.
2. Grow in culture in vitro, often causing malignant transformation in cells from heterologous species.
3. Icosahedral symmetry, 55 nm in diameter, 72 capsomers; VP1-3 forms the viral capsid.
4. Genome circular, monopartite, dsDNA in acircular supercoiled structure and isassociated with histones H2a, H2b, H3, and H4from the host, 5 kb in length, and both DNA strands code for proteins.
5. Replication in nucleus.
6. Viruses released via: **less commonly** transported in cytoplasmic vacuoles to the plasma membrane & bud or **more frequently** released after the cell lysis caused by the cytotoxicity of virus.
7. Resistant to lipid- solvents, acids, 60°C for 30 minutes.

Classification of *Polyomaviridae*

Group I dsDNA

Family: *Polyomaviridae*

Genus: *Polyomavirus*

Species

African monkey polyomavirus, Avian polyomavirus causes **Budgerigar fledgling disease** (BFDPyV) with acute, often fatal generalized infection in young budgerigars, *BK polyomavirus* (BKPLV), *Canary polyomavirus, Chimpanzee polyomavirus, Crow polyomavirus, Goose hemorrhagic polyomavirus, Finch polyomavirus, Hamster polyomavirus, Human polyomavirus 6, Human polyomavirus 7, Human polyomavirus 9, JC polyomavirus* (JCPyV), *KI polyomavirus, Lymphotropic polyomavirus; Mastomys polyomaviru; Merkel cell polyomavirus* (MCPyV), *Murine pneumotropic virus; Murine polyomavirus; Myotis polyomavirus, Orangutan polyomavirus* (Borneo), *Orangutan polyomavirus* (Sumatra), *Rabbit kidney vacuolating virus, California sea lion polyomavirus 1, Simian virus 12, Simian virus 40* (SV-40), *Squirrel monkey polyomavirus, Trichodysplasia spinulosa associated polyomavirus* (TSV), *WU polyomavirus* (WUPyV).

Group II ssDNA virus families

Family 7 : *Parvoviridae*

(L. parvus= small)

General characteristics

1. Non enveloped **smallest** 18-26 nm in diameter**, simplest ssDNA viruses.**
2. Icosahedral symmetry with 60 capsomers. **These viruses are one of the most environmentally resistant viruses.**
3. Genome is ssDNA of 5 kb, either linear, negative-sense, ssDNA in most cases, or of linear, negative-sense and positive-sense ssDNA in up to 50% in some members, palindromic at ends enabling circularization of DNA during replication.
4. Replicate in the nucleus forming intranuclear inclusion bodies. Replicate only **in dividing cells such as marrow, gut and the developing fetus cells.** Genomes contain long terminal palindromic sequences (**serves as a self-primer**), each end fold back on itself to form a **hairpin** useful during replication for **synthesis of plus sense DNA.**
5. Virus released by budding out of the host.
6. Resistant to heat 56^{0}C for more than 60 minutes, also resistant to lipid solvents, pH (3-9). Inactivated by formalin, β – Propiolacton & sodium hypochlorite.

Classification of *Parvoviridae*

Group: Group II ssDNA

Family: *Parvoviridae*

Subfamilies: SF 1: *Parvovirinae* & SF 2: *Densovirinae*

Subfamily 1: Parvovirinae

Genus 1: *Parvovirus;* type species: *Murine minute virus;* causes **Feline panleucopenia, Canine parvovirus-2 infection, Porcine parvovirus infection.**

Genus 2: *Erythrovirus;* type species: B 19 virus.

Genus 3: *Dependovirus;* type species: *Adeno-associated virus 2;* causes **Duck parvovirus infection & Goose parvovirus infection.**

Genus 4: *Amdovirus;* type species: *Aleutian mink disease virus*-causes **Aleutian mink disease.**

Genus 5: *Bocavirus;* type species: *Bovine parvovirus*- causes **Bovine parvovirus infection.**

Subfamily 2: Densovirinae

Genus 1: *Densovirus;* type species: *Junonia coeniadensovirus*

Genus 2: *Iteravirus;* type species: *Bombyx moridensovirus*

Genus 3: *Brevidensovirus;* type species: *Aedes aegyptidensovirus*

Genus 4: *Pefudensovirus;* type species: *Periplanta fuliginosadensovirus*

Family 8 : *Circoviridae*

General characteristics

1. Non enveloped, small 17- 22 nm in diameter, positive sense or ambisense ssDNA viruses.
2. Icosahedral symmetry.
3. Genome is **circular** ss DNA 1.8 to 3.8 kb long, the ends are closed by covalent bonds **forming a circle.**
4. Virus replicates in the nucleus of dividing cells during S phase, replicated through ds intermediates using **rolling-circle replication.**
5. Virus released from the cell by budding.
6. Stable at pH 3-9, & heating at 60°C for 30 minutes.

Classification of *Circoviridae*

Group II ssDNA

Family: *Circoviridae*

Genus 1: *Circovirus;* type species: *Porcine circovirus* Type 1 and 2, other species is *Beak and feather disease virus* (BFDV)-cause Porcine circovirus infection, Beak & feather disease in psitacine birds.

Genus 2: *Gyrovirus;* type species: *Chicken anaemia virus*-causes Chicken anemia.

Unassigned Genus 3: *Anellovirus* includes human virus such as Transfusion transmitted virus or *Torque teno virus.*

Group III ds RNA virus families

Family 9 : *Reoviridae*

(L. reo; r = respiratory, e = enteric, o = orphan) name is derived from respiratory enteric orphan viruses.

General characters

1. Non-enveloped, 60-80 nm in diameter with double capsid, ds RNA viruses.
2. Double layered icosahedral capsid, **outer capsid** 75-80 nm in diameter with **92 capsomers** (T=13) e.g. *Orthoreovirus* & the **inner capsid with 32 capsomers** (*Orbivirus*) & **measures 45 nm in diameter** (T =2).
3. Genome segmented (10, 11, 12 segments) ds RNA, segments from 0.2 to 3.0 kb & genome total size range from 18.2 to 30.5 kb, 10, 11, 12 segments **called L (large), M (medium) and S (small). L encodes λ proteins,** the M encodes for **μ proteins** and the S encodes for **σ proteins, total** 10 to 14 proteins.
4. Replicate in cytoplasm with intracytoplasmic inclusion bodies, the coat not fully uncoated, is resistant to protease digestion by the infected cell.
5. Genetic reassortment readily takes place.
6. Mature virions are formed in the endoplasmic reticulum & released after cell lysis.
7. Resistant to heat, organic solvents.

Classification of *Reoviridae*

There are 15 genera of *Reoviridae* divided in 2009 on basis of the presence of a "turret" or spike protein on the inner capsid into **two subfamilies;**

***Sedoreovirinae* containing the non-turreted virus genera & *Spinareovirinae* containing the spiked or turreted viruses in the family.**

Group III dsRNA

Family: *Reoviridae*

The subfamily 1: *Spinareovirinae* contains 9 genera:

Genus 1: *Aquareovirus;* type species: *Aquareovirus A* (ARV-A).

Genus 2 : *Cypovirus;* type species: *Cypovirus 1* (CPV- 1).

Genus 3: Fijivirus; type species: *Fiji disease virus* (FDV).

Genus 4: *Idnoreovirus;* type species: *Hyposeter exiquae reovirus* (HeRV).

Genus 5: *Mycoreovirus;* type species: *Mycoreovirus 1* (MRV-1).

Genus 6: *Orthoreovirus;* type species: *Mammalian orthoreovirus* (MRV).

Genus 7: *Oryzavirus;* type species: *Rice ragged stunt virus* (RRSV).

Genus 8: *Coltivirus; type specie: Colorado tick fever virus* (CTFV)

Genus 9: *Dinovernavirus;* type species: *Aedes pseudoscutellaris virus.*

The subfamily 2: *Sedoreovirinae* contains 6 genera

Genus 1: *Mimoreovirus;* type species:

Genus 2: *Orbivirus;* type species: *Bluetongue virus* (BTV).

Genus 3: *Phytoreovirus;* type species: *Rice dwarf virus* (RDV).

Genus 4: *Rotavirus*: type species: *Rotavirus A* (RV-A).

Genus 5: *Seadornavius; type species: Kadipiriro virus (KDV).*

Genus 6: *Cardoreoviris; type species: Eriocheir sinensus reovirus.*

Clinical infections in animals are: Genus: *Orbivirus*- **Arthropods- borne infections-**African horse sickness, Blue tongue in sheep, Epizootic haemorrhagic disease in white tailed & mule deer, **cattle, buffaloes,** Palyam virus infection in cattle & sheep, Equine encephalosis, Genus: *Orthoreovirus*- Avian orthoreovirus infection, Genus- *Rotavirus*-Rotavirus infection in farm animals.

Family 10 : *Birnaviridae*

(L. bi = two, rna = ribonucleic acid) are so named as these viruses contain two segments of linear ds RNA.

General characteristics

1. Small, naked, & spherical dsRNA about 70 nm in diameter.
2. Icosahedral symmetry made of **132 capsomers (T=13).**

3. Genome linear dsRNA of **two segments, A (larger) and B (shorter), A** (3.2 kb) encodes viral proteins **VP2, VP3, VP4, and VP5; VP2 protein elicits protective immune response., B** encodes (2.75-2.85kb) encodes **VP1 with RNA polymerase and capping enzyme activities,** the 5'-end of the genome has a cap on both segments & genome-linked protein (VPg).
4. Birnaviruses **replicate in the cytoplasm,**penetrates VIA pep46 that deforms membranes and induces pores, segments A & B encode for 5-6 proteins.
5. Mature virions buds out from the infected cell.
6. Virions stable over a wide pH range and 60 C° for 1 hour, resistant to ether and chloroform.

Classificatinc of *Birnaviridae*

Group III dsRNA

Family: *Birnaviridae*

Genus 1: *Aquabirnavirus*; type species: *Infectious pancreatic necrosis virus* infects salmonids (fish).

Genus 2: *Avibirnavirus;* type species: *Infectious busal disease virus* (IBD-1) causes Infectious busal disease/Gumboro disease.

Genus 3: *Blosnavirus*; type species: *Blotched snakehead virus.*

Genus 4: *Entomobirnavirus*; type species: *Drosophila X vrus*- infect insects.

Two serotypes of IBDV **serotypes 1 & 2, serotype 2 infects chickens and turkeys but does not cause clinical disease or immunosuppression,** but IBDV **1 viruses cause clinical disease in poultry. There exist six antigenic subtypes of IBDV serotype 1,** these antigenic subtypes called **variants, 3 subtypes** Classical IBDV, subclinical IBDV & very virulent vvIBDV exist, latter with **mortality in chicken up to > 70%.**

Group IV (+) ss RNA virus families

Family 11: *Picornaviridae*

(L. pico= very small; rna = ribonucleic acid)

General characteristics

1. Non-enveloped, very small (+) ssRNA viruses measuring 27-30 nm in diameter.

2. Capsid icosahedral symmetry of 60 capsomers made of 4 proteins, **VP1, VP2, VP3, & VP4.**
3. Genome is unsegmented, linear, (+) ssRNA of 7.1-8.9 kb, the genome naked + ssRNA is tightly packed into the capsid, the 3′ end with shorter UTR important in (-) strand synthesis & is polyadenylated, 5′end has a protein **VPg instead of a cap, used as a primer for transcription by RNA polymerase, 5′ end also has Internal Ribosome Entry Site(IRES).**
4. Replicate in cytoplasm, RNA is infectious and serves as both as the genome and viral mRNA.
5. **Viruses are released through cell lysis except Hepatits A, non-lytic and creates a more persistent infection.**
6. Resistant to many organic solvents (ether, chloroform), individual members differ in their susceptibility to pH change.

Classification of *Picornaviridae*

Group IV ss (+) RNA

Order: *Picornavirales*

Family: *Picornaviridae*
Subfamily: *Picornavirinae*

Genus 1: *Enterovirus,* type species: *Poliovirus* (PV), others cause Swine vesicular disease by **(EV-B5)** & *Porcine enterovirus B causes* porcine enterovirus B infection.

Genus 2: *Rhinovirus,* type species: *Human rhinovirus A* (HRV-IA).

Genus 3: Cardiovirus , type species: *Encephalomyocarditis virus* (EMCV) causes Encephalomyocarditis in rodents.

Genus 4: *Aphthovirus,* type species: *Foot-and-mouth disease virus* (FMDV) causes Foot-and-mouth disease, *Equine rhinitis A virus* causes Equine rhinitis.

Genus 5: Hepatovirus, type species: *Hepatitis A virus* (HAV).

Genus 6: Teschovirus, type species: *Porcine teschovirus 1* (PTV-1) causes Teschen disease or Talfan disease in pigs.

Genus 7: *Parechovirus,* type species: *Human parechovirus* (HPeV).

Genus 8: *Erbovirus,* type species: *Equine rhinitis B virus* (ERBV).

Genus 9: *Kobuvirus,* type species: *Aichi virus* (AiV).

Genus 10: *Sapelovirus*, type species; *Porcine Sapelovirus* (PSV).

Genus 11: *Senecavirus*, type species: *Seneca valley virus* (SVV).

Genus 12: *Tremovirus*, type species: *Avian encephalomyelitis virus* (AEV) causes **Avian encephalomyelitis.**

Genus 13: Avihepatovirus: type species; *Duck hepatitis A virus* (DHAV) causes **Duck hepatitis A virus infection.**

Plant picornaviruses fall under the family *Secoviridae.*

Family 12 : *Caliciviridae*

(L. calyx= cup) are so named because these viruses contain cup like depressions on the surface of virions.

General characteristics

1. Non enveloped, small 27-40 nm in diameter, (+) ss RNA viruses.
2. Capsid has icoshedral symmetry (T= 3) with 180 capsomers.
3. Genome isunsegmented, linear +ssRNA of about 7.3 to 8.3 kb, 5′ end has a protein (VPg) covalently linked to genome, whereas 3′-end is polyadenylated.
4. The virus replicates in the cell cytoplasm, virion RNA is infectious and serves as both the genome and viral mRNA.
5. Virus particles are assembled and released by cell lysis.
6. Resistant to ether, chloroform and mild detergents and heat, sensitive to acid pH values.

Classification of *Caliciviridae*

Group IV (+) ssRNA

Order: Picornavirale

Family: *Caliciviridae*

Genus 1: *Vesivirus;* type species: *Vesicular exanthema of swine virus*-causes Vesicular exanthema of swine, *Feline calcivirus* (FCV) infection occurs in cats-kittens 2-6 month old.

Genus 2: *Lagovirus;* type species: *Rabbit hemorrhagic disease virus* causes Rabbit hemorrhagic disease, & European brown hare syndrome.

Genus 3: *Norovirus;* type species: *Norwalk virus.*

Genus 4: *Sappovirus;* type species: *Sapporo virus.*

Genus 5: *Nebovirus;* type species: *Newbury-1 virus, the single species under this genus, subtypes are* Bovine enteric calicivirus, Jena virus & Newbury agent 1. Genogroup III noroviruses(NoVsGIII) and neboviruses are associated with enteric disease in cattle.

Family 13 : *Togaviredae*

(L. toga= cloack or mantle)

General characteristics

1. Enveloped that is closely bound to capsid, 70 nm in diameter, (+) ssRNA viruses
2. Icosahedral capsid symmetry made of 240 monomers (T= 4).
3. Genome is linear, (+) ssRNA of 10-12 kbp, like mRNA, viral RNA 5′ end has cap & 3′ end a tail.
4. Of two genera, *Alpphavirus* & *Rubivirus*, **alphaviruses are arthropod-borne being transmitted by mosquitoes**, while the *Rubivirus* with sole member of *Rubellavirus* is non arthropod-borne.
5. Replication occurs in the cytoplasm of the host cell at the surface of ER.
6. Virus assemble at the endoplasmic reticulum, buds at the endoplasmic reticulum, then transported to the Golgi apparatus, and finally buds from the cell membrane acquiring the envelope.
7. The virus agglutinates goose and chick RBCs.
8. *Alphavirus,* in common with certain members of the *Flaviviridae, Reoviridae, Rhabdoviridae, Bunyaviridae* are termed Arboviruses indicating that they are arthropod- born.

Classification of *Togaviredae*

Group IV +ssRNA

Family: *Togaviridae*

Genus 1: *Alphavirus;* type species: *Sindbis virus* (SINV), other species include, **encephalitis group** like *Eastern equine encephalitis virus* (EEEV), *Western equine encephalitis virus* (WEEV), *Venezuelan equine encephalitis virus* (VEEV), & *Everglades virus (EVEV)*, cause Eastern, Western & Venezuelan equine encephalitis; **arthritis group** include-*Chikungunya virus* (CHIV), *Getah virus* (GETV), *Ross River virus* (RRV), *O'nyong'nyong virus* (ONNV), *Semliki forest virus* (SFV) & others.

Genus 2: *Rubivirus;* type species: *Rubella virus* (RUBV) is the sole species causing **Rubella, an exanthematous disease in humans** (German measles) in children and young adults.

Family 14 : Flaviviridae

(L. flavus= yellow) derived its name from Yellow fever virus.

General characteristics

1. Enveloped bearing peplomers, spherical or pleomorphic 40-60 nm in diameter, (+) ssRNA, a large group.
2. Icosahedral capsids 40-50 nm & consists of a single type of capsid protein.
3. Genome linear, (+) ssRNA 9.7-12 kb long, the virus5′ end has a cap or a genome-linked protein, VPg but hepaciviruses & pestiviruses members of this family are uncapped and encode an internal ribosome entry site. The 3′ end is not polyadenylated.
4. Virus replicates in the cell cytoplasm, uses the host cell's RNA dependant RNA polymerase to replicate.
5. Virus assembly occurs at the ER, then the virion buds at the endoplasmic reticulum, is transported to the Golgi apparatus, and then buds from the cell membrane.
6. Sensitive to heat, detergents & organic solvents.
7. Agglutinate goose red cells.

Classification of *Flaviviridae*

Group IV + ssRNA

Family: *Flaviviridae*

Genus 1; *Flavivirus;* type species; *Yellow fever virus* (YFV), others include: **tick-borne viruses:** *Kyasanur Forest disease virus* (KFDV), *Louping ill virus* (*LIV*), *Powassan virus* (POWV), &*Tick-borne encephalitis virus* (TBEV). **Mosquito-borne viruses:** *Dengue virus* (DENV), *Japanese encephalitis virus* (JEV), *Murray valley encephalitis virus* (MVEV), *St. Louis encephalitis virus* (SLEV), & *West Nile virus* (WNV).**Yellow fever group:** *Wesselsbron virus (WESSV)* & *Yellow fever virus* (YFV).

Genus 2: *Hepacivirus;* type species: *Hepatitis C virus*- the single member.

Genus 3: *Hepatitis G virus* -The GB agent and the hepatitis G virus (HGV).

Genus 4: *Pestivirus;* type species: *Bovine virus diarrhea virus,* others include classical *Swine fever virus* or hog cholera, & *Border disease virus*-contains viruses infecting non-human mammals.

Clinical infections in animals, Genus: *Flavivirus*-Tick-borne diseases-Louping ill, Mosquitoborne diseases-Japanese encephalitis, West Nile disease, Wesselsbrown disease, Israel turkey meningitis, Genus-*Pestivirus*-Border disease, Bovine virus diarrhea, & Classical swine fever.

Family 15: *Coronaviridae*

(L. corona= crown) club shaped peplomers imparting crown-like appearance to the virus.

General characters

1. Enveloped, large, pleomorphic (+) ssRNA viruses 75-160 nm in diameter; have club shaped peplomers projecting from the envelope imparting crown-like appearance to the virus. Toroviruses tubular nucleocapsid is disc or kidney-shaped or rod-shaped, 120-140 nm in diameter.
2. Viruses with coiled **helical nucleocapsid** structure, (+) ssRNA.
3. Genome is monopartite, + ssRNA 27-31kb long, **the largest among RNA virus genomes**. 5′ end capped & 3′ end is polyadenylated. Viral RNA is infectious & acts both as genome & as mRNA.
4. Four structural proteins are: M (EI)- transmembrane glycoprotein; S (E2) peplomer glycoprotein; N nucleoprotein, and in some coronaviruses HE (E3-hemagglutinin-esterase glycoprotein). **The large S (E2)** makes up the club shaped spike or projections, **binds to cellular receptors, causes membrane fusion, and induces the production of neutralizing antibodies**.
5. Replicate in cytoplasm in the rough endoplasmic reticulum and the Golgi.
6. Maturation and assembly occur in the rough endoplasmic reticulum and the Golgi, and virions are released by exocytosis.
7. Sensitive to heat, lipid solvents, some are stable at pH= 3.

Classification of *Coronaviridae*

Group: Group IV (+) ssRNA

Order: Nidovirales

Family: Coronaviridae

Subfamily: Coronavirinae

Genus1: *Alphacoronavirus*: Species: Group 1 coronaviruses include-*Canine coronavirus* (CCoV), *Felinecoronavirus* (FCoV), *Humancoronavirus* (HCoV229E),

Porcine epidermal diarrhea virus (PEDV) and *Transmissible gastroenteritis virus* (TGEV).

Genus 2: *Betacoronavirus*: Group 2 coronaviruses include- *Sars coronavirus* (SARS-CoV), Bovine *coronavirus* (BCoV), *Murine* hepatitis virus (MHV) and *Humancoronavirus* (HCoV-OC43).

Genus 3: *Gammacoronavirus*: Group 3 coronaviriruses- *Infectious bronchitis virus* (IBV), *Turkeycorona virus* (TCoV).

Subfamily: Torovirinae

Genus 1: Bafinivirus: White bream virus (fish nidoviruses).

Genus 2: *Torovirus* includes-*Bovine torovirus* (BToV-Breda), TS: *Equine torovirus* (EToV-Berne) & *Porcine torovirus* (PToV).

Clinical infections in animals, Genus: *Alphacoronavirus*- Canine coronavirus infection, Feline coronavirus infection/Feline infectious peritonitis, Transmissible gastroenteritis, Porcine epidermal diarrhea, Porcine hemagglutinating encephalomyelitis, Genus; *Betacoronavirus* – Bovine coronavirus infection, Genus- *Gammacoronavirus*-Infectious bronchitis, Turkey coronavirus infection, Genus-*Torovirus*- Bovine torovirus infection, Equine torovirus infection, & Porcine torovirus infection.

Family 16 : *Arteriviridae*

(Arteriviridae derived its name from the disease Equine arteritis)

General characteristics

1. Enveloped, small, spherical 40-60 nm in diameter, (+) ss RNA viruses.
2. Icosahedral symmetry & spherical shape.
3. Genome unsegmented, linear, (+) ssRNA of 12-16 kb long, 5′ end has a leader RNA (65-89 bp), also at the 5′ end of each subgenomic RNAs.
4. Replicate in cytoplasm of macrophages and endothelial cells.
5. Virus assembly & budding occurs at membranes of the ER, the intermediate compartments, and/or the Golgi complex, & new virions are released.
6. Sensitive to heat, low PH, lipid solvent, detergent treatment, UV irradiation and many disinfectants.

Classification of *Arteriviridae*

Group IV (+) ssRNA

Order: *Nidovirale*

Family : *Arteriviridae*

Genus: *Arterivirus;* type species: *Equine arteritis virus* (EAV), & other species are *Porcine reproductive and respiratory syndrome virus* (PRRSV), *Lactate dehdrogenase elevating virus* (LDV) of mice and *Simian haemorrhagic fever virus* (SHFV).

Clinical infections in animals, Genus: *Arterivirus*- Equine arteritis, Porcine respiratory & reproductive syndrome, Lactic dehydrogenase elevating virus infection, & Simian hemorrhagic fever.

Family 17 : *Astroviridae*

(G, aster= star) derived its name as they contain unique five- or six-pointed star-like surface structure under electron microscopy.

General characteristic

1. Non-enveloped small 28- 30 nm in diameter (+) ssRNA viruses.
2. Capsid has icoshedral symmetry.
3. Genome is non-segmented, linear, positive sense ssRNA of about 6.8-7.9 kb long; 5′ end of the RNA has no cap & 3′ end has polyadenylated tail.
4. Virus replicates in the cell cytoplasm, (-) ssRNA from the + genomic RNA, then new genomic RNA from (-) RNA. 5. Maturation of the capsid occurs by proteolytic cleavage & then the virus is released by cell lysis.
5. The viruses are resistant to low pH values, & heating at 60°C for 5 minutes.
6. Trypsin is required for cultivation on cell cultures.

Classification of *Astroviridae*

Group IV + ssRNA

Family: *Astroviridae*

Genus 1: *Mamastrovirus;* type species: *Human astrovirus* (HAstV); other species are; *Bovine astrovirus* (BAstV), *Feline astrovirus* (FAstV), *Ovine astrovirus* (OAstV), *Porcine astrovirus* (PAstV), *& Mink astrovirus* (MAstV).

Genus 2: *Avastrovirus;* type species: *Turkey astrovirus* (TAstV); other species are; *Chicken astrovirus* (CAstV), *& Duck astrovirus* (TAstV).

Clinical infections in animals, Genus: *Mamastrovirus* - Bovine astrovirus infection, Feline astrovirus infection, Porcine astrovirus infection, Genus: *Avastrovirus*-Chicken astrovirus infection, Duck astrovirus infection, Turkey astrovirus infection.

Group V (-) RNA virus families

Family 18 : *Orthomyxoviridae*

(G. orthos=straight; myxa= mucus) or classical mucous

General characteristics

1. Enveloped, spherical, elongated or pleomorphic 80-120 nm in diameter, segmented (-) ss viruses. Haemagglutinin (HA) -a trimer- is so called as it agglutinates certain species of RBCs, & neuraminidase (NA), a tetramer spikes project from the envelope.

2. Nucleocapsid has helical symmetry, nucleocapsid (RNA+N); nucleoproteins of different sizes occur with a loop at each end.

3. Genome is segmented (6-8 segments), linear, (-) ss RNA with total genome length of 12-15 kbp, each of the 8 segments is of different length, encodes 10 different polypeptides with different functions, segmented genome facilitate genetic reassortment. Genome sequence has terminal repeated sequences at both ends. 3 polymerase polypeptides, PB1, PB2 & PA are associated with each end of each segment.

4. Replication occurs in the the infected cytoplasm **involving nucleus for RNA replication.**
5. For virus release, eight RNA segments come to the site at plasma membrane, and the virus buds out.
6. Surface projections of glycoproteins spike or peplomers in *Influenzavirus A & B* are of two types: a haemagglutinin (H), responsible for virus attachment and envelope fusion, and a neuraminidase (N) capable of cleaving viral receptors & promoting both virus entry into cells & release from the infected cells.

Classification of *Orthomyxoviridae*

Group V (-) ssRNA

Family: *Orthomyxoviridae*

Genus 1: *Influenzavirus A*; type species: *Influenza A virus* - Infects humans, birds, pigs, horses, dogs, seals & whales. The current circulating serotypes in humans are- H1N1, H1N2 & H3N2; in birds are- H5N1, H7N2, H1N7, H7N3,

H13N6, H5N9, H11N6, H3N8, H9N2, H5N2, H4N8, H10N7, H2N2, H8N4, H14N5, H6N5, H12N5 and others; in pigs are H1N1(classic swine HlNl), avianlike HlNl, H1N2, H3N1, H3N2 (human- and avianlike H3N2), & H2N3; in horses are- H7N7 & H3N8, & in dogs is- H3N8, which is now endemic in birds, horses and dogs.

Genus 2: *Influenzavirus B*; type species: *Influenza B virus*- Infects humans & seal.

Genus 3: *Influenzavirus C*; type species: *Influenza C virus*- Infects humans & pigs.

Genus 4: *Isavirus*; type species:*Infectious salmon anemia virus*- Infects Atlantic salmons.

Genus 5: *Thogotovirus*; type species: *Thogoto virus* & other is *Dhori virus*- Infects mosquito & ticks & mammals including humans.

Clinical infections in animals, Genus: *Infuenzavirus A*- Avian influenza, Swine influenza, Equine influenza, Canine influenza, Genus: *Influenzavirus B* infection, Genus: *Influenzavirus* C infection, Genus: *Thogotovirus* infection.

Influenzavirus A viruses are grouped into subtypes on the basis of their H & N antigens. 16 H antigens & 9 N antigens are recognized. New subtypes of influenza A virus emerge periodically by two mechanisms; point mutation & genetic reassortment.

Point mutations: give rise to antigenic drift in which variation occurs within subtype.

Genetic reassortment: is a more complex process producing antigenic shift, resulting in the development of new subtypes. The frequency of genetic reassortment in birds & pigs can lead to the emergence of virulent influenza virus subtypes which are capable of infecting humans & and initiating pandemics. Many avian subtypes facilitating genetic reassortments with occasional transfer of avian subtypes to pigs where genetic reassortments involving avian & porcine subtypes result in periodic emergence of new virulent subtypes & occasional transfer to humans with pandemics.

Family 19 : *Paramyxoviridae*

(L. para= by the side of; myxa= mucus)

General characters

1. Enveloped, peplomer bearing, spherical or filamentous or pleomorphic 150-200 nm in diameter, (-) ss RNA viruses.

Fusion (F) proteins and **attachment proteins (H/HN/G)** form the spikes on the virion surface. **Matrix proteins (M)** lie inside the envelope & stabilize virus structure.

2. The helical nucleocapsid, nucleocapsid **core** is composed of the genomic RNA, nucleocapsid proteins (NP), phosphoproteins (P) and polymerase proteins.
3. Genome is non-segmented, linear (-) ssRNA 15-19 kb, 5'-end does not contain a covalently attached terminal protein, nor a cap & 3′ end has no poly A.
4. Replicate in the cytoplasm, (-) RNA transcribed into mRNAs, & a (+) RNA template is used to create (-) RNA.
5. Viruses bud from the cell membrane acquiring the envelope.
6. Genetically stable & does not exhibit recombination but some antigenic variation may occurs through mutation, Paramyxoviruses can cause cell-to-cell fusion creating large multinucleated cells called **syncytia**.

Classification of *Paramyxoviridae*

Group V (-)ss RNA

Order: *Mononegavirales*

Family: *Paramyxoviridae*

Subfamily 1: *Paramyxovirinae*

Genus 1: *Respirovirus;* type species: *Sendai virus* (SeV); others include *Human parainfluenza virus* (HPIV1, 3), *Bovine parainfluenza virus* (BPIV-3), *Simian virus* (SV-10) & some of the viruses of the common cold.

Genus 2: *Rubulavirus;* type species: *Mumps virus* (MuV); others include *Human parainfluenza viruses* (HPIV-2, 4), *Simian parainfluenza virus 5* (SPIV-5), *Menangle parainfluenza viruses, Tioman parainfluenza viruses, Tuhoko parainfluenza viruses1, 2 and 3.*

Genus 3: *Morbillivirus;* type species: *Measles virus* (MeV); others include *Rinderpest virus* (RPV), *Canine distemper virus* (CDV), *Phocine distemper virus* (PDV), *Peste Des Petits Ruminants virus* (PPRV).

Genus 4: *Henipavirus;* type species: *Hendra virus* (HeV); others include *Nipah virus* (NiV).

Genus 5: *Avulavirus:* type species: *Newcastle disease virus* (NDV/APMV-1).

Genus 6: TPMV-like parainfluenza viruses;type species: *Tupaia paramyxovirus.*

Subfamily 2: *Pneumovirinae*

Genus 1: *Pneumovirus;* type species *Human respiratory syncytial virus* (HRSV), others include *Bovine respiratory syncytial virus* (BRSV).

Genus 2: *Metapneumovirus;* type species *Avian metapneumovirus, Human metapneumovirus.*

Unassigned viruses

For de Lance virus, Nariva virus, Tupaia paamyxovirus, Salem virus, & j virus.

Clinical infections in animals, Genus: *Respirovirus-* Bovine parainfluenza, Genus: *Rubulavirus-*Porcine rubula virus infection, Genus: *Morbillivirus-*Canine distemper, Rinderpest, Peste des petits ruminants, Genus: *Henipavirus-*Hendra virus infection, Nipah virus infection; Genus: *Avulavirus*: Newcastle disease, Genus- *Pneumovirus-*Bovine respiratory syncytial virus infection, Genus: *Metapneumovirus-*Avian metapneumovirus infection.

Family 20 : *Rhabdoviridae*

(L. rhabdo= rod)

General characteristics

1. Enveloped, characteristic rod shaped & bullet-shaped in vertebrates, 180 nm long & 75 nm wide (-) ssRNA viruses, prominent **spikes, G** on the surface that hemagglutinates RBCs, & inner side is lined by the **matrix protein, M.**
2. Helical **nucleocapsid wound helically inside the core**, two non-structural proteins, L and NS are associated with the nucleocapsid and act as the viral polymerase.
3. Viral genome is unsegmented, linear, (-) ssRNA, about 11-15 kb in size, & do not have a 5' cap or a polyA tail.
4. Virus replication occurs in an Inclusion body within the cytoplasm/ in a portion of the cytoplasm which acts as a **virus 'factory'** and appears as a characteristic cytoplasmic inclusion body- **perinuclear Negri bodies.**
5. Virions are assembled around coiled nucleoprotein core, the ribonucleocapsid interacts with the matrix protein under the plasma

membrane M protein and buds from the plasma membrane, acquiring the M + G proteins.

6. Stable in the pH range of 5- 10, rapidly inactivated by heating at 56^0 C & sensitive to lipid solvents and UV light.

Classification of *Rhabdoviridae*

Group V (-)ssRNA

Order: *Mononegavirales*

Family: *Rhabdovirdae*

Genus 1: *Vesiculovirus;* type species: *Vesicular stomatitis Indiana virus* (VSIV)

Genus 2: *Lyssavirus;* type species: *Rabies virus*(RABV)

Genus 3: *Ephemerovirus;* type species: *Bovine ephemeral fever virus* (BEFV)

Genus 4: *Cytorhabdovirus;* type species: *Lettuce necrotic yellow virus* (LNYV)

Genus 5: *Nucleorhabdovirus;* type species: *Potato yellow dwarf virus* (PYDV)

Genus 6: *Novirhabdovirus;* type species: *Infectious haemapoietic virus* (IHV)

Clinical infections in animals: Genus *Vesiculovirus*- Vesicular stomatitis, Genus *Lyssavirus*-Rabies, Genus *Ephemerovirus*-Bovine ephemeral fever.

Family 21 : *Bornaviridae*

(Named after the town Borna in Germany where the disease was detected as a neurological diease of horses)

General characteristics

1. Enveloped, spherical 70 to 130 nm; an inner matrix protein layer beneath envelope, (-) ssRNA viruses.
2. Helical nucleocapsid; non-lytic, persistent, neurotropic virus.
3. Genome smallest unsegmented, linear (-) ssRNA made of 8.9 kb, encodes 6 proteins called, nucleoprotein N, Phosphoprotein P, Matrix protein M (beneath envelope), glycoprotein G (spike), & Polymerase L.
4. Replicates in nuclei of neural cells- (others *Mononegavirale* replicate in cytoplasm).
5. Nucleocapsid interacts with the matrix protein under the plasma membrane M protein and buds from the plasma membrane, releasing the virion.
6. Sensitive to heat, lipid solvents and low pH values.

Classification of *Bornaviridae*

Group V (-) ss RNA

Order: *Mononegavirales*

Family: *Bornaviridae*

Genus: *Bornavirus;* Type species: *Borna disease virus* causing Bonra disease, an infection of the CNS, fatal in many domestic species, particularly horses. Antibodies reacting with BDV have been found in the sera of human patient with psychiatric disorders and there exists a possible link between infection with the virus and human neurological disorders.

Family 22 : *Filoviridae*
(L. filum= thread-like)
General characteristics

1. Enveloped, pleomorphic-long or **branched or short filaments shaped like a "6", a "U", or a circle measuring up to 14,000 nm in length with uniform** 80 nm diameter, (-) ssRNA viruses.
2. Nucleocapsid is **helical**
3. Genome has one molecule of linear (-) ssRNA, 18-19 kb in length; 3′ end not polyadenylated, & 5′ end is not capped. 4 structural proteins-envelope protein GP (spikes), nucleocapsid protin (NP) binds to the genomic RNA, Nucleocapsid protein VP30, Matrix protein VP40 , & polymerase complex protein (VP 35) & polymerase L.
4. Virus replication occurs in the cytoplasm.
5. The ribonucleocapsid interacts with the matrix protein under the plasma membrane, buds from the plasma membrane, releasing the virion.
6. Cause viral hemorrhagic fever characterised by coagulation abnormalities, Filoviruses are zoonotic & is transmitted to humans from life cycles in animals.
7. Viruses sensitive to heat, acid pH levels, lipid solvents.

Classification of *Filoviridae*

Group: Group V (-) ssRNA

Order: *Mononegavirales*

Family: *Filoviridae*

Genus 1: *Ebolavirus:* Species are *Zaire ebola virus* (ZEBOV), *Sudan ebolavirus* (SEBOV), *Reston ebolavirus* (REBOV), *Côte d'Ivoire ebolavirus* (CIEBOV) & *Bundibugyo ebolavirus.*

Genus 2: *Marburgvirus; Species: Lake Victoria marburgvirus.*

Family 23 : *Arenaviridae*

(L. arena= sand)

1. Enveloped, pleomorphic, spherical 120 nm in diameter with club-shaped surface projections, (-) ssRNA viruses, sandy appearance due to acquired host cell ribosomes.
2. Nucleocapsid structure is helical.
3. Genome (-) ss RNA viruses with **two RNA segments, large L** 7.5 kb & **short** S 3.5 kb.
4. Each arenavirus maintained with a particular rodent causing subclinical, life-long persistent infections with continuous excretion of virus in saliva, urine and feces, a source of inection to humans.
5. The virus replication occurs in the cell cytoplasm & is complex.
6. The ribonucleocapsid interacts with the Z protein beneath the plasma membrane and buds, releasing the virion.

Classification of *Arenaviridae*

Group V (-) ssRNA

Family: *Arenaviridae*

Genus: *Arenavirus*

Group 1: LCMV-Lassa virus (Old World) complex:

Ippy virus, Lassa virus, Lujo virus, Lymphocytic choriomeningitis virus-TS, Mobala virus & Mopeia virus.

Group 2: Tacaribe virus (New World) complex:

Amapari virus, Chapare virus, Flexal virus, Guanarito virus, Junin virus, Latino virus, Machupo virus, Oliveros virus, Paraná virus, Pichinde virus, Pirital virus, Sabia virus, Tacaribe virus, Tamiami virus & Whitewater Arroyo virus.

None of these viruses is pathogenic for domestic animals.

Family 24 : Bunyaviridae

(Bunyamwera, a place in Uganda where the type species Bynyamwera virus was first isolated).

General characteristics

1. Enveloped, spherical medium sized 80-120 nm, surface projections or spikes, (-) ss RNA viruses.
2. Nucleocapsids are elongated with helical symmetry.
3. Genome in **three segments** of linear (-) ssRNA- called Large L-6.8- 12 kb, Medium M 3.2- 4.9 kb, & Small S 1-3 kb with total genome 10.5- 22.7 kbp, or ambisense depending on the genus, terminal sequences of each segment are base-paired due to which, the RNAs form non-covalently closed circles.
4. Virus replication occurs in cytoplasm.
5. Sensitive to heat, acid pH levels, lipid solvents.
6. More than 300 viruses in the family most of them Arboviruses.

Classification of *Bunyaviridae*

Group V (-)ss RNA

Family: *Bunyaviridae*

The family *Bunyaviridae* contains 6 genera:

1. Genus *Hantavirus;* type species: *Hantaan virus:* Diseases Hantanvirus pulmonary syndrome, Korean hemorrhagic fever.
2. Genus *Nairovirus;* type species: *Dugbe virus.*
3. Genus *Orthobunyavirus;* type species: *Bunyamwera virus.*
4. Genus *Phlebovirus;* type species: *Rift valley fever virus.*
5. Genus *Tospovirus;* type species: **Tomato spoted wilt virus- plant virus**
6. Genus *Tenuivirus (unclassified)* plant viruses.

Clinical infections in animals: Genus: *Phlebovirus*- Rift Valley fever, Genus: *Nairovirus*- Nairobi sheep disease, Genus- *Orthobunyavirus*- Akabane disease, Cache valley virus infection.

Group VI (+) RNA virus families -reverse transcribing

Family 25: *Retroviridae*

(L. retro = reverse) viruses contain reverse transcriptase that transcribes DNA from viral RNA template.

General characters

1. Enveloped, labile carrying glycoprotein peplomers, & measure 80-100 nm in diameter RNA-RT viruses, 3 layers-(a) inner **nucleoprotein** containing ++ viral RNA, reverse transcriptase, protease, integrase with helical nucleocapsid, (b) **icosahedral capsid**, (c) **envelope** carrying glycoprotein peplomers.
2. Capsid has icosahedral capsid.
3. Genome is ss (++) RNA duplex, 2 linear RNAs arranged as inverted dimer, each 7-11kb in size with 5′end cap & 3′end poly A, 5′end has long terminal repeats (LTR) & 3′LTR are noncoding regions have promoter & enhancer but are important in replication; host RNA polymerase II converts ssRNA to ds DNA, which is incorporated into the host's genome as a **provirus.**
4. Retroviral common major genes (*gag*, pro, *pol* & *env* genes) encode structural proteins, genes that encode regulatory proteins & control virus expression (*tat, rev & nef* genes), genes that encode virion maturation (*vif & vru*), & genes that encode transcriptional activator proteins (*vpr*).
5. Retrovirus has many copies of RT (DNA polymerase) > after infection, uncoating, release of virion RNA in cell cytoplasm > RT makes viral DNA from viral RNA> cViral DNA strand > ds viral DNA transported to nucleus, inserted into the host-cell chromosome > host-cell RNA polymerase make virus-related RNAs serving as templates for new copies of the viral chromosomal RNA and also as mRNA. The mRNA is translated into viral proteins used to make the virus envelope > new virions assembled & bud from the PM & released.
6. Mutation and recombination occur with high frequency.

Classification of *Retroviridae*

The family contains 7 genera.

Group VI ssRNA-RT

Sufamily 1: *Orthoretrovirinae*

G1: *Alpharetrovirus;* type species: *Avian leukosis virus* (ALV), others are: *Rous sarcoma virus,* (RSV), *Avian carcinoma Mill Hill virus* (ACMHV), & *Avian myeloblastosis virus* (AMV).

G2: *Betaretrovirus;* type species: *Mouse mammary tumor virus* (MMV), *Mason-Pfizer monkey virus* (MFMV) *& Jaagsiekte sheep retrovirus* (JSRV).

G3: *Gammaretrovirus;* type species: *Murine leukemia virus* (MLV), *Feline leukemia virus* (FeLV) *& Porcine Type C oncovirus* (PCOV), *& Reticuloendotheliosis virus* (REV).

G4: *Deltaretrovirus;*type species: *Bovine leukemia virus* (BLV) & *Primate T-lymphotropic virus* (HTLV1, 2, 3).

G5: *Epsilonretrovirus;*type species: It comprises fish tumor viruses-*Walleye dermal sarcoma virus* (WDSV).

(Retroviruses of G1-G5 are called oncogenic retroviruses because they induce neoplastic transformation of cells).

G6: *Lentivirus;* type species: *Human immunodeficiency virus* (HIV-1, 2), *Bovine immunodeficiency virus* (BIV), *Feline immunodeficiency virus* (FeIV), *Equine infectious anemia virus* (EIAV), *Simian immunodeficiency virus* (SIV), *Visna/maedi virus* (VISNA), & *Caprine arthritis encephalitic virus* (CAEV).

Subfamily 2: Spumavirinae

G7: *Spumavirus;*type species: *Simian foamy virus,* contains viruses causing vacuolation of contaminating cultured cells but cause no classical symptoms e.g. *Bovine foamy virus, Feline foamy virus & Equine foamy virus.*

Clinical infections in animals: Genus: *Alpharetrovirus*- Avian leukosis, Ross sarcoma, Genus: *Betaretrovirus*-Jaagsiekte, Mouse mammary tumor, Genus: *Gammaretrovirus*-Feline leukemia, Genus: *Deltaretrovirus*- Bovine leukemia, Genus: *Lentivirus*- Bovine immunodeficiency, Equine infectious anemia, Feline immunodeficiency, Caprine arthritis –encephalitis, Visna-maedi.

Group VII DNA virus families-RT

Family 26 : *Hepadnaviridae*

(Hepar= liver, dna= DNA)

General characters

1. Enveloped, spherical virions with a diameter of about 42 nm DNA viruses-reverse transcribing.
2. Capsid is icosahedric capsid (T=4)
3. Hepadnaviruses genome consists of **two uneven strands of DNA (partially ds & partially ss DNA, circular). (-) DNA strand is complete** & are 3-3.3 kb in size. **(+) DNA strand is** incomplete, is made of 1.7-2.8 kb.

4. Hepadnaviruses replicate in the cell nucleus of hepatocytes, in the nucleus the partially double stranded DNA is 'repaired' by the cell to form acovalently closed complete circular DNA. (-) DNA strand acts as a template > forms +RNA strand (full length) > +RNA is packaged into the viral core in the infected cell cytoplasm > viral reverse transcriptase copies ss (-) viral DNA strand from ss (+) RNA > + ssRNA is degraded > viral DNA pol II forms (+) DNA from (-) DNA template >± ds DNA is packaged into virion before full length +DNA is synthesized, thus (+) DNA remains incomplete.
5. New virus particles acquire lipid from the endoplasmic reticulum of the host cell, and the genome is packaged within these particles, which then bud off from the cell.

Classification of *Hepadnaviridae*

Group VII-Reverse transcribing dsDNA

Family: *Hepdnaviridae*

Genus 1: *Orthohepadnavirus*, type species *Hepatitis B virus.* Other species within the genus include *Ground Squirrel hepatitis B* & *Woodchuck hepatitis B.*

Genus 2: *Avihepadnavirus*, type species: *Duck hepatitis virus.* Other species within the genus include *Heron hepatitis B virus* (HHBV), *Snow goose hepatitis B virus* (SGHBV), *Ross Goose hepatitis B virus* (RGHBV) and *Stork hepatitis B virus* (SHBV).

Hepadnaviruses infect humans-the important hepatitis B virus, herons, ducks, woodchucks, squirrels & recovered from other wild and domestic species such as geese, marsupials and orangutans. Hepadnaviruses are highly host specific & have a predilection for the liver and **produce persistent infections.**

Atypical Particles Associated with Infections

Defective viruses

Defective viruses are those virus particles that lack the full complement of genes necessary for a complete infectious cycle, and hence they need another virus to provide the missing functions; this second virus is called a helper virus. Defective viruses must provide the necessary signals for a polymerase to replicate their genome and for their genome to be packaged but need provide no more. Some defective viruses do more for themselves. Some retroviruses have picked up host cell sequences but have lost some viral functions. These need a closely related virus which retains these functions as a helper. Some defective viruses can use unrelated viruses as a helper. For example, hepatitis delta virus, an RNA virus does not code for its own envelope proteins but uses the envelope of hepatitis B virus, a DNA virus. Some viruses, during infection produce a greater quantity of defective virions than infectious virions. The production of defective particles is a characteristic of some virus species and is believed to moderate the severity of the infection/disease in *vivo*.

Pseudovirions

Pseudovirions are synthetic viruses used to inject genetic material, including DNA and RNA with specific and desired traits into bacterial and eukaryotic cells. Pseudoviruses are closely related to viruses in structure and behavior but lack many characteristics exhibited by true viruses, including the capability to replicate. Sometimes, pseudovirions are produced during viral replication when the host genome is fragmented. Consequently, host DNA fragments are incorporated into the capsid instead of viral DNA. In this way, pseudovirions possess the viral capsid to which antibodies may bind and facilitate attachment and penetration into a host cell, but fail to replicate once they enter the host cell because they lack essential viral genes needed for viral life cycle.

Prions

Although not viral, prions are proteinaceous infectious particles associated with transmissible spongiform encephalopathies (TSE) of humans and animals. **Prions,** collectively called **transmissible spongiform encephalopathies (TSE)** cause neurodegenerative diseases in humans & many animal species by forming aggregates extracellularly in CNS called **plaques or amyloid fibrils,** which disrupt the normal tissue structure, form holes or vacuoles in the neurons tissue giving spongy architecture, astrogliosis, absence of an inflammatory reaction & immune responses, very long incubation period (years), but after symptoms appear the disease progresses rapidly, leading to brain damage with clinical symptoms of behavioral or personality changes, weight loss, convulsion, dementia, ataxia and **death. Prion is used for several, unique group of neurodegenerative diseases, which induce spongiform degeneration in the grey matter of brain, & is fatal**. Prion diseases include **scrapie** of sheep & goat, **bovine spongiform encephalopathy (BSE), feline spongiform encephalopathy (FSE), transmissible mink encephalopathy** (TME), **chronic wasting disease (CWD)** of White-tailed deer, elk mule & **exotic ungulate encephalopathy (EUE)** of nyalaoryx, & greater kudu, & human diseases- **Kuru & Creutzfeldt Jacob disease.**

The name **Prion** was coined in **1982 by Stanley B. Prusiner from** proteinaceous infection particle. Prusiner was awarded the Noble Prize in Physiology or Medicine in 1997 for his research into prions. While the infectious agent was named prion, the specific protein that the prion was composed of is also known as the **Prion Protein (PrP)**, though this protein occur both in infectious and non-infectious forms. The protein that prions are made of (PrP) is found throughout the body, even in healthy people and animals. However, PrP found in infectious material has a different structure and is **resistant to proteases**, the enzymes in the body that can normally break down proteins. **The normal form of the protein** is called **PrP^{C}** (C refers to 'cellular' or 'common' PrP), while the infectious form is called **PrP^{Sc}** (*Sc* refers to **srapie**, a prion disease occurring in sheep. **PrP^{C}** is structurally well-defined but **PrP^{Sc}** is certainly polydspers and defined at a relatively poor level. PrP can be induced to fold into other more-or-less well-defined isoforms in vitro, and their relationship to the form(s) that are pathogenic in vivo is not yet clear. **All known prion diseases affect the structure of the brain or other neural tissue and all are currently untreatable and universally fatal.** Prions are propagated by **transmitting a misfolded protein state.** When a prion enters a healthy organism, it induces existing, properly-folded proteins to convert into the disease-associated, prion form; the **prion acts as a template to guide the misfolding of more protein into prion form.** These newly-formed prions can then go on to convert more prion proteins, thus triggers a chain reaction that produces large amounts of the prion form. **All known prions induce the formation of an amyloid fold,** in which the protein polymerises into an aggregate consisting of **tightly packed β sheets.** Prions and the TSEs of animals are discussed in detail in **Chapter 29.** At postmortem, the brain has large vacuoles in the cortex and cerebellum regions and hence prion diseases are called "spongiform encephalopatlues". Closer examination of brain tissue reveals the accumulation of prion-protein associated fibrils and amyloid plaques. These diseases are characterized by loss of motor control, dementia, paralysis, wasting and eventually death.

Viroids

Viroids are plant pathogens that consist of a short stretch-a few hundred nucleobases of highly complementary, single piece of circular, single-stranded RNA without the protein coat. The smallest discovered is a 220 nucleobase scRNA (small cytoplasmic RNA) associated with the rice yellow mottle sobemovirus (RYMV). In comparison, the genome of the smallest known viruses capable of causing an infection by themselves is around 2 kilobases in size. The human pathogen hepatitis D is similar to viroids. Viroids are naked, low-molecular weight nucleic acids that are extremely resistant to heat, ultraviolet, and ionizing radiation.

Viroids were discovered and given this name by Theodor Otto Diener, a plant pathologist at the Agricultural Research Service in Maryland, in 1971.

Viroid RNA does not code for any protein. The replication mechanism involves RNA polymerase II, an enzyme normally associated with synthesis of mRNA from DNA, which instead catalyzes "Rolling circle" synthesis of new RNA using the viroid's RNA as template. Some viroids are ribozyme, having catalytic properties which allow self-cleavage and ligation of unit-size genomes from larger replication intermediates. The first viroid to be identified was the Potato spindle tuber viroid (PSTVd). Some 33 species have been identified.

Virusoids

Virusoids (also called satellite RNAs) are circular single-stranded RNAs dependent on plant viruses for replication and encapsidation. The genome of virusoids consists of several hundred nucleotides and only encodes structural proteins. Virusoids are similar to viroids in size, structure and means of replication (rolling-circle replication). They depend on a helper virus for replication. Virusoids replicate in cytoplasm via a RNA dependent RNA polymerase. Virusoids, while being studied in virolog, are not considered as viruses but as **subviral particles**. Since they depend on helper viruses, they are classified as satellites. In the virological taxonomy they appear as Satellites/ Satellite nucleic acids/Subgroup 3: Circular satellite RNAs. The term *virusoid* is also sometimes used more generally to refer to all satellites.

Novel virus family - *Mimiviridae*

Mimiviridae is a family of viruses that contains one member, *Mimivirus*. The name *Mimivirus* is derived from "mimicking microbe". It was discovered in 1992 inside a protozoan and is the largest virus known to date, about 400 nm in diameter. The capsid is icosahedral in shape, the virion lacks an envelope, and has a circular dsDNA genome, which is 1.2 Mb in length and contains 1,260 genes. The *Mimivirus* genome sequence was published in 2004.

Table 1.1 : Important discoveries relating to medical and veterinary virology

Date	Discoverer (s)	Discovery (ies)
400 BCE	Hippocrates	father of medicine, important epidemiologic observations on many infectious diseases
1546	G Fracastoro	theory that epidemic diseases are contagious and disseminated by minute particles carried over long distances
1595-1660	S & H Jansen, R Hooke	development of the first compound microscopes and illumination system
1660	Lord Brouncker, C Wren, R Boyle, others	founding of the Royal Society

1668	A van Leeuwenhoek	invention of a simple microscope, observation of bacteria
1690-1907		major yellow fever epidemics in U.S. and throughout the Western hemisphere, recurring every few years
1735	C Linnaeus	development of the hierarchical classification (Classes, Orders, Genera, Species) of all organisms and the binomial nomenclature system
1762	C Bourgelat	founding of L'Ecole Nationale Vétérinaire de Lyon, the first veterinary school in the world
1765	J Morgan, B Franklin	founding of the first medical school in the United States (the University of Pennsylvania)
1765-1775	L Spallanzani	first experiments refuting the theory of the spontaneous generation and the first growth of bacteria in culture
1774	B Jesty	vaccination against smallpox using material from cowpox lesion
1793	B Rush	descriptive account of great yellow fever epidemic in Philadelphia, 1793 (during which he treated up to 120 patients per day), and account of what is considered the first case report on dengue fever (1789, case from 1780)
1796	E Jenner	application of cowpox virus for vaccination against smallpox
1798	U.S. Public Health Service	establishment of the U.S. Public Health Service [first as the Marine Hospital Service (1798-1902), then the Public Health and Marine Hospital Service (1902-1912), and finally as the Public Health Service (1912-present)]
1835-1870s	C Chevalier, J Purkinje, W His, C Minot, A Pfeiffer, others	development of the microtome, crucial to the development of cellular biology and cellular pathology
1835	M Schleiden, T Schwann, others	development of the concept that all organisms are composed of cells

1838>	J Snow, along with J Graunt, W Farr, L Villerme, P Panum, M Pruden, H Biggs, others	father of epidemiology
1840	F Henle	father of the germ theory, first substantial proposal that infectious agents are the cause of many diseases
1840s-1860s	I Semmelweis, O Holmes, J Lister	development of practical methods of hygiene and antimicrobial disinfection
1857>	L Pasteur	father of microbiology
1858	C Darwin	father of evolutionary science, development of the concepts of evolutionary progression, common descent, natural selection
1858-1867	R Virchow	father of pathology, founded the disciplines of cellular (microscopic) pathology and comparative pathology (comparison of diseases common to humans and animals)
1860s	W Henderson, R Paterson	discovery of the inclusion body of molluscum contagiosum virus
1863	A Bache, L Agassiz, B Peirce, B Gould, C Felton, J Henry	founding of the U.S. National Academy of Sciences
1863	C Davaine	first association of a specific infectious organism with a specific disease (*Bacillus anthracis*—anthrax)
1865	G Mendel	father of genetics
1868	J-F Meischer	discovery and characterization of nucleic acids
1868	J Law	father of modern veterinary medicine in the United States
1874	W Osler	father of modern medicine, physician, clinician, pathologist, teacher, diagnostician, bibliophile, historian, classicist, essayist, and author
1876	R Koch	with Pasteur, the founder of microbiology, first incontrovertible proof that a microorganism can cause disease (Bacillus anthracis—anthrax)

1878	L Pasteur, R Koch, others	popularization of the germ theory of disease
1879	S Chaille	father of hygiene and health education in the United States
1880	J Michels, American Association for the Advancement of Science	publication of the journal, *Science*
1880-1897	P Manson, C Laveran, R Ross, G Grassi	discovery of the protozoan etiologic agents of malaria, filariasis and trypanosomiasis, and their arthropod transmission cycles—keys to the discovery of the first human virus, yellow fever virus, and its transmission by mosquitoes
1883>	E Metchnikoff, J Bordet, P Ehrlich, Shiga Kiyoshi, E von Behring	founding of immunology, hematology and chemotherapy
1884	J Henle, R Koch, F Loeffler, C Chamberland	Henle-Koch postulates, criteria for proof of causation of disease
1884	C Chamberland	development of the Chamberland-Pasteur unglazed porcelain ultra-filter and the autoclave
1885	L Pasteur, E Roux	development of rabies vaccine
1886	A Mayer	development of the concept of transmissibility of tobacco mosaic disease and the earliest concept of filterable virus
1887	J Buist, E Cowdry	discovery of the elementary bodies of vaccinia and variola viruses
1887	J Kinyoun	establishment of the National Institute of Allergy and Infectious Diseases, first as the Laboratory of Hygiene of the Marine Hospital Service, then of the U.S. Public Health Service, and in 1955 as the National Institute of Allergy and Infectious Diseases of the National Institutes of Health
1888	Institut Pasteur	founding of the Institut Pasteur at 15 rue du Docteur-Roux, Paris
1888>	F Loeffler, P Roux, A Yersin, E von Behring	discovery of microbial toxins and antitoxins
1892	G Sternberg	discovery of virus neutralization (vaccinia virus)

1892	D Ivanovsky	discovery of tobacco mosaic virus
1893	T Smith, C Curtice, F Kilborne, D Salmon	the first proof of arthropod transmission of disease (agent: *Babesia bigemina*; tick vector: *Boophilus annulatus*) – a key to the discovery of the first human virus, yellow fever virus, and its transmission by mosquitoes
1893	G Sternberg	founding of Walter Reed Army Institute of Research
1895-1929	J Bordet, Bedson, J Bland	discovery of complement and development of the complement-fixation diagnostic test
1898	M Beijerinck [2]	discovery of tobacco mosaic virus
1898	F Loeffler, P Frosch [2]	discovery of foot-and-mouth disease virus (the first virus, the first vertebrate virus, the first picornavirus)
1898	G Sanarelli	discovery of myxoma virus (the first poxvirus)
1881-1898	C Finlay	initial experiments on the mode of transmission of yellow fever virus
1898	H Rose Carter	discovery of the extrinsic incubation period in the mosquito vector of yellow fever virus
1899	P Manson	father of tropical medicine
1899	W Sedgwick, W Welch, H Conn, T Smith, F Novy, E Jordan, E Smith, J Carroll, others	founding of the American Society for Microbiology (then the Society of American Bacteriologists)
1900	W Reed, J Carroll, A Agramonte, J Lazear, C Finlay	discovery of yellow fever virus (the first human virus, the first arbovirus, the first flavivirus) and its transmission cycle
1900	J M'Fadyean, T Edgington, A Theiler	discovery of African horse sickness virus (the first orbivirus)
1900	H. de Vries, C Correns, E von Tschermak	founding of genetics, and rediscovery of Mendel's work
1901	J Rockefeller, W Welch, T Prudden, L Holt, C Herter, H Biggs, T Smith, S Flexner	founding of the Rockefeller Institute for Medical Research (1901), Rockefeller Institute (1958), Rockefeller University (1958)
1901	E Centanni, E Savonuzzi, A Lode, J Gruber	discovery of fowl plague virus (avian influenza virus, the first orthomyxovirus)

1902	A Aujeszky	discovery of pseudorabies virus (the first herpesvirus)
1902	A Borrel	discovery of sheeppox virus
1902	M Nicolle, M Adil-Bey	discovery of rinderpest virus (the first morbillivirus)
1902-1906	J Spruell, A Theiler	discovery of bluetongue viruses
1903	M Dorset, E De Schweinitz	discovery of classical swine fever virus (hog cholera virus, the first pestivirus)
1903	A Negri	discovery of the rabies inclusion body—Negri body
1903	M Remlinger, Riffat-Bay, A di Vestea	discovery of rabies virus (the first rhabdovirus)
1903	A Tiselius	development of electrophoresis
1904	H Vallée, H Carré	discovery of equine infectious anemia virus (the first retrovirus)
1904	W Gorgas	control of yellow fever, allowing construction of the Panama Canal
1905	H Carré, P Laidlaw, G Dunkin	discovery of canine distemper virus
1906	P-L Simond, E Marchoux	first suggestion of transovarial transmission of a virus in its mosquito vector (yellow fever virus, *Aedes aegypti*)
1907	R Harrison	development of the first cell cultures (nerve fibers from frog embryo tissues)
1907	P Ashburn, C Craig	discovery of dengue viruses
1908	V Ellermann, O Bang	discovery of avian leukemia virus (the first leukemia virus)
1909	K Landsteiner, E Popper	discovery of poliovirus (the first enterovirus)
1909	C Levaditi, K Landsteiner	discovery of poliovirus in non-nervous system tissues
1909	R Doerr, K Franz, S Taussig	discovery of sandfly (phlebotomus) fever viruses (the first phleboviruses)
1910>	T Morgan	discovery of the nature and role of the chromosome, and the use of *Drosophila* in genetics research

1911	J Goldberger, J Anderson	discovery of measles virus
1911	P Rous, J Beard	discovery of Rous sarcoma virus (first solid tumor virus)
1911-1934	G von Hevesey, R Schoenheimer, D Rittenberg	development of radioisotopic labeling
1912>	A Carrel, M Burrows, W&M Lewis, H&M Maitland, C Levaditi, H Eagle, G Gey, T Puck, R Hamm, J Enders, T Weller, F Robbins, others	development of many cell and tissue culture methods
1913	E Steinhardt, C Israeli, R Lambert	cultivation of the first virus in tissue culture (vaccinia virus on pieces of rabbit cornea)
1913>	W Sawyer, T Rivers, F Horsfall, M Theiler, R Shope, others	founding of the Rockefeller Foundation (1913) and its international research programs
1914-1938	A Hess, Y Hiro, S Tasaka	discovery of rubella virus (the only rubivirus)
1915-2004	American Public Health Association	publication of the book, *Control of Communicable Diseases Manual*, to date 18 editions
1917-1919	F Twort, F d'Herelle	discovery of bacteriophages
1917	R Montgomery	discovery of Nairobi sheep disease virus (the first nairovirus, the first tick-borne virus)
1918-1919		influenza pandemic, 40-100 million deaths worldwide
1918-1952	A Breinl, J Cleland, E French	discovery of Murray Valley encephalitis virus
1919	A Löwenstein	discovery of herpes simplex virus
1920s	G Ramon	development of the use of formaldehyde to inactivate virus for vaccines and toxins for toxoids, the means for measuring vaccine potency, and the first adjuvants
1921	R Montgomery	discovery of African swine fever virus (the only asfarvirus)
1923	T Svedberg	development of the ultracentrifuge
1925	S Lewis	publication of the inspiring book, *Arrowsmith*

1925>	F Sabin	discoveries of the role of the monocyte and other white blood cells in defense against viral (and bacterial) infections
1925-1952	K Kundratitz, H Ruska, T Weller, M Stoddard	discovery of varicella-zoster virus – chickenpox and zoster
1926	W Cotton, P Olitsky, J Traum, H Schoening	discovery of vesicular stomatitis viruses
1926	F Kraneveld, T Doyle	discovery of Newcastle disease virus
1926	P de Kruif	publication of the book, *Microbe Hunters*, translated into 18 languages
1927	T Rivers	publication of paper differentiating bacteria from viruses, establishing virology as a field distinct from bacteriology, and the beginning of clinical virology
1928	W Sawyer, T Rivers, F Horsfall, M Theiler, R Shope, others	founding of the Rockefeller Foundation Virus Laboratory (RFVL)
1928	F Griffith	discovery of transformation in bacteria, a foundation of molecular genetics
1928>	R Lancefield, E Lennette, others	founding of viral disease diagnostics
1928	T Rivers (ed)	publication of the first major virology book, *Filterable Viruses*
1928	J Verge, N Christoforoni	discovery of feline panleukopenia virus (the first parvovirus)
1928	A Stokes, J Bauer, N Hudson, J Laigret	transmission of yellow fever virus to rhesus macaque
1929	S Nicolau, I Galloway	discovery of Borna virus (the only bornavirus)
1930	R Green, N Ziegler, others	discovery of infectious canine hepatitis virus (the first adenovirus)
1930	M Theiler, J Furth, C Armstrong	development of the mouse as an experimental animal for research on viruses
1930	K Meyer, C Haring, B Howitt	discovery of western equine encephalitis virus (the first alphavirus)
1931	W Elford, C Andrewes	use of graded collodion membranes to determine virion size

1931	R Shope	discovery of swine influenza virus (the first Influenzavirus)
1931	A Woodruff, E Goodpasture, M Burnet, H Cox	development of embryonated hen's eggs as host for viruses
1931	R Daubney, J Hudson, P Garnham	discovery of Rift Valley fever virus
1931	G Kärber	development of the Spearman-Kärber method for estimating fifty percent endpoints
1932	C Little, J Bittner, Staff of Jackson Memorial Laboratory	discovery of mouse mammary tumor virus (Bittner virus)
1932	F Gay, A Sabin, M Holden, W Wright	discovery of B virus
1933	W Smith, C Andrewes, P Laidlaw	discovery of human influenza viruses
1933	R Shope, P Rous, J Beard	discovery of rabbit papillomavirus (the first papillomavirus)
1933	E Ruska, M Knoll	invention of the electron microscope
1933	R Muckenfuss, C Armstrong, H McCordock, L Webster, G Fite	discovery of St. Louis encephalitis virus
	F Soper, H Penna, R Shannon, L Whitman, J Boshell-Manrique	discovery of the jungle cycle of yellow fever virus involving *Haemagogus* species in the Americas and as *Aedes* species in Africa
1933-1954	W Dimmock, P Edwards, E Doll, J Kintner	discovery of equid herpesvirus 1 (EHV-1; equine abortion virus) and equid herpesvirus 4 (EHV-4; equine rhinopneumonitis virus)
1934	C Johnson, E Goodpasture	discovery of mumps virus
1934	A Beckman	development of the electronic pH meter
1934	M Merrill, C Lacaillade, C Ten Broeck	discovery of eastern equine encephalitis virus
1934	M Hayashi, S Kasahara, R Kawamura, T Taniguchi	discovery of Japanese encephalitis virus
1935	W Stanley	purification and crystallization of tobacco mosaic virus
1935	M Theiler	development of yellow fever vaccine

1935	H Zinsser	publication of the inspiring book, *Rats, Lice and History*
1936	F Bawden, N Pirie	discovery that tobacco mosaic virus is comprised of nucleoprotein and that the nucleic acid is RNA
1936	J CuilleCuillé, P-L Chelle	transmission of scrapie to normal sheep by cell-free material from diseased sheep
1936	C Armstrong, T Rivers, E Traub	discovery of lymphocytic choriomeningitis virus (the first arenavirus)
1936	T Dobzhansky	publication of the book *Genetics and the Origin of Species*, seminal in the development of concepts in evolutionary genetics
1936	P Rous, J Beard	induction of carcinomas in other species by rabbit papillomavirus
1936	J Traum	discovery of vesicular exanthema virus of swine (the first calicivirus)
1937	F Beaudette, C Hudson	discovery of avian infectious bronchitis virus (the first coronavirus)
1937	M Theiler	demonstration of persistent CNS infection (Theiler's virus)
1937	T Rivers	criteria for proof of viral disease causation: the Henle-Koch postulates revisited
1937	L Zilber, M Chumakov, N Seitlenok, E Levkovich	discovery of tick-borne encephalitis virus (Russian spring summer encephalitis virus)
1937	E Wollman, E Wollman	discovery of the eclipse period in virus infection (bacteriophage)
1938	L Reed, H Muench	development of the Reed-Muench method for estimating fifty percent endpoints
1938	V Kubes, F Rios, C Beck, P Wyckoff	discovery of Venezuelan equine encephalitis virus
1938	R Doerr, C Hallauer (eds)	publication of the major virology book, *Handbuch der Virusforschung-erste Halfte*
1938	B von Borries, H Ruska, E Ruska	first electron micrograph of a virus (ectromelia virus)

1939	R Doerr, C Hallauer	first international virology journal, *Archiv für die gesamte Virusforschung* (now *Archives of Virology*)
1939	J Hillier, A Prebus	development of first electron microscope in North America at the University of Toronto
1940	K Smithburn, T Hughes, A Burke, J Paul	discovery of West Nile virus
1940	E Mayr	proposal of the widely used definition of species used in systematic
1940s	B McClintock	development of the concept of transposable elements, transposons
1941	G Hirst	discovery of virus hemagglutination, hemagglutination-inhibition, receptor destroying enzyme (neuraminidase) (influenza virus)
1941	N Gregg	discovery of rubella virus congenital abnormalities
1941	W Hammon, W Reeves, colleagues	quantitative study of natural history of arboviruses in vector arthropods (St. Louis encephalitis virus, *Culex tarsalis*)
1941	A Beckman	development of the spectrophotometer (the Beckman DU)
1941	T Anderson	discovery of the variety of bacteriophage morphologies and invention of critical point drying of specimens for electron microscopy
1942	C Huang	development of the quantitative virus neutralization assay (WEE virus and pH color change endpoint)
1942	J Mountain, others	founding of the U.S. Centers for Disease Control and Prevention, first as the Office of National Defense Malaria Control Activities (1942), then the Office of Malaria Control in War Areas (1942), then the Communicable Disease Center (1946), then the National Center for Disease Control (1967), then the Center for Disease Control (1970), then the Centers for Disease Control (1980), finally the Centers for Disease Control and Prevention (1992)

1942>	A Coons, colleagues	development of immunofluorescence
1943-1948	W Earle, K Sanford	development of the L cell line and clone L929 cell line (subcutaneous connective tissue, mouse; one of the first cell lines to be established in continuous culture; clone L929 was the first cloned cell line to be established)
1943	U.S. Army, Camp Detrick	development of military high-containment virology laboratories
1944	K Smithburn, A Haddow	discovery of Semliki Forest virus
1944	O Avery, C MacLeod, M McCarty	identification of DNA as the material of inheritance
1944	E Schrödinger	publication of seminal book, *What is Life?* – a motivation for many scientists, leading to the rise of molecular biology
1945-1953	M Delbrück, S Luria, A Hershey, S Benzer, G Stent	founding of the "Phage School" at the Cold Spring Harbor Laboratory, with "branches" at the California Institute of Technology and the University of California Berkeley
1945>	T Francis, G Hirst, F Davenport, T Eickhoff, G Meiklejohn, E Kilbourne	development of inactivated influenza vaccines
1945-1956	M Chumakov, G Courtois, colleagues	discovery of Crimean-Congo hemorrhagic fever virus (the first nairovirus)
1946	M Delbrück	discovery of genetic recombination (bacteriophage)
1946	K Smithburn, A Haddow, A Mahaffy	discovery of Bunyamwera virus (the first bunyavirus)
1946	J Steele	founder of the field of veterinary public health
1947	F Fenner	experimentation with ectromelia virus in mice and the beginning of viral pathogenesis research
1947-1955	M Burnet, A Gottschalk, E Klenk	discovery of virus receptors
1947-2007	C Clifton, S Raffel	publication of *Annual Review of Microbiology*, 60 volumes

1947	A Beckman	development of the Spinco Model E Analytical Ultracentrifuge
1947	Mettler Instruments AG	development of the first single-pan precision analytical balance
1948	World Health Organization	establishment of the World Health Organization
1948	G Dalldorf, G Sickles	discovery of Coxsackieviruses
1948	K Sanford	culture of single animal cells
1948-1965	T Rivers, F Horsfall, I Tamm	publication of book, *Viral and Rickettsial Infections of Man* (eventually four editions)
1948-1995	American Public Health Association, E Lennette, N Schmidt	publication of book, *Diagnostic Procedures for Virus and Rickettsial Diseases*, Seven Editions
1949	A Beckman	development of the Spinco Model L preparative ultracentrifuge
1949	J Enders, T Weller, F Robbins	development of cell culture methodology for polio, measles and other vaccines, neutralization of poliovirus with immune sera, and demonstration of attenuation of poliovirus neurovirulence with repetitive passage
1949	A Lwoff, L Siminovitch, N Kjeldgaard	discovery of lysogeny and induction (bacteriophage)
1950	L Florio, M Miller, E Mugrage	discovery of Colorado tick fever virus (the first coltivirus)
1950-1960s	M Delbrück, A Hershey, S Luria	discovery of mechanisms of virus replication and genetic variation
1950-1960s	C Mims	development of immunofluorescence in viral pathogenesis research
1951	G Gey	establishment of the HeLa cell line (human cervical adenocarcinoma; named for patient Henrietta Lacks)
1951	L Gross	discovery that murine leukemias and lymphomas caused by viruses are transmitted through the embryo
1951	E Lederberg	discovery of bacteriophage ë
1951	UNIVAC 1 and Ferranti Mark I	development of the first commercial electronic digital computers

1951-1960	L Pauling, J Kendrew, M Perutz	discovery of the structure of proteins using X-ray crystallography
1952	A Hershey, M Chase	biological proof of DNA as the material of inheritance
1952	W Stanley	establishment of the Virus Laboratory at the University of California Berkeley
1952	J Lederberg, N Zinder	discovery of transduction: transfer of genetic information between bacteria by viruses
1952	K Maramorosch	demonstration that some viruses can replicate in both plants and insects
1952	R Dulbecco	development of virus quantification by plaque assay
1953	W Rowe	discovery of human adenoviruses
1953	J Watson, F Crick, M Wilkins, R Franklin	discovery of the structure of DNA
1953	J Murphy, F Bang	discovery of virus release by budding at the cell surface
1953	N Ishida, N Kuroya	discovery of Sendai virus (parainfluenza virus 1)
1953	S Stewart, L Gross, B Eddy	discovery of polyoma virus (the first polyomavirus)
1953	W Plowright	discovery of bovine malignant catarrhal fever virus
1953	S Luria	publication of the major book, *General Virology*
1953	R Billingham, P Medawar, L Brent, F Fenner, M Burnet, R Owens	discovery of immunologic tolerance in virus infections
1953	K Smith	publication of the first major virology review series, *Advances in Virus Research*
1953-1959	A Sabin	discovery of orthoreoviruses (the first reoviruses)
1954	R Dulbecco, P Vogt	development of the concept of the "one-step virus growth curve," "latent period," "burst size," etc. (WEE virus)
1954	J Salk, J Youngner, T Francis	development of inactivated polio vaccine

1954	M Smith	discovery of murine cytomegalovirus
1954	B Sigurdsson	development of the concept of slow viruses (maedi-visna virus, scrapie prion)
1954	G Takatsy	development of microtiter plate technology
1955	G Hirst, L Black, S Luria	publication of the journal, *Virology*
1955-1962	W Joklik	seminal studies in viral genetics: recombination and reactivation (vaccinia virus)
1955>	F Brown	seminal studies on the chemical structure, replication, diagnosis and vaccinology of foot-and-mouth disease viruses
1955	R Taylor, T Hurlbut, T Work, J Kingston, T Frothingham	discovery of Sindbis virus
1955	M Minsky	development of confocal microscopy
1955	H Fraenkel-Conrat, R Williams	reconstitution of tobacco mosaic virus from its protein and nucleic acid
1955	S Benzer	definition of a gene (cis-trans test)
1955	W Schäfer	discovery that fowl plague virus is an influenza virus, and likely zoonotic
1956	J Morris, R Chanock, colleagues	discovery of respiratory syncytial virus (the first pneumovirus)
1956	W Pelon, W Mogabgab, W Price	discovery of human rhinoviruses and numerical nomenclature system
1956	C Friend	discovery of Friend murine erythroblastosis virus
1956	A Gierer, G Schramm, H Fraenkel-Conrat, B Singer	discovery of the infectivity of viral RNA (tobacco mosaic virus)
1956	S Madin, C York, D McKercher	discovery of infectious bovine rhinotracheitis virus
1956	R Ross	discovery of chikungunya virus
1956	R Chanock	discovery of human parainfluenza viruses
1956	M Smith, W Rowe, T Weller	discovery of human cytomegalovirus
1956>	W Plowright	development of rinderpest vaccine
1956	W Coulter	development of first high-throughput flow cytometer

1956-1966	C Hartsough, J Gorham, J Henson, R Leader, G Padgett, F Dixon	discovery of Aleutian disease of mink virus and its relationship to immunologically mediated glomerulonephritis and myeloma
1957	M Burnet, D Talmadge	discovery of clonal selection as the central mechanism in the immune response
1957	A Isaacs, J Lindenmann	discovery of interferons
1957	T Work, F Rodriguez, P Bhatt	discovery of Kyasanur Forest disease virus
1957	H Fraenkel-Conrat, R Williams	first in vitro assembly of a virus (tobacco mosaic virus)
1957	E Doll, J Bryans, W McCollum	discovery of equine arteritis virus (the first arterivirus)
1957	K Lee, J Gillespie, N Underdahl, others	discovery of bovine virus diarrhea virus
1957>	J Enders, M Hilleman, A Gershon, S Katz, S Plotkin, M Takahashi, others	development of vaccines against measles, mumps, rubella, Marek's disease, hepatitis A, hepatitis B, varicella-zoster, adenoviruses
1962>	R Webster	discovery of the link between avian and human influenza viruses and development of the concept that that pandemic virus strains arise via reassortment of genes of various human and non-human strains
1958	M Meselson, F Stahl	discovery of the semi-conservative mode of replication of DNA
1958	E Berger, J Melnick	publication of virology review series, *Progress in Medical Virology*
1958	R Kissling, R Goldwasser	development of rabies immunofluorescence diagnostics
1958>	A Parodi, D Greenway, H Rugiero, I Pirosky, J Zuccarini, E Molinelli, J Maizstegui, others	discovery of Junin virus, the etiologic agent of Argentine hemorrhagic fever, and development of an attenuated live-virus vaccine
1958	D Burkitt	description of Burkitt's lymphoma in African children
1958>	S Krugman	separation of two forms of hepatitis (HBV, HAV) in seminal studies of the natural history of viral hepatitis at the Willowbrook State School

1958	K Åström, E Richardson, J Cavanaugh, G Zu Rhein, B Padgett, D Walker, M Bouteille, L Horta-Barbosa	discovery of progressive multifocal leukoencephalopathy (JC, SV40 viruses – polyomaviruses)
1959	J Gowans	discovery of lymphocyte circulation
1959	A Sabin, H Cox, H Koprowski	development of attenuated live-virus polio vaccine
1959	L Kilham	discovery of murine parvoviruses
1959	S Brenner, R Horne	invention of negative stain electron microscopy
1959	R Porter, G Edelman, A Nisonoff	discovery of the structure and molecular function of antibodies
1959	R Sinsheimer	discovery that a virus may have a single stranded DNA genome (bacteriophage ØX174)
1959	R Yalow, S Berson	development of radioimmunoassays (RIAs)
1959	A Kornberg, S Ochoa	discovery of the mechanisms in the biological synthesis of DNA and RNA
1959- 1962	A Shubladze, K Chzhu-Shan, K Schneweis, W Dowdle	differentiation of herpes simplex viruses 1 and 2
1960	Digital Equipment Corporation	development of the first minicomputer
1960	B Sweet, M Hilleman	discovery of simian virus 40 (SV40)
1960	V Riley, K Rowson, colleagues	discovery of lactate-dehydrogenase elevating virus
1960	W Thompson, B Kalfayan, R Anslow	discovery of La Crosse virus
1960-1970s	G Palade, A Claude, K Porter, C de Duve	description of the fine structure and biochemistry of cellular organelles
1960-1970s	F Dixon, W Weigle, M Oldstone, J Feldman, J Vazquez, R Lerner, others	founding of immunopathology, and the role of viruses in immune complex diseases
1960s>	J Casals, D Clarke, R Shope, R Tesh, J Digoutte, O and C Causey, R Taylor, S Buckley, C Calisher, F Murphy, D Bishop, T Monath, J Dalrymple, B Beaty, C Schmaljohn, many others	discovery, serological grouping and characterization of many arthropod-borne alphaviruses, flaviviruses, bunyaviruses, rhabdoviruses and orbiviruses

1960s	C Mims, R Johnson, N Nathanson, R Blanden, B Fields, M Oldstone, A Haase, D Griffin, F Murphy, others	founding of the modern era of viral pathogenesis research
1960s	R Merrifield	development of solid phase synthesis technology (polypeptides, oligonucleotides, etc.)
1961	F Jacob, J Monod, A Lwoff, S Brenner, F Gros, M Meselson	discovery of messenger RNA, the operon theory, and genetic regulatory mechanisms for control of the synthesis of proteins
1961	J Miller	discovery of the role of the thymus in cellular immunity
1961	I Macpherson, M Stoker	development of BHK-21 cell line
1961	F Crick, S Brenner, J Griffith, L Orgel, L Barnett, R Watts-Tobin	discovery of the triplet coding of DNA (bacteriophage)
1961	U.S. Centers for Disease Control and Prevention	publication of CDC's Morbidity and Mortality Weekly Report (then U.S. Communicable Disease Center)
1961-1966	M Nirenberg, H Khorana, R Holley, S Ochoa, J Matthaei, colleagues	deciphering of the genetic code
1962	Y Yasumura, Y Kawakita	establishment of the Vero cell line (African green monkey kidney epithelial cell, named from "Verda Reno" meaning "green" and "truth" in Esperanto)
1962	A Chovnick, R Dulbecco, J Cairns, G Hirst, A Lwoff, H Rubin, M Stoker	Cold Spring Harbor Symposium on Quantitative Biology: *Basic Mechanisms in Animal Virus Biology*
1962	A Lwoff, R Horne, P Tournier	first comprehensive classification of the viruses based on virion characteristics
1962	L Kraft	discovery of mouse hepatitis virus (lethal intestinal virus of infant mice)
1962	D Caspar, A Klug	discovery of the principles of icosahedral virus structure
1962	P Gomatos, I Tamm	discovery of double-stranded RNA in a virus (reovirus)

1962	A Cosgrove, H Lasher	discovery of infectious bursal disease virus (the first birnavirus)
1962	F Rauscher	discovery of the first virus-induced lymphoid leukemia in mice
1962	J Trentin, Y Yabe, G Taylor	discovery of induction of tumors in hamsters by human adenoviruses
1963	W Downs, C Anderson, L Spence, others	discovery of Tacaribe virus
1964	M Epstein, B Achong, Y Barr	discovery of Epstein-Barr virus and its association with Burkitt's lymphoma
1964	W Jarrett	discovery of feline leukemia virus
1965	K Johnson, N Wiebenga, R McKenzie, P Webb, others	discovery of Machupo virus, the etiologic agent of Bolivian hemorrhagic fever
1965	J Casals, H Hoogstraal, K Johnson, A Shelokov, N Wiebenga, T Work	initial viral disease scientific exchange between U.S. and U.S.S.R. – on hemorrhagic fevers in Eurasia
1965	D Tyrrell, M Bynoe, J Almeida, D Hamre, J Procknow	discovery of human coronaviruses (B814 and 229E)
1965	M Bouteille, T Chen, L Horta-Barbosa, J Sever, others	discovery of subacute sclerosing panencephalitis (measles virus)
1965	R Atchison, J Melnick, colleagues	discovery of adeno-associated viruses
1965	R Valentine, H Pereria, E Norrby	discovery of adenovirus structural elements (penton fibers, etc.)
1965>	B Roizman	seminal studies of the molecular structure and replication and the cell biology of herpes simplex virus
1965-1978	S Kasakura, L Lowenstein, J Gordon, L Maclean, K Smith	discovery and characterization of the first interleukin,
IL-2		
1966	C Gajdusek, C Gibbs, W Hadlow, M Alpers	transmission of the etiologic agent of kuru (the kuru prion), to non-human primates
1966	National Library of Medicine	development of Medline
1966	P Wildy, F Fenner, R Matthews, others	founding of the International Committee on Nomenclature of Viruses (now the International Committee on Taxonomy of Viruses)[3]

1966	H Meyer, P Parkman	development of rubella vaccine
1966>	P Bhatt, R Jacoby, H Morse, A New, others	development of diagnostic virology of laboratory rodents
1966>	M Studdert	seminal studies of equine viruses (herpesviruses, rhinoviruses, others)
1967	B Blumberg, H Alter, A Prince, others	discovery of Australia antigen, hepatitis B virus and the etiology of post-transfusion hepatitis (the first hepadnavirus)
1967	J Kates, B McAuslan	discovery of DNA-dependent RNA polymerase in a virion (vaccinia virus)
1967	W Siegert, R Slenczka, G Martini, R Kissling, R Robinson, F Murphy, others	discovery of Marburg virus (the first filovirus)
1967	U.S. Centers for Disease Control and Prevention	development of civilian high-containment virology laboratories (then U.S. Communicable Disease Center)
1967	B van der Westhuizen, Y Inaba, Y Tanaka, colleagues	discovery of bovine ephemeral fever virus
1967	R Wagner, L Kozloff, N Salzman	publication of the journal, *Journal of Virology*
1967	C Kaplan, P Wildy	publication of the journal, *Journal of General Virology*
1967	J Maizel, U Laemmli	development of SDS polyacrylamide gel electrophoresis of proteins
1967-1969	A Churchhill, P Biggs, B Bermester	discovery of Marek's disease virus (herpesvirus) and development of vaccine
1968	M Ptashne, W Gilbert	identification of repressor genes (bacteriophage, lac operon)
1968	Congressman J Fogarty	founding of the John E. Fogarty International Center for Advanced Study in the Health Sciences at the National Institutes of Health
1968	J Kates, B McAuslan, A Shatkin, J Sipe	discovery of RNA-dependent RNA polymerase in a virion (reovirus)
1968	U.S. Advanced Research Projects Agency	development of the Internet
1968	W and G Henle	association of Epstein-Barr virus with mononucleosis

1968	L Hayflick	development of human diploid cell strains (WI-1 through WI-38)
1968	H-W Doerr	publication of virology review series, *Monographs in Virology*
1968	S Gard, C Hallauer, K Meyer	publication of virology review series, *Virology Monographs*
1968	P Wildy, J Melnick, N Oker-Blom, V Zhdanov	the First International Congress for Virology
1968	T Kelly, W Arber, H Smith, K Wilcox, D Nathans, K Danna	discovery and characterization of first restriction endonucleases, cleaving DNA only at specific sites
1968>	P Vogt, H Hanafusa, C Moscovici, W Okazaki, B Burmester, others	discoveries elaborating the molecular biology of avian retroviruses
1969	R Huebner, G Todaro	development of the viral oncogene hypothesis
1969	S Buckley, J Casals-Ariet	discovery of Lassa virus
1969	C Mebus, N Underdahl, M Rhodes, M Twiehaus	discovery of bovine rotavirus (the first rotavirus)
1969	M Crichton	publication of book, *The Andromeda Strain*, viral science fiction
1970	I Page, W McDermott, I Bennett, C Child, J Comroe, C MacLeod, J Murtaugh, D Wilbur, R Glaser, J Hogness, D Fredrickson, J Shannon, D Hamburg	founding of the Institute of Medicine (IOM) of the U.S. National Academy of Sciences
1970	D Baltimore, A Huang	discovery of RNA-dependent RNA polymerase in an enveloped RNA virion (vesicular stomatitis virus)
1970	H Temin, D Baltimore	discovery of the reverse transcriptase of retroviruses
1970-1973	W Plowright, R Tesh, D Watts	transovarial transmission of viruses by arthropods (African swine fever virus by ticks, vesicular stomatitis Indiana by sandflies and La Crosse virus by mosquitoes)
1970s	P Halonen, others	development of modern rapid clinical diagnostic methods

1970s	S Kalter, R Heberling	development of non-human primate virology
1970s1980s	G Hitchings, G Elion, R Whitley, L Corey, others	development of "rational" drug design" and the antiviral chemotherapeutic, acyclovir, for treatment of herpesvirus infections
1971	P Doherty, R Zinkernagel	discovery of how the cellular immune system recognizes virus-infected cells
1971	P Perlmann, E Engvall, A Schuurs, B van Weemen	invention of enzyme immunoassays—EIAs and ELISAs
1971	T Diener	discovery of viroids (infectious naked RNA molecules)
1971	D Baltimore	Baltimore system of virus classification based on replicative path to mRNA
1971-1982>	G Baer, M Abelseth, M Debbie, G Winkler, F Steck, A Wandeler, others	development of the concept, strategy and programs for oral vaccination of wildlife against rabies
1971>	B Achong, M Epstein, P Luciw, W Heneine, D Neumann-Haefelin, T Folks, others	discovery and characterization of simian foamy virus infection in humans
1971>	M Horzinek	seminal studies of veterinary viruses (bovine, equine, feline viruses)
1972	R Tomlinson	development of e-mail
1972	A Kapikian, colleagues	discovery of Norwalk virus (the first human calicivirus)
1972	P Berg, H Boyer	development of the first recombinant-DNA molecules
1973	S Cohen, H Boyer	development of the technology for manipulation of recombinant DNA molecules, the start of genetic engineering
1973	R Bishop, G Davidson, I Holmes, T Flewett, A Kapikian, others	discovery of human rotaviruses
1973	A Hellman, M Oxman, R Pollack	Asilomar conference and proceedings: *Biohazards in Biological Research*
1973	S Feinstone, A Kapikian, R Purcell	discovery of hepatitis A virus

1973	J Sambrook, colleagues	development of agarose gel electrophoresis of DNA and use of staining with ethidium bromide
1973	D Nathans	completion of the restriction enzyme map of a viral genome (SV40 virus)
1974	G Köhler, C Milstein	development of monoclonal antibodies
1974	F Blattner, P Leder, L Enquist, K Murray, T Maniatis, others	development of phage ë as a viral vector for recombinant DNA technology
1974	T Torsvik, I Dundas, A Wais, others	discovery of viruses of Archaea, many with exceptional morphologies
1974	H zur Hausen	discovery of the association between human papillomavirus infection and cervical cancer
1974-1982	I Tischer, H Gelderblom	discovery of porcine circovirus (the first circovirus)
1975	P Berg, D Baltimore, S Brenner, R Roblin III, M Singer	Asilomar *International Conference on Recombinant DNA Molecules, 1975*
1975	P Sharp, L Chow, R Roberts, T Broker	discovery of RNA splicing and split genes (adenovirus)
1975	Y Cossart, A Field, A Cant, D Widdows	discovery of parvovirus B-19 and its association with aplastic crisis in hemolytic anemia
1975	C Madeley, B Cosgrove, T Lee, J Kurtz	discovery of human astrovirus 1 (the first astrovirus)
1975	B Blumberg, B Larouze, W London, B Werner, J Hesser, I Millman, G Saimot, M Payet	discovery of the relationship of hepatitis B virus with hepatocellular carcinoma
1975	B Moss, A Shatkin	discovery that messenger RNA contains a specific nucleo-tide 5' cap for correct processing during translation (vaccinia, reovirus)
1975	E Southern	development of southern blotting
1976	K Johnson, P Webb, J Lange, F Murphy, S Pattyn, W Jacob, G Van der Groen, P Piot, E Bowen, G Platt, G Lloyd, A Baskerville, colleagues	discovery of Ebola virus

1976	J Bishop, H Varmus	discovery of the cellular origin of retroviral oncogenes
1976	A Evans	special criteria for proof of viral disease causation: the Henle-Koch postulates revisited again
1976	R Rott, C Scholtissek	development of the concept that an optimum constellation of genes determines pathogenicity (influenza viruses)
1976-1977	W Fiers, F Sanger colleagues	first complete sequencing of viral genomes (bacteriophages MS2 and Ö×174)
1977	D Henderson, F Fenner, I Arita, many others	global eradication of smallpox
1977	A Maxam, W Gilbert, F Sanger, colleagues	development of the technology for rapid sequencing of DNA (chain termination (dideoxy) method, and partial cleavage of end-labeled DNA method)
1977	M Rizzetto, J Gerin, M Canese, colleagues	discovery of hepatitis delta virus (the only deltavirus)
1977>	C Woese	recasting of *The Tree of Life*, phylogeny based on mRNA gene sequences
1978	H Lee, P Lee, K Johnson	discovery of Hantaan virus, the etiologic agent of hemorrhagic fever with renal syndrome, Korean hemorrhagic fever
1978	L Carmichael, M Appel	discovery of canine parvovirus (CPV-2)
1978	C Parrish	molecular characterization, structure and phylogeny of canine parvovirus
1978	D Botstein	discovery of restriction-fragment-length polymorphisms (RFLPs), yeast, bacteriophage, humans
1978	A Waterson, L Wilkinson	publication of the book, *An Introduction to the History of Virology*
1978	R Swanson, H Boyer	founding of Genentech, the first biotech company listed on the NY Stock Exchange
1978-1985	S Harrison, M Rossman, N Olson, R Kuhn, T Baker, J Hogle, M Chow, R Rueckert, J Johnson	determination of the atomic structure of a plant virus (tomato bushy stunt virus) and vertebrate viruses (poliovirus, rhinovirus)

1979	L Enquist, M Madden, P Schiop-Stanley, G Vande Woude	development of the technology for cloning viral DNA fragments into phage ë vector (herpes simplex virus)
1979	S Halstead	discovery of the role of immune enhancement in the pathogenesis of dengue hemorrhagic fever and dengue shock syndrome
1980	R Gallo, B Poiesz, M Yoshida, I Miyoshi, Y Hinuma, colleagues	discovery of human T lymphotropic viruses 1 and 2, the first unequivocal human cancer viruses to be identified
1980	E Williams, S Young	discovery that chronic wasting disease of deer and elk is a spongiform encephalopathy and caused by a prion
1980s	S Altman, T Cech	discovery of the catalytic properties of RNA, the ribozyme concept
1981	U.S. Centers for Disease Control and Prevention, Morbidity and Mortality Weekly Report (MMWR)	publication of reports of *Pneumocystis carinii* pneumonia in five previously healthy young men in Los Angeles, and an unusual number of cases of Kaposi sarcoma in gay men – AIDS
1981	V Racaniello, D Baltimore	development of the first infectious recombinant clone of an animal virus (poliovirus)
1981	G Binnig, H Rohrer	development of the scanning tunneling microscope
1981	D Wiley, J Skehel, I Wilson, others	discovery of structure of the influenza virus hemagglutinin
1981	G Stark, W Burnette, R Reiser, H Towbin	invention of western blotting – electrophoretic transfer of proteins from polyacrylamide gels to nitrocellulose sheets and detection with antibody
1981	W Joklik, H Ginsberg, others	founding of the American Society for Virology
1982	S Prusiner	development of the concept of the prion and the etiologic role of prions in spongiform encephalopathies
1982	W Goad	development of GenBank
1982	M Oldstone, Y Sinha, P Lampert, colleagues	development of the concept of virus-induced alterations in cellular homeostasis and luxury functions of infected cells

1982-1997	G Woode, D Reed, M Weiss, F Steck, M Horzinek, M Koopmans, R Glass, R Guerrant, colleagues	discovery of bovine, equine and human toroviruses
1983	F Barre-Sinoussi, J Chermann, L Montagnier, R Gallo, others	discovery of human immunodeficiency virus 1 (HIV1)
1983	M Balayan, colleagues	discovery of hepatitis E virus (the only hepevirus)
1983	M Carruthers, M Matteucci, M Hunkapiller, Applied Biosystems Inc	development of commercial DNA synthesizer technology
1983	A Murray, J Szostack	development of the yeast artificial chromosome – vector to clone large DNA fragments
1984	B Mahy, R Compans	publication of the journal, *Virus Research*
1984	M Hilleman, others, Merck Sharp & Dohme Inc	development of the first recombinant vaccine for humans (hepatitis B vaccine made in yeast)
1985	K Mullis, colleagues, Cetus, Perkin-Elmer	invention of the polymerase chain reaction (PCR)
1985>	B Fields, others	publication of *Fields Virology*, now five editions
1985	bioMérieux, Bio-Rad Genetic Systems, Abbott	development of the first FDA approved HIV antibody tests (EIAs)
1985	N Letvin, R Desrosiers	discovery of simian immunodeficiency virus
1985	F Barin, F Clavel, M Essex, P Kanki, F Brun-Vézinet, others	discovery of human immunodeficiency virus 2 (HIV2)
1985	A Jeffreys	development of DNA fingerprinting (detection of single nucleotide polymorphisms (SNPs) to identify genetic variation)
1985	C Richardson	discovery of bovine spongiform encephalopathy in the United Kingdom
1986	S Kit	development of the first recombinant DNA vaccine for animals (pseudorabies virus, TK-deletion mutant)

1986	R Gallo	discovery of human herpesvirus 6A
1986	N Pedersen, E Ho, M Brown, J Yamamoto	discovery of feline immunodeficiency virus
1987	M St. Clair, S Broder, H Mitsuya, M Fischl, D Richman, Burroughs Wellcome Co, others	development of the first anti-HIV drug approved by the FDA (AZT- zidovudine)
1987	L Hood, A Marion, S Eletr, Applied Biosystems Inc	development of commercial DNA sequencing technology
1987	M Capecchi, M Evans, O Smithies	development of knockout and other genetically manipulated mice
'1987>	M Estes	seminal studies of human gastroenteritis viruses (noroviruses, rotaviruses)
1988	C Lopez, P Pellett, K Yamanishi, T Kurata, colleagues	discovery of human herpesvirus 6B and its association with exanthem subitum
1988	National Library of Medicine	founding of the National Center for Biotechnology Information (NCBI) and the creation of public databases and systems for their use
1988>	M Eigen, C Biebricher, J Holland,E Domingo, E Koonin, A Gibbs, L Villarreal, J de la Torre, R Adino, S Weaver, others	development of modern concepts of the origin of viruses, virus evolution and quasispecies
1988>	A Osterhaus, colleagues	discovery of phocine distemper virus, marine mammal morbilliviruses
1989	M Houghton, Q-L Choo, G Kuo, D Bradley, H Alter, colleagues	discovery of hepatitis C virus
1989	T Brock	discovery of Taq polymerase
1989	S Fodor, I Herskowitz, M Schena, R Davies, P Brown, Affymax Research Institute	development of microarray technology
1989	M van Regenmortel	definition of virus species
1990	U.S. National Institutes of Health, U.S. Department of Energy, others	launching of the Human Genome Project

1990	N Frenkel	discovery of human herpesvirus 7
1991	T Berners-Lee	development of the World Wide Web (WWW)
1991	C Venter, H Smith, colleagues (TIGR)	invention of shotgun cloning methods
1991	G Reyes, J Kim, Genelabs Incorporated	development of SISPA (sequence-independent single primer amplification)
1991	R Salas, N de Manzione, R Tesh, R Rico-Hesse, R Shope, colleagues	discovery of Guanarito virus and its association with Venezuelan hemorrhagic fever
1992	J Smith, C Rupprecht, others	development of rabies genotyping and mapping geographi-c and temporal distribution of virus variants in support of wildlife rabies control programs
1992>	J Lederberg, S Morse, R Shope, S Oaks, M Hamburg, M Smolinski, others	development of the concept of *New, Emerging and Re-emerging Infectious Diseases,* the basis for rebuilding infectious disease research
1993	N Lisitsyn, N Lisitsyn, M Wigler	development of representational difference analysis (RDA)
1993	S Nichol, C Peters, P Rollin, T Ksiazek, colleagues	discovery of Sin Nombre virus and its association with hantavirus pulmonary syndrome
1993	S Falkow	molecular criteria for proof of viral disease causation: the Henle-Koch postulates revisited again
1994	Y Chang, P Moore	discovery of human herpesvirus 8—Kaposi sarcoma herpesvirus
1994	M Schnell, T Mebatsion, K-K Conzelmann	development of reverse genetics for negative-strand RNA viruses, infectious virus derived from cloned cDNA (rabies virus)
1994	T Lisieux Moraes Coimbra, E Nassar, F Pinheiro, A Travassos da Rosa, R Rico-Hesse, J LeDuc, P Jahrling, colleagues	discovery of Sabiá virus and its association with Brazilian hemorrhagic fever
1995	K Murray, P Hooper, A Hyatt, colleagues	discovery of Hendra virus and its reservoir host fruit bats

1995	R Preston	publication of the influential book, *The Hot Zone*
1996	R Will, J Ironside, J Collinge, colleagues	discovery that bovine spongiform encephalopathy prion is the cause of variant Creutzfeldt-Jakob disease in humans
1996	D Fredricks, D Relman	development of sequence-based identification of microbial pathogens: the Henle-Koch postulates revisited again
1996	M Hirsch, D Ho, T Merigan, S Hammer, others	development of HAART treatment for AIDS
1996	L Diatchenko, Y-F Luat, A Campbell, P Siebert, colleagues	development of suppression subtractive hybridization [SSH]
1997	National Center for Biotechnology Information	development of PubMed
1997	T Nishizawa, H Okamoto, colleagues	discovery of torque teno virus (TTV) (anellovirus) and its association with acute hepatitis
1998	A Fire, C Mello	discovery of RNA interference (RNAi, RNA silencing by dsRNA)
1998	L Page, S Brin	development of Google
1999	K Chua, S Lam, W Bellini, T Ksiazek, B Eaton, colleagues	discovery of Nipah virus
2001	B van den Hoogen, A Osterhaus, colleagues	discovery of human metapneumovirus
2001	International Human Genome Project: U.S. Department of Energy, U.S. National Institutes of Health, (F Collins, others; National Human Genome Research Institute (NHGRI), The Wellcome Trust), and Celera Genomics (C Venter, others)	completion and publication of draft version of the 2.9 billion base pair (bp) consensus sequence of the euchromatic portion of the human genome
2001>		anthrax bioterrorism events, beginnings of development of large-scale biodefense research and response programs

2002-2006	I Frazer, J Zhou, S-J Ghim, A Jenson, R Schlegel, R Kirnbauer, D Lowy, J Schiller, R Reichman, W Bonnez, R Rose, Sanofi Pasteur, Merck Sharp & Dohme, GlaxoSmithKline	development of papillomavirus vaccine (cervical cancer)
2002>	E Norrby	series of papers describing the awarding of the Nobel Prizes pertinent to virology
2003	C Urbani, J Peiris, S Lai, L Poon, G Drosten, K Stöhr, A Osterhaus, T Ksiazek, D Erdman, C Goldsmith, S Zaki, J DeRisi, many others	discovery of SARS coronavirus
2003	D Raoult, J-M Claverie	discovery of mimivirus, from amoebae, the largest virus known
2005	J Taubenberger, P Palese, T Tumpey, A Garcia-Sastre, others	1918 influenza virus genome sequenced and the virus reconstructed
2005	R Mahieux, A Gessain	discovery of human T lymphotropic viruses 3 and 4
2005	C Rice, F Chisari, T Wakita	manipulation of virus and cells for the first in vitro hepatitis C virus culture system
2005	J Rothberg, 454 Life Sciences	development of very rapid, very high throughput sequencing (pyrosequencing)
2005	European Centre for Disease Prevention & Control	founding of European Centre for Disease Prevention and Control (ECDC)
2006	T Allander	discovery of human bocavirus (parvovirus)
2008-2015	WHO Global Polio Eradication Initiative	planned global eradication of poliomyelitis

□□□

Chapter 2

Propagation, Purification & Enumeration of Viruses

Contents

Propagation of Viruses

As the viruses do not reproduce independently of living host cells, they cannot be cultured in the artificial media in the same way as bacteria and eukaryotic microorganisms. The cultivation of viruses can be done only in living systems, namely (i) cultivation of animal viruses in laboratory animals, (ii) cultivation of animal viruses in embryonated hosts, and (iii) cultivation of viruses in cell cultures. Viruses must be cultured on a living organism since they cannot reproduce independently.

Cell Culture

Currently cell culture is the most common way to study viruses. It is cheap & economical. Large quantities of virus can be harvested. Cells can be infected synchronously and viruses grown on a large scale, sterility is crucial (fungal or bacteria contamination) which can be easily obtained by adding suitable antibiotics & antifungal agents in the medium.

Types of Cell Culture

- A *primary culture* is defined as the original plating of cells directly obtained from a tissue & grown to a confluent monolayer, without subculturing. Primary culture is the stage of the culture after the cells are isolated from the tissue and proliferated under the appropriate conditions until they occupy all of the available substrate i.e., reach confluence.
- A *cell strain* is defined as a euploid population of cells subcultivated more than once in vitro, lacking the property of indefinite serial passage. If a subpopulation of a cell line is positively selected from the culture by cloning or some other method, this cell line becomes a cell strain. A cell strain often acquires additional genetic changes subsequent to the initiation of the parent line. Cell strains ultimately undergo degeneration and death, also called crisis or senescence.
- *Cell lines*- after the first subculture, the primary culture becomes known as a cell line or subclone. Cell lines derived from primary cultures have a limited life span, they are finite, and as they are passaged, cells with the highest growth capacity predominate, resulting in a degree of genotypic and phenotypic uniformity in the population. Spontaneous transformation or alteration of a cell strain to an immortal cell line can occur at any time during cultivation of the cell strain.
- *Diploid cell lines*-these maintain the dipolid number of chromosomes but can divide up to 100 times (usually from human embryos).

  Continuous cell lines-can be propagated indefinitely; are usually obtained from tumor viruses. Normal cells usually divide only a limited number of times before losing their ability to proliferate, which is a genetically determined event known as senescence; these cell lines are known as finite. However, some cell lines become immortal through a process called **transformation**, which can occur spontaneously or can be chemically or virally induced. When a finite cell line undergoes transformation and acquires the ability to divide indefinitely, it becomes a **continuous cell line**. There exists little resemblance to original cell, abnormal chromosomes (aneupolid), can be tumorigenic primary cell culture.
- *Organ culture*- in vitro culture & growth of organs or parts the organ in which their various tissue components, e.g. parenchyma & stroma, are

preserved both in terms of their structure & functions so that the culture organs resemble closely the concerned organs in vivo are called organ culture.

A Primary Cell Culture

Cell cultures can be cultivated as adherent cell cultures/ monolayer cell cultures or suspension cell cultures.

Primary cell culture is defined as a culture of cells obtained directly from the original tissue, e.g. rabbit, bovine, hamster kidney, chicken embryos & other sources that have been cultivated in vitro for the first time, and that have not been subcultured. Primary cultures contain a mixture of cell types, and they retain the closest resemblance to the tissue of origin. Primary cell cultures can be established from whole animal embryos, or from selected tissues from embryos, newborn animals, or adult animals of almost any species. The most commonly used cell cultures in virology derive from primates, including humans and monkeys; rodents, including hamsters, rats, mice, and birds, most notably chickens.

Pieces of tissue can be placed in growth media, and the cells that grow out are available for culture; this method is known as **explants culture.** Most primary cell cultures have limited lifespan, & after a certain number of population doublings, called the Hayflick limit, cells undergo the process of senescence and stop dividing, while generally retaining viability.

Preparation: Cells to be cultured are obtained by mincing tissue, and dispersing individual cells by treatment with proteases and/or collagenase/ trypsin to disrupt cell-cell interactions and interactions of cells with the extracellular matrix. With the exception of cells from the hemopoietic system, normal vertebrate cells will grow and divide only when attached to a solid surface. Dispersed cells are therefore placed in a plastic flask, tissue culture bottles, dish, the surface of which has been treated to promote cell attachment. The following antibiotics can be aseptically added to liter of media: Amphotericin-2.5 mg, Gentamycin- (50mg/ml solution)- 1.0 ml, Benzyl Penicillin 10000 units & Streptomycin-100 mg.

Cells can be grown either in suspension or adherent cultures. Some cells naturally live in suspension, without being attached to a surface, such as cells that exist in the bloodstream. There are also cell lines that have been modified to be able to survive in suspension cultures, so they can be grown to a higher density than adherent conditions would allow. Adherent cells require a surface, such as tissue culture plastic or microcarrier, which may be coated with extracellular matrix components to increase adhesion properties and provide other signals needed for growth and differentiation. Most cells derived from solid tissues are adherent. Another type of adherent culture is organotypic culture, which involves growing cells in a three-dimensional (3-D) environment as opposed to two-dimensional culture dishes. This 3D culture system is biochemically and physiologically more similar to *in vivo* tissue, but is technically challenging to maintain because of many factors (e.g. diffusion).

Cultivation: Cells are suspended & incubated in a growth medium, buffered nutrient medium in the presence of blood serum, which contains a complex mixture of hormones and factors required for the growth of normal cells. The blood serum may come from a variety or sources, but bovine serum is most commonly used. The cells grown and maintained at an appropriate temperature, gas mixture (typically, 37°C, 5% CO2 for mammalian cells) in a cell incubator, & in most cases added growth medium. Requirements for growth media can vary in pH, glucose concentration, growth factors, and the presence of other nutrients. The growth factors used to supplement media are often derived from animal blood, such as calf serum. One complication of these blood-derived ingredients is the potential for contamination of the culture with viruses or prion. Current practice is to minimize or eliminate the use of these ingredients wherever possible and use chemically defined media, but this cannot always be accomplished.

Alternative strategies involve sourcing the animal blood from countries with minimum BSE/TSE risk, such as Australia and New Zealand, and using purified nutrient concentrates derived from serum in place of whole animal serum for cell culture.

The cells will attach to the surface of the culture dish, and they will divide and migrate until the surface of the dish is covered with a single layer of cells, **a monolayer,** whereupon they will remain viable but cease to divide. If the cell monolayer is "wounded" by scraping cells from an isolated area, cells on the border of the wound will resume division and migration until the monolayer is reformed, whereupon cell division again ceases. Media changes in the case of adherent cultures are done by removing them directly by aspiration, and then they are replaced with fresh media.

These and other observations led to the conclusion that the arrest of division is observed when cells reach confluency that results from cell–cell contact, and it is therefore called **contact inhibition.**

Cell Strains

Starting with the establishment of a secondary culture and until cells either senesce or become transformed, the culture is termed a cell strain, to distinguish it from a primary culture on the one hand, or a transformed, immortal cell line, on the other hand.

- After a limited number of cell generations, usually 20 to 100 depending on the age and species of the original animal, cultured normal cells cease to divide and they degenerate and die, a phenomenon called **crisis or senescence.**
- During culture, cells in a strain retain their original karyotype and are thus called euploid; however, culturing induces profound changes in the composition and characteristics of the cell strain.
- Only a few cell types survive subculturing, so that by the second or third passage typically only one cell type remains in the cell strain.
- Cells in culture can be divided in to three basic categories based on their shape and appearance/ morphology. **Fibroblast-like** cells are bipolar or multipolar, have elongated shapes, and grow attached to a substrate. **Epithelial-like** cells are polygonal in shape with more regular dimensions, and grow attached to a substrate in discrete patches. **Lymphoblast-like** cells are spherical in shape and usually grown in suspension without attaching to a surface.

Two basic cell types, fibroblast-like (elongated, spindle shape) or epithelial-like(a polygonal shape) are shown below:

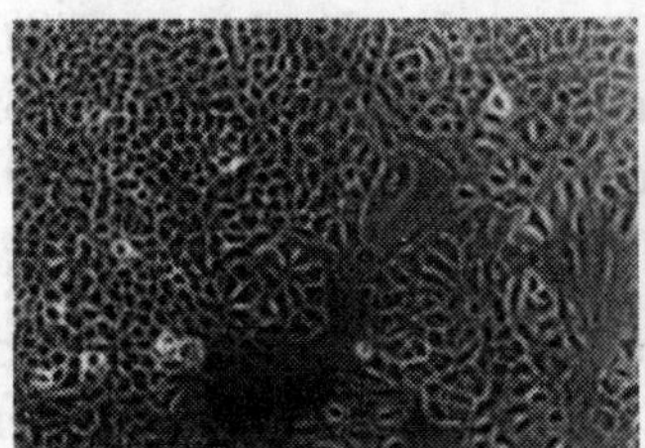

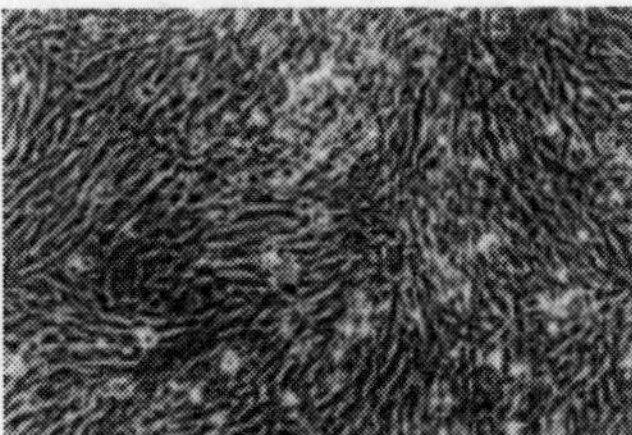

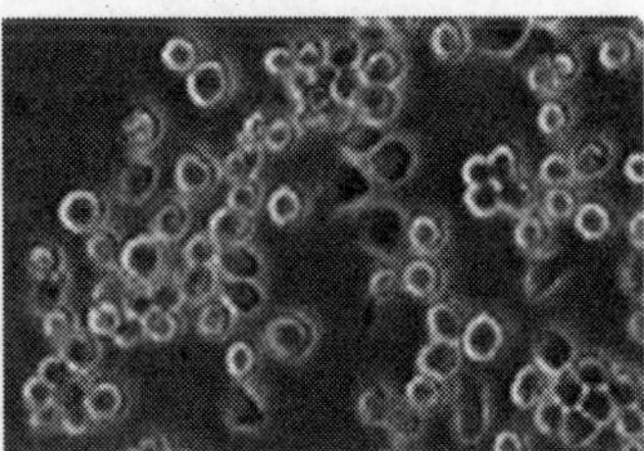

Figure 2.1: Epithelial like growth Fibroblast like growth Lymphoblast like growth

Cell Lines

An established or immortalized cell line has acquired the ability to proliferate indefinitely either through random mutation or deliberate modification, such as artificial expression of the telomerase gene. Numerous cell lines are well established as representative of particular cell types. At any time during the culture of a cell strain, cells in the culture may become transformed, meaning that they are no longer subject to crisis and senescence but can be passaged indefinitely. The monolayer cells are removed and washed with saline solution devoid of calcium and magnesium ions and then added to the dilute solution of EDTA (1: 3000) to chelate intracellular magnesium or calcium ions. After sometime, the loosened cells are shaken and resuspended in growth medium in fresh culture vessels and incubated. The cells are cultivated under 5% CO_2 condition. The cultures of cell obtained are called diploid cell strain. It is extremely difficult to distinguish primary cell and the diploid cell strain. On repeated subculturing, each cell starts multiplying to form separate colony. If each colony is removed and cultivated separately, it forms pure culture. These bunches of cells from single cell is called **clonal cell lines.**

- Immortalization can occur spontaneously during passage of a cell strain, or it can be induced by treatment with chemical mutagens, infection with tumorigenic viruses, or transfection with oncogenes. These immortal lines are usually derived from tumor tissue or by treating a primary cell culture or a diploid strain with a mutagenic chemical or a tumor virus.
- Immortalization is typically accompanied by genetic changes; such cells become aneuploid and not all cells in a culture of a continuous cell line necessarily display the same karyotype.
- Like cell strains, cell lines are usually composed of cells that are either fibroblast-like or epithelial-like in morphology.

Transformation

- Transformed cells are distinguished from normal cells by several properties, which can be grouped into three fundamental types of changes: **immortalization, aberrant growth control, and malignancy.**
- These characteristics of transformed cells are not interdependent. Transformed cell line that is immortalized but still contact- inhibited may be used in a viral transformation assay that measures the further transformation to loss of contact inhibition. When cells in a monolayer are transformed by a tumor virus and lose contact inhibition, they grow on top of a confluent monolayer forming a **focus**, a **heap** or a pile of cells, which is readily distinguishable from the rest of the monolayer.

Growth media for cell culture

Animal cells are more difficult to culture than microorganisms because they require several nutrients and grow only when attached to specially coated surfaces. Despite these difficulties, various types of animal cells, including both undifferentiated and differentiated ones, can be cultured successfully. Rich media are required for culture of animal cells. Nine amino acids referred to as the essential amino acids, cannot be synthesized by adult vertebrate animals and thus must be obtained from their diet. Animal cells grown in culture also must be supplied with these nine amino acids- histidine, isoleucine, leucine, lysine, methionine, phenylalanine, threonine, tryptophan, and valine.

In addition, most cultured cells require cysteine, glutamine, and tyrosine. In the intact animal, these three amino acids are synthesized by specialized cells; for example, liver cells make tyrosine from phenylalanine, and both liver and kidney cells can make glutamine. Animal cells both within the organism and in culture can synthesize the 8 remaining amino acids; thus these amino acids need not be present in the diet or culture medium. The other essential components of a medium for culturing animal cells are vitamins, which the cells cannot make at all or in adequate amounts; various salts; glucose; and *serum*, the noncellular part of the blood.

Serum-containing medium (Eagle's medium) contain essential amino acids- histidine, isoleucine, leucine, lysine, methionine, phenylalanine, threonine, tryptophan, and valine plus cysteine, glutamine, and tyrosine (all at 10^{-4} to 10^{-5} M). Vitamins choline, folic acid, nicotinamide, pantothenate, pyridoxal, and thiamine (all at 1 mg/L); inositol (2 mg/L); riboflavin (0.1 mg/L)SaltsNa$^+$, K$^+$, Ca^{2+}, Mg^{2+}, Cl$^-$, PO_4^{3-}, HCO_3^- glucose 0.9 g/L, & dialyzed serum 5 – 10% of total volume. Defined (serum-free) medium: Amino acids as above plus alanine and asparagine (10^{-4} M), vitamins, salts, glucose as above. Other additions: fatty acids-Linoleic acid, lipoic acid, Nitrogen compounds-Hypoxanthine, thymidine, putrescine, Carbon source-Pyruvate and glucose (0.9 g/L). Trace elements-Cadmium (Cd), manganese (Mn), molybdenum (Mo), nickel (Ni), tin (Sn), vanadium (V), hormones and growth factors, insulin, transferrin, hydrocortisone, fibroblast growth factor, & epidermal growth factor.

The Growth medium is a complete medium with growth supplements already added to Basal medium. Because it is ready for use, growth medium is the most popular cell culture medium requirement. Growth medium kit: for the growth medium kits include basal medium and growth supplements are packaged separately. The Kit format provides researchers the flexibility to adjust supplements as needed.

Basal medium : basal medium is a defined medium that contains essential and nonessential amino acids, vitamins, inorganic salts, organic compounds, and trace elements, but does not contain the growth supplements necessary for cell growth. Growth supplement: growth supplements include cell-specific growth factors, antibiotics, with or without serum. Each growth supplement is optimized for its specific cell type. When the growth supplements are added to the basal medium, it forms the growth medium. Subculture reagent kit: subculture reagents are specially formulated for use with cell applications adherent primary cells. We do not recommend the use of non-cell applications reagents for subculturing procedures. Components are available as a kit or individually:

- HBSS: Hanks Balanced Salt Solution
- Trypsin/EDTA
- Trypsin Neutralizing Solution

Cells are grown and maintained at an appropriate temperature and gas mixture (typically, 37°C, 5% CO_2) for mammalian cells in a cell incubator. Culture conditions vary widely for each cell type, and variation of conditions for a particular cell type can result in different phenotypes being expressed. Besides temperature and gas mixture, the most commonly varied factor in culture systems is the growth medium. Minimum Essential Media (MEM) is patterned after Eagle's Media and is well suited for the growth of mammalian cells. Dulbecco's Modified Eagle Medium (DMEM) is well supported for the growth of a spectrum of mammalian cell lines. RPMI 1640 is an enriched media formulation with extensive applications for mammalian cells. F-10 Nutrient mixture is formulated for the growth of CHO cells and various mammalian lines with serum supplementation. F-12 Nutrient mixture is formulated for single-cell plating of near-diploid CHO cells.

Plating density (number of cells per volume of culture medium) plays a critical role for some cell types. For example, a lower plating density makes granuloma cells exhibit estrogen production, while a higher plating density makes them appear as progesterone-producing theta lutein cells. Adjust concentration to 1- 10 cells / ml growth medium and dispense into tubes or bottles.

Manipulation of cultured cells

As cells generally continue to divide in culture, they generally grow to fill the available area or volume. This can generate several issues: nutrient depletion in the growth media, accumulation of apoptotic /necrotic (dead) cells, cell-to-cell contact can stimulate cell cycle arrest, causing cells to stop dividing, known as **contact inhibition**; cell-to-cell contact can stimulate cellular differentiation.

Among the common manipulations carried out on culture cells are media changes, passaging cells, and transfecting cells. These are generally performed using tissue culture methods that rely on sterile technique. Sterile technique aims to avoid contamination with bacteria, yeast, or other cell lines. Manipulations are typically carried out in a biosafety hood or laminar flow cabinet to exclude contaminating microorganisms. Antibiotics (e.g. penicillin and streptomycin) and antifungals (e.g. amphotericin B) can also be added to the growth media.

As cells undergo metabolic processes, acid is produced and the pH decreases. Often, a pH indicator is added to the medium to measure nutrient depletion.

Media changes

In the case of adherent cultures, the media can be removed directly by aspiration, and then is replaced.

Passaging cells

Passaging or subculture involves transferring a small number of cells into a new vessel. Cells can be cultured for a longer time if they are split regularly, as it avoids the senescence associated with prolonged high cell density. Suspension cultures are easily passaged with a small amount of culture containing a few cells diluted in a larger volume of fresh media. For adherent cultures, cells first need to be detached; this is commonly done with a mixture of trypsin-EDTA; however, other enzyme mixes are now available for this purpose. A small number of detached cells can then be used to seed a new culture.

Virus growth in cultured cells

The culture of viruses requires the culture of cells of mammalian origin as hosts for the growth and replication of the virus. Whole wild type viruses, recombinant viruses or viral products may be generated in cell types other than their natural hosts under the right conditions. After confluent growth of tissue cultures, the monolayrs are first infected with a virus, and then the culture is covered with a thin layer of agar. Viral infection causes cells to lyse, producing localized areas of cell death **(plaques)** that can be detected visually with dyes & counted. Viral infections usually do not always cause cell lysis, but instead may cause cells to undergo micro or macroscopic degenerative cellular changes called **cytopahic effects (CPE)**. Cytoathic effects are morphologic changes induced in individual cells or groups of cells by virus infection. Cytopathic effects may be lethal, but plaques do not always form.

Virus Detection and Titration

After a virus is propogated in either cell culture or in a suitable animal, we need to know the infectivity titre of the virus material obtained. This can be determined in vivo by inoculating increasing dilutions of the virus material to a susceptible host animal such as laboratory mice and based on mortality seen in different dilutions, the **infectivity titer which is the reciprocal of highest dilution showing 50% mortality in the inoculated mice and expressed as LD_{50}/ml** and can be calculated by using either **Reed-Muench or Karber formula.**

Microtitration of viruses

Most of the commonly encountered animal viruses produce characteristic cytopathic effect in one or the other cell lines routinely used in virology laboratories. The infectivity titres of these viruses can conveniently be determined by infecting a particular cell line with increasing dilutions of the virus material and determining the **highest dilution producing cytopathic effect in 50% of the inoculated cells**. The 50% end point dilution which in this case is expressed as $TCID_{50}$/ml can be calculated by using either Reed-Muench or Karber formula.

Calculation of 50% end points

In any biological quantitation, the most desirable endpoint is one representing a situation in which half of the inoculated animals or cells show the reaction (death in the case of animals and CPE in case of cells) and the other half do not. In other words, the endpoint is taken as the highest dilution of the biological material , which produces desired reaction in 50% of the animals or cells. The 50% endpoint can be based on several types of reactions. The most widely used endpoint, based on mortality, is the LD_{50} (50% lethal dose). This terminology can also be applied to other host systems-for example, tissue cultures - in which the $TCID_{50}$ represents the dose that gives rise to cytopathic effect in 50% of inoculated cultures. When computing, if closely-placed dilutions are used and in each dilution large number of animals or cells are used, it may be possible to interpolate a correct 50% end point dilution, but it is neither practical nor economical. Reed and Muench devised a simple method for estimation of 50% endpoints based on the large total number of animals, which gives the effect of using at the 2 critical dilutions between which the endpoint lies, larger groups of animals than were actually included in these dilutions.

Reed & Müench endpoint calculation method:

$$I = \frac{(\text{\% of wells infected at dilution above 50\% - 50\%})}{(\text{\% of wells infected at dilution above 50\% - \% of wells infected at dilution below})}$$

$$\text{50\% endpoint titer} = 10^{\text{log total dilution above 50\%} - (\text{I} \times \log h)}$$

I = Interpolated value of the 50% endpoint (also known as the proportional distance)h = dilution factor

Virus titration by using the plaque assay

To study and quantitate virus infectivity in the laboratory, animal viruses must be propagated in cells and cell lines. One very widely used assay is the **plaque assay**. This method relies upon (1) the use of confluent monolayers of cells which are susceptible to the virus, (2) the induction of a visible cytopathic effect by the virus (i.e., cell killing or cell damage) and (3) the use of a semisolid overlay (usually agar) which prevents virus diffusion from one infected cell to other nearby cells. As a result, small round plaques (clear areas) form in the cell monolayer as the virus replicates. These plaques can be visualized by staining the cells with a vital dye like crystal violet or neutral red. Prepare confluent monolayers of cells, prepare serial 10-fold dilutions (10^1 to 10^7) of virus in chilled maintenance medium (MEM, with 1% serum). Remove culture medium and add 0.2 ml of virus inoculum, starting from the highest dilution. Ensure that a film of medium completely covers the cell sheet. Incubate the plate at 37°C for 1 hour with intermittent rocking of the plate. Remove the inoculum, preferably with a pipette and then add 1.5 ml of agarose overlay medium (growth medium with 0.3% agarose and 2.5% FCS) & ensure that overlay medium has spread evenly over the monolayer, leave at room temperature for 10 mins and then incubate at 37°C. Examine the monolayers daily starting from second day of incubation. Once the plaques have developed, usually by the fourth day post inoculation, count the number of plaques at each dilution, remove the agarose overlay and gently wash the monolayer with PBS. Stain the plate with 0.1% crystal violet solution and count the plaques again. Estimate the virus titre as a plaque forming units per ml (pfu/ml) as follows by counting the number of plaques at an appropriate dilution.

For example :

Number of plaques produced 9

Dilution of virus 1×10^5

Volume of inoculum 0.2 ml

Virus titre $= 9 \times 1\text{x}10^5 \times 1/5$ pfu per ml

$= 4.5 \times 10^6$

Table 2-1 : Cytopathic effects producd by various viruses after growing in cell culture.

SN	Cytopathic effects produced by the viruses	Viruses
1	Nuclear shrinking (pyknosis), proliferation of membanes	Picornaviruses
2	Proliferation of nuclear membanes	Herpesviruse, alphaviruses
3	Vacuoles in cytoplasm	Polyomaviruses
4	Syncytia (cell fusion)	Paramyxoviruses, coronaviruses
5	Migration & breaking of chromosomes	Herpesviruses
6	Rounding up & detachment of cultured cells	Herpesviruses, rhabdoviruses, adenoviruses, picornaviruses

7	Inclusion bodies (virons) in nucleus	Adenoviruses
8	Inclusion bodies (virons) in cytoplasm (Negri bodies)	Rabies virus
9	Factories in cytoplasm (Guarnieri body)	Poxviruses
10	Clumps of ribsomes in the virion	arenaviruses
11	Clumps of chromatin in nucleus	herpesviruses

Hemagglutination assay

EM analysis can be used to directly visualize virus particles. Another method that has been widely used to measure virus particles is the **hemagglutination assay**. This assay takes advantage of the fact that many viruses contain proteins that can bind red blood cells (erythrocytes). Examples of viral proteins with the ability to bind to red blood cells include the influenza virus hemagglutinin (HA) protein, which binds to sialic acid residues on the cell surface. Normally, red blood cells will fall to the bottom of a culture well, forming a sharp dot. However, if viruses are present, the red cells become bound to the virus particles in a lattice or network (this happens because a single virus can bind multiple red blood cells). This lattice then coats the well. The assay is fast (30 minutes).

Viral enzyme assays

As noted previously, one can measure the activity of virally-encoded enzymes such as reverse transcriptase (retroviruses, hepatitis B virus) or viral proteases (encoded by many viruses, and used in protein maturation; these are useful because they have unique cleavage specificities that differ from those used by cellular proteases). Other unique viral enzymes may also be possible substrates for assay development.

Transformation assay

Other assays for virus infectivity include the **transformation assay**, which can be used to determine the titers or the biological activity of non-plaque forming viruses that have the ability to cause cellular growth transformation. Examples of such viruses include retroviruses (.e.g., the Rous sarcoma virus).

Virus neutralization

It is a method in which antibodies are added to a virus preparation, and the infectivity of this preparation is then measured using indicator cells. Typically, a subset of the antibodies produced against any given virus will have the ability to interfere with the interaction between the virus and its host cell receptor. Such antibodies will have the ability to neutralize the infectivity of the virus. Other antibodies may react with the virus, but may fail to prevent it from infecting its target cell. Such antibodies would not have neutralizing activity. Neutralization assays have been very useful in defining **viral serotypes**. For example, poliovirus serotypes were defined serologically, using neutralization assays (i.e., poliovirus type 1 is neutralized by antiserum to type 1 viruses, but not by antiserum to types 2 or 3, and so on). The definition of viral serotypes is a useful tool in terms of classification, and it is also of potential significance in the development of vaccines since one may need to include examples of all the virus serotypes in order to develop an effective vaccine. Thus, both the live-attenuated ("Sabin") and the whole-killed ("Salk") poliovirus vaccines contain mixtures of all three virus serotypes.

Immunostaining

This is a method in which antibodies are used to detect viral proteins in infected tissues or cells. Two basic methods are used. In direct immunostaining, the virus-specific antibody is directly labeled with an indicator molecule, so as to permit its visualization (the indicator molecule is usually either an enzyme such as horseradish peroxidase or a fluorescent molecule such as fluorescein). In indirect immunostaining, the virus-specific antibody is detected using a labeled secondary antibody directed against the first antibody (e.g., a labeled anti-mouse antibody if the initial antibody was a murine monoclonal antibody).

Immunoblotting and immunoprecipitation

These methods allow one to detect specific viral proteins in lysates from infected tissues or cells. In the case of immunoprecipitation, one typically remain pre-labels cells (and proteins) with radioactivity. The cells are then lysed, and the labeled proteins are precipitated out of solution using a specific antibody. The antibody: protein complex is then captured and purified, after which the bound protein is released, for analysis by SDS-polyacrylamide gel electrophoresis (SDS-PAGE). In immunoblot analysis, the proteins are not prelabeled with radioactivity. Instead, the whole cell extract is subjected to SDS-PAGE analysis, so as to separate out the proteins based on their size and other physical properties. The proteins are then transferred to a solid membrane support (often nitrocellulose), either by capillary action, pressure or by electrophoresis. Membranes can then be probed with specific antibodies, and the bound antibodies can be visualized using highly sensitive indicator molecules (for example, enzymes such as horseradish peroxidase).

Enzyme-linked immunosorbent assay (ELISA)

ELISA assays allow the detection of viral antigen or antibody, using a solid-phase assay system. For **antigen capture** ELISA (in which virus protein is measured), a solid matrix (plastic dish) is coated with a capture antibody specific for the viral protein of interest. The virus-containing test sample (e.g., supernatant from a virally-infected cell culture) is then added to the well. After allowing time for the protein to bind to the antibody, the well is washed and a second antibody is then added. This detection antibody is also specific for the virus protein being assayed, and it has an indicator molecule attached to it to allow for quantitative analysis of binding.

Antibody ELISA is a very similar method, except that in this case, one is measuring the amount of antibody directed against a specific virus protein in a sample of serum from an infected person or animal. In this case, the plastic dish is precoated with the virus protein. The antibody-containing test sample (serum) is then added. After incubation and washing, the bound antibody is detected using a secondary antibody that is usually directed against the constant region (Fc) of the specific antibody isotype of interest (most commonly, IgG).

Nucleic Acid Detection

Methods for the detection of viral nucleic acids in clinical and laboratory specimens include Southern blot analysis, in situ hybridization, polymerase chain reaction (PCR) and the use of gene arrays.

Southern blot analysis

It was developed in the 1970s, and it involves the fractionation of DNA with restriction enzymes, followed by transfer of DNA to a solid membrane support and detection of virus-specific sequences using radiolabeled viral nucleic acids.

Northern blot analysis is an analogous method for the detection of RNA sequences. Nucleic acid probes can also be used to detect viral sequences within tissues or individual cells, by using the method of **in situ hybridization.**

Polymerase chain reaction (PCR)

PCR is one of the most widely used methods for detection of viral nucleic acids. In this method, specific oligonucleotides are used to amplify fragments of viral nucleic acid from cell or tissue samples. The method uses a thermostable DNA polymerase, and multiple cycles of amplification, which comprise 3 steps – (1) melting of the double-stranded DNA template, (2) annealing of the oligonucleotide primers to the template and (3) extension of the primers by the thermostable DNA polymerase, thus generating new DNA chains. PCR analysis can also be adapted to the analysis of viral RNA, by including an initial step in which the RNA is converted into DNA, using a reverse transcriptase enzyme. This is referred to as reverse transcription (RT)-PCR.

Real-Time PCR

Methods for the quantitative analysis of nucleic acids using PCR include so-called "real time" PCR methods. This involves the direct measurement of the amount of PCR product produced while the reaction is in progress. Mathematical analysis of the data, and comparison to control reactions containing known amounts of template, allow one to then calculate the amount of input DNA in the initial reaction. Real-time PCR analysis is performed by taking advantage of a process known as fluorescence resonance energy transfer (FRET).

DNA Microassay

Finally, one powerful technology which is becoming increasingly useful in the analysis of viral infections is that of **DNA microarray** technology (aka gene chips). In this method, a high density DNA array is generated, comprising millions of different oligonucleotides spotted onto a solid support. Labeled sample DNA (usually biotinylated) is then added to this microarray, and allowed to anneal. After extensive washing, the bound sample DNA is detected using a fluorescent probe (e.g., streptavidin-phycoerythrin). DNA microarray can be used to probe for specific point mutations in the human genome (e.g., disease associated mutations, or mutations associated with enhanced susceptibility to certain viral infections). It can also be used to detect viruses, and even to detect specific mutations within virus populations – for example, mutations associated with resistance to antiviral drugs.

Other Applications of Cell Culture

It is possible to fuse normal cells with an immortalized cell line to produce monoclonal antibodies. This method is used to produce monoclonal antibodies. In brief, lymphocytes isolated from the spleen (or possibly blood) of an immunized animal are combined with an immortal myeloma cell line (B cell lineage) to produce a hybridoma which has the antibody specificity of the primary lymphoctye and the immortality of the myeloma. Selective growth medium (HA or HAT) is used to select against unfused myeloma cells; primary lymphoctyes die quickly in culture and only the fused cells survive. These are screened for production of the required antibody, generally in pools to start with and then after single cloning.

Cell culture is one of the major tools used in cellular and molecular biology, providing excellent model systems for studying the normal physiology and biochemistry of cells (e.g., metabolic studies, aging), the effects of drugs and toxic compounds on the cells, and mutagenesis and carcinogenesis. It is also used in drug screening and development, and large scale manufacturing of biological compounds, e.g., vaccines, diagnostic agents & therapeutic proteins. The major advantage of using cell culture for any of these applications is the consistency and reproducibility of results that can be obtained from using a batch of clonal cells. Mass culture of animal cell lines is fundamental to the manufacture of viral monoclonal antibodies (mAbs), vaccines and other products of biotechnology.

Biological products produced by recombinant DNA (rDNA) technology in animal cell cultures include enzymes, synthetic hormones, immunobiologicals e.g. mAbs, IL, lymphokines, and anticancer agents. Although many simpler proteins can be produced using rDNA in bacterial cultures, more complex proteins that are glycosylated (carbohydrate-modified) currently must be made in animal cells. An important example of such a complex protein is the hormone erythropoietin. Research in tissue engineering, stem cells and molecular bilogy primarily involves cultures of cells on flat plastic dishes.

Vaccines: Vaccine for polio, measles, mumps, rubella, chickenpox & several animal vaccines are currently made in cell cultures. Due to the H5N1 pandemics threat, research into using cell culture for influenza vaccines is being funded by the USA government. Novel ideas in the field include recombinant DNA-based vaccines, such as one made using human adenovirus (a common cold virus) as a vector, and novel adjuvants.

Human cell lines: include Hela, National cancer Institute's cancer 60 cell lines, ESTDBA database, DU1 45 (prostrate cancer), Incap (prostrate cancer), MCF-7 (breast cancer), MDA-MB-4 38 (breast cancer), PC3 (prostrate cancer), PC3 (prostrate cancer), T47D (breast cancer), TH-2 (acute myeloid leukemia), U87 (glioblastoma), SHSY5 Y Human neuroblastoma cells, cloned from a myeloma, sao-2 cells (bone cancer).

Primate cell lines : includes Vero (African green monkey Clorocebus kidney epithelial cell line initiated in 1962)

Rat tumor cell lines: include GH3 (pituitary cancer), PC12 (pheochromcytoma).

Mouse cell lines : MC3T 3 (embryonic calvarium)

Virus Cultivation in Embryonated Eggs

Prior to the advent of cell culture, animal viruses were propagated only on whole animals or embryonated chicken eggs. The developing chick embryo, 10 to 14 days after fertilization, provides a variety of differentiated tissues, including the amnion, allantois, chorion, and yolk sac, which serve as substrates for growth of a wide variety of viruses, including orthomyxoviruses, paramyxoviruses, rhabdoviruses, togaviruses, herpesviruses, and poxviruses. To prepare the egg for virus cultivation, the shell surface is first disinfected with iodine and penetrated with a small sterile drill. After inoculation, the drill hole is sealed with gelatin and the egg is then incubated. Viruses may be able to region. For convenience, the myxoma virus grows well on the chorioallantoic membrane, poxvirus forms pock on CAM, whereas the mumps virus prefers the allantoic cavity. The infection may produce a local tissue lesion known as pock, whose appearance often is characteristic of the virus. Inoculated eggs are observed for embryo death, embryo cell damage, formation of pocks / lesions on the membrane & for cytopathogenic effect (CPE) or plaques. Figure2-2 depicts the various routes of embryo inoculation for growth of different viruses.

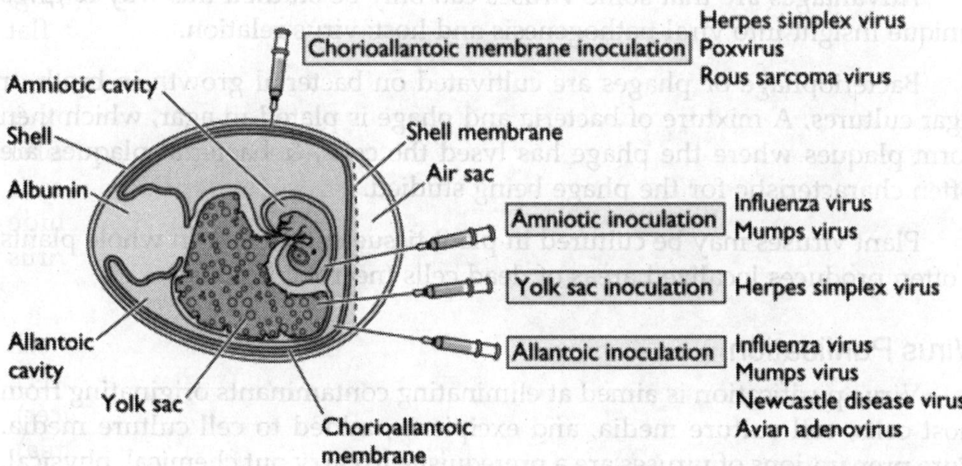

Figure 2.2 : Different routes of inoculation in embryonated eggs for virus cultivation.

Virus Growth in Laboratory Animals

Live animals such as mice, rabbits, guinea pigs & others are used for diagnostic purposes: observed for symptoms of disease & observed for tissue damage. Some viruses cannot be grown in animals. The problem of studying AIDS is slow growth of virus in humans & therefore vaccine trials take a very long to test. Simian AIDS (1986, infects green monkeys) & feline AIDS (1987, domestic cats) are HIV related virus & the disease develops within a few months, hence are good models to study growth of the virus in different tissues. Chimps can be infected with one sub-species of the AIDS virus, viz HIV-1 (genus lentivirus) but no symptoms are produced. Genetically engineered mice strains (containing genes for human T cells & human gammaglobin) developed in 1990 are susceptible to AIDS infection.

Laboratory animals are seldom used for routine cultivation of virus, but they still play an essential role in studies of viral pathogenesis. Suitable living mammals (such as sheep or calves or rabbits) are selected for cultivation of viruses. The selected animals must be healthy and free from any communicable diseases. The specific virus is introduced into the healthy animals. The site of administration varies according to the type of virus, & is allowed to grow in the living animal. At the end of incubation period, the animals are slaughtered and washed thoroughly and viruses are obtained from them.

There are problems in invivo cultivation because: it is inconvenient and expensive, it is not a defined system, leads to generation of escape mutants, & there is problem of animal welfare issues.

Advantages are that some viruses can only be studied this way & gives unique insight into viral pathogenesis and host: virus relation.

Bacteriophage or phages are cultivated on bacterial growth in broth or agar cultures, A mixture of bacteria and phage is plated in agar, which then form plaques where the phage has lysed the cells, & bacterial plaques are often characteristic for the phage being studied.

Plant viruses may be cultured in plant tissue cultures, & in whole plants - often produces localized areas of dead cells (necrotic lesions).

Virus Purification

Virus purification is aimed at eliminating contaminants originating from host cells, cell culture media, and excipients, added to cell culture media. Pure preparations of viruses are a prerequisite to carry out chemical, physical, and other biological studies of viruses. There are several procedures of virus purification that can be used to purify many of the viruses. There are several different purification systems that can be selected for use according to the type of virus. The other purpose of virus purification is to obtain highly concentrated viruses that are biologically active and highly efficient in target gene expression.The clarified extract obtained can be processed by many different methods to obtain the particles of the virus. Some of the methods used are the following:

Differential and gradient centrifugation

- Precipitation with ammonium sulfate
- Denaturation of cellular constituents
- Enzymatic degradation of cellular components

- Virus assays are used to quanitate the number of virions present
- Direct count using electron microscopy
- Hemagglutination assays - needs a standard assay to determine how many virions it takes to cause agglutination
- Gel filtration (agar, agarose, sephadex)
- Crystallization
- Isoelectric precipitation
- Electrophoresis
- Ion exchange chromatography
- Two-phase systems
- Ultracentrifugation
- Centrifugation through density gradient
- Serological methods
- Dry gels
- Microfilters

Plaque assay - determines numbers in terms of plaque foming units per volume

- Biological assays to determine disease or death-infectious dose (ID50), lethal dose – (ID50), respectively.

Gel filtration (agar, agarose, sephadex)

This process is also known as molecular sieve chromatography and is especially useful for those viruses that denature during high-speed centrifugation. The substance to be used as a molecular filter is packed in a column. The smallest molecules enter the gel, while the larger molecules are excluded and pass readily through the column. The separation depends on the gel porosity and the size of the virus particles as well as the cellular components of the cell. The virus is obtained in a volume at least twice the original one, and must be concentrated.

Crystallization

Many viruses and proteins can be precipitated or crystallized due to the action of the salt concentration, especially if great amounts of ammonium sulfate (25%) are added. The resulting precipitate can be concentrated through filtration or low-speed centrifugation. After that, the precipitate can be dissolved in a small volume of buffer solution to obtain a suspension of virus particles. During crystallization, most of the crystallized or precipitated proteins of the host are denatured and cannot be dissolved when they are suspended again in a buffer solution. However, a certain percentage of the host proteins do dissolve with the virus particles.

Isoelectric precipitation

It is also known as precipitation by acidification or by pH change. Viruses are amphoteric molecules (which contain positive and negative charges at the same time). There is a pH value known as the isoelectric point, where the net charge of the molecule becomes zero and will precipitate out of solution. This procedure for concentrating viruses (lowering the pH to their isoelectric point) is most useful for viruses that precipitate at a pH value lower than 4.5, since most host material precipitates at a pH value of 4.8 or 5 and can thus be removed from the preparation before the virus itself is precipitated.

Electrophoresis

This separation method is based on the migration of charged particles or molecules through an electric field. The rate of movement depends on the net charge of the particle or molecule, the potential gradient formed by the electric field, and the resistance of the medium to the movementof the particle or molecule. Electrophoresis in gels (semi-solid medium) of agarose or agarose/ acrylamide can be used for purifying viral preparations, because viruses are charged particles that migrate through an electric field (except at their isoelectric point). However, this technique is not widely used for purifying viruses due to the small quantities that must be used. The electrophoresis in a density gradient column (a liquidmedium, usually sucrose) is more commonly used because a much larger volume can be processed. This method is useful when purifying unstable viruses or viruses that have a sedimentation coefficient similar to that of vegetal components.

Chromatography of ionic exchange

Resins of ionic exchange are synthetic polymers, which are produced as spheres with a certain number of ionizable groups. One of these groups becomes fixed to the polymer and others remain free to be replaced or exchanged. In resins of cationic exchange, the fixed ion is negatively charged (anion) and the positive ion (cation) can be exchanged. The opposite occurs in resins of anionic exchange. According to the charge, molecules in the virus preparation are retained or they pass freely. Although ion exchange chromatography separates molecules with similar electric charges, it is not commonly used to purify viruses because it does not always separate the virus completely and sometimes, the virus remains irreversibly joined to the resin. It is normally used to remove some impurities from the suspension of viruses.

Size-exclusion chromatography (SEC) has been efficiently used for purification of retroviruses since 1970's.

Two-phase systems/ partition chromatography

Virus purification using two liquid phases has been used up to a limited extent. Examples of phase systems are: polyethyleneglycol-dextran and polyethylene glycol-dextran sulfate. Theprocess depends on salt concentration, and in some cases the virus can be concentrated in the phase of the least volume.

Ultracentrifugation

Ultracentrifugation in a fixed angle rotor is the most commonly used method to concentrate viruses. The viral particles sediment against the sloping outer walls of the tube and slide to the bottom to form a "pellet." Generally, this process takes 2 hours or less. Itis important to centrifuge the preparation during the least possible time because sedimentation at high speed is a severe physical process that may damage the virus particles. Immediately after centrifugation, the supernatant (liquid) must be eliminated and the sediment (pellet) resuspended in a small volume of buffer. High-speed preparative centrifugation or ultracentrifugation, using cesium chloride or sucrose gradients, has traditionally been used to process many viral vectors on the laboratory scale. However, this process is labor-intensive, time-consuming and scale-restricted. Additionally, virus particles may suffer a cumulative loss of infectivity during extended period of time required for fractionation of gradients, and they can form aggregates when pelleted onto the bottom of a centrifuge tube.

Centrifugation in density gradients

This technique is most commonly used for final virus purification. Concentrated preparations of virus are carefully layered onto the surface of tubes that contain pre-formed gradients and centrifuged. During the centrifuge run, the virus and the host components move along the gradient at different rates. After centrifugation, the layer containing the virus may be observed under diffuse light as a dense opalescent band and can be collected from the tube by using a hypodermic syringe or using a fractionator of density gradients.

Serological methods

There are two serological methods for concentrating purified viruses and eliminating host contaminants. The first is affinity chromatography. In this case, the virus preparation is passed through a column with antiviral antibodies adsorbed to the solid matrix. Viral particles are caught by the antibodies and remain in the column, while vegetal material is eluted out. Viral particles are subsequently removed from the column by dissociating the virus-antibody complex. This technique has been successfully used in the preparation of highly pure viruses for the production of antibodies.

The second method consists in using antiserum to remove host proteins. The antiserum is prepared by injecting purified host plant proteins into a rabbit. The antiserum is then purified and the gammaglobulin fraction incubated with the viral preparation. The antibody-host protein complex is removed by low speed centrifugation and the viral preparation is separated from the serum soluble proteins by centrifugation with density gradients.

Adsorbent or dry gels

Calcium phosphate is one of the most commonly used adsorbents for the purification of some viruses. Freshly calcium phosphate precipitates is obtained by mixing 1M $CaCl2$ and 0.2M $Na2HPO4$. This precipitate must be washed several times in order to remove residual salts and then it is mixed with the viral preparation. The adsorbent-protein mixture is then separated by centrifugation or filtration. Either host proteins or the virus can be adsorbed. The virus can be eluted under appropriate conditions.

Microfilters

This technique has been widely used for the purification of animal viruses. Systems of filters with pores of different sizes can be arranged so that pre-filtration (to remove the biggest particles that can clog filters with small pores) and virus concentration occur simultaneously. This method is suitable for globular molecules and for inflexible rod-shaped viruses. It is not recommended to use ribbon-shaped flexible molecules, because they can be broken by the torsion force of filtration and their fragments can clog the filters. Another disadvantage is that viruses can stick on the filters of pre-filtration. One way of avoiding virus loss consists in using filters with a pore diameter at least ten times bigger than the size of the virus to be filtered. Membrane-based tangential flow filtration techniques, in particular ultrafiltration and microfiltration, are applicable in the purification and concentration of viruses. They were successfully used for purification. While membrane filtration is a good procedure, there may be problems with membrane fouling, and since separation is based on size differences, large molecular weight impurities are co-concentrated with viral particles, requiring additional purification step(s).

Nanofiltration

Virus removal processes using nanofiltration techniques remove viruses specifically by size exclusion. This type of process is typically used for parvoviruses and other viruses containing a protein coat. A typical HIV virion is 180 nm and a typical parvovirus can vary between 15 and 24 nm, which are very small. One great advantage of filtration, as opposed to methods involving extremes of temperature or acidity, is that filtration will not denature the proteins in the sample. Nanofiltration is also effective for most types of proteins. Since it is not chemically selective, no matter what the surface chemistry of the viral particle is, viral removal processes using nanofiltration techniques will still be effective. Another great advantage of this technique is its ability to be performed on a lab scale and then effectively scaled up to production standards. It is important to consider, however, the fact that the level of removal of the viruses is dependent on the size of the pores of the nanofilter. In some cases, very small viruses will not be filtered out. It is also necessary to consider the possible effects of pressure and flow rate variation. Some of the filters used to perform these types of processes are Planova 15, VAG-300, Viresolve 180, and Viresolve 70TM.

□□□

Chapter 3

Viral Relication, Viral Genetics & Recombination

Contents

The Productive Life Cycle of Animal Viruses

The life cycle of most viruses is designed to maximize the production of progeny virus particles. In general, the details of a viral replication cycle are dictated by the type of nucleic acid carried into the host cell by the infecting virion. Most DNA viruses enter the nucleus where they parasitize the host cell's DNA replication apparatus. There are exceptions, notably the poxviruses encode its own DNA replication machinery, and thus remains in the cytoplasm. Most RNA viruses replicate in the cytoplasm because the enzymes used to replicate viral RNA are virally encoded. The details of each step in the virus life cycle have not yet been fully characterized in case of many viruses, and among the viruses that have been well studied, there is great deal of variation. Therefore a generalized productive life cycle for animal viruses is furnished consisting of the following steps: **adsorption, viral entry, viral movement to the site of replication, & release of the viral genome**.

The life cycle of animal viruses has been developed in large part by studying virus infections under conditions where cell cultures become infected synchronously with the virus in such a way that only a single cycle of infection can occur. Synchronous infection can be achieved by infecting cultures with a high amount of virus, such that all cells within the culture become infected rapidly. To do this, one typically infects cells at a multiplicity of infection of 5 to 10 per cell. One-step growth analysis begins with the addition of virus to cells. After a brief (~1 hour) period of adsorption, the virus inoculum is washed away, and cells are cultured. Aliquots of the cells and the cell-culture fluid are then collected at various time intervals and analyzed for the presence of virus. A typical one-step growth analysis can be divided into several phases **(Figure 3-1)**:

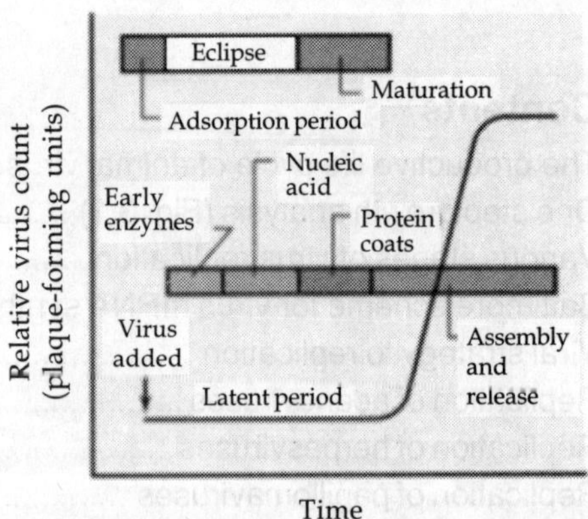

One step growth curve of virus replication

Figure 3.1 : One-Step Growth Analysis

1. *Adsorption* of virus (initial phase).
2. *Eclipse phase.* This lasts for 10-12 hours, and it corresponds to the period during which the input virus becomes uncoated. As a result, no infectious virus can be detected during this time (any infectious virus detected is simply virus that is still stuck on the cell membrane).

3. *Synthetic phase*. This starts around 12 hours post-infection and corresponds to the time during which new virus particles are assembled.
4. *Latent period*. During this period, no extracellular virus can be detected. After ~18 hours, extracellular virus is detected. Ultimately, production will reach a maximum plateau level.

The virus **burst size** (amount of infectious virus produced, per infected cell) can be calculated on the basis of the results from a one-step growth experiment. Burst sizes for viruses typically vary between 10 and 10,000. Viruses vary considerably in terms of the kinetics of their replication and the specifics of their one-step growth curves.

In the case of many animal viruses, the time elapsed from infection to the generation of the first progeny ranges from **several hours to a day.** There are several possible consequences to a cell that is infected by a virus, and ultimately this may determine the pathology of a disease caused by the virus. Often, the burden of producing a large number of virus particles causes the infected cell to die. This lysis of the host cell is called the **viral lytic cycle**, and is an immediate and inevitable consequence of viral reproduction. Lytic infections are caused by virulent viruses, which inherently bring about the death of the cells that they infect, & are able to infect a new cell. Other viruses, in contrast, will **refrain from killing the host cell.** They can establish a **long-term infection of the cell, in which the cell releases a steady stream of viral particles over an extended period of time.** If this continuous production of virus particles does not compromise the health of the host cell, it can live on indefinitely devoting some of its resources to making virions. When enveloped viruses are formed by budding, the release of the viral particles may be slow and the host cell may not be lysed. Such infections may occur over relatively long periods of time and are thus referred to as **persistent infections.** In persistent infections, the virus may go dormant and be reactivated at a later time. The host cell may or may not be destroyed. Some viruses can cause persistent infection in different organs and tissues at the same time. Persistent infections last for long periods, and occur when the primary infection is not cleared by the adaptive immune response. Varicella-zoster virus, measles virus, HIV-1, and human cytomegalovirus are examples of viruses that cause typical persistent infections. A chronic infection is a type of persistent infection that is eventually cleared, while latent or slow infections last the life of the host. Viruses may also cause **latent infections**. Latent infections are a type of persistent infection in which the appearance of disease symptoms does not happen immediately, but follows after a period of time. The virus responsible for the latent infection is **reactivated** at some later point, usually prompted by some type of event such as infection of the host by another virus or physiological changes in the host or various stresses. The effect of a latent infection is that there is a delay between the infection by the virus and the appearance of symptoms. Fever blisters (cold sores) caused by herpes simplex type 1 result from a latent infection; they appear sporadically as the virus emerges from latency, usually triggered by some sort of stress in the host.

Some animal viruses have the potential to change a cell from a normal cell into a tumor cell, the hallmark of which is to grow without restraint. This process is called **transformation.** Viruses that are able to transform normal cells into tumor cells are referred to as oncogenic viruses. Other viruses may cause HIV, Human herpesviruses 6 and 7, and the Epstein-Barr viruses are examples of persistent virus infections that are associated with the immune system. Oncogenic viral infections cause changes in host cells, tuning them into tumor cells. These cancer viruses alter or transform cell properties leading to abnormal cell growth.

Various Stages of Virus Replication

1. Viral Attachment or Adsorption to the Host Cell

Adsorption involves the **binding of virus attachment sites on the viral surface with receptor sites on the host cell cytoplasmic membrane**. For a virus to infect a host cell, that cell must have receptors for the virus on its surface and also be capable of supporting viral replication. These host cell receptors are normal surface molecules involved in routine cellular function, but since a portion of a molecule on the viral surface resembles the chemical shape of the body's molecule that normally bind to the receptor, the virus is able to attach to the host cell's surface. Animal viruses attach to host cells by means of a complementary association between attachment sites on the surface of the virus and receptor sites on the host cell surface. This accounts for specificity of viruses for their host cells. Many different molecules are used as receptors by different viruses, including **cell surface glycoproteins, components of the extracellular matrix, receptors involved in cell signaling and activation, & certain receptors are targeted by several different viruses** (e.g., sialic acid, heparan sulfate proteoglycans, ICAM-1, CAR, CD46, CD4 and certain integrins.

Many viruses also use **coreceptors** to gain entry to cells, i.e., these viruses require the presence of two essential molecules in order to infect their target cells. If either one of these receptors is absent, infection will not occur. The distinction between a **receptor and coreceptor** is a reflection of the sequential nature of virus attachment. Initial interactions with a primary receptor located some distance from the cell membrane may bring the virus into closer proximity with a secondary receptor (coreceptor) that is located much closer to the lipid bilayer. Binding of this coreceptor is often dependent on a **conformational change** in the virus, brought about by the initial interaction between the virus and its primary receptor. Cells lacking receptors for a certain virus are resistant to it and cannot be infected. Attachment can be blocked by antibody molecules that bind to viral attachment sites or to host cell receptors. Since antibodies block the initial attachment of viruses to their host cells, the presence of these antibodies in the host organism is the most important basis for immunization against viral infections.

Common cellular receptors for virus attachment are presented in the table given below.

Table 3.1 : Receptors for selected animal viruses.

Receptors for selected animal viruses Virus	Receptor	Biological Function or Type of Molecule	Coreceptor
Adeno-associated virus	Heparan sulfate	Glycosaminoglycan; part of extracellular matrix	$\alpha_v\beta_5$ integrin
Adenovirus *(subgroups A, C-F)*	CAR (Coxsackie and adenovirus receptor); also used by several coxsackie viruses	Immunoglobulin (Ig)-like	$\alpha_v\beta_5$, $\alpha_v\beta_3$ integrins. Also used by several picornaviruses; binds vitronectin ($\alpha_v\beta_3$)
Epstein-Barr virus	CD21 (aka CR2, complement receptor 2)	Ig-like; complement receptor	MHC class II (HLA-DR) in B cells; ?in epithelial cells.
Herpes simplex virus	Heparan sulfate. Also used by AAV, Dengue, others	Glycosaminoglycan; part of extracellular matrix	HveA, Prr (Herpes virus entry mediator A; *Pvr*-related protein 1).
HIV-1	CD4. Also used by *Human herpesvirus 7.*	Ig-like; role in helper T cell function.	CCR5, CXCR4. Chemo kine receptors.
Influenza virus	Sialic acid. *Also used by reo-, corona- virus.*	Carbohydrate	
Measles virus	SLAM. Some vaccine strains can use CD46; this is also used by *Human herpesvirus 6.*	T/B cell surface protein; involved in cellular activation	
Poliovirus	Pvr (poliovirus receptor, aka CD155)	Ig-like	

Rabies virus	Acetylcholine receptor, NCAM (CD56)	Neuronal receptor or adhesion molecule
Rhinovirus *(major subtypes)*	ICAM-1 (intercellular adhesion molecule 1); also used by some coxsackieviruses	Ig-like; role in cell adhesion
Human cytomegaloviruses (CMV)	MHC-I molecules	MHC-I enable Th8-lymphocytes to recognize Ags during adaptive immunity
Hepatitis B virus (HBV)	IgA receptors	These receptors bind the Abs isotype IgA for transport across cells.

2. Viral Entry into the Host Cell

The **penetration stage** follows attachment. Penetration of the virus occurs either by engulfment of the whole virus, or by fusion of the viral envelope with the cell membrane allowing only the nucleocapsid of the virus to enter the cell. Animal viruses generally do not "inject" their nucleic acid into host cells as do bacteriophages, although occasionally non enveloped viruses leave their capsid outside the cell while the genome passes into the cell.

a. Enveloped viruses

Enveloped viruses enter the host cell in one of two ways:

i. In some cases, the **viral envelope may fuse with the host cell cytoplasmic membrane** and the **nucleocapsid is released into the cytoplasm** and.

ii. Usually they enter by **endocytosis,** whereby the host cell cytoplasmic membrane invaginates and pinches off, placing the virus in an endocytic vesicle.

iii. *Pore formation*. Some non-enveloped viruses like picornaviruses, form pores in the cell membrane. One example is poliovirus, which after binding to its receptor (Pvr) undergoes a conformational change that exposes a hydrophobic domain on the VP1 virion protein. This forms a pore in the cell membrane, through which the viral RNA is then released into the cytosol.

b. Naked viruses

Naked viruses enter the cell in one of two ways:

i. In some cases, interaction between the viral capsid and the host cell cytoplasmic membrane causes a **rearrangement of capsid protein sallowing the viral nucleic acid to pass through the membrane** into the cytoplasm.

ii. Most naked viruses enter by **receptor-mediated endocytosis** whereby the host cell cytoplasmic membrane invaginates and pinches off, placing the virus in an **endocytic vesicle.**

3. Viral Movement to the site of Replication within the Host Cell and Release of the Viral Genome

Some viruses that enter by endocytosis, the **endocytic vesicles containing the virus move within the host cell.** During this process the pH of the endocytic vesicle typically decreases and this enables the virus to leave the endocytic vesicle. Viruses exit the endocytic vesicle through a variety of mechanisms:

a. **Fusion of the viral envelope with the membrane of the endocytic vesicle** enabling the viral nucleocapsid to enter the cytoplasm of the host cell.

b. **Lysis of the endocytic vesicle** releasing the viral nucleocapsid into the cytoplasm of the host cell.

c. The **viral capsid undergoing conformational changes** that forms pores in the endocytic vesicle **enabling the viral genome to enter the cytoplasm** of the host cell.

Before viruses can replicate within the infected host cell, the viral genome needs to be released from the remainder of the virus. This process is sometimes referred to as **uncoating.** In **most viruses with an RNA genome, the viral RNA genome is released from the capsid and enters the cytoplasm** of the host cell where replication generally occurs.

In most cases with **DNA virus genome**, the viral genome enters the nucleus of the host cell through one the mechanisms shown below. Most larger DNA viruses use either a or b to enter the nucleus. Method c is used by some very small DNA whose capsid is small enough to be carried through the nuclear pores. Nuclear localization is dependent on the presence of **nuclear localization signals (NLS)** within the proteins associated with the viral genome.

a. **The viral DNA genome is released from the capsid, enters the cytoplasm** of the host cell, and subsequently **enters the nucleus of the host cell** through the pores in the nuclear membrane.

b. The **capsid of the viruses interacts with the nuclear membrane** of the host cell **enabling the viral DNA genome to enter the nucleus of the host cell** via the pores in the nuclear membrane.

c. The **nucleocapsid of a small DNA virus enters the nucleus** of the host cell and the capsid is subsequently removed releasing the viral DNA genome into the nucleoplasm

This uncoating begins the **eclipse period**, the period during which no intact virions can be detected within the cell. After uncoating and during the replication stage the virus is not infectious.

4. Viral Replication within the Host Cell

The viral genome **directs the host cell's metabolic machinery** (ribosomes, tRNA, nutrients, energy, enzymes, etc.) **to synthesize viral enzymes and viral parts. The viral genome has to both replicate itself and become transcribed into viral mRNA molecules. The viral mRNAs are then be translated by the host cell's ribosomes into viral structural components and enzymes needed for replication and assembly of the virus.**

Baltimore Classification

The **Baltimore classification**, developed by David Baltimore, is a virus classification system that groups viruses into families, depending on their type of genome (DNA, RNA) single-stranded (ss), double-stranded (ds), etc.), & their method of replication. Baltimore system of virus classification provides a useful guide with regard to the various mechanisms of viral genome replication. The central theme here is that **all viruses must generate positive strand mRNAs from their genomes (Figure 3-3)**, in order to produce proteins and replicate themselves. The precise mechanisms whereby this is achieved differ for each virus family.

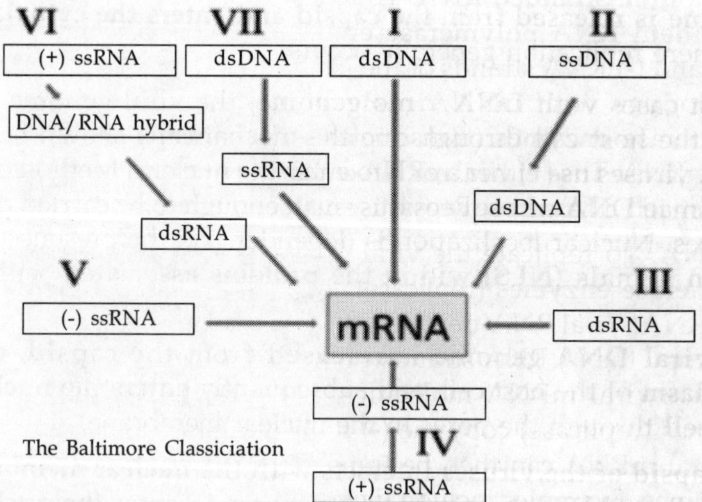

Figure 3.3 : Baltimore scheme for virus mRNA synthesis

Viruses can store their genetic information in seven different types of nucleic acid which are named based on how that nucleic acid eventually becomes transcribed to the viral mRNA:

a. **(+/-) double-stranded DNA**. To replicate the viral genome, **DNA-dependent DNA polymerase** enzymes usually provided by the cell copy both the (+) and (-) DNA strands producing dsDNA viral genomes. To produce viral mRNA molecules, host cell **DNA-dependent RNA polymerase** enzymes copy the (-) DNA strand into (+) viral mRNA. The (+) viral mRNA is then be translated into viral proteins by host cell ribosomes. Examples include most bacteriophages, Papillomaviruses, Polyomaviruses, Adenoviruses, and Herpesviruses.

b. **(+) single-stranded DNA**. To replicate the viral genome, **DNA-dependent DNA polymerase enzymes** usually provided by the cell copy the (+) DNA strand of the genome producing a dsDNA intermediate. DNA-dependent DNA polymerase enzymes, again, usually provided by the cell then copy the (-) DNA strand into ss (+) DNA genomes. To produce viral mRNA molecules, host cell **DNA-dependent RNA polymerase** enzymes copy the (-) DNA strand into (+) viral mRNA. The (+) viral mRNA can then be translated into viral proteins by host cell ribosomes. Examples include Phage M13, Parvoviruses & Circoviruses. Exceptions are small DNA viruses - parvoviruses and papillomaviruses. Note that viruses with no DNA polymerase of their own require actively dividing cells to replicate, since they must use the cellular DNA polymerase (eg, HPVs and parvovirus B19; this has important consequences for pathogenesis).

c. **(+/-) double-stranded RNA**. To replicate the viral genome, **viral RNA-dependent RNA polymerase enzymes (replicase**) copy both the (+) RNA and (-) RNA strands of the genome producing a dsRNA genomes. To produce viral mRNA molecules, **viral RNA-dependent RNA polymerase enzymes** (transcriptase) copy the (-) RNA strand into (+) viral mRNA. The (+) viral mRNA can then be translated into viral proteins by host cell ribosomes. Reoviruses are an example.

d. **(+) RNA**. To replicate the viral genome, **viral RNA-dependent RNA polymerase enzymes (**replicase) copy the (+) RNA genome producing ss (-) RNA. Viral RNA-dependent RNA polymerase enzymes (replicase) then copy the (-) RNA strands producing ss (+) RNA viral genome. To produce viral mRNA molecules, RNA-dependent RNA polymerase enzymes (replicase) copy the (-) RNA strand into (+) viral mRNA. The (+) viral mRNA can then be translated into viral proteins by host cell ribosomes. Examples include Picornaviruses, Calciviruses, Togaviruses, Coronaviruses, Flaviviruses, Astroviruses, Arteriviruses.

e. **(-) RNA**. To replicate the viral genome, **viral RNA-dependent RNA polymerase** enzymes (transcriptase) copy the (-) RNA genome, producing ss (+) RNA. Transcriptase must be **carried into the cell with the virion**. Viral RNA-dependent RNA polymerase enzymes (replicase) then copy the (+) RNA strands producing ss (-) RNA viral genome. The (+) mRNA strands also function as viral mRNA and can then be translated into viral proteins by host cell ribosomes. Examples include Orthomyxoviruses, Paramyxoviruses, Rhabdoviruses, Bornaviruses & Filoviruses.

f. **(+) RNA Retroviruses**. To replicate the viral genome, viral reverse transcriptase enzymes (RNA-dependent DNA polymerases) copy the (+) RNA genome producing ss (-) DNA strands. Viral reverse transcriptase can also function as a DNA-dependent DNA polymerase enzyme and will copy the (-) DNA strands to produce a dsDNA intermediate. Reverse transcriptase must be carried into the cell with the virion. The viral DNA will move to the nucleus where it integrates into the cell's DNA using the viral enzyme integrase which also must be carried into the host cell with the virion. Once in the host cell's DNA, **host cell DNA-dependent RNA polymerase enzymes** then copy the ds (-) DNA strands to produce ss (+) RNA genomes. To produce viral mRNA molecules, host cell DNA-dependent RNA polymerase enzymes copy the ds (-) DNA strand into (+) viral mRNA. The (+) viral mRNA can then be translated into viral proteins by host cell ribosomes. Retroviruses, such as HIV-1, HIV-2, and HTLV-1 are examples.

g. **Partially ds DNA Hepadnaviruses**. To replicate the viral genome **in the nucleus, the partially ds DNA is 'repaired' by the cell to form a** covalently closed complete circular DNA. It then undergoes **transcription by the host cell RNA polymerase II of the pregenomic RNA** (pgRNA) and subgenomic mRNAs, inducing synthesis of all the viral proteins by host cell ribosomes. The viruses replicate in the nucleus of hepatocytes. (-) DNA strand acts as a template to form +RNA strand (full length). +RNA is packaged into the viral core in the infected cell cytoplasm. Viral reverse transcriptase copies ss (-) viral DNA strand from ss (+) RNA & + ssRNA is degraded. Viral DNA pol II forms (+) DNA from (-) DNA template. ±ds DNA is packaged into virion before full length +DNA is synthesized, thus (+) DNA remains incomplete.

As the host cell's ribosomes attach to the viral mRNA molecules, the mRNAs are translated into viral structural proteins and viral enzymes. During the **early phase** of replication, proteins needed for the replication of the viral genome are made and the genome makes thousands of replicas of itself. During the **late phase** of replication, viral structural proteins (capsid and matrix proteins, envelope glycoproteins, etc.) and the enzymes involved in maturation are produced. Some viruses translate mRNA molecules that are transcripts of several genes into one or more large polyproteins. These **polyproteins** are subsequently cut into individual functional proteins by viral enzymes called **proteases.** Other viruses produce monocistronic mRNA molecules, each coding for a separate functional protein.

In the case of **most RNA viruses, replication and assembly occurs in the host cell's cytoplasm.** With DNA viruses, most replication and assembly occurs in the nucleus of the host cell. The viral genome enters the nucleus of the host cell and is transcribed into viral mRNA. The viral mRNA molecules then leave the nucleus through the pores in the nuclear membrane and are translated into viral proteins by the host cell's ribosomes in the cytoplasm. Most of these viral proteins then re-enter the nucleus where the virus assembles around the replicated genomes.

During replication, **viral envelope proteins and glycoproteins coded by the viral genome are incorporated into the host cell's cytoplasmic membrane or nuclear membrane.**

In the case of RNA viruses, all of the enzymes used in genome replication and transcription are viral encoded enzymes different from those of the host cell so these enzymes can potentially be targeted. On the other hand, DNA viruses use the host cell's RNA transcription machinery and DNA replication machinery so these enzymes, shared by the virus and the host cell, cannot be targeted without killing the host cell. Since all viruses use the host cell's translation machinery regardless of genome type, translation can not be targeted in any viruses.

5. Viral Assembly or Maturation within the Host Cell

During maturation, the viral components & enzymes are produced separately and begin to assemble either in the cytoplasm or nucleus. **Capsidis assembled around the viral genome.**

- *Maturation of an enveloped virus*: Its structural proteins have been synthesized by a host cell that appears relatively normal, or that may be damaged. Some viruses (e.g. poliovirus) assemble completely in the cytoplasm, whereas others (e.g. adenoviruses) are predominantly nuclear in location. During maturation, envelope glycoproteins are transported to the host cell's cytoplasmic membrane and the capsid assembles around the viral genome.
- *Maturation of a naked virus*: During maturation, the capsid assembles around the viral genome.

6. Viral Release from the Host Cell

a. Naked viruses

Naked viruses are predominantly released by **host cell lysis**. While some viruses are cytolytic and lyse the host cell more or less directly, in many cases it is the body's immune defenses that lyse the infected cell.

b. Enveloped viruses

With **enveloped viruses**, the host cell may or may not be lysed. The viruses **obtain their envelopes from host cell membranes by budding**. As mentioned above, prior to budding, viral proteins and glycoproteins are incorporated into the host cell's membranes. During budding, the host cell membrane with incorporated viral proteins and glycoproteins evaginates and pinches off to form the viral envelope. Budding occurs either at the outer cytoplasmic membrane, the nuclear membrane, or at the membranes of the Golgi apparatus.

1. Viruses obtaining their envelope from the cytoplasmic membrane are released during the budding process.

2. Viruses obtaining their envelopes from the membranes of the nucleus, the endoplasmic reticulum, or the Golgi apparatus are then released by exocytosis via transport vesicles

Some viruses, capable of causing cell fusion, may be transported from one cell to adjacent cells without being released, that is, they are **transmitted by cell-to-cell** contact whereby an infected cell fuses with an uninfected cell.

As many as **10,000 to 50,000** animal viruses may be produced by a single infected host cell.

Viral Strategy to Replication

The ds DNA viruses

Viral genomic DNA contains necessary information to ensure replication of viral genome, ensures packaging of genomes into virion & alters the structure and or function of the host cell to a greater or lesser degree. i. The virus must make mRNAs that can be translated into viral protein by the host cell translation machinery. ii. The virus needs to replicate its genome. iii. The host enzymes for mRNA synthesis and DNA replication are nuclear, hence a virus avails nuclear enzymes by entering in to the nucleus. Among the dsDNA viruses are: *Adenoviridae, Asfarviridae, Herpesviridae, Poxviridae, Papillomaviridae* & *Polyomaviridae; Adenoviridae, Herpesviridae, Papillomaviridae* & *Polyomaviridae* replicate in the nucleus while *Poxviridae & Asfarviridae* **replicate in the cytoplasm.** The ssDNA viruses, *Parvoviridae & Circoviridae* replicate in the nucleus.

Once the nucleocapsid of genomes of dsDNA virus enters the cell, it proceeds to the nucleus where it mimics the genome of the host cell. Usually, the viral genome is replicated using the **host cell DNA polymerase**, and the viral genome is transcribed by the host cell RNA polymerase. The resulting transcripts carrying information encoding viral proteins is then transported to the cytoplasm and seen as a template by the host cell ribosomes. Some of these newly synthesized viral proteins are used as the protein capsid around newly replicated viral DNA molecules. These new virions are released from the cell, where they target other host cells and trigger new rounds of infection.

However, the dependence of these viruses on the host cell replication machinery creates an awkward situation: the enzymes of DNA replication are generally **not expressed in quiescent cells (cells in G0)**. Most of the cells infected will be in G0 and therefore inhospitable hosts. Some dsDNA viruses, like the herpesviruses or the **Epstein-Barr virus** (responsible for mononucleosis), have large genomes that contain greater than sixty genes. These viruses encode their **own DNA polymerase** and thus ensure their ability to replicate in quiescent cells. Other viruses circumvent this problem by **producing a protein that induces the resting host cell to enter the active cell cycle.** This ensures that the host cell replication enzymes are available for exploitation and reproduction of the virus. This means of producing many virions usually results in host cell death.

When the infected cell is not killed by the virus, the presence of the virus and the viral growth-promoting protein can drive the host cell into **unceasing growth and cell division.** This converts the host cell growth from a normal pattern to a pattern typical of **cancer cells**. The gene that encodes the growth-promoting protein can function as an *oncogene* that acts to ***transform*** the infected cell into a cancer cell.

More than 90% of human cervical carcinomas are associated with infection by human papillomas virus (HPV) a dsDNA virus that infects the lining of the cervix. In order for HPV to create a tumor, the viral genome must perpetuate itself so when the original infected cell divides into many cells, each new cell contains the virus and the viral growth-promoting protein.

The Epstein-Barr dsDNA virus causes infectious mononucleosis (a non-cancerous condition). For reasons that are unclear, the Epstein-Barr virus triggers Burkitt's lymphoma (a childhood tumor) in central Africa, and a tumor of the nasal cavity in Southeast Asia. These tumors are inadvertent by-products of the need to replicate viral DNA. The outgrowth of tumors happens on occasion when virus-infected cells are not eliminated by the completion of the viral lytic cycle.

Single-stranded DNA viruses

Some small viruses carry their genome as ssDNA, these viruses have a simple genome: one gene for a viral nucleocapsid protein and another gene for a DNA replication enzyme. The virus with a ssDNA genome also faces a serious replication problem in the host cell. When introduced into cells, these genomes can not be used to make viral proteins because the only template for transcription is double-stranded DNA. For this reason, the first step after infection is the conversion of the viral ssDNA into dsDNA using host **cell DNA polymerase.** DNA polymerase requires a primer for replication.

In some of these viruses, the **3' end of the viral DNA folds back and forms dsDNA** by base pairing with an internal sequence. In this way, the primer is built into the genome and the 3' end can be extended to create dsDNA that serves as a template for transcription. The resulting transcripts are translated to make the viral proteins, the replicated viral DNA is converted back into a ssDNA genome, and the virion is packaged for export. Canine and feline parvoviruses are members of the ssDNA virus family.

(+) Single-stranded RNA viruses

(+) ssRNA viruses, the virion (genomic) RNA is the same sense as mRNA and so functions as mRNA. This mRNA can be translated immediately upon infection of the host cell. Examples are: picornaviruses, togaviruses & flaviviruses. This viral RNA molecule can be directly translated by the host cell ribosomes to make viral proteins. The host cell does not have a mechanism to replicate RNA (there is no host enzyme that uses RNA as a template for nucleic acid synthesis).

Thus, this genome must **encode a viral enzyme that can replicate the ssRNA genome** as well as the proteins needed for the capsid. In principle, the viral enzyme could convert ssRNA into dsRNA, but that is not what is seen. As **the viral polymerase moves along the (+) stranded RNA template, it elongates a (-) stranded RNA molecule that remains single-stranded.** No hydrogen bonds are formed between the complementary RNA strands. The resulting (-) ssRNA molecules are then used as templates by the viral enzyme for polymerizing new (+) ssRNA molecules destined to serve as the genome in a progeny virion, or as mRNA for viral proteins. Members of this class of virus include many of the common cold viruses as well as poliovirus. Translation of the (+) strand of RNA from the poliovirus results in a large **polyprotein** that is then cut into the separate required viral proteins. Interestingly, the protease needed to cut the polyprotein is part of the polyprotein.

(-) Single-stranded RNA viruses

The largest family of viruses is the (-) ssRNA family of viruses. The virion RNA is negative sense (complementary to mRNA) and must therefore be copied into the complementary plus-sense mRNA before proteins can be made. Thus, besides needing to code for an **RNA-dependent RNA-polymerase,** these viruses also need to package it in the virion so that they can make mRNAs upon infecting the cell. Examples are: orthomyxoviruses, paramyxoviruses & rhabdoviruses.

Their viral RNA genome can not be directly translated, instead the (-) strand is complementary to the viral mRNAs that need to be produced and translated into viral proteins. For reasons that are unclear, nature has created hundreds of different (-) ssRNA viruses ranging from the measles and influenza viruses to the rabies and Ebola viruses. They are all, without exception, lipid-containing viruses. We will illustrate this type of virus through the vesicular stomatitis virus (VSV). After entering a host cell, the VSV (-) strand of RNA faces a problem as with the poliovirus, there is no host enzyme that uses RNA as a template for nucleic acid synthesis. In addition, this (-) stranded RNA is not recognized as a template by the host ribosomes and thus this enzyme can not be directly produced. It solves it by **packaging a viral RNA dependent RNA polymerase along with the (-) ssRNA genome** within the nucleocapsid. Therefore, once inside the cell, the viral polymerase begins to work on the (-) ssRNA making two kinds of (+) stranded viral RNA. Some of this (+) stranded RNA is made as **short viral mRNAs that are then transcribed into viral proteins,** some of it is made as **full length RNA that is then replicated to make the (-) ssRNA genome** that is needed for the progeny virions. Some of the (-) ssRNA viruses have segmented genomes. For example, Ebola virus is thought to have three distinct (-) ssRNAs in it genome, each encoding a separate protein. Members of the influenza viruses have eight different (-) ssRNAs. The life cycle of these viruses is as described above, but each viral RNA is replicated separately, and packaging must be regulated to ensure that each virion receives one of each distinct RNA.

Double-stranded RNA viruses

A small group of viruses carries its genetic information around in the form of double-stranded RNA (dsRNA) molecules. These are members of the reovirus class of viruses. The virion (genomic) RNA is double stranded and so cannot function as mRNA; thus these viruses also need to package an **RNA polymerase** to make their mRNA after infection of the host cell. Example: reoviruses

Their genomes have ten distinct dsRNAs and virions of this class lack lipid membranes. The virions carry an **RNA polymerase** that transcribes the dsRNA into (+) ssRNA. These transcripts can serve as mRNA that is then translated into the necessary viral proteins or they can act as a template for (-) strand synthesis and be converted back into a dsRNA genome for packaging.

(+) ssRNA retroviruses

After entering the cell, the (+) strand of RNA is not associated with ribosomes, even though it has all the attributes of mRNA. Instead, the virion RNA is used as a template to make a DNA copy of the viral genome. This copying of RNA into DNA is foreign for the host cell and must be carried out by a viral enzyme that is packaged in virion. The viral enzyme, called ***reverse transcriptase*** carries out this process. The terms "reverse" and "retro" imply a mechanism that is the opposite of that normally operating in all cells. The usual flow of information in a cell is from DNA to RNA, not from RNA to DNA. The initial product of reverse transcription is an RNA:DNA hybrid double helix. The RNA portion of this hybrid is degraded and reverse transcriptase copies the remaining DNA strand into dsDNA. These processes take place **in the cytoplasm.** Once the viral dsDNA is synthesized, it is transported into the nucleus where it is inserted and covalently linked to the host chromosomal DNA. The viral DNA that is integrated into the host genome is called a *provirus*, and it is indistinguishable from the host cell genes. In effect, the retrovirus has created a version of the viral genome that has all the attributes of a cellular gene found in the host. The integrated provirus can now be transcribed by the host cell into (+) RNA that is transported to the cytoplasm and used either as mRNA in viral protein synthesis, or as the genome for new progeny viruses.

The Translation Problem

Eucaryotic host cell translation protein synthesis machinery in general uses monocistronic mRNAs and so there is a problem in making more than one type of protein from a single mRNA. RNA viruses have **several solutions** to this problem: the virus makes **multiple monocistronic mRNAs**, the virus makes **primary transcripts which are processed by the host splicing machinery to give more than one monocistronic RNA**, the viral mRNA acts as a monocistronic transcript. A large polypeptide (called a **polyprotein**) is made which is then cleaved into separate proteins - thus, one initial translation product is processed to give rise to multiple proteins. This happens, for example, in picornaviruses. The viral mRNA has special features which enable ribosomes to bind internally instead of (or as well as) at the 5′ end.

Genome size of RNA viruses

RNA viruses tend to have a relatively small genome; this is probably because the lack of RNA error correction mechanisms puts a limit on the size of RNA genomes. The result of having a small genome is that RNA viruses tend to code for only a few proteins. These will include a polymerase which can copy RNA into a complementary nucleic acid (either RNA or, as in the case of retroviruses, DNA) and a viral attachment protein.

Description of stages of replication of both DNA & RNA viruses representing the 7 groups are mentioned below.

Replicaion of Adenoviruses

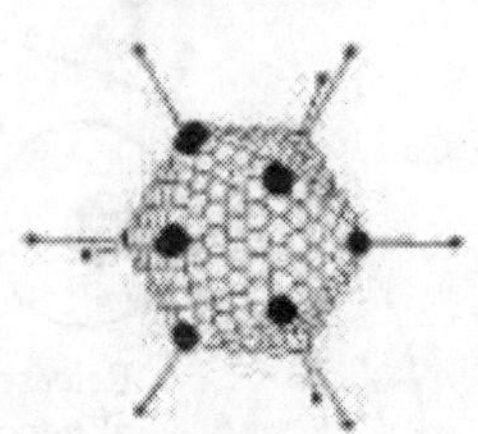

Non-enveloped, 80-100 in diameter, genome 36-44kb, the ds DNA is linear, associated with virally coded, basic proteins in virion, adenoviruses **code for their own DNA polymerase and DNA packaging proteins**, they use host factors in addition to viral protein for DNA replication, and they use **host RNA polymerase and RNA modification systems** and so nucleic acid synthesis needs to be in the nucleus.

Adsorption and penetration

The knob domain of the fiber protein binds to 2 types of cell receptors-CD46 for the group B human adenovirus serotypes, and the coxsackie virus & adenovirus receptor (CAR) for all other serotypes. The virus is engulfed by endocytosis. The virus appears to be able to lyze endosomes. Uncoating occurs in steps, & DNA is released into the nucleus at a nuclear pore **(Figure 3 -4)**.

Early phase

Immediate early and early mRNAs are transcribed from the viral DNA. Transcription of the Adenovirus genome is regulated by virus-encoded trans-acting regulatory factors. Products of the immediate early genes regulate expression of the early genes. Early genes are encoded at various locations on both strands of the DNA. Multiple protein products are made from each gene by alternative splicing of mRNA transcripts. Adenovirus **uses host cell RNA polymerase** and early mRNAs are transcribed from scattered regions of both strands. Multiple promoters result in more flexible control. mRNAs are processed by host cell capping, methylation, polyadenylation and sometimes splicing enzyme systems, they are then exported to the cytoplasm and translated.

The early proteins include those needed for transcription (E1A protein is needed for transcription of the other early genes); as a result these other genes are sometimes referred to as delayed early genes and E1A is referred to as an immediate early gene, are needed for adenovirus DNA synthesis includes DNA polymerase & alter expression of host cell genes. This includes genes whose products interfere with the host anti-viral response and/or interfere with cell cycle regulation

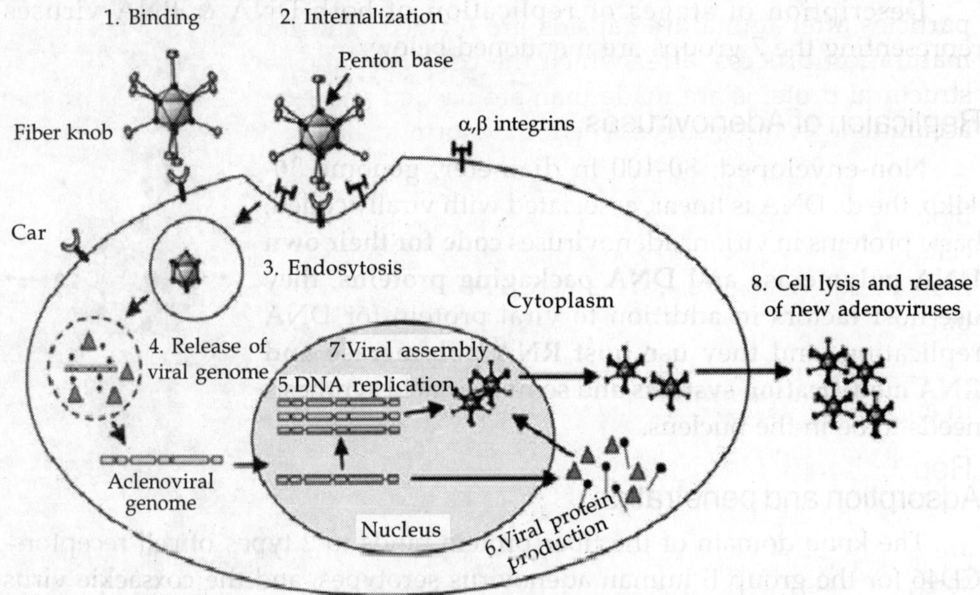

Figure 3–4 : Stages of adenovirus replication cycle.

Late phase

DNA replication

Adenovirus encodes its own **DNA polymerase**, which is one of the early proteins. The DNA is replicated by a strand displacement mechanism. There are no Okasaki fragments, both strands are synthesized in a continuous fashion.

DNA polymerases cannot initiate synthesis *de novo*, **they need a primer.** In the case of adenovirus, the virally coded **terminal protein acts as a primer**. It is thus found covalently linked to the 5' end of all adenovirus DNA strands.

Late transcription

Late mRNAs code predominantly for structural proteins and there is one major late promoter. The primary transcript is processed to generate various monocistronic mRNAs. There are two types of cleavage of primary transcript:

i. to generate various 3' ends which are then polyadenylated
ii. for intron removal

It is not understood how this process is controlled such that the correct amounts of each mRNA are made. Probably the virus makes more mRNAs and proteins than are needed for virion assembly, so precise control may not be necessary.

Assembly of adenovirus particles occurs in the nucleus. DNA enters the particles after immature capsids are formed. The capsids then undergo a maturation process, after which the cells lyse and virions leak out. More structural proteins are made than are needed and excess structural proteins accumulate in the nucleus where they form inclusion bodies.

Adenovirus can induce transformation: a change in the morphological, biochemical or growth parameters of the cell, which may or may not result in cells which are able to produce tumours in experimental animals. **E1A** can immortalize primary cells in vitro. **E1B** does not transform cells on its own, but "cooperates" with E1A to stably transform cells.

E1A + E1B are necessary for full transformation and tumour formation in animals.

Replication of Herpesviruses

Enveloped, icosahedral, virions 180-200nm, genome linear, dsDNA, there are no obvious blocks of early or late genes, they are more independent than some of the smaller viruses.

Adsorption and penetration

Many herpesviruses, including herpes simplex virus, can **fuse** directly with the cell plasma membrane causing partial uncoating. Capsids are transported towards the nucleus and the DNA passes into the nucleus.

Early phase

In herpesviruses there is no apparent organization of the genome into blocks for either early or late transcription. Early transcription i.e. mRNAs made during this phase are the α and β mRNAs. Herpesviruses use **host RNA polymerase**. However, a virion tegument protein (VP16) enters the nucleus upon infection and is important as part of the transcription factor complex recognized by the host RNA polymerase. The virus uses host mRNA modification enzymes. Firstly, α-mRNAs are transcribed. These are the **immediate early mRNAs** and are exported to the cytoplasm and translated into á -proteins, & transported into nucleus where they enable the β -promoters to be used by the host RNA polymerase.

β -mRNAs are transcribed by **host RNA polymerase.** β -genes are still early since they are transcribed prior to DNA synthesis.

Therefore, alpha-genes are called "immediate early" and beta-genes are called "early". β-proteins are involved in gene expression regulation. They decrease α alpha-gene expression and are needed for γ gene expression. They are also involved in various aspects of DNA synthesis; for example, herpes β -genes code for a variety of proteins including: DNA polymerase, DNA binding proteins, thymidine kinase & ribonucleotide reductase.

Late phase

DNA replication

Herpesviruses code for several proteins, & DNA polymerase, that are needed for DNA replication. DNA replication is accompanied by a lot of recombination. The replicated DNA is present as long concatameric molecules (tandem repeats of the genome linked head-to-tail). These are cleaved to genome-size lengths when the DNA is packaged into the virion. Some herpesviruses (e.g. herpes simplex virus) have a genome structure in which two parts of the genome can invert relative to each other, others do not. Late transcription:

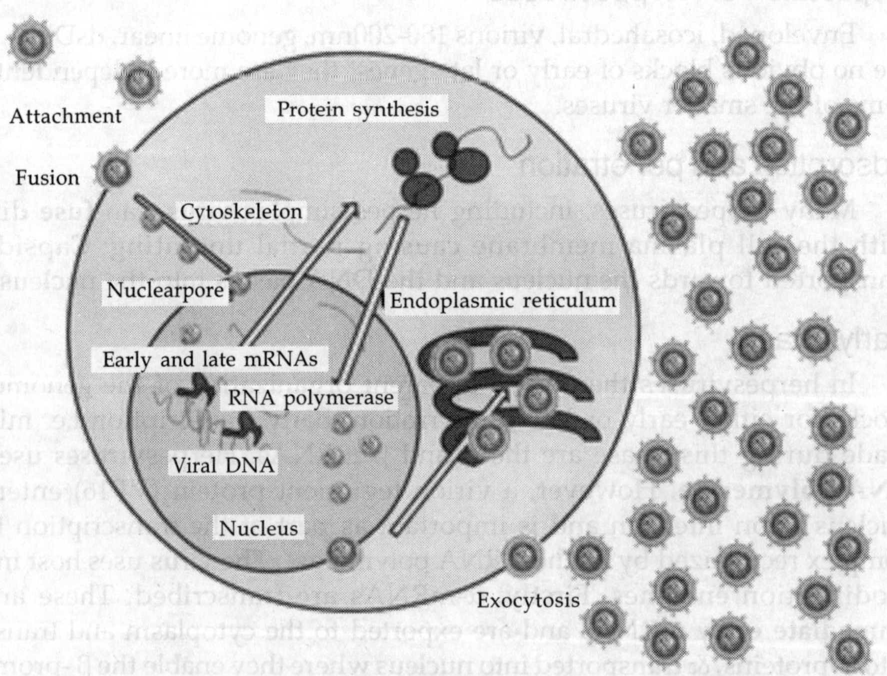

Figure 3.5 : Stages of herpesvirus replication cycle

Late transcription occurs after DNA replication. γ mRNAs are made and are translated in the cytoplasm, & are predominantly structural. There is decreased expression of β genes in the late stage. This is probably due to down-regulation of transcription of β genes by one of the γ proteins.

Assembly

Assembly occurs in the nucleus. A capsid is formed and the DNA enters the capsid. The capsids acquire an envelope by budding through areas of the **inner nuclear membrane** which have viral membrane proteins inserted into them **(Fig 3-5)**. These areas have tegument proteins associated with the inner face of the inner nuclear membrane. The virus envelope then fuses with the outer nuclear membrane and the de-enveloped nucleocapsid is delivered into the cytoplasm, where it acquires a more mature tegument. It then becomes re-enveloped by budding into Golgi-derived vesicles and is then released. The late protein required for transcription of immediate early mRNAs in the next round of infection is packaged in the virion. Excess structural proteins accumulate in nucleus, often form inclusion bodies.

In order to establish **latency,** the virus enters sensory neurons, which are non-dividing, and replicates infrequently. Latency-associated transcripts (LAT) are the only mRNAs that are expressed during latency, and these proteins serve to help the neuron survive initial infection. LAT are also required to establish and maintain viral latency and for the virus to be reactivated from latency.

Replication of Papillomaviruses

Papillomaviruses are non-enveloped, small: 40-60nm, icosahedral: circular, ds DNA is associated with cell histones, major capsid protein is VP1, with lesser amounts of VP2, VP3, & are difficult to grow in culture.

Papillomaviruses gain access to keratinocyte stem cells through small wounds, known as microtraumas, in the skin or mucosal surface. Interactions between L1 and sulfated sugars on the cell surface promote initial attachment of the virus. The virus is then able to get inside from the cell surface via interaction with a specific receptor, likely via the alpha-6 beta-4 integrin, and transported to membrane-enclosed endosomes. The capsid protein L2 disrupts the membrane of the endosome, allowing the viral genome to escape and traffic, along with L2, to the cell nucleus.

Viral Persistence

After successful infection of a keratinocyte, the virus expresses E1 and E2 proteins, which are for replicating and maintaining the viral DNA as a circular episome. The viral ongogenes E6 and E7 promote cell growth by inactivating the tumor suppressor proteins p53 and pRb. Keratinocyte stem cells in the epithelial basement layer can maintain papillomavirus genomes for decades.

Production of progeny virus

The expression of the viral late genes, L1 and L2, is exclusively restricted to differentiating keratinocytes in the outermost layers of the skin or mucosal surface. The increased expression of L1 and L2 is typically correlated with a dramatic increase in the number of copies of the viral genome. Since the outer layers of stratified squamous epithelia are subject to relatively limited surveillance by cells of the immune system, it is thought that this restriction of viral late gene expression represents a form of immune evasion.

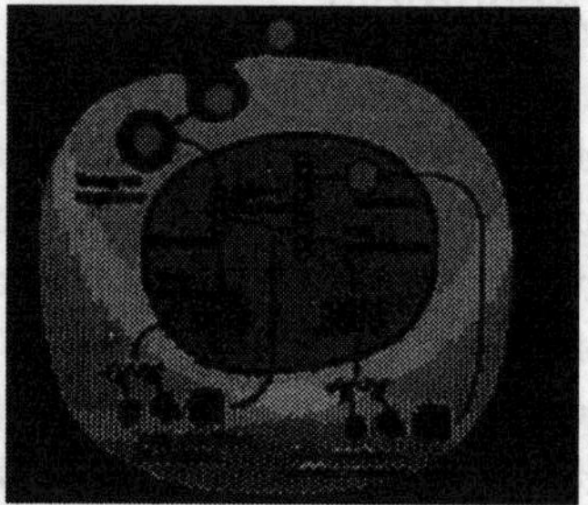

Figure 3-6 : Stages of papillomavirus replication cycle

New infectious progeny viruses are assembled in the cell nucleus. Papillomaviruses have evolved a mechanism for releasing virions into the environment. Other kinds of non-enveloped animal viruses utilize an active lytic process to kill the host cell, allowing release of progeny virus particles. Often this lytic process is associated with inflammation, which might trigger immune attack against the virus. Papillomaviruses exploit desquamation as a stealthy, non-inflammatory release mechanism.

Cancer

Several types of human papillomaviruses (HPVs) have been identified that cause specific types of cancers. The etiology of cancer of the cervix has been linked to a high preponderance of HPV16. The role of these virus infections has been established 1) by the regular presence of HPV DNA in the respective tumor biopsy specimens, 2) by the demonstration of viral oncogene expression (E6 and E7) in tumor material, 3) by the identification of transforming properties of these genes, 4) by the requirement for E6 and E7 expression for maintaining the malignant phenotype of cervical carcinoma cell lines, 5) by the interaction of viral oncoproteins with growth-regulating host-cell proteins, and 6) by epidemiologic studies pointing to these HPV infections as the major risk factor for cervical cancer development. Also, a major proportion of anal, perianal, vulvar, and penile cancers appear to be linked to the same HPV infections. In addition, close to 20% of oropharyngeal cancers contain DNA from the same types of HPV. Recent evidence also points to a possible role of other HPV infections in squamous cell carcinomas of the skin. Modifications in host-cell genes, most likely engaged in the control of

HPV gene expression in proliferating cells, emerge as important events in HPV-mediated carcinogenesis.

Replication of Polyomavirses

Polyomaviruses are non-enveloped, small (~40nm diameter), icosahedral, small circular genome ~5kb the possessing early and late genes, replicate in the nucleus. Depending on the host cell, they can either transform the cell or replicate the virus and lyze the cell. Early and late functions, multiple use of the same DNA sequence-alternative splicing, overlapping reading frames, multifunctional protein (T antigen), virus codes for a very limited number of proteins, & host cell provides RNA synthesis machinery, RNA modification machinery, DNA synthesis machinery, & histones for packaging DNA are the features of these viruses.

Life cycle

Attachment, penetration & uncoating

Viral capsid proteins interact with cell surface receptors and penetration is via endocytosis. Cellular receptors for polyomaviruses are sialic acid residues of gangliosides. The attachment of polyomaviruses to host cells is mediated by viral protein 1 (VP1) via the sialic acid attachment region. Virions are transported to the nucleus and uncoated. DNA and associated histones enters nucleus through a nuclear pore.

Production of viral mRNAs & proteins

Gene expression is divided into early and late phases. **Early genes** encode enzymes and regulatory proteins needed to start viral replication.**Late genes** encode structural proteins, & proteins needed for assembly of the mature virus.

Early phase of lytic cycle

The early promoter is recognized by **host RNA polymerase II** (SV40 contains a strong enhancer). Post transcriptional RNA modification (capping, methylation, polyadenylation, splicing etc.) is carried out by host enzymes. The early transcript (primary transcript) is made and then undergoes alternative processing, resulting in the mRNAs for the small T and large T antigens (these proteins have common amino-termini but different carboxy-termini). The mRNAs are translated in the cytoplasm.

Late phase of lytic cycle

The late phase starts with the onset of viral genome replication.

DNA replication

SV40/polyoma DNA replication occurs in the nucleus. **Large T antigen is needed for DNA replication. This binds to the origin of replication.** Polyomaviruses **use the host cell DNA polymerase**, which recognizes the viral origin of replication if the T antigen is present. DNA replication is bidirectional-there are two replication forks per circular DNA genome and replication involves leading/lagging strands, Okasaki fragments, DNA ligase etc. This process of DNA replication is very similar to that which occurs in the host cell - which is not surprising as the virus is using mainly host machinery except for the involvement of the T antigen. Host histone complexes with the newly made DNA.

Late mRNAs are made after DNA replication as a lot of newly made viral DNA is now available as template. Early mRNAs are still transcribed, but at a very much lower rate. T antigen is involved in controlling increased transcription from the late promoter and decreased transcription from early promoter. It also interacts with host proteins and changes the properties of the host cell, thus playing a role in cell transformation and tumor formation.

VP1, VP2, and VP3 are made from same primary transcript which undergoes differential splicing. This results in the reading frame for VP1 being different from that for VP2 and VP3. Thus, one region of the DNA can code for two different amino acid sequences according to which reading frame is used. This is another way that viruses can use a short stretch of DNA to code for more than one protein sequence.

Assembly

VP1, 2 and 3 mRNAs are translated in the cytoplasm, the proteins are transported to nucleus, and capsids assemble with DNA (and cell histones) inside the capsid. Large numbers of capsids accumulate in the nucleus and form inclusion bodies. Virions are released by cell lysis.

Cytoplasmic DNA viruses

Replication of Poxviruses

Poxviruses are enveloped, large virions with large genome, dsDNA viruses, & the virus has unusual capabilities compared to other viruses. Poxviruses may be possible agents of bioterrorism, & are used in new techniques of vaccine development such as genetically-engineered vaccinia virus. Two distinct infectious virus particles, the intracellular mature virus (IMV) and the extracellular enveloped virus (EEV) can initiate infection. Poxviruses replicate in the cytoplasm. This means that they must provide their own mRNA and DNA synthetic machinery. Vaccinia is the most intensively studied member of the poxvirus family.

Adsorption and penetration

The virus binds to cell surface receptors. The binding of the virion is determined by several virion proteins and by glycosaminoglycans (GAGs) on the surface of the target cell or by components of the extracellular matrix. It enters cells via endocytosis or by direct fusion of the virus with the plasma membrane. The virus is then released into the cytoplasm, minus its membrane.

Early phase & early transcription

After the initial phase of uncoating has occurred, the virus can make a limited number of mRNAs-the immediate early mRNAs. The poxvirus has virally coded **DNA-dependent RNA polymerase** to make their RNAs. "Naked" vaccinia DNA which has had all the protein removed is thus not infectious, since it will have no RNA polymerase associated with it, and nothing can happen in the vaccinia life cycle without the vaccinia RNA polymerase since no RNA or proteins can be made.

Poxvirus mRNAs are capped, methylated and polyadenylated just like standard eucaryotic mRNAs, but host cell mRNAs are modified in the nucleus and vaccinia replicates in the cytoplasm. Since Vaccinia is cytoplasmic, these modifications must be carried out by **virally-coded** enzymes. The modifying enzymes are packaged in virions and thus those mRNAs made immediately upon infection can be modified. So far, no spliced mRNAs have been reported for vaccinia. One of the immediate early mRNA translation products is an **uncoating enzyme**. This allows further uncoating of the vaccinia DNA and more genes can now be transcribed - the early genes are now all expressed. Poxviruses are exceptional in that they code for an uncoating protein which has to be made in the newly infected cell before uncoating can be completed.

Virus production "factories" are seen in the cytoplasm - sites of vaccinia virus replication. The early proteins are involved in DNA replication, RNA transcription, RNA modification and uncoating. They also include a few structural proteins.

Late phase

DNA synthesis

DNA synthesis occurs in "factories" and uses an unusual mechanism.

Late transcription and translation

This is a complex process. Some late proteins are made throughout the late phase, but others only at the beginning of late phase. Some early proteins are not synthesized once DNA replication commences while other early proteins are made during late as well as early phases. Thus, there is complex control of which proteins are made by vaccinia and when they are made. This means that there are controls other than just early/late controls.

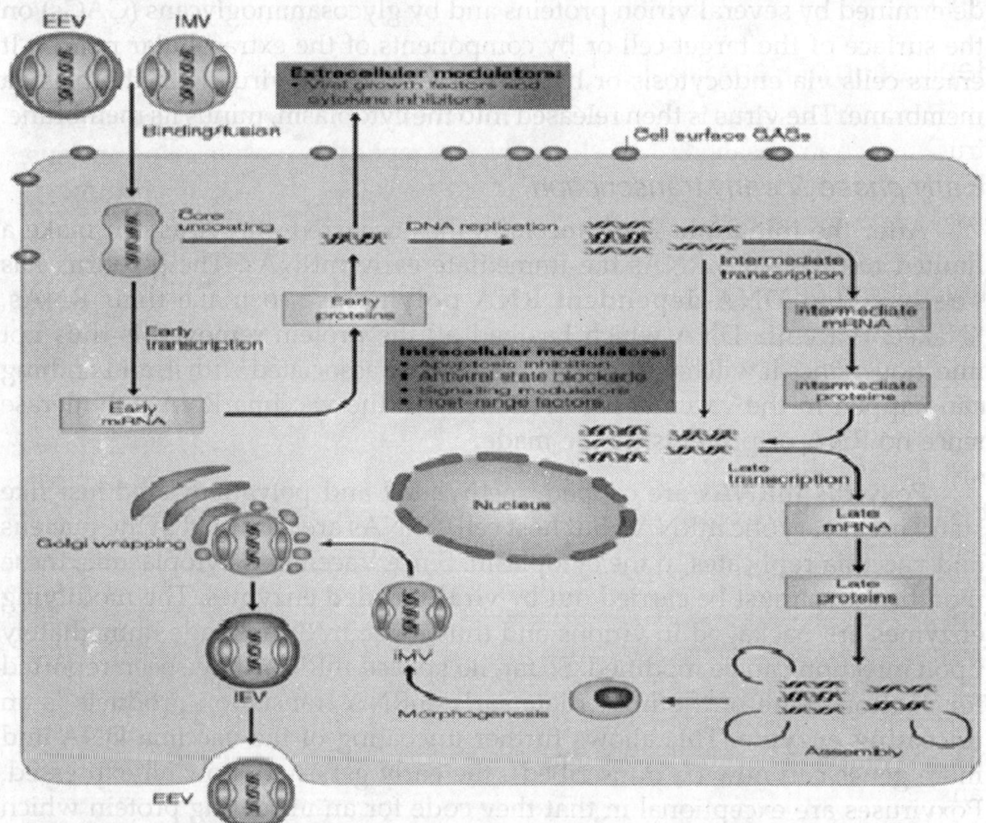

Figure 3.7 : Stages of poxvirus replication cycle

Assembly

Assembly occurs in "factories" in the cytoplasm. The new, immature virus particles acquire a membrane while in the cytoplasm - the exact mechanism is not fully understood but it seems that the virus gets "wrapped" by cellular membranes. The initial intracellular mature virus (IMV) is transported via microtubules and is wrapped with Golgi-derived membrane, after which it is referred to as an intracellular enveloped virus (IEV). The IEV fuses to the cell surface membrane to form cell-associated enveloped virus (CEV), which is either extruded away from the cell by actin-tail polymerization or is released to form free EEV. EEV might also form by direct budding of IMV, therefore bypassing the IEV form. The older idea that a membrane is formed directly from lipids rather than from a pre-existing membrane is not correct. There is a gradual maturation of enveloped particles. The virus is usually released by host cell disintegration, but some may get out by budding through membranes (in which case they have an extra membrane). Both forms appear to be infectious. The exact mechanism by which the virus gets out of infected cells may depend on host cell type.

Replication of Parvoviruses

Parvoviruses are non-enveloped, very small 18 to -25nm diameter, ss DNA viruses, have an icosahedral capsid, and DNA replication occurs in the nucleus. Human parvovirus B-19 replicates in dividing cells–primarily in erythrocyte progenitors in the bone marrow.

Attachment, penetration

Parvoviruses bind to a sialic acid-bearing cell surface receptor. Penetration into the cytoplasm is mediated by a phospholipid A2 activity carried on the amino-terminal peptide of the capsid VP1 polypeptide. Once in the cytoplasm, the intact virus is translocated to the nucleus prior to uncoating. Transcription only initiates when the host cell enters S-phase under its own cell cycle control, at which time the cell's replication machinery converts the incoming single strand into a duplex transcription template, allowing synthesis of mRNAs encoding the non-structural proteins, NS1 and NS2. The mRNAs are transported out of the nucleus into the Cytoplasm where the host ribosomes translate them into viral proteins. Viral DNA replication proceeds through a series of monomeric and concatemeric duplex intermediates by a unidirectional strand-displacement mechanism that is mediated by components of the cellular fork, aided and orchestrated by the viral NS1 polypeptide. NS1 also transactivates an internal transcriptional promoter that directs synthesis of

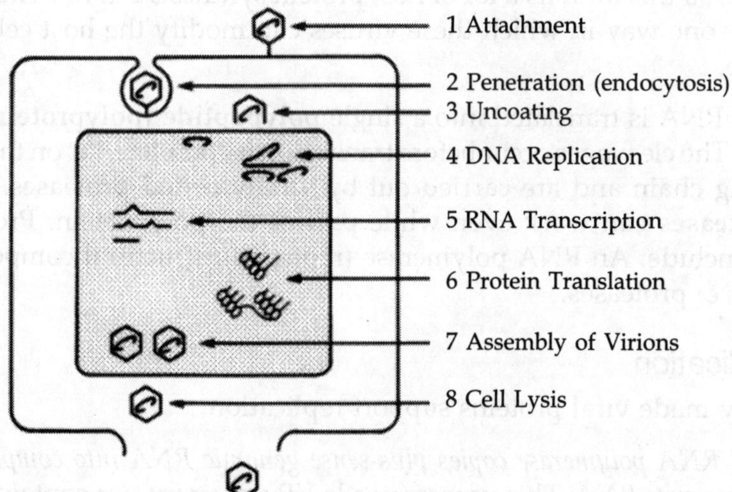

Figure 3-8 : Stages of parvovirus replication cycle

the structural VP polypeptides. Once assembled capsids are available, replication shifts from synthesizing duplex DNA to displacement of progeny single strands, which are typically negative-sense and are packaged in a 3'-to-5' direction into preformed particles within the nucleus. Mature virions may be released from infected cells prior to cell lysis, which promotes rapid transmission of the virus, but if this fails then the virus is released at cell lysis.

Replication of Picornaviruses

These are small (28nm), naked icosahedral, (+) ss RNA viruses, polyadenylated. It functions as mRNA immediately upon infection. Prototype member: poliovirus.

Adsorption and penetration

The genome RNA has a protein on the 5' end that is used as a primer for transcription by RNA polymerase. A viral protein recognizes a receptor on the host cell membrane. Binding to the receptor causes a conformational change in the viral capsid proteins, and myristic acid are released, & form a pore in the cell membrane through which RNA is injected. The mRNA is now available for translation.

Synthesis of viral proteins

Poliovirus virion RNA functions as an mRNA but does not have the methylated cap structure of eucaryotic mRNAs, but it has the **internal ribosome entry site or IRES** which enables ribosomes to bind without having to recognize a 5' methylated cap structure. Most host cell translation is cap-dependent, so this inhibits a lot of host protein synthesis but not viral protein synthesis - one way in which these viruses can modify the host cell to their advantage.

The mRNA is translated into a single **polypeptide (polyprotein)**, which is cleaved. The cleavages occur before translation is complete, i.e. on the nascent or growing chain and are carried out by virally coded proteases. Some of these **proteases** can work even while part of the polyprotein. Products of cleavage include: An RNA polymerase (replicase), structural components of the virion, & proteases.

RNA replication

Newly made viral proteins support replication.

1. *Viral RNA polymerase copies plus-sense genomic RNA into complementary minus-sense RNA*: This process needs VPg or precursor containing VPg, Viral RNA polymerase (replicase) & certain host proteins. VPg may act

as a primer for RNA synthesis; this would explain why it is at the 5' end of all newly synthesized RNA molecules.

2. New minus sense strands serve as template for new plus sense strands. Again, poliovirus RNA polymerase and VPg are needed. VPg is linked to the 5' ends of the new plus sense strands that functions as a primer.

The new plus strand has three alternative fates:

i. It may serve as a template for more minus strands

ii. It may be packaged into progeny virions.

iii. It may be translated into polyprotein (in this case VPg is usually removed prior to translation).

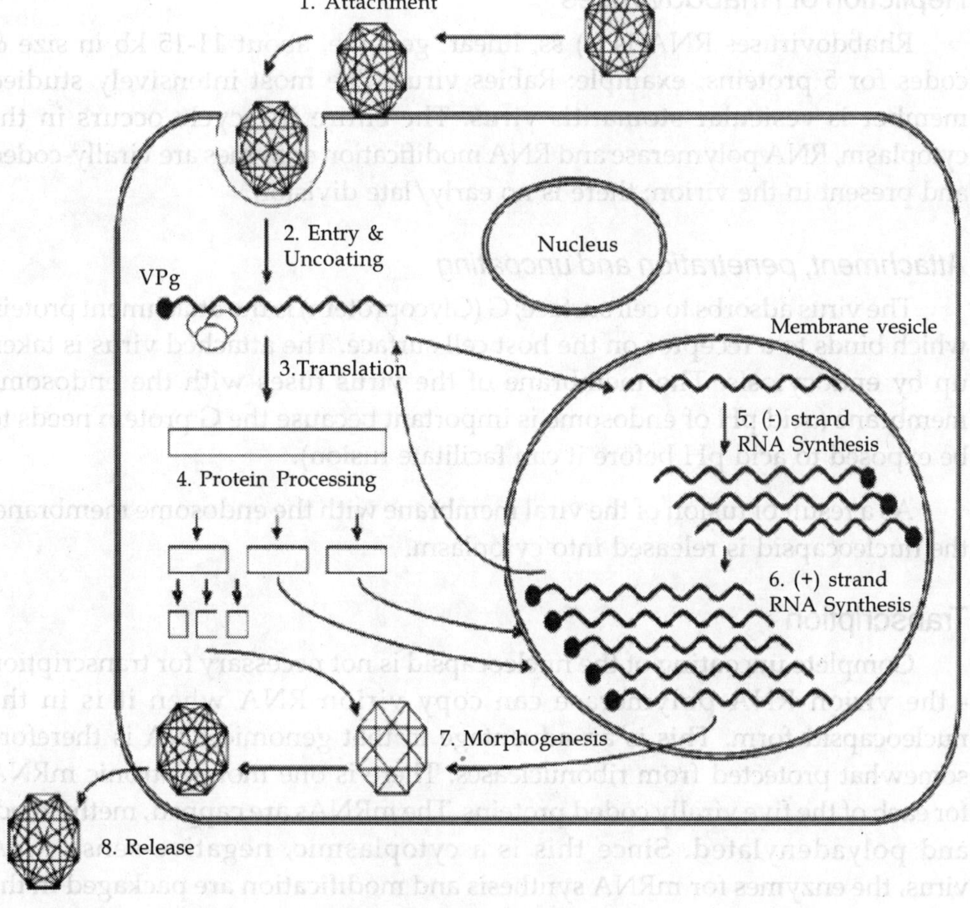

Figure 3.9 : Stages of picornavirus replication cycle

Assembly

When sufficient plus-sense progeny RNA and virion proteins have accumulated, assembly begins. Particles assemble with VPg-RNA inside and 3 proteins in the capsid -VP0,1 and 3. VP0 is then cleaved to VP2 and VP4 as the virions mature and these mature virions are infectious. Virions are released following **cell lysis**. Excess capsids are formed and inclusion bodies may be seen in the cytoplasm.

The entire life cycle occurs in the cytoplasm; there is no division into early and late gene expression.

Non-Segmented Negative Strand Viruses

Examples are: rhabdovirus , paramyxoviruses

Repliction of Rhabdoviruses

Rhabdoviruses RNA is (-) ss, linear, genome, about 11-15 kb in size & codes for 5 proteins, example: Rabies virus. The most intensively studied member is vesicular stomatitis virus. The entire life cycle occurs in the cytoplasm, RNA polymerase and RNA modification enzymes are virally-coded and present in the virion; there is no early/late division.

Attachment, penetration and uncoating

The virus adsorbs to cell surface; G (Glycoprotein) is the attachment protein which binds to a receptor on the host cell surface. The attached virus is taken up by endocytosis. The membrane of the virus fuses with the endosome membrane (acid pH of endosome is important because the G protein needs to be exposed to acid pH before it can facilitate fusion).

As a result of fusion of the viral membrane with the endosome membrane, the nucleocapsid is released into cytoplasm.

Transcription

Complete uncoating of the nucleocapsid is not necessary for transcription - the virion RNA polymerase can copy virion RNA when it is in the nucleocapsid form. This is an advantage in that genomic RNA is therefore somewhat protected from ribonucleases. There is one monocistronic mRNA for each of the five virally coded proteins. The mRNAs are capped, methylated, and polyadenylated. Since this is a cytoplasmic, negative-sense RNA virus, the enzymes for mRNA synthesis and modification are packaged in the virion.

Translation

The mRNAs are translated on host ribosomes and all five viral proteins made at the same time. There is no distinction between early and late functions.

RNA replication

RNA replication is the process by which new copies of genome-length RNAs are made. RNA replication occurs in the cytoplasm and is carried out by the viral RNA polymerase. The full length plus strand is coated with nucleocapsid protein as it is made (mRNAs are not coated with this protein, which would interfere with the host protein translation machinery.

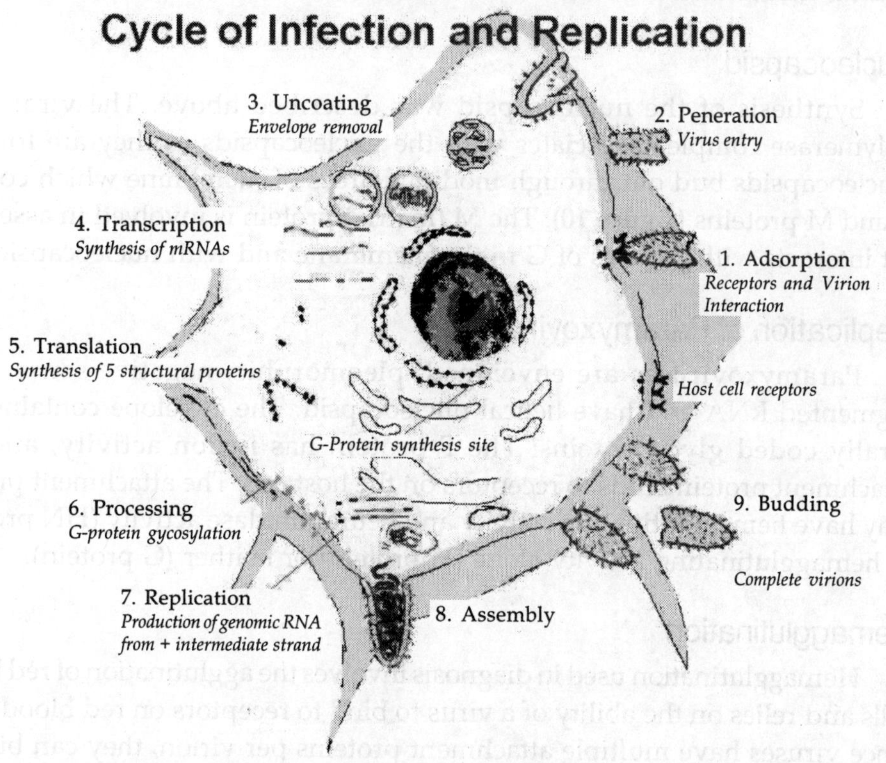

Figure 3.10 : Stages of rhabdovirus replication cycle.

The new positive strand is copied into full length minus strand, which is also coated with nucleocapsid protein as it is made. Since the viral RNA polymerase synthesizes mRNAs (transcription) and full-length RNA (replication), it is also sometimes called a transcriptase or a replicase. New negative strands may: i. be used as templates for the synthesis of more full length plus strands, ii. be used as templates for the synthesis of more mRNAs & iii. be packaged into virions.

Assembly

The virus consists of the envelope and the nucleocapsid:

Envelope

Transmembrane proteins are made on ribosomes bound to the **endoplasmic reticulum**. They are inserted into the endoplasmic reticulum membrane as they are made, glycosylated in the endoplasmic reticulum and pass through the Golgi body where substantial modification of the carbohydrate chains occurs. They are then transported, in vesicles, to the appropriate cell membrane; in the case of vesicular stomatitis virus, this is the plasma membrane.

Nucleocapsid

Synthesis of the nucleocapsid was described above. The viral RNA polymerase complex associates with the nucleocapsids as they are formed. Nucleocapsids bud out through modified areas of membrane which contain G and M proteins **(figure 10)**. The M (matrix) protein is involved in assembly - it interacts with patches of G in the membrane and with nucleocapsids.

Replication of Paramyxoviruses

Paramyxoviruses are enveloped, pleomorphic, negative-sense, non-segmented RNA and have helical nucleocapsid. The envelope contains two virally coded glycoproteins: The F protein has fusion activity, and the attachment protein binds to receptors on the host cell. The attachment protein may have hemagglutinating activity and neuraminidase activity (HN protein) or hemagglutinating activity alone (H protein) or neither (G protein).

Hemagglutination

Hemagglutination used in diagnosis involves the agglutination of red blood cells and relies on the ability of a virus to bind to receptors on red blood cells. Since viruses have multiple attachment proteins per virion, they can bind to more than one red blood cell and so they can serve to link red blood cells into a network. Inactivated virus can still hemagglutinate as long as its attachment proteins are intact. If someone has antibodies to a viral hemagglutinin, the antibodies will binds to the attachment protein and prevent its binding to the red blood cells. The serum of that person will inhibit the agglutination reaction by the virus to which they have antibodies - but not by other hemagglutinating viruses. This can be used to determine which hemagglutinating virus a person has been exposed to.

Hemadsorption

During infection, the viral attachment protein will be inserted into the plasma membrane of the infected cell. If the viral attachment protein can bind to red blood cells, the infected cell will bind red blood cells because it has the viral attachment protein on its surface - this is called hemadsorption. In the clinical laboratory, this may enable virally-infected cells to be detected at an early stage in infection, and may allow detection of viruses which do not visibly damage the cell.

Adsorption and penetration

The H (N)/G protein recognizes receptors on cell surface. The F protein facilitates fusion between membranes at physiological pH, so although paramyxoviruses can be taken up by endocytosis, they also often enter the cell by direct fusion with the plasma membrane **(figure 13)**. Because the F protein functions at physiological pH, this can result in syncytia being formed in paramyxovirus infections.

Transcription, translation and replication of RNA

Events inside the cell are very similar to rhabdoviruses. Viral multiplication occurs in the cytoplasm. The viral RNA polymerase uses the nucleocapsid as a template. The RNA polymerase does not need a fully uncoated nucleocapsid.

Viral mRNAs are transcribed; these are capped, methylated and polyadenylated. Since this is a negative-strand RNA virus, RNA polymerase and RNA modification enzymes are packaged in the virion. The viral mRNAs are translated to give viral proteins. There is no distinction between early and late functions in gene expression.

Viral RNA replication involves full length plus strand synthesis. This is used as a template for full length minus strand. Both full length strands are coated with nucleocapsid protein as they are made.

New full length minus strands may serve as templates for replication, or templates for transcription, or they may be packaged into new virions.

Assembly

Both viral glycoproteins (i.e. attachment protein and F protein) are translated as transmembrane proteins and transported to the cell plasma membrane. M (matrix) protein enables nucleocapsids to interact with the regions of the plasma membrane which have the glycoproteins inserted. The virus buds out through membrane.

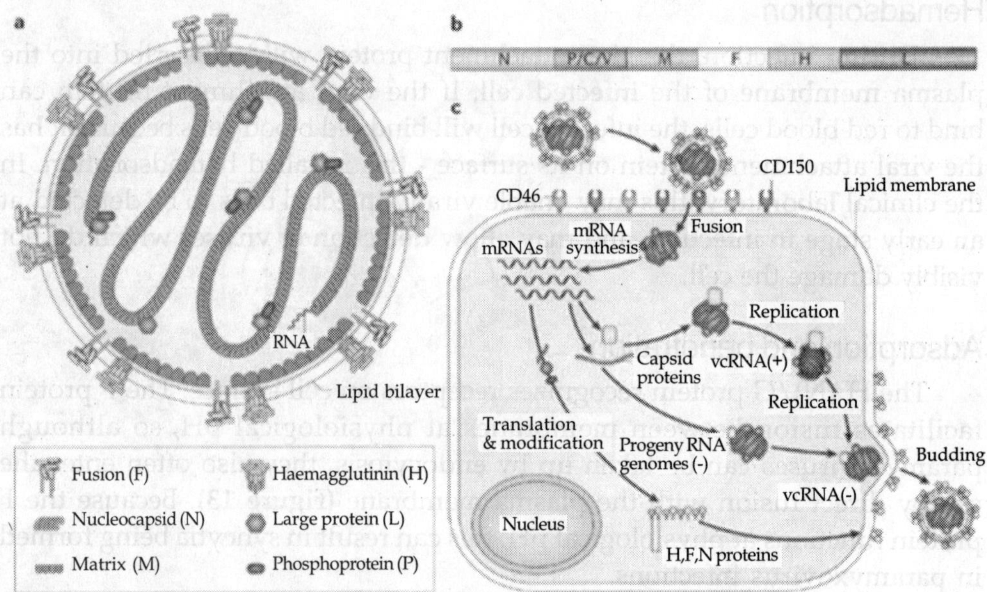

Figure 3.11 : Stages of paramyxovirus replication cycle

Role of neuraminidase

In those paramyxoviruses which have it, the neuraminidase may facilitate release. In these viruses, sialic acid appears to be an important part of the receptor. The neuraminidase removes sialic acid (neuraminic acid) from the cell surface. Thus, since sialic acid will have been largely removed from the cell surface and the progeny virions, neither will have functional receptors, so progeny virions will not stick to each other or to the cell they have just budded out from (or any other infected cell). They will therefore be able to diffuse away until they meet an uninfected cell.

The neuraminidase may also help during infection since, if the virus binds to sialic acid residues in mucus, it would not be able to bind to a receptor on a cell and infect that cell. But if the sialic acid in the mucus is eventually destroyed, the virus will be freed and may then reach a receptor on the cell surface.

Activation of the F protein

The F protein needs to be cleaved before it can function in facilitating fusion when the virus binds to another cell. This is a late event in maturation.

Segmented Negative Strand Viruses

Orthomyxoviruses, Bunyaviruses (include Hantavirus genus) & Arenaviruses.

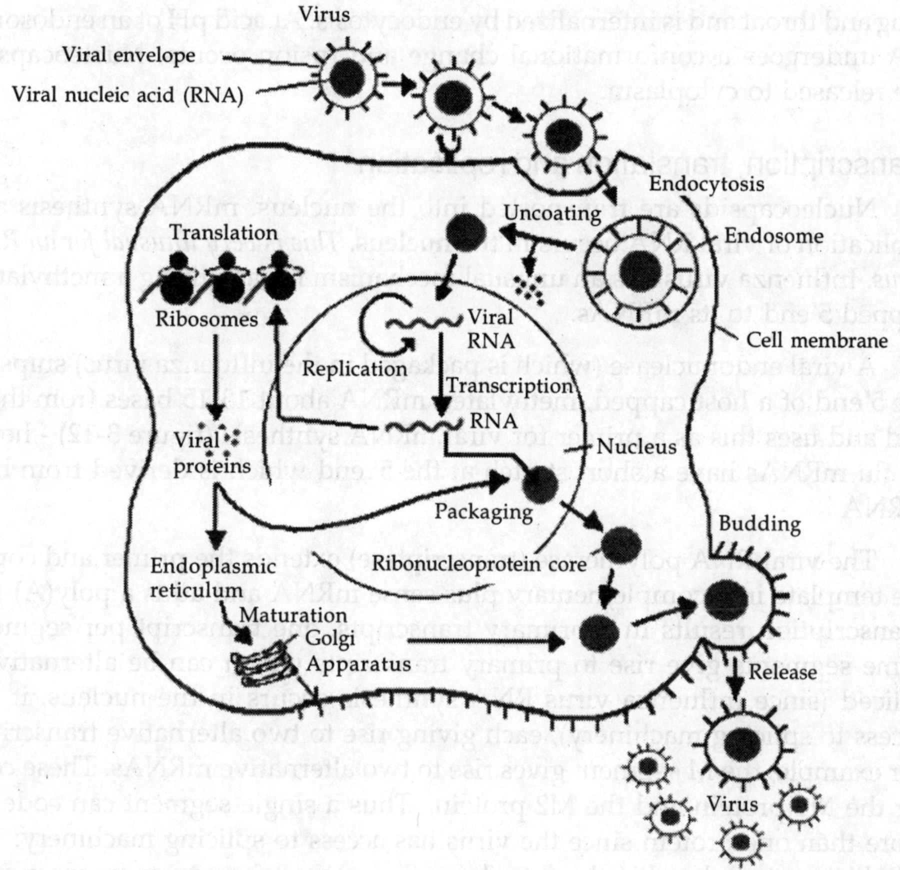

Figure 3.12 : Stages of orthomyxovirus replication cycle

Replication of Orthomyxoviruses

There are three Genera of *Influenzavirus: A, B and* C. Influenzavirus A is most intensively studied and influenzaviruses A and B are the most important in human disease. Influenza viruses are pleomorphic virions. They have negative-sense, single-stranded RNA and an RNA genome that is **segmented.** There are eight RNA segments in influenza A. The nucleocapsid is helical **(figure 19).** Virions contain RNA polymerase packaged within the virus particle. These viruses are enveloped and have two membrane glycoproteins: HA - hemagglutinin - this is the attachment and fusion protein, & NA - neuraminidase - this is important in release. It removes sialic acid from proteins of the virus and the host cell.

Adsorption and penetration

The virus adsorbs to a cell through interactions between its hemagglutinin glycoprotein and sialic acid sugars on the surfaces of epithelial cells in the lung and throat and is internalized by endocytosis. At acid pH of an endosome, HA undergoes a conformational change and fusion occurs. Nucleocapsids are released to cytoplasm.

Transcription, translation and replication

Nucleocapsids are transported into the nucleus. mRNA synthesis and replication of viral RNA occurs in the nucleus. *This is very unusual for an RNA virus.* Influenza virus has an unusual mechanism for acquiring a methylated, capped 5′end to its mRNAs.

A viral endonuclease (which is packaged in the influenza virus) snips off the 5′end of a host capped, methylated mRNA about 13-15 bases from the 5' end and uses this as a primer for viral mRNA synthesis (figure 3-12) - hence all flu mRNAs have a short stretch at the 5' end which is derived from host mRNA.

The viral RNA polymerase (transcriptase) extends the primer and copies the template into complementary plus sense mRNA and adds a poly(A) tail. Transcription results in 8 primary transcripts, one transcript per segment. Some segments give rise to primary transcripts which can be alternatively spliced (since influenza virus RNA synthesis occurs in the nucleus, it has access to splicing machinery), each giving rise to two alternative transcripts. For example, the M segment gives rise to two alternative mRNAs. These code for the M1 protein and the M2 protein. Thus a single segment can code for more than one protein since the virus has access to splicing machinery. The mRNAs are translated in the cytoplasm. Transmembrane proteins are moved to the plasma membrane while proteins needed for RNA replication are transported to the nucleus.

Replication of RNA

RNA replication occurs in the nucleus using a virus-coded enzyme (this may be same as the RNA polymerase involved in transcription of mRNAs, or a modified version). A full length, exact complementary copy of virion RNA is made - this plus sense RNA is probably coated with nucleocapsid protein as it is made. Full length plus strand RNA is then used as a template for full-length minus strand synthesis; again the new minus strand is probably coated with nucleocapsid protein as it is made. New minus strands can be used as templates for replication, mRNA synthesis, or packaged.

Assembly

This occurs at the plasma membrane. Nucleocapsids are transported out of the nucleus while envelope proteins are transported via the Golgi body to the plasma membrane. The M1 protein interacts with both nucleocapsid and a modified region of the plasma membrane which contains the glycoproteins HA and NA. Virus then buds out through the host cell.

HA needs to be cleaved before it can promote fusion. Cleavage occurs as the virus leaves the cell or in the extracellular fluid. The requirement for cleavage affects which tissues can produce infectious virus. The cleaved protein needs to then undergo a conformational change, usually caused by exposure to a acidic endosome environment when t infects the next cell, before it cause fusion.

NA probably helps the virus leave the cell by removing sialic acid from receptors. NA may also help the virus penetrate mucus to reach epithelial cells of the respiratory tract by enabling it to dissociate from sialic acid-containing receptors in the mucus by destroying them. The neuraminidase does not prevent the virus infecting new cells because endocytosis is presumably faster than receptor removal. There are similarities and differences between the Paramyxovirus family and the Orthomyxovirus family, members of both are enveloped, both contain negative sense, single stranded RNA, have helical nucleocapsids. However, the two families are very different. There is no immunological relationship between the two families.

Double Stranded RNA Viruses

Reoviridae

Reoviruses have icosahedral symmetry and a multiple layered capsid-inner and outer capsid, RNA is double stranded, with 10-12 segments. There are some significant differences in the life cycle of members of the reovirus family and of the rotavirus family. Due to their clinical importance in humans, we shall focus on rotaviruses.

Replication of Rotaviruses

(rota = wheel (from appearance of virions in the electron-microscope)

Adsorption, penetration and uncoating

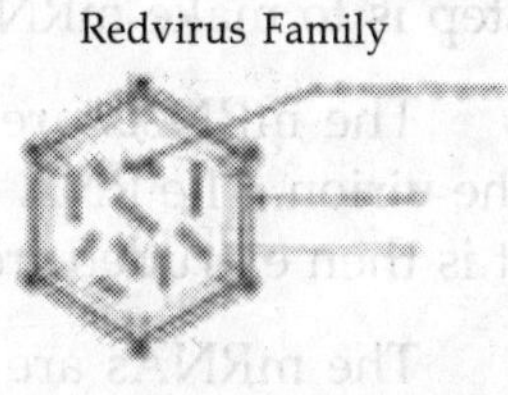
Redvirus Family

The virus enter cells by receptor mediated endocytosis and form a vesicles known as an endosome. Proteins in the third layer (VP7 and the VP4 spike) disrupt the membrane of the endosome, creating a difference in the calcium concentration. This causes the breakdown of VP7 trimer into single protein subunits, leaving the VP2 and VP6 protein coats around the viral dsRNA, forming a double-layered particle (DLP). The eleven dsRNA strands remain within the protection of the two protein shells and the viral RNA-dependent RNA polymerase creates mRNA transcripts of the double-stranded viral genome. In the cytoplasm, the virion RNA is copied by the viral RNA polymerase **while still in a nucleocapsid** that has fewer proteins associated with it than are associated with the virion.

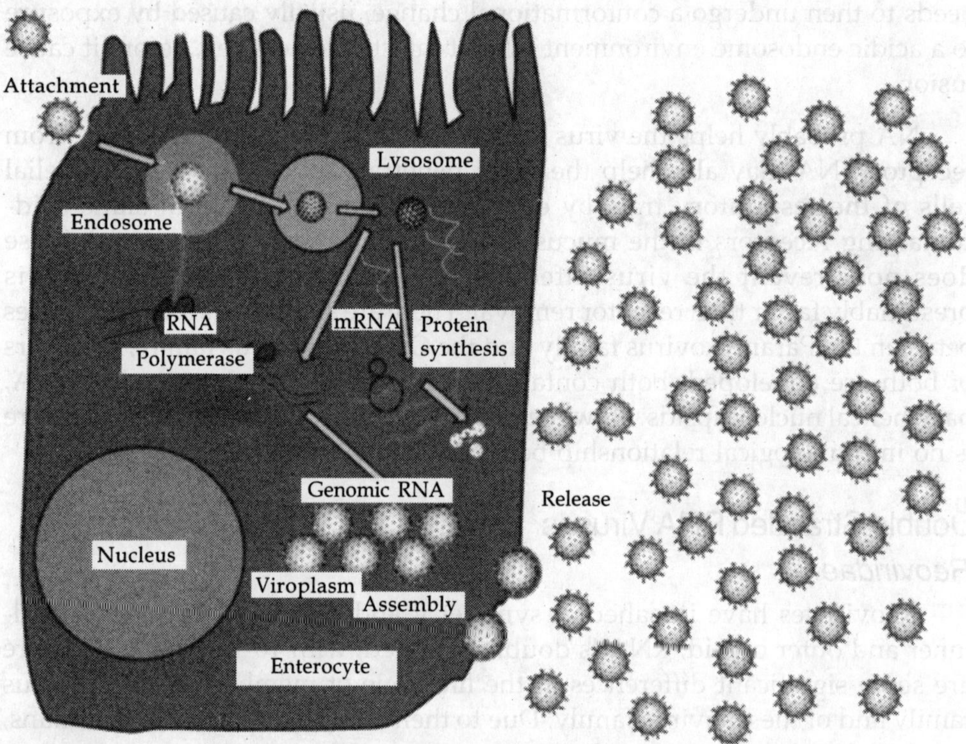

Figure 3.13 : Stages of rotavirus replication cycle

Transcription and translation

Double stranded RNA does not function as an mRNA and so the initial step is to make mRNA (transcription).

The mRNAs are made by virally-coded RNA polymerase packaged in the virion. The RNA is capped and methylated by virion packaged enzymes. It is then extruded from the vertices of the capsid.

The mRNAs are translated and the resulting viral proteins assemble to form an immature capsid. The mRNAs are packaged into the immature capsid and are then copied within the capsid to form double stranded RNAs (It is not known how the virus ensures that each particle gets one copy of the 11 different mRNAs) (figure 3.13). More mRNAs are now made by the newly formed immature capsids.

Assembly

More proteins are made and eventually the immature capsids bud into the lumen of the endoplasmic reticulum. In doing so, they acquire a transient envelope which is lost as they mature. This is a very odd feature of the rotaviruses.

Release

This probably occurs via cell lysis.

Replication of Retroviruses

Retroviruses are enveloped, labile carrying glycoprotein peplomers, measure 80-100 nm in diameter RNA-RT viruses, 3 layers-(a) inner **nucleoprotein** containing ++ viral RNA, reverse transcriptase, protease, integrase with helical nucleocapsid, (b) **icosahedral capsid**, (c) **envelope** carrying glycoprotein peplomers.

For retroviral entry, the envelope glycoprotein gp120, present on the surface of viral particles as gp41/gp120 trimers recognizes the primary receptor CD4. This interaction leads to conformational changes in both CD4 and gp120 and to the recruitment of coreceptors belonging to the chemokine receptor family, mainly CXCR4 and CCR5. A second interaction then takes place between gp120 and one of these coreceptors, which triggers new conformational shifts in the envelope glycoproteins. These sequential conformational changes finally lead to the dissociation of gp120 from gp41, and to the transition of gp41 to its fusogenic conformation. Entry of virions into the cell is achieved by insertion of the gp41 fusion peptide into the target membrane, resulting in the fusion of viral and cellular membranes and the release of the viral core in the cytoplasm. After entering the cell, the (+) strand of RNA is not associated with ribosomes, even though it has all the attributes of mRNA. Instead, the virion RNA is used as a template to make a DNA copy of the viral genome. This copying of RNA into DNA is foreign for the host cell and must be carried out by a viral enzyme that is packaged in virion. The viral enzyme, called *reverse transcriptase* carries out this process. The terms "reverse" and "retro" imply a mechanism that is the opposite of that normally operating in all cells. The usual flow of information in a cell is from DNA to RNA, not from RNA to DNA. The initial product of reverse transcription is an RNA:DNA hybrid double helix. The RNA portion of this hybrid is degraded and reverse transcriptase copies the remaining DNA strand into dsDNA. These processes take place in the cytoplasm. Once the viral dsDNA is synthesized,

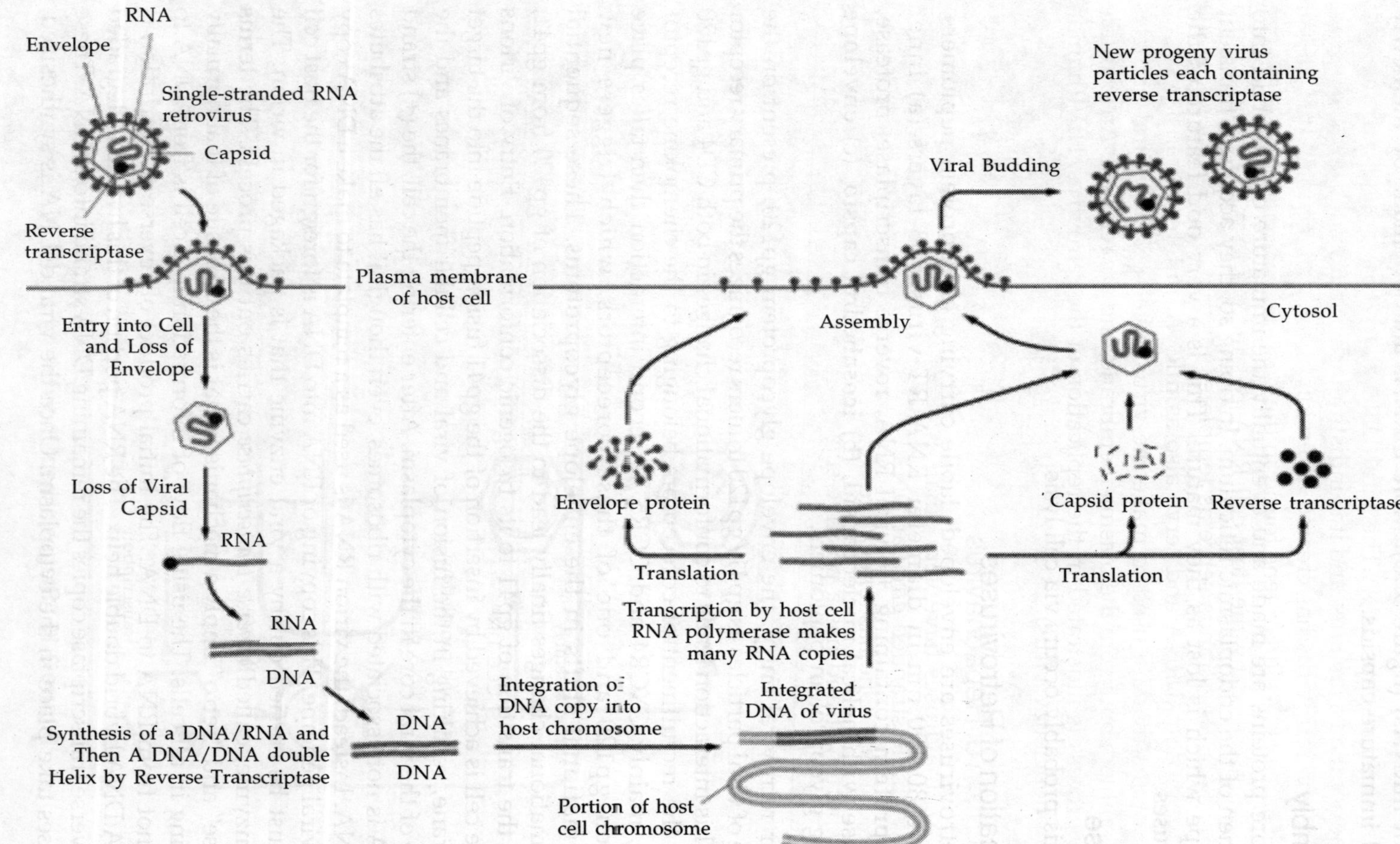

Figure 3.14: Stages of retroviral replication cycle

it is transported into the nucleus where it is inserted and covalently linked to the host chromosomal DNA.The viral DNA that is integrated into the host genome is called a *provirus,* and it is indistinguishable from the host cell genes. In effect, the retrovirus has created a version of the viral genome that has all the attributes of a cellular gene found in the host. The integrated provirus can now be transcribed by the host cell RNA polymerase to make virus-related RNA. These RNA strands serve as templates for making new copies of the viral chromosomal RNA and serve also as mRNA. mRNA is translated into viral proteins that are used to make the virus envelope. New viral particles are assembled, bud from the plasma membrane, and are released. An example of this process is illustrated in the replication of the retrovirus, HIV (human immunodeficiency virus).

Replication of Hepadnavirus

Hepadnaviruses have very small genome of partially double-stranded, partially single stranded circular DNA. The genome consists of two uneven strands of DNA. One has a negative-sense orientation & is complete, and the other, shorter, strand has a positive-sense orientation.

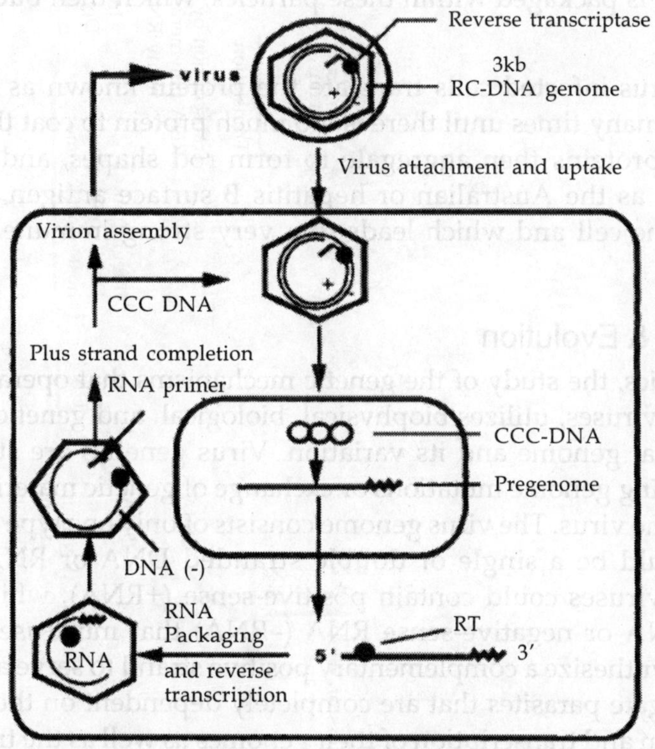

Figure 3.15 : Stages of hepadnavirus replication cycle.

The replication involves an RNA intermediate. Three main open reading frames are encoded (ORFs) and the virus has four known genes which encode the core protein, the virus polymerase, surface antigens (preS1, preS2, and S) and the X protein. The X protein is thought to be non-structural; however, its function and significance are poorly understood.

Replication

Hepadnaviruses replicate through an RNA intermediate (which they transcribe back into cDNA using reverse transcriptase. The reverse transcriptase becomes covalently linked to a short 3- or 4-nucleotide primer. Most hepadnaviruses will only replicate in specific hosts, and this makes experiments using in vitro methods very difficult.

The virus binds to specific receptors on cells and the core particle enters the cell cytoplasm. This is then translocated to the nucleus, where the partially double stranded DNA is 'repaired' by the cell to form a complete circle of DNA. It then undergoes transcription by the host cell RNA polymerase and the transcript is translated by host cell ribosomes. New virus particles are formed, which acquire lipid from the endoplasmic reticulum of the host cell, and the genome is packaged within these particles, which then bud off from the cell.

Hepadnavirus-infected cells translate the protein known as the virus surface antigen many times until there is too much protein to coat the virions formed. These proteins then aggregate to form rod shapes, and it is this antigen, known as the Australian or hepatitis B surface antigen, which is released from the cell and which leads to a very strong immune response from the host.

Viral Genetics & Evolution

Viral genetics, the study of the genetic mechanisms that operate during the life cycle of viruses, utilizes biophysical, biological, and genetic analyses to study the viral genome and its variation. Virus genetics are studied by either investigating genome mutations or exchange of genetic material during the life cycle of the virus. The virus genome consists of only one type of nucleic acid, which could be a single or double stranded DNA or RNA. Single stranded RNA viruses could contain positive-sense (+RNA), which serves directly as mRNA or negative-sense RNA (-RNA) that must use an RNA polymerase to synthesize a complementary positive strand to serve as mRNA. Viruses are obligate parasites that are completely dependent on the host cell for the replication and transcription of their genomes as well as the translation of the mRNA transcripts into proteins. Viral proteins usually have a structural function, making up a shell around the genome, as well as may contain some enzymes that are necessary for the virus replication and life cycle in the host cell. Animal viruses play an important role as tools in molecular and cellular biology research.

RNA viruses exploit all known mechanisms of genetic variation to ensure their survival. Distinctive features of RNA virus replication include high mutation rates, high yields, and short replication times. These mutation rates affect every aspect of virus biology and are at least a hundred-fold higher than those estimated for DNA viruses. RNA viruse having rapid mutation rate, is an advantage since these viruses will evolve constantly and rapidly, and thus evade the defensive responses of e.g. the human immune system. As a consequence, RNA viruses replicate as complex and dynamic mutant swarms, called viral quasispecies. A mutation refers to a change in the nucleic acid sequence of a virus. The virus having a mutation is referred to as a mutant. The change caused by mutation is based on comparison with the reference virus. After comparision with the reference virus, strains (wild types of the same virus), types (serological or biological), and variants (phenotypically different from wild type where genetic reason is unknown are identified. Mutation rates at defined genomic sites are affected by the nucleotide sequence on the template molecule as well as by environmental factors. In vitro hypermutation reactions offer a means to explore the functional sequence space of nucleic acids and proteins. The evolution of a viral quasispecies is extremely dependent on the population size of the virus that is involved in the infections. Repeated bottleneck events lead to average fitness losses, with viruses that harbor unusual, deleterious mutations. In contrast, large population passages result in rapid fitness gains, much larger than those so far scored for cellular organisms. Fitness gains in one environment often lead to fitness losses in an alternative environment. An important challenge in RNA virus evolution research is the assignment of phenotypic traits to specific mutations. Recent evidence suggests the existence of critical thresholds for the expression of phenotypic traits. Epidemiological as well as functional and structural studies suggest that RNA viruses can tolerate restricted types and numbers of mutations during any specific time point during their evolution. Viruses occupy only a tiny portion of their potential sequence space. Such limited tolerance to mutations may open new avenues for combating viral infections.

Mutation rate in RNA viruses is characterized by very high mutation rates compared to DNA viruses, because viral RNA polymerases **lack the proof-reading ability of DNA polymerase.** This is one reason why it is difficult to make effective vaccines to prevent diseases caused by RNA viruses. Retroviruses also have a high mutation rate even though their DNA intermediate integrates into the host genome, and is thus subject to host DNA proof reading once integrated, because errors during reverse transcription are embedded into both strands of DNA before integration. Some genes of RNA virus are important to the viral replication cycles and mutations are not tolerated. For example, the region of the hepatitis C virus genome that encodes the core protein is highly conserved, because it contains an RNA structure involved in an internal ribosome entry site

Mutations are neutral events that can be acted upon by natural selection. If the mutation enhances the survival transmission and replication of the organism, it has a selective advantage. If the mutation is detrimental to the growth and survival, the organism is eventually eliminated from the population. If the mutation does not alter the survivability or its phenotype, then the mutation may not be easily detected. **Mutations occur by two different mechanisms, spontaneous mutation and induced mutation.**

Among the viruses, DNA viruses replication within the nucleus are more genetically stable than RNA viruses; the **spontaneous mutation rate is 10^{-8} to 10^{-11} per incorporated nucleotide.** In DNA viruses reduced rate of mutation is due to the fact that DNA polymerases have some error correction ability. There are error correction mechanisms in the host cell for DNA repair, which do not exist for RNA viruses.

Among RNA viruses, the viruses are very less genetically stable, with a **spontaneous mutation rate of 10^{-3} to 10^{-4} per incorporated nucleotide** because viral RNA polymerases lack the proof-reading ability of DNA polymerase. RNA polymerases typically lack error correction ability.

Viruses undergo genetic change by several mechanisms: Genetic drift where individual bases in the DNA or RNA mutate to other bases. Antigenic shift is where there is a major change in the gene. Spontaneous mutations are endogenous, being the result of DNA or RNA polymerase errors or the result of incorporation of naturally occurring tautomeric forms of nucleotides.

Mutants

Spontaneous Mutations

These arise naturally during viral replication: e. g. due to errors by the genome - replicating polymerase or as a result of the incorporation of tautomeric forms of the bases. Published mutant frequencies yield a wide range of mutation rates per genome per replication, mainly because mutational targets have usually been small and, thus, poor samples of the mutability of the average base. Nevertheless, there is a clear central tendency for lytic RNA viruses (poliomyelitis, vesicular stomatitis, and influenza A) to display rates of spontaneous mutation of approximately 1 per genome per replication. This rate is some 300-fold higher than previously reported for DNA-based microbes. Lytic RNA viruses thus mutate at a rate close to the maximum value compatible with viability. Retroviruses, however, mutate at an average rate about an order of magnitude lower than lytic RNA viruse. ssDNA viruses tend to more genetically stable than RNA viruses. There are error correction mechanisms in the host cell for DNA repair, but probably not for RNA. However, Some RNA viruses are remarkably invariant in nature. Probably these viruses have the same high mutation rate as other RNA viruses, but are so precisely adapted for transmission and replication that fairly minor changes result in failure to compete successfully with parental (wild-type) virus.

Induced Mutation by Physical or Chemical Means

Induced mutations are exogenous, it is due to either using chemical mutants like nitrous oxide that acts directly on bases and modify them or by incorporating already modified bases in the virus genome by adding these bases as substrates during virus replication. Physical agents such as ultra-violet light and x rays can also be used in inducing mutations. Genotypically, the induced mutations are usually point mutations, deletions, and rarely insertions. Exposure to mutagens (chemical or radiation) profoundly increases the mutation rate for a given virus. Whereas chemical mutagens act either directly on the bases or indirectly by enhancing mispairing. Ultra violet radiation can induce the formation of pyrimidine dimers; ionizing radiation can damage DNA directly by breaking chemical bonds or indirectly by forming free radicals that in turn damage DNA.

1. *Chemical agents*: e .g .nitrous acid acting directly on bases, e.g. nitrous acid.
2. Agents acting indirectly such as base analogs which mispair more frequently than normal bases thus generating mutations.
3. *Physical*: Agents such as UV light or X-rays

There occurs many phenotypes that are generated as the result of mutation. Some of the more common mutations are mentioned below.

Genotypic classification of mutants

Point mutantions-is due to one base being replaced by another; this is the most common type of mutation. Most point mutations are silent. Less frequent are mutation of one or more nucleotides.

Insertion/deletionmutation- is due to insertion or deletion of one or small or large block of nucleotides. Suck mutation, if small revert back, otherwise not.

Quasispecies- sometimes mutation confers selective advantage for positive selection of the mutant virus. Non lethal mutations rarely accumulate in the genome of RNA viruses resulting in, genetically diverse populations of viruses around consensus sequence.

Suppresser mutation- the phenotypic expression mutation may be reversed by a back mutation in the affected nucleotide but may also be reverted by suppression mutation.

Phenotypic classification of mutants

Conditional lethal mutants- refer to a viral mutant that can replicate under some permissive conditions but not under other restrictive or nonpermissive conditions, the parent (wild type) strain is being able to replicate under both conditions.

Temperature sensitive mutants- will grow at low temperature at 31^0 C but not at higher temperature at 39° C; wild type grows both at 31 and 39 degrees C. Probably the altered protein cannot maintain a functional conformation at the elevated temperature. Temperature sensitive mutants have been useful in the development of live intranasal vaccine.

Host range mutants are most commonly studied whose replication is blocked in certain hosts or will only grow in a subset of the cell types in which the wild type virus will grow - such mutants provide a means to investigate the role of the host cell in viral infcction

Plaque mutants- may produce a different plaque in cell monolayer culture, either larger or smaller than in the wild type virus; often these mutants exhibit altered pathogenicity.

Antibody escape mutants- become resistant to presence of neutralizing antibody against wild type or show variant properties; these are important in causing persistent infection.

Nonsense (amber) mutations-is point mutations that result in the formation of a translational stop codon at a position where an amino acid is incorporated in the wild type protein. Consequently, the protein is truncated and frequently nonfunctional. This type of common nonsense mutation is to the UAG codon, called amber.

Attenuated mutants- After replication several viral mutants cause much milder symptoms compared to the wild type; these viruses are said to be attenuated. Such attenuated strains have an important role in vaccine development.

Antigenic drift

Antigenic drift is a result of accumulation of point mutations (single bases substitutions) & has been identified as the mechanism associated with the antigenic variation observed with influenza viruses and may be the mechanism associated with the variability observed with rhinoviruses.

Interactions between Two Viruses

If viral infections occur in nature as well as in culture with **two or more different viruses simultaneously**, these are called as mixed infections. Such infection can result in new viral combinations, and thus new variants of the virus. The following are some of the interactions that can occur during mixed infections.

Complementation

When complementation occurs during a mixed viral infection, one of the two viruses is deficient in a particular gene product. The virus without this protein is unable to transmit and replicate; thus a defective vius particle results. In a mixed infection, if the second virus makes up the product & thus complements the defect, the defective particle is capable of completing the transmission and replication processes. Usually, complementation occurs with the human Hepatitis D virus. The virus is defective in a surface antigen that is provided by Hepatitis B in mixed infections, allowing the replication of the Hepatitis D life cycle to be completed.

Reassortment

Reassortment occurs when there is mixing of the genetic material of two similar viruses that are infecting the same cell. Reassortment of a virus has a segmented genome. Human viruses characterized with segmented genomes are RNA viruses, e.g. orthomyxoviruses, reoviruses, arenaviruses, & bunyaviruses. Reassortment may play an important role in nature in generating novel reassortants and has also been useful in laboratory experiments. Reassortment is a non - classical kind of recombination.

Exchange of Genetic Material Materials in Viruses

Recombination

Besides mutation, new genetic variants of viruses also arise through exchange of genetic material by recombination and reassortment. Genetic recombination is the process by which a strand of DNA is broken and then joined to the end of a different DNA molecule. This can occur when viruses infect cells simultaneously and studies of viral evolution have shown that recombination has been rampant in the species studied. This type of recombination is almost exclusively reserved to DNA viruses and retroviruses. RNA viruses that do not have a DNA phase rarely use this mechanism. Recombination usually enables a virus to pick up genetic material from similar viruses and even from unrelated viruses and the eukaryotic host cells. Exchange of genetic material with the host is especially common with retroviruses. Reassortment is a non-classical kind of recombination that occurs if two variants of a segmented virus infect the same cell. The resulting progeny virions may get some segments from one parent and some from the other. All known segmented virus that infect humans are RNA viruses. The process of reassortment is very efficient in the exchange of genetic material and is used in the generation of viral vaccines especially in the case of influenza live vaccines. The ability of viruses to exchange genetic information through recombination is the basis for virus-based vectors in recombinant DNA technology and hold great promises in the development of **gene** therapy.

Classic recombination: There is breaking of covalent bonds within the nucleic acid, exchange of genetic information, and reforming of covalent bonds. Such break/join recombination is common in DNA viruses or those RNA viruses which have a DNA phase e.g. retroviruses. The host cell has recombination systems for DNA.

But recombination is very rare in RNA viruses because there are probably no host enzymes for RNA recombination. In picornaviruses there is a form of very low efficiency recombination. The mechanism is different from the standard DNA mechanism, and is probably a copy kind of mechanism in which the polymerase switches templates while copying the RNA. Recombination also occurs in the coronaviruses; but the mechanism is different from the situation with DNA and probably is a consequence of the unusual way in which RNA is synthesized in this virus. There is no evidence for recombination in the negative stranded RNA viruses giving rise to viable viruses.

Various uses for recombination techniques

Recombination in viruses is used for **mapping genomes-**the further apart two genes are, the more likely it is that there will be a recombination between them. **Marker rescue:** DNA fragments from wild type virus can recombine with mutant virus to generate wild type virus - this provides a means to assign a gene function to a particular region of the genome. This also provides a means to insert foreign material into a gene. Recombination also enables a virus to pick up genetic information from viruses of the same type and occasionally from unrelated viruses or even the host genome as in case of retroviruses.

Reassortment

Some viruses have segmented genome and if two variants of the same virus infect a single cell, progeny virions can result with some segments from one parent, some from the other. This is limited to viruses with segmented genomes so far the only human viruses characterized with segmented genomes of RNA viruses e.g. orthomyxoviruses, reoviruses, arenaviruses & bunyaviruses. Reassortment plays an important role in nature in generating novel reassortants and has also been useful in laboratory experiments. It has also been exploited in assigning functions to different segments of the genome. For example, in a reassorted virus, if one segment comes from virus A and the rest from virus B, we can see which properties resemble virus A and which to virus B.

Reassortment is a non-classical kind of recombination. However the mechanism of assortment occurring in birds & pigs has been implicated in the appearance of new, highly virulent influenza virus strains causing influenza pandemics in humans throughout the 20th century.

Multiplicity reactivation

In case of DNA viruses, if the viruses are inactivated with UV irradiation, there occurs reactivation if we infect cells with the inactivated virus at a very high multiplicity of infection. This occurs since inactivated viruses cooperate each other; probably complementation allows viruses to grow initially, as genes inactivated in one virion may still be active in one of the others. As the number of genomes present increases due to replication, recombination can occur, resulting in new genotypes, and sometimes regenerating the wild typevirus.

Defective Viruses

Defective viruses lack the full component of genes required for a complete infectious cycle, hence they need another virus to provide the missing functions; this second virus is called a helper virus. Defective viruses usually provide the signals for a polymerase to replicate their genome and for their genome to be packaged but need provide no more.

Some retroviruses pick up host cell sequences but lose some viral functions. These need a closely related virus which retains these functions as a helper. But some defective viruses can use unrelated viruses as a helper, e. g. hepatitis delta virus; an RNA virus fails to code its envelope proteins but uses the envelope of hepatitis B virus.

Defective interfering particles

The replication of the helper virus is less effective than if the defective virus is not present; the defective particle is competing with the helper for the functions that the helper provides. This phenomenon is known as interference, and defective particles which cause this phenomenon are known as "defective interfering" particles. Probably the defective interfering particles can modulate natural infections.

Phenotypic mixing

In case two different viruses infect a cell, progeny viruses may contain coat components derived from both parents and so they will have coat properties of both parents. This is called phenotypic mixing, but there is no change in genetic material. The progeny virions will be determined by which parental genome is packaged and not by the nature of the envelope. This may occur between related viruses, e.g. different members of the picornaviruses, or between genetically unrelated viruses, e.g. rhabdoviruses and paramyxoviruses. In some case a coat is that of another virus, e.g. a retrovirus nucleocapsid in a rhabdovirus envelope. This kind of phenotypic mixing is sometimes referred to as pseudotype. The pseudotype will show the adsorption-penetration-surface antigenicity characteristics of the rhabdovirus but on infection, behaves as a retrovirus and produce progeny retroviruses. This results in pseudotypes having an altered host range/ tissue tropism on a temporary basis

Applied Genetics

The vaccine Flumist used for influenza virus involves some of the genetic principles mentioned above. The vaccine is trivalent containing 3 strains of influenza virus. These viruses are cold adapted strains that can grow well at 25^{0}C and in the upper respiratory tract where it is cooler but they grow poorly in the warmer lower respiratory tract. These viruses are attenuated strains and less pathogenic than wild-type virus caused by multiple changes in the various genome segments.

Antibodies to the influenza virus surface proteins, HA and NA are important in protection against infection. The HA and NA change from year to year. The vaccine technology uses reassortment to generate reassortant viruses which have six gene segments from the attenuated, cold-adapted virus and the HA and NA coding segments from the virus which is likely to be a problem in the up-coming influenza season. This vaccine is a live vaccine and is given intranasally as a spray and can induce mucosal and systemic immunity.

A live, attenuated reassortant vaccine has recently been approved for rotaviruses (RotaTeq from Merck). Another attenuated vaccine, Rotarix (Glaxo), is in development.

Gene therapy

Gene therapy is based on the premise of using viruses with no pathogenic properties, but retains their ability to selectively interact with and transmit their genes as well as any genetically-engineered genes into specific host cells and tissues. Retroviruses are an excellent means for gene delivery into target host cells. The genome of dsDNA is stable and readily integrated into the host genome. The viruses are engineered in such a manner that once the genome has been integrated into the genome they cannot replicate. Often this means using helper viruses to aid in the initial uptake of the engineered virions by the host cells by complementation. The limitation of this method of gene therapy is that in some cases the gene in question needs to be present in all cells of the host and not just a select group of cells or tissues. Retroviruses have been used in gene therapy for incorporation of the adenine deaminase (ADA) gene into the immune cells of patients with an ADA immunodeficiency. In addition to retroviruses, some other viruses currently being studied as potential vectors for gene therapy include the adenoviruses, adeno-associated viruses, parvoviruses and herpesviruses.

Viruses and Cancer

A limited number of DNA viruses are associated with certain types of human neoplasia, while a variety of RNA viruses, or retroviruses cause tumors in animals. The main viruses associated with human & animal cancers are human & bovine papillomaviruses, hepatitis B and hepatitis C viruses, Epstein-Barr virus, Marek's disease virus, human T-lymphotropic virus, Kaposi sarcoma-associated herpesviruses (KSHV) and Merkel cell polyomavirus. The mode of virally-induced tumors can be divided into two, *acutely-transforming* or *slowly-transforming*. In case of RNA retroviruses; the infected cell of acutely transforming viruses, the viral particles carry a gene that encodes for an overactive oncogene called viral-oncogene (v-onc), and is transformed as soon as v-onc is expressed. In contrast, in slowly-transforming viruses, the virus genome is inserted, especially as viral genome insertion is an obligatory part of retroviruses, near a proto-oncogene in the host genome. The viral promoter or other transcription regulation elements in turn cause overexpression of that proto-oncogene, which in turn induces uncontrolled cellular proliferation. Because viral genome insertion is not specific to proto-oncogenes and the chance of insertion near that proto-oncogene is low, slowly-transforming viruses have very long tumor latency compared to acutely-transforming viruses, which already carry the viral oncogene.

Hepatitis viruses, including hepatitis B and hepatitis C virus can induce a chronic viral infection that leads to liver cancer in 0.47% of hepatitis B patients per year (especially in Asia, less so in North America), and in 1.4% of hepatitis C carriers per year. Liver cirrhosis, whether from chronic viral hepatitis infection or alcoholism, is associated with the development of liver cancer, and the combination of cirrhosis and viral hepatitis presents the highest risk of liver cancer development. Worldwide, liver cancer is one of the most common and most deadly cancers due to a huge burden of viral hepatitis transmission and disease.

Advances in cancer research have made a vaccine designed to prevent cancer. The hepatitis B vaccine is the first vaccine that has been established to prevent cancer (hepatocellular carcinoma) by preventing infection with the causative virus. In 2006, the US Food & Drug Administration approved a human papillomavirus vaccine, called Gardasil. The vaccine protects against four HPV types, which together cause 70% of cervical cancers and 90% of genital warts. In March 2007, the US Centre for Disease Control and Prevention (CDC) Advisory Committee on immunization Practices (ACIP) officially recommended that females aged 11–12 receive the vaccine, and indicated that females as young as age 9 and as old as age 26 are also candidates for immunization.

Viruses seem able to cause cancer in three ways: Presence of the viral DNA may disrupt normal host DNA function, viral proteins needed for virus replication may also affect normal host gene regulation, & the virus may serve as a vector for oncogene insertion.

DNA viruses

Human papillomavirus (HPV), a DNA virus, causes transformation in cells through interfering with tumor suppressor proteins such as p53. Interfering with the action of p53 allows a cell infected with the virus to move into a different stage of the cell cycle, enabling the virus genome to be replicated. Forcing the cell into the S phase of the cell cycle could cause the cell to become transformed. Some types of HPV increase the risk of cervical cancer. Kaposi sarcoma-associated herpesvirus (KSHV or HHV-8) is associated with Kaposi's sarcoma, a type of skin cancer.

Eptein-Barr virus (EBV or HHV-4) is associated with four types of cancers. Merkel cell polyomavirus is associated with the development of Merkel cell carcinoma. Human cytomegalovirus (CMV or HHV-5) is associated with mucoepidermoid carinoma and possibly other malignancies.

In many cases, tumor viruses do not cause cancer in their native hosts but only in dead-end species. For example, adenoviruses do not cause cancer in humans but become tumorigenic when infected into certain rodent species, such as Syrian hamsters. Some viruses are tumorigenic when they infect a cell and persist as circular episomes or plasmids, replicating separately from host cell DNA (Epstein Barr virus and Kaposi sarcoma-associated herpesvirus). Other viruses are only carcinogenic when they integrate into the host cell genome as part of a biological accident, such as polyomaviruses and papillomaviruses. Some RNA viruses have also been associated such as the hepatitis C virus as well as human T-lymphotropic virus (HTLV-1).

- *Adenovirus/ Mastadenovirus* causes solid tumour in Hamsters (not in natural hosts).
- *Alphaherpesvirinae /Mardivirus:* Marek's disease virus causes T cell lymphomatosis in fowls.
- *Papillomavirus/*Bovine papillomavirus 1, 2 cause carcinomas in intestinal tract & bladder when grazing land is infected with Bracken. BPV-4 also causes carcinoma of intestine & bladder.
- *Hepadnavirus/ Orthohepadnavirus*-Woodchuk hepatitis viruses cause hepatocellular carcinoma in woodchuck.
- *Avihepadnavirus*-Duck hepatitis virus causes hepatocellular carcinoma in ducks.
- *Retrovirus/Alpharetrovirus*:
- Avian leukosis viruses cause leukosis- lymphoma, leukemia, osteopetrosis, & nephroblastoma in fowls.
- Rous sarcoma virus causes sarcoma in fowls.
- Avian erythroblastosis virus causes erythroblastosis in fowls.
- *Betaretrovirus*-Mouse mammary carcinoma virus causes mammary carcinoma in mice.
- *Gammaretrovirus*- Feline leukemia virus causes leukemia in cats.
- *Deltaretrovirus*: Bovine leukemia virus causes B cell leukemia in cattle.
- Deltaretrovirus: Ovine pulmonary carcinoma virus/Jaagsiekte virus causes pulmonary adenocarcinoma in sheep.
- *Flaviviridae/Hepacivirus*- Hepatitis C virus causes hepatocellular carcinoma in humans.

❐❐❐

Chapter 4

Virus-Cell Interactions and Viral Pathogenesis

Contents

Virus-Cell Interactions

Outcome of interaction between viruses and their host cells depends on host capacity to inhibit or limit viral infection, & virus ability to shutdown or evade host defenses. During infection a battle ensues in which both host and viral genomes must each be protected to maintain their genetic integrity.The interaction of virus with cellular components during the replication process influences how viruses cause disease. If virus succeeds, the infection & viral replication may take place. Hence, it is important to understand the mechanisms of virus–host interactions, as this information can prove useful in symptomatic treatment of viral infections and aid in the design of antiviral vaccines. Further, since viruses rely almost entirely on the host cell machinery for their propagation, these studies throw light about our own cells and the basic mechanisms of gene expression and immunity. Understanding principles of viral replication machinery and viral genetics is prerequisite for understanding complex interaction between the virus and the host cell responses during viral infection. The virus-host cell interaction at the cellular level and progression of a particular viral infection determines disease pathogenesis and clinical manifestations.

Viral infection may be **productive** i.e. virus is able to replicate effectively in a permissive host cell; that host cell allows virus replication. Cells that support viral replication are called **permissive**. Infections of permissive cells are usually **productive** because infectious progeny virus is produced. Most productive infections are called **cytocidal (cytolytic)** because they kill the host cell. Infections of nonpermissive cells yield no infectious progeny virus and are called **abortive**. When the complete repertoire of virus genes necessary for virus replication is not transcribed and translated into functional products, the infection is referred to as **restrictive**. In **persistent** and in some transforming infections, viral nucleic acid may remain in specific host cells indefinitely; progeny virus may or may not be produced. Alternatvely, infection may be **nonproductive**; the virus failing to replicate in that host.

There are **four possible primary effects of viral infection on a host cell:** i. most infections cause no apparent cellular pathology or morphological alteration; ii cause cytopathic effect (cell rounding, detachment, syncytium formation, etc.), iii. cell lysis or cell death & iv. malignant transformation.

In most cases, the disturbances of bodily function that are manifested as the signs and symptoms of viral disease result from the direct effects of viruses on cells. Knowledge of the morphologic, physiologic, biochemical, and immunologic effects of viruses on cells is essential in understanding the virus-cell interaction of viral diseases that help in developing accurate diagnostic procedures and effective treatment.

Virus-host cell interactions (**Table 4-1**) may produce either 1) cytocidal (cytolytic) infections, in which production of new infectious virus kills the cell; 2) persistent infections, in which the virus or its genome resides in some or all of the cells without killing most of them; or 3) transformation, in which the virus does not kill the cell, but produces genetic, biochemical, physiologic, and morphologic changes that may result in the acquisition of malignant properties. The type of virus infection and the virus-induced effects on cells are dependent on the virus, the cell type and species, and often the physiologic state of the cell.

Table 4.1 : Types of virus-cell interactions

Type of infection	Effects on cells	Virion release	Effects on cells Morpholoical	Biochemical	Physiological	Genetic	Examples
Cytocidal							
Productive	Death	Yes	+	+	+	DNA degradation	Alphaherpesviruses, reoviruses, enteroviruses
Abortive	Variable	No	±	+	+	Mutate	Many viruses
Persistent productive	No CPE	Yes	+	±	±	-	Pestiviruses, arenaviruses, Rabies virus, most retroviruses
Persistent nonprodutive	No	No, can be induced	-	-	-	Mutate	CDV in brain
Latent	Survive	-	-	-	-	Mutate	Herpesviruses
Chronic	Variable	+	variable	+	+	Mutate	Borna disease virus
Transforming DNA	Survival	-	+	+	+	Mutate	Polyomavirus, papilloviruses
Transforming RNA	Survival	±	+	+	+	Mutate	Muine, avian leukosis, Sarcoma viruses.

Cytocidal Infections

Infection by cytocidal viruses is usually associated with changes in cell morphology, in cell physiology and sequential biosynthetic events. Certain viruses cause cell death during viral replication by several factors. Viruses causing cell death include reoviruses, poxviruses, picornaviruses, paramyxoviruses & rhabdoviruses. The most common cause of cell death is the inhibition of cellular synthesis of biomolecules, such as proteins as during the replication cycle, the virus induces the cellular machinery to manufacture largely viral products rather than those the of cell. Consequently, the cellular products necessary for the survival of the cell are not present or present in too low a quantity to maintain its viability. Secondly, there is accumulation of viral structural proteins, RNA & DNA in excess, which can be toxic for the cells. During virus release, some viruses induce apoptosis of the host cell. Inhibition of the synthesis of cellular macromolecules causes damage to lysosomal membranes and subsequent release of hydrolytic enzymes causing cell death. Many of these changes are necessary for efficient virus replication. Morphologic Effects: The changes in cell morphology caused by infecting virus are called cytopathic effects (CPE). Common examples are rounding of the infected cell, fusion with adjacent cells to form syncytia (polykaryocytes), and the appearance of nuclear or cytoplasmic inclusion bodies. Inclusion bodies may represent either altered host cell structures or accumulations of viral components.

Effects on Cell Physiology: The interaction of virus with the cell membrane and/or subsequent events, (for example, *de novo* synthesized viral proteins) may change the physiological parameters of infected cells, including movement of ions, formation of secondary messengers, and activation cascades leading to altered cellular activities.

Effects on Cell Biochemistry: Many viruses inhibit the synthesis of host cell macromolecules, including DNA, RNA, and protein. Viruses may also change cellular transcriptional activity, and protein-protein interactions, promoting efficient production of progeny virus. For some viruses, specific cellular biochemical functions may be stimulated in order to enhance virus replication.

Genotoxic Effects: Following virus infection, breakage, fragmentation, rearrangement and/or changes in the number of chromosomes may occur.

Biologic Effects: Virus-specified proteins may alter the cell's antigenic or immune properties, shape, and growth characteristics.

Non Cytopathic Viral Infections

Some viruses induce various types of cytopathic effect (CPE) including morphologic changes in cells resulting from virus infection. Sometimes infected cells have an altered cell membrane which is capable of fusing with its neighbor cell. Altered membrane is the result of the insertion of viral proteins during the replication cycle. Fusion of adjacent cells causes generation of a multinucleate cell or **syncytia**. Syncytia formation is characteristic for many enveloped viruses, such as herpesviruses and paramyxoviruses, HPV, BK virus,

Respiratory syncytial virus, & Cytomegalovirus. Often the multinucleate cells are large and are called multinucleate giant cells. The cell membrane is altered with regard to its permeability, allowing influxes of various ions, toxins, antibiotics, etc. CPE is also observed as the disruption of the cytoskeleton, leading to a rounded up appearance of the infected cell; cells are either lysed or form syncytia. Characteristic CPE in clinical specimens is used as diagnosis for viral infection and CPE is also used for the plaque assay used in viral enumeration. Some virus infection of cells like poxviruses and rabies virus is characterized by the formation of cytoplasmic inclusion bodies, discrete areas containing viral proteins or viral particles. Such inclusions have a characteristic location and appearance within an infected cell, depending upon the virus.

Some noncytocidal viral infections, e.g. Alphaherpesviruses produce lytic infecton in epith cells, but also enter sensory nerve ganglia to produce latent infection in neuronal perikaya. Viral DNA is present as circular episomal & viral replication is restricted in nondividing neurons. However, under certain stresses, they are reactivated & are triggered producing productive viruses & transmission to susceptible animals.

Persistent Infections

Some viruses evolved the ability to remain in specific cells for long periods of time. In persistent viral infection, there are no CPE changes, little cellular metabolic disturbance, cells divide & simultaneous produce infectious virions. Such persistent infections typically occur in viruses like pestiviruses, arenaviruses, rabies virus & most retroviruses. These infections include: latent, chronic, and slow virus infections. The type of persistent infection usually influences the extent of cellular changes.

Latent infections are characterized by restricted expression of the episomal or integrated virus genome. The viral genomic product(s) are associated with few, if any, changes in the latently infected cell.

In **Chronic infection,** the cellular effects are usually the same as those of acute cytocidal infections, except that production of progeny may be slower, intermittent or limited to a few cells. The long-term cellular changes may result in severe disease, immune suppression or may trigger immune responses to damage, or undamage cells or tissues.

Slow Infection type of virus-cell interaction is characterized by a prolonged incubation period, without significant morphological and physiological changes of infected cells. A slow progression of cellular injury may take years and is followed by extensive cellular injury and disease.

Transforming Infections

DNA or RNA tumor viruses may mediate multiple changes that convert a normal cell into a malignant one. RNA tumor viruses usually transform cells to a malignant phenotype by integrating their own genetic material into the cellular genome and may also produce infectious progeny. DNA tumor virus infections are often cytocidal; thus transformation is associated with abortive or restrictive infections in which few viral genes are expressed.

Stages of transformation involve at least two processes: first, the cell gains the capacity for unlimited cell division (immortalization), and second, the immortalized cells acquire additional heritable genetic changes by which the cell is able to produce a tumor in an appropriate host. Mechanism of oncogenic transformation occurs by two general patterns by which cell transformation may be accomplished: 1) the tumor virus may introduce and express a so-called transforming gene in the cells or 2) the tumor virus may alter the expression and (or) coding capacity of preexisting cellular genes. After development of a malignant phenotype the relevant segment(s) of the viral genome may or may not be retained in the transformed cells, depending on the mechanism of transformation. These mechanisms are not mutually exclusive, and both may occur in the same cell.

Cytocidal Infections Description

Morphologic and structural effects

Infection of permissive cells with virus leads to productive infection and often results in cell death (cytocidal, cytolytic infection). The first effects of the replication of cytocidal viruses to be described were the morphologic changes known as cytopathic effects. Cultured cells that are infected by most viruses undergo morphologic changes, which can be observed easily in unfixed, unstained cells by a light microscope. Some viruses cause characteristic cytopathic effects; thus, observation of the cytopathic effect is an important tool for virologists concerned with isolating and identifying viruses from infected animals or humans.

Many types of cytopathic effects occur. Often the first sign of viral infections is rounding of the cells. In some diseased tissues, **intracellular structures** called **inclusion bodies** appear in the nucleus and/or cytoplasm of infected cells. Inclusion bodies were identified by light microscopy in smears and stained sections of infected tissues. Their composition can often be clarified by electron microscopy. Intracytolasmic inclusions are observed in cells infected with poxviruses, reoviruses, paramyxoviruses & rabies virus. Intranuclear inclusions are seen in the cells infected with hepesviruses, adenoviruses & parvovaviruses. **Canine distemper virus & porcine cytomegalovirus** may produce both intrcytoplasmic & intranuclear inclusion bodies. In an adenovirus infection crystalline arrays of **adenovirus** capsids accumulate in the nucleus to form an inclusion body. Inclusions may alternatively be host cell structures altered by the virus. For example, in **reovirus**-infected cells, virions associate with the microtubules, giving rise to a crescent-shaped perinuclear inclusion. Infection of cells by other viruses causes specific alterations in the cytoskeleton of cells. For example, extensive changes in cellular intermediate filaments in relation to formation of viral inclusions may be observed after cytomegalovirus infection. Some characteristics of inclusion bodies produced by various viruses are listed in **Table 4.2**.

Table 4.2: Intracytoplasmic and intranuclear viral inclusion bodies.

Viruses	Intracytoplasmic inclusion bodies	Intranuclear inclusion bodies
Adenoviruses (ICH)	-	Cowdry type A
Herpesviruses	+ cytomegalovirus	Cowdry type A
Parvoviruses	-	Cowdry type A
Paramyxoviruse (CDV, measles)	+	Cowdry ype A
Poxviruses	Guarnieri bodies	-
Rhabdoviruses (rabies virus)	Negri bodies	-
Reoviruses	+	-

A particularly striking cytopathic effect of some viral infections is the formation of syncytia, or polykaryocytes, which are large cytoplasmic masses that contain many nuclei (*poly*, many; *karyon*, nucleus) and are usually produced by fusion of infected cells. The mechanism of cell fusion during viral infection probably results from the interaction between viral gene products and host cell membranes. Cell fusion may be a mechanism by which virus spreads from infected to uninfected cells.

Effects on cell physiology

Pathogenesis of virus infections suggests a close correlation between cellular physiologic responses and the replication of some viruses. The physiological state of living cells has a significant effect on the outcome of the virus infection, since the host cell provides the synthetic machinery, key regulatory molecules, and precursors for the newly synthesized viral proteins and nucleic acids. The optimal intracellular environment for virus replication develops through events that begin to take place with attachment of virus to the cell membrane. Binding of virus to the cell membrane receptors may be followed by cascades of events that are associated with biochemical, physiological and morphological changes in the cells. The virus receptor is a cell membrane component that participates in virus binding, facilitates viral infection, and is a determinant of virus host range, as well as tissue tropism. Some viruses recognize more than one cellular receptors namely, in case of HIV, & adenoviruses; and the binding is a multistage process. Multiple receptors may act together either to modulate each other's activity or to contribute complementary functions.

Other virus-associated alterations in cell physiology are related to insertion of viral proteins or other changes in the cell membrane. One example is the leaky cell membrane that appears after infection with picornaviruses or Sindbis virus; the change in intracellular ion concentrations that results from the leaky membrane may favor translation of the more salt-stable (e.g., Na^+ or K^+) viral mRNA over cellular, mRNA. These and other effects may be maintained or modified by immediate early and/or early viral gene products (e.g., changes in transcription and protein levels of cell cycle regulatory molecules). **Figure 4-3** demonstrates the interaction between different viruse with their cellular receptors.

Table 4.3 : Cellular receptors during virus-cell interaction.

Family	Virus	Receptors on target cells
Adenoviridae	Human adenovirus-2	Integrin αVβ3
Herpesviridae	Bovine herpesvirs1 & 4	Heparin sulfate
Poxviridae	Vaccinia virus	Epidermal growth factor receptor1
Polyomaviridae	Polyomavirus	Sialic acid with oligsaccharides
Parvoviridae	Canine parvovirus-2	Sialic acid with oligsaccharides
Reoviridae	Reovirus B	Sialic acid with oligsaccharides & β Adrenergic receptorst
Picornaviridae	FMDV	Integrins
Togaviridae	Sindbis virus	Laminin receptor
Orthomyxoviridae	Influenza A viruses	Sialic acid with oligosaccharides
Paramyxoviridae	Parainfluenza viruses	Sialic acid with oligosaccharides, gangliosides
	Coxsackie B viruses	Decay-accelerating factor

	Echoviruses	Decay-accelerating factor & integrins
	Rhinovirus	ICAM-1
Rhabdoviridae	Rabies virus	Acetylcholine Rcpt &gangliosides, phospholipids
Arenaviridae	LCMV	100kDa glycoprotein
Retroviridae	Feline Immunodeficiency virus	CD4 & coreceptors
	HIV-1	CD4 & other coreceptors

Effects on cell biochemistry

Virus binding to the cell membrane in concert with immediate early (IE proteins of herpesviruses), early non-structural proteins (E-6, E-7 of HPVs) or virion components (e.g., ICP0, ICP4, VP16 of herpes simplex virus, penton protein of adenoviruses) may mediate a series of biochemical changes that optimize the intracellular milieu for use of cellular synthetic machinery, low molecular weight precursors for productive virus replication or to achieve latency, chronic, slow or transforming infection. For example, studies of transcriptional regulation of viral genes and post-transcriptional modification of gene products (splicing, polyadenylation of RNA) demonstrate that the nature of the basic biochemical processes for virus replication are similar to the mechanisms used to regulate expression of cellular genes. Viruses have sequence motifs in their nucleic acid for binding of known transcriptional regulators of cellular origin. Thus, promoter regions of regulatory and structural proteins for many viruses contain contiguous binding sites for a large array of identifiable mammalian cellular transcription factors (e.g., NFê B, Sp1, CRE/B, AP-1, Oct-1, NF-1). These cellular transcription factors in concert with regulatory viral proteins are involved in activation or repression of viral and cellular genes to develop latent, persistent, transforming virus infections, as well as to produce progeny virus. Most cellular transcription factors must be activated prior to binding to their specific recognition (consensus) sequences. The biochemical events may include phosphorylation, dephosphorylation, disassociation (from inhibitory subunit) and dimerization. These activation processes can be accomplished as a result of the cascade of events initiated by the virus and cell receptor interaction. Events associated with these cascades may include, for example, formation of secondary messengers (phosphatidyl inositols, diacylglycerols, cAMP, cGMP, etc.), activation of protein kinases, and ion (e.g., Ca^{2+}) influxes.

To maintain cell activation processes, viruses have evolved unique mechanisms to regulate these cellular processes, adapting their proteins to interact with cellular proteins. Examples include the association of early virus gene products (e.g., E-6, E-7 of papillomaviruses; IE proteins of herpesviruses; SV40 T antigen) with the Rb tumor suppresser protein which results in liberation of the E2F transcription factor that is required for modification (activation/inhibition) of cellular biochemical pathways, for synthesis of viral DNA, or initiation of cellular apoptotic processes (programmed cell death).

In some cases the virus directly incorporates cellular biochemical regulatory strategies by triggering the cells to overproduce and excrete regulatory molecules (e.g., transforming growth factors, tumor necrosis factors, interleukins), which may activate in an autocrine fashion cellular biochemical cascades involved in virus (e.g., HIV, herpesviruses, papillomaviruses) replication, maintenance of or reactivation from a latent state, or maintaining a transformed phenotype. On the other hand, these soluble cellular regulatory molecules may inhibit biochemical reactions of immune cells in a paracrine manner to compromise elimination of infected cells.

Inhibition of cellular macromolecule synthesis may result from virus infection and provide an advantage for synthesis of virus proteins and nucleic acids in the absence of competing synthesis of cellular products. This inhibition occurs in characteristic ways. In poliovirus or herpes simplex infections, for example, selective inhibition of host protein synthesis occurs prior to the maximal synthesis of viral proteins. In some cases, viral products inhibit both protein and nucleic acid synthesis. Purified adenovirus penton fibers significantly decrease the synthesis of host protein, RNA, and DNA. Total inhibition of host macromolecular synthesis also may occur when excess viral products accumulate in the cell late in the viral replicative cycle. Some picornaviruses specify a protein that causes cell damage independent of the viral proteins that inhibit cell macromolecular synthesis. Cellular mRNA may be degraded. For example, in influenza virus and herpes simplex virus infections, cellular mRNA stops binding with ribosomes to form polyribosomes; only virus-specific mRNA is bound, giving viral mRNAs a selective advantage. Cell DNA synthesis is inhibited in most cytolytic virus infections. This may be achieved by virus-induced apoptosis or by a decrease in cellular protein synthesis. Reoviruses and some herpesviruses may be exceptions in that they cause a decrease in cell DNA synthesis before a substantial decline in cellular protein synthesis occurs. Direct degradation of host DNA is seen in vaccinia virus infections due to a virion-associated DNase.

Genotoxic effects

Chromosome damage may be caused directly by the virus particle or indirectly by events occurring during synthesis of new viral macromolecules

(RNA, DNA, protein). The chromosome damage may or may not be repaired, and in either case, it may or may not be compatible with survival of the infected cell. When the cell survives, the virus genome may persist within the cell, possibly leading to continued instability of cellular genomic material or to altered expression of cellular genes (e.g., cellular oncogenes). Virus-induced genomic instability appears to be associated with accumulation of mutations and related to the process of cell immortalization and oncogenic transformation.

Biologic effects

The biologic consequences of virus infection results from the biochemical, physiological, structural, morphological and genetic changes. In productive infections virus-induced biological modifications of the cell may be closely related to the efficiency of virus replication or to the recognition of these cells by the immune system. For cells that are persistently infected, the cellular changes caused by the virus could lead to disease (e.g., subacute sclerosing panencephalitis after measles infection), cellular genetic damage (e.g., hepatitis B virus), immortalization (e.g., Epstein-Barr virus), or malignant transformation (e.g., HTLV-1, HTLV-2, hepatitis B virus). The wide variety of these effects of virus infection points to the complex interaction between the viruses and their host cell.

Relation of cellular effects to viral pathogenesis

Although most of the events that damage or modify the host cell during lytic infection are difficult to separate from viral replication, the effects are not always linked directly to the production of progeny virions. For example, changes in cell size, shape, and physiologic parameters may occur before progeny virions or even many virus proteins, are produced. These alterations in cell structure and function may be important aspects of the pathogenesis of a number of viral infections. For example, through their cellular effects many viruses (rotaviruses, caliciviruses, and Norwalk viruses) induce gastrointestinal symptoms (ranging from mild alteration in absorption of ions to severe watery diarrhea). Cytocidal viral infections (e.g., herpesviruses, togaviruses, flaviviruses, bunyaviruses) of the central nervous system are related to necrosis, inflammation or phagocytosis by supporting cells. Rubella virus infections are associated with demyelination without neural degeneration. The long-term effects of persistent virus infections may also be related to such progressive diseases as atherosclerosis and demyelination in multiple sclerosis.

Persistent Infections

In a persistent infection the virus is not eliminated from all of the host tissues after initial infection or the acute phase of disease. The several types of persistent infection [chronic, slow, latent, and transforming) differ in the mechanisms controlling their pathogenesis. In **chronic infections,** a limited number of cells (in the target organs) are infected. These infected cells may demonstrate a cytopathic effect, synthesize virus macromolecules, and release infectious virus. The spread of infection is limited by host factors such as humoral and cell-mediated immune responses, interferons and other nonspecific inhibitors. **Slow infections** induced by conventional (e.g. measles) are characterized by long incubation periods (years), preceding the onset of clinical symptoms. In **latent infections,** infectious virus is seldom detected between clinical episodes of disease. Few cells are infected, and virus expression and replication are extensively restricted. Common features of latent infection are their ability to reactivate in response to various environmental stimuli (e.g., heat, ultraviolet irradiation), and **immune suppression** brought on by heterologous virus infection (e.g., HIV) or chemotherapy, often associated with organ transplantation. In transforming persistent infections, infectious virus (RNA tumor viruses) may or may not be released, but as a result of heritable genetic changes to cellular genes, acquisition of a viral oncogene, or the effect of integrated viral sequences, the cells undergo alterations that result in malignant phenotypes.

Responses to persistent infections

Autoimmune injury and other forms of cell damage may occur during persistent infections. Budding virions and viral peptides associated with the cell membrane change the antigenic characteristics of the cell so that the immune system may recognize it as foreign. The cell then may be attacked by the humoral and cellular immune systems of the host and may die, even if it was infected by a noncytocidal virus. The immune response also may cause formation of circulating antigen-antibody complexes involving viral antigens. These complexes may deposit (e.g., in the glomeruli) and elicit inflammation by activating the classical pathway of complement. The long-term association of the virus with specific target cells may lead to altered function or responses; this type of mechanism is thought to be responsible for the progressive neurologic disease associated with slow virus infections such as Kuru, Creutzfeldt-Jakob disease, or subacute sclerosing panencephalitis.

Transforming Infections

The term oncogenic transformation refers to the process through which control of cell proliferation is genetically modified, so that the cell becomes cancerous. In the context of virus-cell interactions, the cells can also undergo various types of heritable changes that result in biochemical, antigenic, morphologic, and physiologic alterations, called non-oncogenic transformation.

Transforming virus host cell interactions

DNA viruses induce transformation only under conditions that restrict virus replication and permit survival of infected cells (e.g., in noncytolytic infections of selected cell types or animal hosts, or in infection with incomplete virions). Under such conditions, immediate early (e.g., EBNAs of Epstein-Barr virus) or early proteins (e.g., SV40 "T" or polyoma middle "t" antigen) are usually present, but infectious progeny virions are seldom produced. In contrast, because RNA tumor virus replication is usually noncytocidal, they can cause oncogenic transformation in permissive cells or in their natural hosts, and viral products may be produced whether or not virus is released.

Current data indicate that transformation of a cell involves at least two components: first, the cell gains the capacity for unlimited cell division **(immortalization)**, and second, the immortalized cells acquire the ability to produce a tumor in an appropriate host. Some viral genes that can immortalize cells include T antigens of papovaviruses (e.g., polyoma, JC, SV40), early proteins (e.g., E6, E7) of papillomaviruses, and Epstein-Barr virus (e.g. EBNA-5). In these cases, the viral proteins may interact and inactivate one or more cellular tumor suppresser proteins (e.g., Rb, p53), resulting in a significantly impaired cell cycle regulation. During the perturbed cell cycling, accumulation of mutations may occur either spontaneously or as an effect of other agents (virus, chemical, radiation) in cellular oncogenes (e.g., H-*ras*, K-*ras*; c-*myc*), in anti-oncogenes (e.g., p53, Rb), or in other cellular genes. *In vivo*, the history of malignancies also suggests a multiple process of cellular evolution, involving cumulative genetic changes, selection of rare cells that have the ability to invade, metastasize, and avoid immune surveillance. The number of mutations supporting an oncogenic transformation is estimated to range from six to more. Virus infections may contribute both to immortalization and to the accumulation of mutations in growth related cellular genes during oncogenic processes.

Non Specific Host Defenses

Humans & animals have evolved a highly complex host defense system to combat a wide variety of pathogens, but developing a remedy for most of the viral infections still remains a great challenge as viruses evolve very rapidly as well as produce a variety of proteins that thwart host defenses. These features provide viruses with strategies to evade almost any hurdle imposed by the host defenses to block their replication.

Viruses & the diseases associated with them are the major cause of human & animal morbidity and mortality. When a virus infects a host, the latter tries to eliminate it by nonspecific defense mechanisms (anatomical barrier, cellular components, natural killer cells and interferons) & by stimulating both nonspecific & antigen-specific immune effector mechanisms, while the virus tries to subvert one or more of these mechanisms to prolong its own lifespan. Virus infections are characterized by high and rapid rate of viral replication, production of large numbers of progeny particles, rapid generation times, generation of high mutation rates, viruses hiding within cells & generating new variants in very short periods of time. Besides their small size, all viruses have only two common features, a genetic programme-either DNA or RNA, and a protein coat to protect this genetic information and aid in its transfer from one host to another. Small size necessitates a small genome, which is the reason for its being obligate intracellular parasites.

Most viral infections are **limited by nonspecific defenses**, which restrict initial virus multiplication to manageable levels, initiate recovery from established infections that is then completed by a combination of these early nonspecific and subsequent antigen-specific immune defenses, and enable the host to cope with the peak numbers of virus that, if presented as the infecting dose, could be lethal.

Some nonspecific defenses exist **independent of infection like** genetic factors, anatomical barriers, nonspecific inhibitors in body fluids & phagocytosis. **Others like fever, inflammation, & interferon are produced by the host in response to infection.** All nonspecific defenses begin to act before the specific defenses response develops. The fact that viruses **replicate intracellularly** and the ability of some viruses to spread by inducing cell fusion **partly protect viruses** against such extracellular defenses as neutralizing antibody, phagocytosis & nonspecific inhibitors.

However, because they replicate within the cell, viruses are vulnerable to intracellular alterations caused by host responses to infection. Nonspecific responses that **alter the intracellular environment include** fever, inflammation, & interferon. These multiple defenses function with great complexity because of their interactions with one another. This complexity is compounded by the varying effectiveness of the defenses that results from the diversity of viruses, hosts, and sites and stages of infection.

Most viral infections are limited in the beginning by host defenses that are antigen nonspecific. Nonspecific defenses act immediately than specific defenses. Some of these host defenses are always in place like anatomical barrier, nonspecific inhibitors, & phagocytosis; others are evoked by the infection such as (fever, inflammation & interferon).

Anatomic barriers

Anatomic barriers are located at body surfaces namely skin and mucosa or within the body such as endothelial cells and basement membranes. The dead cells of the epidermis and any live cells that may lack viral receptors resist virus penetration and do not permit virus replication. However, this barrier is easily breached, for example, by animal bites (rabies virus), insect bites (togaviruses), and minor traumas (wart virus), increased permeability, replication of virus in endothelial cells, or by transportation of virus in leukocytes. At mucosal surfaces, only the **mucus layer** stands between invading virus and live cells. They are partly effective in preventing virus spread.

Membrane receptors

The host range of the virus depend on the presence of appropriate receptors on the cell membrane (Table 4-3). If a host lacks the receptor for a virus or if the host cells lack some component necessary for the replication of a virus, the host will be resistant to that virus. Mice lack receptors for polio viruses and thus are resistant to polio virus, & humans are resistant to plant and many animal viruses.

Mucus

The mucus layer forms a physical barrier that entraps foreign particles and carries them out of the body; it also contains nonspecific inhibitors. The **mucus barrier is not absolute**, however, since **sufficient quantities of many viruses can overwhelm it and infect by this route**. In fact, most viruses use mucous surfaces as the portal of entry and initial replication site.

Ciliated epithelium

The ciliated epithelium drives the mucociliary elevator & can help diminish infectivity of certain viruses. Ciliated activity has been shown to be important in respiratory infections since; lack of the activity of this system causes an increased infection rate with a given virus.

Within the Body

Anatomic barriers to virus spread are formed by the **layer of endothelial cells that separates blood from tissues** (e.g., the blod barrier). Under normal conditions, these barriers have a low permeability for viruses unless the virus can penetrate them by replicating in the capillary endothelial cells or in circulating leukocytes. These internal barriers may explain, in part, the high level of viremia required to infect organs such as brain, placenta & lungs.

Nonspecific inhibitors

Body fluids and tissues normally contain **soluble viral inhibitors**. These inhibitors mostly prevent viral attachment, some directly inactivate viruses, and others act intracellularly and a few act by inhibiting virus replication. But these inhibitors are overwhelmed by sufficient number of virus. They vary **chemically** (lipids, polysaccharides, proteins, lipoproteins & glycoproteins and in the **degree of viral inhibition** and **types of viruses affected.**

In the gastrointestinal tract, some susceptible viruses are inactivated by acid, bile salts, and enzymes.

Whereas **most inhibitors block only one or a few viruses, some** have a **broad antiviral spectrum**. Although the **effectiveness of the inhibitors** has not been fully established *in vivo*, their importance as host defense is suggested by their antiviral activity in tissue culture, in vitro & by the direct correlation between the degree of virulence of some viruses & their degree of resistance to certain inhibitors. Examples are the serum and mucus inhibitors of influenza viruses during experimental infections. However, even sensitive viruses may overwhelm if infecting dose of the virus is high. Therefore, the presence of these inhibitors may explain the relatively high dose of virus required to initiate infection *in vivo*, compared with the dose needed in cell cultures.

Phagocytosis

The information available suggests that **phagocytosis is less effective against viral infections than against bacterial infections.** However, few of the factors that control uptake of virions or infected cells by phagocytes and their digestion by lysosomal enzymes have been studied systemically. Different viruses are affected differently by the various phagocytic cells. Some viruses are not engulfed, whereas others are engulfed but may not be inactivated. In fact, some viruses, such as human immunodeficiency virus (HIV), may even multiply in the phagocytes (e.g., macrophages), which may serve as a persistent reservoir of virus. The virulence of several strains of HIV and herpesviruses correlates with their ability to multiply in macrophages. **Infected macrophages may carry virus across the blood-brain barrier.** Cytomegalovirus has been reported to replicate in granulocytes.

Macrophages seem to be more effective against viruses than are **granulocytes**, and some viruses seem to be more susceptible to phagocytosis than others. Macrophages & polymorhonuclear leukocyte can afford imptannt protection by markedly reducing the viremia caused by virus strains susceptible to phagocytosis.

Viruses may stimulate macrophages to produce **monokines**, which can reduce viral multiplication. For example, macrophage-produced alpha interferon (**IFN-a**) inhibits viral multiplication both **directly** and also **indirectly** by activating natural killer cells.

Interleukin 1 (IL-1), produced by macrophages, **can interfere with viral multiplication in a number of ways:** by inducing T lymphocytes to produce interleukin-2, which in turn induces gamma interferon, which can induce alpha and beta interferons; by inducing the production of beta interferon (IFN-β) by fibroblasts and epithelial cells; by inducing fever, which inhibits viral replication; by enhancing macrophage-mediated cytolysis of infected cells; and by inducing production of tumor necrosis factor (TNF), which inhibits virus multiplication both directly & indirectly by inducing interferon & other cytokines & augmentating inflammation, phagocytosis & cytotoxic activity.

Depending on the situation, **macrophages** therefore **acting as phagocytes** may reduce the number of viruses, help spread the infection, augment or depress immune defenses, or have little effect.

NK Cells/other cells

The principal effector cells of the innate immune system are monocytes/ macrophages, dendritic cells (DC), natural killer (NK) cells, and NK-T cells. These effector cells recognize **pathogen-associated molecular patterns**, e.g., viral proteins, CpG DNA, or double-stranded viral RNA, via a variety of so-called **pattern recognition receptors**, which include **Toll-like receptors, NK cell receptors, and mannose-binding receptors**. These cells then release a variety of proinflammatory cytokines and chemokines, which recruit inflammatory cells to the site of infection and initiate inflammation and antiviral responses. These soluble mediators also activate macrophages, NK cells, and DC. Viral infections are usually accompanied by NK cell activation. Activated NK cells kill virus-infected cells and serve as an immediate source of interferon (IFN-γ). An important event is the induction of type I (α and β) IFN. Although almost all cell types can produce these IFN, a specialized cell type, precursor plasmacytoid DC, produces 1000-fold more of these cytokines and is called the natural IFN-producing cell. IFNs also increase expression of major histocompatibility complex (MHC) class I and II antigens and of costimulatory molecules on the surface of so-called antigen-presenting cells (APC). Activation of the innate immune system plays an instructive role (adjuvant effect) for the induction of virus-specific, adaptive immune responses. In general, exogenous viral particles and viral antigens are phagocytosed and/ or endocytosed by APC. They are then degraded in lysosomes, and immunogenic peptides are presented in association with MHC class II antigens to naïve CD4+ T cells. NK cells and macrophages also kill virus-infected cells in association with virus-specific antibodies. NK cells kill antibody-coated, virus-infected cells via antibody-dependent, cell-mediated cytotoxicity

(ADCC). Virus-specific ADCC plays a significant role in killing virus-infected cells, especially against human immunodeficiency virus (HIV) and herpesviruses. Macrophages and polymorphonuclear leukocytes can engulf antibody-coated pathogens as well as virus-infected cells and/or kill them via reactive oxygen species, nitric oxide, and activated caspases.

NK cells may kill virus-infected cells without help from antibodies. These cells, however, usually do not recognize any viral antigen or viral peptide per se. Their effector function is controlled by a complex system of inhibitory & activating NK cell receptors and coreceptors. They kill target cells unless inhibited by the engagement of inhibitory receptors by their cognate ligands on the target cells. The most important inhibitory receptors include killer cell Ig-like receptors (KIR), NKG2/CD94A, and Ig-like transcripts (ILT), which bind to classical and nonclassical MHC class I antigens; also called human leukocyte antigen (HLA)-A, -B, -C, -E, and -G (Table 1). It is noteworthy that most of the KIR recognize HLA-C & inhibit NK cells. A down-regulation of the MHC antigens on the surface of virus-infected cells usually makes them susceptible to NK cell-mediated killing. Despite their different mechanisms of recognition of virus-infected cells, NK cells and CTL represent the most important cytolytic cells leading to the elimination of tumor and virus-infected cells from the host. Patients with low NK cell activity are more susceptible to reoccurrences with herpes simplex type 1 virus. NK cells recognize virus infected cells & kill such cells. Importantly, NK cell recognition of virus infected cells is not MHC-restricted or antigen specific. NK cells, therefore kill cells infected with different viruses. Besides the above, NK cells IFN-γ and Il-2 can enhance the activities of NK cells.

Defense Mechanisms Evoked by Infection

Fever

Viral replication is influenced strongly by temperature. Fever can be induced during viral infection by at least three independent endogenous pyrogens: interleukins-1 and 6, interferon, prostaglandin E2, and tumor necrosis factor.

Even a modest increase in fever can cause strong inhibition: a temperature rise from 37°C to 38°C drastically decreases the yield of many viruses. This phenomenon has been observed in tissue culture as well as in many experimental and natural infections. Artificial induction of fever reduces mortality in mice infected with viruses. Artificial lowering of the temperature during infection may increase mortality, as in suckling mice infected with coxsackieviruses and taken away from the warmth of their mother's nest. Fever also augments the generation of cytotoxic T lymphocytes.

Several observations suggest strongly that fever reduces virus multiplication during human viral infections.

Retrospective studies have shown that the **incidence** and **severity** of **paralysis** among children infected with polioviruses were significantly greater in patients **treated with antipyretic drugs** (e.g., aspirin) than in untreated children. Also consistent with these findings is the observation that virus strains that replicate best at fever temperature are usually virulent, whereas virus strains that replicate poorly at fever temperature are usually low in virulence and therefore often are used as live virus vaccines.

Temperatures as low as 33°C are normal at body surfaces exposed to air; viruses that infect these sites and replicate optimally at these temperatures establish only local infections **that do not spread to deeper tissues, where the body temperature is higher**. For example, rhinovirus that cause common colds replicate optimally at 33°C to 34°C; however, they are inhibited at 37°C. An interesting question is whether this temperature increase is important for recovery from coryza. The same general considerations of temperature probably apply to other human viral infections such as measles, rubella, and mumps, although, unfortunately, suitable and controlled studies have not been conducted. Nevertheless, available information suggests that antipyretic drugs be used conservatively.

Inflammation

Several antiviral mechanisms are generated by the local inflammatory response to virus-induced cell damage or to virus-stimulated mediators such as activated complement. The **major components of the inflammatory process** are: circulatory alterations, edema, leukocyte accumulation and perhaps prostaglandins A and J. These result in elevated local temperature, reduced oxygen tension in the involved tissues, altered cell metabolism, and increased levels of CO2 and organic acids.

All of these alterations, which occur in a cascading and interrelated fashion, drastically reduce the replication of many viruses. For example, the altered energy metabolism of the infected and surrounding cells, as well as the accumulating lymphocytes, can generate local hyperthermia. At superficial sites where the temperature is normally lower, hyperthermia can also be generated by hyperemia during the early stages of inflammation. As inflammation progresses, hyperemia become passive, thereby greatly reducing blood flow & decrease oxygen tension. Two factors account for this decrease in oxygen tension: **limited influx of erythrocytes, and lower diffusion of oxygen through edema fluid.** In turn, the decreased oxygen tension **causes less ATP production, thus reducing the energy available for viral synthesis** and increasing anaerobic glycolysis, which increases **the accumulation of CO_2 and organic acids in the tissues.** These acid catabolites may **decrease the local pH to levels that inhibit the replication of many viruses.** Local acidity also may increase by accumulation and subsequent degradation of the leukocytes in the affected area. It is possible that other less well-defined factors are also significant.

Therefore, the local inflammation resulting from viral infection clearly activates several metabolic, physiochemical & physiological changes; acting individually or together, these changes interfere with virus multiplication. Although further animal and human studies are required, this interpretation is supported by the finding that anti-inflammatory drugs **(corticosteroids)** often increase the severity of infection in animals. Therefore, these drugs should be used with caution in treating viral diseases.

Interferon

The most important type in natural infections is **directed by the host cells themselves**. These infected cells may respond to viral infection by producing **interferon**, an antiviral protein, which can react with uninfected cells to render them resistant to infection by a wide variety of viruses.

The important role played by **interferon as a defense mechanism** against viruses is clearly documented by **three types** of experimental and clinical observations. For many viral infections, a strong correlation has been established between interferon production and natural recovery; inhibition of interferon production or action enhances the severity of infection; and treatment with interferon protects against infection.

In addition, the interferon system is one of the earliest appearing of known host defenses, **becoming operative within hours of infection.** Clinical studies of interferon and its inducers have shown protection against certain viruses, including hepatitis B and C viruses, papovaviruses, rhinoviruses, and herpes simplex virus.

There are three types of interferon-**alpha, beta, and gamma** that differ both structurally and antigenically and have molecular weights ranging from 16,000 to 45,000. Interferons are secreted **by the cell into the extracellular fluids.** Usually virus induced interferon is produced at about the same time as the virus progeny are released by the infected cell thus protecting neighbouring cell from the spreading virus.

The three known types of interferon are induced by different stimuli.

Alpha interferon is induced by foreign cells, virus-infected cells, tumor cells, bacterial cells, and viral envelopes that stimulate mostly circulating dendritic cells and to a lesser degree monocytes and B lymphocytes to produce it.

Beta interferon is induced by viral and other foreign nucleic acids in most body cells (fibroblasts, epithelial cells, and macrophages).

Gamma interferon is produced (along with other lymphokines) by T lymphocytes induced by foreign antigens to which the T lymphocytes have been presensitized. Mitogens for T cells may mimic this induction. **Gamma interferon has several unusual properties: (1)** it exerts **greater immunomodulatory activity, including activation of macrophages,** than the other interferons; **(2)** it exerts **greater lytic effects** than the other interferons; **(3)** it **potentiates the actions of other interferons; (4)** it **activates cells** by a mechanism significantly different from that of the other interferons; and **(5)** it **inhibits intracellular microorganisms other than viruses** (e.g., rickettsia).

Inducers of interferon react with cells to derepress the interferon gene(s). This leads to the production of mRNA for interferon. The mRNA is translated into the interferon protein, which is secreted into the extracellular fluid, where it reacts with the membrane receptors of cells. The interferon-stimulated cells derepress genes for effector proteins (AVP) that establish antiviral resistance and other cell changes. The activated cells also stimulate contacted cells to produce AVP by a still unknown mechanism.

Interferon does not inactivate viruses **directly**. Instead, **it prevents viral replication in surrounding cells by reacting with specific receptors** on the cell membranes **to derepress** cellular genes that encode intracellular effector antiviral proteins, which must be synthesized before virus replication can be inhibited.

Alpha and beta interferons both bind to the same type of membrane receptor; **gamma interferon** binds to a different receptor. The **antiviral proteins** probably inhibit viral multiplication by inhibiting the synthesis of essential viral proteins, but **alternative or additional inhibitory mechanisms** (e.g. inhibition of transcription and viral release) also occur.

Viral protein synthesis may be inhibited by several biochemical alternatives of cells which can inhibit viral relication at different steps.

It has been shown that the antiviral state may be transferred from interferon-treated cells to adjacent untreated cells without the continued presence of interferon; this transfer mechanism may further simplify & spread the activity of the interferon system. The **interferon system is nonspecific in two ways**: various viral stimuli induce the same type of interferon, and the same type of interferon inhibits various viruses.

On the other hand, the interferon molecules are mostly specific in its action for the animals species in which it was induced: interferon produced by animals or humans generally stimulates antiviral activity only in cells of the same or closely related families (e.g., human interferon protects human and monkey cells, but not chicken cells).

Interferon during natural infection

The importance of interferon in the response to certain natural virus infections **varies.** Much depends on the effectiveness of the virus in stimulating interferon production & on its susceptibility. Interferon **protects solid tissues during virus infection;** it is also **disseminated through the bloodstream during viremia,** thereby **protecting distant organs** against the spreading infection. **Cells protected against viral replication may eliminate virus by degrading the virus genome.**

Viral Strategy to Evade Host Defense Mechanisms:

The antiviral state induced by IFN-α & IFN-β types of IFNs is characterized by inhibition of viral replication, inhibition of protein synthesis, degradation of mRNA and induction of apoptosis. This is an important impediment to a virus's ability to replicate itself; and needs to be overcome in some way for a virus to ensure its survival.

Some highly virulent viruses (e.g. poliovirus) rapidly inhibit cellular RNA and protein synthesis, and thus interfere with the ability of cells to produce IFN; others offer more subtle regulation. An overview shows that DNA viruses generally target the IFN mediated signal transduction; the cellular PKR and RNase L enzymes that form the effector arm of IFN responses are also popular targets with many viruses. Viruses have developed various strategies to subvert host's antiviral responses to ensure their own replication and survival as shown in Table 4-1.

Antagonism with other cytokines

Interferons are not the only cytokines targetted by viral products. Viruses have developed elaborate forms of molecular mimicry whose only purpose appears to be to circumvent cytokine-mediated host defenses (Table 4-5). Many viruses can direct the synthesis of proteins that can either neutralize cytokines or inhibit their synthesis.

Table 4-4 : Molecular mechanisms developed by viruses to inhibit interferon actions

Virus	Virus product	Specific target	Mechanism of action
Adenovirus	Ela protein	Signal transduction	Blocks INF signaling
	VA RNA	PKR	Blocks activation
Vaccinia	E L protein	PKR	Blocks ds RNA
Epstein-Barr virus	EBNA 2 protein	Signal transduction	Blocks signaling
	EBER RNA	PKR	Blocks activation
Myxoma virus	M-T7 protein	INF-ã	Neutralizes INF-ã
Hepatitis B virus	Terminal protein	Signal transduction	Blocks signaling
Herpes simplex virus	2-5(A) analogues	RNAse L	Blocks activation
HIV-1 virus	Tat protein	PKR	Degrades PKR
	TAR RNA	PKR	Blocks activation
Reovirus	Sigma 3 protein	PKR	Binds ds RNA
Hepatitis C virus	E2 glycoprotein	PKR	Blocks activation

Table 4-5 : Proteins encoded by viruses that inhibit cytokine action

Virus	Product	Mechanism of action
Epstein-Barr virus	BCRFI (viral RL-10 which inhibits synthesis of INF-α which binds to & signals through the human IL-10 receptor)	Inhibits synthesis of INF- ã, Il-2, IL-1, TNF; it facilitates EBV replication by promoting B cell growth& transformation.
Poxvirus	Cytokine response modifier (crmA), a protease inhibitor.	Inhibits proteolytic activation of IL-1β by IL-1β converting enzyme (ICE) & thus blocks apoptosis induced by CTLs, TNF or Fas.
Vaccinia & cowpox virus	Array of cytokine receptors	Bind & block the activity of α, β, γ, INF, TNF, IL-1.

Evading host's NK cell responses

NK cells can kill certain virus-infected and tumor cells without prior activation and sensitization. Apart from killing virus-infected cells, NK cells play an important role in immune regulation by secreting immunologically important cytokines and chemokines, e.g., including IFN-, TNF-, macrophage-inflammatory protein-1 (MIP-1), and MIP-1ß. The NK cell-secreted IFN and TNF- may also control viral replication by noncytolytic mechanisms. NK cells and mature DC reciprocally activate each other. NK cells are usually activated in early phases of a viral infection, & activated NK cells are important in killing virus-infected cells, especially before the generation of virus-specific CTL and antibodies. NK cells activity is controlled by a diverse array of **activating and inhibitory receptors and coreceptors,** which bind different ligands present on the surface of a target cell and send activating and inhibitory signals to the NK cell. The balance between the inhibitory and activating signals determines whether the NK cells would kill the target cell or be inhibited from killing it. The most important ligands, which bind inhibitory receptors on NK cells and inhibit their activity, are MHC class I antigens, especially HLA-C and -E. Most body cells and tumor cells usually express ligands for some activating NK cell receptors. NK cells would kill these cells by default unless they are inhibited by the engagement of their inhibitory receptors. The presence of MHC class I antigens on the surface of a cell usually makes it resistant to NK cell-mediated killing.

As NK cells could play an important role in controlling virus replication, viruses have evolved many strategies to evade host's NK cell responses (Table4 -6). Moreover, certain viruses encode proteins, which are MHC class I homologues and can inhibit NK cell activation. The HCMV encodes MHC class I -chain homologue UL18, which can complex with ß2m and bind endogenous peptides. It is resistant to down-regulation by the viral proteins US2, -3, -6, and -11. Similarly, the MCMV encodes a MHC class I homologue, m144, which confers protection from NK cell effector functions, even when classical MHC class I antigens are down-regulated from the surface of the virus-infected cells. In vivo studies have shown that m144-expressing MHC class I-deficient lymphoma cells can inhibit activation and accumulation of NK at the site of immune challenge. Finally, viruses may induce de novo expression of certain MHC antigens and inhibit NK cell functions. For example, HIV induces HLA-G and HLA-E on the surface of HIV-infected cells. Both molecules act as ligands for certain inhibitory NK cell receptors.

Viruses usually down-regulate the expression of MHC class I on the surface of the infected cells to escape antiviral CTL. However, this MHC down-regulation usually makes them susceptible to NK cell-mediated killing. Many viruses, therefore, have evolved the strategy to differentially down-regulate MHC class I antigens. They down-regulate HLA-A and -B but not HLA-C and -E. As HLA-A and -B mainly present virus-derived antigenic peptides to CTL, their down-regulation protects virus-infected cells from CTL-mediated killing. Conversely, HLA-C and -E mainly act as ligands for inhibitory NK cell receptors by maintaining their normal expression on the surface of virus-infected cells; viruses tend to maintain their resistance to NK cells. This way, these viruses can evade CTL and maintain resistance of the virus-infected cell to NK cells.

The viruses may also evade NK cell responses by increasing the expression of HLA-E. For its expression on the cell surface, this nonclassical HLA molecule needs peptides derived from the signal sequences of HLA-G and many HLA-A, -B, and -C allotypes. The HCMV protein UL-40 acts as a source of the peptides that can bind HLA-E. Thus, by supplying a source of HLA-E-specific peptides, UL-40 stabilizes the expression of HLA-E on the surface of HCMV-infected cells. HLA-E inhibits NK cell activation by interacting with the inhibitory receptor CD94/NKG2A.

Table 4-6 : Viral strategies to evade NK cell responses

Virus	Virus protein	Effect on infected cells	Effect on NK cells
EBV	EBNA-1	Novel peptides for HLA-A, -B	NK cell activation via KIR3DL
HCMV	Pp65		NK cell activation via NKp30
	UL 40	HLA-E	NK cell activation via NKG2A
	UL 18		NK cell activation via ILT-2
	UL 141	CD155 (PVR)	NK cell activation via DNAM-1,CD96(TACTILE)
	UL 16	ULBP1, -2; MIC-B	NK cell activation via NKG2D
MCMV	m157		Binds LY49I, NK cell activation
	m 155	H60	NK cell activation via NKG2D
	m 152	H60, Rae-1	Do
	m 145	MULT-1	Do
HCV	E2		NK cell activation via CD81
HIV-1	nef	HLA-A, -B but not of HLA-C,-E	Maintenance of NK
KSHV	K5	HLA-A, -B but not of HLA-C, -E	

Table 4-7 : Viral products that interfere with host defenses.

Host defense affected	Virus	Virus product	Mechanism
Interferon	EBV	EBERS (small RNAs)	Blocks protein kinase activation
	Vaccinia	eIF-2 alpha homologue	Prevents phosphorylation of eIF-2 alpha by protein kinase

Complement	Vaccinia	Homologues of C′ control proteins	Blocks complement activation
Cytokines	Shope fibroma virus	TNF receptor	Competes for TNF and blocks function
	EBV	IL-10 homolog	Reduces IFN-gamma function
MHC Class I	CMV	Early protein	Prevents transport of peptide-loaded MHC
	Adenovirus	E3	Blocks transport of MHC to surface
Apoptosis	Adenovirus	14.7K	Inhibits capsases
	EBV	Bcl-2 homolog	Anti-apoptotic
NK cells	HCMV	UL-18	MHC homolog inhibits NK cells

Virus Modulation of Cell Death

Programmed cell death (PCD) or **apoptosis** is a process in which cells are induced to commit suicide. It occurs during embryogenesis, tissue differentiation, aging or tumour regression. Apoptosis can be triggered by a variety of external and internal stimuli which include viral infection, growth factor withdrawal and DNA damage. It is an effective way for the organism to sacrifice a few infected cells to limit the spread of infection, or cells with damaged DNA to preserve the overall genetic integrity. Cells undergoing apoptosis show DNA laddering, chromatin condensation and break-up into small, membrane-wrapped pieces (apoptotic bodies). These apoptotic bodies are engulfed by nearby phagocytic cells, e.g. macrophages and thus the entire scavenging action takes place without induction of an inflammatory response. It is noteworthy that NK and CTL use apoptosis as the principal mechanism for killing virus-infected cells. They do so by releasing certain cytotoxic molecules, such as TNF-, **perforin, and granzymes**, as well as by engaging DR on the surface of the virus-infected cells. It is noteworthy that the granzyme B, which is released by CTL and NK cells and is endocytosed by the target cells, can activate several caspases directly.

Viruses encode various proteins to modulate apoptosis to their own advantage (Table 4-7). They inhibit premature apoptosis of the virus-infected cells (before replication of the virus has occurred). After completion of the viral replication, viruses may promote apoptosis to disseminate progeny virus without causing inflammatory responses. Viral anti-apoptotic strategies also help the virus evade CTL and NK cell-mediated killing of the virus-infected cells.

Viral Pathogenesis

Viral pathogenesis deals with the interaction between a virus and its host. The scope of pathogenesis is the stepwise progression of infection from virus entry through dissemination to shedding, the defensive responses of the host and the mechanisms of virus clearance or persistence. Pathogenesis also encompasses the disease processes that result from infection, variations in viral pathogenicity and the genetic basis of host resistance to infection or disease. Understanding how viruses spread from the initial site of infection to become systemic and cause symptoms in a host is an important aspect of viral pathogenesis.

Interactions between a virus and its host include: i. virus entry, ii. virus spread, iii. virus localization or tropism, iv. virus shedding, v. virus transmission, vi. virus factors - virulence, & vii. host factors- resistance/ susceptibility.

1. Virus Entry:

Common pathways of virus entry include the following:

1. Skin and mucous membranes
2. Respiratory tract
3. Oropharynx and gastrointestinal tract
4. Genitourinary tract
5. Transcutaneous and intravenous injection

Various viruses adopt different routes to enter their hosts, & some viruses enter through more than one routes; **Table** 4-8, 9, 10,11,12,13, 14 depicts routes employed by viruses to enter their hosts.

Entry through skin & mucous membrane

Skin outer layer is made of dead, keratinized cells-stratified squamous epithelium of epidermis that is very protective & cannot support viral infection, epidermis is not vascularized & it is difficult for infection to spread. Beneath the epidermis, dermis and subdermal tissue is highly vascularized & it is easy for infection to spread, therefore usually only a local infection can occurs. Although skin is a good barrier, skin is broken by trauma, abrasion, scratch, insect bite, needle etc. Skin may be penetrated by viruses as a result of: mechanical trauma (HPV, HIV, HSV, HBV, poxvirus), by injection (HBV, HIV), by the bite of an infected insect (arboviruses) or by the bite of an infected animal (rabies). Some viruses such as papillomaviruses, poxviruses and herpes simplex viruses will replicate in cells of the skin or mucous membranes. Most viruses that replicate in the skin grow in the germinal cells, and papillomaviruses have a selective tropism for these cells & produce proliferative lesions. Poxviruses and herpes simplex viruses also replicate in fibroblasts and macrophages in the dermis. Infections with these viruses are initiated at breaks in the epithelium. Mucous membranes represent a minimal physical barrier to infection but are bathed in mucus that contains immunoglobulin and provides protection by virtue of its viscous nature.

Following infection, generally viruses do not multiply locally but are carried away from site of infection by bloodstream (HBV, arboviruses) or migration along nerves (rabies). A list of viruses entering through skin is shown in Figure 4-8.

Table 4-8 : Virus entry through skin & mucosa

Family/Genus	Virus	Routes
Herpesviridae	Several herpesviruses	Minor abrasions
Papillomaviridae	Many papillomaviruses	Do
Picornaviridae	Swine vesicular disease virus	Do
Poxviridae	Cowpox, bovine paplar stomatitis, Swinepox, orf, pseudocowpox, fowl pox	Do
Rhabdoviridae	VSV	Do
Poxviridae	Fowlpox, myxoma swinepox viruses	Bite of arthropod/ mechanical
Retroviridae	Equine infectious anemia	Do
Rhabdviridae	VSV	Do
Asfarviridae	ASFV	Arthropod bite-biological transmission
Bunyaviridae	*Phlebovirus* –RVFV; *Nairovirus*-Nairobi sheep disease virus	Do
Flaviviridae/Flavivirus	Almost all members	Do
Reoviridae/Orbivirus	Bluetongue, African horse sickness	Do
Rhabdoviridae	Bovine ephemeral fever virus, VSV	Do
Togaviridae/Alphavirus	All members	Do
Retroviridae/Lentivirus	Feline immunodeficiency virus	Bite of vertebrate
Rhabdoviridae	Rabies virus	Do

Papillmaviridae	Most of the member viruses	Infected needles, equipments
Polyomaviridae	Most of the member viruses	Do
Flaviviridae/Pestiivirus	CSFV, BVD	Do
Retroviridae/Lentivirus /Delta	Equine infectious anemia, BLV	Do
Herpesviridae	IBR virus, Equine herpesvirus 1	Via Conjunctiva
Adenoviridae/Mastade-novirus	Canine adenovirus-1, 2	Do

Entry through respiratory tract

Respiratory tract provides huge absorptive surface area (140m) & there is high turnover; at resting ventilatory rate (6L/min) samples environment. A layer of mucus (traps the virus) produced by goblet cells and ciliated epithelial cells clear the respiratory tract of foreign bodies. In spite of protective system, respiratory infection is most common; viruses attach to respiratory tract by specific receptors present on upper & lower respiratory tract. Infection is initiated either by virus contained in aerosols that are inhaled by the recipient host or by virus that is contained in nasopharyngeal fluids and is transmitted by hand-to-hand contact. Aerosolized droplets are deposited at different levels in the respiratory tract depending upon their size: those over 10 μm diameter are deposited in the nose, those 5-10 μm in the airways and those <5 μm in the alveoli. There are phagocytic cells in the respiratory lumen. The temperature of the respiratory tract modify infection, Rhinovirus replicates at 33ºC (nose = URT) while Influenza virus replicates at 37ºC (alveola = LRT). In respiratory tract once deposited, the virus must bypass several effective barriers to initiate infection. Most respiratory viruses initiate infection by replicating in epithelial cells lining the alveoli or the respiratory tree. Several viruses remain localized (rhinoviruses, adenoviruses, & influenza viruses), other viruses become systemic (FMD, CD, RP, CSFV & NDV). Table 4-9 depicts viruses that enter through respiratory tract.

Table 4.9 : Virus entry through respiratory tract

Family	Virus	Disease
Adenoviridae/ Mastadenovirus, Aviadenovirus	Animal adenoviruses	Mainly respiratory disease
Calciviridae	Feline calicivirus	Do
Coronaviridae	Avian infectious bronchitis virus	Do

Herpesviridae	Herpesviruses of several animals	Do
Orthmyxoviridae	Swine influenza, horse influenza	Do
Paramyxviridae	Parainfluenza & res syncytial viruses	Do
Picornaviridae	Rhinoviruses of animals, FMD	Do
Arenaviridae	LCM virus	Causes systemic disease
Herpesviridae	Pseudorabies, BMCFV, Marek's disease virus	Do
Flaviridae	Swine fever virus	Do
Orthomyxoviridae	Avian influenza viruses	Do
Paramyxoviridae	CDV, RPV	Do

Entry through the oropharynx and gastrointestinal tract

The oropharynx and gastrointestinal tract is an important portal of entry for many viruses. Intestinal host defenses include acidic stomach, alkaline intestine, digestive enzymes, detergents, phagocytes, mucous, & IgA. These conditions are very hostile for most viruses (especially enveloped). Virus survival depends on acid stability & resistance to bile salts inactivation by proteolytic enzymes. Enteric viruses may invade the host in a variety of sites from the oral cavity to the colon. Viruses causing intestinal infections include: enteroviruses, rotaviruses and caliciviruses. Entry via GI tract may involve local infection (rotavirus, coronavirus and adenovirus) or invasion of the host to produce systemic illness (enteroviruses, hepatitis A) due to invasion of tissues underlying the mucosal layer. Some viruses may be taken up by the M cells overlying the Peyers patches. Most enteric viruses, such as rotaviruses, caliciviruses, toroviruses & astroviruses cause diarrhea in animals. Enteric viruses infect the epithelium of the small or large intestine but some enteroviruses, such as poliovirus, also can replicate in the lymphoid tissue of the gut and nasopharynx. Parvovirus reaches intestinal tract cells following viremia. Table 4-10 shows viruses favouring intestinal tract for entry.

Entry through genitourinary tract

Nature of cervical mucus, the pH of vaginal secretions and the chemical composition of urine all play a role in host defenses. Several viruses cause sexually transmitted disease, which is usually acquired by exposure to virus containing secretions. HIV, herpes simplex (mostly HSV II), BHV-1, EqHV-3, papillomaviruses (genital warts) & hepatitis B virus infection is initiated either by penetration through breaks in the skin or by direct invasion of the superficial epithelium of the mucous membranes. Some sexually transmitted viruses, such as hepatitis B and human immunodeficiency virus (HIV) may be introduced directly into the circulation via breaks in skin and membranes by exposure to contaminated blood or semen. Viruses using genital tract for entry are presented in Table 4-11.

Table 4.10 : Virus entry through intestinal tract

Family	Virus	Disease
Astroviridae	Astroviruses of animals	Diarrhea
Coronaviridae/ Coronavirus	Enteric coronaviruses, mouse hepatitis virus	Diarrhea
Coronaviridae/Torovirus	Bredavirus	Diarrhea
Flaviviridae	Bovine virus diarrhea	Diarrhea
Parvoviridae	Feline panleukopenia virus, Canine parvovirus	Diarrhea
Reoviridae/ Rotavrus	Rotavirus diarrhea in young animals	Diarrhea
Adenoviridae/ Mastadenovirus Aviadenovirus	Adenoviruses of many animals	Systemic disease
Calciviridae/Vesivirus	Vesicular exanthema of swine	Do
Picornaviridae/ Enterovirus	Enteroviruses of many animals	Do

Table 4.11 : Virus entry through genital tract

Family	Virus	Disease
Arteriviridae	Equine arteritis virus	Genital infection
Herpesviridae/many viruses	IBRV, herpesviruses of many animals	Do
Paillomaviridae	Bovine papillomaviruses	Do

Entry through transcutaneous and intravenous injection

Although the skin is a formidable barrier, mechanical injection that breaches the barrier is a 'natural' route of entry for many viruses. Some viruses that infect by this mechanism are: Arboviruses (insect bite), Rabies virus (dog bite), & Hepatitis B, HCV (intravenous inoculation). Arboviruses are those animal viruses that are maintained in nature by a cycle that involves an insect vector and a vertebrate host. When the infected vector takes a blood meal, virus contained in the salivary gland is injected into the host. Examples are

Dengue, RRV, MVE etc. Rhabdoviruses-rabies is the only virus that is maintained in many of its natural cycles by the bite of a sick animal. Following transcutaneous and intramuscular injection, the virus may either enter the processes of peripheral nerves directly or replicate in striated muscle. It can then cross the neuromuscular junction and spread along peripheral nerves to the central nervous system. Injection or transfusion in case of HBV, HCV, HIV viruses may be transmitted accidentally by repeated use of contaminated needles, injection of a virus contaminated therapeutic substance, or transfusion with virus-contaminated blood or blood products. The agents most frequently involved are those that produce persistent viremia, such as hepatitis B, C or D, cytomegalovirus and human immunodeficiency virus. Following injection, virus appears to be widely disseminated, rapidly reaching those cells for which it has a tropism.

In viremic infections, some viruses cross placenta & reach fetal circulation. Among these viruses, some cause fetal death, resorption, abortion, stillbirth, mummification, infertility or congenital defects. Included among these viruses are Akabane virus, bovine leukemia virus, BT virus, IBV, BVDV in cattle; EHV-1, pseudorabies virus, hog cholera virus, & canine hepesvirus etc (Table: 4-12).

Entry through lymphoreticular & haematopoietic system

Viruses that infect cells of lymphoreticular & haematopoietic system include filoviruses, arenaviruses, hantaviruses, certain bunyaviruses (RVFV), & VEEV. Viruses infecting cells of immune system is present in Table 4-13.

Other organs

Rift valley fever & ICH causes severe hepatitis, togaviruses & coxsackievirus infect muscle cells, & CAEV infect synovial cells to cause arthritis.

Virus Spread

Once infection is established at the site of entry, most viruses spread locally by cell-to-cell transmission of infection. **Local infection** refers to viral replication at the site of inoculation. **Disseminated infection** refers to virus spread and infection/disease at site distant from virus inoculum. **Systemic dissemination** occurs if disseminated virus infects multiple organs. Some viruses remain localized near their site of entry whereas others spread widely. Breach of physical and immune barriers leads to disseminated infection. Basement membrane is barrier to subepithelial tissues, but is compromised by inflammation (host) or destruction (viral replication).

Table 4.12 : Virus infecting fetuses

Family	Virus	Animal	Symptoms
Arenaviridae	LCM virus	Mice	Lifelong inaparent carrier state & shedding
Arteriviridae	Equine arteritis virus	Horses	Feta death & abortion
Bunyaviridae/Bunyavirus	Akabane virus	Cattle	Fetal death, abortion, stillbirth, congenital defects
Bunyaviridae/Phlebovirus	Rift Valley fever virus	Sheep	Fetal death, abortion
Bunyaviridae/Nairovirus	Nairobi sheep disease virus	sheep	Fetal death, abortion
Flaviviridae/Pestivirus	BVDV	Cattle	Fetal death, abortion, congenital defects, inapparent with lifelong carrier state & shedding
Flaviviridae/Flavivirus	JEV	Swine	Fetal death, abortion
Flaviviridae/Pestivirus	Swine fever virus	Swine	Fetal death, abortion, congenital defects, inaparent carrier & shedding
Herpesviridae/Varicellovirus	IBR virus	Cattle	Fetal death, abortion
Herpesviridae/Varicellovirus	Pseudorabies virus	Swine	Fetal death, abortion
Parvoviridae/Parvovirus	Swine parvovirus	Swine	Fetal death, abortion, mummification, stillbirth, infertility
Parvoviridae/Parvovirus	Feline panleukopenia	Cat	Cerebral hypoplasia
Parvoviridae/Parvovirus	Rat virus	Rat	Fetal death
Picornaviridae/ Enterovirus	Avian encephalomyel itis virus	Chicken	Congenital defects, fetal death
Reoviridae/Orbivirus	Bluetongue virus	Cattle	Fetal death, abortion, congenital defects
Reoviridae/Orbivirus	Bluetongue virus	Sheep	Fetal death, abortion, congenital defects
Retroviridae/Deltaretrovirus	Bovine leukemia virus	Cattle	Inapparent, leukemia
Retroviridae/ Gammaretrovirus	Feline leukemia virus	Cat	Inapparent, leukemia, fetal death

Table 4.13 : Viruses infecting cells of immune system

Cells	
B lymphocytes	Equine herpesvirus-2, EB virus, IBD virus, Murine leukemia virus, Simian type D retrovirus.
T lymphocytes	Feline leukemia virus, Feline immunodeficiency virus, HIV-1, 2, Simian immunodeficiency virus.
Monocytes	CDV, Caprine arthritis-encephalitis virus, CMV, Influenza viruses, LCM-mice& hamsters, Lactose dehydrogenase virus in mice, Maedi/visna virus-sheep, parainfluenza viruses-cattle, humans, other species, & VEE virus.
Dendritic cells	HIV-1, 2, LCM virus-hamsters, mice
Stromal cells of lymphoreticular tissues	Cytomegalovirus- several host species, Borna disease virus-horse, rabbit, cat

One determinant of dissemination is the pattern of viral release from polarized epithelial cells. Viruses that are released only at the apical surface of infected cells tend to remain localized, whereas those that are released at the basal surface tend to disseminate.

Usually, the first step in dissemination of the infection is the transport of virus via the efferent lymphatic drainage from the initial site of infection to the regional lymph nodes, either as free virions or in virus-infected phagocytic cells. Then the most important route of dissemination is the **blood circulation**, which can potentially carry viruses to any site in the body. This is known as **viremia**. There are several sources of viremia. Virus may enter the blood with the efferent lymphatic flow, or may be shed from infected endothelial cells or circulating mononuclear leucocytes. Viruses can circulate free in the plasma phase of the blood ('plasma' viremia). Virus may get into the bloodstream by direct inoculation - e.g. Arthropod vectors, blood transfusion or I.V. drug abuse. The virus may travel free in the plasma (togaviruses, enteroviruses, parvoviruses), or in association with red cells (orbiviruses), platelets (HSV), lymphocytes (EBV, CMV) or monocytes (BTV, feline leukemia, CDV, Beta & gammaherpesviruses, lentiviruses). Primary viraemia usually proceeds and is necessary for spread to the blood stream, followed by more generalized, higher titer secondary viremia as the virus reaches other target tissues or replicates directly in blood cells. Viruses may be associated with cells ('cell-associated' viremia). Once the host has developed circulating antibody, plasma virus is very rapidly neutralized, and virus-antibody complexes are formed, facilitating removal by sessile macrophages. Exceptions are instances in which the infected host is 'tolerant' of the viral antigens and fails to develop enough antibodies to clear viremia. Example is chronic hepatitis B. Tissue invasion from the blood may occur. There are several ways in which a virus might cross the vascular wall, but the precise mechanism for penetrating the blood-tissue barrier is unknown in most instances.

Tissue Invasion: 1. In many tissues viruses can pass between capillary/endothelial cell junctions. 2. Virus may be transported through endothelial cells by endocytosis, translocation of virus-containing vesicles and subsequent release by exocytosis at the basal surface of the endothelial cells.

Neural spread

Some viruses can disseminate by spreading along peripheral nerves. This is important for rabies, several herpesviruses, Borna disease, pseudorabies, & BHV-5 infection. Viruses enter neurons by mechanisms similar to those involving entry into other cell types. Spread to nervous system is preceded by primary viraemia. In some cases, spread occurs directly by contact with neurons at the primary site of infection, in other cases via the bloodstream. Once in peripheral nerves, the virus can spread to the CNS by axonal transport along neurons (classic - HSV). Viruses can cross synaptic junctions since these frequently contain virus receptors, allowing the virus to jump from one cell to another. The uncoated nucleocapsid is then carried passively along axons or dendrites, by fast axoplasmic flow. After the transport process the virus may replicate in the perikaryon, but this is a much slower process and is not required for neural spread.

Localization or Tropism

One of the salient features that distinguish viruses is their localization within the animal host. Tropism is the ability of a virus to replicate in particular cells or tissues, & is controlled partly by the route of infection but largely by the interaction of a virus attachment protein (V.A.P.) with a **specific receptor molecule on the surface of a cell,** and has considerable effect on pathogenesis. Many V.A.P.'s and virus receptors are now known (Table 4-3). If tissue has receptor for a virus, then that virus could attach and potentially infect. But there are very few instances where receptor is the only determining factor for viral tropism. For example, receptor for influenza virus is sialic acid (ubiquitous in body), but the virus only infects respiratory cells. CD4 is the receptor for HIV-1: parallels tropism, but still requires co-receptor for virus entry. Cell proteins are involved in viral transcription. JC Papovavirus only replicates in oligodendrocytes. Viral enhancer is involved in DNA-dependent RNA synthesis; it is only active in oligodedrocytes. Cell proteases in Influenza virus play a role: HA (hemaglutinnin receptor) must be cleaved by serine proteases in order to be infectious.

Clara cells in respiratory tract secrete protease, "Tryptase Clara" which cleaves HA of influenza virions & the virion is released by nearby respiratory epithelial cells. What about then influenza virions spread to liver? Can't infect liver because there are no clara cells to secrete and activate HA on basolateral surface of respiratory tract or at liver. The names of individual viral diseases often reflect the organs or tissues that are involved: glandular fever, hepatitis & encephalitis. Localization of infection or **viral tropism** is regulated both by viral dissemination and by cellular susceptibility.

Viral dissemination

The localization of a virus is determined at several phases of infection: penetration at the portal of entry, systemic spread by viremia or the neural route, & invasion of local organs or tissues. Most viruses are quite selective in the cell types that are infected in vivo and this selectivity plays a significant role in viral pathogenesis.

Virus Shedding

Acute viral infections are characterized by brief periods of intensive virus shedding into respiratory aerosols, feces, urine or other bodily secretions or fluids. Shedding may occur in the gastrointestinal tract via feces (enteric viruses), respiratory tracts via mucus, saliva, sneezing, eating & drinking (BHV-1, paramyxoviruses, some coronaviruses); skin (cowpox, vaccinia, papillomaviruses & herpesviruses), urinary tract in the urine (ICHV, FMDV, RPV, arena viruses), mucous membranes, oral and genital fluids (equine arthritis virus), semen and milk (caprice arthritis encephalitis virus, mouse mammary tumor virus), blood (arthropod-borne viruses) and urine. Persistent viruses are often shed at relatively low titers, but this may be adequate for transmission over the prolonged duration of infection.

Modes of Transmission

- Inhalation of aerosolized virus.
- Direct person-to-person contact (oral-oral, genital genital, oral-genital or skin-skin).
- Indirect person-to-person transmission via blood or contaminated needles.
- Common source transmissions via contaminated water, food products or biologicals such as blood products & vaccines.

In the cycle of infection, the period during transmission of the viral agent from one host to the next is when the virus is exposed to the environment and therefore most vulnerable. The major division is between direct transmission, which is essentially immediate, and indirect transmission, which is delayed. Direct (essentially immediate) transmission occurs by contact (touching, kissing, sexual intercourse etc.), & by large droplet at limited distance.

Indirect transmission is vehicle-borne, indirect contact through fomites, other inanimate objects and biological substances (water, milk, urine, stool etc.).

Vector-borne transmission is either mechanical without multiplication or biological with multiplication in the vectors, & dusts and air-borne droplet nuclei (aerosols).

Virulence of viruses

Virulence refers to the ability of a virus strain or isolate to cause illness or death in an infected host, relative to other isolates or variants of the same agent. That is, different strains of a given virus may vary in their ability to cause disease. Virulence is not an absolute property of a virus strain but depends on the dose of virus, the route of infection and the age, gender and genetic susceptibility of the host. The conventional measure of viral virulence is the ability to produce disease in the host, using as an endpoint either death or some specific symptoms caused by the infection.

Virulence refers to capacity of virus to cause disease. Avirulent/ Attenuated virus is infectious but causes no disease or reduced disease. We can quantify virulence: e.g. how much virus is needed to kill half of animals, cause paralysis in half of animals, "mean time to death," etc. Quantification of virulence helps determine and measure treatment outcomes.

What makes viruses virulent? Goal of virology is to understand the genes of virus and host that determines virulence. Most genes are identified by mutation (delete or disrupt gene-then determine if virulence is present or absent). There are four classes of genes affecting virulence via different mechanisms: Enhancer that helps in viral replication, Modification of host defense mechanisms enable viral spread in host, & have intrinsic cell killing effects.

Genes affecting viral replication. Take first gene affecting growth in cell culture and in vivo. If we mutate gene to create attenuated virus and it slows growth in cell culture and also in live mouse, then you don't care much. If a 2nd gene is mutated and it grows well in cell culture but not well in a live mouse, then this is the type of gene to target in vaccines/therapies etc.

Genes that modify host defense mechanisms; non specific host response involves release of cytokines to recruit immune cells. **Virokines** are proteins that mimic cytokines and try to block cytokine actions. Virokines mimic the action of cytokines; increases host cell proliferation and virus production. **Viroceptors** causes cytokine decoys & antibodies or complement scavenger. **Pox virusesVCP (Vaccinia Complement Control** Protein) abrogates complement mediated attack on viral infected cells; they are homolog of C4-BP that inactivates C4b, a critical player in the complement cascade.

TNF Viroceptors; TNF is proinflammatory cytokine that activates immune networks. Soluble TNF-receptor homology encoded by poxviruses can enable TNF secreted by host cell and dampen subsequent immune response. IL-4: "Super-" pox is Th2 cytokine which suppresses Th1 (cell-mediated) immunity. Mousepox engineered to express IL-4 becomes extremely virulent. Herpesviruses gE/gI glycoprotein can act as Fc receptors; prevent effector functions of antiviral antibodies produced by the host.

"*Super antigens*-Inhibit complement cascade activation; inhibit MHC-1/ Ag presentation. These genes are not needed for growth in culture, but are only virulent because of evading host response. Toxic viral proteins cause cell death, e.g. NSP4 glycoprotein of rotavirus, an enterotoxin causes gastroenteritis by increasing intracellular Ca+ and in young mice, causes increase in chloride secretion causing diarrhea. Probably it triggers signal transduction pathway resulting in ion imbalance.

Injury from viral infections

Cytolytic viruses have different mechanisms of cell injury/death; they inhibit host protein and RNA synthesis, cause loss of membrane integrity causing leakage of enzymes & degradation. Syncytium formation is the fusion of host and virus membranes. These viruses induce apoptosis—programmed cell death.

Non-cytolytic viruses do not cause cell injury/death. There are 3 mechanisms to do so: symptoms are due to host immune response mediated by CD8 cells, CD4 cells, phagocytes, etc. Example is coxsackieviruses and dengue virus, in which damage is due to free-radicals. **Cellular-based immune response:** Coxsackievirus infection leads to damage of heart tissue (myocarditis) that is due to host response (and damage) mediated by CD8 cells. Nl CTL job is to lyse and clear virus infected cells.

Perforin, enzyme is involved in cell lysis. Perforin KO mice have significantly less myocarditis.

Antibody-based immune response damage is seen in dengue virus, a mosquito-borne virus (Carribbean, Africa, C/S Amer, SE Asia) which has 4 serotypes. Primary infection is usually asymptomatic, may cause acute, febrile illness, usually self-limiting (50 million infections/yr)/14,000 primary infections. Dengue Hemorrhagic Fever (DHF) is severe & life-threatening. Patients produce antibodies to the infecting virus, & the patient are protected against the same virus, but not protected against 3 other serotypes. In secondary infection with a different serotype, the patient is not protected from it. However, it does mount a memory antibody response to the first serotype you encountered. This immune response enhances infection of immune cells by other serotypes. Memory antibodies bind monocytes via FC regions. Virus binds antibodies, then enter monocytes and induces release of cytokines causing dengue shock syndrome.

Free radical-induced cell injury is mediated by superoxide and nitric oxide produced during inflammatory responses. Nitric oixide synthase enzyme produced in virally infected tissues converts arginine to NO induced by IFN. Low concentration of NO is protective; high concentration causes tissue damage. High concentration reacts with superoxide to produce peroxynitrite which is much more reactive/damaging to tissues than O2- or NO. Treat infected animals with NO synthase inhibitors.

Host determinants of susceptibility and resistance

The outcome of the virus-host interaction is determined in part by host variables that can be conveniently considered under 2 categories:

- Physiological factors
- Genetic determinants

Physiological factors

The host response to a viral infection is influenced by a variety of physiological variables such as age, sex, stress and pregnancy, all of which have been shown to affect the outcome of infection with some viruses.

Genetic factors

Studies with inbred animals have shown that the outcome of infections often varies in different strains of mice, and show that genetic factors influence the inheritance of susceptibility to viral infection. Among the many viruses that are known to infect the human liver, hepatitis B virus (HBV) and hepatitis C virus (HCV) are unique because of their prodigious capacity to cause persistent infection, cirrhosis, and liver cancer. HBV and HCV are noncytopathic viruses and, thus, immunologically mediated events play an important role in the pathogenesis and outcome of these infections. The human gastrointestinal and respiratory tracts harbor the largest number and greatest diversity of microorganisms in the body. Proximity to the external environment makes these tissues especially vulnerable to pathogens and allergens, so it is not surprising that mucosal tissue contains the greatest immunological activity and number of immune cells, cytokines, and secondary lymphoid tissues. Causes of mucosal immune dysfunction include microbial infections, dietary indiscretions such as excess refined sugars and lack of fiber, allergies and food intolerances, indiscriminant and overuse of oral antibiotics, disruption of lipid and fatty acid metabolism, and aging. All of these etiologies, most a product of modern lifestyle, can result in dysfunctional mucosal immunity and may even be responsible for a wide range of chronic diseases.

The complement system functions as an immune surveillance system that rapidly responds to infection. Activation of the complement system by specific recognition pathways triggers a protease cascade, generating cleavage products that function to eliminate pathogens, regulate inflammatory responses, and shape adaptive immune responses. However, when deregulated, these powerful functions can become destructive and the complement system has been implicated as a pathogenic effector in numerous diseases, including infectious diseases.

Evasion of immune surveillance includes

- antigenic variation.
- immune tolerance, causing a reduced response to an antigen, may be due to genetic factors, pre-natal infection, molecular mimicry.
- restricted gene expression.
- down-regulation of MHC class I expression, resulting in lack of recognition of infected cells e.g. Adenoviruses.
- down-regulation of accessory molecules involved in immune recognition e.g. LFA-3 and ICAM-1 by EBV.
- infection of immunocompromised sites within the body e.g. HSV in sensory ganglia in the CNS.
- direct infection of the cells of the immune system itself e.g. Herpes viruses & retroviruses (HIV) - often resulting in immunosuppression.

Clearance

Example - Influenza virus:

Two mechanisms allow influenza virus to alter its antigenic constitution:

- *Antigenic Drift*: The gradual accumulation of minor mutations (e.g. nucleotide substitutions) in the virus genome which result in subtly altered coding potential and therefore altered antigenicity, resulting in decreased recognition by the immune system. This process occurs in all viruses all the time, but at greatly different rates, e.g. RNA viruses >>> DNA viruses. In response, the immune system constantly adapts by recognition of and response to novel antigenic structures - but is always one step behind. In most cases however, the immune system is eventually able to overwhelm the virus, resulting in clearance.

- *Antigenic Shift*: Is a sudden and major change in the antigenicity of a virus due to recombination of the virus genome with another genome of a different antigenic type. This process results initially in the failure of the immune system to recognize a new antigenic type, giving the virus the upper hand.

□□□

Chapter 5

Antiviral Immunity

Contents

Non Specific Host Defenses

Viruses are small, obligate intracellular parasites which cause infection by invading cells of the body and multiplying within them. Within their life cycle, they have a relatively short extracellular period, prior to infecting the cells, and a longer intracellular period during which they undergo replication. The immune system has mechanisms which can attack the virus in both these phases of its life cycle, and which involve both non-specific and specific effector mechanisms. The immune responses to viral infection comprise innate and adaptive defenses. In viral infections the host innate immune system is meant to act as a first line of defense to prevent viral invasion or replication before more specific protection by the adaptive immune system is generated. The innate immune response functions continuously in a normal host without exposure to any virus. Most viral infections are controlled by the innate immune system. However, if viral replication outpaces innate defenses, the adaptive response must be mobilized. Humans & animals have evolved a highly complex host defense system to combat a wide variety of pathogens. All living organisms have developed several kinds of mechanisms to protect themselves from invasion by exogenous microorganisms, including viruses. Although the production of neutralizing antibodies and activation of cytotoxic T lymphocytes (CTL) or natural killer (NK) cells are essential for a specific and effective antiviral immune response, other host cells also possess some immune mechanism to prevent viral infection. Although multiple cytokines and chemokines are produced by several kinds of host cells in viral infection, type I IFNs (INF α, & INF β) are the principal cytokines involved in the antiviral response. Developing a remedy for most of the viral infections still remains a great challenge as viruses evolve very rapidly as well as produce a variety of proteins that thwart host defenses. These features provide viruses with strategies to evade almost any hurdle imposed by the host defenses to block their replication. An outline of innate immune response & specific acquired immune responses are presented in Table 5-1.

Viruses & the diseases associated with them are the major cause of human & animal morbidity and mortality. When a virus infects a host, the latter tries to eliminate it by nonspecific defence mechanisms (anatomical barrier, cellular components, natural killer cells and interferons) & by stimulating both nonspecific & antigen-specific immune effector mechanisms, while the virus tries to subvert one or more of these mechanisms to prolong its own lifespan. Virus infections are characterized by high and rapid rate of viral replication, production of large numbers of progeny particles, rapid generation times, generation of high mutation rates, viruses hiding within cells & generating new variants in very short periods of time. Besides their small size, all viruses have only two common features, a genetic programme-either DNA or RNA, and a protein coat to protect this genetic information and aid in its transfer from one host to another. Small size necessitates a small genome, which is the reason for its being obligate intracellular parasites.

Table 5.1 : Nonspecific host defenses

Nonspecific resistance	Prevention of entrance to the body	Physical barrier	Skin barrier Mucous membranes One-way valves
		Removal by washing	Washing of the eyes Washing of the mouth Washing of the respiratory tract Washing of the urogenital tract Antimicrobials of the skin
		Chemical barrier	Lysozyme made by the body Gastric juices
	Inhibition within the body	---	Leukocytosis Phagocytosis Inflammation Fever Complement Interferon NK cells
Specific resistance	Cellular arm of the immune system	CD_4 T cells & CD_8 T cells	Cellular immune responses
	Antibodies	B cells	Humoral immune responses

Most viral infections are **limited by nonspecific defenses,** which restrict initial virus multiplication to manageable levels, initiate recovery from established infections that is then completed by a combination of these early nonspecific and subsequent antigen-specific immune defenses, and enable the host to cope with the peak numbers of virus that, if presented as the infecting dose, could be lethal.

Some nonspecific defenses exist **independent of infection like** genetic factors, anatomical barriers, nonspecific inhibitors in body fluids & phagocytosis. **Others like fever, inflammation, & interferon are produced by the host in response to infection**. All nonspecific defenses begin to act before the specific defense resonses develop. The fact that viruses **replicate intracellularly** and the ability of some viruses to spread by inducing cell fusion **partly protect viruses** against such extracellular defenses as neutralizing anibody, phagocytosis & nonspecific inhibitors. However, because they replicate within the cell, viruses are vulnerable to intracellular alterations caused by host responses to infection. Nonspecific responses that **alter the intracellular environment include** fever, inflammation, & interferon. These multiple defenses function with great complexity because of their interactions with one another. This complexity is compounded by the varying effectiveness of the defenses that results from the diversity of viruses, hosts, and sites and stages of infection.

Most viral infections are limited in the beginning by host defenses that are antigen nonspecific. Nonspecific defenses act immediately than specific defenses. Some of these host defenses are always in place like anatomical barrier, nonspecific inhibitors, & phagocytosis; others are evoked by the infection such as (fever, inflammation & interferon). In the case of many threats to an individual's well being, specific defenses [e.g., antibodies & cellular immunity] do not need to be called on because the body is adequately protected by its nonspecific defenses-those that act against any type of invading agent. Often such defenses perform their function before specific body defense mechanisms are activated."

Non-specific host defenses include: (i) Physical barrier, (ii) Chemical barrier, (iii) Cellular defences, (iv) Inflammation, (v) Fever, & (vi) Molecular defenses.

Physical Barriers (mucous membranes)

Physical barriers act to prevent pathogens from entering the body, they include the skin and mucous membranes, include the viscous mucous that covers mucous membranes, giving these membranes their name, movement of substances out of the body additionally serve as physical barriers, including the movement of mucous out of the lungs, the movement of urine down the urethra and out of the body, vomiting, diarrhea, and even the movement of blood out of a wound. Usually physical barriers do a good job of preventing pathogens from entering the body. However, some pathogens are capable of breaching these physical barriers, and sometimes physical barriers are not functional or are not as present as one would otherwise hope (e.g., cuts in the skin, drying out of mucous membranes, not voiding one's bladder when necessary, etc.); for example: A number of viruses specifically infect mucous-membranes or via them {e.g., polio virus (intestine), chickenpox (lungs)} & a number of viruses infect via skin abrasions (e.g., warts, smallpox, herpes, hepatitis B, HIV).

Anatomic Barriers

Anatomic barriers are located at body surfaces namely skin and mucosa or within the body such as endothelial cells and basement membranes. The dead cells of the epidermis and any live cells that may lack viral receptors resist virus penetration and do not permit virus replication. However, this barrier is easily breached, for example, by animal bites (rabies virus), insect bites (togaviruses), and minor traumas (wart virus), increased permeability, replication of virus in endothelial cells, or by transportation of virus in leukocytes. At mcosal surfaces, only the **mucus layer** stands between invading virus and live cells. They are partly effective in preventing virus spread.

Membrane receptors

The host range of the virus depend on the presence of appropriate receptors on the cell membrane (Table 4-3). If a host lacks the receptor for a virus or if the host cells lack some component necessary for the replication of a virus, the host will be resistant to that virus. Mice lack receptors for polio viruses and thus are resistant to polio virus, & humans are resistant to plant and many animal viruses.

Mucus

The mucus layer forms a physical barrier that entraps foreign particles and carries them out of the body; it also contains nonspecific inhibitors. The **mucus barrier is not absolute**, however, since **sufficient quantities of many viruses can overwhelm it and infect by this route**. In fact, most viruses use mucous surfaces as the portal of entry and initial replication site.

Ciliated epithelium

The sticky mucous lining of the nose and nasal passages acts as a filter, trapping bacteria and air-borne dirt particles. The mucus is then moved by the action of hair-like cilia either to the front of the nose where it can be blown out, or to the back of the nose where it enters the throat and is swallowed. The ciliated epithelium drives the mucociliary elevator & can help diminish infectivity of certain viruses. Ciliated activity has been shown to be important in respiratory infections since lack of the activity of this system causes an increased infection rate with a given virus.

Within the Body

Anatomic barriers to virus spread are formed by the **layer of endothelial cells that separates blood from tissues** (e.g., the blood barrier). Under normal conditions, these barriers have a low permeability for viruses unless the virus can penetrate them by replicating in the capillary endothelial cells or in circulating leukocytes. These internal barriers may explain, in part, the high level of viremia required to infect organs such as brain, placenta & lungs.

Nonspecific inhibitors

Body fluids and tissues normally contain **soluble viral inhibitors.** These inhibitors mostly prevent viral attachment, some directly inactivate viruses, and others act intracellularly and a few act by inhibiting virus replication. But these inhibitors are overwhelmed by sufficient number of virus. They vary **chemically** (lipids, polysaccharides, proteins, lipoproteins & glycoproteins) and in the **degree of viral inhibition** and **types of viruses affected.**

In the gastrointestinal tract, some susceptible viruses are inactivated by acid, bile salts, and enzymes.

Whereas **most inhibitors block only one or a few viruses, some** have a **broad antiviral spectrum.** Although the **effectiveness of the inhibitors** has not been fully established *in vivo,* their importance as host defense is suggested by their antiviral activity in tissue culture, in vitro & by the direct correlation between the degree of virulence of some viruses & their degree of resistance to certain inhibitors. Examples are the serum and mucus inhibitors of influenza viruses during experimental infections. However, even sensitive viruses may overwhelm if infecting dose of the virus is high. Therefore, the presence of these inhibitors may explain the relatively high dose of virus required to initiate infection *in vivo,* compared with the dose needed in cell cultures.

Phagocytosis

Phagocytosis is the engulfing of debris or pathogens by the phagocytes (neutrophils and the macrophages). Phagocytosis occurs in four steps. The phagocyte must first find the pathogen or cell debris meaning that it comes into physical contact with it (chemotaxis). The phagocyte must then chemically adhere to the pathogen (adherence). Next, the pathogen is ingested (endocytosed into a phagosome). Finally, the pathogen is digested intracellularly (digestion).

The information available suggests that **phagocytosis is less effective against viral infections than against bacterial infections.** However, few of the factors that control uptake of virions or infected cells by phagocytes and their digestion by lysosomal enzymes have been studied systemically. Different viruses are affected differently by the various phagocytic cells. Some viruses are not engulfed, whereas others are engulfed but may not be inactivated. In fact, some viruses, such as human immunodeficiency virus (HIV), may even multiply in the phagocytes (e.g., macrophages), which may serve as a persistent reservoir of virus. The virulence of several strains of HIV and herpesviruses correlates with their ability to multiply in macrophages. **Infected macrophages may carry virus across the blood-brain barrier.** Cytomegalovirus has ben repoted to replicate in granulocytes.

Macrophages seem to be more effective against viruses than are **granulocytes**, and some viruses seem to be more susceptible to phagocytosis than others. Macrophages & polymorhonuclear leukocyte can afford important protection by markedly reducing the viremia caused by virus strains susceptible to phagocytosis.

Viruses may stimulate macrophages to produce **monokines**, which can reduce viral multiplication. For example, macrophage-produced alpha interferon (**IFN-a**) inhibits viral multiplication both **directly** and also **indirectly** by activating natural killer cells.

Interleukin 1 (IL-1), produced by macrophages, **can interfere with viral multiplication in a number of ways:** by inducing T lymphocytes to produce interleukin-2, which in turn induces gamma interferon, which can induce alpha and beta interferons; by inducing the production of beta interferon (IFN-b) by fibroblasts and epithelial cells; by inducing fever, which inhibits viral replication; by enhancing macrophage-mediated cytolysis of infected cells; and by inducing production of tumor necrosis factor (TNF), which inhibits virus multiplication both directly & indirectly by inducing interferon & other cytokines & augmentating inflammation, phagocytosis & cytotoxic activity.

Depending on the situation, **macrophages** therefore **acting as phagocytes** may reduce the number of virus spread limiting the infection, augment or depress immune defenses, or have little effect.

Defense Mechanisms Evoked by Infection

Fever

Viral replication is influenced strongly by temperature. Fever can be induced during viral infection by at least three independent endogenous pyrogens: interleukins-1 and 6, interferon, prostaglandin E2, and tumor necrosis factor.

Even a modest increase in fever can cause strong inhibition: a temperature rise from 37°C to 38°C drastically decreases the yield of many viruses. This phenomenon has been observed in tissue culture as well as in many experimental and natural infections. Artificial induction of fever reduces mortality in mice infected with viruses. Artificial lowering of the temperature during infection may increase mortality, as in suckling mice infected with coxsackieviruses and taken away from the warmth of their mother's nest. Fever also augments the generation of cytotoxic T lymphocytes.

Several observations suggest strongly that fever reduces virus multiplication during human viral infections.

Studies have shown that the **incidence** and **severity** of **paralysis** among children infected with polioviruses were significantly greater in patients **treated with antipyretic drugs** (e.g., aspirin) than in untreated children. Also consistent with these findings is the observation that virus strains that replicate best at fever temperature are usually virulent, whereas virus strains that replicate poorly at fever temperature are usually low in virulence and therefore often are used as live virus vaccines.

Temperatures as low as 33°C are normal at body surfaces exposed to air; viruses that infect these sites and replicate optimally at these temperatures establish only local infections **that do not spread to deeper tissues, where the body temperature is higher**. For example, rhinovirus that cause common colds replicate optimally at 33°C to 34°C; however, they are inhibited at 37°C. An interesting question is whether this temperature increase is important for recovery from coryza. The same general considerations of temperature probably apply to other human viral infections such as measles, rubella, and mumps, although, unfortunately, suitable and controlled studies have not been conducted. Nevertheless, available information suggests that antipyretic drugs be used conservatively.

Complement

Complement refers to a variety of highly prevalent blood proteins that are involved in the nonspecific defenses against especially bacterial pathogens. The effects of complement action are extensive, varied, and most easily understood in the context of their mechanism of action. Complement action occurs by either of two molecular pathways termed "classical" and "alternative". The classical pathway involves the binding of specific antibody to bacterial cells while the alternative pathway involves the binding of non-specific complement molecules to bacterial cells; that is, the alternative pathway involves molecules that preferentially bind to bacterial cells, but not by bonding to specific molecules that are unique to a particular pathogen (e.g., as antibodies do). Regardless of the mechanism of initiation, the result of complement activation includes: opsonization, inflammation, & attack complexes. A great advantage of the complement system to host defenses is that, once activated, the reaction cascade occurs rapidly."Opsonization is the complement or antibody mediated adherence of pathogens to phagocytes which stimulates phagocytosis. Thus, one effect of complement adherence to a pathogen is the stimulation of the phagocytosis of the pathogen. **Membrane attack complexes-an** even more direct consequence of complement binding to a pathogen is the formation of holes in the pathogens' cell membranes. The formation of these holes is mediated via membrane attack complexes. Most viruses do not fix complement by the alternative route. However, the interaction of a complement-fixing antibody with a virus infected cell or with an enveloped virus can result in the lysis of the cell or virus. Thus, by interfacing with the specific immune system, complement also plays a role in resistance to viral infections.

Inflammation

Several antiviral mechanisms are generated by the local inflammatory response to virus-induced cell damage or to virus-stimulated mediators such as activated complement. The inflammation of tissues is a defensive response that serves to protect damaged tissues against infection (or a worsening of an existing infection). The four indications of the occurrence of localized inflammation are: warming of the area, reddening of the area, swelling of the area, pain in the area (e.g., to touch). The goal of inflammation is to kill pathogens (kill), remove tissue debris (clean), and repair damaged tissue (repair). Inflammation results from local histamine release from damaged cells which causes vasodilatation (a widening of blood vessels), an increase in blood flow to the area that accounts for the warming, swelling, and redness associated with inflammation. The chemicals produced upon cellular injury, along with inducing inflammation, additionally attract neutrophils and ultimately attract wandering macrophages. The **major components of the inflammatory process** are: circulatory alterations, edema, leukocyte accumulation and perhaps prostaglandins A and J. These result in elevated local temperature, reduced oxygen tension in the involved tissues, altered cell metabolism, and increased levels of CO2 and organic acids.

All of these alterations, which occur in a cascading and interrelated fashion, drastically reduce the replication of many viruses. For example, the altered energy metabolism of the infected and surrounding cells, as well as the accumulating lymphocytes, can generate local hyperthermia. At superficial sites where the temperature is normally lower, hyperthermia can also be generated by hyperemia during the early stages of inflammation. As inflammation progresses, hyperemia become passive, thereby greatly reducing blood flow & decrease oxygen tension. Two factors account for this decrease in oxygen tension: **limited influx of erythrocytes, and lower diffusion of oxygen through edema fluid.** In turn, the decreased oxygen tension **causes less ATP production, thus reducing the energy available for viral synthesis** and increasing anaerobic glycolysis, which increases **the accumulation of CO_2 and organic acids in the tissues.** These acid catabolites may **decrease the local pH to levels that inhibit the replication of many viruses.** Local acidity also may increase by accumulation and subsequent degradation of the leukocytes in the affected area. It is possible that other less well-defined factors are also significant.

Therefore, the local inflammation resulting from viral infection clearly activates several metabolic, physiochemical & physiological changes; acting individually or together, these changes interfere with virus multiplication. Although further animal and human studies are required, this interpretation is supported by the finding that anti-inflammatory drugs **(corticosteroids)** often increase the severity of infection in animals. Therefore, these drugs should be used with caution in treating viral diseases.

Viral Interference and Interferon

Generally, **infection by one virus renders host cells resistant to other, superinfecting viruses**. This phenomenon, called viral interference, occurs frequently in cell cultures and in animals including humans. Although interference occurs between most viruses, it may be limited to homologous viruses under certain conditions. Some types of interference are caused by competition among different viruses for critical replicative pathways, extracellular competition for cell surface receptors, & intracellular competition for biosynthetic machinery and genetic control. Similar interference may result **from competition** between defective (nonmultiplying) and infective viruses that may be produced concurrently.

The most important type in natural infections is **directed by the host cells themselves**. These infected cells may respond to viral infection by producing **interferon**, an antiviral protein, which can react with uninfected cells to render them resistant to infection by a wide variety of viruses.

Interferon

The important role played by **interferon as a defense mechanism** against viruses is clearly documented by **three types** of experimental and clinical observations. For many viral infections, a strong correlation has been established between interferon production and natural recovery; inhibition of interferon production or action enhances the severity of infection; and treatment with interferon protects against infection. In addition, the interferon system is one of the earliest appearing of known host defenses, **becoming operative within hours of infection.** Clinical studies of interferon and its inducers have shown protection against certain viruses, including hepatitis B and C viruses, papovaviruses, rhinoviruses, and herpes simplex virus.

Interferon Production and Types

Interferon **is produced *de novo* by cellular protein synthesis.**There are three types of interferon-**alpha, beta, and gamma** (INF α, INF β & INF γ) that differ both structurally and antigenically and have molecular weights ranging from 16,000 to 45,000. Both α-interferon and β-interferon are secreted by virus-infected cells; these molecules bind to other body cells, stimulating those cells to produce antiviral proteins, which act to interfere with the subsequent viral replication of those cells. Gamma-interferon differs in that it is secreted by uninfected immune system cells (stimulated by the binding of these cells to pathogen antigens) and has a broader effect (i.e., in addition to stimulating the production of antiviral proteins). Interferons are used as treatments for certain viral diseases and some cancers. Interferons are secreted **by the cell into the extracellular fluids**. Usually virus induced interferon is produced at about the same time as the virus progeny are released by the infected cell thus protecting neighbouring cell from the spreading virus. The three known types of interferon are induced by different stimuli.

INF α is induced by foreign cells, virus-infected cells, tumor cells, bacterial cells, & viral envelopes that stimulate mostly circulating dendritic cells and to a lesser degree by monocytes & B lymphocytes to produce it.

INF β is induced by viral and other foreign nucleic acids in most body cells (fibroblasts, epithelial cells, and macrophages).

INF γ is produced along with other lymphokines by T lymphocytes induced by foreign antigens to which the T lymphocytes have been presensitized. Mitogens for T cells may mimic this induction. INF γ **has several unusual properties:(1)** it exerts **greater immunomodulatory activity, including activation of macrophages**, than the other interferons; **(2)** it exerts **greater lytic effects** than the other interferons; **(3)** it **potentiates the actions of other interferons; (4)** it **activates cells** by a mechanism significantly different from that of the other interferons; and **(5)** it **inhibits intracellular microorganisms other than viruses** (e.g., rickettsia).

Inducers of interferon react with cells to depress the interferon gene(s). This leads to the production of mRNA for interferon. The mRNA is translated into the interferon protein, which is secreted into the extracellular fluid, where it reacts with the membrane receptors of cells. The interferon-stimulated cells derepress genes for effector proteins (AVP) that establish antiviral resistance and other cell changes. The activated cells also stimulate contacted cells to produce AVP by a still unknown mechanism.

Interferon **occurs without apparent stimulation** in the plasma of patients with autoimmune diseases (such as rheumatoid arthritis, disseminated lupus erythematosus and pemphigus) and in patients with advanced HIV infection.

In these cases, an **interferon antigenically identical to interferon alpha** is present but which, unlike the latter, is partially inactivated at pH 2 (acid-labile interferon alpha). This interferon is synergistic combination of interferon alpha (acid labile) & interferon beta (acid stable). Consequently, **acid treatment**

reduces the interferon activity by inactivating the synergistic interferon gamma.

Mechanism of Action

Interferon does not inactivate viruses **directly**. Instead, **it prevents viral replication in surrounding cells by reacting with specific receptors** on the cell membranes **to derepress** cellular genes that encode intracellular effector antiviral proteins, which must be synthesized before virus replication can be inhibited. INF α & INF β both bind to the same type of membrane receptor; INFγ binds to a different receptor. The **antiviral proteins** probably inhibit viral multiplication by inhibiting the synthesis of essential viral proteins, but **alternative or additional inhibitory mechanisms** (e.g., inhibition of transcription and viral release) also occur. **Viral protein synthesis may be inhibited** by several biochemical alternations of cells which can inhibit viral replication at different steps. It has been shown that the antiviral state may be transferred from interferon-treated cells to adjacent untreated cells without the continued presence of interferon; this transfer mechanism may further simplify & spread the activity of the interferon system. The **interferon system is nonspecific in two ways**: various viral stimuli induce the same type of interferon, and the same type of interferon inhibits various viruses. On the other hand, the interferon molecule is mostly specific in its action for the animal species in which it was induced: interferon produced by animals or humans generally stimulates antiviral activity only in cells of the same or closely related families (e.g., human interferon protects human and monkey cells, but not chicken cells).

Interferon during natural infection

The importance of interferon in the response to certain natural virus infections **varies**. Much depends on the effectiveness of the virus in stimulating interferon production & on its susceptibility. Interferon **protects solid tissues during virus infection**; it is also **disseminated through the bloodstream during viremia**, thereby **protecting distant organs** against the spreading infection. **Cells protected against viral replication may eliminate virus by degrading the virus genome.**

NK Cells

The principal effector cells of the innate immune system are monocytes/ macrophages, dendritic cells (DC), natural killer (NK) cells, and NK-T cells. NK cells are a subset of lymphocytes found in the blood and tissues, which lack antigen specific surface receptors (TcR or immunoglobulin receptors). NK cells do not express the characteristic cell surface markers that define T cells and B cells, and so NK cells represent a distinct lineage of lymphocytes. NK cells possess the ability to recognise and lyse virally infected cells and certain tumour cells. Whilst not showing antigen specificity, they clearly exhibit some degree of selectivity in targeting "abnormal" cells for lysis. It has been shown recently that the expression of "self" MHC molecules inhibits NK lysis of target cells.The main advantage that NK cells have over antigen-specific lymphocytes in antiviral immunity is that there is no "lag" phase of clonal expansion for NK cells to be active as effectors, as there is with antigen-specific T and B lymphocytes. Thus NK cells may be effective early in the course of viral infection, and may limit the spread of infection during this early stage, while antigen-specific lymphocytes are being recruited and clonally expanded. These effector cells recognize **pathogen-associated molecular patterns**, e.g., viral proteins, CpG DNA, or double-stranded viral RNA, via a variety of so-called **pattern recognition receptors**, which include **Toll-like receptors, NK cell receptors, and mannose-binding receptors**. These cells then release a variety of proinflammatory cytokines and chemokines, which recruit inflammatory cells to the site of infection and initiate inflammation and antiviral responses. These soluble mediators also activate macrophages, NK cells, and DC. Viral infections are usually accompanied by NK cell activation. Activated NK cells kill virus-infected cells and serve as an immediate source of interferon-(IFN-γ). An important event is the induction of type I (α and ß) IFN. Although almost all cell types can produce these IFN, a specialized cell type, precursor plasmacytoid DC, produces 1000-fold more of these cytokines and is called the natural IFN-producing cell. IFNs also increase expression of major histocompatibility complex (MHC) class I and II antigens and of costimulatory molecules on the surface of so-called antigen-presenting cells (APC). Activation of the innate immune system plays an instructive role (adjuvant effect) for the induction of virus-specific, adaptive immune responses. In general, exogenous viral particles and viral antigens are phagocytosed and/ or endocytosed by APC. They are then degraded in lysosomes, and immunogenic peptides are presented in association with MHC class II antigens to naïve CD4+ T cells. NK cells and macrophages also kill virus-infected cells in association with virus-specific antibodies. NK cells kill antibody-coated, virus-infected cells via antibody-dependent, cell-mediated cytotoxicity (ADCC). Virus-specific ADCC plays a significant role in killing virus-infected cells, especially against human immunodeficiency virus (HIV) and herpesviruses. Macrophages and polymorphonuclear leukocytes can engulf antibody-coated pathogens as well as virus-infected cells and/or kill them via reactive oxygen species, nitric oxide, and activated caspases.

NK cells may kill virus-infected cells without help from antibodies. These cells, however, usually do not recognize any viral antigen or viral peptide. Their effector function is controlled by a complex system of inhibitory and activating NK cell receptors and coreceptors. They kill target cells unless inhibited by the engagement of inhibitory receptors by their cognate ligands on the target cells. The most important inhibitory receptors include killercell Ig-like receptors (KIR), NKG2/CD94A, and Ig-like transcripts (ILT), which bind to classical and nonclassical MHC class I antigens; also called human leukocyte antigen (HLA)-A, -B, -C, -E, and -G (Table 1). Most of the KIR recognize HLA-C and inhibit NK cells. **A down-regulation of the MHC antigens on the surface of virus-infected cells usually makes them susceptible to NK cell-mediated killing.** Despite their different mechanisms of recognition of virus-infected cells, NK cells and CTL represent the most important cytolytic cells leading to the elimination of tumor and virus-infected cells from the host. Patients with low NK cell activity are more susceptible to reoccurrences with herpes simplex type 1 virus. NK cells recognize virus infected cells & kill such cells.Nk cell recognition of virus infected cells is not MHC-restricted or antigen specific. NK cells therefore kill cells infected with different viruses. Besides the above, NK cells mediate ADCC and can kill virus infected cells by this mechanism. IFN-γ and Il-2 can enhance the activities of NK cells.

Recognition of Viral Nucleic Acids & other Viral Products

Recognition of viral nucleic acids with **pattern recognition receptors** (PRRs) is the first step to induce innate immune system. Pattern recognition receptors (PRRs) are engaged to detect specific viral components such as viral RNA or DNA or viral intermediate products and to induce type I interferons (IFN α & INF β) and other pro-inflammatory cytokines in the infected cells and other immune cells. Recently these innate immune receptors and their unique downstream pathways have been identified. Here, their roles in the innate immune response to virus infection, discrimination between self and viral nucleic acids and inhibition by virulent factors, & some recent advances in the coordination between innate and adaptive immune activation are being described.

Viral infections are detected by sensor molecules, which initiate innate antiviral responses, including the activation of type I interferons (IFNα & INFβ) and proinflammatory cytokines. These cytokines are responsible for not only inhibiting viral replication in infected cells but also regulating the induction of adaptive immunity, leading to the swift eradication of viruses. Recent advances in the identification of pathogen receptors in the innate immune system have revealed that distinct types of multiple pattern recognition receptor (PRR) families, including Toll-like receptors (TLRs), RIG-I-like receptors (RLRs) and NOD-like receptors (NLRs), contribute significantly to viral detection by sensing viral proteins and nucleic acids, leading to induction of cytokines and type I interferons (IFN á & INFâ /sensors play a role in the detection of viral nucleic acids in different ways. **Toll-like receptors (TLRs) detect viral DNA or RNA in endosomal compartments in immune cells, retinoic acid inducible gene-I (RIG-I)**-like receptors **(RLRs)** recognize **viral RNA in the cytoplasm**, and DNA sensors detect cytoplasmic viral DNA. Since these sensors have to exclusively recognize viral infections. Recently RNA polymerase III **(Pol III) was shown to transcribe some viral DNAs into RNA for detection by RIG-I, leading to IFN induction.** Another novel mechanism of **viral DNA recognition unveiled,** leading to proinflammatory cytokine production, involves the **PYHIN family member AIM2**.

Type I interferons (IFNs), central mediators in the antiviral innate immunity, are responsible for induction of cytokines and chemokines that disrupt virus replication. Production of type I IFN is the key response to viral infection. Recent studies indicated that there are at least two distinct pathways for the induction of type I IFN by viral infection. Toll-like receptors (TLRs) are extracellular and endosomal PRRs for microbial pathogens whereas **retinoic acid inducible gene-I(RIG-I) and melanoma differentiation-associated gene 5 (MDA5) are novel intracellular PRRs for viral dsRNA.** The distinct mechanisms inducing type I IFNs through TLRs and RIG-I/MDA5 pathways are being described.

Previously after discovery of type I IFNs in 1957, long ds RNA formed during replication of many viruses was thought to be responsible for type I IFN induction, and for decades ds RNA-activated protein kinase (PKR) was thought to be the receptor. Recently, this picture has dramatically changed. It now became evident that not PKR but two members of the Toll-like receptor (TLR) family, TLR7 and TLR9, and two cytosolic helicases, RIG-I and MDA-5, are responsible for the majority of type I IFNs induced upon recognition of viral nucleic acids. **TLR4 recognizes viral components at the cell surface, TLR3, TLR7, TLR8, and TLR9 recognize viral nucleic acids on endosomal membrane**. After ligand recognition, these members activate their intrinsic signaling pathways and induce type I interferon. Based on the recent progress in the field, we now know that TLR7, TLR9, and RIG-I do not require long ds RNA for type I IFN induction.

Type I IFNs include multiple IFN α isoforms, a single IFN β, and other members, such as IFN-e, -j, -x and so on. In contrast to type II IFN (IFN γ), is exclusively produced by T cells and NK cells, type I IFNs can be produced by all nucleated cells in response to virus infection. Type III IFNs, comprised of IFN-k1, k2 and k3, have also recently been identified. These IFNs each have different receptors but share downstream signaling molecules and regulate the same genes. IFNs have pleiotropic functions. They increase the expression of intrinsic proteins including TRIM5a, Fv, Mx, eIF2a and 20–50 OAS, and induce apoptosis of virus-infected cells and cellular resistance to viral infection. In addition, **they activate NK cells and dendritic cells (DC) and induce the activation of the adaptive immune system.** The expression of type I IFN and cytokine genes is regulated by an intracellular signaling pathway that is activated by germline-encoded PRRs. These receptors recognize molecular patterns specific to microorganisms, such as viral genome nucleic acids. Nucleic acids such as DNA and RNA are essential components of all living organisms, so discrimination between self and non-self nucleic acids is essential especially in virus infection. Recent advances in research into innate immunity have revealed that this discrimination relies, to a great extent, on PRRs including Toll-like receptors (TLRs), **retinoic acid-inducible gene I (RIG-I)-like receptors (RLRs),** and **nucleotide-binding oligomerization domain (NOD)-like receptors(NLRs)**. The current understanding of innate immune recognition of viruses and discrimination between self and viral nucleic acids, provide some recent advances in coordination between innate signaling and adaptive immune activation are described below.

Endosomal TLRs in DCs

Several viruses utilize host endocytic pathways at the cell entry phase or budding, so they are inevitably surveyed by endosomal innate immune sensors. Endosomal TLRs, including TLR3, TLR7, TLR8 and TLR9, share the property of being activated by nucleic acids. Their expression can be increased by type I IFNs but their distribution is restricted. LR7 and TLR9 are highly expressed in **plasmacytoid DCs (pDCs)** which are expert cells known to produce a large amount of type I IFNs in response to virus infection. TLR3 is expressed more widely, but is mainly expressed on conventional DCs (cDCs). The function of TLR8 is not clearly known yet. Recently endoplasmic reticulum (ER) protein **UNC93B1** turned out to be essential for trafficking of TLR7 and TLR9 from ER to endosome. A recent report suggests that TLR-sorting to the ligand may utilize autophagy, which is a cellular process for recycling cytosolic compartments and, in the case of pDC, eliminating exogenous pathogen. Although cytoplasmic vesicular stomatitis viruses (VSV) in pDC are thought to be trapped by autophagosome expressing ATG5 and detected by TLR7 in lysosomes for a type I IFN response, in non-immune cells ATG5 suppresses the type I IFN response by interaction with caspase recruitment domains (CARDs) presented by RIG-I and IFN β promoter stimulator-1 (IPS-1).

Endosomal recognition of viral RNA by TLRs

TLR7 recognizes several kinds of RNA viruses, including orthomyxoviruses in pDCs. TLR7 signals through a TIR domain containingadapter, myeloid differentiation factor 88 (MyD88). Upon exposure to its ligand, MyD88 forms a complex with interleukin-1-receptor (IL-1R)-associated kinase-4

(IRAK-4), IRAK-1, tumor necrosis factor-receptor associated factor 3 (TRAF3), TRAF6, Ikka and IRF-7. Following the formation of this signaling complex, IRF7 and nuclear factor-kappa B (NF-jB) are activated, which results in the production of type I IFNs and cytokines). TLR3 recognizes double-stranded (ds)RNA and triggers a signaling pathway via a TIR domain-containing adapter inducing IFN-b (TRIF) (also known as TICAM-1). TRIF associates with TRAF3 and TRAF6 via TRAF-binding motifs which exist in its N-terminal portion and also with receptor interacting protein (RIP) 1 and RIP3 via RIP homotypic interaction motif (RHIM). TRAF6 and RIP1 activate NF-jB while TRAF3 activates TRAF family member-associated NK-jB activator (TANK)-binding kinase 1(TBK1) and inducible IjB kinase (IKK-i). Activation of these pathways triggers antiviral responses. TLR3 also activates the phosphatidylinositol-3 kinase (PI3K) pathway. Tyrosine phosphorylation of TLR3 induces PI3K recruitment to the receptor and subsequent activation of Akt leads to activation of IRF-3. **TLR3 plays an important role in the pathogenesis of RNA virus infections** in vivo. For example, TLR3 deficient mice are resistant to infection with West Nile virus and influenza virus. In both cases inflammatory responses are decreased in TLR3 deficient mice, which suggest that an excess production of cytokines is rather harmful for the survival of mice.

Intracellular recognition of viral RNA by RLRs

Recently, three homologous DExD/H box RNA helicases, **RIG-I**, melanoma differentiation-associated gene 5 **(MDA5) and LGP2**, were identified as cytoplasmic sensors of virus RNA, named here as **RIG-like receptors (RLRs)**. RIG-I and MDA5 play a major role in recognition of RNA viruses in cDCs, macrophages and fibroblasts. RIG-I binds 50-triphosphorylated single-stranded (ss) RNA and short dsRNA and stimulates production of type I IFNs. By contrast, MDA5 preferentially recognizes longer-dsRNA, including synthetic poly-IC. RIG-I recognizes a variety of RNA viruses including influenza virus, VSV and Japanese encephalitis virus (JEV) while MDA5 recognizes picorna family such as encephalomyocarditis virus (EMCV), Theiler's virus and Mengo virus. Therefore, RIG-I and MDA5 deficient mice are highly susceptible to VSV and EMCV, respectively. In addition it was indicated that the antiviral protein RNase L, which can cleave and turn a single stranded portion of not only viral but also self RNA into preferentially ds RNA, is a ligand for RIG-I and MDA5. The CARDs of RIG-I and MDA5 are responsible for initiating the signaling pathway. Both RIG-I and MDA5 associate with an adapter protein IPS-1 also known as MAVS, VISA or CARDIF, which also contains an N-terminal CARD. IPS-1 localizes on the outer mitochondrial membrane. The IPS-1 CARD interacts with that of RIG-I or MDA5. IPS-1 then associates with TRAF3, followed by activation of TBK1 and Ikk-i. These kinases phosphorylate IRF3 and IRF7 and induce type I IFN production. IPS-1 also interacts with Fas-associated death domain-containing protein (FADD) and leads to activation of NF-jB through cleavage of caspase-8/-10.

Differential role of TLRs and RLRs in antiviral responses

Occasionally both TLR and RLR are engaged for sensing the same dsRNA or ssRNA. Normally dsRNA does not exist in host cells but in virus infection it is detected as not only a viral structure but also as a byproduct of viral replication. dsRNA activates macrophages and dendritic cells via TLR3 to secrete pro-inflammatory cytokines, especially IL-12. However, type-I IFNs are produced by virus-infected cells such as fibroblasts by TLR3 independently. MDA5 recognizes synthetic dsRNA, poly-IC, and the ssRNA virus, EMCV, which generates dsRNA during replication, and induces the type-IIFN response. Poly-IC is neither capable of inducing an innate immune response nor of working as an adjuvant in TRIF/ IPS-1 double knockout mice. In contrast to dsRNA, ssRNA abundantly exists not only in pathogens but also in host cells. ssRNA is recognized by TLR7 (or TLR8 in humans) and RIG-I in a cell-type specific manner. Although TLR7 and TLR8 recognize GU of AU rich sequences of ssRNA viruses such as influenza virus and HIV, through TLR7 expressing cells such as pDC, or TLR8 expressing cells such as myeloid DC or monocytes, it is unclear whether its sequence specificity is dependent on the receptor or the cell. In contrast to TLR7, RIG-I is expressed in most cell types. As described previously, RIG-I recognizes 50-triphosphorylated ssRNA. In the case of influenza A virus infection, its negative-sense ssRNA genome is recognized by TLR7 expressed in pDCs and a signal is transmitted through its adaptor protein MyD88. On the otherhand, it is recognized by RIG-I ubiquitously expressed in most cell types, such as fibroblasts or cDCs in vitro, and probably by the alveolar macrophage in vivo, via its adaptor protein IPS-1. In mouse lungs after intranasal infection of influenza virus both TLR7/ MyD88 and RIG-I/IPS-1 pathways concurrently control the type-I IFN response.

Endosomal and intracellular recognition of viral DNA

TLR9 recognizes unmethylated DNA with a CpG motif (CpGDNA) and DNA viruses, including herpes simplex virus (HSV)-1, HSV-2 and cytomegalovirus (CMV) in pDCs. TLR9 shares the adapter protein MyD88 and the downstream signaling pathway with TLR7. cDCs and macrophages also respond to CpG-DNA and produce small amounts of IFN-β through IRF-1 activation rather than IRF-3 or IRF-7 activation. Recently, it was reported that genomic DNA of viruses, such as adenovirus, vaccinia virus and HSV, could be also recognized in a TLR9-independent manner, using an as yet unknown recognition mechanism in the cytoplasm. In this case, DNA which has entered the cytoplasm activates the infected cells via TBK1 and IRF3. Actually the source of DNA is not restricted to viruses; but it can also come from bacteria and damaged host cells. The activity of this DNA is more potent in ds right-hand B-form DNA than in left-handed Z-form DNA, while ssDNA displays no activity. In addition, DAI (also known as ZBP1 or DLM1) which contains two Z-DNA binding domains, was shown to be a potential cytoplasmic DNA sensor. However, DAI KO mice induced a normal type I IFN response in vitro and in vivo after B-DNA stimulation and also indicated DNA-vaccine-induced adaptive immune responses, suggesting its role is redundant. **Potential cytoplasmic DNA sensors still remain to be elucidated.**

The recognition of viral components at the cell surface

In addition to the endosomal TLRs, **TLR2 and TLR4** have also been suggested to be involved in recognition of viruses. TLR2 has been shown to detect components of measles virus, HSV and hepatitis C virus (HCV), while TLR4 produces a response to retrovirus and respiratory syncytial virus (RSV). While viral proteins recognized by these surface TLRs trigger pro-inflammatory responses, their contribution to either protective or pathological immune responses largely depends on the type of virus, route of infection, and other host factors.

NLRs mediates innate immune activation by intracellular viral nucleic acids

NLR proteins are comprised of three motifs, C-terminal LRRs, central nucleotide-binding domain and N-terminal signaling domain containing CARDs, and Pyrin domain or baculovirus IAP repeats. Cryopyrin/NALP3 was shown to recognize both ssRNA and dsRNA of viral origin or their synthetic versions and to induce caspase-1 activation via apoptosis-associated speck-like protein containing a caspase-activating and recruitment domain (ASC). In addition, some NLRs participate in nucleic acid-mediated innate immune activation through caspase-1 activation and NF-jB activation towards IFN-I production via a synergistic pathway activated by NOD2.

Discrimination between self and viral nucleic acids

The innate immune systems for virus sensing described above miraculously detect the invasion of pathogens such as viruses, but are silent in normal conditions. As dsRNA generated by viral replication and virus DNA rich in CpG motifs are not normally found in our body, it is easy to consider that our innate immune system recognizes them as foreign molecules. In contrast to these nucleic acids, ssRNA abundantly exists not only in pathogens but also in host cells. It is, therefore, essential for the host to detect and discriminate viral ssRNA from self ssRNA. However, the mechanism of this robust discrimination is not fully understood. For example, although the 50 triphosphate on many ssRNAs of viruses is absent from mRNA and transfer RNA but is found in ribosomal RNA, which abundantly exists in host cells, only the 50 triphosphate on viruses can induce RIG-I activation. Recently RNase L activation in infected host cells was shown to generate small self RNAs which can induce an innate immune response via RLRs. In addition, it is known that TLR7/8 and TLR9 also recognize host RNA and DNA. Therefore, it is necessary for absolute discrimination by the host innate immune system to recognize some additional factors such as the methylation state, certain sequences and intracellular localization of RNA, or restricted endosomal expression of TLRs for viral recognition where host nucleic acids have limited access.

Virulent factor for inhibition of host immune responses

Viruses have developed several kinds of immune evasion strategies to proliferate within host cells. Their main target is the type I IFN response. Viruses can inhibit type I IFNs by many strategies i.e. inhibition of IFN synthesis, interference of IFN receptor signaling and so on. For example, vaccinia virus E3L and influenza virus NS1 which possess a dsRNA-binding site are thought to inhibit type I IFN production through dsRNA sequestration. As E3L also possesses a DNA-binding site, it might sequester viral DNA from host DNA sensing. NS1 protein was also indicated to inhibit the function of IPS1 and RIG-I. Viruses without such abilities to suppress the host type I IFN responses are generally low pathogenic and available for vaccine strains.

Adaptive immunity against viruses through innate immune signaling pathway

Recent advances in the understanding of innate immunity show that the activation of the innate immune system is essential for subsequent adaptive immune responses including specific antibody production and CTL activation which play a key role in protection against virus infection. A recent report indicated that the adaptive immune response elicited by inactivated whole influenza virus vaccine containing viral ssRNA was strictly governed by the **TLR7/MyD88** pathway, but not by the RIG-I/IPS-1 pathway, although both pathways concurrently controlled the innate immune response. However, the innate immune response elicited by a DNA vaccine containing CpG-DNA was dependent on TBK1, but not on the TLR9/MyD88 pathway. These findings suggested that the innate immune pathway engaged for protective immunity against virus infection was different according to the source of antigen.

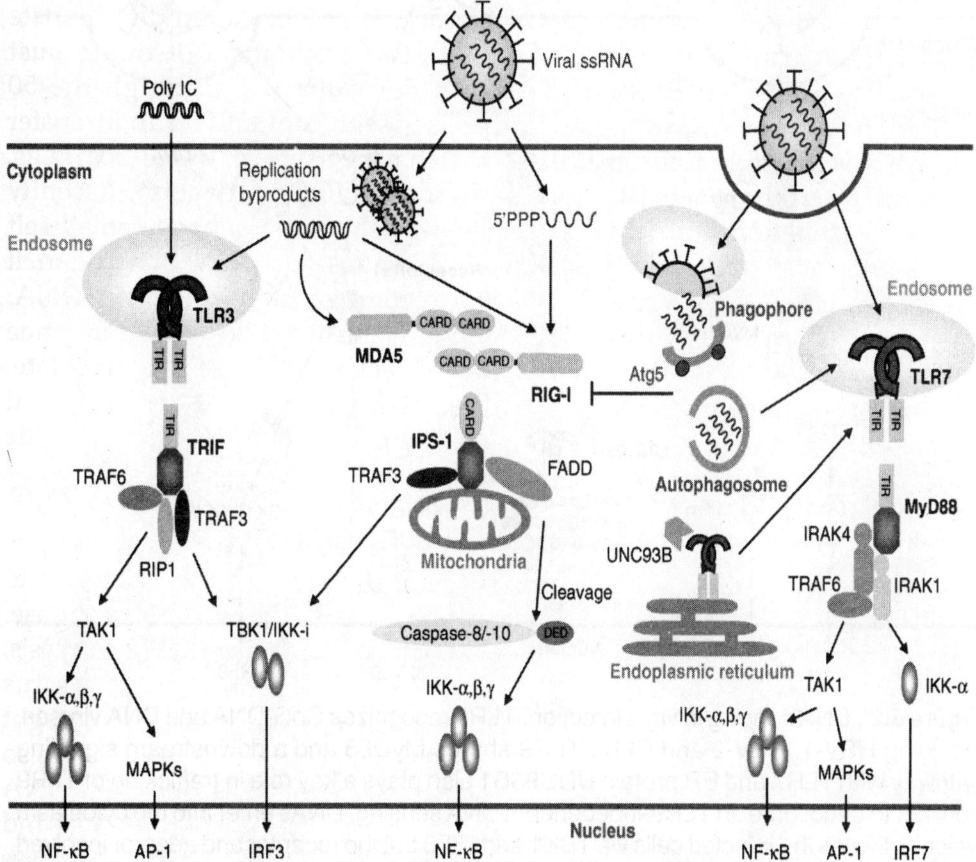

Figure 5.1 : RNA sensing in virus infection. TLR3 recognizes dsRNA and triggers a signaling pathway via a TRIF. TRIF associates with TRAF3, TRAF6 and RIP1. TRAF6 and RIP1 activate NF-kB and AP-1 while TRAF3 activates TBK1/IKK-i and is followed by a type I IFN response. Both RIG-I and MDA5 associate with an adapter protein IPS-1. IPS-1 localizes on the outer mitochondrial membrane and the CARD of it interacts with that of RIG-I or MDA5. IPS-1 associates with TRAF3 which induces the production of type I IFNs and FADD which induces activation of NF-kB. TLR7 signals through MyD88. MyD88 forms a complex with IRAK-4, IRAK-1, TRAF3, TRAF6, Ikka and IRF-7 and this complex is recruited to the TLR by ligand stimulation. Downstream of this signaling complex, IRF7 and NF-kB are activated and this is followed by the production of type I IFNs and cytokines. ER protein UNC93B1 plays a key role in trafficking of TLR7 from ER to endosome, but the triggers are unknown. In the case of VSV recognition in pDC, the virus is trapped by autophagosome expressing ATG5 and detected by TLR7 in the lysosome for production of a type I IFN response. Moreover in non-immune cells ATG5 suppresses the type I IFN response via RIG-I or IPS-1 inhibition. Yellow rectangles (TIR, CARD) indicate protein–protein interaction regions for downstream signaling.

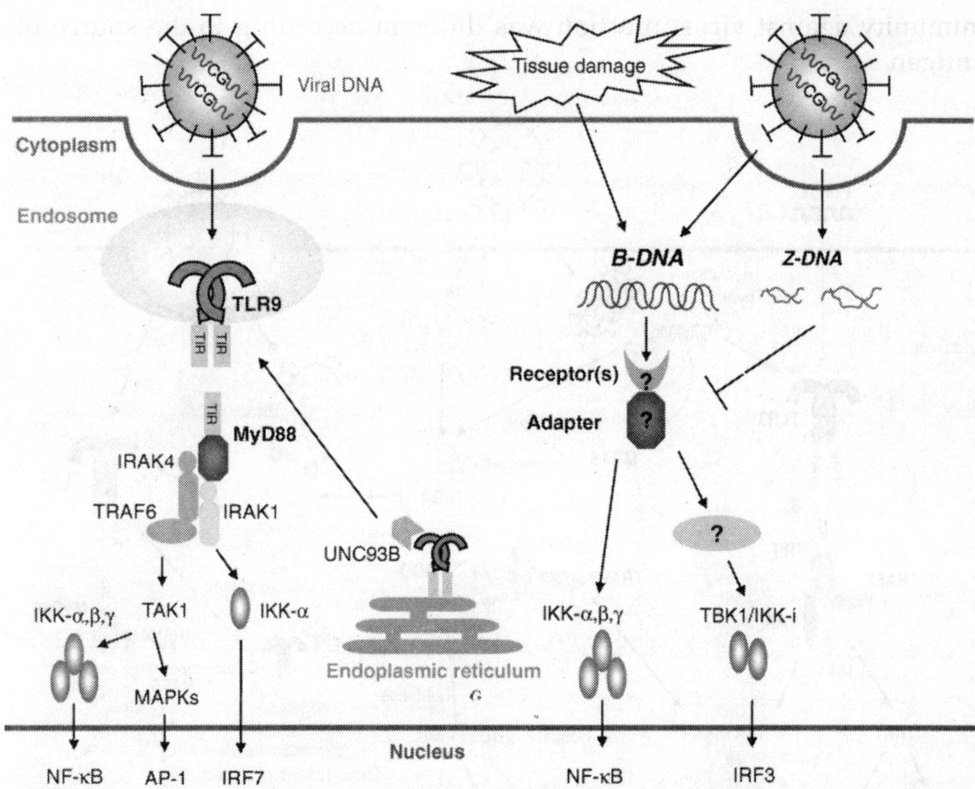

Figure 5.2 : DNA sensing in virus infection. TLR9 recognizes CpG-DNA and DNA viruses, including HSV-1, HSV-2 and CMV. TLR9 shares MyD88 and a downstream signalling pathway with TLR7 and ER protein UNC93B1 also plays a key role in trafficking of TLR9 from ER to endosome. In TLR9-independent DNA sensing, DNAs enter into the cytoplasm which activates the infected cells via TBK1 and IRF3 but the receptor and adaptor involved are still unknown. Their activities are more potent in ds right-hand B form DNA than in left-handed Z-form DNA.

These findings have illustrated the recent progress in understanding how a host discriminates between viruses and self components by innate immune receptors and elicits an inflammatory response involving type I IFNs and other cytokines. Elucidating such mechanisms in detail is essential for not only the development of a clinical approach such as nucleic acid-based immunotherapy and TLR based vaccine adjuvant but also the understanding of the pathogenesis of diverse viral diseases.

Adaptive Immune Response

The adaptive defense consists of antibodies and T lymphocytes, often called the humoral response *and the* cell mediated response. The term 'adaptive' refers to the differentiation of self from non-self, and the tailoring of the response to the particular foreign invader. The ability to shape the response in a virus-specific manner depends upon communication between the innate and adaptive systems. This communication is carried out by cytokines that bind to cells, and by cell-cell interactions between dendritic cells and lymphocytes in lymph nodes. This interaction is so crucial that the adaptive response cannot occur without an innate immune system.

The cells of the adaptive immune system are lymphocytes; B cells and T cells. B cells, which are derived from the bone marrow, become the cells that produce antibodies. T cells, which mature in the thymus, differentiate into cells that either participate in lymphocyte maturation, or kill virus-infected cells. Both humoral and cell mediated responses are essential for antiviral defense. The contribution of each varies, depending on the virus and the host. Antibodies generally bind to virus particles in the blood and at mucosal surfaces, thereby blocking the spread of infection. In contrast, T cells recognize and kill virus infected cells.

A key feature of the adaptive immune system is *memory*. Repeat infections by the same virus are met immediately with a strong and specific response that usually effectively stops the infection with less reliance on the innate system. When we say we are immune to infection with a virus, we are talking about immune memory. Vaccines protect us against infection because of immune memory. The first adaptive response against a virus, called the primary response often takes days to mature. In contrast, a memory response develops within hours of infection. Memory is maintained by a subset of B and T lymphocytes called memory cells which survive for years in the body. Memory cells remain ready to respond rapidly and efficiently to a subsequent encounter with a pathogen. This so-called secondary response is often stronger than the primary response to infection. Consequently, childhood infections protect adults, and immunity conferred by vaccination can last for years.

B cells & T cells, which play vital role in preventing viral infections, are briefly described below.

B Cells & Humoral Immunity

B cells bear the B cell receptor (BCR) or membrane bound-immunoglobulin (mIg) for antigen recognition, produce antibodies against antigens that play a role in the humoral immune response, perform the role of APCs and eventually develop into memory B cells after activation by antigen. B cells are an essential component of the humoral adaptive immunity. B cells are produced in the either the bursa of Fabricus in birds or bone marrow in the vertebrates where they also mature. There are up to 10^9 B cell clones produced due to somatic recombination between several hundred V_L & V_H gene segments;

such diversity in B cell clones are capable to recognize each & every type of possible antigen. V region genes of H chain are made of variable genes (V gene), diversity genes (D genes) and joining genes (J genes) situated widely apart on a chromosome. There are multiple copies of V, D & J genes. Similar is the case with V region genes of L chain but it lacks D genes. C region is made by C gene and there is usually one copy for each isotype (IgM, IgD, IgG, IgE & IgA) and one each for kappa or lambda L chain. Somatic mutation adds to diversity. Million of clones of lymphocytes having different combination of V region genes on mIgM are produced, each clone of lymphocytes having similar binding site on mIgM for an antigen that recognizes only one epitope of Ag. The binding site on mIgs on one clone of B cells differs from that of a second clone. Each B cell possesses approximately $1.5x10^5$ immunoglobulin molecules having the same binding site, & all B cells derived from the same clone possess mIgs of the same specificity that differ from that of a second clone of B cells. Each B cell clone surface immunoglobulins recognize antigens in their native & soluble form. The bound antigen molecules are engulfed into the B cell by receptor mediated endocytosis. The antigen is digested into fragments, which are then displayed at the cell surface with a class II histocompatibility molecule. Helper T cells specific for this structure (i.e., with complementary TCRs) bind the B cell and secrete lymphokines that stimulate the B cell to enter the cell cycle and develop, by repeated mitosis, into a **clone** of cells with identical BCRs. Most of antigen activated B cells differentiate into plasma cells that secrete antibodies; firstly IgM that switch to IgG, IgA, IgE & IgE into blood that bind the same epitope that elicited proliferation in the first place. A small minority survives as memory cells that can recognize only the same epitope years after its production.

B cells express the following important surface markers. **(a) CD45 (CD220)** is present on B cells & their precursors with several isoforms. It is a tyrosine phosphatase that plays a role in antigen receptor-mediated signaling. **(b) CD40** that plays a role in T-dependent B cells activation, it interacts with the ligand 40 L expressed on T helper cells. (c) **B-7-1 or CD80 & B7-2 or CD86** are important B cell surface molecules that act as costimulator for T cells & interact with CD28 & CTLA-4 on T cells. (d) CR1 (CD35) & CR11 (CD21) are receptors for C3b & C3d respectively, & form coreceptor complex with CD19 & CD81 to deliver an activating signals to B cells. (e) MHC II molecules on B cells allow the cells to act as APC that displays peptide Ags to T helper cells.

A molecule of immunoglobulin is made of 2 identical light chains (L chains) & 2 identical heavy chains (H chain) i.e. L_2H_2 that are linked together by disulfide bonds. N-terminal of an immunoglobulins molecules forms Fab (fraction antigens binding) that binds to its specific Ags, while the carboxyl terminal forms Fc (fragment crystallizable) that interacts with various cells to perform biological effector functions of an antibody. Each L and H chain is divided into variable region (V region) and constant region (C region). It is variability of sequence of amino acids in the V region that determines the specificity of mIg on each B cell.

Antibody is described here in relation to its role in antiviral immunity. The most effective type of antiviral antibody is neutralizing antibody - this is antibody which binds to the virus, usually to the viral envelope or capsid proteins, and which blocks the virus from binding and gaining entry to the host cell. Only epitopes on molecules involved in the release of the viral genome into the cells are targets of neutralization. In influenza viruses, only the HA and not the NA are targets for neutralization. In polioviruses, all antigenic sites recognizable on the capsid are targets for neutralization, because the capsid is a unit for releasing the nucleic acid. For adenoviruses, the main targets are the hexons rather than the pentons, as the hexons are strongly interconnected and work together for the release of the viral DNA. Occasionally, Abs bound to non-neutralizing epitopes can be detected by neutralization in the presence of complement, whereby the viral envelope is attacked by the complement cascade. Virus specific antibodies may also act as opsonins in enhancing phagocytosis of virus particles - this effect may be further enhanced by complement activation by antibody-coated virus particles. In addition, in the case of some viral infections, viral proteins are expressed on the surface of the infected cell. These may act as targets for virus-specific antibodies, and may lead to complement-mediated lysis of the infected cell, or may direct a subset of natural killer cells to lyse the infected cell through a process known as antibody-directed cellular cytotoxicity (ADCC). At mucosal surfaces like the respiratory and gastrointestinal tracts, virus infection may induce the production of specific antibodies of the IgA isotype, which may be protective against infection at these surfaces. This is the basis of immunization with the current oral polio vaccine. Not all antibodies to viruses are protective, however, and in certain cases antibody to the virus may facilitate its entry into a cell through Fc receptor-mediated uptake of the antibody coated particle. Such antibodies are called enhancing antibody. Antibody is most effective at an early stage of viral infection, before the virus has gained entry to its target cell; antibody is relatively ineffective in primary viral infections, due mainly to the lag phase in antibody production. Neutralizing antibody is an effective form of protective immunity against viral infections at the time of infection or during viremia as witnessed by the success of many viral vaccines, which work by stimulating virus-neutralising antibody responses. Neutralizing antibodies inhibit the ability of a virus to invade the cells and to replicate; they interfere with the viral attachment, penetration, or uncoating & they are able to damage the viral envelope with the aid of complement-classical pathway. Virus specific antibodies may also act as opsonins in enhancing phagocytosis of virus particles - this effect may be further enhanced by complement activation by antibody-coated virus particles. In addition, in the case of some viral infections, viral proteins are expressed on the surface of the infected cell. These may act as targets for virus-specific antibodies, and may lead to complement-mediated lysis of the infected cell, or may direct a subset of natural killer cells to lyse the infected cell through a process known as antibody-directed cellular cytotoxicity (ADCC).

i. Killed virus preparations elicit antibodies predominantly directed against the surface of the virions. These Abs have neutralizing and HI activities against the virions as well as CF and precipitating activities against the Ags of the viral coat. ii. Live virus preparations elicit antibodies against all the viral antigens, including both external and internal antigens.iii. Immunization with internal components of the virions produces CF and precipitating Abs active only toward the Ags of these components. iv. Immunization with peptides reproducing segments of virion proteins elicit Abs, the properties of which depend both on the protein and the specific sequences reproduced.

T Cells & Cellular Immunity

T cell mediate cell mediated immune responses, originate in the bone marrow but mature in thymus & acquire TCR to recognize Ag peptides presented by MHC class I & II molecules, circulate through blood, lymph & secondary lymphoid organs & are recruited at the sites of infection to destroy the Ags. Two subsets of T cells are $CD4^+$ T helper cells & $CD8^+$ cytotoxic T cells that perform different functions. T cells acquire TCR that does not recognize soluble or free Ags as with B cells, but recognize only peptide Ags complexed with self-MHC molecules presented by APC or by target cells like virus infected cells, altered self cells & graft cells. Along with TCR, T cells express surface molecules like CD3, CD4 or CD8. αβ T cells on the basis of their TCR constitute major population (90-99%) of T cells. During developmental maturation in the thymus, the following developmental changes in T cells take place. (i) Acquisition of αβTCR, CD3, CD4 or CD8 molecules (ii) positive selection, & (iii) negative selection (iv) recirculation & homing. Other features of T cells are (v) activation of T helper cells & cytotoxic T lymphocytes, (vi) effector & memory T cells & (vi) important surface molecules on T cells.

Precursors of T cells migrate to the cortex of the thymus. At this time they have neither a complete TCR nor either CD4 or CD8 & thus are called "double-negative" or **DN** cells. In the cortex of the thymus, they begin to form a TCR; synthesize both CD4 and CD8, hence they are "double-positive" or **DP** cells.

The cortical cells of the thymus express a wide variety of small molecules, usually a peptide of 6–8 amino acids derived from body proteins; that is, "self" proteins such as proteins within the cytosol serum proteins; i.e., proteins circulating in the blood and lymph nestled in a histocompatibility molecule encoded by the MHC. Most of the cells (~97%) will produce a TCR that does not bind to any of the peptide-MHC molecules present on the surface of the cortical cells. Unless they can try again with a new TCR, these cells die by neglect/by apoptosis. Those remaining cells whose TCR have bound a peptide antigen presented in **class II** MHC molecule stop expressing CD8 and become $CD4^+$ T cells. It is these cells that become T1 cells playing role in cell-mediated immune responses; & are the helper cells for cytotoxic T lymphocytes (CTLs) or Th2 helper cells for **B cells**. Those remaining cells whose TCR has bound a peptide antigen presented in **class I** MHC molecule stop expressing CD4 and become $CD8^+$ T cells. Both sets of cells are said to have undergone **positive selection.**

After positive selection, these cells migrate to the **medulla** of the thymus. There, those cells whose TCR binds very strongly to complexes of self-peptide and self-MHC are destroyed by apoptosis. This process of **negative selection** is important as it eliminates cells that might otherwise mount an autoimmune attack. It is one of the ways in which **tolerance** to self antigens is achieved. The cells whose TCRs bind antigen at an affinity below the threshold that trigger apoptosis are free to leave the thymus and migrate throughout the immune system (lymph nodes, spleen, etc.). It is this population that mounts immune responses against foreign antigens. A TCR that binds self-peptide/self-MHC with low affinity may well bind a foreign-peptide in self MHC with high affinity.

T cells acquire T cell antigen receptors (TCR), which is made of heterodimeric peptide chains; made of α and β peptide chains. T cells with α and β TCR are called ab **TCR^+ T cells** that constitute about **90-95%** of total T cells population. Each chain has a variable (V) region and a constant (C) region. The V regions each contain 3 **hypervariable regions** that make up the antigen-binding site on the cell surface for antigen recognition. Presence of TCR on their surface enables T cells to distinguish between self and non-self antigens. T cells recognize only small peptide fragments of antigen complexed with self-MHC molecules. T cells become tolerant to the self-Ags but initiate immune responses against the non-self or foreign Ags.

V domain for α chain is encoded by V & J gene segments while V domain for β chain is encoded by V, D & J gene segments. Any a chain may combine with any β chain to generate αβ TCR and thus **more than 10^9 clones of αβ TCR can be produced**, each capable of recognizing only one Ag. (c) T cells acquire important co-stimulatory receptors like CD3, CD4 or CD8 concerned with **signal transmission.** T cells also acquire essential **surface homing receptors,** which enable them to migrate from lymphatic to blood circulation (lymphocyte trafficking).

Two subsets-T helper (T_H) cells and cytotoxic T (T_C) cells of αβ T cells have been divided on the basis of **possession of CD4 or CD8 coreceptors** respectively on their surface. **αβ T cells with CD4** molecules restrict TCR recognition of exogenous Ag peptides in the context of self class II MHC molecules displayed on Ag presenting cells (macrophages, dendritic cells, and B cells); these cells are called helper T cells (T_H cells). T_H cells help or regulate cellular and humoral immune responses. The second subpopulation of αβ T cells having CD8 coreceptors on their surface are **called cytotoxic T cells (Tc cells) that restrict TCR recognition of foreign endogenous Ag peptides in the context of class I MHC** molecules presented on the surface of the target cells including all nucleated cells. Tc cells are involved in **direct killing of the virus infected and the altered cells.**

Helper T cells (CD4$^+$ T cells subsets: CD4+ helper T cell subsets are: T_H1, T_H2 and T_HO cells. Th1 are inflammatory cells, secrete IL-2, Interferon γ & Interferon β & GM-CSF, mediate delayed type hypersensitivity, promote IgG2a production & play a role in cell-mediated immune response. T_H cells become activated when they are presented with peptide antigen by MHC class II molecules that are expressed on the surface of Antigen presentation cells (APCs- dendritic cells, phagocytic macrophages and B cells). **(a) T_H1 cells are activated by the following events:** (a) interaction of TCR -antigen peptide whereby mRNA for cytokines IL-2 is produced and T cells change from G0 phase to G1 phase and then into S phase of cell synthesis, (b) CD2 interacts with B7-2 (CD 86) ligands on macrophage leading to formation of transcription factor CD 28 RC that stabilizes mRNA of IL-2 gene. (c) CD 40-CD40L interaction takes place when CD40 receptors on APC bind to its ligands CD40L on the activated T cells causing T cells to divide. The activated T_H1 cells secrete **IFN-γ and IL-2 that activate macrophages and Tc cells.** The stimulated macrophages secrete **nitric oxide that kills intracellular located bacteria.** Activated Tc cells turn into **effector cytotoxic T lymphocytes** that kill virus infected or altered cells. Hence **T_H1 cells are central to cell mediated immunity.**

T_H2 cells help B cells to divide & differentiate into antibody producing plasma cells and memory B cells. T_H 2 cells are stimulated by IL-4 secreted possibly by mast cells, basophils and certain CD4$^+$ T cells in the beginning of infection, and supplemented later by IL-10 secreted by the macrophages. The **activated T_H2 cells secrete IL-4, IL-5 and IL-10 that stimulate B cells to divide and transform into plasma cells that secrete antibodies** in the blood and body fluid, or into memory B cells that induce secondary immune responses, which are central to humoral immunity.

T_H1 & T_H2 cells are counter suppressive to each other. IFN-γ production by T_H1 cells suppresses T_H2 cell activity and thus prevents humoral immunity. T_H2 cells produce IL-4 that suppresses T_H1 cell activity and thus inhibits cellular immunity. **CD8⁺ cytotoxic T cells** are the second subset of T cells that recognize foreign peptide Ags produced within the cells (endogenous), for example, **multiplying viral antigens in the cytosol attach to class I MHC molecules and then peptide-MHC complex** is presented on the target cells that are recognized by Tc cells. Other examples include viral Ags synthesized in the cytosol of the infected cells, transplanted cells showing mismatched MHC molecules, and altered cells possessing altered peptide, each of these Ag peptides attachés to class I MHC molecule and displayed on the cell surface for recognition by T_C cells. There is a direct contact between target cells & CTLs. Activated T_C cells are transformed into effector T cells called cytotoxic T lymphocytes that kill the target cells directly through secretion of **perforins and granzymes or by apoptosis**. Perforin makes a whole in the target cells causing its lysis; CTLs also destroy virally infected cells and tumor cells, and are also implicated in transplant rejection. These cells recognize their targets by binding to antigen associated with MHC class I, which is present on the surface of nearly every cell of the body. **Tc cells also consist of two subsets: Tc1 and Tc2 cells that secrets cytokines similar to T_H1 and T_H2 cells respectively**. Some Tc cells secrete cytokines that suppress the activity of B cells or Tc cells.

$CD8^+$ T cells

The best understood $CD8^+$ T cells are **cytotoxic T lymphocytes (CTLs)**.

CD8+ T cells can, in principle, recognize (and exert their antiviral effects upon) almost any infected cell; thus CD8+ T cells are the foot soldiers of the immune response, engaging in hand-to-hand combat against viruses within cells. In contrast, CD4+ T cells are unable to recognize the majority of infected cells (which do not express MHC class II), and so they seem unlikely to play a direct role in eradicating the microbe; these cells instead orchestrate the antiviral campaign. However, cytolytic activity is not always the primary means by which CD8+ T cells control virus infections, and it plays little part in eradicating vaccinia, Semliki Forest and vesicular stomatitis viruses, rotaviruses, coxsackieviruses and HBV. In these, and other, cases, CD8+ T cells can control virus infection by a non-lytic mechanism; they can secrete cytokines, such as interferon-gamma and tumour necrosis factor (TNF), which can directly reduce virus replication, and may even 'cure' infected cells by inactivating virus replication in the absence of cell death. They secrete molecules that destroy the cell to which they have bound. If the target cell is infected with a virus, the cell is usually destroyed before it can release a fresh viruses able to infect other cells. An example will show the beauty and biological efficiency of this mechanism. Every time you get a virus infection, say influenza virus, the virus invades certain cells of your body-cells of the respiratory passages. Once inside, the virus subverts the metabolism of the cell to make more viruses. This involves synthesizing a number of different macromolecules encoded by the viral genome. In due course, these are assembled into a fresh crop of virus particles that leave the cell (often killing it in the process) and spread to new target cells. Except while in transit from their old homes to their new, the viruses work inside the cells safe from any antibodies that might be present in blood, lymph, and secretions. But early in the process, infected cells display fragments of the viral proteins in their surface class I molecules. CTLs specific for that antigen will be able to bind to the infected cell and often will be able to destroy it before it can release a fresh crop of viruses. In general, the role of the $CD8^+$ T cells is to monitor all the cells of the body, ready to destroy any that express foreign antigen fragments in their class I molecules.

The nature of the adaptive immune response can clearly determine whether a virus infection is cleared or causes damage to the host. However, an uncontrolled or inappropriate adaptive response can also be damaging. A complete understanding of how viruses cause disease requires an appreciation of the adaptive immune response.

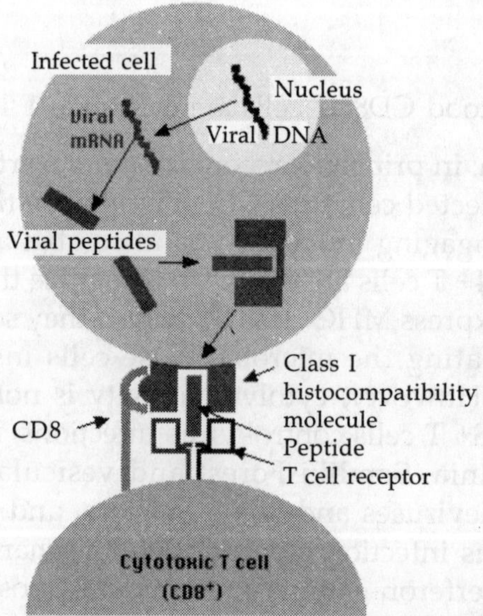

Figure 5.3: Recognition of antigen peptide by CD8 T cells

Host response to viral pathogens relies heavily on T cells

With intracellular parasites, viruses and some microorganisms, cytotoxic T cells are particularly important. After activation, cytotoxic T cells attacked infected host cells killing them. The response to a viral infection is quite different from that seen in a bacterial infection. Viral infections are intracellular for the most part. This has two implications. First, much of the damage is going to occur inside infected cells. Second, elimination of the infection is going to require destruction of host cells. Therefore, the immune system needs a method of discriminating virally infected cells from healthy cells. Fortunately our bodies have just such a mechanism and it involves the MHC I molecules. In general, cell-mediated immunity is much more important for clearing a viral infection. Figure 5-4 summarizes the hosts response to infection with influenza virus.

An immune defense against a viral infection is more dependent on T cells and less dependent on antibodies. Cytotoxic T cells are important in killing virally infected cells. In step (1) influenza virus enters the cell and begins to replicate (2). Viral proteins fill the cytoplasm (3). Most go on to form influenza virus and escape (4). The presence of viral proteins in the cytoplasm also causes the production of α-interferon (5). Some viral proteins are degraded and end up being displayed in MHC I molecules (6). Passing T_c cells will test the MHC I molecule presenting foreign antigen and a fraction will be activated by it. Activated T_c cells are directed to differentiate into cytotoxic T cells by T_H1 cells. Activated cytotoxic T cells then attack other virally infected cells displaying viral antigens in the MHC I molecules that the T cells react to. Viral antigens are also presented to B cells producing antibodies in a similar fashion. These antibodies attack free virus, agglutinating it and making it available for phagocytosis (9).

Influenza virus is a good example to study because it illustrates many of the salient points of viral infection and is also an important human pathogen. However, the specific response of the immune system is dependent upon the particular pathogen. Many of the mechanisms that we describe here come into play in other viral infections, but the exact response is always unique to the particular viral agent.

Virus begins to replicate and viral proteins accumulate in the infected cell. Some of these proteins are degraded by host cell machinery and the peptide fragments are transported into the endoplasmic reticulum, where they combine with newly synthesized MHC I molecules. The MHC I molecules loaded with foreign viral antigens now find their way to the surface of the cell. The infected cell also begins to produce and secrete α-interferon. This notifies surrounding cells of viral infection and induces them to produce compounds that interfere with viral replication making further infection more difficult.

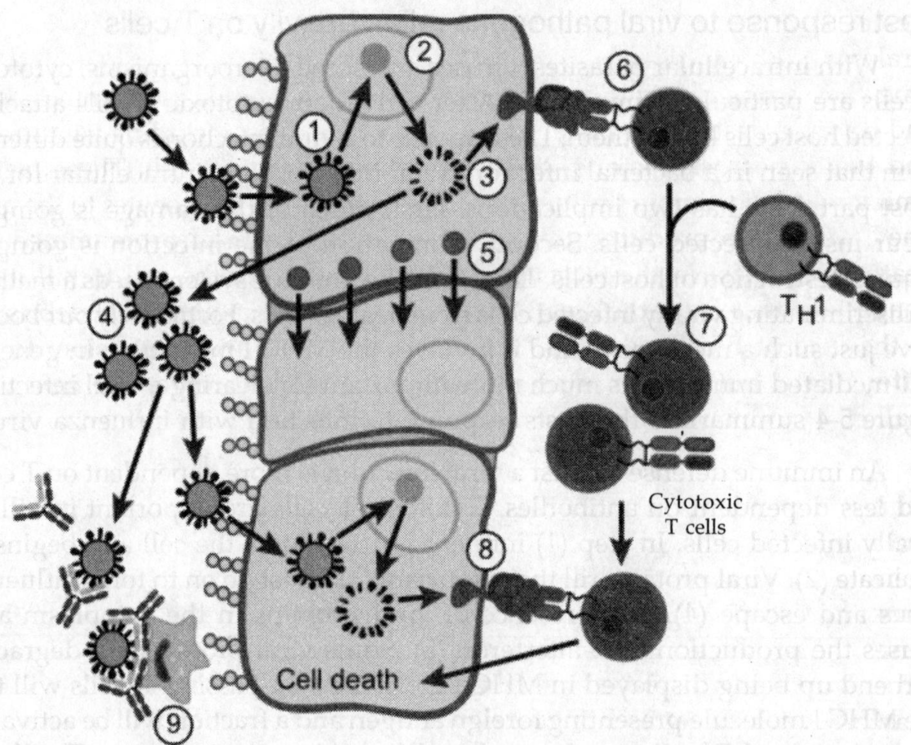

Figure 5.4 : Immune response to influenza infection

Virally infected cells begin to release flu virus particles into the surrounding tissues. The presence of viral particles and the death of virally infected cells begin the process of inflammation. This causes the characteristic redness, soreness and swelling in the back of the throat and the induction of fever observed in influenza. At this point, macrophages and dendritic cells take up viruses and viral debris, process them and add to MHC II molecules for presentation to T helper cells. T_H1 cells detect the presented antigen and those that match are activated and begin to secrete IL-2, which has several effects on other T and B cells responding to the infection.

Mucous secretion from the intensifying inflammation begins to cause a runny nose and coughing. The release of interferon and IL1 contribute to the aches and fever associated with influenza. As the concentration of virus increases in the body, these symptoms intensify.

Cytotoxic T cells (T_c cells) roaming in the tissues encounter infected cells presenting viral antigens in their MHC I molecules. Those that have TCRs that respond to the antigen are activated to begin clonal expansion and develop into active cytotoxic cells under the influence of the T_H1 cells. During the next encounter with a virally infected cell, these cells again recognize the viral antigen being presented in an MHC I molecule using their TCR, but this time, they are activated to attack the cell. The T_c cell binds to the infected cell and begins a destructive cycle. A number of cytokines, including γ-interferon and tumor necrosis factor (TNF), are secreted by the T_c cell. These factors limit viral replication in the target cell and also attract phagocytes to the area. The T_c cells also produce molecules that elicit a form of programmed cell death (apoptosis) in the target cell, essentially telling the cell to kill itself. Phagocytes that enter the area then clean up any remaining viral debris. As in the case of B cells, some of the T_c cells of the clonal expansion do not differentiate, but remain as memory cells in preparation for the next viral challenge by this viral strain.

The importance of CTL in the clearance of virus infection has been demonstrated in a wide variety of viral infections in both laboratory animals and in man. In addition, adoptive transfer of virus-specific CTL in mice has been shown to protect the recipient against infections with the virus. As with virus-specific antibody responses, however, not all CTL responses to virus are beneficial to the host, and in some cases the tissue destruction caused by the virus-specific CTL is greater than the damage done by the virus itself; and example of this would be the fulminant hepatitis associated in a small proportion of cases with infection with hepatitis B virus, in which the liver damage is caused by virus-specific CTL rather than directly by the virus.

Phagocytized virus is also presented to T_H2 cells that respond by activating in a manner identical to that described earlier. Virally infected cells also stimulate B cells that respond by clonal expansion and differentiation into plasma cells, resulting in the formation of antibodies against viral antigens. Antibodies are commonly raised against hemagglutinin and neuraminidase, two proteins on the outer surface of the virus. In most viral infections, antibody is not as important as in bacterial infections, but it does have several consequences. Antibodies bound to virus cause them to agglutinate, precipitate them out of solution and slow their spread through the body. Many effective antibodies block the receptor site of the virus and prevent its attachment to new host cells. These types of antibodies are especially useful in stopping subsequent infections by the same virus. Antibodies attached to virus also assist phagocytes in the efficient uptake of viral particles.

Free virus in the body is eliminated by the action of antibodies and phagocytes and the activated T_c cells destroy any virally infected cells. As the load of virus present in the body decreases, T suppressor cells help the immune response abate. After infection, subsequent attack by this strain of influenza virus is prevented by the action of T and B memory cells.

AIDS patients lose their CD4⁺ T cells

AIDS provides a vivid illustration of the importance of $CD4^+$ T cells in immunity. The human immunodeficiency virus (**HIV**) binds to CD4 molecules and thus is able to invade and infect $CD4^+$ T cells. As the disease progresses, the number of $CD4^+$ T cells declines below its normal level of about 1000 per microliter (µl). A partial explanation for this may be the unceasing efforts of the patient's $CD8^+$ T cells to destroy the infected $CD4^+$ cells. However, it turns out that only a small fraction of the patients $CD4^+$ T cells are infected at any given time. Also **uninfected** $CD4^+$ cells are induced to commit suicide by apoptosis. When the number of $CD4^+$ T cells drops below 400 per microliter, the ability of the patient to mount an immune response declines dangerously. Not only does the patient become hypersusceptible to pathogens that give all of us grief but also to microorganisms, especially viruses and fungi, that normally inhabit our tissues without harming us. These **opportunistic infections** can be fatal.

Chronic viral infections eventually take hold because they wear the immune system out, a phenomenon immunologists describe as **exhaustion.** But exhausted immune cells can be revived after the introduction of fresh Th cells. Their findings provide support for an emerging strategy for treating chronic infections by infusing immune cells back into patients after a period of conditioning. Antigen-specific CD4 T cells help rescues exhausted CD T cells during chronic viral infection. Immune responses against LCMV are driven by CD8 or "killer" T cells, which destroy virus-infected cells in the body. But a few weeks after exposure to LCMV, the mice develop a chronic infection that their immune systems cannot shake off, similar to when humans are infected by viruses like HIV and hepatitis C. Researchers infused CD4 helper T cells from uninfected mice, in mice chronically infected with LCMV. After the infusion, the CD8 cells in the infected mice revived and the levels of virus in their bodies decreased by a factor of four after a month. The helper cells drove the CD8 or "killer" T cells that were already in the infected mice to emerge from exhaustion and re-engage. The cell-based treatment was especially effective when combined with an antibody that blocks the molecule PD-1, which appears on exhausted T cells and inhibits their functioning. There was ten-fold reduction in virus, sometimes to undetectable levels. The antibody against PD-1 helps the exhausted killer T cells to revive, and enhances the function of the helper T cells as well. The combination reduced viral levels by roughly ten-fold, and made the virus undetectable in some mice. The helper cells were all genetically engineered to recognize LCMV, a difference between mouse experiments and potential clinical application. But it may be possible to remove helper T cells from a human patient and stimulate them so that all the cells that recognize a given virus grow. The molecule

PD-1 was previously identified by Ahmed and colleagues as a target for therapy designed to re-activate exhausted immune cells. Antibodies against PD-1 have been undergoing tests in clinical studies against hepatitis C and several forms of cancer.

Passive Immunity

Passive immunity refers to the transfer of antibodies from a donor in which they were produced to a recipient for temporary immunity. Passive immunity can be achieved through transfer of immune serum or via colostrums or yolk. Significant transplacental transfer of antibodies is found in primates, but does not occur in domestic animals. Passive immunity in domestic mammals comes via the colostrums, with its high concentration of antibodies, and the more than normally pervious epithelium of the neonate's intestinal epithelium. In birds maternal antibody is transferred to the yolk, from where the developing chick embryo absorbs it from about day 11 of incubation. **Passive immunization** is transient immunization produced by the introduction into the system of pre-formed antibody or specifically sensitized lymphoid cells. The persons/animals immunized is protected only as long as these antibodies remain in his blood and are active usually from 4 to 6 weeks. For example, passive immunization in case of CDV, canine parvovirus, feline panleukopenia hog cholera & other severe diseases immediately protects them against these viral diseases.

Maternal immunity

It is the immunity that is acquired by the neonate by transplacental transfer of immunoglobulins or from ingestion of colostrum or via the yolk sac in the case of birds. The placentation of all animals precludes trans-placental transfer of immunoglobulin. Passive transfer of maternal immunity is effected by the transfer of immunoglobulilns present in high concentration in the first milk, colostrum, through the intestine of the newborn. The success of this transfer is dependent upon the time after birth that colostrum is ingested (physiologically 24-36 hours, but effectively for adequate transfer, 8 hours after birth) and on the mass of immunoglobulin ingested which is determined by the concentration of immunoglobulin in colostrum and the amount of colostrum ingested.

Colostrum contains a high level of IgG for several days after parturition. Following ingestion, colostral IgG molecules are absorbed unchanged across the intestinal mucosa for the first 1 to 2 days in cattle, dog, pig and horse and for up to 4 days in the sheep and goat. IgA is also present in colostrum but is not translocated to the circulation of the suckling animal to any extent; it may provide some local gut immunity. Natural passive immunity is important because it protects young animals during first few weeks of life, & because length of maternal immunity should be considered when designing vaccination schedule.

Failure of passive transfer results in a significant increase in risk for neonatal viral infection. Neonates that fail to acquire serum concentrations of IgG_1 greater than 10 mg/ml are at significantly higher risk of septicemic, enteric and respiratory diseases. Failure of passive transfer occurs as a result of neonates sucking the dam or acquiring colostrum by artificial feeding too late in the absorptive process, or by receiving too little colostrum or receiving colostrum with low immunoglobulin concentration.

Antibodies can be transferred from mothers to fetus and young ones either through placenta or through colostrums and milk. There are four types of placenta which determine the transfer or antibodies to its off springs in man and various animals.

(i) Haemochorial placenta: it is present in humans and primates in which the maternal blood is in direct contact with the trophoblasts. Such placenta favours transfer of maternal IgG antibodies to the foetus, but IgM, IgA and IgE are not transferred.

(ii) Endotheliochorial placenta: Such placentas are present in dogs and cats in which chorionic epithelium contact directly with the endothelium of maternal capillaries. Such placenta remains with the endothelium of maternal capillaries; such placenta allows only small proportion of IgG (5-10%) from mothers to young ones but major portion are obtained from colostrum.

(iii) Syndesmochorial placenta: such placentas are present in the ruminants in which the chorionic epithelium lies in direct contact with uterine tissues. Only IgGl is transferred.

(iv) Eptheliochorial placenta: This type of placenta is present in horses and pigs wherein fetal chorionic epithelium is opposed to uterine epithelium. There is no transfer of Igs from the mother to the fetus via such placenta. Young ones get antibodies through colostrum which is rich in IgG.

Colostrum is rich in IgG and IgA antibodies and some amount of IgE. The predominant antibodies are IgG which represent 65 to 90% of the total antibodies. IgA is present in minor concentration but it is also significant. Soon as the colostrums production ceases, it is replaced by milk production. In humans and primates IgA is the predominant antibodies in the colostrum and in milk both. In horses and pigs IgG is the predominant antibody in the colostrum but IgA is predominant antibody in milk. Ruminants contain IgGl as predominant antibodies in both milk and colostrum. Milk contains only 30% of IgG and 10% of IgA derived from the serum while the rest is produced locally in the udder. In contrast, colostrum contains all the IgG and IgMs from the serum and half IgA from the serum and rest is produced locally in the udder.

Absorption of Colostrum

When newborn animals suckle colostrum, the colostrum proteins are not cleaved in the intestine because power of proteolysis has not been developed. Moreover, there is presence of trypsin inhibitors in colostrum and hence colostrum reaches the general circulation.

(i) The immunoglobulins bind to FcRN receptors present in the epithelial cells of the intestine of newborns. The receptor FcRN consist of class I b MHC heterodimer comprising heavy alpha chains and beta-2 microglobulin and resembles Fc receptors in the chicken. The bond immunoglobulins are taken up by pinocytosis and cross the epithelial cells, enter lacteals and intestinal capillaries and lastly it reaches in the general circulation. In this way newborns get adequate quantity of maternal immunoglobulin.

(ii) The young ones of different species differ in their capability to absorb immunoglobulins. All immunoglobulins are absorbed without selectivity. However, in horses and pigs, selective absorption of immunoglobulins occur. Mainly IgG is absorbed to selectivity in case species contain free secretary component in the intestinal tract due to which IgA bind to these secretary component that prevent its absorption.

(iii) Permeability of intestine for the colostrum immunoglobulins vary in young ones of different species of animals. The intestinal permeability for colostrum proteins in highest just after birth which gradually declines in 6 hours and is extremely low after 24 hours. This is because the intestinal cells responsible for absorption power. Calves, foals and other young ones should be fed a minimum of 1 liter of colostrum by 6 hours of birth. If there is good management, the level of immunoglobulins particularly IgG parallel those in the adult between 12 to 24 hours after birth. When absorption of colostrum stops, the level of immunoglobulins declines due to catabolism.

(iv) There is proteinuria that occurs during colostral absorption from intestine, this happens because beta lactoglobulin and other polypeptides are very small and excreted in the urine. At the same time the glomeruli of the newborns are permeable to the macromolecules and as such calves contain intact immunoglobulins in urine. As soon as the absorption of colosturm stops, proteinuria also terminates. Colostrum antibodies do not allow active synthesis of that type of immunoglobulins by the negative feedback mechanism.

(v) When milk replaces colostrum, the milk also contains high quantity of IgA in ruminants and IgA in neutropenic because proleolytic enzyme is poor during first few weeks; immunoglobulin remain present throughout the intestine. Gradually, digestion increases with increased production of proteolytic enzymes as such immunoglobulin is broken except IgA. Only secretory IgA is left which protects the young ones from pathogens entrance through intestine and they are also protected against septicemic diseases.

(vi) If some young ones fail to absorb colostrum or milk resulting in deficiency. The lambs which fail to get colostrum are neutropenic which reduces phagocytosis and inflammatory reaction. The failure of absorption of colostrum may be due to the following reasons: (a) Production of poor quality of colostrum by the mothers. This usually happens when there is premature birth with weak offsprings. (b) Inadequate absorption by the newborns. This condition arises either due to multiple birth in sheep and pigs and weak offsprings. (c) Failure of absorption in the intestine. If young ones, e.g. foals possess less than 4mg/ml, they may contract bacterial infections and a level of 200mg/dl get life threatening infections; such young ones should be fed 2-3 liter of colostrum either from the mare or from the frozen stock by tube. Similarly, calves possessing less than 10 mg/ml of their serum at 24 to 48 hours of age, succumb to infections. As such the calves are fed commercial colostrum to protect them from pathogenic E. coli, (k 99), Coronavirus and Rotavirus. Colostrum also contains lymphocytes including T. cells having CD4/CD8 ratio of about 0.57 (normal 0.8). These lymphocytes of colostrum survive for 36 hours in intestine. These lymphocytes carry immunity along with these lymphocytes.

What is the function of γδ T cells?

The role of γδ T cells is still something of a mystery. Situated as they are at the interfaces between the external and internal worlds, they may represent a first line of defense against invading pathogens. Their response does seem to be quicker than that of αβ T cells. Curiously, many of the antigens to which γδ T cells respond are found not only on certain types of invaders (e.g., *Mycobacterium tuberculosis*) but also on host cells that are under attack by pathogens. Knockout mice that cannot make γδ T cells are slower to heal injuries to their skin. They are also much more susceptible to skin cancers than normal mice. Perhaps immune surveillance is one of the functions of ãä T cells.

Viral-Induced Immunopathology

Besides the beneficial effect of humoral & cellular innate immune responses, viral-induced immunopathology causes tissue damage resulting from the immune response to a virus. Viral immunopathology is a consequence of various immunologic interactions, such as formation of antibody-antigen complexes, tissue damage due to cytotoxic Tcells, antibody or complement. Fixation of complement by immune complexes can result in the release of vasoactive amines, recruitment of inflammatory cells and subsequent damage to host tissue. Some viruses such a lymphocytic choriomeningitis virus produce large amounts of immune complexes in the circulation which lodge in the vascular beds and in the kidneys where they fix complement and result in tissue damage. Other examples of viruses that cause these effects are: measles, respiratory syncytial virus, dengue and serum hepatitis virus. Such tissue damage depends on the type and location of immunopathology can be characteristic of a particular viral infection. For examples, anterior uveitis is due to antigen-antibody complexes deposit in the eye, inducing local inflammation, and result in anterior uveitis. Immune-complexes remaining in circulation deposit in the kidney, resulting in the some kidney damage-glomerular nephritis as seen during the recovery stage of infectious canine hepatitis infections. In case of LCM induced choroiomeningitis caused by an arenavirus infection in mice, results in CNS damage from the destruction of virus infected cells by cytotoxic T lymphocytes. In old-dog encephalitis in case of canine distemper virus (paramyxovirus) is also the result of a cell-mediated immune response to persistent virus infection. Infants infected with cytomegalovirus have circulating immune complexes that are deposited in the kidneys and joints resulting in pathology such as arthritis and glomerular nephritis. Another example is fatal hemorrhagic shock syndrome associated with dengue virus infection. In this instance fixation of complement by circulating immune complexes results in release of products of the complement cascade leading to sudden increased vascular permeability, shock and death. There are many other examples.

In case of Woodchuck hepatitis and Duck hepatitis B Infections (Hepadnavirus), most of the liver damage is caused by the continuous action of $CD8^+$ T lymphocytes in killing infected hepatocytes rather than by the action of the virus itself. In respiratory viral infection ciliated epithelia are destroyed, & columnar epithelia are denuded. Many viruses like rotaviruses, coronaviruses, toroviruses, calciviruses, & astroviruses producing diarrhea cause shortening of intestinal villi. IBDV infection in chicks results in atrophy of bursa of Fabricius with immunosuppression & subsequent bacterial infection. FIV infection damages B cells inviting wide range of bacterial infection. There are several viral infections in which macrophages &

lymphocytes infiltration in the tissue occur with resultant cytokines that induce inflammation causing progression of disease. For examples, Aleutian mink disease (macrphages) causes arthritis & glomerulonephritis. EIAV in horses (macrophages) causes anemia, vasculitis & glomerulonephritis. These immune responses can be perturbed by direct virus infection of immunocompetent cells, and effective responses may produce tissue damage for example by immune complex formation and T cell-mediated destruction of infected cells. This virus immunopathology assumes particular importance when the virus itself is relatively non-cytopathic and in the case of persistent infections.

Virus Strategies to Induce Immunosuppression

Some of the viral infections are characterized by immunosuppress and in doing so are able to establish infection. Immunosuppression occurs during the course of both cytolytic or noncytolytic viral infection. Many viruses by suppressing immune responses overcome or minimize host defenses. A number of viruses have been found to encode proteins that interfere at various levels with specific or nonspecific host defenses. These proteins enable the virus to replicate more efficiently amidst antiviral host defenses by evading them. The evasion of host immunity is advantageous to the virus at several levels. In case of widespread immunity in a host population, a new virus can evade the preexisting immunity and thus persist in the population without getting eliminated. Evasion of immunity also increases viral pathogenicity in the individual host. The virus e.g. may grow to higher titres in the host and thus increase its chances of transmission to a naïve recipient. Several viruses avoid detection and elimination by the immune system and are able to persist in the host. This brings us to the point of acute versus persistent viral infections, situations important for understanding the pathogenic nature of different viruses. There are many infections, e.g. herpes, hepatitis B and C, in which the virus is not eliminated from the host, but persists for months, years or even the lifetime of the host. This is in contrast to acute infections, such as poliomyelitis or influenza, in which the virus is eliminated from the host within a few weeks. In a persistent infection, the virus either (a) continues to multiply and hence remains demonstrable, resulting in a chronic infection, or (b) may survive in some non-infectious form, as a latent infection with a potential for future reactivation.

Some viruses are able to evade the immune system of the host by various means: infection of immunologically privileged sites, antigenic variability of virions, inhibition of INF-β, decrease in MHC class I expression, inhibition of peptide processing, and expression of immune system homologous structures. Immunologically privileged sites include parts that do not come directly into contact with the circulation and are therefore normally segregated from the immune system, e.g. the brain, the testis and prostate, the retina of the eye, and hamster cheek pouches. Since epitope recognition, antigen-specific lymphocyte expansion and antibody production form the basis of adaptive immunity, these are the very steps targeted by pathogens for successfully persisting in the host.

i. Infection of immunocytes

Many persistent viruses infect lymphocytes (B or T cells) and monocytes and either destroy these immunocytes by cytolytic mechanisms or alter their functions. Examples are the herpes simplex virus (HSV), Epstein-Barr virus (EBV), CMV, poliovirus, measles virus, & IBDV.

ii. Destruction of specialized antigen-presenting cells

Blood monocytes, tissue macrophages and dendritic cells comprise a principal cellular element in the clearance and inactivation of most viral pathogens. These cells are a major target and infectious reservoir for many persistent viruses, e.g. lentiviruses (such as HIV), & cytomegaloviruses. Destruction of macrophages following viral infection results in a generalized immunosuppression against most immunogens, affecting both antibody and T cells. This mechanism appears to be the reason for late immune failure in AIDS.

iii. Induction of tolerance

Some viruses can infect the thymus & cause clonal deletion of maturing virus specific T cells. This results in the virus being viewed as self by the immune system, without any generalized immunosuppression. Such a mechanism for viral persistence has been demonstrated experimentally for lymphocytic choriomeningitis virus (LCMV) and hepatitis B virus (HBV).

Strategies to Evade Antibody Responses

Viruses carry proteins on their surface that are critical for binding to target cells and for entry into these cells. These proteins, which are so important for the viral life cycle, are obvious targets for the host antibody response. The host produces neutralizing antibodies targeted to these proteins. Many persistent viruses respond by altering immunogenic regions of these proteins to escape the neutralizing antibodies (Table 5-2).

i. Antigenic variation

The polymerases of RNA viruses lack proof-reading function, resulting in high mutation rates & the gradual accumulation of minor mutations in viral proteins. Point mutations in the envelope glycoprotein result in escape from neutralizing antibodies, e.g. neuraminidase and hemagglutinin of influenza virus and gp120 of HIV. In HIV-1 there is epitope changes in intracellular proteins such as Gag, Pol & Nef (Table 5-2).

ii. Antigenic shift

This strategy is used by viruses with segmented genomes, e.g. the influenza virus genome is made up of 8 RNA segments. During coinfection of a single cell by two viruses, the segments from both infecting viruses can reassort resulting in the emergence of a new strain which will not be recognized by previously-formed antibodies, & can thus establish infection in individuals previously exposed to influenza virus (Table 5.2).

iii. Down-regulation of viral protein expression

The intracellular localization of a virus facilitates it to escape antibody responses. Although antibodies can detect viral antigens expressed on the cell surface, many viruses delay displaying their proteins on the cell surface until late in the infective cycle. Others down-regulate the expression of surface glycoproteins, in comparison with other nonsurface viral proteins.

Strategies to evade interferon production

Viruses have developed a various mechanisms to interfere with interferon response. Examples of interference with various portions of this response follow and are summarized in Table 5-3.

Strategies to evade NK cells responses

Viruses adopt several mechanisms to cause inhibition of NK cell activation and destruction of infected cells. Inhibition can be furnished by modification of expression of ligands on the surface of the infected cell either by increased expression of inhibitory ligands, expression of viral mimics of inhibitory ligands or decreased expression of activating ligands, inhibition of cytokines such as Interferon-γ (IFN-γ) or IL-18, viral molecules that competitively bind IL-18 receptors or disruption of the release of effector molecules like perforins and granzymes as depicted in Table 5-B.

Strategies to evade Cytotoxic T cells responses

CTLs identify virally infected cells if viral peptides are presented by MHC-1 molecules on the cell surface; MHC-1 molecule processed through degradation by polyubiquitination, processed in proteasomes where they are sectioned into small peptides 8-10 amino acids long, which enter the ER via a transporter associated with antigen processing (TAP), then from the ER into the Golgi complex and out to the plasma membrane where it can be detected by passing CTL. At all steps along this pathway, viruses have developed mechanisms to stop or delay this process sufficiently for viral replication to occur.

Table 5.2 : Virus mechanisms to evade some host defenses

Viral evasion	Mechanism	Viruses
Infection of immune cells	Destruction & immunosupression	IBD, cytomegalovirus, FIV, feline panleukopenia virus, HIV.
	Infection of macrophages	LDEV, ASFV.
Infection of non permissive cells	fail to express viral genes	Papillomaviruses in basal epith, herpesviruses in ganglion, lentiviruses in lymphocytes.
Evasion by cell to cell transfer	Transfer by cell fusion	Equine infectious anemia virus (EIAV), DV, herpesviruses.
Non expression of viral Ags on cell membrane	Causes restricted viral gene expression	Herpesviruses in ganglion neurons, lentiviruses in lymphocytes & macrophages.
Growth in immune sequestrated sites	Replication in sites inaccessible to immune cells	Rabies virus in muscle cells, peudorabies & rabies virus in neurons.
Immunological tolerance	Induces clonal anergy	BVDV, hog cholera virus, arenaviruses.
Evasion of neutralizing antibodies	Large amount of viral proteins produced that soaks Abs	Ebola & Marburg viruses, Lassa virus & arenaviruses.
	Viral proteins masked by glycoproteins or carbohydrates	Ebola & Marburgviruses, Rift Valley fever virus & arenaviruses.
Production of nonneutralizing antibodies	Produce low affinity or non neutralizing Abs against undesirable epitopes	Aleutian mink disease virus, ASFV, LCMV
Enhancing antibodies	Abs attached to virus increase macrophages infection	Cytomegalovirus, LDEV, FIPV, dengue viruses
Viral genome integration into host cell genome	Provirus DNA integration	Retroviruses
Antigenic changes	Mutation causes antigenic variants	Maedi-visna, EIAV, Influenza viruses
	Recombination between viral segments results in new subtypes	Influenza A viruses

Table 5.3 : A Virus mechanisms to evade IFN production

Virus	Gene / Gene product	Function
Adenovirus	E1A	Suppression of IKK, Prevents formation of ISGF3
African Swine Fever Virus	A238L	IkB homologue
Ebola Virus	VP35	dsRNA binding protein, Blockage of IRF3
Hepatitis C Virus	NS3-4A	Cleavage of MAVS
Human Cytomegalovirus	pp65	Blocks phosphorylation of IRF3
Human Papillomavirus	E6	Blocks phosphorylation of IRF3
	E7	ISGF3 blocker
Influenza Virus	NS1	dsRNA binding protein
	Unknown	Inactivation of PKR
	Unknown	Inactivation of PKR
Japanese Encephalitis Virus	NS5	JAK-STAT blocker
Myxoma virus	M-T7	Soluble INF-γ receptor
Paramyxovirus	V protein	Binds MDA-5, STAT1 Degradation
Rabies virus	P protein	JAK-STAT blocker Blocks phosphorylation of IRF3
Reovirus	σ3	dsRNA binding protein
Simian virus 5	V Protein	STAT1 Degradation
Vaccinia virus	B18R	Soluble INF-α receptor

Table 5.4 : Virus mechanisms to evade NK cell activation

Cowpox Virus	P35	Chemokine binding protein
Ectromelia Virus	P13	Binds IL-18, blocks IFN-γ expression
Human Cytomegalovirus	UL-16	Retains ULBP1, -2 & MICB intracellularly, prevents NKG2D recognition
	UL-18	Binds inhibitory LIR-1 receptor
	US-28	Sequesters CC chemokines
	UL-40	Loads HLA-E, Maintains HLA-E on infected cells
	UL-142	Decreases MICA
Hepatitis B Virus	HB surface AG	Decreases: number of NK cells, activation, TRAIL expression

Hepatitis C Virus	E2	Binds CD81 – Decreases IFN-γ, impairs cytotoxic granule release, CD16
	Hep C core Protein	Increases MHC-1 expression
	Core 35-44	HLA-E stabilization
Human Immunodeficiency Virus	NEF	Decreases HLA-A,-B maintains HLA-C, -, E, Decreases MICA, ULBP-2
	P24	Stabilizes HLA-E expression
Human Papillomavirus	E6,E7	Antagonistic binding of IL-18Rα, Binds IL-18, blocks IFN-γ expression
Kaposi's Sarcoma Herpes Virus	K-5	Down regulates expression B7-2, ICAM-1
Murine Cytomegalovirus	Gp40	Down regulates surface expression RAE-1 glycoproteins
	M131/129	Chemokine homologue, inhibits NK function
	M144	MHC-1 mimic
	M155	Down regulates H60
	M157	Binds inhibitory Ly49I receptor in sensitive 129/J mice
Molluscum contagiosum virus	MC53L MC54L	Binds IL-18, blocks IFN-γ expression
	MC080R	MHC-1 homologue unable to bind peptide

Table 5.5 : Virus mechanisms to evade MHC-1 expression

Adenovirus	E3/19K	Retention of MHC-1 in ER
African Swine Fever Virus	Unknown	Dispersion of trans-Golgi network, slowing of MHC-1 to plasma membrane
Bovine Papillomavirus	E5	Retention of MHC-1 in Golgi, repression of MHC-1 gene promoter
Cowpox virus	Unknown early gene	Retention of MHC-1 in ER
Human Cytomegalovirus	pp65	HLA-DR segregation and destruction, phosphorylation of 72-kDa transcription factor
	US2	Destruction of MHC-1 heavy chains

	US3	Retention of MHC-1 in ER
	US6	Inhibition of TAP
	US11	Destruction of MHC-1 heavy chains
Human immunodeficiency virus	Nef	Endocytosis of MHC-1 and CD4
	Tat	Repression of MHC-1 gene promoter
	Vpu	Destabilization of newly synthesized MHC-1
	Unknown	Inhibition of TAP
Human Papillomavirus	E7	Repression of MHC-1 gene promoter, repression of TAP gene promoter
Herpes Simplex Virus	ICP-47	Inhibition of TAP
Kaposi's Sarcoma Herpes Virus	K3 K5	Targets MHC-1 for degradation
Murine Cytomegalovirus	gp37/40	Retention of MHC in ER/Golgi
	gp48	Targets MHC for degradation
Murine Herpesvirus	mK3	Targets MHC-1 for degradation
Myxoma virus	m153R	MHC-1 internalization and degradation
Porcine Reproductive and Respiratory Syndrome virus	Unknown	Down regulation of MHC-1 expression
Vaccinia virus	UL49.5	Inhibition of TAP

□□□

Chapter 6

Control of Viral Diseases, Vaccines & Vaccination Policy

Contents

Control of Viral Infections and Diseases

Viral diseases cause distress to man and animals and the most worrying ones are those that are difficult to control. Human immunodeficiency virus (HIV) continues to spread in an uncontrolled manner. How viruses are transferred ? Viruses are carried by infected people or animals and excreted in discharges such as those from the nose, gut and reproductive fluids. The control of viruses blocks this transfer. Control measures for viruses include:

1. *Quarantine* : Separate the infected persons or animals with signs suspicious of an acute viral disease such as rash, vesicles, vomiting with diarrhoea & other symptoms.

2. *Import controls :* Include blocking animal imports from a country such as one infected with foot and mouth disease virus (FMDV) or avian influenza.

3. *Notification* : There are many notifiable diseases of man & animals including HIV, measles, mumps and rubella and those of animals include FMDV, swine fever and rabies. Anyone who suspects a notifiable disease must contact the national authorities. The authorities inform the World Health organisation (WHO) or World organisation for animal health (formerly the OIE). These organisations publicise the global spread of diseases.

4. *Slaughter* : Culling the infected animal or herd is essential. Viruses require living cells to multiply and this is halted by the death or slaughter of an animal.

5. *Decontamination* : Washing and disinfecting hands, clothing and equipment is very important. Disposing of dead bodies in a safe manner like incineration or burial in lime prevent spread of the pathogen. Treatment of waste water and chlorination of water is essential. Personal hygiene is utmost required, e.g. not coughing over people and washing hands after toilet and before food preparation.

   Sanitation and Vector Control : Several early approaches to virus control deserve recognition even though they are less dramatic than vaccination. One approach is the avoidance of viral exposure. This is an effective means of preventing the transmission of HIV-1, which is spread through sexual contact and exposure to blood of infected individuals. Blood bank testing, e.g, for hepatitis B surface antigen and for antibodies to HIV-1, HIV-2, HTLV-I, and hepatitis C, also avoids exposure by identifying and discarding blood units contaminated with these infectious agents.

Control of nonhuman viral reservoirs is another early, worthwhile approach. Unfortunately, few opportunities exist for practical application. The most notable success was the control, and in some cases, the elimination of rabies in some countries through removal of stray dogs, quarantine of incoming pets, and vaccination of domestic animals.

Another approach of enormous contemporary and historic importance is **vector control**. Transmission of viral disease by the bite of an arthropod vector was first demonstrated by Walter Reed and his associates, with their discovery that yellow fever was transmitted by mosquitoes. At the turn of the century, yellow fever was a disease of major consequence in the Americas and Africa. By immediately applying Reed's discovery, Gorgas mounted the anti-*Aedes aegypti* campaign in Havana that marked the beginning of the conquest of epidemic yellow fever. In dealing with the arthropod-borne diseases such as St. Louis encephalitis, any procedure that reduces vector populations or limits the access of the arthropod to humans or animals has potential value. These procedures include draining swamps, applying insecticide, screening homes, and using insect repellant or protective clothing. The last of the older approaches is to improve sanitation. This method is applicable in a limited way to diseases whose epidemiology involves fecal-oral transmission. The well-known link between the discharge of raw sewage into tidal waters, contamination of shellfish, and type A hepatitis is an example of a situation readily reversible by improved sanitary practices.

6. *Isolation* : Avoiding multiple close contacts such as in crowded housing is essential. A secure farm will also exclude other animals and visitors that might transfer the virus.
7. *Treatment* : Antiviral drugs are used for only a few viruses because they are expensive, often have side effects and they select for resistant viruses. They exist for HIV, hepatitis B, hepatitis C, herpes simplex, respiratory syncytial virus and influenza of man. Antiserum to rabies soon after a bite from a suspect is recommended.
8. *Other measures* : The guaranteed means to prevent viral infection are to prevent exposure, which is achieved by only allowing those animals without evidence of previous exposure to the farm. Adopting restricted contact is called as "closed herds". For maintaining closed herd status, all replacement animals and show animals should be isolated from the remaining animals for at least 2 - 3 weeks. These animals are closely examined for clinical signs and tested serologically/ virologically for evidence of exposure. This type of preventing exposure through restricted contact is quite effective in areas where suspected viruses are relatively uncommon; it is impractical in areas where these viruses are endemic.

Basic to controlling viral infections and diseases are adoption of good hygienic management practices. Various type s of **stress factors** play pivotal roles in predisposing animals to infection and in the spread of disease; the stresses associated with **poor nutrition, overcrowding, and housing with improper ventilation** are important. Hence, management measures include preventative measures to **protect the fetus and the newborn.** The viruses that cause mild or inapparent infections in adult animals may cause abortions or serious disease in neonates (e.g. parvovirus in swine). It is therefore desirable to restrict the contact of pregnant animals and newborns from other animals; also required is to insure that the newborn receives **colostrum**, which contains antibodies that would confer protection during the first weeks of life. Proper management also require restricting contact between different species of animals, as some viruses cause inapparent infections in one species but severe disease in others, e.g. **pseudorabies** virus, which causes subclinical infections in older pigs but is frequently fatal in piglets, sheep, dogs and cats. Regular cleaning and disinfection, the use of clean coveralls and footbaths, are essential to prevent the spread of viruses by fomites during disease outbreaks. During a disease outbreak, all animals should be quarantined and, if indicated, treated symptomatically. For instance: the necessary supportive therapy, as fluid replacement in severe cases of diarrhea is desired. Compulsorily use of aqueous sodium chlorite solution/ other disinfection is required. Using antibiotics may be recommended to prevent secondary bacterial infection.

Vaccination : Majority of viral diseases in humans & animals are being controlled by prophylactic use of vaccines that protect against infection and disease. These vaccines exist for many viruses such as mumps, measles, rubella and yellow fever & several viral disease in animals. They are made of a living harmless strain of the virus or of dead or inactivated virus. They induce antibodies, cytotoxic T cells and clones of memory cells but only to the vaccine virus. In many instances, viral disease prevention can be accomplished through vaccination. While vaccination doesn't necessarily prevent infection, the previous "priming" of the host's immune system allows for a quick response and clearance of the virus before disease occurs or mild disease of shorter duration. Indeed, vaccination is the most effective and cost-benefit among all preventive measures in animal health.

Veterinary Viral Vaccines

The major goals of veterinary vaccines are to improve the health and welfare of companion animals, increase production of livestock in a cost-effective manner, and prevent animal-to-human disease transmission from both domestic animals and wildlife. These diverse aims have led to different approaches to the development of veterinary vaccines from crude but effective whole-pathogen preparations to molecularly defined subunit vaccines,

Table 6.1 : Common commercial available antiviral disinfectants

Disinfectant	Examples	Uses	Comments
Alcohol	Ethyl, isopropyl	Hands, thermometers	Moderately virucidal at 70 - 80 %; ethanol is preferable
Chlorhexidine	Hibitane, Nolvasan	Many uses including examination tables, cages, other surfaces	Tolerant to the presence of organic compounds, body fluids, etc.; expensive
Detergent iodophores	Betadine, Wescadine, Redene	Drinking water, food and utensils, dairies, spot disinfection	Action based release of iodine & detergent action; less affected by high protein; expensive
Ethylene dioxide		For heat sensitive materials	Available as a compressed gas at 10% with 90% CO_2, otherwise toxic and explosive
Formaldehyde	Formalin	Laundry & bedding surfaces; as a vapor for other surfaces	Low power of penetration; irritating hypersensitivity occurs
Glutaraldehyde	Cidex	Cold sterilization of instruments with lenses	2% solution buffered with sodium bicarbonate; virucidal (10 min., pH 7.5 - 8.5); expensive
Phenol derivatives	Lysol, Dettol, Staphene, Sudol	Hands, examination tables, cages, other surfaces	2.5% aqueous solution; efficacy dependent on concentration and temperature; high protein decreases effectiveness
Quaternary ammonium compounds	Zephiran, Roccal, Savlon	Zephiran (benzylkonium chloride) used for cleaning wounds	Not effective against many viruses; high protein decreases effectiveness
Sodium hypochlorite	Chlorox, Chlorize	Same as detergent iodophores	Highly effective, rapid action; high protein decreases effectiveness; irritating; inexpensive

genetically engineered organisms or chimeras, vectored antigen formulations, and naked DNA injections. The final successful outcome of vaccine research and development is the generation of a product that will be available in the market or that will be used in the field to achieve desired outcomes. Successful veterinary viral vaccines have been produced against several viral pathogens, which in many ways have led the field in the application and adaptation of novel technologies. These veterinary viral vaccines have had, and continue to have, a major impact not only on animal health and production but also on human health through increasing safe food supplies and preventing animal-to-human transmission of infectious diseases. The continued interaction between animals and human researchers and health professionals will be of major importance for adapting new technologies, providing animal models of disease, and confronting new and emerging infectious diseases.

The criteria for successful animal or veterinary vaccines can be very different from those for human vaccines depending on the animal groups under consideration. For example, criteria for companion animal vaccines are similar to those for human vaccines in that the health and welfare of the individual animal are primary concerns. The main objective of livestock vaccines, on the other hand, is to improve overall production for the primary producers, and the cost-benefit resulting from vaccination is the bottom line for this industry. Vaccination against zoonotic or food-borne infections is aimed at reducing or eliminating the risk for the consumer and in some cases to improve the productivity of the individual animal. Vaccination of wildlife is generally considered only with respect to infections that are transmittable to humans (zoonotic diseases), although welfare concerns are of increasing importance.

While veterinary vaccines comprise only approximately 23% of the global market for animal health products, the sector has grown consistently due mainly to new technological advances in vaccine development, the continuous development of drug resistance by pathogens, and the emergence of new diseases. Apart from improving animal health and productivity, veterinary vaccines have a significant impact on public health through reductions in the use of veterinary pharmaceuticals and hormones and their residues in the human food chain. This will be an increasing impetus for activity with the more stringent requirements of regulatory agencies and consumer groups, particularly in the major markets of Europe and the United States. For example, the use of antibiotics in animal production has already been severely restricted, and the European Union has recently banned the use of coccidiostats for poultry. In addition, vaccines contribute to the well-being of livestock and companion animals, and their use is favored by the growing animal welfare lobby.

The process of developing veterinary vaccines has both advantages and disadvantages over human vaccine development. On the one hand, the potential returns for animal vaccine producers are much less than those for human vaccines, with lower sales prices and smaller market sizes, resulting in a much lower investment in research and development in the animal vaccine area than in the human vaccine area, although the complexity and range of hosts and pathogens are greater. For example, the market size for the recently launched human vaccine (**Gardasil**) against papillomavirus and cervical cancer is estimated to be greater than 1 billion U.S. dollars, while the most successful animal health vaccines (e.g., against foot-and-mouth disease [FMD] virus in cattle and *Mycoplasma hyopneumoniae in* pigs) enjoy a combined market size that is 10 to 20% of this figure. On the other hand, veterinary viral vaccine development generally has less stringent regulatory and preclinical trial requirements, which can make up the largest cost in human vaccine development, and a shorter time to market launch and return on investment in research and development. In contrast to human vaccine development, veterinary scientists are also able to immediately perform research in the relevant target species. This is an obvious advantage over human vaccine development, as experimental infections, dose-response studies, and challenge inoculations need not be carried out in less relevant rodent models.

Immunity acquired through natural infection can take on several forms depending on the type and life cycle of the pathogen. Vaccines may be used to prevent clinical signs of disease after infection or to help control, eliminate, or even eradicate an infection at the population level (e.g., the expected global **eradication of rinderpest** virus through vaccination). Both vaccine effectiveness and mechanism of action may vary depending on the required outcome. New technologies to achieve the selective induction of effective immune responses in the development of new vaccines are becoming available to vaccine researchers. Notwithstanding the scientific advances, the single factor that determines the success of an experimental vaccine is its successful commercialization and/or use in the field. This outcome requires a combination of basic research, commercial imperatives, local requirements, and global perspectives depending on the particular disease under investigation. These four aspects are represented here which will concentrate on recent advances in veterinary vaccines that have reached the market place or are actively produced by veterinary institutes for use by local farming communities.

When an animal (or human) is vaccinated, it contains a small amount of a virus under the skin of the animal. This organism that gets injected is generally a non-harmful strain of the virus that is protecting the animals from (live vaccine) or a killed form of the actual wild-type, disease-causing virus.

The injection may contain live organisms (live vaccine); inactivated organisms, incapable of replicating in the body (killed vaccine) or just little bits of the organisms: specific proteins or sugars (termed antigens) that the immune system will recognize as foreign to the body (subunit vaccines-are a form of killed vaccine). As will be discussed in the killed vaccine section, killed vaccines and subunit vaccines are generally less immune-stimulatory than live vaccines and so additives (termed adjuvants) which enhance the immune system's response to the vaccine are generally added to the killed vaccines to improve their effect.

The immune mechanisms that can act to protect animals against invading viruses that infect non-antigen-presenting cells can be killed by cytotoxic T cells (CTL) that recognize pathogen-derived epitopes presented in conjunction with major histocompatibility complex (MHC) class I on infected cells or by antibody-dependent lysis or opsonization of infected cells expressing pathogen molecules. Extracellular pathogens, or intracellular pathogens on their way to infect other cells, can be attacked by specific circulating antibodies and either killed by lysis or agglutination or phagocytosed by macrophages and neutrophils. Both antibody and CTL induction requires help from pathogen-specific CD4 helper T cells that are activated after interaction with pathogen-derived epitopes presented in conjunction with MHC class II molecules on the surface of MHC class II+ antigen-presenting cells. If pathogens infect antigen-presenting cells, they can be killed directly by CD4 T cells as well as CD8 CTL through the induction of mediators such as gamma interferon (IFN-γ), reactive oxygen and nitrogen species, and indoleamine 2,3-dioxygenase (IDO). Toxins released by pathogens can be neutralized by circulating antibodies, thereby decreasing clinical signs of infection.

General Immunological Principles

- B cells antigen receptors predominantly sees 3-Dimensional conformations.
- T cells sees processed antigen in association with MHC molecules again as a 3-D conformation.
- In an Antigen Presenting Cell, such as a macrophage, non-infectious proteins are endocytosed and degraded in lysosomes to peptides (endosomal pathway), some of which bound specifically to MHC II molecules & recognized by Th cells. In contrast, if an agent such as a virus infected the macrophage, some newly synthesized viral antigens are likewise degraded in the cytoplasm to peptides (the cytoplasmic pathway), but these are associated with class I MHC molecules & are detected by Tc cells.

The role of different components of the immune response to infection

Antibody has 3 important functions

- It is the only means to prevent an infection by neutralization of viral infectivity. The generation of protective Ab has usually been the only response measured by vaccine developers. Generally neutralizing Ab reacts with just a few epitopes on one or two surface antigens of the infecting agent. It is ineffective if the protective epitopes are subject to pronounced antigenic drift.
- Infected cells which express viral antigen on their cell surface may be lysed by 2 antibody-dependent mechanisms - (a) complement pathway, or (b) antibody-dependent cell cytotoxicity.
- Antibody may facilitate the removal of debris (a scavenging mechanism)

The function of effector T cells : Particular Tc cells, is to clear an infection. Although antibody can contribute to recovery from infection, T cells are the main mechanism for achieving this. The most important feature of CMI, in direct contrast to Ab, is that it responds to many peptides from an agent. Some come from proteins that are not subject to antigenic variation. This broad T cell response is an important mechanism for overcoming antigenic variation of an agent and the genetic variability of the host population. Although such an agent may bypass the protection afforded by a preformed Ab after vaccination, the cell-mediated immune response allows most animals to recover from an acute infection. Infectious agents causing chronic persistent infections have found a way of escaping a cell-mediated immune response. The mechanisms include;

- Generation of cells that escape a cell-mediated immune response.
- Down regulation of MHC production in infected cells so that they are not recognized and destroyed by T cells.
- Infection of cells in immunoprivileged sites such as the brain.

The typical events that occurs after an acute virus infection is as follows;-

- Virus replicates in the lungs, reaches maximum titres in 4-5 days, and decreases thereafter. About 12 days virus can no longer be recovered.
- Effector Tc cell activity reaches a maximum activity after 6-8 days, becomes undetectable after 14 days. Tc memory cells reach their highest level 2-6 weeks after infection and remain constant or decrease only slowly.

- The number of Ab producing cells, producing first IgM then IgG and IgA peak at about 6 weeks and then steadily decline. Maximum B cell memory is found 10-15 weeks after infection but decreases thereafter but some are present at 18 months.

Both Ab-secreting and memory B cells are present after infection. In contrast Tc activity is generated only whilst infectious virus is present. Memory T cells persist but require further exposure to infectious virus for reactivation.

Requirements of a vaccine

To be effective a vaccine should be capable of eliciting the following:

- Activation of Antigen-Presenting Cells to initiate antigen processing and producing interleukins.
- Activation of both T and B cells to give a high yield of memory cells.
- Generation of Th and Tc cells to several epitopes, to overcome the variation in the immune response in the population due to MHC polymorphism.
- Persistence of antigen, probably on dendritic follicular cells in lymphoid tissue, where B memory cells are recruited to form antibody-secreting cells that will continue to produce antibody.

Live vaccines fulfill these criteria par excellence. Neutralizing antibodies are very important. Subunit vaccines induce poor immune responses and several doses with adjuvant are required to get an adequate response. The two main functions of the adjuvant antigen are to keep the antigen at or near the injection site and to activate antigen-presenting cells to achieve effective antigen processing and interleukin production. Vaccines composed simply of one T-cell epitope and one B-cell epitope is unlikely to be effective.

General Principles

The most successful immunization programs have been those directed against viral diseases such as smallpox, poliomyelitis and measles in humans & rinderpest in animals. Before embarking on any vaccination program, the need for a vaccine in a community must be evaluated. An epidemiological assessment of the incidence and severity of an infection will determine whether it is worth preventing. No vaccine is completely safe and potential benefits from immunization should be weighed against the risk of side effects. Two ingredients are needed for a successful immunization program.

1. A safe and effective vaccine
2. An appropriate strategy with adequate vaccine coverage

The strategy required depend on whether the aim of the program is **eradication, elimination or containment.** Eradication is the complete extinction of the organism in question. In elimination, the disease disappears but the organism remains. Containment is the control of the disease to the point at which it no longer constitutes a public health problem.

When eradication or elimination is the aim, mass immunization in early life of both sexes is usually necessary. In practice, it is very difficult to achieve 100% coverage and the success of the program depends on the ability of the vaccine to interrupt transmission of the wild virus, thereby protecting the unvaccinated. When containment is the aim, selective immunization of those most at risk is normally sufficient. The usual indications for selective immunization are travel, occupational risk, outbreak control and for individuals at special risk of severe illness. Herd immunity plays little part, as the virus continues to circulate widely among the unvaccinated. In theory, selective immunization is less expensive than mass immunization. In practice, it is not always easy to identify and vaccinate those most at risk and mass immunization may be an easier option.

Vaccination policy

- Varies between different countries
- Maternal antibodies are present up to 6 months after birth, which may interfere with the induction of an effective immune response against the vaccine by the infant. This should be duly taken into account when formulating a vaccination policy.

Different Types of Vaccines

Whole virus vaccines, either live or killed, constitute the vast majority of vaccines in use at present. However, recent advances in molecular biology had provided alternative methods for producing vaccines. Listed below are the possibilities;-

- Live whole virus vaccines
- Killed whole virus vaccines
- Subunit vaccines;- purified or recombinant viral antigen
- Recombinant virus vaccines
- Anti-idiotype antibodies
- DNA vaccines

Types of Vaccines

There are six basic types of vaccine in use today

Killed vaccines

These are preparations of the normal (wild type) infectious, pathogenic virus that has been rendered non-pathogenic, usually by chemical treatment such as with formalin or other chemicals that cross-links viral proteins. Most killed vaccines contain an adjuvant system, whose purpose is to stimulate an immune response. Without an adjuvant, the body is less likely to produce an effective response to the disease antigen.

Attenuated vaccines

These are live virus particles that grow in the vaccine recipient but do not cause disease because the vaccine virus has been altered (mutated) to a non-pathogenic form. Attenuation is usually achieved by passage of the virus in foreign host such as embryonated eggs or tissue culture cells. From among the many mutant viruses that exist in a population (especially so in RNA viruses), some will be selected that have a better ability to grow in the foreign host (higher virulence). These tend to be less virulent for the original host. To produce the Sabin polio vaccine, attenuation was only achieved with high inocula and rapid passage in primary monkey kidney cells. The virus population became overgrown with a less virulent strain (for humans) that could grow well in non-nervous (kidney) tissue but not in the central nervous system. Non-virulent strains of all three polio types have been produced for the vaccine. They activate all phases of immune system. They elicit humoral IgG and local IgA. They raise an immune response to all protective antigens. Inactivation, such as by formaldehyde in the case of the Salk vaccine, may alter antigenicity. They offer more durable immunity and are more cross-reactive. Thus, they stimulate antibodies against multiple epitopes which are similar to those elicited by the wild type virus. They cost less to produce. They give quick immunity in majority of vaccines. In the cases of polio and adenovirus vaccines, administration is easy. These vaccines are easily transported in the field. They can lead to elimination of wild type virus from the community.

Subunit vaccines

These are purified components of the virus, such as a surface antigen that induce protective immune response. Injected peptides which are much smaller than the original virus protein raise an IgG response but there is a problem with poor antigenicity. This is because the epitope may depend on the conformation of the virus as a whole.

Anti-idiotype vaccine

An antigen binding site in an antibody is a reflection of the three-dimensional structure of part of the antigen that is of a particular epitope. This unique amino acid structure in the antibody is known as the idiotype which can be thought of as a mirror of the epitope in the antigen. Antibodies (anti-idiotype) can be raised against the idiotype by injecting the antibody into another animal. This gives us an anti-idiotype antibody and this therefore mimics part of the three dimensional structure of the antigen, that is, the epitope. This can be used as a vaccine. When the anti-idiotype antibody is injected into a vaccinee, antibodies (anti-anti-idiotype antiobodies) are formed that recognize a structure similar to part of the virus and might potentially neutralize the virus. This happens: Anti-idiotype raised against antibodies to hepatitis B virus S antigen elicits anti-viral antibodies.

Recombinant DNA techniques

Virus proteins have been expressed in bacteria, yeast, mammalian cells, and viruses. E. Coli cells were first to be used for this purpose but the expressed proteins were not glycosylated, which was a major drawback since many of the immunogenic proteins of viruses such as the envelope glycoproteins, were glycosylated. Nevertheless, in many instances, it was demonstrated that the non-glycosylated protein backbone was just as immunogenic. Recombinant hepatitis B vaccine is the only recombinant vaccine licensed at present.

An alternative application of recombinant DNA technology is the production of hybrid virus vaccines. The best known example is vaccinia; the DNA sequence coding for the foreign gene is inserted into the plasmid vector along with a vaccinia virus promoter and vaccinia thymidine kinase sequences. The resultant recombination vector is then introduced into cells infected with vaccinia virus to generate a virus that expresses the foreign gene. The recombinant virus vaccine can then multiply in infected cells and produce the antigens of a wide range of viruses. The genes of several viruses can be inserted, so the potential exists for producing polyvalent live vaccines. HBsAg, rabies, HSV and other viruses have been expressed in vaccinia.

DNA vaccines

These are usually several harmless viruses into which a gene for a (supposedly) protective antigen has been spliced. The protective antigen is then made in the vaccine recipient to elicit an immune response.

These vaccines are based on the deliberate introduction of a DNA plasmid into the vaccinee. The plasmid carries a protein-coding gene that transfects cells *in vivo* at very low efficiency and expresses an antigen that causes an immune response. These are often called DNA vaccines but would better be called DNA-mediated or DNA-based immunization since it is not the purpose to raise antibodies against the DNA molecules themselves but to get the protein expressed by cells of the vaccinee. Usually, muscle cells do this since the plasmid is given intramuscularly. It should be noted that the plasmid does not replicate in the cells of the vaccinee, only protein is produced.

It has also been shown that DNA can be introduced into tissues by bombarding the skin with DNA-coated gold particles. It is possible to introduce DNA into nasal tissue in nose drops. In the case of the gold bombardment method, one nanogram of DNA coated on gold produced an immune response. One microgram of DNA could potentially introduce a thousand different genes into the vaccinee.

Whole Inactivated or Killed Viral Vaccines Details

Killed viral vaccines are generally more stable and do not pose the risk of reversion to virulence compared to live vaccines, but their inability to infect cells and activate cytotoxic T cells makes them much less protective. These were the easiest preparations to be used as vaccine. The virus preparation was simply inactivated. The outer virion coat should be left intact but the replicative function should be destroyed. To be effective, non-replicating virus vaccines must contain much more antigen than live vaccines that are able to replicate in the host. Preparation of killed vaccines may be inactivated by heat or chemicals. The chemicals used include formaldehyde or beta-propiolactone. The traditional agent for inactivation of the virus is formalin. Excessive treatment can destroy immunogenicity whereas insufficient treatment can leave infectious virus capable of causing disease. Soon after the introduction of inactivated polio vaccine, there was an outbreak of paralytic poliomyelitis in the USA due to the distribution of inadequately inactivated polio vaccine. This incidence led to a review of the formalin inactivation procedure and other inactivating agents are now available, such as Beta-propiolactone. Consequently, they generally require strong adjuvants and several injections to induce the required level of immunity and are usually effective in controlling only clinical signs rather than infection. Inactivated adjuvanted vaccines also pose a greater risk of causing **autoimmune diseases, allergic disorders, and vaccine injection site sarcomas.** Viral inactivation is commonly achieved through heat or chemicals (e.g., formaldehyde, thiomersal, ethylene oxide, and β-propriolactone). The higher production cost and need for adjuvants make these vaccines more expensive to manufacture. Inactivated viral vaccines for a wide range of viral diseases have been available for several decades and are still being developed for some recently emergent diseases. For example, a one-dose inactivated porcine circovirus type 2 (PCV2) vaccine has recently been licensed in the United States for the prevention of postweaning multisystemic wasting syndrome in pigs **(Table 6-2B)**. Much of the recent research in this area has concentrated on the development of improved adjuvanted formulations to overcome the effects of maternal antibodies on young animals.

Inactivated vaccines for several viral diseases need to be continuously adapted to contain the appropriate serotypes, as exemplified by equine influenza virus vaccines. Vaccines for equine influenza virus, mostly inactivated, have been available since the 1960s. The most important equine subtypes are H7N7 and H3N8, although H7N7 has not been detected for several decades and is no longer included in vaccines, at least in Europe and the United States. Conversely, vaccination against H3N8 has been less effective, possibly due to antigenic drift, and there are now considered to be two distinct lineages, European and United States, and vaccines therefore tend to contain both. Over the years, improvements have been attempted, and more potent adjuvants have been used. Several European vaccines now produce high antibody responses that last for up to 1 year. Until recently, equine influenza virus vaccines produced in the United States have been considered to be of limited efficacy and sometimes lacking the relevant H3N8 strains.

You are probably by now wondering, "If killed vaccines (inactivated or subunit) have all of the antigens needed in order to induce an immune protective response and they do not replicate in the animal and cause disease, why don't we just use killed vaccines all the time?" When we inject a killed (or subunit) vaccine into the body, it does not replicate. It just stays in one spot for the immune system to 'kill'. Without replication of the virus, the immune system does not get exposed to the massive amounts of antigen generated by live viruses when they replicate. This results in poorer humoral immunity (fewer memory B cells and smaller amounts of antibody that don't last in the body as long) and poorer cell mediated immunity (not as many memory T cells waiting by to target the next wild-type virus that comes along). The only way that the humoral and cell-mediated immunity can be improved is by:

1. Putting massive quantities of killed virus into each inactivated vaccine. This increases the amount of antigen available for the immune system to recognize, but increases the risk of allergic reactions and also local, inflammatory injection site reactions.
2. Adding adjuvants which are designed to increase the effectiveness of the immune response to that vaccine. These adjuvants are not all benign and, being highly immune-stimulatory, they can increase the risk of

allergic reactions, anaphylaxis, injection site reactions and even feline vaccination associated fibrosarcomas.

Killed vaccines - benefits

1. Unlikely to cause disease in immunocompromised or pregnant or newborn animals (though the response to vaccination in immunosuppressed individuals might be low).
2. Do not tend to cause the same relative immunosuppression and vulnerability to other diseases that the live vaccines do.
3. They store for longer periods.

What are the contraindications of killed virus vaccines?

Because killed virus vaccines do not invade and replicate within the cells of animals, they are unlikely to cause disease in immunosuppressed animals or pregnant animals or newborn animals (neonates) that failed to get their colostrum. In fact, many of the killed vaccines have, as part of their recommendations sheet, a statement saying that they are safe for use in animals which are pregnant or which have immunodeficiencies.

- The one major issue with the use of killed vaccines in immunocompromised animals is that, even though these vaccines might be safe to give to immunodeficient animals, if an animal has a poor immune system will it actually be able to respond to the vaccine in order to gain protective immunity? It is possible that vaccines given to immunosuppressed patients and FIV cats (ones which already have proven immunodeficiency and low T cell counts) may be doing very little.
- Other situations in which a killed vaccine might be ineffective (due to a poor immune response) include animals with a fever and animals with subnormal temperatures. Obviously, if these animals were also sick (already diseased), the vaccine might even be unsafe (contraindicated) to use.
- *Unwell animals*. When an animal is vaccinated, lots of white blood cells are consumed in fighting the vaccine 'infection'. These white cells (especially the non-antigen-specific 'soldier' cells) are thus not available for use elsewhere in the body, should another infection arise somewhere. If an animal is unwell or brewing an infection somewhere, then all of its immune cells will already be invested in battling the infection or trauma already afflicting the animal. If you then go and vaccinate this animal, cells will need to be diverted away from the site of disease to the vaccine

site. This loss of 'troops' from the site of disease could well result in the disease becoming worse since there are less cells available to fight it. (Note - this immune-suppressive effect of vaccination is nowhere near as much of an issue with killed vaccines as it is for live vaccines.).

- Sick animals with a fever.
- Sick animals with a subnormal / low temperature.
- Animals that have had previous allergic reactions to killed or subunit vaccines should not be given the same ones again.

Note: some killed vaccine labels indicate that they are unsafe to use in pregnant bitches (e.g. some of coronavirus vaccines, some of the leptospira vaccines). This contraindication is probably not due to the infectious organism (after all, it is dead), but some other component of the vaccine (e.g. an adjuvant chemical) that is unsafe for fetuses.

Conventional Live Attenuated Viral Vaccines Details

A live vaccine is vaccine containing whole, live viruses. These viruses are non-virulent strains of virus which are very closely related to the wild-type, disease-causing viruses that we are trying to protect our animals against. These viruses have many of the exact same antigens (proteins/sugars that the immune system must recognize as foreign to trigger an attack) present on their surface that the disease causing organisms do and, as a result, the antibodies and memory T and B cells created following the vaccination will be able to protect the animal against the dangerous viral organisms that bear those same surface antigens.

When these vaccine viruses are injected into the animal, they multiply within the cells and tissues of the animal, growing to large populations. They do multiply: greater numbers of viral particles mean that the immune system will be exposed to greater volumes of viral vaccine antigens. A greater immune response will be triggered to 'kill' off these millions of viral antigens and the end result will be higher levels of protective antibodies floating through the blood and greater numbers of memory T and B cells waiting to protect the body in the face of attack with a real, disease causing organism.

It is because of this greater immunoprotective response to the live vaccines, that live attenuated vaccines are preferred over killed-type vaccines for immunizing normal animals where possible. The avirulent viruses may not replicate as fast or they might not access cells as quickly as the wild-type viruses and, thus, they will not have had as much chance to cause severe disease by the time the immune system evoke immune responses (around 2 weeks for a naive immune system).

How do manufacturers make viruses non-harmful for the purposes of vaccination?

Scientists design these avirulent strains of virus for vaccines in many ways:

1. Selecting strains that preferentially grow in (have adapted to) the cells of animal species different to the one we are vaccinating (e.g. using viruses that like mouse cells more than dog cells) - i.e. they are less adapted to and thus less able to cause disease in the dog cells.
2. Storing the viruses for a long time (aged viruses are less adept at causing disease).
3. They can also now use fancy technologies such as putting parts of the DNA of the infectious-disease virus (the parts that code for the viral antigens that the immune system needs to recognize to protect the body against wild-type viruses) into the 'body' of a different species of avirulent live carrier virus such that, the antigens of the infectious disease virus will be produced (and exposed to the animal immune system) by the carrier virus when it replicates.
4. Use of a related virus from another animal - the earliest example was the use of cowpox to prevent smallpox. The origin of the vaccinia viruses used for production is uncertain.
5. Administration of pathogenic or partially attenuated virus by an unnatural route - the virulence of the virus is often reduced when administered by an unnatural route. This principle is used in the immunization of military recruits against adult respiratory distress syndrome using enterically coated live adenovirus type 4, 7 and 21.
6. Passage of the virus in an "unnatural host" or host cell - the major vaccines used in man and animals have all been derived this way. After repeated passages, the virus is administered to the natural host. The initial passages are made in healthy animals or in primary cell cultures. There are several examples of this approach: the 17D strain of yellow fever was developed by passage in mice and then in chick embryos. Polioviruses were passaged in monkey kidney cells and measles in chick embryo fibroblasts. Human diploid cells are now widely used such as the WI-38 and MRC-5. The molecular basis for host range mutation is now beginning to be understood.
7. Development of temperature sensitive mutants - this method may be used in conjunction with the above method.
8. Sometimes, just inoculating the animal with a live, semi-virulent virus in a site of the body that is different to the one the organism usually

favours for replication, can result in a protective immune response and minimal clinical side effects. For example, the feline respiratory viruses (feline herpes, feline calicivirus) preferentially infect the cells of the respiratory tract. When they infect these cells, they cause disease (cat-flu). If the viruses are placed in a vaccine and injected into the skin (a site they would not normally attack), the immune system will attack them and acquire immunity towards the wild-type, disease-causing cat-flu viruses, but the cat should not exhibit signs of disease towards the vaccine.

However, they can pose a risk of residual virulence and reversion to pathogenic wild types as well as provide a potential source of environmental contamination in few cases. Although modern regulatory processes require data to provide assurance on these issues, problems in the field can arise. This was highlighted during a program to control **porcine respiratory and reproductive syndrome (PRRS) in Denmark.** This disease first emerged in North America in the late 1980s and spread quickly in Europe in the early 1990s. The two main types of PRRS virus, European and North American, are only 55 to 80% identical at the nucleotide level and cause distinguishable serological responses. Following vaccination with the live, attenuated North American PRRS vaccine against the European PRRS virus type present in Denmark in 1996, the vaccine virus reverted and spread within vaccinated herds as well as from vaccinated to nonvaccinated herds, leaving both virus types in the Danish pig population.

What are the contraindications of live virus vaccines?

Because live virus vaccines do invade the cells of animals and replicate, it is possible for them to cause disease eventually, should the immune system not come along at some point to destroy them. After all, endless viral replication, even of avirulent strains of virus, will eventually prove harmful. As explained above, these viruses do cause cell damage during replication in the body, it is just that they do it so much slower and less effectively than the wild-type viruses do (consequently, the 1-2 week delay in immune response that occurs when a normal, but naive immune system first meets a live vaccine virus will not usually be a problem - the avirulent viruses should not get a chance to do a lot of damage in this period of time).

Live virus vaccines are considered unsafe in animals in which an immune system response is unlikely to be forthcoming or normal. These include:

- Animals with proven genetic immunodeficiencies (i.e. born without certain functional parts of the immune system).

- Animals with acquired immunodeficiencies - this includes animals on chemotherapy; cats with FIV (no T cells) and animals with bone marrow suppression and low white blood cell counts.
- *Unwell animals* : When an animal is vaccinated, lots of white blood cells are consumed in fighting the vaccine 'infection'. These white cells (especially the non-antigen-specific 'soldier' cells) are thus not available for use elsewhere in the body, should another infection arise somewhere. If an animal is unwell or brewing an infection somewhere, then all of its immune cells will already be invested in battling the infection or trauma already afflicting the animal. If you then go and vaccinate this animal, cells will need to be diverted away from the site of disease to the vaccine site. This loss of 'troops' from the site of disease could well result in the disease becoming worse due to there being less inflammatory cells available to fight it.
- Animals with a fever (some immune cells will not respond normally to an antigen in the presence of fever making vaccination, at best, ineffective and, at worst, harmful).
- Animals with a subnormal / low temperature.
- Newborn animals that did not get their colostrum. Although live vaccines are fine for use in animals over 4 weeks (which have a functional, though naive immune system) and newborn animals protected by their mother's colostrum, newborn animals (termed neonates) unprotected by maternal antibodies have a greatly reduced immune response (not much better than the late-stage fetus) and live vaccines may produce disease in them.

Animals that have had previous allergic reactions to live vaccines should not be given the same once again.

Because many of these viruses like to replicate in rapidly-dividing cells, they will tend to preferentially infect tissues where cells are dividing quickly. This includes the dividing cells of fetuses. Live vaccines have the potential to cause birth-defects, abortion and stillbirth and are contraindicated in pregnant bitches and queens.

Live vaccines - benefits

1. More amplified and longer lasting humoral and cell mediated immune responses - resulting in better, longer lasting immune protection.
2. More rapid induction of immunity.

3. Only a small amount of viral material needs to be injected because it replicates in the body. Less viral material means a reduced risk of allergic and injection site reactions.
4. New vaccines produced can achieve long-lasting antibody (12 months - 3 years) after only a single dose.
5. No adjuvants required, reducing the risks of allergic and injection site reactions.
6. Live vaccines can be produced that can be given by routes other than injection (e.g. intranasal vaccines). This means that vaccines can potentially be tailored to induce immunity in the areas of the body where immune protection will be most effective (e.g. immunity in respiratory system to protect against respiratory viruses.)
7. From a company viewpoint, they cost less to produce (this cheaper price might then, hopefully, be passed onto veterinarians and then pet owners).
8. Attenuated viral strains are also obtained by inducing random mutations and selecting for reduced virulence. As the live organism can still infect target cells, these vaccines can replicate and induce both cellular and humoral immunity and generally do not require an adjuvant to be effective. Live products also offer the advantage of ease of administration, potentially in drinking water, intranasally, intraocularly, etc. Live virus vaccines are prepared from attenuated strains that are almost or completely devoid of pathogenicity but are capable of inducing a protective immune response. They multiply in the human host and provide continuous antigenic stimulation over a period of time, Primary vaccine failures are uncommon and are usually the result of inadequate storage or administration. Another possibility is interference by related viruses as is suspected in the case of oral polio vaccine in developing countries.

Live vaccines - potential problems

1. Because the virus is alive, it has to be stored carefully or the virus can die and become ineffective.
2. Potential to cause disease in immunocompromised or pregnant animals.
3. Certain live vaccines can cause severe complications: e.g. live rabies vaccines can cause fatal neurological disease in some dogs and cats.
4. Vaccines that have not been produced properly and undergone adequate quality control may contain virulent organisms which could produce severe disease (this is very rare).

5. Some live vaccines, if given by the wrong route, can cause severe illness (e.g. injectable cat flu vaccine viruses that accidentally get inhaled by a cat will produce marked signs of cat-flu and intranasal Bordetella vaccine viruses that get injected can cause liver damage and death of the animal).
6. Live vaccines tend to 'take up the time' of a lot of the body's white blood cells, leaving fewer white blood cells available to fight other infections. This relative immunosuppression may leave the body less defended and thus more vulnerable to other diseases during the period of time that the vaccine is present. This is less of a problem with killed vaccines.
7. A lack of preservatives in these vaccines means that their shelf life might be shorter. As with the first vaccine for human smallpox, most live veterinary viral vaccines induce mild infections with live organisms derived from non target host.

Live vs Dead vaccines

Feature	Live	Dead
Dose	low	high
no. of doses	single	multiple
need for adjuvant	no	yes
Duration of immunity	many years	less
antibody response	IgG,	IgA, IgG
CMI	good	poor
Reversion to virulence	possible	not possible

Because live vaccines replicate inside host cells, bits of virus antigen are presented to the cell surface and recognized by cytotoxic cells.

Potential safety problems

Live vaccines

1. Under attenuation
2. Mutation leading to reversion to virulence
3. Preparation instability
4. Contaminating viruses in cultured cells
5. Heat labiality
6. Should not be given to immunocompromized or pregnant patients
7. Live vaccines of certain viruses can (i). induce reactivation, (ii) be oncogenic in nature
8. Different routes of administration of vaccines (e.g. intranasal vaccines).

Some of the live attenuated vaccines can be given by routes other than subcutaneous (under the skin) or intramuscular (into the muscles) injection. The use of alternative routes of administration is designed to

1. Improve the protective immune response of the animal by inducing protective immunity at the very places in the body that certain viruses and bacteria are likely to target (e.g. the respiratory viruses attack the respiratory tract: intranasal vaccines are great at inducing protective immunity in the respiratory tract).
2. Reduce the side effects of the vaccine by either slowing the rate of uptake of the antigens (e.g. intranasal vaccines are taken into the body more slowly than injectable vaccines, thus reducing the risk of allergic reaction) or by administering the vaccine viruses to an area of the body that they do not typically grow in (thus reducing the disease-causing effects of some of the strains of live vaccine viruses).
3. Improve the ease of administration (some animals don't mind intranasal or conjunctival vaccines as much as needles).

Intranasal Vaccines

Intranasal vaccines are the most common alternative route of vaccine administration encountered in veterinary practice. Intranasal vaccines are avirulent, live virus strains that are given up the nostrils of the animal using a special applicator. The vaccine virus coats the cells lining the upper respiratory tract (nasal passages, throat and trachea) and replicates in these cells. The immune cells present in the respiratory tract attack these viruses (and/or bacteria), inducing a protective immune response that tends to remain within or near the respiratory tract (e.g. protective antibodies actually get secreted onto the surface of the respiratory tract cells during this immune response to the vaccine).

When a wild-type, pathogenic, respiratory virus (e.g. kennel cough, cat-flu) comes along, it will usually access the body via the respiratory route (these organisms are usually inhaled by a potential 'host' when another, infected animal coughs: each cough contains millions of aerosolized infectious particles). If the animal has received an intranasal vaccine previously, the lining of its respiratory tract will be coated with protective antibodies and the regional, respiratory-system lymph nodes will contain hundreds of memory cells all primed to recognize the antigens contained on the invading respiratory viruses. As soon as the invading viruses and bacteria reach the respiratory tract, these antibodies and memory cells will react and kill them off, a response that will be so much quicker than that seen with an injectable vaccine because, with intranasal vaccination, the immune defenses produced are located in the same region as the invading pathogens. As a result, the invading viruses will not get the opportunity to damage many cells and clinical signs of disease should not occur or, if they do, they should be very mild.

Diseases for which intranasal vaccines are available: kennel cough (Bordetella, parainfluenza +/- the respiratory form of canine adenovirus).

- Cat flu (feline herpes virus, feline calicivirus, feline Bordetella).
- In the USA, Heska has brought out an intranasal vaccine that contains panleukopenia (a gut organism).
- In the USA, Canada and Europe, Pfizer has brought out an intranasal vaccine against feline coronavirus - a common virus that is a precursor to the development of the highly fatal disease, FIP.

Despite such drawbacks of live viral vaccines, or some killed vaccines have played a major role in successful viral disease control and eradication. For example, the virtual eradication of rinderpest virus from the globe is widely believed to have been critically dependent on the use of the "Plowright" vaccine. This is an attenuated vaccine produced from the Kabete O strain passaged 90 times in tissue culture. The vaccine virus was recently found to have attenuating mutations in most of its genes, none of which are sufficiently debilitating to induce strong pressure for reversion. Although there are examples of stable attenuations from a single point mutation in the polymerase gene, the high rate of spontaneous mutations of RNA viruses increases the risk for reversion to virulence. Safe live viral vaccines are therefore likely to require a number of attenuating mutations distributed throughout the genome. Live attenuated viral vaccines have played pivotal role in controlling viral infections in animals.

Table 6.2A : Companion animal viral vaccines

Product	Description
ECLIPSE 3	A modified live virus vaccine for immunization of cats, 9 weeks of age or older, against **feline rhinotracheitis, calicivirus, and panleukopenia viruses.**
ECLIPSE 3+ FELV	A combination vaccine consisting of a modified live virus vaccine to help prevent diseases caused by **feline rhinotracheitis, calici, and panleukopenia viruses and a tissue culture derived feline leukemia virus**, Subgroups A and B vaccine as an aid in the prevention of lymphoid tumors caused by, and diseases associated with, feline leukemia virus (FeLV) infection.

ECLIPSE 4	A modified live virus and chlamydia vaccine for immunization of cats and kittens against **feline rhinotracheitis, calici, panleukopenia viruses and chlamydia**.
ECLIPSE 4 + FELV	A combination vaccine consisting of a modified live virus and chlamydia vaccine for the vaccination of healthy cats as an aid in the prevention of disease caused by **feline rhinotracheitis, calici, and panleukopenia viruses and *Chlamydia psittaci* and a tissue culture derived feline leukemia virus**, Subgroups A and B vaccine as an aid in the prevention of lymphoid tumors caused by, and diseases associated with, feline leukemia virus (FeLV) infection.
FEVAXYN FELV	A tissue culture derived **feline leukemia virus**, Subgroups A and B vaccine. Used as an aid in the prevention of lymphoid tumors caused by, and diseases associated with, **feline leukemia virus (FeLV) infection.**
FVR C	A modified live virus vaccine for the vaccination of healthy cats 8 to 9 weeks of age or older as an aid in the prevention of disease caused by **feline rhinotracheitis and calici viruses.**
FVR C-P VACCINE	A combination modified live and killed virus **Feline Rhinotracheitis-Calici-Panleukopenia Vaccine vaccine**. For vaccination of healthy cats 8 to 9 weeks of age or older as an aid in the prevention of disease caused by **feline rhinotracheitis, feline calici and feline panleukopenia** viruses.
GALAXY CV	A killed virus vaccine containing **feline enteric coronavirus.** Recommended for the vaccination of healthy dogs as an aid in the prevention of disease caused by **canine coronavirus infection.**
GALAXY D	Modified live Canine Distemper virus vaccine. Contains **Onderstepoort-type Canine Distemper strain**. For the vaccination of healthy dogs 9 weeks and older.
GALAXY DA2PPV	A modified live virus vaccine for the vaccination of healthy dogs, 6 weeks of age and older, as an aid in the prevention of disease caused by **canine distemper virus, adenovirus type 1 (hepatitis) and adenovirus type 2 (respiratory disease), canine parainfluenza virus, and canine parvovirus.**
GALAXY DA2PPV+CV	A modified live virus vaccine for the vaccination of healthy dogs, 6 weeks of age and older, as an aid in the prevention of disease caused by **canine distemper virus, adenovirus type 1 (hepatitis), adenovirus type 2 (respiratory disease), canine parainfluenza virus, and canine parvovirus.**

GALAXY DA2PPVL	A modified live virus vaccine which is combined with inactivated *Leptospira canicola* and *L. icterohaemorrhagiae* bacterin for the vaccination of healthy dogs, 6 weeks of age or older, as an aid in the prevention of disease caused by **canine distemper virus, adenovirus type 1 (hepatitis), adenovirus type 2 (respiratory disease), canine parainfluenza virus, canine** parvovirus, and leptospirosis.
GALAXY DA2PPVL+CV	A combination vaccine of a modified live virus vaccine (to prevent **canine distemper, adenovirus type 2, hepatitis, parainfluenza, parvovirus) with inactivated *Leptospira canicola* and *Leptospira icterohaemorrhagiae*** bacterin (to prevent leptospirosis) and killed virus vaccine containing feline enteric coronavirus (to prevent canine coronavirus). For the vaccination of healthy dogs nine weeks of age or older.
GALAXY PV	A modified live virus vaccine containing a CPV Type 2b strain for the vaccination of healthy dogs, 6 weeks of age and older, as an aid in the prevention of disease caused by **canine parvovirus.**
INTRATRA-TRACC3/ADT	A modified live **Canine Adenovirus Type 2-Parainfluenza-*Bordetella Bronchiseptica* Vaccine.** For the vaccination of dogs **intranasally.**
NOBIVAC DHP	A live vaccine for the immunization of dogs against canine distemper (CDV), canine contagious hepatitis caused by **canine adenovirus type 1 (ICH), canine parvovirus disease (CPV) and respiratory disease caused by canine adenovirus type 2 (CAV2).**
NOBIVAC DHPPI	A live vaccine for the immunization of dogs against canine distemper (CDV), canine contagious hepatitis caused by **canine adenovirus type 1 (ICH), canine parvovirus disease (CPV) and respiratory disease caused by canine parainfluenza (CPi) and canine adenovirus type 2 (CAV2).**
NOBIVAC KC	A live intranasal vaccine for the immunization of dogs against ***Bordetella bronchiseptica* and Canine parainfluenza virus** for periods of increased risk to reduce clinical signs induced by *B. bronchiseptica* and Canine parainfluenza virus and to reduce shedding of Canine parainfluenza virus.
NOBIVAC PUPPY DP	A live vaccine for the active immunization of young puppies against **canine distemper and canine parvovirus disease.**
NOBIVAC RABIES	An inactivated vaccine for the immunization of **dogs, cats, cattle, sheep, goats, foxes, ferrets and horses**, and in principle all healthy mammals against **Rabies.**

NOBIVAC TRICAT	A live vaccine for the immunization of cats against **feline viral rhinotracheitis, feline calicivirus and feline panleucopenia viral infections.**
PANAGEN	A non-adjuvanted killed virus vaccine for the vaccination of healthy cats 8 to 9 weeks of age or older as an aid in the prevention of disease caused by **feline panleukopenia virus**.
RABDOMUM 1 VACCINE	A vaccine prepared from cell-culture grown, chemically-inactivated rabies virus. For the **annual vaccination of dogs and cats against rabies.**
RABDOMAN VACCINE	A vaccine prepared from cell-culture-grown, chemically-inactivated rabies virus for the vaccination of healthy **dogs, cats, cattle and sheep as an aid in the prevention of rabies.**

Table 6.2B : Veterinary viral vaccines marketed by Intervet, 2009

Product Intervet 2009	Description
AE+POX	A combination live virus vaccine against Avian Encephalomyelitis and Fowl Pox. For the vaccination of healthy chickens 10 weeks and older.
AVA-BRON-HN-63	A combination Newcastle disease and Infectious Bronchitis vaccine. Contains Newcastle La Sota strain and IB Massachusetts serotype. For the revaccination of healthy chickens 4 weeks of age or older previously vaccinated with mild ND and IB vaccines.
AVA-POX-CE	A live virus vaccine against Fowl Pox. For the vaccination of healthy chickens and turkeys between 8 and 18 weeks of age.
AVIMUNE-ARK	A live virus vaccine against Infectious Bronchitis. Contains IB Arkansas serotype. For the vaccination of healthy chickens one day of age or older.
BOVILIS BOVIPAST RSP BOVIGRIP	An inactivated vaccine containing BRSV (strain EV 908), PI-3-virus (strain SF-4 Reisinger) and *Mannheimia haemolytica*. Contains aluminium hydroxide and Quil A as adjuvants. For the immunization of cattle against the main respiratory disease pathogens.
BOVILIS BVD	An inactivated vaccine for the immunization of cattle against Bovine Viral Diarrhoea virus (BVDV). Also for use in pregnant cows and heifers to prevent infection of the foetus with BVDV. The vaccine contains cytopathogenic BVD virus strain C86 in an aluminium salts adjuvant.

BOVILIS IBR	A live freeze dried vaccine containing Bovine Herpesvirus type 1 strain INT 1 for the immunization of cattle against Infectious Bovine Rhinotracheitis.
BOVILIS IBR MARKER INAC	An inactivated marker vaccine against infections with Bovine Herpesvirus type 1 in cattle. Bovine Herpesvirus type 1 (BoHV-1) is the causative agent of Infectious Bovine Rhinotracheitis (IBR).
BOVILIS IBR MARKER LIVE	A live attenuated marker vaccine against infections with Bovine Herpesvirus type 1 in cattle. Bovine Herpesvirus type 1 (BoHV-1) is the causative agent of Infectious Bovine Rhinotracheitis (IBR).
BOVILIS LACTOVAC C	A multivalent inactivated vaccine containing antigens of rotavirus, coronavirus and *E.coli*. Aluminium hydroxide and Quil A are used as adjuvants. The vaccine is indicated for the immunization of pregnant cows and heifers to reduce the severity and duration of diarrhea caused by these infectious agents in neonatal calves.
BOVILIS QARAT	An inactivated vaccine for use in cattle as an aid in the control of respiratory disease caused by infectious bovine rhinotracheitis virus, bovine parainfluenza 3 virus, bovine viral diarrhea virus and bovine respiratory syncytial virus infections. The vaccine contains antigens in an aluminium salt adjuvant.
BOVILIS RHINOBRON	An inactivated marker vaccine containing BoHV-1 in an aluminium hydroxide adjuvant for the immunization of cattle against Infectious Bovine Rhinotracheitis.
BROILERBRON B1	A combination live virus vaccine prepared from a mild Connaught Massachusetts type Infectious Bronchitis virus and a B_1 strain Newcastle virus. For vaccination of healthy broilers or initial vaccination of healthy replacement chickens at one day of age or older to prevent IB and ND.
BROILERBRON N-ARK B1	A combination live virus vaccine against Newcastle disease and Infectious Bronchitis. Contains B_1 strain of Newcastle and IB strains Massachusetts and Arkansas. For vaccination of healthy broilers or initial vaccination of healthy replacement chickens one day of age or older.
BROILERBRON N-79	A combination live virus vaccine against Newcastle disease and Infectious Bronchitis. Contains B_1 and La Sota Newcastle strains and IB strain Massachusetts. For vaccination of healthy broilers or initial vaccination of healthy replacement chickens at 2 weeks of age or older.
BROILERBTRAKE-M	A modified live virus vaccine against Infectious Laryngotracheitis. For vaccination of healthy chickens 4 weeks of age or older.

BURSA-VAC 3	A live virus vaccine against Infectious Bursal Disease. Contains an intermediate classic IBD strain. For vaccination of healthy chickens at one day of age or older.
BURSA-VAC 51	A live virus vaccine containing a carefully selected strain of bursal disease virus grown in chicken embryos and combined with stabilizing agents. For vaccination of healthy chickens 2 weeks of age or older against Infectious Bursal Disease caused by standard and variant bursal disease viruses.
Circumvvennt R PCV	An inactivated vaccine containing a killed baculovirus vector carrying protective antigen against Porcine Circovirus 2 (PCV2) in Microsol Diluvac Forte® adjuvant. The vaccine is for the immunization of pigs against PCV2 infection.
DECTAV FMD DOE	An inactivated oil adjuvanted vaccine for the immunization of pigs, cattle, buffalo, sheep and goats against Foot and Mouth Disease (FMD). FMD strains included in the vaccine are dependent on the local situation where the vaccine is required.
ECLIPSE 3	A modified live virus vaccine for immunization of cats, 9 weeks of age or older, against feline rhinotracheitis, calici, and panleukopenia viruses.
ECLIPSE 3 +FELV	A combination vaccine consisting of a modified live virus vaccine to help prevent diseases caused by feline rhinotracheitis, calici, and panleukopenia viruses and a tissue culture derived feline leukemia virus, Subgroups A and B vaccine as an aid in the prevention of lymphoid tumors caused by, and diseases associated with, feline leukemia virus (FeLV) infection.
ECLIPSE 4	A modified live virus and chlamydia vaccine for immunization of cats and kittens against feline rhinotracheitis, calici, panleukopenia viruses and chlamydia.
ECLIPSE 4+FELV	A combination vaccine consisting of a modified live virus and chlamydia vaccine for the vaccination of healthy cats as an aid in the prevention of disease caused by feline rhinotracheitis, calici, and panleukopenia viruses and *Chlamydia psittaci* and a tissue culture derived feline leukemia virus, Subgroups A and B vaccine as an aid in the prevention of lymphoid tumors caused by, and diseases associated with, feline leukemia virus (FeLV) infection.
ENDFLUENCE-2	An inactivated vaccine containing type A Swine Influenza Viruses, subtypes H1N1 and H3N2. Microsol Diluvac Forte® is the adjuvant. The vaccine is for the prevention of swine Influenza infections caused by subtypes H1N1 and H3N2 in pigs.
ENTEROVAX	A modified live vaccine containing an avian reovirus (tenosynovitus biotype). For use in healthy chickens to aid in

the prevention of reovirus induced tenosynovitis (viral arthritis) by spray or drinking water administration.

EQUINE PREQUENZA An inactivated vaccine containing purified antigens of the hemaglutinin (HA) of both European and American type of Newmarket equine A/2 influenza virus in a saponin-based adjuvant. The vaccine is for the immunization of horses against equine influenza.

FELVAXYN FELV A tissue culture derived feline leukemia virus, Subgroups A and B vaccine. Used as an aid the prevention of lymphoid tumors caused by, and diseases associated with, feline leukemia virus (FeLV) infection.

FVR C A modified live virus vaccine for the vaccination of healthy cats 8 to 9 weeks of age or older as an aid in the prevention of disease caused by feline rhinotracheitis and calici viruses.

FVR C –P VACCINE A combination modified live and killed virus Feline Rhinotracheitis-Calici-Panleukopenia Vaccine vaccine. For vaccination of healthy cats 8 to 9 weeks of age or older as an aid in the prevention of disease caused by feline rhinotracheitis, feline calici and feline panleukopenia viruses.

GALAXY CV A killed virus vaccine containing feline enteric coronavirus. Recommended for the vaccination of healthy dogs as an aid in the prevention of disease caused by canine coronavirus infection.

GALAXY D Modified live Canine Distemper virus vaccine. Contains Onderstepoort-type Canine Distemper strain. For the vaccination of healthy dogs 9 weeks and older.

GALAXY DA2PPV A modified live virus vaccine for the vaccination of healthy dogs, 6 weeks of age and older, as an aid in the prevention of disease caused by canine distemper virus, adenovirus type 1 (hepatitis) and adenovirus type 2 (respiratory disease), canine parainfluenza virus, and canine parvovirus.

GALAXY DA2PPV + CV A modified live virus vaccine for the vaccination of healthy dogs, 6 weeks of age and older, as an aid in the prevention of disease caused by canine distemper virus, adenovirus type 1 (hepatitis), adenovirus type 2 (respiratory disease), canine parainfluenza virus, and canine parvovirus.

GALAXY DA2PPVL A modified live virus vaccine which is combined with inactivated *Leptospira canicola* and *L. icterohaemorrhagiae* bacterin for the vaccination of healthy dogs, 6 weeks of age or older, as an aid in the prevention of disease caused by canine distemper virus, adenovirus type 1 (hepatitis), adenovirus type 2 (respiratory disease), canine parainfluenza virus, canine parvovirus, and leptospirosis.

GALAXY DA2PPVL +CV	A combination vaccine of a modified live virus vaccine (to prevent canine distemper, adenovirus type 2, hepatitis, parainfluenza, parvovirus) with inactivated *Leptospira canicola* and *Leptospira icterohaemorrhagiae* bacterin (to prevent leptospirosis) and killed virus vaccine containing feline enteric coronavirus (to prevent canine coronavirus). For the vaccination of healthy dogs nine weeks of age or older.
GALAXY PV	A modified live virus vaccine containing a CPV Type 2b strain for the vaccination of healthy dogs, 6 weeks of age and older, as an aid in the prevention of disease caused by canine parvovirus.
GUARDDIAN SCOURS VACCINE	Bovine rotavirus-coronavirus vaccine, killed virus, *Clostridium perfringens* types C & D-*Escherichia coli* bacterin-toxoid. For use in healthy heifers and cows as an aid in the prevention of neonatal calf diarrhea and enterotoxemia.
INTRA-TRAC 3 ADT	A modified live Canine Adenovirus Type 2-Parainfluenza-*Bordetella Bronchiseptica* Vaccine. For the vaccination of dogs intranasally.
JENCINE 3	Modified live Bovine Rhinotracheitis-Virus Diarrhea-Parainfluenza$_3$ vaccine. For the vaccination of healthy cattle as an aid in the prevention of disease caused by infectious bovine rhinotracheitis (IBR), bovine virus diarrhea (BVD) type 1 and type 2 and bovine parainfluenza$_3$ (PI3).
JENCINE 4	Modified live virus vaccine for the vaccination of healthy cattle as an aid in the prevention of disease caused by infectious bovine rhinotracheitis (IBR), bovine virus diarrhea (BVD) type 1, bovine parainfluenza$_3$ (PI3), bovine respiratory syncytial virus (BRSV) and BVD type 2.
J JENCINE 4+ L5	Modified live virus and bacterin vaccine. For vaccination of healthy cattle as an aid in the prevention of disease caused by infectious bovine rhinotracheitis (IBR), bovine virus diarrhea (BVD) types 1 and 2, bovine parainfluenza$_3$ (PI3), and bovine respiratory syncytial virus (BRSV) and for protection against clinical disease caused by *L. canicola, L. grippotyphosa, L. hardjo, L. icterohaemorrhagiae*, and *L. pomona.*
LT-IVAX	A modified live virus vaccine against Fowl Laryngotracheitis. For use in chickens four weeks of age or older.
MAXIVAC EXCELL3	An inactivated virus vaccine for use in healthy pigs 5 weeks of age or older as an aid in the prevention of disease associated with swine influenza virus subtypes H1N1 and H3N2.
MAXIVAC PLATINUM	An inactivated virus vaccine indicated for use in healthy pigs 5 weeks of age or older as an aid in the prevention of pneumonia caused by *Mycoplasma hyopneumoniae* and in the reduction of disease due to swine influenza virus type A, H1N1 and H3N2.

NASALGEN IP	Modified live Bovine Rhinotracheitis-Parainfluenza$_3$ vaccine. For the vaccination of healthy cattle as an aid in the prevention of disease caused by infectious bovine rhinotracheitis and parainfluenza$_3$ virus.
NEWCASTLE CLONED N-79	A live virus Newcastle vaccine containing B_1 Type, clone-selected LaSota Strain. For revaccination of healthy chickens 2 weeks of age or older, and healthy turkeys 3 weeks of age or older, which have previously received mild Newcastle vaccination.
NEWCASTLE DISEASE VACCINE N-63	Live Newcastle virus vaccine containing B_1 Type, LaSota Strain. For revaccination of healthy chickens 2 weeks of age or older, which have previously received a mild Newcastle vaccination.
NOBILIS AE + POX	Live vaccine containing an Avian Encephalomyelitis virus strain and a Fowl Pox virus strain for the immunization of chickens against AE and Fowl Pox infection.
NOBILIS AE 1143	Live vaccine containing an Avian Encephalomyelitis virus strain. For immunization of chickens against Avian Encephalomyelitis infection.
NOBILIS CAV P4	Live attenuated vaccine for the immunization of chickens against Chicken Anaemia Virus infection.
NOBILIS COR4+IB+ ND+EDS	Inactivated vaccine for the immunization of chickens against Infectious Bronchitis, Newcastle Disease, Egg Drop Syndrome and Infectious Coryza (serotypes A, B, C and B variant). In a water-in-oil emulsion.
NOBILIS CORVAC	Trivalent inactivated vaccine for the immunization of chickens against Infectious Coryza infection (serotypes A, B and C). In a water-in-oil emulsion.
NOBILIS CORYZA	Trivalent inactivated vaccine for the immunization of chickens against Infectious Coryza infection (serotypes A, B and C). In an aluminium hydroxide gel.
NOBILIS DUCK PLAGUE	Live vaccine for the immunization of ducks against Duck Virus Entritis (Duck Plague).
NOBILIS EDS	Inactivated vaccine for the immunization of chickens against Egg Drop Syndrome '76 in a water-in-oil emulsion.
NOBILIS G + ND	Inactivated combined vaccine for the immunization of chickens against Gumboro Disease (Infectious Bursal Disease) and Newcastle Disease in a water-in-oil emulsion.
NOBILIS G + ND + EDS	Inactivated combined vaccine for the immunization of chickens against Gumboro Disease (Infectious Bursal Disease), Newcastle Disease and Egg Drop Syndrome '76 in a water-in-oil emulsion.

NOBILIS GUMBORO 228E	Live vaccine for the immunization of chickens against Infectious Bursal Disease (Gumboro).
NOBILIS GUMBORO BROILER	A live vaccine for the immunization of broilers and pullets and for the primary vaccination of future breeding stock against Infectious Bursal Disease. The vaccine contains Infectious Bursal Disease virus strain 228 TC.
NOBILIS GUMBORO D78	Live vaccine for the immunization of chickens against Infectious Bursal Disease (Gumboro).
NOBILIS GUMBORO INAC	Inactivated vaccine for the of chickens to protect offspring against Gumboro Disease (Infectious Bursal Disease) in a water-in-oil emulsion.
NOBILIS IB + G + ND	An inactivated combined vaccine for the immunization of breeding chickens against Infectious Bronchitis (serotype Massachusetts), Gumboro Disease (Infectious Bursal Disease) and Newcastle Disease to convey passive immunity to offspring. The active components are IB strain M41, Gumboro strain D78 and ND Clone 30 in a water-in-oil emulsion.
NOBILIS IB + ND	inactivated combined vaccine for the immunization of chickens against Infectious Bronchitis (serotype Massachusetts) and Newcastle Disease in a water-in-oil emulsion.
NOBILIS IB + ND - EDS	Inactivated combined vaccine for the immunization of chickens against Infectious Bronchitis (serotype Massachusetts and D207/strain D274 and related strains), Newcastle Disease and Egg Drop Syndrome '76 in a water-in-oil emulsion.
NOBILIS IB 4/91	Live vaccine for the immunization of chickens against Infectious Bronchitis.
NOBILIS IB D274	A live vaccine for the immunization of future layer and breeder chickens against Infectious Bronchitis serotype D207.
NOBILIS IB H120	Live vaccine for the immunization of chickens against Infectious Bronchitis.
NOBILIS IB MA5	Live vaccine for the immunization of chickens against against Infectious Bronchitis serotype Massachusetts.
NOBILIS IB MULTI + G + ND	Inactivated combined vaccine for the immunization of chickens against Infectious Bronchitis (serotype Massachusetts and D207/ strain D274 and related strains), Gumboro Disease (Infectious Bursal Disease) and Newcastle Disease in a water-in-oil emulsion.
NOBILIS IB MULTI + ND	Inactivated combined vaccine for the immunization of chickens against Infectious Bronchitis (serotypes Massachusetts and

	D207/ strain D274 and related strains) and Newcastle Disease in a water-in-oil emulsion.
NOBILIS IB MULTI + ND + EDS	Inactivated combined vaccine for the chickens against Infectious Bronchitis (serotype Massachusetts and D207/ strain D274 and related strains), Newcastle Disease and Egg Drop Syndrome '76 in a water-in-oil emulsion.
NOBILIS IB3 + G + ND	Inactivated combined vaccine for the immunization of chickens against Infectious Bronchitis (serotype Massachusetts, D207/ strain D274, D212/ stain D1466 and related strains), Gumboro Disease (Infectious Bursal Disease) and Newcastle Disease in a water-in-oil emulsion.
NOBILIS IB3 + ND	Inactivated combined vaccine for the immunization chickens against Infectious Bronchitis (serotype Massachusetts, D207/ strain D274, D212/ strain D1466 and related strains) and Newcastle Disease in a water-in-oil emulsion.
NOBILIS ILT	Live vaccine for the immunization of chickens against Infectious Laryngotracheitis.
NOBILIS INFLUENZA H5N2	Inactivated vaccine for the immunization of chickens against Avian Influenza virus type A, subtype H5 in a water in oil emulsion.
NOBILIS INFLUENZA H9N2	Inactivated vaccine for the immunization of chickens against Avian Influenza virus type A, subtype H9 in a water in oil emulsion.
NOBILIS MA5 + CLONE 30	A live vaccine for the immunization of chickens against Infectious Bronchitis serotype Massachusetts (strain Ma5) and Newcastle Disease (strain Clone 30). Active components are IB strain Ma5 and ND strain Clone 30.
NOBILIS MA5 + HITCHNER	Live vaccine for the immunization of chickens against Infectious Bronchitis and Newcastle Disease.
NOBILIS MAREK THV LYO	Live freeze dried vaccine for the immunization of chickens against Marek's Disease based on the Turkey Herpes Virus (THV).
NOBILIS MAREXINE CA126	Live vaccine for the immunization of chickens against Marek's Disease, vaccine based on the Turkey Herpes Virus (THV).
NOBILIS MAREXINE CA126 + SB1	Live vaccine for the immunization of chickens against Marek's Disease, based on the Turkey Herpes Virus and SB1 strain.
NOBILIS ND + EDS	Inactivated combined vaccine for the immunization of breeder chickens against Newcastle Disease and Egg Drop Syndrome '76 in a water-in-oil emulsion.

NOBILIS ND BROILER	Inactivated vaccine for the immunization of day-old chicks against Newcastle Disease in a water-in-oil emulsion.
NOBILIS ND C2	Live vaccine for the immunization of chickens against Newcastle Disease.
NOBILIS ND CLONE 30	A live vaccine for the immunization of chickens against Newcastle Disease.
NOBILIS ND HITCHNER	Live vaccine for immunization of chickens against Newcastle Disease.
NOBILIS ND LASOTA	Live vaccine for the immunization of chickens against Newcastle Disease.
NOBILIS NEWCAVAC	Inactivated vaccine for the immunization of chickens against Newcastle Disease in a water-in-oil emulsion.
NOBILIS OVO-DIPHTHERIN	Live vaccine for immunization of chickens against Fowl Pox.
NOBILIS PARAMYXO P201	Inactivated vaccine for the immunization of pigeons against Paramyxovirus Disease in a water-in-oil emulsion.
NOBILIS REO + IB + G + ND	Combined inactivated vaccine for the immunization against Avian Reovirus infections, Infectious Bronchitis (Massachusetts type), Infectious Bursal Disease and Newcastle Disease in chickens in a water-in-oil emulsion.
NOBILIS REO 1133	Live vaccine for the immunization of chickens against Reovirus infections.
NOBILIS REO 2177	Live vaccine for the immunization of chickens against Reovirus infectios, which can be given simultaneously with Marek's vaccines.
NOBILIS REO INAC	Inactivated vaccine for the immunization of breeding stock chickens against Avian Reovirus to protect their offspring in a water-in-oil emulsion.
NOBILIS RHINO CV	Live vaccine for the immunization of chickens against Avian Rhinotracheitis caused by Avian Pneumovirus infections.
NOBILIS RISMAVAC	Live vaccine for the vaccination of chickens against very virulent Marek Disease challenge.
NOBILIS RISMAVAC + CA126	Live vaccine for the immunization of chickens against very virulent Marek Disease challenge, containing both Turkey Herpes Virus strain and the Rispens strain.
NOBILIS RT + IB MULTI + G + ND	Combined inactivated vaccine for the immunization of breeder and layer chickens against Infectious Bronchitis (serotype Massachusetts and D207 (strain D274 and related strains) and

	against Newcastle Disease, Infectious Bursal Disease and Avian Pneumovirus in a water-in-oil emulsion.
NOBILIS RT + ND	Combined inactivated vaccine for the immunization of breeder and layer chickens against Newcastle Disease and Avian Pneumovirus in a water-in-oil emulsion.
NOBILIS RT INAC	Inactivated vaccine for the immunization of layer chickens against Avian Pneumovirus virus infection in a water-in-oil emulsion.
NOBILIS RT+IBMULTI +ND+EDS	Combined inactivated vaccine for the vaccination of breeder and layer chickens against Avian Pneumovirus, Infectious Bronchitis (serotype Massachusetts and D207 (strain D274 and related strains), Newcastle Disease and Egg Drop Syndrome in a water-in-oil emulsion.
NOBILIS RTV 8544	Live vaccine for the immunization of chickens against Avian Rhinotracheitis caused by Avian Pneumovirus infections.
NOBILIS TRT	Live vaccine for the immunization of turkeys against Turkey Rhinotracheitis caused by an Avian Pneumovirus.
NOBILIS TRT + ND	A combined inactivated vaccine for the immunization of turkeys against Newcastle Disease and Turkey Rhinotracheitis (caused by Avian Metapneumovirus) in a water-in-oil emulsion.
NOBILIS TRT INAC	Inactivated vaccine for the vaccination of chickens against Avian Influenza virus type A, subtype H5 in a water in oil emulsion to enhance immunity.
NOBIVAC DHP	A live vaccine for the immunization of dogs against canine distemper (CDV), canine contagious hepatitis caused by canine adenovirus type 1 (ICH), canine parvovirus disease (CPV) and respiratory disease caused by canine adenovirus type 2 (CAV2).
NOBIVAC DHPPI	A live vaccine for the immunization of dogs against canine distemper (CDV), canine contagious hepatitis caused by canine adenovirus type 1 (ICH), canine parvovirus disease (CPV) and respiratory disease caused by canine parainfluenza (CPi) and canine adenovirus type 2 (CAV2).
NOBIVAC KC	A live intranasal vaccine for the immunization of dogs against *Bordetella bronchiseptica* and Canine parainfluenza virus for periods of increased risk to reduce clinical signs induced by *B. bronchiseptica* and Canine parainfluenza virus and to reduce shedding of Canine parainfluenza virus.
NOBIVAC PUPPY DP	A live vaccine for the active immunization of young puppies against canine distemper and canine parvovirus disease.

NOBIVAC RABIES	An inactivated vaccine for theimmunization of dogs, cats, cattle, sheep, goats, foxes, ferrets and horses, and in principle all healthy mammals against Rabies.
NOBIVAC TRICAT	A live vaccine for the immunization of cats against feline viral rhinotracheitis, feline calicivirus and feline panleucopenia viral infections.
ORALVAX HE	A live virus vaccine containing a turkey avirulent Type II avian adenovirus of pheasant origin recommended for use in healthy turkeys 6 weeks of age or older as an aid in the prevention of hemorrhagic enteritis through vaccination by the drinking water method.
PANAGEN	A non-adjuvanted killed virus vaccine for the vaccination of healthy cats 8 to 9 weeks of age or older as an aid in the prevention of disease caused by feline panleukopenia virus.
PIGEON	A live virus vaccine prepared from a strain of Pigeon Pox Virus. For the vaccination of healthy broilers and roasters by the wing web method at four weeks of age against Fowl Pox.
PORCILIS AD BEGONIA	A live attenuated vaccine for the immunization of pigs against Aujeszky's disease virus infections (Pseudorabies). The vaccine based on the virus strain NIA-3(tk- and gE-). Diluvac Forte® is used as a diluent. The gE deletion allows field infections to be differentiated from vaccination responses.
PORCILIS CSF LIVE	A live vaccine for the immunization of pigs of pigs as an aid in protection against Hog Cholera (classical swine fever). The vaccine contains live attenuated classical swine fever virus strain GPE-.
PORCILIS ERY & PARVO	An inactivated combination vaccine containing inactivated Porcine Parvo virus strain 014 and an inactivated lysate of *E. rhusiopathiae*, strain M2 (serotype 2), dissolved in Diluvac Forte as adjuvant. For the immunization of sows and gilts, as an aid to the control of swine erysipelas and for the protection of embryos and foetuses against PPV infection.
PORCILIS PARVO	An inactivated vaccine for the immunization of sows and gilts for the protection of embryos and foetuses against Porcine Parvo Virus infection. The vaccine contains inactivated PPV strain 014. The active component is dissolved in Diluvac Forte®.
PORCILIS PESTI	An inactivated water-in-oil emulsion marker vaccine for the immunization of pigs to priotect against Classical Swine Fever. The vaccine contains the CSFV-E2 antigen. The corresponding test kit makes it possible to differentiate between marker vaccine vaccinated and infected animals.

PORCILIS PRRS	A live vaccine for the immunization of pigs against Porcine Reproductive and Respiratory Syndrome. The vaccine contains PRRS virus strain DV dissolved in Diluvac Forte.
Porcilis® PCV	An inactivated vaccine containing a killed baculovirus vector carrying protective antigen against Porcine Circovirus 2 (PCV2) in Microsol Diluvac Forte® adjuvant. The vaccine is for the immunization of pigs against PCV2 infection.
PREVENILE	A vaccine to prevent viremia and aid in the prevention of disease and encephalitis caused by West Nile Virus infection in horses.
PROSYSTEM RCE	A live vaccine for the vaccination of pregnant sows and gilts as an aid in the prevention of rotaviral diarrhea, enterotoxemia and colibacillosis in nursing piglets. Contains two major Rotavirus serotypes, four major *E. coli* pilus antigens (K88, K99, F41 and 987P) and *C. perfringens* type C toxoid.
PROSYSTEM TREC	A live vaccine for the vaccination of pregnant sows and gilts as an aid in the prevention of rotaviral diarrhea, TGE enterotoxemia and colibacillos infections in nursing piglets. Contains TGE, two major Rotavirus serotypes, four major E. coli plus antigens and C. perfringens type C toxoid.
PRV/MARKER GOLD	Modified live virus pseudorabies vaccine. For the immunization of healthy pigs 3 days of age or older as an aid in the prevention of disease caused by pseudorabies virus, including the respiratory form of the disease.
RABDOMUN 1 VACCINE	A vaccine prepared from cell-culture grown, chemically-inactivated rabies virus. For the annual vaccination of dogs and cats against rabies.
RABDOMUN VACCINE	A vaccine prepared from cell-culture-grown, chemically-inactivated rabies virus for the vaccination of healthy dogs, cats, cattle and sheep as an aid in the prevention of rabies.
RABDOMUN VACCINE FOR CATTLE	Inactivated rabies vaccine for the prevention of rabies in cattle.
SHOR-BRON-D	Modified live Infectious Bronchitis virus vaccine. Contains IB strain Delaware Type, 072 Strain. For vaccination of healthy chickens 2 weeks of age or older.
TENO-VAXIN	Live tenosynovitis vaccine containing reovirus strain S-1133. For vaccination of healthy chickens 10 to 17 weeks of age as an aid in control and prevention of reovirus-induced tenosynovitis (viral arthritis) in broiler breeders.
TRACHIVAX	Modified live Fowl Laryngotracheitis Vaccine. For vaccination and revaccination of chickens by eyedrop method.

UNIVAX PLUS	Live Bursal Disease vaccine. Contains two strains of Bursal Disease virus. For the vaccination of chickens one day of age by subcutaneous route of administration or by drinking water at 2 weeks or older.
UNIVAX-BD	Live Infectious Bursal Disease vaccine. For use in 18 to 19 day old embryonated chicken eggs or chickens at 1 day of age by subcutaneous route of administration and by drinking water at 1 week or older.
VISTA 3 SQ	A live vaccine for the immunization of non-pregnant cattle, 3 months of age or older, as an aid in the control of diseases caused by infectious bovine rhinotracheitis (IBR) virus and bovine virus diarrhea (BVD) virus (Types 1 and 2).
VISTA 5 L5 SQ	A live vaccine for cattle containing modified-live cultures of bovine rhinotracheitis (IBR) virus; bovine virus diarrhea (BVD) virus (Types 1 and 2); parainfluenza$_3$ virus (PI$_3$) and bovine respiratory syncytial virus (BRSV) and inactivated cultures of *Leptospira canicola, L. grippotyphosa, L. hardjo, L. icterohaemorrhagiae*, and *L. Pomona*.
VISTA 5 SQ	A modified-live vaccine for the immunization of non-pregnant cattle at the age of 3 months and older to prevent diseases caused by infection with bovine rhinotracheitis (IBR) virus and bovine virus diarrhea (BVD) virus (Types 1 and 2); bovine parainfluenza 3 virus (PI-3) and bovine respiratory syncytial virus (BRSV).
VISTA IBR SQ	A live vaccine for the immunization of non-pregnant cattle, 3 months of age or older, as an aid in the prevention of disease caused by infectious bovine rhinotracheitis (IBR) virus. The vaccine contains modified-live cultures of bovine rhinotracheitis (IBR) virus in a freeze dried form.
VISTA ONCE SQ	A modified live vaccine for the immunization of cattle, 3 months of age or older, as an aid in the control of disease caused by infectious bovine rhinotracheitis (IBR) virus and bovine virus diarrhea (BVD) virus (Types 1 and 2); parainfluenza3 virus (PI3) and bovine respiratory syncytial virus (BRSV) and as an aid in the control of respiratory disease caused by *Mannheimia haemolytica* and *Pasteurella multocida*.

Table 6.2C : Veterinary viral vaccines marketed by Pfizer, Animal Health, USA 2009

Scientific Name	Trade name	Date licensed
Bovine Respiratory Syncytial Virus Vaccine, Modified Live Virus.	Bovi-Shield BRSV	Prior to 2000
Bovine Rhinotracheitis-Virus Diarrhea-Parainfluenza 3-Respiratory Syncytial Virus Vaccine, Modified Live Virus.	Bovi-Shield Gold FP 5	2006-12-18
Bovine Rhinotracheitis-Virus Diarrhea-Parainfluenza 3-Respiratory Syncytial Virus Vaccine, Modified Live Virus, Leptospira Canicola, Grippotyphosa, Hardjo, Icterohaemorrhagiae, Pomona Bacterin.	Bovi-Shield Gold FP 5 L5	2005-05-17
Bovine Rhinotracheitis-Virus Diarrhea-Parainfluenza 3-Respiratory Syncytial Virus Vaccine, Modified Live & Killed Virus, Leptospira Canicola-Grippotyphosa-Hardjo-Icterohaemorrhagiae-Pomona Bacterin.	Cattlemaster 4 + L5	Prior to 2000
Bovine Rhinotracheitis-Virus Diarrhea-Parainfluenza 3-Respiratory Syncytial Virus Vaccine, Modified Live & Killed Virus.	Cattlemaster Gold FP 5	2006-05-30
Bovine Rhinotracheitis-Virus Diarrhea-Parainfluenza 3-Respiratory Syncytial Virus Vaccine, Modified Live & Killed Virus, Campylobacter Fetus-Leptospira Canicola-Grippotyphosa-Hardjo-Icterohaemorrhagiae-Pomona Bacterin.	Cattlemaster 4 + VL5	Prior to 2000
Bovine Rhinotracheitis-Virus Diarrhea-Parainfluenza 3-Respiratory Syncytial Virus Vaccine, Modified Live Virus.	Bovi-Shield Gold FP 5	2011-08-15
Bovine Rhinotracheitis-Virus Diarrhea-Parainfluenza 3-Respiratory Syncytial Virus Vaccine, Modified Live Virus, Haemophilus Somnus Bacterin.	Resvac 4 Somubac	1990-11-08
Bovine Rhinotracheitis-Virus Diarrhea-Parainfluenza 3-Respiratory Syncytial Virus Vaccine, Modified Live Virus.	Bovi-Shield Gold 5	2010-12-02
Bovine Rhinotracheitis-Virus Diarrhea-Parainfluenza 3-Vaccine, Modified Live Virus.	Bovi-Shield Gold 4	2010-12-02
Bovine Rhinotracheitis-Parainfluenza 3-Vaccine, Modified Live Virus.	TSV 2	Prior to 2000
Bovine Rhinotracheitis-Parainfluenza 3-Vaccine, Modified Live Virus.	Bovi-Shield IBR-PI3	Prior to 2000
Bovine Rhinotracheitis-Parainfluenza 3-Respiratory Syncytial Virus Vaccine, Modified Live Virus.	INFORCE 3	2011-07-11

Bovine Rhinotracheitis-Virus Diarrhea-Parainfluenza 3-Respiratory Syncytial Virus Vaccine, Modified Live & Killed Virus, Leptospira Canicola-Grippotyphosa-Hardjo-Icterohaemorrhagiae-Pomona Bacterin.	Cattlemaster Gold FP 5 L5	2008-04-03
Bovine Rhinotracheitis-Virus Diarrhea-Parainfluenza 3-Respiratory Syncytial Virus Vaccine, Modified Live Virus, Campylobacter Fetus-Leptospira Canicola-Grippotyphosa-Hardjo-Icterohaemorrhagiae-Pomona Bacterin.	Bovi-Shield Gold FP 5 VL5	2004-12-17
Bovine Rota-Coronavirus Vaccine, Killed Virus, Clostridium Perfringens Type C-Escherichia Coli Bacterin-Toxoid.	ScourGuard 4KC	2008-01-17
Bovine Rotavirus-Coronavirus Vaccine, Modified Live Virus.	Calf-Guard	1986-12-31
Canine Coronavirus Vaccine, Killed Virus Firstdose CV	Firstdose	1989-06-28
Canine Distemper-Adenovirus Type 2-Parainfluenza-Parvovirus Vaccine, Modified Live Virus.	Vanguard Plus 5	Prior to 2000
Canine Distemper-Adenovirus Type 2-Coronavirus-Parainfluenza-Parvovirus Vaccine, Modified Live and Killed Virus, Leptospira Canicola-Grippotyphosa-Icterohaemorrhagiae-Pomona Bacterin. For dogs 6 weeks of age or older. Give 1 ml IM or SQ. Give 3 doses, each 3 weeks apart. If primary vaccination is given after 9 weeks of age, give 2 doses, 3 weeks apart. Annual revaccination with a single dose is recommended. Not for pregnant bitches. Requires mixing. Order syringes separately.	Vanguard Plus 5 L4 CV	2007-05-17
Canine Distemper-Adenovirus Type 2-Parainfluenza-Parvovirus Vaccine, Modified Live Virus, Leptospira Canicola-Grippotyphosa-Icterohaemorrhagiae-Pomona Bacterial Extract.	Vanguard Plus 5 L4	2007-05-17
Canine Distemper-Adenovirus Type 2-Parainfluenza Vaccine, Modified Live Virus.	Vanguard DAP or DA2P	Prior to 2000
Canine Distemper-Adenovirus Type 2-Coronavirus-Parainfluenza-Parvovirus Vaccine, Modified Live & Killed Virus.	Vanguard Plus 5/CV	1998-05-01
Feline Leukemia Vaccine, Killed Virus.	Leukocell 2	Prior to 2000
Feline Panleukopenia Vaccine, Modified Live Virus.	Felocell FPV	2002-11-20
Feline Rhinotracheitis-Calici-Panleukopenia-Chlamydia . Psittaci Vaccine, Modified Live Virus and Chlamydia.	Felocell 4 or Felocell CVR-C	1987-03-27
Feline Rhinotracheitis-Calici Vaccine, Modified Live Virus.	Felocell FVR C (IN) or Felomune CVR	1985-12-31

Feline Rhinotracheitis-Calici-Panleukopenia Vaccine, Modified Live Virus.	Felocell 3 or Felocell CVR	1989-12-31
Feline Rhinotracheitis-Calici Vaccine, Modified Live Virus.	Felocell FVR/FCV	2002-11-19
Parvovirus-Swine Influenza Vaccine, H1N1 and H3N2, Killed Virus Erysipelothrix Rhusiopathiae-Leptospira Bratislava-Canicola-Grippotyphosa-Hardjo-Icterohaemorrhagiae-Pomona Bacterin.	Flusure XP/Farrowsure GOLD B	2010-11-02
Parvovirus Vaccine, Killed Virus, Erysipelothrix Rhusiopathiae-Leptospira Bratislava-Canicola-Grippotyphosa-Hardjo-Icterohaemorrhagiae-Pomona Bacterin.	Farrowsure GOLD B	2009-03-24
Parvovirus Vaccine, Killed Virus.	Parvo-Vac	Prior to 2000
Parvovirus Vaccine, Killed Virus, Erysipelothrix Rhusiopathiae-Leptospira Bratislava-Canicola-Grippotyphosa-Hardjo-Icterohaemorrhagiae-Pomona Bacterin.	Farrowsure B	Prior to 2000
Porcine Circovirus Vaccine Type 1-Type 2 Chimera, Killed Virus.	Fostera PCV	2011-08-10
Swine Influenza Vaccine, H1N1 & H3N2, Killed Virus.	Flusure XP	2008-12-05
Swine Influenza Vaccine, H1N1 & H3N2, Killed Virus, Mycoplasma Hyopneumoniae Bacterin.	Flusure XP/Respisure	2010-08-06
Swine Influenza Vaccine, pH1N1, Killed Virus.	Flusure Pandemic	2011-01-13
Rabies Vaccine, Killed Virus Target Group: Dogs, cats, sheep, cattle.	Defensor 3	1993-08-12
Rabies Vaccine, Killed Virus Target Group: Dogs, cats.	Defensor 1	1993-05-12
Avian Encephalomyelitis-Fowl Pox Vaccine, Live Virus.	AE Pox Vac	Prior to 2000
Avian Encephalomyelitis Vaccine, Live Virus.	AE Vac	Prior to 2000
Bursal Disease Vaccine, Live Virus.	Bursine 2	do
Bursal Disease-Reovirus Vaccine, Standard & Variant, Killed Virus.	Poulvac Maternavac IBD-Reo	2008-09-23
Fowl Laryngotracheitis Vaccine, Modified Live Virus.	Laryngo Vac	Prior to 2000
Newcastle-Bronchitis Vaccine, B1 Type, Lasota Strain, Mass. Type, Live Virus.	LS Mass II	Prior to 2000

Table 6.2D : Equine veterinary viral vaccines marketed by Merial

MERIAL Equine Vaccines - vaccines that fight against dangerous equine diseases, including

RECOMBITEK EQUINE WEST Nile Virus Vaccine. Horses exposed to the West Nile Virus can develop devastating neurological symptoms and risk death in severe cases. The virus continues to be unpredictable in its location, having spread throughout the United States since 1999. RECOMBITEK® Equine West Nile Virus (WNV) vaccine was proven 100% effective in preventing viremia after the primary vaccination course in a clinical trial, can be used to booster previously vaccinated horses with a single dose and lasts throughout the entire mosquito season. Available only through your veterinarian.

Equine POTOMAVAC® + IMRAB® is a combination vaccine that provides powerful protection against two potentially fatal diseases in horses: Potomac horse fever and rabies. Equine POTOMAVAC + IMRAB can be administered to healthy horses and foals 3 months of age and older. After the primary vaccination and booster, annual revaccination is needed.

MERIAL® IMRAB® Bovine Plus: Horses are at risk of becoming infected with the rabies virus because they are often kept in environments that overlap with wildlife habitat. When a horse contracts rabies, the results are devastating. MERIAL® IMRAB® Bovine Plus can be administered to **healthy horses and foals 3 months of age and older**. Horses should be revaccinated annually.

IMRAB® the world's leading rabies vaccine, offers rapid protection from rabies. Because equine housing tends to overlap with wildlife, horses are at risk of contracting rabies. When that occurs, the results can be devastating. Talk to your veterinarian about rabies vaccination for your **horses**.

Table 6.2E : Equine veterinary viral vaccines marketed by Merial

PreveNile® WEST NILE VIRUS VACCINE LIVE FLAVIVIRUS CHIMERA For the vaccination of healthy horses to prevent viremia and as as an aid in the prevention of disease and encephalitis caused by West Nile virus infection.	**Flu Avert® I.N. vaccine.** EQUINE INFLUENZA VACCINE Modified Live Virus - For Intranasal Use Only For the vaccination of healthy horses, 11 months of age or older, as an aid in the reduction of clinical disease and viral shedding caused by equine influenza viruses of both the American and Eurasian lineages.
Encevac® with Havlogen®* ENCEPHALOMYELITIS VACCINE EASTERN AND WESTERN, KILLED VIRUS For vaccination of healthy horses against Eastern and Western Equine Encephalomyelitis.	**Encevac®-T with Havlogen®*** ENCEPHALOMYELITIS VACCINE EASTERN AND WESTERN, KILLED VIRUS TETANUS TOXOID For vaccination of healthy horses, 6 months of age or older, against Eastern and

Western Equine Encephalomyelitis and Tetanus.

Encevac® T+VEE with Havlogen®*
ENCEPHALOMYELITIS VACCINE EASTERN, WESTERN AND VENEZUELAN, KILLED VIRUS TETANUS TOXOID
For vaccination of healthy horses, 6 months of age or older, against Eastern, Western and Venezuelan Equine Encephalomyelitis and Tetanus.

Prestige® II with Havlogen®*
EQUINE RHINOPNEUMONITIS - INFLUENZA VACCINE KILLED VIRUS
For vaccination of healthy horses, 6 months of age or older, as an aid in the control of respiratory disease caused by Equine Influenza Virus and Equine Herpesvirus and as an aid in the reduction of EHV-1 and EHV-4 virus shedding and Influenza Virus shedding. DOI shown to be 6 months for Equine Influenza Virus.

Prodigy® with Havlogen®*
EQUINE RHINOPNEUMONITIS VACCINE KILLED VIRUS
For vaccination of healthy horses 6 months of age or older, as an aid in the prevention of abortion and respiratory disease associated with EHV-1 infection.

Encevac® TC-4 with Havlogen®*
ENCEPHALOMYELITIS - INFLUENZA VACCINE EASTERN AND WESTERN, KILLED VIRUS TETANUS TOXOID
For vaccination of healthy horses, 6 months of age or older, as an aid in the prevention of Eastern and Western Equine Encephalomyelitis and Tetanus, and as an aid in the reduction of virus shedding and control of respiratory disease caused by Equine Influenza Virus. DOI shown to be 6 months for Equine Influenza Virus.

Prestige® with Havlogen®*
EQUINE RHINOPNEUMONITIS VACCINE
KILLED VIRUS
For vaccination of healthy horses, 6 months of age or older, as an aid in the control of respiratory disease caused by EHV-1 and EHV-4 and as an aid in the reduction of EHV-1 and EHV-4 virus shedding.

Prestige® V with Havlogen®*
ENCEPHALOMYELITIS - RHINOPNEUMONITIS - INFLUENZA VACCINE EASTERN AND WESTERN, KILLED VIRUS TETANUS TOXOID
For vaccination of healthy horses, 6 months of age or older, as an aid in the prevention of Eastern and Western Encephalomyelitis and Tetanus, as an aid in the control of respiratory disease caused by Equine Influenza Virus and Equine Herpesvirus and as an aid in the reduction of EHV-1 and EHV-4 virus shedding and Influenza Virus shedding. DOI shown to be 6 months for Equine Influenza Virus.

Super-Tet® with Havlogen®*
TETANUS TOXOID
Purified Tetanus Toxoid for vaccination of healthy horses, cattle, swine and sheep, 6 months of age or older, against Tetanus.

Encevac® TC-4 + VEE with Havlogen®*
ENCEPHALOMYELITIS - INFLUENZA VACCINE EASTERN, WESTERN, AND VENEZUELAN, KILLED VIRUS TETANUS TOXOID
For vaccination of healthy horses, 6 months of age or older, as an aid in the prevention of Eastern, Western and Venezuelan Equine Encephalomyelitis and Tetanus, and as an aid in reduction of virus shedding and the control of respiratory disease caused by Equine Influenza Virus. DOI shown to be 6 months for Equine Influenza Virus.

Table 6.2F : Veterinary viral vaccines marketed by Fort Dodge

Fel-O-Vax LVK: Fel-O-Vax LV-K (killed virus) is recommended for the vaccination of healthy cats 10 weeks of age or older to protect against diseases caused by feline leukemia virus.

DOSE: Inject one 1 ml dose IM or SC using aseptic technique. Repeat in 3 to 4 weeks. Annual revaccination with a single dose of vaccine is recommended. Thimerosal, neomycin, polymyxin B and amphotericin B added as preservatives.

Fel-O-Vax PCT: killed vaccine for IM or SC vaccination of healthy cats and kittens 8 weeks of age or older, as an aid in the prevention of disease caused by feline rhinotracheitis, calici and panleukopenia viruses.

DOSE: Vaccinate healthy cats 8 weeks of age or older with one 1 ml dose, followed by a second 1 ml dose 3 to 4 weeks later. Inject IM or SC. Cats vaccinated less than 12 weeks of age should be given an additional 1 ml dose of vaccine at 12 to 16 weeks of age. Annual revaccination with a single dose of vaccine is recommended. Vaccination of pregnant queens has shown no deleterious effect. Thimerosal, neomycin, polymyxin B and amphotericin B added as preservatives.

Rabvac 1: Rabvac 1 is a killed virus vaccine for the vaccination of healthy dogs and cats against rabies. This vaccine meets the one year duration of immunity requirements for dogs & cats.

Dogs and Cats: Inject one 1 ml dose SC or at one site in the thigh IM at 3 months of age or older. Revaccinate one year later and annually thereafter.

Fel-O-VaxPCT+CailiciVax: Fel-O-Vax PCT + CaliciVax, by Fort Dodge Labs, is a killed virus for protection against panleukopenia (cat distemper), calicivirus and rhinotracheitis. Protects against new hemorrhagic calicivirus strain VS-FCV. For cats 8 to 10 weeks of age, or older.

DOSE: Inject one 1 ml dose SC using aseptic technique. Repeat in 3 to 4 weeks. Annual revaccination with a single dose of vaccine is recommended.

Fel-O-Guard Plus 3: For SC vaccination of healthy cats, eight weeks of age or older, as an aid in the prevention of disease caused by feline rhinotracheitis, calici and panleukopenia viruses.

Fel-O-Guard Plus 4: For SC vaccination of healthy cats, eight weeks of age or older, as an aid in the prevention of disease caused by feline rhinotracheitis, calici, panleukopenia viruses and feline Chlamydia psittaci.

Fel-O-VaxIV + CaliciVax: Fel-O-Vax IV + CaliciVax, by Fort Dodge Labs, is a killed virus for protection against panleukopenia (cat distemper), calicivirus, rhinotracheitis and chlamydia. Protects against new hemorrhagic calicivirus strain VS-FCV. For cats 8 to 10 weeks of age, or older. Give SC & repeat in 3-4 weeks. Annual revaccination is recommended. Safe for pregnant queens. Ready to use liquid.

Duramune Adult 3: It is a USDA-licensed vaccine with 3-year virus challenge data against a trio of deadly canine diseases: canine distemper (CDV), canine adenovirus (CAV-2), and canine parvovirus (CPV). The vaccine is particularly well suited as a booster for adult dogs if an extended vaccination interval program is being used.

Fel-O-Guard Plus 4 + LvK: For SC vaccination of healthy cats, eight weeks of age or older, as an aid in the prevention of disease caused by feline leukemia, rhinotracheitis, calici, panleukopenia viruses and feline Chlamydia psittaci.

DURAMUNE MAX PV: For SC vaccination of healthy dogs 6 weeks of age or older as an aid in the prevention of disease caused by canine parvovirus. DOSE: Inject one 1 ml dose SC using aseptic technique. A recommended vaccination schedule should start at or about 6 weeks of age. The presence of maternal antibody is known to interfere with the development of active immunity. Puppies should be revaccinated every 2 to 3 weeks until they are at least 12 weeks of age. All dogs over 12 weeks of age should initially receive 1 dose of vaccine and a second dose 2 to 3 weeks later. Annual revaccination with one dose is recommended.

DURAMUNE MAX PC: Modified live and killed virus for SC vaccination of healthy dogs 6 weeks of age or older as an aid in the prevention of disease caused by canine coronavirus and canine parvovirus. DOSE: Inject one 1 ml dose SC using aseptic technique. A recommended vaccination schedule should start at or about 6 weeks of age. The presence of maternal antibody is known to interfere with the development of active immunity. Puppies should be revaccinated every 2 to 3 weeks until they are at least 12 weeks of age. All dogs over 12 weeks of age should initially receive one dose of vaccine and a second dose 2 to 3 weeks later. Annual revaccination with one dose is recommended.

DURAMUNE Cv-K: For vaccination of healthy dogs six weeks of age or older as an aid in the prevention of disease caused by canine coronavirus. Dosage and Administration: Dogs, inject one 1 ml SC or IM using aseptic technique. All dogs over 12 weeks of age should initially receive one dose of Duramune Cv-K and a second dose 2 to 3 weeks later. Annual revaccination with one dose is recommended. A recommended vaccination schedule should start at or about 6 weeks of age. The presence of maternal antibody is known to interfere with the development of active immunity. Puppies should be revaccinated every 2 to 3 weeks until they are at least 12 weeks of age.

Rabvac 3TF: Rabvac 3 TF is a killed virus vaccine for the vaccination of healthy dogs, cats and horses against rabies. This vaccine meets the three year duration of immunity requirements for dogs and cats.

DURAMUNE MAX 5: Canine Distemper-Adenovirus Type 2-Parainfluenza-Parvovirus Vaccine Modified Live Virus for subcutaneous vaccination of healthy dogs 6 weeks of age or older as an aid in the prevention of disease caused by canine distemper, infectious canine hepatitis, canine adenovirus type 2, canine parainfluenza and canine parvovirus.

NEOPAR® NeoTech Canine Parvovirus vaccine, modified live virus U.S. Vet. Lic. No.: 472. Overrides moderate to high antibody levels such as those found in puppies having maternal antibodies or in dogs from pre-existing vaccination. It can be used successfully as a booster for a pre-existing vaccination. Inject 1 ml SC or IM into healthy dogs. Administer the initial dose at or about 42 days of age. Because there is potential for maternal antibody to interfere with the immune response to the original vaccination, **NeoVac® DA2**: It is a high antigenic Mass vaccine that will override maternal antibodies, enabling for an earlier protection age. NeoVac® DA2's stabilized formula is safe in that there is no shedding of the distemper virus. Inject 1 dose (1 ml) SCy into healthy dogs that are at least 42 days of age. Puppies should be revaccinated every 14 to 28 days until 16 weeks of age. Dogs over 16 weeks require only a single 1 ml dose. Revaccinate annually with one dose.

Fluvac Innovator®: For vaccination of healthy horses against the infectious respiratory disease equine influenza. Protects against the type A_2 Equine Influenza strain. Killed vaccine includes thimerosal, neomycin, and polymyxin B as preservatives. Administer 1ml IM only and repeat the dose in 3 to 4 weeks. Administer annually thereafter.

Revaccinate every 14 to 21 days until the dog is 18 weeks of age. Dogs over 18 weeks should receive a single dose (1 mL). Revaccinate annually with one dose.

NEOVAC® D: It is a high antigenic mass vaccine that will override maternal antibodies, enabling for an earlier protection age. NEOVAC® D's stabilized formula is safe in that there is no shedding of the distemper virus. Studies have shown that NEOVAC® D is completely safe for not only Canines but Ferrets as well. Administer only one dose (1 ml) for initial vaccination of susceptible animals. Inject 1 dose (1 ml) SC into healthy dogs that are at least 42 days of age. Puppies should be revaccinated every 14 to 28 days until 16 weeks of age. Dogs over 16 weeks require only a single 1 ml dose. Revaccinate annually with one dose.

DIVA (differentiating infected from vaccinated animals) Vaccines or "Marker Vaccines"

For several viral infections of livestock, effective conventional vaccines are available but cannot be used, as they would interfere with disease surveillance based on serological testing and may result in the loss of a country's disease-free status. A classic example is FMD in cattle. Although inactivated FMD vaccines have been available for many years and are quite effective in controlling clinical disease, they are not used in FMD-free countries, as this would compromise this status and hence international trade. Nevertheless, conventional vaccines have reduced the prevalence of disease in enzootic areas, and in a recent outbreak in The Netherlands, vaccination was used to reduce the spread of the disease, although the vaccinates were subsequently slaughtered to enable the rapid reestablishment of the FMD-free status of the country. The ability to identify and selectively delete genes from a pathogen has allowed the development of **"marker vaccines"** that, combined with suitable diagnostic assays, allow **differentiating infected from vaccinated animals (DIVA)** by differentiation of antibody responses induced by the vaccine (no antibodies generated to deleted genes) from those induced during infection with the wild-type virus. Such DIVA vaccines and their companion diagnostic tests are now available or in development for several diseases including infectious bovine rhinotracheitis (IBR), pseudorabies, classical swine fever (CSF), and FMD, as detailed below.

Simplified representation of the reverse genetic approach used to construct the chimera vaccine Poulvac FluFend i AI H5N3 RG to protect poultry against the pathogenic H5N1 virus. The HA gene was removed from an H5N1 virus (from a recent Asian outbreak), inactivated by removing the polybasic amino acid sequences, and combined with the NA gene from an H2N3 virus onto an H1N1 "backbone" virus. An immunoassay able to specifically detect antibodies against N3 and N1 proteins could be used for DIVA (i.e., N3+ N1- indicates vaccinated, and N3- N1+ indicates infected).

IBR, caused by bovine herpesvirus type 1 (BHV-1) infection of cattle, and pseudorabies (Aujeszky's disease) in pigs have been identified internationally as being candidates for eradication from national herds, and so there has been an impetus for the development of DIVA vaccines and diagnostics. The demand for a marker (DIVA) vaccine for IBR in Europe was met by the development of a glycoprotein E (gE)-deleted vaccine using conventional methodology. The gE protein is not essential for viral replication, but it plays a major role in intercellular spread, particularly along nerves. Specific diagnostic tests based on gE deletion have been developed using both gE-blocking enzyme-linked immunosorbent assay (ELISA) techniques and PCR amplification.

Deletion of the gE gene has also been used to enable a DIVA approach for an Aujeszky's disease vaccine. The gene for thymidine kinase is also deleted in some formulations (e.g., Suvaxyn Aujesky), adding to the degree of attenuation. These deletion vaccines have been available since the 1980s, and their use has contributed to disease control and eradication in the United States and several European countries.

CSF is on the World Organization for Animal Health list of notifiable diseases and is one of the most important contagious diseases of pigs worldwide. In its classical clinical form, it is an acute hemorrhagic disease accompanied by high fever, depression, anorexia, and conjunctivitis. Morbidity and mortality are both very high and may reach 100%. However, it can also present as a subacute, chronic, or even subclinical condition. Countries in which the disease is enzootic tend to vaccinate with a very effective live, attenuated vaccine, while those that are free of disease do not. Two subunit vaccines based on the viral envelope glycoprotein E2 produced in a baculovirus/insect cell system, formulated in a water-in-oil adjuvant, and accompanied by discriminatory ELISA tests are available. These vaccines will allow a DIVA approach to emergency vaccination and disease control in the case of new outbreaks, although these have not yet been used widely in the field and appear to be less protective than conventional live, attenuated CSF vaccines.

As there are now major doubts about the sustainability of "stamping-out" policies in areas of high animal population density, there is considerable investment in DIVA vaccine approaches for FMD. Subunit antigen approaches to vaccination have been largely ineffective, as they present only a limited number of epitopes to the animal's immune system, and multiple antigens are generally required for protection. Current research is focused largely on combinations of capsid proteins, including empty capsid delivered by various expression systems, and the development of sensitive tests (ELISA) for antibodies against nonstructural proteins. Other diseases for which a DIVA approach is highly desirable but currently unavailable include bluetongue virus in cattle, Newcastle disease virus and avian influenza virus in poultry, bovine viral diarrhea, and equine viral arteritis.

Molecularly Defined Subunit Vaccines

The development of synthetic peptides that might be useful as vaccines depends on the identification of immunogenic sites. Several methods have been used. The best known example is foot and mouth disease, where protection was achieved by immunizing animals with a linear sequence of 20 amino acids. Synthetic peptide vaccines would have many advantages. Their antigens are precisely defined and free from unnecessary components which may be associated with side effects. They are stable and relatively cheap to manufacture. Furthermore, less quality assurance is required. Changes due to natural variation of the virus can be readily accommodated, which would be a great advantage for unstable viruses such as influenza.

But synthetic peptides do not readily stimulate T cells. It was generally assumed that, because of their small size, peptides would behave like haptens and would therefore require coupling to a protein carrier which is recognized by T-cells. It is now known that synthetic peptides can be highly immunogenic in their free form provided they contain, in addition to the B cell epitope, T- cell epitopes recognized by T-helper cells. Such T-cell epitopes can be provided by carrier protein molecules, foreign antigens or within the synthetic peptide molecule itself.

Synthetic peptides are not applicable to all viruses. This approach did not work in the case of polioviruses because the important antigenic sites were made up of 2 or more different viral capsid proteins so that it was in a concise 3-D conformation. Examples of purified subunit vaccines include the HA vaccines for influenza A and B, and HBsAg derived from the plasma of carriers.

Advantages of defined viral antigens or peptides include

1. Production and quality control simpler
2. No NA or other viral or external proteins, therefore less toxic.
3. Safer in cases where viruses are oncogenic or establish a persistent infection
4. Feasible even if virus cannot be cultivated.

Disadvantages

1. May be less immunogenic than conventional inactivated whole-virus vaccines
2. Requires adjuvant
3. Requires primary course of injections followed by boosters
4. Fails to elicit CMI.

Identification of the protective viral antigens potentially allows their isolation and/or recombinant production so that they can be administered as safe, nonreplicating vaccines. However, as isolated antigens generally induce poor protective immunity, subunit vaccines usually require repeated administration with strong adjuvants, making them less competitive. Notwithstanding these limitations, there are some examples of effective subunit vaccines.

PCV2 is considered to be the major pathogen in the etiology of postweaning multisystemic wasting syndrome in pig. A recombinant baculovirus producing the protective ORF2 protein of PCV2 has recently become available as a vaccine for pigs.

Dow Agro Sciences successfully registered the first plant-based vaccine for Newcastle disease virus in poultry in the United States in 2005. Recombinant viral HN protein was generated in plant cell lines via Agrobacterium transformation and could successfully protect chickens from viral challenge. This process was a proof-of-concept exercise designed to test regulatory feasibility, and the product is now on the market.

Genetically Engineered Viral Vaccines

The availability of complete DNA sequences and a better understanding of gene function have allowed specific modifications or deletions to be introduced into the viral genome, with the aim of producing well-defined and stably attenuated live or inactivated viral vaccines.

Gene-deleted vaccines

Glycoprotein I and/or glycoprotein X against pseudorabies allowed a DIVA approach and control of Aujeszky's disease in swine; however, the potential for recombination between pseudorabies virus strains has raised concern. Similarly, thymidine kinase deletion in BHV-1 vaccines has been associated with latency and reactivation after treatment with dexamethasone, and deletion of multiple genes has been proposed in order to improve safety.

Chimera vaccines

An interesting development in genetically engineered viral vaccines is the production of **chimera viruses** that combine aspects of two infective viral genomes. A chimera PCV1 & 2 vaccine has the immunogenic capsid gene of PCV2 cloned into the backbone of the nonpathogenic PCV1 and induces protective immunity to wild-type PCV2 challenge in pigs. A further sophistication of this approach is a recently developed vaccine against avian influenza virus (Poulvac FluFend), where the hemagglutinin (HA) gene has been removed from an H5N1 virus, inactivated by removing the polybasic amino acid sequences, and combined with the NA gene from an H2N3 virus onto an H1N1 "backbone" virus. A vaccine containing the resultant inactivated H5N3-expressing virus administered in a water-in-oil emulsion protects chickens and ducks against the highly pathogenic H5N1 strain.

Live Flavivirus chimera vaccine

Live Flavivirus chimera vaccine against West Nile virus (WNV) in horses (PreveNile) was registered in the United States in 2006. In this chimera vaccine, the structural genes of the attenuated yellow fever YF-17D backbone virus have been replaced with structural genes of the related WNV. The resulting chimera vaccine expresses the PreM and E proteins of WNV, while the nucleocapsid (C) protein, nonstructural proteins, and nontranslated termini responsible for virus replication remain those of the original yellow fever 17D virus. After a single shot, the vaccine stimulates both cell-mediated and humoral responses without causing any clinical illness or spreading to sentinel horses and provides protection against WNV challenge for up to 12 months (PreveNile package insert). A similar vaccine could be a candidate for a human WNV vaccine.

Live viral vector vaccines

Poxviruses including vaccinia virus, fowlpox virus, and canarypox virus have been used as vectors for exogenous genes, as first proposed in 1982, both for the delivery of vaccine antigens and for human gene therapy. Poxviruses can accommodate large amounts of foreign genes and can infect mammalian cells, resulting in the expression of large quantities of encoded protein. For example, **modified vaccinia virus Ankara is a highly attenuated strain** produced by several hundred passages of the virus in chicken cells. Modified vaccinia virus Ankara lacks about 10% of the vaccinia virus genome, including the ability to replicate in mammalian cells.

A particular success story has been the development of an **oral recombinant vaccinia-rabies vaccine** in bait for wild carnivores such as foxes in Europe and foxes, raccoons, and coyotes in the United States. Rabies is caused by a negative-stranded *Rhabdoviridae* RNA virus transmitted mainly via saliva following a bite from an infected animal. The main source of infection for humans is domestic reservoir species including dogs and cats. There are seven rabies virus genotypes, all of which, excluding type 2, produce similar effects in humans. Rabies can infect most if not all mammals. The virus enters the central nervous system, causing an encephalomyelitis that is always fatal once symptoms develop. Worldwide, the disease causes many thousands of human deaths each year. One type of oral vaccine is in the form of a bait containing a recombinant vaccinia virus vector expressing the protective glycoprotein G of rabies virus. After several years of vaccination campaigns against fox rabies virus in several Western European countries, rabies could be eliminated from its wildlife terrestrial reservoir, as exemplified by the successful elimination of terrestrial rabies virus from Belgium and France.

The canarypox virus vector system ALVAC has been used as a platform for a range of veterinary vaccines including **WNV, canine distemper virus, feline leukemia virus, rabies virus, and equine influenza virus**. Canarypox virus was originally isolated from a single pox lesion in a canary and serially passaged 200 times in chicken embryo fibroblasts and serially plaque purified under agarose (Merial bulletin TSB-4-0019-FTB). Canarypox viruses and fowlpox viruses have the advantage of being more host restricted than vaccinia virus. While they produce an abortive infection in mammalian cells, canarypox virus recombinants still effectively express inserted foreign genes. Several veterinary viral vaccines have been produced using the ALVAC vector system. Most notably, a novel equine influenza virus vaccine using the canarypox vector to express the hemagglutinin genes of the H3N8 Newmarket and Kentucky strains has recently been registered in the European Union (**Proteq-Flu**) and the United States (**Recombitek**). It contains a polymer adjuvant (Carbopol; Merial Ltd.), and through the induction of both cell-mediated and humoral immunity, it is claimed to produce sterile immunity 2 weeks after the second of two doses. The new vaccine is also designed to protect horses against the highly virulent N/5/03 American strain of equine influenza virus and to prevent the virus from spreading through the elimination of viral shedding.

Trovac AI H5 is a recombinant fowlpox virus expressing the H5 antigen of avian influenza virus. This product has had a conditional license for emergency use in the United States since 1998 and has been widely used in Central America, with over 2 billion doses administered. As the vaccinated birds will not develop antibodies against matrix protein/ nucleoprotein, this vaccine can also be used with a DIVA approach.

Several vaccines are available based on inactivated adjuvanted formulations for equine herpesvirus type 1 and equine herpesvirus type 4, equine herpesviruses that are major causes of abortion and respiratory disease. None of these vaccines are considered to provide complete clinical or virological protection. A canarypox virus-vectored vaccine containing the genes for gB, gC, and gD has been developed, but the latest reports suggested that it did not completely protect against challenge.

Use of an attenuated viral pathogen

A further application of vectored vaccines is the **use of an attenuated viral pathogen as** the vector, with the aim of inducing protection against two diseases, as with the live recombinant vaccine against both Marek's disease virus (MDV) and infectious bursal disease virus (IBDV) in chickens (Vaxxitek HVT + IBD). MDV is a highly contagious neoplastic disease of poultry caused by gallid herpesvirus type 2, while IBDV replicates in the bursa of Fabricius, the primary lymphoid organ in birds, and causes a serious immunosuppressive condition in poultry flocks worldwide. Turkey herpesvirus (HVT) is nonpathogenic in chickens but confers cross-protection against MDV and has traditionally been used in live vaccines against MDV. The new vaccine is based on a recombinant parent HVT virus expressing the VP2 gene of IBDV and can be given to embryonated eggs or 1-day-old chicks without interference from maternally derived antibodies. Data from large-scale field trials for this vaccine have not yet been reported, but those studies may encounter difficulties in maintaining high efficacy. This is because these tightly regulated recombinant vaccines cannot easily adapt to meet the emergence of very virulent strains of both IBDV and MDV, apparently induced by the comprehensive numbers of vaccinations performed against these diseases.

Chimera avian influenza virus vaccines have also recently been produced on a backbone of an existing, attenuated Newcastle disease virus vaccine strain. Both Asian H5N1 and the pathogenic H7N7 strain, responsible for the chicken influenza virus outbreak in The Netherlands in 2003, were produced as chimeras with the Newcastle disease virus strain. This chimera vaccine induced strong protection against the respective wild-type influenza virus as well as against Newcastle disease virus.

Presentation of immunogenic proteins and peptides

Proteins separated from virus particles are generally much less immunogenic than the intact particles. This difference in activity is usually attributed to the change in configuration of a protein when it is released from the structural requirements of the virus particle. Many attempts have been made to enhance the immunogenic activity of separated proteins.

Adjuvants

Used to potentiate the immune response.

1. Functions to localize and slowly release antigen at or near the site of administration.
2. Functions to activate APCs to achieve effective antigen processing or presentation

Materials that have been used include;

1. Aluminum salts
2. Mineral oils
3. Mycobacterial products, e.g. Freund's adjuvants

Immunostimulating complexes (ISCOMS)

1. An alternative vaccine vehicle
2. The antigen is presented in an accessible, multimeric, physically well defined complex
3. Composed of adjuvant (Quil A) and antigen held in a cage like structure
4. Adjuvant is held to the antigen by lipids
5. Can stimulate CMI
6. Mean diameter 35nm

Immunization and Herd Immunity

The following questions should be asked when a vaccination policy against a particular virus is being developed.

1. What proportion of the population should be immunized to achieve eradication.
2. What is the best age to immunize?
3. How is this affected by birth rates and other factors?
4. How does immunization affect the age distribution of susceptible individuals, particularly those in age-classes most at risk of serious disease?
5. How significant are genetic, social, or spatial heterogeneities in susceptibility to infection?
6. Hoe does this affect herd immunity?

A basic concept is that of the basic rate of the infection R_0. for most viral infections, R_0 is the average number of secondary cases produced by a primary case in a wholly susceptible population. Clearly, an infection cannot maintain itself or spread if R_0 is less than 1. R_0 can be estimated from as B/(A-D);B = life expectancy, A = average age at which infection is acquired, D = the characteristic duration of maternal antibodies.

The larger the value of R_0, the harder it is to eradicate the infection from the community in question. A rough estimate of the level of immunization coverage required can be estimated in the following manner: eradication will be achieved if the proportion immunized exceeds a critical value pinc = 1-1/ R_0. Thus the larger the R_0, the higher the coverage is required to eliminate the infection. Thus the global eradication of measles, with its R_0 of 10 to 20 or more, is almost sure to be more difficult to eradicate than smallpox, with its estimated R_0 of 2 to 4. Another example is rubella and measles immunization in the US. Rubella (A = 9 years) has an Ro roughly half that of measles (A = 5 years) and indeed rubella has been effectively eradicated in the US while the incidence of measles have declined more slowly.

Why do we not require 100% coverage to eradicate an infection? Immunization has both a direct and indirect effect. The susceptible host population is reduced by mass immunization so that the transmission of infection has become correspondingly less efficient and eventually, the infection will be unable to maintain itself.

Anti-Idiotype Vaccines

An antigen binding site in an antibody is a reflection of the three-dimensional structure of part of the antigen that is of a particular epitope. This unique amino acid structure in the antibody is known as the idiotype which can be thought of as a mirror of the epitope in the antigen. Antibodies (anti-idiotype) can be raised against the idiotype by injecting the antibody into another animal. This gives us an anti-idiotype antibody and, therefore, mimics part of the three dimensional structures of the antigen, that is, the epitope. This can be used as a vaccine. When the anti-idiotype antibody is injected into a vaccinee, antibodies (anti-anti-idiotype antiobodies) are formed that recognize a structure similar to part of the virus and might potentially neutralize the virus. This happens: Anti-idiotype vaccines raised against antibodies to hepatitis B virus S antigen elicit anti-viral antibodies.

DNA Vaccines

Recently, encouraging results were reported for DNA vaccines whereby DNA coding for the foreign antigen is directly injected into the animal so that the foreign antigen is directly produced by the host cells. In theory these vaccines would be extremely safe and devoid of side effects since the foreign antigens would be directly produced by the host animal. In addition, DNA is relatively inexpensive and easier to produce than conventional vaccines and thus this technology may one day increase the availability of vaccines to developing countries. Moreover, the time for development is relatively short which may enable timely immunization against emerging infectious diseases. In addition, DNA vaccines can theoretically result in more long-term production of an antigenic protein when introduced into a relatively **nondividing tissue, such as muscle**. The first clinical trials using injections of DNA to stimulate an immune response against a foreign protein began for HIV in 1995. Four other clinical trials using DNA vaccines against influenza, herpes simplex virus, T-cell lymphoma, and an additional trial for HIV were started in 1996.

The technique that is being tested in humans & animals involves the direct injection of plasmids - loops of DNA that contain genes for proteins produced by the organism being targeted for immunity. Once injected into the host's muscle tissue, the DNA is taken up by host cells, which then start expressing the foreign protein. The protein serves as an antigen that stimulates immune responses and protective immunological memory.

Enthusiasm for DNA vaccination in humans is tempered by the fact that delivery of the DNA to cells is still not optimal, particularly in larger animals. Another concern is the possibility, which exists with all gene therapy, that the vaccine's DNA will be integrated into host chromosomes and will turn on oncogenes or turn off tumor suppressor genes. Another potential downside is that extended immunostimulation by the foreign antigen could in theory provoke chronic inflammation or autoantibody production.

DNA Uptake Mechanism

DNA vaccines are being developed that consist of gene segments of infectious organisms. They are injected directly into cells for the production of the desired immunizing antigens. **Intradermal injectors** are used to deliver the DNA directly to the dendritic cells of the dermis. This system induces antibody and cell mediated immunity with a single injection and provides prolonged immunity. A DNA vaccine is being tested for feline leukemia virus. A DNA vaccine licensed with the USDA has been developed to protect horses against viremia caused by West Nile virus. WNV infection, caused by a flavivirus belonging to the Japanese encephalitis virus complex, is enzootic in parts of Africa and Asia. It was first detected in 1999 in the US in an outbreak involving birds, horses, and humans in New York, subsequently spreading rapidly to many states.

When DNA uptake and subsequent expression was first demonstrated *in vivo* in muscle cells, it was thought that these cells were unique in this ability because of their extensive network of T-tubules. Subsequent research revealed that other cells (such as keratinocytes, fibroblasts and epithelial Langerhans cells) could also internalize DNA. Two theories are currently popular - that *in vivo* uptake of DNA occurs non-specifically, in a method similar to phagocytosis or pinocytosis, or through specific receptors. These might include a 30kDa surface receptor, or macropgage scavenger receptors. The 30kDa surface receptor binds very specifically to 4500-bp genomic DNA fragments (which are then internalized) and is found on professional APCs and T-cells. Macrophage scavenger receptors bind to a variety of macromolecules, including polyribonucleotides, and are thus also candidates for DNA uptake. Receptor mediated DNA uptake could be facilitated by the presence of polyguanyl sequences. Further research into this mechanism might seem pointless, considering that **gene gun delivery systems, cationic liposome packaging, and other delivery methods** bypass this entry method, but understanding it might be useful in reducing costs (e.g. by reducing the requirement for cytofectins), which will be important in the food animals industry.

Antigen presentation by bone marrow-derived cells

Studies using chimeric mice have shown that antigen is presented by bone-marrow derived cells, which include dendritic cells, macrophages and specialized B cells called professional antigen presenting cells (APC). After gene gun inoculation to the skin, transfected Langerhans cells migrate to the draining lymph node to present antigen. After IM and ID injections, dendritic cells have also been found to present antigen in the draining lymph node and transfected macrophages have been found in the peripheral blood. Besides direct transfection of dendritic cells or macrophages, cross priming is also known to occur following IM, ID and gene gun deliveries of DNA. Cross priming occurs when a bone marrow-derived cell presents peptides from proteins synthesised in another cell in the context of MHC class 1. This can prime cytotoxic T-cell responses and seems to be important for a full primary immune response.

Role of the target site

IM and ID delivery of DNA initiate immune responses differently. In the skin, keratinocytes, fibroblasts and Langerhans cells take up and express antigen, and are responsible for inducing a primary antibody response. Transfected Langerhans cells migrate out of the skin (within 12 hours) to the draining lymph node where they prime secondary B- and T-cell responses. In skeletal muscle, on the other hand, striated muscle cells are most frequently transfected, but seem to be unimportant in mounting an immune response. Instead, IM inoculated DNA "washes" into the draining lymph node within minutes, where distal dendritic cells are transfected and then initiate an immune response. Transfected myocytes seem to act as a "reservoir" of antigen for trafficking professional APCs.

Delivery methods

DNA vaccines have been introduced into animal tissues by a number of different methods.

The two most popular approaches are **injection of DNA in saline, using a standard hypodermic needle, and gene gun delivery**. A schematic outline of the construction of a DNA vaccine plasmid and its subsequent delivery by these two methods into a host is illustrated at Scientific America. Injection in saline is normally conducted IM) in skeletal muscle, or intradermally (ID), with DNA being delivered to the extracellular spaces. This can be assisted by electroporation; by temporarily damaging muscle fibres with myotoxins such as bupivacaine; or by using hypertonic solutions of saline or sucrose. Immune responses to this method of delivery can be affected by many factors, including needle type, needle alignment, speed of injection, volume of injection, muscle type, and age, sex and physiological condition of the animal being injected.

Gene gun delivery, the other commonly used method of delivery, ballistically accelerates plasmid DNA (pDNA) that has been adsorbed onto gold or tungsten microparticles into the target cells, using compressed helium as an accelerant.

Alternative delivery methods have included aerosol instillation of naked DNA on mucosal surfaces, such as the nasal and lung mucosa, and topical administration of pDNA to the eye and vaginal mucosa. Mucosal surface delivery has also been achieved using cationic liposome-DNA preparations, biodegradable microspheres, attenuated Shigella or Listeria vectors for oral administration to the intestinal mucosa, and recombinant adenovirus vectors.

The method of delivery determines the dose of DNA required to raise an effective immune response. Saline injections require variable amounts of DNA, from 10 μg-1 mg, whereas gene gun deliveries require 100 to 1000 times less DNA than intramuscular saline injection to raise an effective immune response. Generally, **0.2 μg - 20 μg** are required, although quantities as low as 16 ng have been reported. These quantities vary from species to species, with mice, for example, requiring approximately 10 times less DNA than primate. Saline injections require more DNA because the DNA is delivered to the extracellular spaces of the target tissue (normally muscle), where it has to overcome physical barriers (such as the basal lamina and large amounts of connective tissue, to mention a few) before it is taken up by the cells, while gene gun deliveries bombard DNA directly into the cells, results in less "wastage".

Another approach to DNA vaccination is expression library immunization (ELI). Using this technique, potentially all the genes from a pathogen can be delivered at one time, which may be useful for pathogens which are difficult to attenuate or culture. ELI can be used to identify which of the pathogen's genes induce a protective response. This has been tested with *Mycoplasma pulmonis*, a murine lung pathogen with a relatively small genome, and it was found that even partial expression libraries can induce protection from subsequent challenge.

The first clinical trials using injections of DNA to stimulate an immune response against a foreign protein began for HIV in 1995. Four other clinical trials using DNA vaccines against influenza, herpes simplex virus, T-cell lymphoma, and an additional trial for HIV were started in 1996.

Enthusiasm for DNA vaccination in humans & animals is tempered by the fact that delivery of the DNA to cells is still not optimal, particularly in larger animals. Another concern is the possibility, which exists with all gene therapy, that the vaccine's DNA will be integrated into host chromosomes and will turn on oncogenes or turn off tumor suppressor genes. Another potential downside is that extended immunostimulation by the foreign antigen could in theory provoke chronic inflammation or autoantibody production. Immunization of animals with naked DNA encoding protective viral antigens would in many ways be an ideal procedure for viral vaccines, as it not only overcomes the safety concerns of live vaccines and vector immunity but also promotes the induction of cytotoxic T cells after intracellular expression of the antigens. Furthermore, DNA vaccines are very stable and do not require a cold chain. While DNA vaccination of large animals has not been as effective as initially demonstrated in mice, several groups have obtained significant improvements in immune responses using innovative technologies such as specific targeting of the vaccine antigen to antigen-presenting cells, priming-boosting with stimulating CpG oligodeoxynucleotides, and in vivo electroporation of DNA.

Table 6.3 : Comparison of T-Dependent Antibody Responses raised by DNA Immunizations, Protein Inoculations and Viral Infections

	Method of Immunization		
	DNA Vaccine	**Recombinant protein**	**Natural Infection**
Amount of inducing antigen	ng	μg	(ng-μg)
Duration of Ag presentation	several weeks	< 1 week	several weeks
Kinetics of Ab response	slow rise	rapid rise	rapid rise
Number of inoculations to obtain high avidity IgG and migration of ASC to bone marrow	one	two	one
Ab isotype (murine models)	C′-dependent or C′-independent	C′-dependent	C′-independent

Considerable research into DNA vaccines for fish viruses, where this approach seems to be particularly effective, has been ongoing. Notably, the first DNA vaccine for an edible species (Apex-IHN) was registered in 2005 in Canada to protect Atlantic salmon from **infectious hematopoietic necrosis (IHN)**. IHN disease is enzootic in wild salmon populations and can cause devastating outbreaks in farm-raised salmon that have had no prior exposure. The DNA vaccine encodes a surface glycoprotein of IHN virus and is administered intramuscularly.

A DNA vaccine to protect horses against viremia caused by **WNV (West Nile-Innovator DNA)** received a license from the USDA at approximately the same time as the fish DNA vaccine. WNV infection is caused by a flavivirus belonging to the Japanese encephalitis virus complex. It is enzootic in parts of Africa and Asia but was first detected in the United States in 1999 in an outbreak involving birds, horses, and humans in New York, and it subsequently spread rapidly to many states. The DNA plasmid codes for the WNV outer coat proteins and is administered with a proprietary adjuvant. The vaccine was, however, produced as part of a building-platform technology rather than as a commercial product, as the manufacturer already has a WNV vaccine on the market.

The success of these two DNA vaccines may be due more to good fortune than to any specific technological advances, as DNA uptake into fish muscle seems to be unusually efficient (99), and the WNV viral protein may be particularly effective because it naturally produces highly immunogenic virus-like particles. It is likely that a wider application of DNA vaccines will require further improvements and optimization for each host-pathogen combination.

Interest is gaining for the use of **plant-made vaccines for veterinary purposes,** with regulatory authorities sanctioning delivery of either crude extracts or minimally processed plant materials to animals for medicinal purposes. We highlight current research directions and challenges in the development of **plant-made veterinary vaccines against foot-and-mouth disease, avian influenza and Newcastle disease**; each considered restrictive to international trade in animals.

Increasingly, a number of rationally designed and subunit vaccines are reaching the market, called "second-generation" viral vaccines (Table: 6.4).

Table 6.4 : Second-generation licensed/commercialized veterinary viral vaccines

Target pathogen	Target animal	Brand name(s)	Distributor	Characteristic(s)
PCV2	Pigs	Porcilis-PCV2	Intervet	Inactivated baculovirus expressed PCV2 ORF2 protein; adjuvanted
PCV2	Pigs	Suvaxyn PCV2	Fort Dodge	Inactivated PCV1-2 chimera; adjuvanted
Pseudorabies virus	Pigs	Suvaxyn Aujeszky	Fort Dodge	gE- and thymidine kinase-deleted marker vaccine
Classical swine fever virus	Pigs	Porcilis Pesti	Intervet	Baculovirus recombinant E2 protein without emulsion
Classical swine fever virus	Pigs	Bayovac CSF E2	Bayer Leverkusen	Baculovirus recombinant E2 protein without emulsion
BHV-1	Cattle	Bovilis IBR Marker	Intervet	Live or inactivated gE-deleted marker vaccine

Equine influenza virus	Horses	PROTEQ-FLU (European Union), Recombitek (United States)	Merial	Canarypox virus-vectored vaccine
WNV	Horses	PreveNile	Intervet	Live flavivirus chimera vaccine
WNV	Horses	West Nile-Innovator DNA	Fort Dodge	DNA vaccine
WNV	Horses	RECOMBITEK equine WNV	Merial	Canarypox virus-vectored vaccine
MDV (HTV) and IBDV	Poultry	Vaxxitek HVT+IBD	Merial	Live recombinant chimera virus expressing VP2 gene of IBD on HTV virus
Newcastle disease virus	Poultry	NA	Dow Agro Sciences	HN recombinant produced in plant cell lines (registered but not on market)
Newcastle disease virus	Poultry	Vectormune FP-ND	Biomune	Fowlpox virus vectored
Avian influenza virus (H5N1) and NDV	Poultry		Intervet	Chimera virus on NDV backbone; field trials in 2007
Avian influenza virus	Poultry	Poulvac FluFend I AI H5N3 RG	Fort Dodge	Chimera H5N3 virus, inactivated in oil-based adjuvant
Avian influenza virus	Poultry	Trovac AI H5	Merial	Fowlpox virus-vectored H5
Rabies virus	Wildlife, canines	Raboral	Merial	Vaccinia virus recombinant
Rabies virus	Cats	Purevax Feline Rabies	Merial	Canarypox virus-vectored vaccine
Rabies virus	Cats	PUREVAX Feline Rabies	Merial	Canarypox virus-vectored vaccine
Feline leukemia virus	Cats	EURIFEL FeLV	Merial	Canarypox virus-vectored vaccine

Canine parvovirusl	Dogs	RECOMBITEK Canine Parvo	Merial	Modified live virus
Canine coronavirus	Dogs	RECOMBITEK Corona MLV	Merial	Modified live virus
Canine distemper virus	Dogs	RECOMBITEK rDistemper	Merial	Canarypox virus-vectored vaccine (HA and F antigens)
Canine distemper virus	Fur animals	PUREVAXFerre t Distemper	Merial	Canarypox virus-vectored vaccine
IHN virus	Salmon	Apex-IHN	Novartis (Aqua Health)	DNA vaccine

There have been anecdotal reports of oseltavir (Tamiflu) reducing disease severity and hospitalization time in canine parvovirus infection. The drug may limit the ability of the virus to invade the crypt cells of the small intestine and decrease gastrointestinal bacteria colonization and toxin production. Lastly, recombinant feline interferon omega (rFeIFN-ω), produced in silkworm larvae using a baculovirus vector, has been demonstrated by multiple studies to be an effective treatment.

Modulation of the immune responses

Cytokine modulation

For a vaccine to be effective, it must induce an appropriate immune response for a given pathogen, and the ability of DNA vaccines to polarise T-cell help towards TH1 or TH2 profiles, and generate CTL and/or antibody when required, is a great advantage in this regard. This can be accomplished by modifications to the form of antigen expressed (i.e. intracellular vs. secreted), the method and route of delivery, and the dose of DNA delivered. However, it can also be accomplished by the co-administration of plasmid DNA encoding immune regulatory molecules, i.e. cytokines, lymphokines or co-stimulatory molecules. These "genetic adjuvants" can be administered in a number of ways:

- as a mixture of 2 separate plasmids, one encoding the immunogen and the other encoding the cytokine;
- as a single bi- or polycistronic vector, separated by spacer regions; or
- as a plasmid-encoded chimera, or fusion protein.

In general, co-administration of pro-inflammatory agents (such as various interleukins, tumor necrosis factor, and GM-CSF) plus TH2 inducing cytokines increase antibody responses, whereas pro-inflammatory agents and TH1 inducing cytokines decrease humoral responses and increase cytotoxic responses (which is more important in viral protection, for example). Co-stimulatory molecules like B7-1, B7-2 and CD40L are also sometimes used.

This concept has been successfully applied in topical administration of pDNA encoding IL-10. Plasmid encoded B7-1 (a ligand on APCs) has successfully enhanced the immune response in anti-tumour models, and mixing plasmids encoding GM-CSF and the circumsporozoite protein of P. yoelii (PyCSP) has enhanced protection against subsequent challenge (whereas plasmid-encoded PyCSP alone did not). It was proposed that GM-CSF may cause dendritic cells to present antigen more efficiently, and enhance IL-2 production and TH cell activation, thus driving the increased immune response. This can be further enhanced by first priming with a pPyCSP and pGM-CSF mixture, and later boosting with a recombinant poxvirus expressing PyCSP. However, co-injection of plasmids encoding GM-CSF (or IFN-γ, or IL-2) and a fusion protein of *P. chabaudi* merozoite surface protein 1 (C-terminus)-hepatitis B virus surface protein (PcMSP1-HBs) actually abolished protection against challenge, compared to protection acquired by delivery of pPcMSP1-HBs alone.

The advantages of using genetic adjuvants are their low cost and simplicity of administration, as well as avoidance of unstable recombinant cytokines and potentially toxic, "conventional" adjuvants (such as alum, calcium phosphate, monophosphoryl lipid A, cholera toxin, cationic and mannan-coated liposomes, QS21, carboxymethyl-cellulose and ubenimix). However, the potential toxicity of prolonged cytokine expression has not been established, and in many commercially important animal species, cytokine genes still need to be identified and isolated. In addition, various plasmid encoded cytokines modulate the immune system differently according to the time of delivery. For example, some cytokine plasmid DNAs are best delivered after the immunogen pDNA, because pre- or co-delivery can actually decrease specific responses, and increase non-specific responses.

Immunostimulatory CpG motifs

Plasmid DNA itself appears to have an adjuvant effect on the immune system. Bacterially derived DNA has been found to trigger innate immune defence mechanisms, the activation of dendritic cells, and the production of TH1 cytokines. This is due to recognition of certain CpG dinucleotide sequences which are immunostimulatory. CpG stimulatory (CpG-S) sequences occur twenty times more frequently in bacterially derived DNA than in eukaryotes. This is because eukaryotes exhibit "CpG suppression" – i.e. CpG dinucleotide pairs occur much less frequently than expected. Additionally, CpG-S sequences are hypomethylated. This occurs frequently in bacterial DNA, while CpG motifs occurring in eukaryotes are all methylated at the cytosine nucleotide. In contrast, nucleotide sequences which inhibit the activation of an immune response (termed CpG neutralising, or CpG-N) are over represented in eukaryotic genomes. The optimal immunostimulatory sequence has been found to be an unmethylated CpG dinucleotide flanked by two 5′ purines and two 3′ pyrimidines. Additionally, flanking regions outside this immunostimulatory hexamer must be guanine-rich to ensure binding and uptake into target cells.

The innate system works synergistically with the adaptive immune system to mount a response against the DNA encoded protein. CpG-S sequences induce polyclonal B-cell activation and the upregulation of cytokine expression and secretion. Stimulated macrophages secrete IL-12, IL-18, TNF-α, IFN-α, IFN-β and IFN-γ, while stimulated B-cells secrete IL-6 and some IL-12.

Manipulation of CpG-S and CpG-N sequences in the plasmid backbone of DNA vaccines can ensure the success of the immune response to the encoded antigen, and drive the immune response toward a TH1 phenotype. This is useful if a pathogen requires a TH response for protection. CpG-S sequences have also been used as external adjuvants for both DNA and recombinant protein vaccination with variable success rates. Other organisms with hypomethylated CpG motifs have also demonstrated the stimulation of polyclonal B-cell expansion. However, the mechanism behind this may be more complicated than simple methylation – hypomethylated murine DNA has not been found to mount an immune response.

Most of the evidence for the existence of immunostimulatory CpG sequences comes from murine studies. Clearly, extrapolation of this data to other species should be done with caution – different species may require different flanking sequences, as binding specificities of scavenger receptors differ between species. Additionally, species such as ruminants may be insensitive to immunostimulatory sequences due to the large gastrointestinal load they exhibit. Further research may be useful in the optimisation of DNA vaccination, especially in the food animal industry.

Alternative boosts

DNA-primed immune responses can be boosted by the administration of recombinant protein or recombinant poxviruses. "Prime-boost" strategies with recombinant protein have successfully increased both neutralising antibody titre, and antibody avidity and persistence, for weak immunogens, such as HIV-1 envelope protein. Recombinant virus boosts have been shown to be very efficient at boosting DNA-primed CTL responses. Priming with DNA focuses the immune response on the required immunogen, while boosting with the recombinant virus provides a larger amount of expressed antigen, leading to a large increase in specific CTL responses.

Additional methods of enhancing DNA-Raised immune responses

Formulations of DNA

The efficiency of DNA immunization can be improved by stabilising DNA against degradation, and increasing the efficiency of delivery of DNA into antigen presenting cells. This has been demonstrated by coating biodegradable cationic microparticles (such as poly (lactide-co-glycolide) formulated with cetyltrimethylammonium bromide) with DNA. Such DNA-coated microparticles can be as effective at raising CTL as recombinant vaccinia viruses, especially when mixed with alum. Particles 300 nm in diameter appear to be most efficient for uptake by antigen presenting cells.

If vaccines are to reliably prevent disease, they must be developed, produced and quality-controlled according to very strict regulations and procedures. Veterinary viral vaccine registrations are governed by different rules in different countries, but these rules all emphasize that the quality of the raw materials, the cells, eggs, animals or plants that are used in production, need to be carefully controlled. The veterinary vaccine business is also very cost-conscious. Emphasis over the last 5–10 years has therefore been to develop culture systems that minimize labor and sterility problems and thus provide for reliable and cost-effective production. Implementing these often more complex systems in a production environment takes considerable effort, first in scale-up trials and further down the line in convincing production personnel to change their familiar system for something new and possibly untried. To complete scale-up trials successfully, it is absolutely necessary to understand the biochemistry of the cells and the influence of the virus on the cells under scale-up and later production conditions. Once a viral product can be produced on a large scale, it is imperative that the quality of the end-product is controlled in an intelligent way. One needs to know whether the end-product performs in the animal as was intended during its conception in the research and development department. The development of the appropriate tests to demonstrate this plays an important role in the successful development of a vaccine.

Passive Prophylaxis

The use of immunoglobulin preparations remains a mainstay of passive prophylaxis (and occasionally of therapy) for viral illnesses. Passive immunoprophylaxis is most often recommended in one of these situations: (1) when exposure has occurred, or is expected to occur very soon, and time does not allow for vaccination and the development of an adequate post-vaccination immune response; (2) when no effective vaccine exists; (3) when an underlying illness precludes a satisfactory response to vaccination. Although once derived exclusively from animal sources, most immunoglobulins are now manufactured from human sources.

Standard immunoglobulin is produced by pooling plasma obtained from thousands of donors and contains antibodies to a number of common viruses. Specific immunoglobulins are produced from donors with high titers of antibodies to specific viruses, often selected following immunization with the relevant vaccine. Ig may prevent or modify infection with hepatitis A virus if administered in a dose of 0.02 ml/kg within 14 days after exposure. Measles infection may be prevented or modified in a susceptible person if Ig is given in a dose of 0.25 ml/kg within 6 days after exposure. Special forms of Ig include tetanus Ig (TIg), hepatitis B Ig (HBIg), rabies Ig (RIg), rubella Ig, CMV Ig (IV), botulism Ig (IV), and investigational varicella-zoster Ig (VariZIg). These are obtained from donors known to have high titers of antibody against the organism in question. Ig must be given only in the manner for which it is recommended (i.e. IM must be given intramuscularly, IV must be given intravenously). The dose varies depending on the clinical indication. Adverse reactions include pain at the injection site, headache, chills, dyspnea, nausea, and anaphylaxis, although all but the first are rare.

Passive transfer of colostral immunoglobulins has long been accepted as imperative to optimal calf health. Many factors, including timing of colostrum ingestion, the method and volume of colostrum administration, the immunoglobulin concentration of the colostrum ingested, and the age of the dam have been implicated in affecting the optimization of absorption. The practice of colostrum pooling, the breed and presence of the dam, and the presence of respiratory acidosis in the calf also may affect passive transfer. Various tests have been reported to accurately measure passive transfer status in neonatal calves. The radial immunodiffusion and the enzyme-linked immunosorbent assay (ELISA) are the only tests that directly measure serum IgG concentration. All other available tests including serum total solids by refractometry, sodium sulfite turbidity test, zinc sulfate turbidity test, serum gamma-glutamyl transferase activity, and whole blood glutaraldehyde gelation estimate serum IgG concentration based on concentration of total globulins or other proteins whose passive transfer is statistically associated with that of IgG. Many previously accepted truisms regarding passive transfer in calves should be rejected based on the results of recent research.

Neonatal dairy animals are born agammaglobulinemic and must obtain immunoglobulins (Ig) during the period of macromolecular transport within the first 24 h of life. Maternal colostrum has been the traditional source of Ig and recommendations for provision of 2 L of colostrum in two separate feedings within the first 24 hr are widespread. However, high levels of neonatal mortality and evidence of persistence of failure of passive transfer in calves indicates that too many calves consume too little Ig from colostrum or are unable to efficiently absorb IgG. Further, recent research has suggested that methods of collecting, handling and feeding of colostrum promote the transmission of biologically and economically important diseases such as Johne's. Several approaches to improving passive transfer and reducing risk of disease transmission have been proposed, including feeding larger amounts (4 L) of colostrum at the first feeding, pasteurization of colostrum and feeding exogenous sources of Ig. Colostrum supplements and colostrum replacers are products containing <100 or =100 g of IgG per dose, respectively. Sources of colostrum include lacteal secretions (milk, whey or colostrum), blood and eggs (using chicken IgY). Research suggests that the efficiency of IgG absorption varies markedly by product, method of processing and source of Ig. Immunoglobulins derived from egg and supplements containing IgG from lacteal secretions are poorly absorbed by calves. Conversely, highly concentrated IgG from blood or colostrum appear to be well absorbed. More highly concentrated products (colostrum replacers) appear to have better efficiency of absorption than supplements. Immunoglobulins can also be provided to the animal following cessation of macromolecular transport (closure) as a source of local, intestinal immunity. There is firm evidence that IgG initially absorbed from colostrum into the bloodstream is resecreted into the intestinal by crypt cells. These IgGs assist in reducing the incidence and severity of many different types of gastrointestinal infections, including enteropathogenic *Escherichia coli*, rotavirus and *Cryptosporidium parvum*. Sources of IgG for oral administration following closure are similar to that of colostrum supplements; however, variation in efficacy of products depending on source is different from that of colostrum supplements and replacers. Chicken egg IgY and IgG derived from colostrum and blood all appear to be effective, but degree of effectiveness depends on the specificity of Ig against specific pathogens.

Antiviral Chemotherapy

Antiviral chemotherapeutic agents can be divided into three categories: virucidal agents, antiviral agents, and immunomodulators. Virucidal agents directly inactivate intact viruses. Although some of these agents have clinical usefulness (e.g., topical treatment of warts with podophyllin, which destroys both virus and host tissues), most virucides have not demonstrated therapeutic value. Immunomodulators such as interferons that alter the host immune responses to infection could, in principle, be protective, and several are under investigation.

Antiviral agents

These inhibit viral replication at the cellular level, interrupting one or more steps in the life cycle of the virus. These agents have a limited spectrum of activity and, because most of them also interrupt host cell function, they are toxic to various degrees. The emergence of drug resistant viruses may occur during clinical use that further limits the effectiveness of various antivirals.

A number of antiviral agents with demonstrated effectiveness are now available. Antiviral drugs interfere with the life cycle of the virus by preventing: viral entry in the host cell, viral replication in the host cell or egress of newly produced virus. Since antiviral agents act **directly on the virus** and do not rely on the hosts' immune system, as is the case with vaccines, a **potent antiviral could provide instant protection**. By abolishing one or more stages of its life cycle, the spread of the virus, and hence the disease, may be reduced or even halted.

These antiviral agents improve the clinical course of disease, but typically have important limitations especially as therapeutics for chronic or latent infections. For example, the four nucleoside analog drugs now available for the therapy of HIV-1 do not prevent the ultimate worsening of disease. The concept of a targeted approach is now practical since information concerning the structure and replication of viruses and the spatial configuration and function of their proteins is available. Such data may be useful in identifying specific target sites for antiviral agents.

Drugs that target viral processes must penetrate host cells; in doing so, they are likely to negatively impact normal pathways of the host. Antiviral drugs are characterized by a narrow therapeutic margin. Therapy is further complicated by viral latency, i.e, the ability of the virus to incorporate its genome in the host genome, with clinical infection becoming evident without re-exposure to the organism. In vitro susceptibility testing must depend on cell cultures, which are expensive. More importantly, in vitro inhibitory tests do not necessarily correlate with therapeutic efficacy of antiviral drugs. Part of the discrepancy between in vitro and in vivo testing occurs because some drugs require activation (metabolism) to be effective.

Only a few agents have been found to be reasonably safe and effective against a limited number of viral diseases, and most of these have been developed in humans. Few have been studied in animals, and widespread clinical use of antiviral drugs is not common in veterinary medicine. Only a selection of the more promising agents and their purported attributes are briefly discussed.

Most antiviral drugs interfere with viral nucleic acid synthesis or regulation. Such drugs generally are nucleic acid analogs that interfere with RNA and DNA production. Other mechanisms of action include interference with viral cell binding or interruption of virus uncoating. Some viruses contain unique metabolic pathways that serve as a target of drug therapy. Drugs that simply inhibit single steps in the viral replication cycle are virustatic and only temporarily halt viral replication. Thus, optimal activity of some drugs depends on an adequate host immune response. Some antiviral drugs may enhance the immune system of the host.

Amantadine, and its derivative rimantadine, is synthetic antiviral agents that appear to act on an early step of viral replication after attachment of virus to cell receptors. The effect seems to lead to inhibition or delay of the uncoating process that precedes primary transcription. Amantadine may also interfere with the early stages of viral mRNA transcription. Amantadine at usual concentrations inhibits replication of different strains of influenza A virus, influenza C virus, Sendai virus, and pseudorabies virus. It is almost completely absorbed from the GI tract, and ~90% of a dose administered is excreted unchanged in the urine over several days (human data). The main clinical use has been to prevent infection with various strains of influenza A viruses. However, in humans, it also has been found to produce some therapeutic benefit if taken within 48 hr after the onset of illness. Amantadine and its derivatives may be given by the PO, intranasal, SC, IP, or aerosol routes. It produces few side effects, most of which are related to the CNS; stimulation of the CNS is evident at very high doses.

Pleconaril works against rhinovirus, which causes the common cold, by blocking a pocket on the surface of the virus that controls the uncoating process. This pocket is similar in most strains of rhinoviruses and enteroviruses, which can cause diarrhea, meningitis, conjunctivitis, and encephalitis.

A variety of **pyrimidine nucleosides** (both halogenated and nonhalogenated) effectively inhibit the replication of herpes simplex viruses with limited host-cell toxicity. The exact mechanism of action of these compounds appears to reflect substitution of pyrimidine for thymidine, causing defective DNA molecules. **Idoxuridine** (IDU) is effective for the treatment of herpesvirus infection of the superficial layers of the cornea (herpesvirus keratitis) and of the skin, but is toxic when administered systemically.

Trifluridine, also an **analog of deoxythymidine**, is currently the agent of choice for the treatment of herpesvirus keratitis in humans. The other antiviral pyrimidine nucleosides have not been used clinically to any notable extent.

Vidarabine, or araA, purine nucleoside has proved to be effective antiviral and is used as systemic agents. Two of these antiviral drugs deserve special mention. **Vidarabine, or araA,** is used topically for ocular herpes and systemically for herpetic encephalitis as well as for neonatal herpesviral infections. This drug is an adenosine derivative that is phosphorylated by cellular enzymes to a triphosphate compound that inhibits many viral and human DNA polymerases and thus DNA synthesis. Herpesviral enzymes are ~20-fold more susceptible to the drug compared with host DNA. **Vidarabine** is administered IV in large volumes of fluid and is rapidly inactivated. It may produce bone marrow suppression and CNS side effects when high blood levels are reached.

Acyclovir (acycloguanosine) represents a new generation of antiviral agents, mainly because of its unique mechanism of action. This **purine nucleoside** is phosphorylated more efficiently by virus-induced thymidine kinase compared with host thymidine kinase. Once in the triphosphate form, it is a better substrate and inhibitor of viral, compared with host, DNA polymerase. Binding to DNA polymerase is irreversible. Once incorporated into viral DNA, the DNA chain is terminated. Acyclovir is relatively safe (probenecid renders the drug safer) and is useful against a variety of infections caused by DNA viruses, especially the herpesvirus family. However, resistance is increasing. Acyclovir is unable to eliminate latent infections. It is available as an ophthalmic ointment, a topical ointment and cream, an IV preparation, and various oral formulations. The first successful antiviral, acyclovir, is a nucleoside analogue, and is effective against herpesvirus infections. The first antiviral drug to be approved for treating HIV, ***zidovudine*** **(AZT)**, is also a nucleoside analogue.

An improved knowledge of the action of reverse transcriptase has led to better nucleoside analogues to treat HIV infections. One of these drugs, **Lamivudine,** has been approved to treat hepatitis B, which uses reverse transcriptase as part of its replication process. Researchers have gone further and developed inhibitors that do not look like nucleosides, but can still block reverse transcriptase.

Another target being considered for HIV antivirals include **RNase H** - which is a component of reverse transcriptase that splits the synthesized DNA from the original viral RNA.

The prodrug **deoxyacyclovir** is more readily absorbed from the GI tract than acyclovir. Another similar antiviral purine nucleoside analog is **ganciclovir, a synthetic guanine** that is effective against human cytomegalovirus. Its mechanism of action is similar to that of acyclovir.

Ribavirin is a synthetic triazole nucleoside (an **analog of guanosine**) with a broad spectrum of activity against many RNA and DNA viruses, both in vitro and in vivo. Susceptible viruses include adenoviruses, herpesviruses, orthomyxoviruses, paramyxoviruses, poxviruses, picornaviruses, rhabdoviruses, rotaviruses, and retroviruses. Viral resistance to ribavirin is rare. The action of ribavirin involves specific inhibition of viral-associated enzymes, inhibition of the capping of viral mRNA, and inhibition of viral polypeptide synthesis. It is well absorbed, widely distributed in the body, eliminated by renal and biliary routes as both parent drug and metabolites, and has a plasma half-life of 24 hr in humans. It does not have a wide margin of safety in domestic animals. Toxicity is manifest by anorexia, weight loss, bone marrow depression and anemia, and GI disturbances. It has been successfully administered by topical, parenteral, oral, and aerosol routes. Efficacy depends on the site of infection, method of treatment, age of the animal, and the infecting dose of virus. Results of human influenza studies with ribavirin have been equivocal.

Zidovudine (azidothymidine, AZT) is a **thymidine analog**. Within the virus-infected cell, the 3¢-azido group is used by retroviral reverse transcriptase and incorporated into DNA transcription, preventing viral replication. The shared mechanism of action is inhibition of RNA-dependent DNA polymerase (**reverse transcriptase**). This enzyme is responsible for conversion of the viral RNA genome into double-stranded DNA before it is integrated into the cell genome. Because these actions occur early in replication, the drugs tend to be effective for acute infections but are relatively ineffective for chronically infected cells. Cellular á-DNA polymerases are inhibited only at concentrations 100-fold greater than those necessary to inhibit reverse transcriptase, thus rendering this drug relatively safe to host cells. Cellular ã-DNA polymerase, however, is inhibited at lower concentrations.

AZT is effective against a variety of retroviruses at low concentrations. Resistance to AZT is associated with point mutations resulting in amino acid substitutions in the reverse transcriptase. Prolonged use of AZT can facilitate viral resistance. The risk of resistance also appears to correlate with CD4 cell count and the state of infection. Viral susceptibility to AZT may return after the drug has been discontinued for a period of time. Little information regarding the disposition of AZT is available in animals. Granulocytopenia and anemia are the major adverse effects of AZT in human patients. The risk of toxicity increases in human patients with low (CD4) lymphocyte counts, high doses, and prolonged therapy. Granulocyte colony-stimulating factor is indicated for management of granulocytopenia. CNS side effects are more likely as therapy is begun. The risk of **myelosuppression** is increased by drugs that inhibit glucuronidation or renal excretion and may be increased in cats.

Studies in cats regarding the efficacy of AZT (10-20 mg/kg, bid for 42 days) for feline leukemia virus infection indicated that AZT prevents retroviral infection if administered immediately after viral exposure and may reduce replication if administered to previously infected animals. Serum-neutralizing antibodies developed in some of the infected cats, and the cats became resistant to subsequent viral challenge. There was no altered progression of disease in cats when treatment was withheld until 28 days after infection, although the level of viremia was much lower than in untreated cats. AZT appeared to be nontoxic in uninfected cats, although 3 of 12 infected kittens became anorectic and icteric and were vomiting after 40 days of treatment. AZT may cause Heinz body anemia. CBC should be performed on cats receiving AZT.

Several drug classes continue to be investigated mainly because of their in vitro antiviral activities. Their potential clinical usefulness remains obscure in most instances. Included among these agents are **thiosemicarbazones, guanidine, benzimidazoles, arildone, phosphonoacetic acid, rifamycins and other antibiotics,** and several natural products.

Transcription: Once a virus genome becomes operational in a host cell, it then generates messenger RNA (mRNA) molecules that direct the synthesis of viral proteins. Production of mRNA is initiated by proteins known as transcription factors. Several antivirals are now being designed to block attachment of transcription factors to viral DNA.

Translation / antisense drugs: Genomics has not only helped find targets for many antivirals, it has provided the basis for an entirely new type of drug, based on "antisense" molecules. These are segments of DNA or RNA that are designed as complementary molecule to critical sections of viral genomes, and the binding of these antisense segments to these target sections **blocks the operation of those genomes.** A **phosphorothioate antisense drug named fomivirsen** has been introduced, used to treat opportunistic eye infections in AIDS patients caused by cytomegalovirus, and other antisense antivirals are in development. An antisense structural type that has proven especially valuable in research is **morpholino antisense.** Morpholino oligos have been used to experimentally suppress many viral types: caliciviruses, flaviviruses (including WNV), dengue, HCV, & coronaviruses.

Translation / ribozymes: Yet another antiviral technique inspired by genomics is a set of drugs based on ribozymes, which are enzymes that will cut apart viral RNA or DNA at selected sites. In their natural course, ribozymes are used as part of the viral manufacturing sequence, but **these synthetic ribozymes are designed to cut RNA and DNA at sites that will disable them.**

A ribozyme antiviral to deal with hepatitis C has been suggested, and ribozyme antivirals are being developed to deal with HIV. An interesting variation of this idea is the use of genetically modified cells that can produce custom-tailored ribozymes. This is part of a broader effort to create genetically modified cells that can be injected into a host to attack pathogens by generating specialized proteins that block viral replication at various phases of the viral life cycle.

Protease inhibitors: Some viruses include an enzyme known as a protease that cuts viral protein chains apart so they can be assembled into their final configuration. HIV includes a protease, and so considerable research has been performed to find "protease inhibitors" to attack HIV at that phase of its life cycle. Protease inhibitors became available in the 1990s and have proven effective, though they can have unusual side effects, for example causing fat to build up in unusual places. Improved protease inhibitors are now in development.

Protease inhibitors have also been seen in nature. A protease inhibitor was isolated from the **Shiitake mushroom** (Lentinus edodes). The presence of this may explain the Shiitake mushrooms noted antiviral activity in vitro.

Assembly:Rifampicin acts at the assembly phase.

Release phase: The final stage in the life cycle of a virus is the release of completed viruses from the host cell, and this step has also been targeted by antiviral drug developers. Two drugs named **zanamivir (Relenza) and oseltamivir (Tamiflu)** that have been recently introduced to treat influenza prevent the release of viral particles by blocking a molecule named neuraminidase that is found on the surface of flu viruses, and also seems to be constant across a wide range of flu strains.

Vaccination Schedule against Viral Diseases in Animals

Cattle Vaccination Schedule

Maintaining an effective animal health program is an essential part of a successful dairy enterprise. Good animal health is vital for maximum production since cattle must be healthy to reach their performance potential. Dairy cows need to be healthy to obtain maximum benefits from good feeding. Recommended dairy cattle vaccination programs depend upon the type of operation and the area of vaccination.

Livestock are vaccinated to reduce the economic losses associated with disease. It is usually less expensive to prevent than treat a disease. Many effects of diseases are obvious, such as abortion, diarrhea and respiratory disease. Most diseases can be subtle, showing no outward signs, but can significantly reduce efficiency of production. Vaccination is a tool that can be used very effectively to help reduce the incidence of disease in a cow herd. As with all tools, vaccinations must be administered correctly to get the full benefit. Proper timing, route of administration, dosage, and type of vaccine are paramount to preventing disease. Beef quality assurance guidelines should be followed whenever vaccines or medications are administered.

Vaccination stimulates the animal's immune system to produce protective antibodies that will help eliminate the invading disease organisms from the animal's body. There are many vaccine products available on the market. Most of the products on the market today are high quality and should work well if they are used properly. If the vaccine is purchased over the counter, make sure to read the enclosed instructions regarding the disease organisms that the product contains and how the product should be administered.

Preventing Disease in the Cow and Passing Immunity to Calves

Some cow vaccinations are given to protect the cow from diseases that affect her directly. Other vaccines are given to develop immunity in her unborn calf, which later protects it from diseases such as rotavirus, coronavirus agents that cause scours in newborn calves. The need for specific vaccinations of this type may vary depending on the disease prevalence in a given area and the age of the calf when a disease will potentially occur. A third category of vaccines affect the cow directly by preventing disease and affect the calf indirectly by preventing abortion. Examples of diseases these vaccines protect against are viral diseases like infectious bovine rhinotracheitis (IBR) and bovine viral diarrhea (BVD).

The most common vaccines on the market are either killed or modified-live. In general, most killed vaccines must be administered twice, two to four weeks apart. It takes approximately four to six weeks after the initial vaccination before the animal's body will be able to respond to exposure to disease. A modified-live vaccine contains the disease organism that has been altered so that it may reproduce but not make the animal sick. The animal can respond to a modified-live vaccine more quickly and only one vaccination is required. Modified-live vaccines are not recommended for pregnant animals since they may give the animal a mild case of the disease and potentially lead to abortion in pregnant cows. Yearly boosters are usually recommended for both modified-live and killed vaccines. There are many new products on the market that are exceptions with regard to frequency of administration. It is critical to read the instructions carefully and follow them.

The age of the animal and its state of production are also considered. Prior to two months of age, the calf's immune system is immature and cannot respond very well to vaccination. In addition to this, if the calf has received adequate colostrum, the protective antibodies in the milk may actually interfere with a good response to vaccination. Except for scours or the rare outbreak of a respiratory disease, the best time to begin vaccinating calves is **after three months of age.** Most dairy producers will vaccinate **heifer calves at four to six months of age, then boost annually.**

Reproductively cows and bulls will be at highest risk for reproductive diseases prior to and during the breeding season. A specific time span is needed to develop protection once the animal has been vaccinated. Vaccination of breeding animals **30 to 60 days prior to breeding season** would be optimal for the prevention of reproductive diseases. The best protection against diseases that affect the newborn calf can be found in the colostrum or "first milk." Vaccination of the cow 30 to 60 days prior to calving will help with the production of high quality colostrum.

Table 6.5 : Vaccination schedule against viral diseases in cattle

Family/virus	Vaccine	Vaccine schedule	Revaccination
Herpesviridae/ IBR	Combined vac for IBR, BVD & PI3; & marker vac for IBR are available	Vaccination at 4-6 and 12-16 months.	Yearly
Flaviviridae/BVD	Do	Vaccination at 4-6 and 12-16 months.	Yearly
Parmyxoviridae/ PI 3	Do	Parainfluenza-3 (PI3)	Yearly
IBR-BVD-PI3	Intranasal vaccine-live attenuated	Intranasal IBR & PI3 at 1-2 wks; repeat with BVD at 4-6 mths and 12-16 mths.	As required
Herpesviridae/Resp iratory syncytial virus (BRSV)	Live attenuated	Vaccination at 4-6 and 12-16 months	Yearly
Picornaviridae/ FMD	Bovilis FMDV Clovax (MVDV O, A, Asia1), BEI inactivated, concentrated, emulsified in mineral oil.	At 4 wks, 1 booster after 6 mths.	Yearly
Reoviridae/Rotavir us diarrhea	Inactivated vaccine	Vaccinate heifers (twice 30 days before calving)	Each pregnancy

Coronaviridae /Coronavirus diarrhea	Inactivated vaccine	Do	Each pregnancy
IP3, reovirus, adenoviruses	Inactivated vaccine	6 weeks, 3 months & 7 months	Yearly
Rhabdoviridae/ Rabies	Defendor-3 (Pfizer), contin uous, DAPPR (Intervet) & RABVAC3 (Fort Dodge)	3 months, yearly	Three yearly

Vaccination Schedule in Sheep & Goats

Vaccinations are an integral part of a flock health management program. They provide cheap insurance against viral diseases that commonly affect sheep and goats. To confer passive immunity to lambs and kids through the colostrum, ewes and does should be vaccinated 2 to 4 weeks prior to parturition. Females giving birth for the first time should be vaccinated twice in late pregnancy, about four weeks apart.

Maternal antibodies will protect lambs and kids for about two months, if offsprings have ingested adequate colostrum. Lambs/kids should receive their first vaccination when they are 6 to 8 weeks old, followed by a booster 2 to 4 weeks later.

Lambs and kids whose dams were not vaccinated can be vaccinated with some success at two to three days of age and again in two weeks. However, later vaccinations will be more successful since colostral antibodies interfere with vaccinations at very young ages.

A better alternative may be to vaccinate offspring from non-vaccinated dams at 1 to 3 weeks, with a booster 3 to 4 weeks later. Lambs and kids whose dams were not vaccinated should be given vaccine at the time of docking, castrating, and disbudding, especially if elastrator bands are used. Rams and bucks should be boostered annually.

There is a vaccine for sore mouth (contagious ecthyma, orf), a viral skin disease commonly affecting sheep and goats. It is a live vaccine that causes sore mouth lesions at a location (on the animal) and time of the producer's choosing. Ewes should be vaccinated well in advance of lambing. To use the vaccine, a woolless area on the animal is scarified, and the re-hydrated vaccine is applied to the spot with a brush or similar applicator. Ewes can be vaccinated inside the ear or under the tail. Lambs can be vaccinated inside the thigh.

Because the sore mouth vaccine is a "live" vaccine and sore mouth is highly contagious to humans, care must be taken when applying the vaccine. Gloves should be used. Flocks which are free from sore mouth should probably not be vaccinated because the vaccine will introduce the virus to the flock/ premises. Once sore mouth vaccination is begun, it should be continued yearly. Though the risk to sheep and goats is usually minimal, rabies vaccination may be considered if the flock is located in a rabies-infected area and livestock have access to wooded areas or areas frequented by raccoons, skunks, foxes, or other known carriers of rabies. Frequent interaction with livestock may be another reason to consider vaccinating.

Table 6.6 : Vaccination schedule against viral diseases in sheep & goats

Family/disease	Vaccine	Vaccine schedule	Revaccination
Reoviridae/Bluetongue	Polyvalent live attenuated	At 3-6 mths-two doses at 3 weeks interval	Yearly
Poxviridae/Sheeppox	Live attenuated	At 3 months of age	2 years
Poxviridae/Orf virus	Live attenuated	At 2-3 months of age	none
Picornaviridae/FMD	Inactivated	At 3-4 mnth of age, booster after 6 mnths	Yearly
Paramyxoviridae/ Peste Des Petits Ruminants	Live attenuated freeze dried vaccine	1ml sc	-

Table 6.7 : Vaccination schedule against viral diseases in pigs

Family/disease	Vaccine	Vaccine schedule	Revaccination
Herpesviridae/Pseudo rabies	Attenuated	All ages 2 injection at 4 wk intervals	6 months
Parvoviviridae/Porcine parvovirus		Two doses at 4 wk intervals before mating	Before mating
Circoviridae/PCV2	Porcilis PCV2 (Intervet) Inactivated baculovirus expressed PCV2 protein; adjuvanted Suvaxyn (FD)	Piglets 2-4 weeks	One injection each gestation

Flaviviridae/ Hog cholera	Attenuated, polyvalent	At 8 wk age	None
Picornaviridae/Porcine encephalomyocarditis	Killed vaccine	At 4 wk age	6 months
Picornaviridae /Porcine enterovirus	Inactivated vaccine	A vaccine is used to control the disease.	-
Coronaviridae/ transmissible porcine gastroenteritis	Inactivated, attenuated & recombinant vaccines are available	Killed vaccine to sow orally before furrowing or SC/IM subunit vaccine protects piglets with clostral Abs till weaning.	Before furrowing
Reoviridae/Porcine rotavirus	Inactivated vaccine used	Protects from diarrhea	Before furrowing
Arteriviridae/Porcine reproductive & respiratory syndrome	Attenuated/inac tivated vaccines are used	Piglets at 3 wks or sows and gilts 3-6 wks prior to breeding.	Before furrowing
Orthomyxoviridae/ swine influenza	Inactivated vaccine	Two doses at 4 wks interval	yearly

Vaccination schedule against viral diseases in horses: The schedule below is a suggested vaccination schedule and is based on generally accepted veterinary practices. Infectious disease control programs in conjunction with vaccinations are important in maximizing the health, productivity and performance of your horse. Schedules for stallions should be consistent with the vaccination program of the adult horse population on the farm and modified according to risk.

Vaccination schedule in dogs & cats against viral diseases

Vaccination plays an important role in maintaining the health and well-being of animals. The introduction of modified live vaccines has greatly reduced the incidence of several canine and feline diseases that are often fatal.

Here, we discuss issues relating to use of 'core vaccines' in dogs and cats. The term 'core vaccines' is used to refer to vaccines that protect animals from severe, life-threatening diseases that have world-wide distribution. Non-core vaccines are required by only those animals that are at risk from those specific diseases, due to their geographic location, local environment or lifestyle.

Table 6.8 : Vaccination schedule against viral diseases in horses

Family/disease	Vaccine	Vaccine schedule	Revaccination
Herpesviridae/equine abortion vius1EqHV1	Attenuated vaccine	At 3 mths-3 doses with 2 & 6 mnths interval	yearly
Herpesviridae/equine abortion vius EqHV1+ E qHV4	Killed vaccine	At 10 wk age; 3 doses with 1 6 mths intervals	Yearly
Arteriviridae/Equine areritis virus	Attenuated vaccine	Colts intended to be breeding stallions: One dose at 6 to 12 months of age	yearly
Reoviridae/ African horse sickness virus	Attenuated polyvalent vaccine	At 6-8 mths of age	2-3 years
Togaviridae/Eastern, Western & Venezuelan viruses	Attenuated	First dose: 3-4 months, Second dose: 4-5 months Third dose: 5-6 months	Annual spring
Flaviviridae/West Nile virus	PROTEQ-FLU (European Union), Recombitek (United States)	First dose: 3-4 months Second dose: 1 month later (plus 3rd dose at 6 months in areas at risk)	Annual in areas of risk
Orthomyxoviridae /Equine influenza viruses	Inactivated vaccine	First dose: 6 months Second dose: 7 months Third dose: 8 months, then at 3-month intervals.	Annual or at the time of risk.
Rabies	Inactivated vaccine	Foals born to non-vaccinated mares: First dose: 3 to 4 months Second dose: 12 months. Foals born to vaccinated mares: First dose: 6 months, Second dose 7 months, Third dose: 12 months	2-3 yr interval

Vaccination regimes for dogs and cats have developed from years of research and practical experience by veterinarians in industry and in practice.

Current vaccination programs for dogs and cats recognize that most pups and kittens are protected by maternally derived antibodies (MDA) up to about 8 to 12 weeks of age. For strong immunity, it is important that the animal receives at least two fully effective vaccinations. MDA can interfere with vaccination, but it is advisable to vaccinate young animals as soon as MDA levels decline. Because the decline in the level of MDA varies between animals, three initial vaccinations are generally recommended, timed to ensure that the animal is fully protected.

A typical puppy/kitten program consists of an initial primary course of vaccination followed by a 12-month booster to ensure ongoing immunity. Subsequent revaccinations are given at intervals of 12 months, or longer if this is consistent with the manufacturer recommendations. There are several registered products on the market that have been formulated specifically as longer-term vaccines and proven to provide at least 3 years protection. Apart from these, all other dog vaccines, and all cat vaccines, have been registered with data that support only a 12-month vaccination interval.

Table 6.9 : Vaccination schedule against viral diseases in dogs

Family/disease	Vaccine	Vaccine schedule	Revaccination
Adenoviridae/infectious canine hepatitis virus 1 & 2	Live attenuated CAV2 givs protection to both CAV1 & CAV2; mixed with CDV, CPV & canine parainfluenza vaccines, e.g. DA2 PPV & DA2PPVL+CV.	Puppies 6-**12 week old,** usually mixed with the CDV, CPV& canine parainflueza virus within the first months of life.	Yearly
Parvoviridae/ canine parvovirus	Attenuated live vaccine, singly or with multivalent Pfizer's DHPP (distemper, hepatitis, parainfluenza, parvovirus) vaccine.	At 8 wk Ist DHPP, 11-12 wk or after 3-4 wk-2nd DHPP & 14-15 wk or after 3-4 wk final DHPP	One to three years intervals
Paramyxoviridae/ canine distemper	Do	Do	Do
Parainfluenza virus 3	Do	Do	Do
Coronaviridae/ Canine coronavirus	Killed vaccine	9-16 wk, 3 doses at 3 wk intervals	Yearly
Rabies	Killed vaccine	20 weeks or older, then 1 yr later	Every 2-3 yr

Table 6.10 : Vaccination schedule against viral diseases in cats

Family/disease	Vaccine	Vaccine schedule	Revaccination
Parvoviridae/ feline panlekopenia	Live attenuated with multivalent FVCRP (Feline rhinotracheitis, feline calicivirus & feline panleukopenia) vaccine.	3 shots; at 8-9 wk Ist FVRCP, at 12-13 wk-2nd FVRCP & at 14-15 wk final FVRCP.	Yearly
Herpesviridae/ Feline rhinotracheitis FHV1)	Do	Do	Do
Caliciviridae/ feline calcivirus	Do	Do	Do
Retroviridae/Feline leukemia virus	Subunit vaccine	At 9 wk, 2 doses at 3-15 wk intervals	Yearly
Rabies	Merial Purevac	12 wk or older, then 1 yr later	Yearly or every 3 yr

Table 6.11 : Vaccination schedule against viral diseases in poultry

Family/disease	Vaccine	Vaccine schedule	Revaccination
Broilers			
Paramyxoviridae/N DV/RDV	Live attenuated/ avirulent F or K	1-7 days/ oculonasal	
Coronaviridae/Infect ious bronchitis	Do	3-4 wks in drinking water	
Birnaviridae/Infectio us bursal diseae	Do	18-21 days in drinking water	
Herpesviridae/ Marek's disease	Do	3 days before hatching in ovo/5-10 days or 18-21 days in drinking water.	
Broilers/ layers/breeders			
Herpesviridae/ Marek's disease	Do	Day 1-IM	
Paramyxoviridae/N DV/RDV		Day 1, 3 weeks IM, then on 1-7days oculonasal, 3-4 wks, 8 wks, 16-18 wks, 40th wks in drinking water	

Coronaviridae/Infectious bronchitis	3 week, 8 weeks, 14-16 weeks in drinking water
Birnaviridae/Infectious bursal diseae	3 weeks, 16 weeks in drinking water
Poxviridae/Fowl pox	6-8 week, 18-20 weeks (Prick)
Avian encephalomyelitis	Drinking virus
Egg drop syndrome virus	3 week in drinking water
ILT	16 week IM
Turkey breeders	
NDV	3 wks, 6 wk in drinking water, & 12 wk, & 24 wk IM
Paramyxovirus 3	At 12 wk & 244 wk IM
Duck viruses	
Duck plague	9 wks SC, 14-18 wks IM, 14 wks eye drop
Duck hepatitis	2-4 wks, 8 wks & 16 wks IM or SC

Table 6.12 : Broiler Breeder Vaccination Program (Intervet Schering Plough Animal Health)

Age	Disease	Vaccine strain	Route	Vaccine
Hatchery	Marek's	HVT+SB1	SC/in ovo	
	Marek's+LT	HVT+SB1+LT	SC/in ovo	Innovax®-ILT-SB
	Marek's+ND	HVT+ND	SC/in ovo	Innovax-ND
	Marek's+ND	HVT+SB1+ND	SC/in ovo	Innovax®-ND-SB
	Marek's	Rispens	SC/in ovo	Rismavac®
		HVT/Rispens Strain	SC/in ovo	Ris-Ma®
	IBD	Classic Mild Strain	SC/in ovo	Univax-BD®
		Variant Strain	SC/in ovo	89/03®
	Reovirus	2177 Strain	SC	2177®
	Coccidiosis		Spray	Coccivac®-D
2 weeks	ND, IBV	B1 Type, B1 Strain, Mass/Conn	Water/Spray	Triplevac®

		B1 Type, B1 Strain, Mass/Ark	Spray	Trivac-Ark®
		B1 Type, LaSota Strain-Mass Type/Holland	Water/Eyedrop	Broilerbron®-H N-79
	IBD	Classic Mild Strain	Water	Univax®-BD
		Cloned Intermediate Strain	Water	Clonevac® D-78
		Blend of 2 Intermediate Strains	Water	Univax® Plus
		Classic Strain	Water	Bursa-Vac®
	Reovirus	1133 Strain	Water	Enterovax®
3-4 weeks	IBD	Classic Mild Strain	Water	Univax-BD
		Cloned Intermediate Strain	Water/Spray	Clonevac D-78
		Blend of 2 Intermediate Strains	Water	Univax Plus
	Reovirus	1133 Strain	Water	Enterovac
5 weeks	ND/IBV	B1 Type, B1 Strain, Mass/Conn	Water/Spray	Triplevac
		B1 Type, LaSota Strain, Mass/Conn	Spray	Combovac-30
		B1 Type, B1 Strain, Mass/Ark	Water/eye drop	Trivac-Ark
		B1 Type, LaSota Strain-Mass Type/Holland	Water/eye drop	Broilerbron-H N-79
		B1 Type, LaSota Strain, Mass/Conn	Water	Polybron® N-63
	Reovirus	1133 Strain	Water	Interovac
6-8 weeks	Reovirus	1133 Strain	Water	Enterovax
	IBD	Classic Mild Strain	Water/Spray	Univax-BD
		Cloned Intermediate Strain	Water	Clonevac D-78
		Blend of 2 Intermediate Strains	Water	Univax Plus
10 weeks	AE/Fowl Pox	Calnek Strain of AE U.S. Field Isolate	Wing web	Tremvac-FP

	CAV	U.S. Field Isolate	Wing-web	CAV-VAC®
	LT	Live Virus, TCO	Eye drop	LT-Ivax®
		Live Virus, CEO	Water/eye drop	Trachivax®
	Fowl cholera	PM-1	Wing-web	PM-Onevax®-C
		M-9 Strain, Heddleston Type 3-4 Cross	Wing-web	M-Ninevax®-C
	IBD/REO	IBD-Standard, Delaware A & E, GLS REO-1733 & 2408	IM/SC	BreederVac-Reo-Plus®
		Clostridium Perfringens Type A	IM/SC	Clostridium Perfringens Type A, Toxoid
15 weeks	ND/IBV	B1 Strain, Mass/Conn	Water/Spray	Triplevac
		B1 Type, LaSota Strain	Water/Spray	Combovac-30
		B1 Type, B1 Strain, Ark	Spray	Trivac-Ark
		B1 Type, LaSota Strain-Mass Type/Holland	Water/eye drop	Broilerbron-H N-79
		B1 Type, LaSota Strain, Mass/Conn	Water	Polybron N-63
18-20 weeks	Fowl Cholera	PM-1	Wing web	PM-Onevax-C
		M-9 Strain, Heddleston Type 3-4 Cross	Wing web	M-Ninevax-C
	IBD/Reo	IBD-Standard, Delaware A & E, GLS REO-1733 & 2408	IM/SC	BreederVac-Reo-Plus
		IBD-Standard, Delaware E, GLS, & AL-2 REO-1733 & 2408	IM	Bursamate-Plus®
	IBD/Reo/ND/IBV	IBD-Standard, Delaware E, GLS, & AL-2 REO-1733 & 2408 NDV & IB (Mass Type)	IM/SC	BreederVac-IV-Plus®
		Clostridium Perfringens Type A	IM/SC	Clostridium Perfringens Type A, toxoid
		Respiratory Vaccination		

2 & 5 weeks	Arkansas	Spray	Mildvac®-Ark
	Delaware 072	Water/Spray	Shor-Bron®-D
	Georgia 98	Spray	Mildvac-GA-98™

The use of BreederVac-IV-Plus is recommended when the progeny is given recombinant ND vaccine.

Mildvac-Ark, Shor-Bron-D, and Mildvac-GA-98 can be included in the vaccination program if these variant strains of IB have been identified as a problem.

□□□

Chapter 7

Laboratory Diagnosis of Viral Infections

Contents

In general, viral diagnostic tests can be grouped into 3 categories:

1. direct detection,
2. indirect examination (virus isolation), and
3. serology

In direct examination, the clinical specimen is examined directly for the presence of virus particles, virus antigen or viral nucleic acids. In indirect examination, the specimen is inoculated into cell culture, eggs or animals to grow the virus: this is called virus isolation. Serology constitutes by far the bulk of the work of any virology laboratory. A serological diagnosis can be made by the detection of rising titres of antibody between acute and convalescent stages of infection, or the detection of IgM. In general, the majority of common viral infections can be diagnosed by serology. The specimen used for direction detection and virus isolation is very important. A positive result from the site of disease would be of much greater diagnostic significance than those from other sites. For example, in the case of herpes simplex encephalitis, a positive result from the CSF or the brain would be much greater significance than a positive result from an oral ulcer, since reactivation of oral herpes is common during times of stress.

1. Direct Examination of Spcimen

i. Electron Microscopy for morphology/immune electron microscopy
ii. Light microscopy- histological appearance - e.g. inclusion bodies
iii. Antigen detection- immunofluorescence, ELISA etc.
iv. Molecular techniques for the direct detection of viral genomes

2. Indirect Examination

i. Cell Culture - cytopathic effect, haemadsorption, confirmation by neutralization, interference, immunofluorescence etc.
ii. Eggs pocks on CAM - haemagglutination, inclusion bodies
iii. Animals disease or death confirmation by neutralization.

3. Serology

Detection of rising titres of antibody between acute and convalescent stages of infection, or the detection of IgM in primary infection.

Classical Techniques	Newer Techniques
i. Complement fixation tests (CFT)	1. Radioimmunoassay (RIA)
ii. Haemagglutination inhibition tests	2. Enzyme linked immunosorbent assay (EIA)
iii. Immunofluorescence techniques (IF)	3. Particle agglutination
iv. Neutralization tests	4. Western Blot (WB)
v. Single Radial Haemolysis	5. Recombinant immunoblot assay (RIBA), line immunoassay (Liatek) etc.

Direct Examination

Direct examination methods are often also called rapid diagnostic methods because they can usually give a result either within the same or the next day. This is extremely useful in cases when the clinical management of the patient depends greatly on the rapid availability of laboratory results e.g. diagnosis of RSV infection in neonates, or severe CMV infections in immuno-compromised patients. However, it is important to realize that not all direct examination methods are rapid, and conversely, virus isolation and serological methods may sometimes give a rapid result. With the advent of effective antiviral chemotherapy, rapid diagnostic methods are expected to play an increasingly important role in the diagnosis of viral infections.

Electron Microscopy (EM)

Virus particles are detected and identified on the basis of morphology. A magnification of around 50,000 is normally used. EM is now mainly used for the diagnosis of viral gastroenteritis by detecting viruses in feces e.g. rotavirus, adenovirus, astrovirus, calicivirus and Norwalk-like viruses, coronaviruses, and parvoviruses. Occasionally it may be used for the detection of viruses in vesicles and other skin lesions, such as herpesviruses, poxviruses and papillomaviruses. The sensitivity and specificity of EM may be enhanced by immune electron microscopy, whereby virus specific antibody is used to agglutinate virus particles together and thus making them easier to recognize, or to capture virus particles onto the EM grid. The main problem with EM is the expense involved in purchasing and maintaining the facility. One drawback is that at least 10^5 to 10^6 virus particles per ml in the sample are required for visualization. Therefore the observer must be highly skilled. In the technique of negative contrast EM, distilled water lysates of clinical specimens are "stained" with a solution of heavy atoms. Specimen preparation and EM examination usually can be completed within 30 minutes. With the availability of reliable antigen detection and molecular methods for the detection of viruses associated with viral gastroenteritis, EM is becoming less widely used.

Light Microscopy

Replicating virus often produce histological changes in infected cells, called cytopathic effects. These changes may be characteristic or non-specific. Viral inclusion bodies are basically collections of replicating virus particles either in the nucleus or cytoplasm. Examples of inclusion bodies include the Nnegri bodies and cytomegalic inclusion bodies found in rabies and CMV infections respectively. Although not sensitive or specific, histology serves as a useful adjunct in the diagnosis of certain viral infections.

Antigen Detection

Immunoflurescence test

Viral antigen detection includes immunofluorescence testing of nasopharyngeal aspirates for respiratory viruses e.g.. RSV, flu A, flu B, and adenoviruses, detection of rotavirus antigen in feces, the pp65 CMV antigenaemia test, the detection of HSV and VZV in skin scrapings, and the detection of HBsAg in serum. The fluorescent antibody (FA) test detects viral antigens in infected cells with specific antiviral antibody that has been labeled with a fluorescent dye (fluorescein isothiocyanate). FA tests are performed on frozen sections of tissues, blood smears, tissue imprints, scrapings or in cell cultures. Results are available often in less than one hour, and they are accurate provided that the antibody is specific and specimens are in moderately good condition.

Two types of FA techniques exist: **direct FA and indirect FA**. In the direct FA test, the antiviral antibody is labeled, & the labeled antibody is then used to detect viral antigens in cryostat sections of tissues, scrapings, blood smears, etc. In indirect FA test, either the sample is first reacted with an unlabeled antiviral antibody, incubated for antigen-antibody interaction-for one hour, the sample is washed and then incubated with a labeled antibody directed against IgG of the species against which unlabeled antiviral antibody was prepared. The labeled anti-antibody will attach itself to the viral-bound unlabeled antibody, & fluorescence is observed and the test is considered positive.

Direct FA test is quicker to perform and there is availability of direct FA conjugates. Indirect FA test is more sensitive and specific, & only one labeled antibody is required if all antiviral antibodies are prepared in a single species. FA test is the most useful test for routine viral diagnosis because several FA conjugates are available for detecting viruses; Conjugates for detecting viruses of dogs, cats & other animals are available commercially.

Another FA test, Immunofluorescence test is used to detect and measure antibody in which cell cultures with a virus, is infected and then spot microscope slides is prepared with these infected cells. Specific sera are then tested for specific antibody by reacting them with the infected cells followed by a reaction with the anti-species IgG conjugate. Those spots that fluoresce indicate sera that are positive for the presence of specific antibodies.

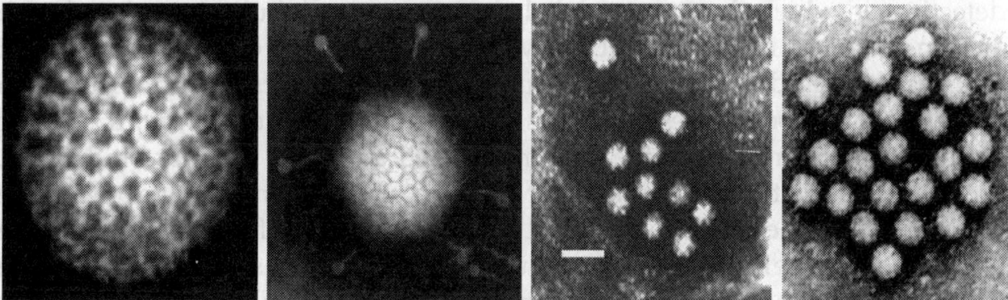

Figure 7.1 : Electronmicrographs of viruses commonly found in stool specimens from patients suffering from gastroenteritis. From left to right: rotavirus, adenovirus, astroviruses, Norwalk-like viruses. (Courtesy of Linda M. Stannard, University of Cape Town).

Immunoperoxidase

The immunoperoxidase technique is used to detect viral antigen in clinical materials and cell cultures; it is similar to the FA test. But in this case the antibody is conjugated to an enzyme (horseradish peroxidase or alkaline phosphatase) rather than to a fluorescent compound. The enzyme is bound to the antibody, but it remains active and, when provided with its substrate, reacts and gives a color reaction. This test has the benifit that it does not require a fluorescence microscope, and it is especially useful for locating viral antigens in histopathologic lesions.

Enzyme-linked immunosorbent assay (ELISA)

ELISA assays allow the detection of viral antigen or antibody, using a solid-phase assay system. For **antigen capture** ELISA (in which virus protein is measured), a solid matrix (plastic dish, polystyrene tube, microtiter plate) specific antibody is first adsorbed to the surface of a polystyrene tube, microtiter plate. The virus-containing test sample (e.g., supernatant from a virally-infected cell culture) is then added to the well. After allowing time for the protein to bind to the antibody, the well is washed and a second antibody is then added. This detection antibody is also specific for the virus protein being assayed, and it has an indicator molecule attached to it to allow for quantitative analysis of binding. If the virus is present, it binds to the adsorbed antibody. After washing, specific antiviral antibody labeled with an enzyme (usually alkaline phosphatase or horseradish peroxidase) is added. The labeled antibody reacts with the complex, creating a "sandwich effect". Following washing, the substrate for the enzyme is added, resulting in a color reaction. In some tests visual interpretation is done, but greater sensitivity is obtained by spectrophotometric analysis.

Different variations of ELISA include **competitive ELISA** for antibody detection, in which the enzyme labeled anti-gammaglobulin is replaced with enzyme-labeled antiviral antibody. The subsequent color development following the addition of the enzyme substrate is inversely proportional to the level of antibody present in the test sample. In other words, if specific antibody has been bound, the enzyme-labeled antibody will not bind. Thus, positive tests are those with no color reaction or less than that of appropriate controls. The **kinetic ELISA** is used for the detection of antibody to canine Lyme disease, feline leukemia virus, feline infectious peritonitis, feline toxoplasmosis, and bovine herpesvirus 1. In the kinetic ELISA, the reaction is continuously monitored over a period of time, rather than being stopped after a predetermined amount of time.

Latex agglutination (LA)

LA tests are used to detect antigen or antibody & are similar in principle to bacterial agglutination in that latex particles coated with antibody will agglutinate when mixed with the specific antigen and thus identifying it. Alternatively, the latex particles can be coated with antigens and used to detect antibody. These tests are easy to perform and provide results within minutes. Commercial kits for use are available for the detection of antibody to some diseases and for detection of some viruses.

Viral Genome Detection

Techniques based on the detection of viral genome are commonly called as **molecular methods.** It is often said that molecular methods are the future direction of viral diagnosis. However in practice, although the use of these methods is increasing, the role played by molecular methods in a routine diagnostic virus laboratory is still small compared to conventional methods. Classical molecular techniques such as **Dot-blot and Southern-blot** depend on the use of specific DNA/RNA probes for hybridization. The specificity of the reaction depends on the conditions used for hybridization. These techniques may allow for the quantification of DNA/RNA present in the specimen. However, it is often found that the sensitivity of these techniques is not better than conventional viral diagnostic methods.

Nucleic acid detection

Methods for the detection of viral nucleic acids in clinical and laboratory specimens include **Southern blot analysis, in situ hybridization, polymerase chain reaction** (PCR) and the use of **gene arrays**.

Southern blot analysis was developed in the 1970s, and it involves the fractionation of DNA with restriction enzymes, followed by transfer of DNA to a solid membrane support and detection of virus-specific sequences using radio labeled viral nucleic acids. A **Southern blot** is a method routinely used in molecular biology for detection of a specific DNA sequence in DNA samples. Southern blotting combines transfer of electrophoresis-separated DNA fragments to a filter membrane and subsequent fragment detection by probe hybridization. The method is named after its inventor, the British biologist Edwin Southern. Other blotting methods (i.e., Western blot, Northern blot, Eastern blot, South-western blot) that employ similar principles, but using RNA or protein, have later been named in reference to Edwin Southern's name.

Northern blot analysis is an analogous method for the detection of **RNA sequences**. Nucleic acid probes also detect viral sequences within tissues or individual cells, by using **in situ hybridization**. In this case like Southern and Northern hybridization in stead of extracting the nucleic acid and transferring it to a nitrocellulose membrane, intact cells or tissue sections on a microscope slide are probed. This technique has little use in routine diagnostic, yet is very valuable for research and pathogenesis studies.

Dot blot hybridization is like Southern and Northern blot & may be used both to detect DNA and RNA. The nucleic acid in this case is placed onto nitrocellulose in an apparatus that focuses the individual spots into concentrated areas, similar to a microtiter plate.

Restriction enzyme analysis

Restriction enzyme analysis identifies specific viruses using restriction endonucleases to cut the genomic sequences of viruses. Due to mutations and/or genetic variability at potential cleavage sites in some viral strains, it leads to different patterns of fragments when they are separated in an agarose gel. Such analysis is called **restriction fragment length polymorphism (RFLP)** and has been used to characterize and to compare among field isolates of a given virus. Since this technique needs large amounts of purified viral DNA, a set of restriction enzymes to cleave the DNA, the ability to separate the resulting DNA fragments by electrophoresis, and a method of documenting the results. Cleavage of the genome of viruses with large genomes, like cytomegalovirus, may yield 20 to 50 DNA bands, while viruses with smaller genomes, such as adenoviruses, usually yield only five to ten DNA bands. A limitation of the method is that the presence of a mutation cannot be detected unless that mutation happens to fall within the recognition sequence of the restriction endonuclease being used for digestion of the DNA. Also use of different restriction enzymes will optimize the probability of detecting mutations in a particular genome or portion of a genome.

Radioimmunoassay

Radioimmunoassay systems are not usually used in veterinary diagnostic laboratories. The two basic radioimmunoassay (RIA) systems are **liquid phase** and **solid phase**; in liquid phase system, the antigen-antibody complexes are precipitated by subsequent addition of anti-gammaglobulin. The precipitate is collected by centrifugation and dried. The amount of radioactivity in the precipitate compared to the total radioactivity is a quantitative measure of the antigen-antibody reaction. The labeling is done with ^{125}I, and any one of the three components can be labeled.

The solid phase system coats the antibody to the inside of a polystyrene tube and then reacted with antigen. The specimen is added to a polystyrene tube previously coated with antiviral antibody. Given the antigen is present, it attaches to the bound antibody. Following rinsing, ^{125}I labeled antiviral antibody is added, which reacts with the complex giving a "sandwich effect". The tube is washed and the amount of radioactivity is determined.

Polymerase chain reaction (PCR)

PCR is one of the most widely used methods for detection of viral nucleic acids. In this method, specific oligonucleotides are used to amplify fragments of viral nucleic acid from cell or tissue samples. The method uses a thermostable DNA polymerase, and multiple cycles of amplification, which comprise 3 steps: (1) melting of the double-stranded DNA template, (2) annealing of the oligonucleotide primers to the template and (3) extension of the primers by the thermostable DNA polymerase, thus generating new DNA chains. PCR analysis can also be adapted to the analysis of viral RNA, by including an initial step in which the RNA is converted into DNA, using a reverse transcriptase enzyme. This is referred to as reverse transcription **(RT)-PCR.**

Real-Time PCR

Methods for the quantitative analysis of nucleic acids using PCR include real time PCR methods. This involves the direct measurement of the amount of PCR product produced while the reaction is in progress. Mathematical analysis of the data, and comparison to control reactions containing known amounts of template, allow one to then calculate the amount of input DNA in the initial reaction. Real-time PCR analysis is performed by taking advantage of a process known as fluorescence resonance energy transfer (FRET). Real-time PCR, also called quantitative real time polymerase chain reaction (Q-PCR/qPCR/qrt-PCR) or kinetic polymerase chain reaction (KPCR), is a laboratory technique based on the PCR, which is used to amplify and simultaneously quantify a targeted DNA molecule. For one or more specific sequences in a DNA sample, Real Time-PCR enables both detection and quantification. The quantity can be either an absolute number of copies or a relative amount when normalized to DNA input or additional normalizing genes.

The procedure follows the general principle of polymerase chain reaction; its key feature is that the amplified DNA is detected as the reaction progresses in real time. This is a new approach compared to standard PCR, where the product of the reaction is detected at its end. Two common methods for detection of products in real-time PCR are: (1) non-specific fluorescent dyes that intercalate with any double-stranded DNA, and (2) sequence-specific DNA probe consisting of oligonucleotides that are labeled with a fluorescent reporter which permits detection only after hybridization of the probe with its complementary DNA target. Frequently, real-time PCR is combined with reverse transcription to quantify mRNA and Non-coding RNA in cells or tissues.

DNA microassay

A **DNA microarray,** commonly known as **gene chip, DNA chip, or biochip** is a collection of microscopic DNA spots attached to a solid surface. Scientists use DNA microarrays to measure the expression levels of large numbers of genes simultaneously or to genotype multiple regions of a genome. Each DNA spot contains picomoles (10^{-12} moles) of a specific DNA sequence, known as probes (or reporters). These can be a short section of a gene or other DNA element that are used to hybridize a cDNA or cRNA sample (called *target*) under high-stringency conditions. Probe-target hybridization is usually detected and quantified by detection of fluorophore-, silver-, or chemilumiminescence-labeled targets to determine relative abundance of nucleic acid sequences in the target. DNA microassay technology, which is becoming increasingly useful in the analysis of viral infections. In this method, a high density DNA array is generated, comprising millions of different oligonucleotides spotted onto a solid support. Labeled sample DNA (usually biotinylated) is then added to this microarray, and allowed to anneal. After extensive washing, the bound sample DNA is detected using a fluorescent probe (e.g., streptavidin-phycoerythrin). DNA microarray can be used to probe for specific point mutations in the human genome (e.g., disease associated mutations, or mutations associated with enhanced susceptibility to certain viral infections). It can also be used to detect viruses, and even to detect specific mutations within virus populations, for example, mutations associated with resistance to antiviral drugs.

Newer molecular techniques such as the, **ligase chain reaction** (LCR), **nucleic acid based amplification** (NASBA), and **branched DNA** (bDNA) depend on some form of amplification, either the target nucleic acid, or the signal itself. bDNA is essentially a conventional hybridization technique with increased sensitivity. However, it is not as sensitive as PCR and other amplification techniques. PCR is the only amplification technique which is in common use. PCR is an extremely sensitive technique: it is possible to achieve a sensitivity of down to 1 DNA molecule in a clinical specimen. However, PCR has many problems, the main among which is contamination, since only a minute amount of contamination is needed to give a false positive result. In addition, because PCR is so sensitive compared to other techniques, a positive PCR result is often very difficult to interpret as it does not indicate the presence of disease. This problem is particular great **in the case of latent viruses such as CMV**, since latent CMV genomes may be amplified from the blood of healthy individuals. Despite all this, PCR is being increasingly used for viral diagnosis, especially as the cost of the assay comes down and the availability of closed automated systems that could also perform quantification (Quantitative PCR) e.g. real-time PCR and Cobas Amplicor systems. Other amplification techniques such as LCR and NASBA are just as susceptible to contamination as PCR but that is ameliorated to a great extent by the use of proprietary closed systems. It is unlikely though that other amplification technique will challenge the dominance of PCR since it is much easier to set up an house PCR assay than other assays.

Virus Isolation

Cell cultures, eggs, and animals may be used for isolation. However eggs and animals are difficult to handle and most viral diagnostic laboratories depend on cell culture only. There are 3 types of cell cultures: **Primary cells** - e.g. Monkey Kidney. These are essentially normal cells obtained from freshly killed adult animals. These cells can only be passaged once or twice. **Semi-continuous cells** - e.g. Human embryonic kidney and skin fibroblasts. These are cells taken from embryonic tissue, and may be passaged up to 50 times. **Continuous cells** - e.g. HeLa, Vero, Hep2, LLC-MK2, and BGM. These are immortalized cells i.e. tumour cell lines and may be passaged indefinitely.

Primary cell cultures are widely acknowledged as the best cell culture systems available since they support the widest range of viruses. However, they are very expensive and it is often difficult to obtain a reliable supply. Continuous cells are the most easy to handle but the range of viruses supported is often limited.

Identification of Growing Virus

The presence of growing virus is usually detected by: **Cytopathic Effect (CPE)** - may be specific or non-specific e.g. HSV and CMV produces a specific CPE, whereas enteroviruses do not. **Haemadsorption** - cells acquire the ability to stick to mammalian red blood cells. Haemadsorption is mainly used for the detection of influenza and parainfluenzaviruses. Confirmation of the identity of the virus may be carried out using neutralization, haemadsorption-inhibition, immunofluorescence, or molecular tests.

Problems with cell culture

The main problem with cell culture is the long period (up to 4 weeks) required for a result to be available. Also, the sensitivity is often poor and depends on many factors, such as the condition of the specimen, and the condition of the cell sheet. Cell cultures are also very susceptible to bacterial contamination and toxic substances in the specimen. Lastly, many viruses will not grow in cell culture at all e.g. Hepatitis B and C, diarrhoeal viruses, parvovirus etc.

Rapid culture techniques

Rapid culture techniques are available whereby viral antigens are detected 2 to 4 days after inoculation. Examples of rapid culture techniques include shell vial cultures and the CMV DEAFF test. In the CMV DEAFF test, the cell sheet is grown on individual cover slips in a plastic bottle. After inoculation, the bottle then is spun at a low speed for one hour (to speed up the adsorption of the virus) and then incubated for 2 to 4 days. The cover slip is then taken out and examined for the presence of CMV early antigens by immunofluorescence.

The role of cell culture (both conventional and rapid techniques) in the diagnosis of viral infections is being increasingly challenged by rapid diagnostic methods, i.e. antigen detection and molecular methods. Therefore, the role of cell culture is expected to decline in future and is likely to be restricted to large central laboratories.

Serology

Serology forms the mainstay of viral diagnosis. This is what happens in a primary humoral immune response to antigen. Following exposure, the first antibody to appear is IgM, which is followed by a much higher titre of IgG. In cases of reinfection, the level of specific IgM either remains the same or rises slightly. But IgG shoots up rapidly & earlier than in a primary infection. Many different types of serological tests are available. The serologic tests commonly used in veterinary diagnostic laboratories for diagnosis of viral infections are:

serum neutralization (SN) tests; hemagglutination inhibition (HI) tests; agar gel immunodiffusion (AGID) tests and enzyme linked immunosorbent assays (ELISAs). With some assays such as ELISA and RIA, one can look specifically for IgM or IgG, whereas with other assays such as CFT and HAI, one can only detect total antibody, which comprises mainly IgG. Some of these tests are much more sensitive than others: ELISA and radioimmunoassays are the most sensitive tests available, whereas CFT and HAI tests are not so sensitive. Newer techniques such as ELIAs offer better sensitivity, specificity and reproducibility than classical techniques such as CFT and HAI. The sensitivity and specificity of the assays depend greatly on the antigen used. Assays that use recombinant protein or synthetic peptide antigens tend to be more specific than those using whole or disrupted virus particles. Usually, dilutions of serum are made & tested, and results are interpreted as the reciprocal of the highest dilution in which antiviral activity is noted. The results of serum collected during the acute phase of illness are compared with results of serum collected during convalescence- 14 - 21 days apart. Diagnosis is confirmed if a four-fold increase in titers is noted between these paired samples.

Microplate ELISA: coloured wells indicate reactivity. The darker the colour, the higher the reactivity.

Criteria for Diagnosing Primary Infection

A significant rise in titre of IgG/total antibody between acute and convalescent sera - however, a significant rise is very difficult to define and depends greatly on the assay used. In the case of CFT and HAI, it is normally taken as a four-fold or greater increase in titre. The main problem is that diagnosis is usually retrospective because by the time the convalescent serum is taken, the patient had probably recovered.

Presence of IgM - EIA, RIA, and IF may be used for the detection of IgM. This offers a rapid means of diagnosis. However, there are many problems with IgM assays, such as interference by rheumatoid factor, re-infection by the virus, and unexplained persistence of IgM years after the primary infection.

Seroconversion - This is defined as changing from a previously antibody negative state to a positive state e.g. seroconversion against HIV following a needle-stick injury, or against rubella following contact with a known case.

A single high titre of IgG (or total antibody) : This is a very unreliable means of serological diagnosis since the cut-off is very difficult to define.

Criteria for diagnosing re-infection/re-activation

It is often very difficult to differentiate re-infection/ re-activation from a primary infection. Under most circumstances, it is not important to differentiate between a primary infection and re-infection. However, it is very important under certain situations, such as rubella infection in the first trimester of pregnancy: primary infection is associated with a high risk of fetal damage whereas re-infection is not. In general, a sharp large rise in antibody titres is found in re-infection whereas IgM is usually low or absent in cases of re-infection/re-activation.

Virus neutralization

It is a method in which antibodies are added to a virus preparation, and the infectivity of this preparation is then measured using indicator cells. The antibodies produced against any given virus will have the ability to interfere with the interaction between the virus and its host cell receptor. Such antibodies will have the ability to neutralize the infectivity of the virus. Other antibodies may react with the virus, but may fail to prevent it from infecting its target cell. Such antibodies would not have neutralizing activity. Neutralization assays have been very useful in defining **viral serotypes**. For example, poliovirus serotypes were defined serologically, using neutralization assays (i.e., poliovirus type 1 is neutralized by antiserum to type 1 viruses, but not by antiserum to types 2 or 3, and so on). The definition of viral serotypes is a useful tool in terms of classification, and it is also of potential significance in the development of vaccines since one may need to include examples of all the virus serotypes in order to develop an effective vaccine. Thus, both the live-attenuated ("Sabin") and the whole-killed ("Salk") poliovirus vaccines contain mixtures of all three virus serotypes.

Dilutions of test serum are made in microtiter plates, followed by the addition of an equal volume of virus suspension diluted to contain approximately 100 to 300 infective doses (an infectious dose is the minimum number of virus particles needed to establish infection). Following an incubation of serum & virus for 1 - 2 hours at room temperature (some systems use 37°C or even 4°C), indicator cell cultures are added. Plates are sealed, incubated at 37°C, and observed daily for development of viral CPE. The presence of specific antibody in the test serum inhibits the production of this CPE.

The VN test is also used to identify unknown viral isolates in essentially the same manner as described above. The only difference is that the antibody is known and the virus is unknown. If a specific antibody inhibits the development of CPE of the unknown virus, then identification is accomplished.

Hemagglutination Inhibition (HI) Test

HI test is like VN tests except that the viral activity being inhibited is hemagglutination. HI tests are useful for measuring antibody to those hemagglutinating viruses that either replicate poorly in cell culture or produce little or no discernible CPE, e.g. type A influenza viruses of most animal species, Newcastle disease virus of birds, and porcine parvovirus. HI tests are performed in microtiter plates when dilutions of test sera are made, followed by the addition of an equal volume of virus suspension diluted to contain approximately 4 to 8 HA units (a HA unit is the highest dilution of the viral sample that causes complete hemagglutination). The appropriate RBC suspension is then added and the plates are gently mixed and allowed to incubate for 1-2 hours at 4°C. Presence of specific antibody in the test serum will inhibit agglutination of RBCs and the RBCs will settle out in a well-defined "button" fashion. Agglutinated cells will settle out in a thin layer over the entire bottom of the test well, or in a rough, irregularly fringed button. Usually test sera contain nonspecific inhibitors of agglutination and it ought to be adsorbed with RBCs prior to testing.

Complement Fixation Test

Complement fixation (CF) test is used to detect and measure antibody, it is useful in the diagnosis of acute or recent viral infections, because they primarily detect IgM, the first immunoglobulin class to appear to infection. CF test uses viral antigens, guinea pig serum complement, and an indicator system of "sensitized" sheep RBCs. Reacting with antibody directed against them sensitizes the sheep RBCs. This anti-sheep RBC antibody is referred to as hemolysin and is prepared in rabbits. In this case antigen and complement are each titrated and diluted. If no specific antibodies are present in the serum under test, the complement is free to react with the sensitized RBCs, causing lysis. Alternatively if sufficient antibody is present, the specific antigen-antibody complexes will have bound the complement and no lysis of the RBCs will occur.

Immunodiffusion

Immunodiffusion is used to detect antibody or antigen; two most commonly used techniques of immunodiffusion are the double-diffusion plate system and immunoelectrophoresis. These tests are performed in a semi-solid medium using agar or agarose gel. In immunoelectrophoresis, the antigen is electrophoretically fractionated prior to an overlay of antibody. In both methods, the antigen and antibody diffuse against each other forming a line of precipitation where they react.

The double-diffusion plate system is the more commonly used diagnostic test, e.g. the "Coggins test" for equine infectious anemia.

Immunodiffusion test can be made more sensitive by using a radioactive label, which will permit the detection of antigen-antibody reactions not visible to the naked eye. In this test the radioactive label is usually iodine (^{125}I), and either the antigen or antibody can be labeled. Labeling occurs by ^{125}I coupling to the amino acid tyrosine. The tests are read by covering the plates or slides with an x-ray film that records the radioactive-precipitation lines.

Protection Tests

Protection tests are used for identification of viruses if other less involved means are not available. This involves the production of either active or passive immunity in an animal or animals followed by challenge with the agent in question. In case of the identification of hog cholera virus, both injecting anti-hog cholera serum with blood or spleen suspension from the animal suspected for hog cholera. If it is hog cholera virus, the passive immunity provided by the anti-hog cholera serum would protect the pig from the challenge dose. The test uses unprotected pig control, which would contract hog cholera infection.

Limitations of serological diagnosis

How useful a serological result is depends on the individual virus. For viruses such as rubella and hepatitis A, the onset of clinical symptoms coincides with the development of antibodies. The detection of IgM or rising titres of IgG in the serum of the patient would indicate active disease. However, many viruses often produce clinical disease before the appearance of antibodies such as respiratory and diarrhoeal viruses. So in this case, any serological diagnosis would be retrospective and therefore will not be very useful. There are also viruses which produce clinical disease months or years after seroconversion e.g. HIV and rabies. In the case of these viruses, the mere presence of antibody is sufficient to make a definitive diagnosis.

There are a number of problems associated with serology: long time is required for diagnosis for paired acute and convalescent sera. Mild local infections such as HSV genitalis may not produce a detectable humoral immune response. Extensive antigenic cross-reactivity between related viruses e.g. HSV and VZV, Japanese B encephalitis and Dengue, may lead to false positive results. Immunocompromised patients often give a reduced or absent humoral immune response. Patients with infectious mononucleosis and those with connective tissue diseases such as SLE may react non-specifically giving a false positive result. Patients given blood or blood products may give a false positive result due to the transfer of antibody.

Antibody in the CSF

In a healthy host, there should be little or no antibodies in the CSF. Where there is a viral meningitis or encephalitis, antibodies may be produced against the virus by lymphocytes in the CSF. The finding of antibodies in the CSF is said to be significant when ratio between the titre of antibody in the serum and that in the CSF is less than 100. But this does depend on an intact blood-brain barrier. The problem is that in many cases of meningitis and encephalitis, the blood-brain barrier is damaged, so that antibodies in the serum can actually leak across into the CSF. This also happens where the lumbar puncture was traumatic in which case the spinal fluid would be blood stained. Hence, one should really check the integrity of the blood-brain barrier before making a definite diagnosis. One way to check the integrity of the blood brain barrier is to use a surrogate antibody that most individuals would have, such as measles virus, since most people would have been vaccinated. So the patient's serum and CSF for measles antibody are tested. If the blood-brain barrier is intact, there should be little or no measles antibodies in the CSF.

Collection and Dispatch of Diagnostic Specimens

For the laboratory diagnosis of an animal viral disease, it is most important to collect the proper samples. Each of the samples may be taken from animals or the environment for a variety of purposes, such as disease diagnosis, disease surveillance, health certification or monitoring the response to treatment or vaccination. The samples collected should be appropriate for the intended purpose, and adequate in number and amount to provide statistically valid results. Diagnostic laboratories require the submission of appropriate samples that arrive at the laboratory in good condition. For disease diagnosis, the tissues sampled should be representative of the condition being investigated and the lesions observed. Samples should be taken with care, to avoid undue stress or injury to the animal or danger to the operator. Where appropriate, samples should be collected aseptically, and care should be taken to avoid cross contamination between samples. The samples should be carefully packaged, labeled, and transmitted to the laboratory by the fastest practicable method, with the appropriate temperature control. There are specific requirements for the packaging and shipping of infectious substances, including diagnostic specimens that must be followed. If material is sent to a laboratory in another country, this laboratory should be consulted in advance to ensure that it is willing to receive the material and to obtain the appropriate import licence. All samples should be accompanied by a letter or submission form, which includes the name and address of the submitter, the origin of the material, the relevant history, animal identification and corresponding specimens, and the tests requested. The viral diagnosis of clinical illness depends to a large extent upon the kind and condition of specimens sent for examination. Several laboratory tests are for specific disease agents, an adequate clinical history must accompany all submissions. Such clinical history will permit laboratory staff to perform additional tests if requires. As most laboratories supply a specimen submission form that should be completed with the available pertinent data. The veterinarian should supply as complete a history as possible in absence of form. Interested veterinarians should personally contact the diagnostic laboratory if they have any questions.

Animals

Preferably samples should be collected from live, sick animals or if possible, animals should be sent directly to the diagnostic laboratory for complete necropsy examination. If more animals are affected, then more than one animal should be sent. Samples should be packaged in leak-proof insulated containers with sufficient ice or cold packs but it should not be frozen for necropsy.

Tissues

Probably it is best to collect a set of tissues prior to thorough examination; including lung, kidney, liver, spleen, small intestine, large intestine, and mesenteric lymph nodes. Tissues from brain or head may be collected if CNS involvement is suspected. Any abnormalities noticed in tissues while examining should be collected- usually a portion of these tissues should be placed in leak-proof plastic bags and placed under refrigeration. It is required to patch tissues separately, but in case of intestine, it should be separated from other tissues to prevent contamination. These collected samples should be brought directly to the laboratory, or shipped under refrigeration by over-night mail, bus, or courier service. Many viruses produce unique microscopic lesions, small pieces of each tissue should be placed in ten percent buffered formalin for histopathologic examination. In case of brain longitudinal half of the brain ought to be submitted, but the specimens should not be frozen.

Feces

In case of feces, it should be collected from acutely ill animals and placed in leak-proof containers. A saturated swabs are adequate for many individual virologic examinations, several milliliters or grams of feces permit a more complete diagnostic work-up including bacteriologic and parasitologic examinations. Fecal samples should be submitted to the laboratory using cold packs as coolant.

Swabs

In case of respiratory tract infections, swab should be collected from nasal and ocular regins for isolating viruses. Similarly, genital swab may be collected from the reproductive tract including vagina, penis mucosa, semen etc. from acutely ill animals and placed directly into screw-capped tubes containing a viral transport medium. It is also useful to collect swabs from vesicular lesions selecting fresh vesicles that myy be ruptured and the swab saturated with the exuding fluid. 2 g of affected epithelial tissue as aseptically as possible and placed in 5 ml phosphate buffered glycerine or Tris-buffered tryptose broth virus transport medium at pH 7.6 is needed. Thse swabs should be collected both for virus isolation and one for electron microscopy. While swab for virus isolation should be placed in viral transport medium and the swab for electron microscopy should be placed in a screw-capped tube containing one or two drops of distilled water. Animals showing advanced lesions should also be swabed & sent.

Commercially, several viral transport media are available that maintain the viability of viruses during shipment to the laboratory. Usually these transport media are balanced salt solutions containing high protein content and antibiotics to prevent bacterial overgrowth. Several laboratories provide their own transport medium to practicing veterinarians upon request.

Slides

Many of the diseases can be diagnosed by examining slides prepared from blood and tissues. Usually, blood smears are sent for diagnosing feline leukemia, while blood smears and conjunctival scrapings are used to diagnose canine distemper. In case of suspected herpesvirus, conjunctival scrapings are particularly useful for diagnosing infections in cats. Slides from liver, spleen, and lungs are especially useful for diagnosing chlamydia and herpesvirus infections of psittacine birds. Care should be taken that slides should have required cells to allow thorough examination but should not be so thick as to cause difficulty in staining. A blunt instrument like scalpel may be used to scrape the conjunctiva. If the eyes are matted, it be cleaned and flushed before scraping the conjunctiva. Before dispatching, the slides should be air-dried and sent to the laboratory in slide holders to prevent breakage.

Serum

Blood samples should be collected in sterile tubes containing no anticoagulants. These should be submitted to the laboratory in specially designed holders to avoid breakage. Blood samples should not be frozen or allowed to overheat. If samples cannot be delivered to the laboratory within a reasonable time, serum should be removed and refrigerated or frozen.

Milk

Milk samples should be taken after cleansing and drying the tip of the teat, the use of antiseptics should be avoided. The initial stream of milk should be discarded and a tube filled with the next stream(s), a sample of bulk tank milk can be used for some tests. Milk for serological tests should not have been frozen, heated or subjected to violent shaking. If there is going to be a delay in submitting them to the laboratory, preservatives can be added to milk samples that are being collected for serological testing.

□□□

Part 2 : Pathogenic Viruses

Chapter 8

Characteristics and Diseases Caused by Group 1 Double Stranded DNA Adenoviruses (Family Adenoviridae)

Contents

Characteristics of Adenoviruses

Adenoviruses (G. adeno=gland) was first isolated in 1953 in cell culture of adenoid tissues from children, hence the name. Adenoviruses are medium sized, spherical, nonenveloped icosahedral viruses measuring 90–100 nm in diameter. The virus genome consists of a nucleocapsid and a double-stranded linear DNA genome of about 26 -45 Kbp that allows the virus to carry 22 to 40 genes. Virions have **icosadehdral symmetry** made of 252 capsomers-240 **"hexons" + 12 "pentons"** at vertices of icosahedron with 2-3-5 symmetry. From each of 12 vertices of the capsid project **unique fibres** 9-31 nm in length with **knob at the end** wich are antigenically different from others. **Fibres attach to the host cells via the coxsackie-adenovirus receptors** on the surface of the host cell and are also type specific hemagglutinins. Some characteristic features of adenoviruses are that they are widespread in nature, infect birds, many mammals and man & **can undergo latent infection in lymphoid tissues, & becoming reactivated some time later**. Several types have oncogenic potential. The scientist in 2010 revealed that human adenovirus is made of around 1 million amino acid residues and weighs around 15 MDa. In 1962, some adenoviruses were shown to cause tumours in rodents that caused a considerable interest. Adenovirus oncogenesis appears to be associated with abortive infections.

Adenoviruses are transmitted mainly by coughed-out droplets, by contact with an infected person, or by virus particles left on objects such as towels and faucet handles, some with gastroenteritis via stools or through sexual practices, and through water in swimming pools. Heat and bleach will kill adenoviruses on objects.

Adenoviruses are resistant to trypsin and lipid solvents, moderately resistant on premises, are stable to chemical or physical agents and adverse pH conditions, allowing for **prolonged survival outside the body and water.**

The virus genome

Adenovirus genome is linear, non-segmented double-stranded DNA measuring 26 and 45 Kbp that enables the virus to carry 22 to 40 genes. The viruses are mainly dependent on the host cells for survival and replication. The viral genome 3′ & 5′ ends have "inverted terminal repeats & the 5′ ends of the linear DNA have **terminal 55 kDa protein** that are used as **primers** in viral replication. The dsDNA encodes more than 30 proteins. The viral genome contains early **(E) genes & late (L) genes. Early genes** on 3′-5′ strand include **E1a, E1b & E3** & on 5′-3′ strand are **E2b, E2a & E4. The late genes** contain **L1 to L4 on** 3′-5′ strand. Early genes express non-structural & regulatory proteins essential for DNA synthesis, & the important ones are DNA-dependent–DNA polymerase & replicase. Late genes express structural proteins for capsid proteins & other viral components. Among 10 structural proteins, **3 polypeptides make 1 hexon, 1 makes up penton base & 1 forms fibre glycoprotein (Fig 8-1)** & other 5 proteins remain inside. **Pentons & fibres determine type specific antigenicity & elicit neutralizing antibodies,** while hexons determine **type specificity** as well as group specificity, the latter provide basis for the test to determine adenoviruses.

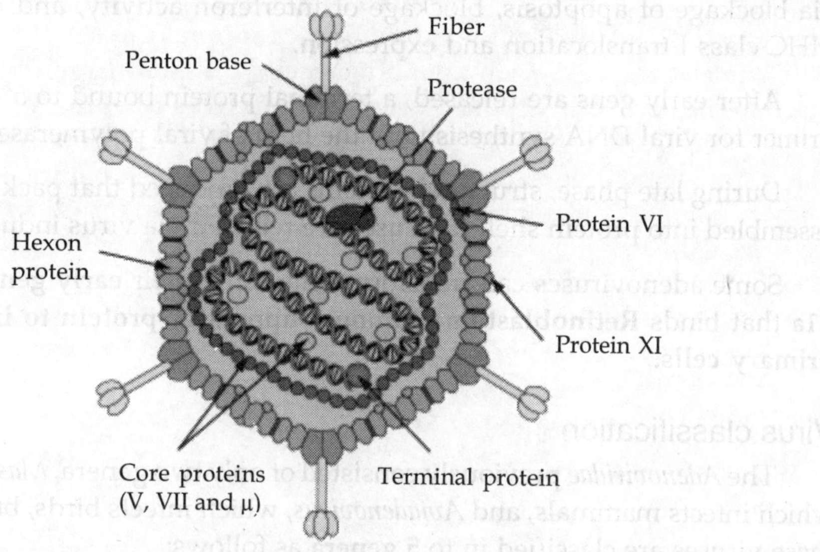

Figure 8.1 : Morphology of Adenovirus

Virus replication

Viral DNA replication, mRNA transcription and virion assembly occur in the nucleus,using the host's replication machinery causing the formation of **basophilic and / or acidophilic intranuclear inclusions**. Adenoviruses entery involves 2 steps betweenthe virus and the host cell. Firstly, the **knob domain of the fiber protein binds to 2 types of cell receptors- CD46 for the group B human adenovirus serotypes, and the coxsackievirus adenovirus receptor (CAR) for all other serotypes.** In a secondary interaction a specialized motif in the penton base protein interacts with α-integrin molecule whereby virions are endocytosed via clathrin-coated pits. Virus enters host cells within an endosome, the endosome acidifies resulting in dissociation of capsid components & the virus is released into the cytoplasm. The cellular microtubules carry virions to the nuclear pore whereby the adenovirus particle dissembles. Viral DNA is released, enters the nucleus via the nuclear pore & the **DNA associates with histone molecules**.

Viral gene expression can occur now and new virus particles are generated. There are **two phases of virus replication: an early phase and a late phase**, & in both phases primary transcripts are generated which are alternatively spliced to monocistronic mRNAs as per the host's ribosomes that translate them into proteins. The early genes express mainly non-structural, regulatory proteins with **3 goals**: to alter host proteins for DNA synthesis; to activate other virus genes like the virus-encoded DNA polymerase; and to avoid premature death of the infected cell by the host-immune defenses via blockage of apoptosis, blockage of interferon activity, and blockage of MHC class I translocation and expression.

After early gens are released, a terminal protein bound to 5′ end acts as primer for viral DNA synthesis with the help of viral polymerase.

During late phase, structural proteins are produced that pack viral DNA, assembled into protein shell & viruses are released via virus induced lysis.

Some adenoviruses can transform cells using their **early gene products, E1a** that binds **Retinoblastoma tumour suppressor protein to immortalize primary cells.**

Virus classification

The *Adenoviridae* previously consisted of only two genera, *Mastadenovirus*, which infects mammals, and *Aviadenovirus*, which infects birds, but presently these viruses are classified in to **5 genera** as follows:

Virus group: Group 1 ds DNA

Family: *Adenoviridae*

Genus 1: *Mastadenovirus;* type species: *Human adenovirus C;* other importance species are

Genus 2: *Aviadenovirus;* type species: *Fowl adenovirus A*

Genus 3: *Atadenovirus;* type species: *Ovine adenovirus D* Genus 4: *Siaadenovirus;* type species: *Frog adenovirus*

Genus 5: *Ichtadenovirus;* type species: *Sturgeon adenovirus A*.

Table 8-1 presented below depicts classification of *Adenoviridae* & briefly mentions diseases caused by the virus species in humans, animals & birds.

Table 8.1 : Classification of *Adenoviridae* & diseases caused by the member viruses in humans & animals.

Genera of *Adenoviridae*	*Species*	Serotypes	Diseases caused
G1. *Mastadenovirus*	*Human adenovirus A*	HAdV 12, 18, 31	
	Human adenoviru B	HAdV 3, 7, 11, **14**, 16, 21, 34, 35, 50	*Human adenovirus B* **(HAdV)** causes **respiratory infection & conjunctivitis in humans: HAdV14 is an emerging disease, rarely with fatality.**
	Human adenovirus C: TS	HAdV 1, 2, 5, 6	**HAdV C mainly causes respiratory disease.**
	Human adenovirus D	HAdV 8, 9, 10, 13, 15, 17, 19, 20, 22, 23, 24, 25, 26, 27, 28, 29, 30, 32, 33, 36, 37, 38, 39, 42, 43, 44, 45, 46, 47, 48, 49, 51, 53, 54	*Human adenovirus D* **(HAdV-D)** some of them cause **conjunctivitis & tonsillitis like streptococcal infection.**
	Human adenovirus E	HAdV 4	
	Human adenovirus F	HAdV 40, 41	*Human adenovirus E* **(HAdV-E)** causes **gastroenteritis in humans.**
	Human adenovirus G	HAdV 5, 2	
	Bovine adenoirus A	BAdV 1	Subclinical infection in bovines
	Bovine adenoirus B	BAdV 3	Do
	Bovine adenoirus C	BAdV 10	Do
	Canine adenovirus	**CAdV 1**	*Canine adenovirus-1* (CAdV-1) **causes infectious canine hepatitis (ICH) in dogs, foxes, wolves, coyotes & bear worldwide. Infectious canine hepatitis (ICH) is a viral, highly contagious generalized disease in dogs, foxes, wolves, coyotes & bear worldwide. The disease is characterized by depression, marked leukopenia, prolonged bleeding time, fever, vomiting, diarrhea, and discharges from the nose and eyes; a viremia with secondary localization and replication in the liver and kidney; main tissue changes involve the endothelium and hepatic cells**

		with damaged endothelium resulting in widespread **petechial hemorrhages, centrolobular necrosis** in liver with typical adenoviral IN inclusion bodies being observed in Kupffer cells and parenchymal cells. **Circulating immune complexes** in the glomeruli causes glomerulonephritis, & recovered dogs develop corneal opacity (blue eye) as a result of local immune complex deposition.
Do	**CAdV 2**	*Canine adenovirus-2* **(CAdV-2)** causes **kennel cough** or infectious laryngotracheitis in dogs characterized bya harsh, dry hacking / coughing, retching, sneezing, snorting, gagging or vomiting in response to slight pressure of the trachea or after excitement or exercise. Fever varies from case to case. The disease last from 10-20 days and can rebreak when the dog is put into a stress which puts stress on the dog's immune system.
Equine adenovirus A	EAdV 1	*Equine adenovirus A* **(EAdV-1)** causes mild upper respiratory tract symptoms in equines, which is severe & often with fatality in immunosuppressed **Arabian foals.**
Equine adenovirus B	EAdV 2	Subclinical infection in equine
Ovine adenovirusA	OAdV 2, 3, 4, 5	Subclinical infection in ovines
Ovine adenovirusB	OAdV 1	Subclinical infection in ovines
Porcine adenovirus A	PAdV 1, 2, 3	Subclinical infection in pigs
Porcine adenovirus B	PAdV 4	Do
Porcine adenovirus C	PAdV 5	Do
T: *Ovine adenovirus C*	OAdV 6	Subclinical
T: *Goat adenovirus*	GAdV 2	Subclinical
T; Simian adenovirus	SAdV 1 through 20	Adenoviruses of monkeys

	T: *Guinea pig adenovirus*	GPAdV 1	Subclinical
G2: *Aviadenovirus*	TS: *Fowl adenovirus A* (Fowl adenovirus 1/CELO)	FAdV 1 (CELO, chicken embryo lethal orphan virus)	*Fowl adenovirus A* **(FAdV-1/CELO, chicken embryo lethal orphan virus) causes a widespread but inapparent infection. CELO virus also causes Quail bronchitis, which is a highly contagious, often fatal respiratory disease of bobwhite quail-both wild and in captivity. The disease is of major economic significance to game bird breeders and has a worldwide distribution. Symptoms include respiratory distress, coughing, sneezing, rales, and lacrimation, loose, watery droppings in some acutely affected older birds, conjunctivitis, mild to severe tracheitis, airsacculitis, hepatitis, and gaseous distention of the intestines. Multiple pale, pinpoint foci of necrosis are seen in the liver and mottling and enlargement of the spleen are common lesions in the infected birds. Mortality may reach 100% in birds <2 wk old but is usually <25% in birds >4 wk old.**
	Fowl adenovirus B	FAdV 5	*Fowl adenovirus B* **(FAdV- 5)** & many types cause **inclusion body hepatitis in young chickens** characterized bydepression, inappetance, ruffled feathers & pallor of comb and wattles. PM lesions include liver swollen, yellow, mottled with petechiae and ecchymoses, kidneys and bone marrow pale, blood thin, & bursa and spleen small. **Microscopically - basophilic IN inclusions** are observed. Infected birds remain carriers for a few weeks. Transmission is via vertical or lateral means or by fomites. Immunosuppression caused, e.g. due to early IBD challenge or congenital CAV infection may result in the disease.

	Fowl adenovirus C	FAdV 4, 10	Subclinical
	Fowl adenovirus D	FAdV 2, 11, 12, 3, 9, 8	Subclinical
	Fowl adenovirus E	FAdV 6, 7, 8a, 8b	Subclinical
	Gooose adenovirus	GsAdV 1, 2, 3	Subclinical
	T: *Duck adenovirus B*	DAdV 2	Subclinical
	T: *Pigeon adenovirus*	PiAdV 1	Subclinical
	T: *Turkey adenovirus*	TAdV 1, 2	Subclinical
G3: *Atadenovirus*	TS: *Ovine adenovirus D*	OAdV 7, Isolate 287	Subclinical
	Goat adenovirus 1	GAdV 1	Subclinical
	Duck adenovirus A (Duck adenovirus1 /EDSV)	DAdV 1/ EDSV, egg drop syndrome virus	*Duck adenovirus A* **(DAdV-1/ EDSV, egg drop syndrome virus)** **occurs mostly in broiler chickens of 5-6 wk age & quails. The first symptom is usually a loss of color in pigmented eggs, followed by thin-shelled, soft-shelled, and shell-less eggs. The shells may be rough or "chalky." Shell-less eggs are not always found, as they may be eaten by the birds. Egg production usually drops 10% to 40%. Ducks and geese are the natural hosts, but has also been isolated from coots and grebes, and Abs are present in many avian species: gulls, owls, storks, swans, guinea fowl, and pigeons.**
	Bovine adnovirus D	BAdV 4, 5, 6	Subclinical
	Bovine adnovirus E	BAdV 6	Subclinical
	Bovine adnovirus F	BAdV 7	Subclinical
G4: *Siadenovirus*	TS: *Frog adenovurus*	FrAdV	Adenoviruses of frogs
	Turkey adenovirus A	TAdV-A	Subclinical
	Avian adenovirus	TAdV-3	*Turkey adenovirus A* / Avian adenovirus splenomegaly virus

	splenomegal y virus		TAdV-3 causes adenovirus splenomegaly in chickens. Gross lesions seen are splenomegaly and splenic mottling. Histologic lesions include splenic reticuloendothelial cell hyperplasia with IN inclusions. Lymphocytic degeneration is observed in the lungs of most chickens. Lung hemorrhage and edema with endothelial disruption and congestion of pulmonary arterioles are found less frequently. The splenic lesions in the chickens are similar to those seen in turkeys naturally infected with hemorrhagic enteritis, and the lung lesions resembled those seen in pheasants naturally infected with marble spleen disease.
	Marble spleen disease virus	Do	Marble spleen disease virus (TAdV-3) also causes marble spleen disease in pheasants of 3-8 months of age. Onset is acute, with dyspnea, asphyxiation, and sudden death due to pulmonary congestion and edema. Mortality is commonly 2-3% but can reach 15%. Secondary bacterial infections occur due to immunosuppression.
	Turkey hemorrhagic enteritis virus	Do	Turkey hemorrhagic enteritis virus (TAdV-3) also causes hemorrhagic enteritis in young turkey poults 4-16 wk old. Symptoms in outbreaks with highly virulent pathotypes include depression, pallor, and bloody droppings. Acute mortality ranges from <1% to 60% with an average of 10-15% over a 2-week period. Surviving birds develop a transient immunosuppression related to the lymphotrophic, lymphocytopathic nature of the virus causing secondary bacterial infections.
G5: *Ichtadenovirus*	TS: *Sturgeon adenovirus A*		

Abbreviation: TS= type species; T = tentative classification

Again, each genus is subdivided into species & each species can have one to several serotypes. In case of humans adenoviruses, there are 56 recognized human adenovirus types (HAdV-1 to 56) in seven species (Human adenovirus A to G) as follows:

A: 12, 18, 31; **B**: 3, 7, 11, **14**, 16, 21, 34, 35, 50, 55; **C**: 1, 2, 5, 6; **D**: 8, 9, 10, 13, 15, 17, 19, 20, 22, 23, 24, 25, 26, 27, 28, 29, 30, 32, 33, **36**, 37, 38, 39, 42, 43, 44, 45, 46, 47, 48, 49, 51, 53, 54, 56; **E**: 4; **F**: 40, 41; G: 52

Adenovirus Clinical Manifestations in Humans and Animals

Clinical Infecton in Humans

Most clinical infections with human adenoviruses include: 1. Upper respiratory tract infection, 2. Conjunctivitis, tonsillitis like streptococcal throat, 3. Ear infection, or croup, 4. Gastroenteritis, 5. Bronchitis in children or pneumonia, 6. Whooping cough like symptoms in babies, 7. Viral meningitis or encephalitis or 8. Hemorrhagic cystitis in rare condition. The disease is severe in immunodeficient persons while others recover.

Different serotypes are associated with different clinical conditions namely:

Respiratory diseases are mainly caused by the species HAdV-B and C

Conjunctivitis is mainly caused by the species HAdV-B and D

Gastroenteritis is mainly caused by the species HAdV-F types 40, 41, HAdV-G type 52.

Adenovirus B serotype 14 (AdV14) cause potentially fatal infection in humans. According to the CDC, outbreaks have been identified in four states within USA with ten identified deaths since May, 2006.

Adenovirus Clinical Manifestations in Animals

Genus: *Mastadenovirus;*

Infectious Canine Hepatitis

Infectious canine hepatitis **(ICH)** is a viral, highly contagious generalized disease in dogs, foxes, wolves, coyotes & bear worldwide. The disease is characterized by depression, marked leukopenia, prolonged bleeding time, fever, vomiting, diarrhea, and discharges from the nose and eyes; a viremia with secondary localization and replication in the liver and kidney. Main tissue changes involve the **endothelium and hepatic cells** with damaged endothelium resulting in widespread **petechial hemorrhages, centrolobular necrosis** in liver with typical adenoviral IN inclusion bodies being observed in Kupffer cells and parenchymal cells. **Circulating immune complexes** in the glomeruli causes glomerulonephritis, & recovered dogs develop corneal opacity (blue eye) as a result of local immune complex deposition.

Etiolgy: ICH is caused by *Canine adenovirus-1* **(CAD-1)**, which is closely related to *Canine adenovirus-2* **(CAD-2)**, which causes kennel cough or infectious laryngotracheitis.

Occurrence

Infectious canine hepatitis was first discovered by Rubarth in Sweden in 1947. It occurs worldwide, though it is rare in the United States, and mostly affects young dogs under 1 year of age, though it can affect adults. Most cases occur in wild or unvaccinated dogs.

Hosts susceptible

Dogs less than one year of age are most often affected, & the virus also infects wild and captive foxes causing encephalitis, wolves, coyotes and bears, but not ferrets. Other carnivores may get subclinical infections.

Transmission

Dog contract CAV-1 through direct or in direct contact with infected saliva, urine, or feces either with dog's mouth or nose. Even a dog dish that has been licked clean can carry the virus. The tonsils and lymph nodes are the first body parts affected. Even after recovery, the dog can shed the virus in his urine for up to 9 months.

Pathogenesis

The incubation period is **4-9 days**. Oronasal infection is followed by replication in tonsils and Peyer'spatches, other lymphatic tissues and viremia. Virus then replicates in vascular endothelial cells in many organs like liver, kidneys, spleen, lungs, and eyes in dogs, and in hepatocytes, endothelial cells of renal glomeruli and the cornea and uvea. Besides causing acute disease, persistent infection of the kidneys and immune complex formation can lead to glomerulonephritis. Immune complexes also may cause corneal and uveal inflammation (blue eye). Persistently infected dogs may shed virus in their urine for up to 6 months. During the acute phase of illness, prior to the onset of circulating antibody, uveitis occurs that is related directly to effects of viral growth in vascular endothelium, and in reticuloendothelial elements of the anterior uvea. The severe iridocyclitis with corneal opacification that occurs in clinically recovered dogs possess characteristics of the Arthus-type of ocular hypersensitivity. With the advent of immune response, the virus is eliminated 10 days after infection, & most dogs recover. But the virus may persist in the kidney that excretes the virus for more than 6 months.

Clinical symptoms & lesions

This disease can cause variable signs and symptoms which can range from mild to severe manifestations. In mild cases, infected dog shows a mild fever, moderate lethargy, and slight loss of appetite. In this case, the dog usually recovers in about two days.

Some of the common symptoms in dogs with ICH are: fever more than 104°F lasting 1-6 days in dogs under 1 year of age, nausea, vomiting, sore throat, coughing, loss of appetite, jaundice, abdominal pain and enlargement, swollen lymph nodes, swelling of tonsils, head, neck, or trunk, weight loss, pale tongue, gums, and nose, drinking and urinating a lot (polydispsia), light colored stool, seizures, difficulty in clotting blood, decreased clotting time as displayed by bleeding around the teeth or spontaneous hematomas in the mouth & cloudiness of eye **("hepatitis blue eye")** in 25% of cases, and usually in dogs under 6 months old.

In severe cases, dogs can develop a **biphasic fever** for 1-6 days, pass bloody diarrhea or bloody vomit, tuck up their belly from pain associated with the liver, become sensitive to light, refuse to eat, and may display any of the above symptoms. Death can occur within a few hours. The fatal form of the disease results in a sudden onset of severe symptoms. Bleeding from the nose and gums, enlarged abdomen due to fluid leaking from the liver, bloody diarrhea and vomit, seizures due to central nervous system association, disorientation, coma, and death may occur. Pets may die suddenly without any obvious illness. Infectious canine hepatitis is most severe and the mortality rate is highest in young dogs.

PM lesions: Endothelial damage results in "paint brush" hemorrhages on the gastric serosa, lymph nodes, thymus, pancreas, & subcutaneous tissues. Hepatic cell necrosis produces a variegated color change in the liver, the gall bladder wall may be edematous and thickened; & edema of the thymus may be found. Grayish white foci may be seen in the cortex of kidney.

Diagnosis

Collection of clinical samples for various tests include: liver, spleen, kidney, blood, urine, nasal swabs and paired serum samples.

1. *Presumptive diagnosis*: Clinical signs, gross and microscopic lesions, **IN inlusions in hepatocytes**, endothelial cells, and Kupffer cells furnish first hand diagnosis. Infected dogs show a low white blood cell count and elevated liver enzymes.
2. *Virus isolation*: ICH virus is cultivated in cell cultures of canine origin for which liver is less suitable for virus recovery than other vital organs.

3. *Virus antigen detection*: Immunofluorescence can detect antigen in frozen liver sections or in a tissue or culture using a fluorescent dye.
4. *Antibody detection*: ELISA detects antibodies in a fecal sample. A rising titer of antibodies employing hemagglutination inhibition or virus neutralization tests is supportive of a diagnosis.

Treatment & prevention

Treatment of ICH is done according to the symptom & includes use of a broad spectrum antibiotic to check bacterial infections. IV fluids along with a dextrose solution may be provided to rehydrate the dog. Blood transfusion may be necessary in severely ill dogs to replenish lost blood. The cloudiness of the eye will usually take care of itself, but an ointment may be given to relieve the dog from eye pain and light sensitivity. A fasting period may be instituted, followed by a light diet consisting of small, frequent meals.

Even after recovery, the pet can shed the virus in his urine for up to 9 months. After recovery from the condition, the liver will completely recover, but long-term kidney damage and prolonged eye cloudiness or glaucoma may result as a delayed inflammatory response. But, the pet will have lifelong immunity to the virus. Disinfection of contaminated areas with a bleach or iodine solution kills the virus.

Vaccination

Modified-live virus vaccines are used and are often combined with other vaccines; attenuated CAV-1 vaccines produce transient unilateral or bilateral opacities of the cornea, and the virus may be shed in urine. Hence, CAV-2 attenuated live virus strains, which provide cross protection against CAV-1, are usually used as they do not produce corneal opacities or uveitis, and the virus is not shed in urine. CAV-2 is much safer, and will help dog build immunity against both CAV-1 & CAV-2 (kennel cough). Vaccine is given when puppies are **9-12 week old**. A combination modified live vaccine containing canine distemper, adenovirus type 1 & 2, canine parvovirus vaccine & canine parainfluenza virus (**Galaxy DA2PPV**-Intervet) & is given to puppies within the first months of life. Give 1 ml dose IM or SC, with a second dose in 2-4 weeks. Annual revaccination is recommended thereafter. Some young dogs may require a third dose, depending on their age when the first vaccination was given. This vaccine also combines with coronavirus and leptospirosis designated as **Galaxy DA2PPV+CV** (CD+Adenovius 2+Parvovirus+canine PI3+ Coronavirus) 1ml SC or IM at 6 weeks of age or older. Repeat at 2 to 4 week intervals until the dog is 12 weeks of age. A minimum of two doses is required for primary immunization. Annual revaccination with one dose is recommended. **Galaxy DA_2PPVL** modified live virus vaccine which is combined with inactivated *Leptospira canicola* and *L. icterohaemorrhagiae* bacterin. Dose & schedule as above. Vanguard plus 5, Vanguard plus 5/CV & Vanguard Plus 5 L4-Pfizer are similar vaccines.

Kennel Cough or Infectious Tracheobronchitis

Kennel cough or infectious laryngotracheitis is a highly contagious disease in canine characterized by inflammation of the upper respiratory tract, a harsh, dry hacking /coughing, retching, sneezing, snorting, gagging or vomiting in response to slight pressure on the trachea or after excitement or exercise. Fever varies from case to case. The disease lasts from 10-20 days and can rebreak when the dog is put into a stress which puts stress on the dog's immune system.

Etiology: It is caused by*Canine adenovirus*-2 **(CAD-2).** Other viral and bacterial causes are *Bordetella bronchiseptica,* Canine adenovirus, canine parvovirus & canine parainfluenza virus contribute to the disease. Exposure to crowded and/or poorly ventilated conditions found in many kennels and shelters, cold temperatures, exposure to dust and/or cigarette smoke & ravel-induced stress are some of other factors.

Occurrence

The disease is found worldwide and will infect a very high percentage of dogs in their lifetime.

Hosts susceptible

Dogs particularly puppies housed in close confinement like veterinary hospitals or kennels

Transmission

Kennel cough are spread through the air by infected dogs sneezing and coughing. It can also spread through contact with contaminated surfaces, such as the ground, toys, and sidewalks and through direct contact. It is highly contagious, even days or weeks after symptoms disappear. A dog can carry the infection causing virus and bacteria for as long as three months after catching the infection.

Clinical symptoms

Symptoms include a harsh, dry hacking/coughing, retching, sneezing, snorting, gagging or vomiting in response to light pressing of the trachea or after excitement or exercise. Many owners describe the cough as having a 'honking sound.' A watery nasal discharge may also be present. With mild cases, dogs continue to eat and be alert and active. Many times, there is a recent history of boarding or coming in contact with other dogs. In more severe cases, the symptoms may progress and include lethargy, fever, inappetence, pneumonia, and in very severe cases, even death. The majority of **severe cases** occur in immunocompromised animals, or **young unvaccinated puppies**. The disease can last from 10-20 days and can rebreak when the dog is put into a stressful situation which puts stress on the dog's immune system.

Diagnosis

Usually no attempt is made to isolate canine adenovirus 2. A presumptive diagnosis of kennel cough is usually based on clinical signs and history. CAD-2 may be cultivated in cell cultures of canine origin, producing characteristic CPE. Virus is identified by virus neutralization with specific antiserum and/or by immunofluorescence assay.

Treament & prevention

Many times, prednisone is given to help reduce the severity and frequency of the cough, bronchodilators like aminophylline or cough suppressants may also be used. In more severe cases where the animal is not eating, running a fever, or showing signs of pneumonia, antibiotics are often used. Steroids or cough suppressants are not usually recommended because of the risk of immunosuppression with steroids and the need to continue to clear extra fluid or mucous in pneumonia patients. Bronchodilators and even aerosol therapy can be used.

Vaccination

Prevention is by vccination for canine adenovirus, distemper, parainfluenza, and Bordetella. The avirulent live vaccines contain *B. bronchiseptica,* with modified live CPIV and CAV-2 (**INTRA-TRAC 3 ADT-**INTERVET) is administered intranasally, dose is 0.5 ml of rehydrated vaccine and have the benefit of being effective in the face of maternal antibodies. This effectiveness in the face of colostral immunity makes their use in young dogs more appealing as reimmunization may not be required. An initial vaccination should be given at 6-8 week and repeated twice at 3- to 4-week intervals until the dog is 14-16 week old. Revaccination should be performed annually. In kennels, the best prevention is to keep all the cages disinfected. Most kennels will not board dogs without proof of vaccination.

Equine Adenovirus A Infection

Equine adenovirus A (EAdV-1) causes widespread subclinical or mild upper respiratory tract symptoms in equines especially in foals, but a severe & often fatal infection in immunosuppressed foals/ Arabian foals.

Occurrence

EAdV-1 infection occurs in horses worldwide.

Hosts susceptible

Equines but foals & immunocompromised foals are severely infected.

Transmission

Transmission mainly occurs by aerosol droplets. The virus enters in to the host through the upper respiratory mucosa or conjunctiva.

Clinical symptoms

Clinical signs in most horses include mild upper respiratory tract infection, cough, conjunctivitis, mild and transient fever, diarrhea & mild bilateral nasal discharge.

Clinical signs in Arab foals are severe interstitial and bronchopneumonia with muffled normal airway sounds and extensive adventitious noises. Other symptoms are cough, ocular/nasal discharge, fever, ulcerated oral mucosa & diarrhea. In Arabian foals, the disease severity is due to a combined immunodeficincy resulting from a genetic defect.

Diagnosis

Collection of clinical samples includes nasal and ocular swabs, and lung tissue.

1. *A presumptive diagnosis*: It is based on clinical symptoms, IN inclusion bodies in conjunctival scrapings and tissue sections of lung and various other tissues.
2. *Virus isolation*: The virus can be isolated in in cell cultures of equine kidney producing typical adenovirus cytopathic effects, & IN inclusions.

Treatment & prevention

Due to the ubiquity of the virus, it is difficult to avoid infection.

Genus: *Aviadenovirus:*

Quail Bronchitis

Quail bronchitis is a naturally occurring, highly contagious, often fatal respiratory disease of bobwhite quail-both wild and in captivity. Symptoms include respiratory distress, coughing, sneezing, rales, and lacrimation, loose, watery droppings in some acutely affected older birds, conjunctivitis, mild to severe tracheitis, airsacculitis, hepatitis, and gaseous distention of the intestines. Multiple pale, pinpoint foci of necrosis are seen in the liver and mottling and enlargement of the spleen are common lesions in the infected birds. Mortality may reach 100% in birds less than 2 weeks old but is usually less than 25% in birds older than 4 week old. The disease is of major economic significance to game bird breeders and has a worldwide distribution. It is a serious disease on certain farms where quails are pen-raised, and **when quails of different ages are maintained on the same premises.**

Etiology: *Fowl adenovirus A* (FAdV-1/CELO, chicken embryo lethal orphan virus) is the causative agent of quail bronchitis.

Occurrence

Quail bronchitis, an important disease of domestic and wild bobwhite quails occurs worldwide.

Hosts susceptible

Mostly young Bobwhite quails are susceptible to this acute to chronic disease. The virus also infects chickens and turkeys. It has been isolated from chicken eggs but does not produce a recognizable disease in chickens or turkeys.

Transmission

The virus is spread by airborne route. It is highly contagious and spreads rapidly through multiple-age units. Other avian species, particularly chickens, may be carriers.

Pathogenesis

Pathogenesis of quail bronchitis virus was studied after inratracheal infection in 1 week old bobwhite quails.Virus was first isolated from the lung 2 hours post inoculation (PI), from cecal tonsils and bursa of Fabricius 4 hours PI, and from spleen and liver 8 hours PI. Tissue virus titers were highest on days 4 to 6 hrs PI, corresponding with the severity of histologic lesions. Viral inclusions were present in tracheal mucosal epithelium by day 2 PI. On day 3 PI, tracheal epithelium was deciliated, formed an irregular luminal border, and had more frequent inclusions. On days 4 and 5 PI, tracheal epithelium was partially desquamated, but there were minimal leukocytic infiltrates.

Bronchiolar epithelium underwent similar changes, but the leukocytic infiltration was more intense and included lymphocytes and heterophils. There was extension of leukocytic infiltrates into surrounding lung that was most extensive on day 3 PI. Hyperplasia of splenic macrophages was first identified on day 2 PI and peaked by day 5 PI.

Clinical signs

The incubation period is a 2-7 days. Clinical signs include coughing, sneezing, huddling, depression, lacrimation, conjunctivitis, tracheitis and neurological signs (tremors and paralysis). Clinical signs also include loose, watery droppings, which are common in some acutely affected older birds. Mild to severe tracheitis, airsacculitis, hepatitis, and gaseous distention of the intestines may be seen. Multiple pale, pinpoint (3 mm) foci of necrosis in the liver and mottling and enlargement of the spleen are common lesions in the infected birds. Mortality may reach 100% in birds less than 2 week old, but is usually less than 25% in birds more than 4 week old.

PM lesions: include mucous in the trachea or bronchi, air sacs, cloudy corneas, and sinusitis. Foci in liver, spleen mottled and swollen spleen, and reddened lungs are consolidated, and atrophy of bursa of Fabricius can be seen.

Diagnosis

Collection of clinical specimens includes whole birds killed in acute cases.

1. *Presumptive diagnosis*: A first hand diagnosis is based on the clinical signs, high mortality, & lesions. Histopathologic lesions of tracheitis and bronchitis & IN inclusions are helpful.
2. *Virus isolation*: The virus is easily isolated from the respiratory tract of acutely affected birds, from fecal samples, intestine, liver, and occasionally the bursa of Fabricius. The virus is isolated in cell cultures of chicken embryonic liver or kidney, or by the inoculation of chicken embryos via the yolk sac requiring many passages to cause death of embryos. Dead embryos exhibit necrotic foci in the liver and urate accumulation in the mesonephrons. The virus is also identified by neutralization tests.

There are no commercial vaccines available. Prevention is by strict sanitary measures to prevent introduction of the virus.

Treatment & prevention

Therapy consists of supportive care; broad-spectrum antibiotics are used to control secondary bacterial infections. Biosecurity and sanitation are helpful to control the disease, and to date no vaccine is available. Prevention remains the principal means of control.

Inclusion Body Hepatitis

Inclusion body hepatitis in young chickens is characterized by depression, inappetance, ruffled feathers & pallor of comb and wattles. PM lesions include liver swollen, yellow, mottled with petechiae and ecchymoses, kidneys and bone marrow pale, blood thin, & bursa and spleen small. **Microscopically - basophilic IN inclusions** are observed.

Etiology: *Fowl adenovirus B* **(FAdV- 1)** & many types cause inclusion body hepatitis in young chickens. There are 12 serotypes of AAV, the most common viruses isolated in cases of IBH belong to serotypes 4 and 8. These viruses are capable of producing the disease without the immunosuppressive effects of infectious bursal disease & other immunosuppressive agents. But, the association with immunosuppressive viruses such as IBDV and chicken anemia virus result in a more severe disease.

Occurrence

IBH, which most often affects young chickens, occurs infrequently worldwide.

Hosts susceptible

The disease usually occurs in broilers that are 3 to 4 weeks of age, although clinical signs can be detected in affected flocks as early as 7 days of age.

Transmission

Infected birds remain carriers for a few weeks. Transmission is via vertical or lateral means or by fomites. Vertical transmission has been described in progeny from breeder flocks infected with serotypes 4 and 8. Horizontal transmission has also been demonstrated; young chicks in contact with infected chicks can die of peracute IBH. Chicks and young chickens are commonly affected. Infection with some strains of AAV may result in minimal hepatic disease; however, if birds have been infected with immunosuppressive viruses (IBD, CAV, Marek's disease), the clinical disease becomes evident. Immunosuppression caused due to early IBD challenge or congenital CAV infection may result in the disease.

Clinical symptoms & lesions

The disease usually occurs in broilers that are 3 to 4 weeks of age, although clinical signs can be detected in affected flocks as early as 7 days of age. The first sign of IBH is severe stunting and unevenness in the flock. As the disease progresses, affected birds look very sick, exhibit signs of extreme depression and refuse to eat or move although overall morbidity is usually low. Abnormal wing feathering ("helicopter wings") can also be seen in affected birds. Winter and spring are the most common seasons for the disease to occur, & recurring infections occurred in 2 or 3 successive flocks on the same farm.

Mortality increases in the third week and ranges from severe to moderate. Mortality usually peaks and abates in the span of 7 to 10 days, but the subsequent unevenness in the flock persists until the birds are moved to the processing plant. Subsequent culling of small birds by the grower adds to the mortality total, which averages 10%, with severely affected flocks approaching 20% mortality. Sudden mortality usually is seen in chickens <6 week old and as young as 4 days of age. Mortality normally ranges from 2-40%, especially when birds are <3 week of age. However, there have been outbreaks in which mortality has reached 80%. Mortality rates also vary depending on the pathogenicity of the virus and coinfection with other viral or bacterial agents. Signs associated with diseases caused by other pathogens (eg, bacteria, fungi, or viruses) commonly occur if birds are immunosuppressed.

Gross liver lesions of IBH; the primary liver lesion is an enlarged, pale or yellow and friable liver with hemorrhagic patches forming a soccer ball pattern in sections of the liver or uniformly throughout the entire organ. In some birds hydropericardium, consisting of clear, yellow fluid around a slightly enlarged heart is seen. Severe swelling and edema of the proventriculus is commonly observed in affected birds and flocks. Birds with deeply yellow skin and body fat can be found. Kidneys may be pale and enlarged, and rarely hemorrhagic lesions may be observed in the pancreas.

Diagnosis

Collection of clinical samples includes whole sick, live birds.

1. *Presumptive diagnosis*: This is usually based on macroscopic liver lesions and microscopic examination of characteristic intranuclear inclusion bodies in hepatocytes. Histopathology of affected livers shows areas of necrosis in which liver cells contained numerous enlarged nuclei filled with basophilic IN inclusion bodies, which were also seen in sections of pancreas but not seen in the proventriculus.

2. *Virus isolation*: virus is isolated on the chorioallantoic membrane of chicken embryos or in avian kidney cell cultures and identified by the virus neutralization test. Since disease is widespread in distribution; isolation of virus is not attempted.

Agar gel immunodiffusion tests using Group 1 AAV antigen were positive on livers from infected embryos. Serotyping was carried out on several isolates.

Treatment & prevention

Although no specific treatment for IBH is available, many IBH flocks were treated with sulfa drugs for treatment and prevention of secondary infections due to *E. coli.*

Disinfection of built-up litter with Virkon-S to prevent recurrence in subsequent flocks was also used with mixed results. Heating of affected houses to 110+F between flocks was ineffective in preventing recurrence of IBH.

Vaccination

Vaccines against IBH are not commercially available in the USA but in other countries **both live and inactivated vaccines are used to control the syndrome using serotypes 4 and 8.** Primary breeders with stringent biosecurity practices sometimes use autogenous inactivated vaccines to ensure the transfer of maternal immunity from breeding flocks to their progeny. In Australia, a live vaccine given via drinking water was developed for breeders between 10-14 weeks of age. In other countries, including Mexico, Pakistan, and Peru, **inactivated vaccines are routinely used to vaccinate breeders and broilers.** When breeders are properly vaccinated, antibodies generated by the vaccine are transmitted to the progeny, providing protection against field infections and clinical disease. Broilers are vaccinated at less than 10 days of age when their parents either do not have serotype-specific adenovirus antibodies or maternal antibody transmission is erratic due to improper vaccination procedures that result in a substantial number of unvaccinated birds.

Genus: *Atadenovirus:*

Egg Drop Syndrome

Egg drop syndrome is a viral disease that occurs mostly in broiler chickens of 5-6 wk age & quails. The first symptom is usually a loss of color in pigmented eggs, followed by thin-shelled, soft-shelled, and shell-less eggs in apparently healthy birds. It has been recognized worldwide, except in the USA. The shells may be rough or "chalky." Shell-less eggs are not always found, as they may be eaten by the birds. Egg production usually drops 10% to 40%.

Etiology: The disease is caused by *Duck adenovirus A* (DAdV-1)/ EDSV, egg drop syndrome virus). The virus has one serotype but at least 3 genotypes: 1 associated with classical EDS, 1 with ducks in the UK, and 1 with EDS in Australia. EDS virus also differs from other avian adenoviruses by strongly agglutinating avian RBC.

Occurrence

EDS has been recognized worldwide, except in the USA. Duck adenovirus A occurs in ducks and geese. Egg drop syndrome occurs in Europe, Asia, Africa, and Latin America, but has not been seen in the U.S. or Canada. Respiratory disease in goslings has been reported only from Hungary.

Hosts susceptible

Egg drop syndrome has been reported in chickens and Japanese quails. Ducks and geese are the natural hosts for duck adenovirus A. This virus has also been isolated from coots and grebes, and antibodies have been found in many avian species including gulls, owls, storks, swans, guinea fowl, and pigeons. Clinical disease has been reported in chickens, quails, and geese. Turkeys can be infected experimentally but remain asymptomatic. The respiratory disease in goslings occurs between 4 and 20 days of age. All ages and breeds of chickens are susceptible, although the disease tends to be most severe in heavy broiler-breeders or brown egg producers.

Transmission

EDSV can be transmitted vertically in eggs; both the interior and the exterior of the egg contain virus. Chicks hatched from infected eggs may excrete the virus immediately. More often, the virus remains latent until the bird becomes sexually mature; it is then excreted in both eggs and droppings.

EDS horizontal transmission occurs mainly by the oral route; the infected birds excrete the virus in the feces. But, respiratory disease in goslings was reproduced by intratracheal administration of the virus. Duck adenovirus A can also be spread on/in fomites including water. Some outbreaks have been attributed to contact with wild birds or water contaminated by feces from wild birds. Iatrogenic transmission is possible by needles.

Pathogenesis

There are three types of EDS: **Classical EDS, endemic EDS & sporadic EDS.** Following horizontal or experimental infection, EDS virus grows to low titers in the nasal mucosa, followed by viremia. The virus then replicates in lymphoid tissue, and then massive replication occurs for about 8 days in the oviduct, especially in the pouch shell gland region. Changes in the egg shell occur coincidentally. Both the exterior and interior of eggs produced between 8-18 days after infection contain virus. A copious exudate in the lumen of the oviduct is rich in virus, and this contaminates the droppings. There is little, if any, growth in the epithelial cells of the intestine. Chicks hatched from infected eggs may excrete virus and develop antibody. More often, the virus remains latent, and antibody does not develop until the bird starts to lay, at which time the virus reactivates and grows in the oviduct, repeating the cycle.

Clinical symptoms & lesions

The incubation period for EDS is variable. Mature, experimentally infected, Rhode Island Red hens produced abnormal eggs from 10 to 24 days post-inoculation. Birds infected vertically can remain asymptomatic until they begin laying eggs. In experimentally infected goslings, the incubation period for respiratory disease is 3 to 4 days.

The major symptoms in affected chickens and quail are a variable decrease in egg production and the production of abnormal eggs. In naive flocks, the first symptom is usually a loss of color in pigmented eggs, followed by thin-shelled, soft-shelled, and shell-less eggs. The shells may also be rough or chalky. Shell-less eggs are not always found, as they may be eaten by the birds. Egg production usually drops 10% to 40%; however, eggs that are suitable for hatching/ setting remain fertile and hatch as usual. Although transient diarrhea and dullness may be seen before the egg shell changes occur, infected birds generally remain healthy. Flocks with some pre-existing immunity usually experience a series of small disease episodes, with minimal symptoms. The overall effect is a small drop in production or a failure to achieve predicted production targets. Outbreaks of egg drop syndrome usually last 4 to 10 weeks. A 10% to 40% drop in egg production can be expected in naive chicken flocks; in flocks with some immunity, the decrease may be 2% to 4%. In two outbreaks in quail, the decrease in egg production was 10% and 50%. Deaths are not expected in either species.

Until recently, geese were thought to be asymptomatic. However, in 2001, a severe acute respiratory disease associated with duck adenovirus A was reported in naturally infected goslings in Hungary. The disease affected goslings between 4 and 20 days of age. The symptoms included anorexia, depression, sneezing, coughing, dyspnea, and rales. This disease could be reproduced by intratracheal administration of duck adenovirus A to 1-day-old goslings without pre-existing antibodies. As of January 2006, this disease has not been reported in ducks. Respiratory disease has been reported in 4 to 20 day old domesticated geese. This disease was seen only in very young birds from a naive flock; its rarity may be explained by the high prevalence of antibodies in goose populations and the presence of maternal antibodies in young birds during the period of susceptibility. In goslings with respiratory disease, the mortality rate was 5% to 7%.

PM lesions in EDS are minimal and are confined to the reproductive tract of hens with inactive ovaries, atrophy of the oviducts, and edema and white exudates in the uterus (shell gland). Laid eggs may be paler than normal, rough, thin-shelled, soft-shelled, or shell-less. Histopathologic changes seen in the oviduct and uterus (shell gland) include severe degeneration and desquamation of the epithelial cells, atrophy of the uterine glands, and infiltration of heterophils, lymphocytes, and plasmacytes. IN inclusion bodies may be seen in the epithelial cells of the uterus, isthmus, and vaginal gland region.

Respiratory disease in goslings showed a plug of gelatinous to firm, white, opaque material in the trachea. Edema and slight congestion were seen in the trachea and lungs. Other reported lesions include ecchymoses on the epicardium and mottling in the liver. Acute tracheo-bronchitis and circumscribed catarrhal pneumonia were observed in experimentally infected birds. Histopathologic abnormalities included fibrin and cellular debris in the tracheal and bronchial lumina; the epithelium was hyperplastic and metaplastic. The superficial cells contained swollen nuclei with amphophilic inclusion bodies. The lungs were congested and contained lympho-histiocytic and heterophil granulocytic infiltration in the septae and in the lumina of the small air spaces.

Diagnosis

1. *Presumptive diagnosis*: Clinical symptoms, poor egg shell quality and a decrease in egg production by visibly healthy flock, or a small decrease in egg yields or a failure to reach expected production levels.are strongly suggestive of EDS.

   Respiratory disease caused by duck adenovirus A may be suspected in young goslings from naive flocks. Decreased production and poor shell quality can also occur in case of infectious bronchitis, Newcastle disease or avian influenza; but, birds with these diseases usually become ill.

2. *Virus isolation*: EDS virus is isolated in embryonated duck or goose eggs, and in cell cultures, in cell lines including duck and chick embryo liver, duck kidney, and fibroblast cells. The virus may be isolated directly from the reproductive tract of affected hens or from abnormal eggs or live hens; from the shell gland of these hens when they produce abnormal eggs.

3. *Viral antigen detection*: Viral antigens can be detected with PCR or antigen-capture ELISA techniques. In some studies immunofluorescence has been used.

4. *Serology*: Serologic tests include hemagglutination inhibition using fowl RBC, ELISA, and serum neutralization. The double immunodiffusion test has also been used.

Treatment & prevention

There is no treatment for EDS. The classical form has been eradicated from primary breeders. The endemic form in breeders can be controlled by washing and sanitizing incubators and egg trays before reuse. In layers, molting will restore egg production. Prevention is through the control of vertical transmission. Endemic EDS is associated with the egg-packing stations, as contaminated egg trays can be a major factor in spread. Virus is also present in fecal material, so hygienic procedures are required. Washing and disinfecting plastic egg trays before use can control the endemic form. The sporadic form can be prevented by separating chickens from other birds, especially water fowl. Sanitary precautions are taken, and potentially contaminated water should be chlorinated before use. Quarantine and disinfection are necessary, as Duck adenovirus A is contagious by either direct or indirect contact.

These viruses are resistant to many commonly used disinfectants & relatively tolerant of heat and pH changes. Iodophor and aldehyde disinfectants can be effective if they are allowed to contact the virus for prolonged periods. Composting infected chicken carcasses for 20 days completely inactivates the virus.

Vaccination

Inactivated vaccines with oil adjuvant are available. These vaccines decrease virus shedding but do not prevent infection. The vaccines are given during the growing phase **at 14-18 weeks**, and can be combined with other vaccines such as for NDV. **NOVILIS RT+IB MULTI+ND+ EDS** (INTERVET) is a combined inactivated vaccine for the vaccination of breeders & layers against Avian pneumovirus, IB (MassachusettsD207), ND in a water-in-oil emulsion. The best results will be obtained if vaccination with inactivated vaccine takes place 6 or more weeks after administration of the live primer but in no circumstances should this be carried out earlier than 4 weeks after priming. Inject each bird: 0.5 ml IM or SC. EDS Sentinel birds are frequently placed along with vaccinated chickens to detect the presence of virus in the flock. Sentinel chickens will become serologically positive on hemagglutination inhibition test.

Genus: *Siadenovirus*

Adenovirus Splenomegaly in Chickens

Splenomegaly in chickens is characterized by splenomegaly and splenic mottling, & splenic reticuloendothelial cell hyperplasia with IN inclusions. Lymphocytic degeneration is observed in the lungs of most chickens. Lung hemorrhage and edema with endothelial disruption and congestion of pulmonary arterioles are found less frequently. The splenic lesions in the chickens are similar to those seen in turkeys naturally infected with hemorrhagic enteritis, and the lung lesions resembled those seen in pheasants naturally infected with marble spleen disease.

Etiology: *Turkey adenovirus A*/ Turkey adenovirus-3 **(TAdV-3)** under the genus *Siadenovirus* remains associated with 3 specific entities in different hosts; splenomegaly in chickens (Avian adenovirus splenomegaly virus), marble spleen disease in pheasants (Marble spleen disease virus), & hemorrhagic enteritis in turkey (Turkey hemorrhagic enteritis virus).

Avian adenovirus splenomegaly was initially reported in 1979 from USA. It is usually a subclinical disease, but one report shows mortality associated with pulmonary edema. Adenovirus splenomegaly is characterized by enlargement of the spleen, pulmonary oedema & congestion. It is observed in broiler breeders at the age of 20-45 weeks. Its course is peracute or acute. The mortality could go up to 8 - 9%. The most typical lesions are splenomegaly, mottled or marble-like appearance of the spleen, edema or hyperaemia of lungs. Chickens, 6-week-old were orally infected with TAdV-3 adenovirus isolate previously obtained from chickens exhibiting splenomegaly in commercial broiler flocks. The primary gross lesions found were splenomegaly and splenic mottling. Histologic lesions included splenic reticuloendothelial cell hyperplasia with intranuclear inclusions. Lymphocytic degeneration was seen in the lungs of most chickens examined. Lung hemorrhages and edema with endothelial disruption and congestion of pulmonary arterioles were found less frequently. The splenic lesions in the chickens were similar to those seen in turkeys naturally infected with hemorrhagic enteritis, and the lung lesions resembled those seen in pheasants naturally infected with marble spleen disease.

Marble Spleen Disease in Pheasants

Marble spleen disease (MSD) is an acute, respiratory disease in pheasants of 3-8 months of age, characterized by acute onset, depression, enlarged mottled spleens, dyspnea, asphyxiation, and sudden death due to pulmonary congestion and edema. Mortality is commonly 2-3% but can reach 15%. Secondary bacterial infections occur due to immunosuppression.

Etiology: It is caused by *Turkey adenovirus- 3*/Marble spleen disease virus **(TAdV-3)**. Infection with less virulent pathotypes in host may go undetected until secondary bacterial infections begin to develop as a result of viral-induced immunosuppression.

Occurrence

Marble spleen disease is geographically widespread and considered endemic in areas where pheasants are raised commercially. Morbidity usually approaches 100% for marble spleen disease.

Hosts susceptible

Pheasants of **3-8 months of age** are susceptible. Pheasants more than 4 week of age are resistant to infection due to age-related resistance or due to the presence of maternal antibody.

Transmission

The usual route of infection is oral, and virus is often introduced onto previously uninfected premises via personnel or equipment contaminated with infectious feces. As infection begins to cycle through a flock, **large quantities of virus are shed in the feces**, which facilitate rapid spread through susceptible birds. The virus may survive under moist conditions (ie, in litter) well beyond the refractory period.

Clinical symptoms & lesions

Marble spleen disease affects pheasants 3-8 months of age. There occurs acute onset, depression, **bloody droppings**, dyspnea, asphyxiation, and sudden death occurring as a result of pulmonary congestion and edema.

PM lesions : include hemorrhages in the gut, liver, gizzard and proventriculus and anemia. An enlarged mottled spleen and free blood in the intestines can be seen. Lung edema and congestion are also evident in MSD. Grayish-tan, mottled, and enlarged spleens are characteristic. **Intranuclear inclusions** are seen in the reticuloendothelial cells of the affected tissue. Mortality is commonly 2-3% but can reach 15%. Secondary bacterial infections as a result of immunosuppression have also been observed.

Histopathologic exam of the infected pheasants reveals flooding of the atria and tertiary bronchi with fibrin and RBC, as well as generalized **vascular congestion and focal necrosis** are often seen in the lung. As with hemorrhagic enteritis, this response may be anaphylactic in nature, with the **lung being considered the target shock organ** in the pheasant. Splenomegaly with lymphoreticular hyperplasia and lymphoid necrosis also occur and are the characteristic lesions for which marble spleen disease is named. Basophilic intranuclear inclusions may be found in a variety of tissues excluding the GI tract with the highest concentration of virus again being found in the spleen.

Diagnosis

Presumptive diagnosis: A first hand diagnosis of marble spleen disease is based on clinical signs, gross lesions & histopathology with intranuclear inclusion bodies in the reticuloendothelial (RE) cells of the spleen.

Serology: The presence of seroprecipitating virus in the spleen is detected by agar gel immunodiffusion test. To determine marble spleen disease is a predisposing factor in cases of bacterial respiratory disease or septicemia, or to verify a primary diagnosis, acute and convalescent sera (3 weeks apart) can be tested using either agar gel immunodiffusion or ELISA. In pheasants with acute respiratory disease, differential diagnoses include Newcastle disease, avian influenza, and in the case of birds reared in confinement, gaseous toxins. Agar gel precipitin (AGP) test and ELISA are used to measure antibody.

Treatment & prevention

There is no specific treatment available for MSD but supportive care, strict sanitation and good management practices are helpful in reducing mortalities and limiting the spread of an epizootic. Antibiotics are used to control bacterial infection. In addition to good biosecurity, prevention hinges on the vaccination of birds.

Vaccination

Vaccincs are used in water at about **4-5 weeks of age.** Commercially available tissue culture products and crude splenic preparations containing **avirulent isolates produce life-long protection**. Due to potential for interaction with other agents, including live vaccines, regular disease monitoring and careful integration of marble spleen disease vaccines into flock vaccination protocols is encouraged. Intuitively, vaccines should not be administered to birds exhibiting signs of illness or within 2 weeks of any other vaccination.

Haemorrhagic Enteritis of Turkey

Haemorrhagic enteritis is an **acute gastroentestinal disorder affecting young turkey poults 4-16 weeks old. Symptoms in** outbreaks with highly virulent pathotypes include depression, pallor, and bloody droppings. Acute mortality ranges from less than 1% to 60% with an average of 10-15% over a 2-week period. Surviving birds develop a transient immunosuppression related to the lymphotrophic, & lymphocytopathic nature of the virus causing secondary bacterial infections, e.g, colibacillosis, in 10-14 days after initial exposure to the virus causing a second peak in mortality. In less virulent outbreaks, the clinical picture is characterized by lesions associated with bacterial respiratory disease or septicemia, e.g., fibrinopurulent pneumonia, air sacculitis, pericarditis, peritonitis, perihepatitis, hepatomegaly, and splenomegaly. Concomitant or prior exposure to NDV, *Bordetellaavium* or *Mycoplasma* spp exacerbates the problem.

Etiology: The disease is caused by *Turkey adenovirus- 3*/Turkey hemorrhagic enteritis virus (THEV). Several viral pathotypes appear to exist that differ slightly at the DNA level but are indistinguishable serologically. All strains of THEV are serologically indistinguishable, although there are naturally occurring avirulent strains of THEV that replicate efficiently in turkeys without the intestinal hemorrhage or mortality is associated with more virulent strains.

Occurrence

Hemorrhagic enteritis is geographically widespread and considered endemic in areas where turkeys are raised commercially.

Hosts susceptible

The virus affects young turkey poults 6-12 week old. Turkeys younger than 2–4 weeks of age are resistant to clinical HE. This age-related resistance is expressed in the presence or absence of maternal antibodies against HEV.

Transmission

The usual route of infection is oral, and virus is introduced into previously uninfected premises via personnel or equipment contaminated with infectious feces. As infection begins to cycle through a flock, large quantities of virus are shed in the feces, which facilitate rapid spread through susceptible birds. Morbidity usually approaches 100%.

Clinical symptoms & lesions

In commercial flocks, hemorrhagic enteritis affects **turkeys 6-12 wk of age.** In outbreaks caused by highly virulent pathotypes, clinical signs include depression, pallor, and bloody droppings. Acute mortality ranges from less than 1% to 60% with an average of 10-15% over a 2-week period. Birds that survive the acute phase experience a transient immunosuppression related to the lymphotrophic, lymphocytopathic nature of the virus. This results in secondary bacterial infections, e.g., colibacillosis) ~10-14 days after initial exposure to the virus. Thus, a second peak in mortality, potentially overlapping the first, may be seen. In less virulent outbreaks, lesser mortality may actually dominate the clinical picture. The second wave of mortality often lasts 2-4 weeks and is characterized by lesions commonly associated with bacterial respiratory disease or septicemia e.g., fibrinopurulent pneumonia, airsacculitis, pericarditis, peritonitis, perihepatitis, hepatomegaly, and splenomegaly. Concomitant or prior exposure to Newcastle disease virus, *Bordetella avium & Mycoplasma* spps is known to exacerbate the problem. Similar multiple agent interactions have been implicated in mortality associated with the use of vaccines for hemorrhagic enteritis.

The virus causes **intranuclear inclusions** in the reticuloendothelial cells. Field data and laboratory studies indicate that THEV causes immunodepression in the humoral as well as the cellular immune functions of turkeys. The mechanism of immunodepression is not known. The main **gross lesions** were splenomegaly and hemorrhagic contents in the gut. The **histological lesions** were intranuclear inclusion bodies in **large mononuclear cells** in many visceral organs and in reticular cells around the sheathed arteries of the spleens and varying degrees of lymphocytic hyperplasia in most tissues. The inclusions were frequently present in areas of the lymphocytic hyperplasia. The large mononuclear cells with the inclusions frequently showed a degenerative change.

Diagnosis

Presumptive diagnosis: A presumptive diagnosis of virulent outbreaks of haemorrhagic enteritis is based on clinical signs, gross lesions, & by histopathology with intranuclear inclusions in the reticuloendothelial cells and the presence of seroprecipitating virus in the spleen as determined by agar gel immunodiffusion.

PCR is used to detect haemorrhagic enteritis viral DNA in tissue in selected laboratories. To determine whether haemorrhagic enteritis is a predisposing factor in cases of bacterial respiratory disease or septicemia, or to verify a primary diagnosis, acute and convalescent sera, 3 week apart can be tested using either agar gel immunodiffusion or ELISA. In turkeys, differential diagnoses include colibacillosis, pasteurellosis, paratyphoid, and erysipelas. Reticuloendotheliosis or lymphoproliferative disease should be considered when lymphoreticular hyperplasia is the predominant lesion. GI lesions without splenic involvement should evoke consideration of other viral, bacterial, parasitic, and toxic enteritis of turkeys.

Treatment & prevention

Virulent outbreaks of hemorrhagic enteritis have been successfully treated and controlled by SC injection of exposed birds with 0.5-1.0 ml of antiserum obtained from recovered flocks. Antibiotics are used to control bacterial infection.

Vaccination

In addition to good biosecurity, & sanitary measures, prevention is based on the use of **vaccines administered in the water at about 4-5 weeks of age. Commercially available tissue culture products and crude splenic preparations containing avirulent isolates produce life-long protection.** Most vaccinate at 4.5 to 5.5 weeks of age, using a mild vaccine. **ORALVAX HE** (Intervet) is a live vaccine containing Type II avian adenovirus of pheasant origin which is vaccinated to 6 weeks or older turkeys to prevent hemorrhagic enteritis in turkeys. Distribute 2000 doses of vaccine in water as used by 2000 turkeys and 5000 doses of vaccine in water as used by 5000 turkeys. Provide ample watering space so that all of the turkeys can drink easily. By taking 10-20 sera before vaccination and 10-20 sera two weeks following vaccine administration, the ELISA results give an excellent comparison to equip management with the tools to measure flock readiness. Due to potential for interaction with other agents, including live vaccines, regular disease monitoring and careful integration of hemorrhagic enteritis vaccines into flock vaccination protocols is encouraged. Vaccines should not be administered to birds exhibiting signs of illness or within 2 weeks of any other vaccination.

□□□

Chapter 9

Characteristics and Diseases Caused by Group I Double-Stranded DNA Asfarviruses (Family *Asfarviridae*)

Contents

Characteristics of Asfarviruses

Asfarviridae name is derived from the acronym: **A**frican **s**wine **f**ever **a**nd **r**elated viruses; the family contains only one genus, *Asfivirus* & type species, *African swine fever virus*that causes African swine fever. Thevirions of *Asfarviridae* are large, **enveloped**, spherical measuring 175-215 nm in diameter. The virus consists of an **icosahedral capsid**& a cylindrical core enclosing viral genome made of linear ds DNA 170-190 kb. Capsid has a diameter of 172-191 nm & exhibits icosahedral symmetry (T=189-217) corresponding to 1892-2172 capsomers each measuring 13 nm in diameter. Virus is maintained in two cycles- **sylvatic cycle** involving inapparent infection between warthogs & bushpigs & *Ornithodorus* ticks; &**domestic cycle** initiated either by the bite of the infected ticks or infection among domestic pigs through direct contact, blood, tissues & secretions & excretions of the infected animals or through indirect means. **Asfaviruses are the only DNA viruses which are arboviruses being transmitted by ticks.** Four **markers of ASFV include hemadsorption,**

virulence, plaque size & antigenicity. Buffy coat cells from the infected animal hemadsorb pig RBCs.

ASF is highly **resistant** to wide range of pH & temperature & other environmental conditions. The virus can survive for a year and a half in blood stored at 4°C, 11 days in feces at room temperature, and at least a month in contaminated pig pens, remain infectious for 150 days in boned meat stored at 4°C, 140 days in salted dried hams, and several years in frozen carcasses.

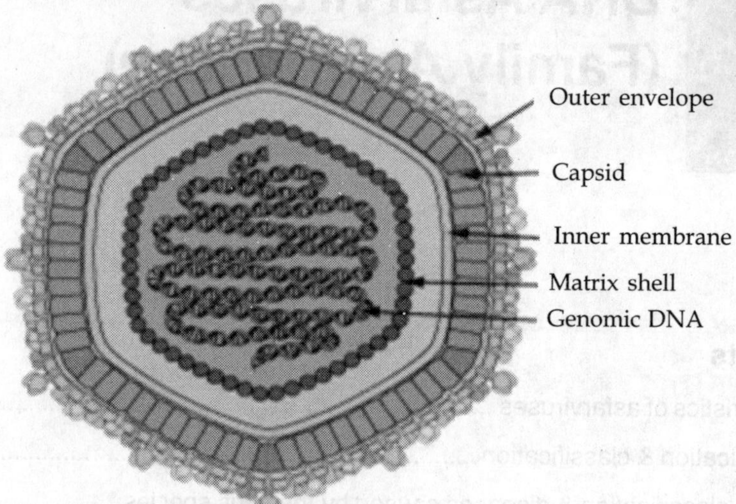

Figure 9.1 : Morphology of Asfivirus

The virus genome

The genome is not segmented & consists of linear dsDNA genome of 170-190 kb. The genomic end sequences are complementary. The genome guanine + cytosine content are 39 %. The genome sequence has termini with hairpin structure. The genome has terminally redundant sequences wih reiterated inverted terminal sequences which are tandemly repeated. The viral genome encodes both non-structural proteins and structural proteins.The genome encodes for at least 151 Open reading frames & 151 proteins. The genome encodes enzymes required for replication and transcription of the dsDNA.

Virus replication

Virus replication occurs in the host cells. The Virus enters host cells through receptor mediated endocytosis followed by fusion of virus membrane with the endocytic vesicle membrane & release of DNA genome into the cytoplasm. Thereafter **early viral genes** are transcribed followed by replication of the DNA genome in the cytoplasm. After DNA replication, **late viral genes** are transcribed as well as structural proteins are formed. Assembly of the icosahedral capsid occurs on modified membranes of the endoplasmic reticulum. Polyproteins form the core shell between the internal membrane and the nucleocapsid core. Outer membrane is gained as particles bud from the plasma membrane.

Virus classification

Group: Group I dsDNA viruses

Family: *Asfarviridae*

Genus: *Asfivirus;* Type species: *African swine fever virus*

Asfarviral Clinical Manifestations in Pigs

Asfivirus causes African swine fever.

Table 9-1: Details of *Asfivirus* showing species, isolates & types.

Family	Genus	Species (Italics)	Types
Asfarviridae	*Asfivirus*	*African swine fever virus*	
		African swine fever virus - Ba71V	ASF- Ba71V
		African swine fever virus- LIL20/1	ASF- LIL20/1
		African swine fever virus- E70, isolate MS44	ASF-E40/MS44
		African swine fever virus- E70, isolate MS16	ASF-E40/MS16
		African swine fever virus-LIS57	ASF-LIS57

African Swine Fever

African swine fever is a highly contagious viral disease of domestic pigs & wild boars characterized hy haemorrhagic fever, rapid spread; and having serious socioeconomic effects in international trade of pigs or pig products and food security. There is initial thrombocytopenia & disseminated vascular coagulation causing hemorrhages, serous exudation, infarction & local edema & engorgement of tissues. The mortality rate depends on the virulence of the isolates, virulent isolates in peracute & acute cases induces about 100% mortality; subacute isolates, 70-80% mortality in young pigs but less than 20% in older animals & 2-3% mortality in chronic cases in endemic areas. ASF is a notifiable disease by the World Health Organization (OIE).

Etolology: African swine fever is caused by *African swine fever virus* (ASFV), that don't contain diffirent antigenic types, but distinct genotypes have been identified using restriction enzyme analysis of the genomes of viruses obtained from different geographic areas. Among 5 genotypes, American & European genotypes of ASFV do not differ much but African genotypes differ.

Occurrence

African swine fever was generally prevalent and endemic in the majority of the countries of Sub-Saharan Africa & in Sardinia (Italy) until 1957 when the disease was reported in Portugal in 1960 & in Spain. The disease became established in the Iberian peninsula and sporadic outbreaks occurred in 1971 in France, Belgium and other European countries during the 1980s. In 1978 ASF outbreaks occurred in Malta, Sardinia, Brazil, Dominican Republic & Haiti. Since then Spain and Portugal eradicated the disease by 1990s through a slaughter policy. In 1970s ASFV crossed the Atlantic Ocean & outbreaks were reported in some Caribbean islands, Cuba and the Dominican Republic. Recently outbreak of ASFV occurred in 2007 in Georgia and spread to the neighbouring countries of Armenia, Azerbaijan & Russia. Outbreaks of ASF again occurred in 2010 in Russia, Armenia & Chad & FAO has declared ASF to be a global threat.

Hosts susceptible

African swine fever affects members of the pig family including domesticated swine, European wild boars, warthogs, bushpigs, giant forest hogs, and peccaries. Clinical infections occur only in domesticated pigs of all ages & breeds, feral pigs and European wild boars. But warthogs, bush pigs and giant forest hogs suffer only inapparent infection; these species are thought to be the reservoirs for the virus in Africa. Other species that may carry the virus asymptomatically include the collared peccary and the white-lipped peccary (*Tayassu albirostris*), both found in America. *Ornidorus spp* ticks get infected from viremic warthog pigs by bite during blood feeding & transmit the virus to domestic pigs. This is followed by maintenance of the virus among domestic pigs via contact with sicks & their blood, tissues & all secretions & excretions.

Transmission

African swine fever virus is maintained in two types of cycles; 1.**Sylvatic cycle & 2. Domestic cycle. In sylvatic cycle** warthogs & bushpigs act as the natural reservoirs & they suffer inapparent infection while the soft ticks of the *Ornithodoro moubata* complex act both as biological carriers & virus vectors. *Ornithodorus* Spp ticks get infected through blood feeding from young viremic warthogs. Thereafter the virus is maintained in wart hog- associated ticks through trans-stadial, transovarian & sexual means from male to female transmission for years. Ticks involved in Africa are *O. moubata* but in some areas where *O. mobata* is absent, *O savignyi* are involved. In Europe *vector ticks are O. erraticus* but in America most *Ornithodorus* Spp that feed on pigs are vectors & in Caribbean countries, vectors are *O. puertoricensis* & *O. coriaceus.* 2. **In endemic areas,** the virus is maintained for more than 5 yrs in these ticks; hence when the ticks come in vicinity of domestic pigs carried by wart hogs or their carcases or when wart hogs mix with domestic pigs, occasional outbreaks of ASF occur. 3. **In domestic cycle** that involves clinical infection in pigs of local breeds, the virus once introduced, transmission occurs through direct or indirct contact. The infected pigs' blood, tissues, all secretions, excretion & feces contain the virus. 4. In Spain & Portugal there is emergence of less virulent virus where some **recovered pigs remain as persistently infected viremic carriers** & they serve to infect other pigs. 5. In some areas like mountainous Sardina source of spread is movement of pigs in previously infected areas, or introduction of infected pigs to healthy herds or feeding of herds with waste meat containg food from infected pigs. 6. Infection among domestic pigs also takes place via infected pens, fomites, by contaminated feed & water & feeding of uncooked garbage. 7. ASFV is very resistant to pH, temp, putrefaction, heat & dryness, chilled garbage survival for 6 months aid to high risk of infection.

Pathogenesis

Domestic pigs get infection via oronasal route, virus initially multiplies in pharyngeal mucosa, tonsils & regional lymph nodes & then virus spread to the blood stream causing viremia. The virus then spread to & replicates in the cells of RBCs, endothelial cells, leukocytes & macrophage lineages of other lymph nodes, spleen, lung, liver, kidneys & bone marrow causing secondary prolonged viremia. There is destruction of monocytes –macrophages, lymphocytes death by apoptosis causing **leucopenia, necrosis of megakryocytes**, vascular damage namely degeneration of vascular endothelium, thrombocytopenia & disseminated intravascular coagulation. Extensive hemorrhages are mediated by the combined mechanism of necrosis of megakaryocytes causing thrombocytopenia, disseminated intravascular coagulation & extensive destruction of monocytes & macrophages. These result in hemorrhages in many organs, serous exudation, infarction, pulmonary edema, engorged spleen, petechiae & echymotic hemorrhages. Lymphopenia is caused by lymphocytes death, mainly T cells death by apoptosis as well as monocytes- macrophages death & **associated immunodeficiency**. Although there are 4 forms of clinical manifestations- **peracute, acute, subacute & chronic**, but all clinical forms show **extensive hemorrhages**, which is a presumptive diagnosis. While virulent viruses produce renal hemorrhages due to vascular endothelial cell damage but moderately virulent viruses cause hemorrhages due to increased vascular permeability.

ASFV crosses placenta & replicates in fetal tissues & causes abortion of pregnant sows.

Clinical symptoms & lesions

Incubation period is 5-15 days, followed by one or usually more of these forms of disease:

Peracute form of ASF is caused by virulent virus strains resulting in some pigs found suddenly dead, or near death.

Acute form shows high fever-40.5^{0}C that persists for 4 days, anorexia and inactivity & extreme weakness to hind quarters. Areas of cyanotic blotching-red or blue skin discoloration appear on the ventral chest or abdomen, tips of ear or tail, or distal limbs. Sick animals may develop diarrhea, vomiting, coughing, breathing difficulty and the pregnants abort. Fatality rate is up to 100%. **Recovered pigs usually become lifelong carriers of the virus.**

Subacute form cases are observed with moderately virulent virus infection in which the affected pigs become mildly ill, but pregnant sows may abort. There may be intermittent fever seen for one month, followed by recovery in majority of cases. Case fatality varies from 30-70%. Recovered pigs excrete the virus up to six weeks of infection.

Chronic form cases show episodes of fever with illness but there is reduced growth, stunting or emaciation. Necrotic patches of skin or chronic skin ulcers may be seen. Sick pigs become prone to secondary infections, pneumonia and lameness/arthritis. Although disease lasts for two to five months but mortality is less than 30%.

PM lesions

PM lesions in **acute form** depend on the virus virulence. Usually hemorrhages are seen in the gastrohepatic and renal lymph nodes. There are pinpoint hemorrhages of the renal cortex, also in medulla and pelvis of kidneys & on the mucous membranes of larynx and bladder and on visceral surfaces of organs.

Also seen are congestive splenomegaly, oedematous areas of cyanosis in hairless parts, cutaneous ecchymoses on the legs and abdomen, & excess of pleural, pericardial and/peritoneal fluid. There are petechiae in the mucous membranes of the larynx and bladder, and on visceral surfaces of organs. Besides the above, oedema in the mesenteric structures of the colon and adjacent to the gall bladder & wall of gall bladder are seen.

In **chronic form,** there are usually focal caseous necrosis and mineralization of the lungs. Lymph nodes are seen enlarged. **Histologically,** diagnostic lesions are **destruction of mononuclear phagocytic system, megakaryocytes, tonsilar crypt cells, renal cells, hepatocytes & endothelial cells.** There are lymphocytic karyorrhexis in lymphoid tissues. Pinpoint hemorrhages are seen in the cortex, medulla and pelvis of the kidneys. Lymph nodes are enlarged and hemorrhages may be seen in the gastrohepatic and renal lymph nodes. Ecchymoses are usually seen in the skin of the legs or abdomen. The spleen is often enlarged and there can be excess fluid in the abdominal, pleural and pericardial cavities. Oedema of the gall bladder and mesentery of the colon is unique to ASF. In chronic cases, lungs may show focal lesions of caseous necrosis and even mineralization.

Diagnosis

1. *Presumptive diagnosis* is usually made on the basis of clinical symptoms and pathologic lesions.

2. *Virus isolation*: Samples for virus isolation include blood, tissues from spleen, kidney or lymph nodes. Samples are inoculated on to pig macrophages obtained from bone marrow or lung washing. Many strains of ASF virus adsorb pig RBCs; the presence of virus in cell cultures is confirmed by **hemadsorption**; when pig RBCs are added to to the culture, RBCs are attracted to the surface of the infected cells, to which they cling and form "rosettes", a phenomenon known as hemadsorption. The virus may also be injected into susceptible pigs & unvaccinated and vaccinated against classical swine fever virus to confirm that it infects pigs and cause disease. Some ASFV strains do not cause hemadsorption but dead cells in the culture will become obvious after a few days. The cultured virus is then characterized to determine the strain.

3. *Virus antigen detection*: Viral antigens can be demonstration by direct immunofluorescence test on suspected tissues.

   PCR detects viral genetic material & is a sensitive test & can be **performed in putrefied samples** that cannot be used for virus isolation and antigen detection.

4. *Antibody detection*: Serological tests: Group-specific tests detect antibodies on serum from recovering pigs, 8-21 days after infection. **ELISA** is considered useful test for detecting antibodies to ASF virus; other tests are indirect fluorescent antibody test, **immunoblotting (confirmatory**

test), & counter immunoelectrophoresis test is used only for screening of large groups.

Treatment & prevention

Currently there exists no treatment or vaccine. Presently scientists are working on using CD^8+ T cells from avirulent ASFV isolates to induce immunity. In disease free countries, all garbage fed to pigs should be cooked, unprocessed meat should be heated to at least 70ºC for 30 minutes to inactivate the virus. Disposal of waste food from aircraft or ships coming from the infected countries & efficient sterilization of garbage are practiced.

Eradication in the infected countries is done by slaughter of infected and in-contact animals, & disposal of carcasses. Strict quarantine is practiced as ASFV survives for long periods on fomites and in the environment. **Sodium hypochlorite** and some iodine and quaternary ammonium compounds are effective for sanitation. Vectors ticks should be controlled with acaricides. In endemic countries contact between pigs and soft tick vectors are avoided & wandering of pigs is prevented.

□□□

Chapter 10

Characteristics and Diseases Caused by Group 1 Double Stranded DNA Herpesviruses (Family *Herpesviridae*)

Contents

Characteristics of Herpesviruses

Herpesviridae (G. herpein= to creep) name is derived from the Greek word **herpein** ("to creep"), meaning to the latent, recurring & lytic infections caused by the viruses. *Herpesviridae* belongs to the order *Herpesvirales* (created in **2008 by the ICTV**) & comprises large, diverse group of DNA viruses that infect amphibians, reptiles, birds & mammals including humans and a wide variety of animal hosts. Herpesviruses are divergent with regard to wide occurrence, genome sequence, proteins, & biological properties, but are similar in overall virion structure and genome organization. Virions are spherical to pleomorphic & measure 150nm-200nm in size having linear dsDNA genome of about 120-230kbp long and contains 60 to 120 genes. A typical virion consists from outside within of: an envelope, a proteinous tegument, & an icosahedral capsid surrounding the DNA genome in the core. To elaborate the four structures: core consists of a single linear molecule of dsDNA in the form of a torus. Capsid surrounds the core & has an **icosahedral symmetry (T= 16)** with a 100 nm diameter made of 162 capsomers. Tegument lie between the capsid & the envelope & is made of an amorphous, sometimes asymmetrical & consists of viral enzymes, some of which are needed to take control of the cell's chemical processes and subvert them to virion production, some of which defend against the host cell's immediate responses, & others of unknown function. Envelope is the outer layer of the virion and is composed of altered host membrane and a dozen unique viral glycoproteins. They appear in electron micrographs as short spikes embedded in the envelope.

There are 4 biological properties of herpesviruses; 1. These viruses express a large number of enzymes needed for metabolism of nucleic acid, like thymidine kinase for DNA synthesis, like DNA helicase/primase and for processing of proteins e.g. protein kinase. 2. The virus replicates in the nucleus, hence viral genome synthesis and capsid assembly takes place in the nucleus. 3. When productive viral infection occurs, there is cell death. 4. Herpesviruses can form a **latent state in their host and reactivate on cellular stress; during latency the viral genome is maintained in the nucleus as circular episomes with limited expression of viral genes.**

The strategies of herpesvirus infections depend upon three mechanisms. 1. The virion invades the host cell & turns off host protein synthesis and release viral DNA into the nucleus rapidly where replication and virion production start. 2. Herpesviruses thwart the host immune attack by inhibiting splicing of mRNA, blocking presentation of antigenic peptides on the cell surface & blocking the apoptosis (cell death) induced by viral gene expression. 3. Herpesviruses become latently infected, is able to hide their bare, circularized genome in the nucleus of lymphoma and central nervous system cells and then return to productive infection months, even years later on various stresses.

These latent infections are mostly benign, but can be very serious to newborns and immunosuppressed hosts.

The virus genome

The genome of herpesviruses is non-segmented, contains one molecule of double-stranded **DNA 120-230kbp** long and contains 60 to 120 genes. Guanine + cytosine base content is 31% to 75%. Genes are of two types, essential & dispensable genes. While the essential genes regulate transcription and are needed for virion, the dispensable genes are required for virus infection, promote cell-to-cell spread, defend the virus from the host's immune system, and make the cellular environment ideal for virus production. Termini have direct and inverted terminal repeats on all herpesvirus genomes. As herpesviruses replicate inside the nucleus, they use both the host's transcription machinery and DNA repair enzymes to support a large genome with complex genes. The genes like the eukaryotic genes are not arranged in operons, and in most cases have individual promoters but unlike eukaryotic genes, very few herpesvirus genes are spliced.

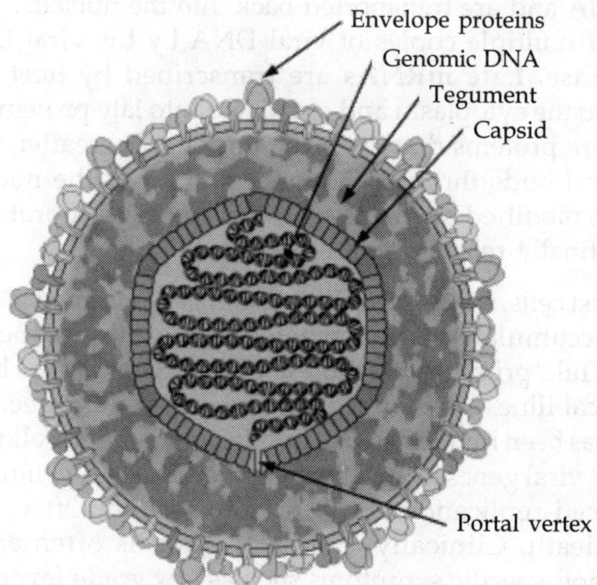

Figure 10.1 : Morphology of a herpesvirus

Herpesviruses provide a subject for intense research activities that include understanding multiple functions of many herpesvirus genes, unraveling the mechanisms for establishing, maintaining and reactivating latency, interactions between viral and host proteins and details of the variety of mechanisms involved in gene regulation & as potential vectors for application to several problems in human health. HSV-1 provide large segments of the genome to replace with genes of choice namely it's affinity for sensory nerves allows it to target gene therapy to the central nervous system, while its capacity for cell destruction could be a powerful weapon for selective destruction of cancer cells. An HSV-1 vector could be engineered to express antigens that induce immunity against a variety of infectious agents.

Virus replication

Herpesviruses **replicate in the nucleus** of the infected host cells with intranuclear inclusions are the characteristic feature. Infection is initiated when a virion attaches via glycoprotein gB, gC & gD to the cell surface sialic acid receptors of the host cells. Then, the viral & cell membranes fuse, virion is internalized, dismantled & capsid is released into the cytoplasm. Viral capsid is transported to the nuclear pore where the viral DNA enters in to the nucleus. Within the nucleus, transcription of early genes expression ensues. During symptomatic infection, infected cells transcribe lytic viral genes. Transcription of early viral mRNA occurs by host polymerase II, transported into the cytoplasm and translated into early proteins, which are involved in replication of the viral DNA and are transported back into the nucleus. This is followed by synthesis of multiple copies of viral DNA by the viral DNA-dependent DNA polymerase. **Late mRNAs** are transcribed by host polymerase II, transported into the cytoplasm and translated into late proteins which include structural & core proteins that enter the nucleus. Thereafter, assembly of the virus occurs and buds through the inner lamella of the nuclear membrane which has been modified by the insertion of herpes glycoproteins, throughout the Golgi and finally released at the plasma membrane.

In some host cells, a small number of viral genes termed latency-associated genes (LAT) accumulate instead whereby the virus can persist in the cell indefinitely. While primary infection is often accompanied by a self-limited period of clinical illness, long-term latency is symptom-free. Reactivation of latent viruses has been implicated in a number of diseases. Following activation, transcription of viral genes from latency-associated LAT to multiple lytic genes lead to enhanced replication and virus production. Often, lytic activation leads to cell death. Clinically, lytic activation is often accompanied by emergence of non-specific symptoms such as low grade fever, headache, sore throat, malaise, and rash as well as clinical signs such as swollen or tender lymph nodes and immunological findings such as reduced levels of natural killer cells.

Virus classification

Group: Group I ds DNA

Order: *Herpesvirales*

Family: *Herpesviridae*

Subfamily 1: *Herpesvirinae*: Members of *Alphaherpesvirinae* are neurotropic, i.e. they infect nervous system tissues, have a short reproductive cycle of about 18 hours with efficient cell destruction and variable host range, The viruses of this subfamily establish **latent infections in neural cells,** most herpesviruses of veterinary importance are found in the genus *Varicellovirus.*

G1: *Simplexvirus;* type species: *Human hepesvius 1* or Herpes simplex virus.

G2: *Varicellovirus;* type species: *Human hepesvirus 3* or Varicella-zoster virus.

G3: *Mardivirus;* type species: *Gallid herpesvirus 2*

G4: *Iltovirus;* type spcies: *Gallid herpesvius1*

Subfamily 2: *Betaherpesvirinae*: Members of *Betaherpesvirinae*are lymphotropic, have a long reproductive cycle, restricted host range, the infected cells become enlarged (cytomegalo), & the viruses may become latent in secretory glands & lymphoreticular cells.

G1: *Cytomegalovirus* ; type species: *Human herpesvius 5*

G2: *Muromegalovirus;* type species: *Murid herpesvirus 1*

G3: *Roseolovirus* ; type species: *Human herpesvirus 6*

G4: *Proboscivirus;* Elephantid herpesvirus1: TS

Subfamily 3: *Gammaherpesvirinae*: Members of *Gammaherpesvirinae* are also lymphotropic and specific for either T or B lymphocytes. If lymphocytes are infected, viral expression is minimal, some replicate in the epithelial cells & fibroblasts with cell lysis, & several species can lead to neoplastic transformation of lymphocytes.

G1: *Lymphocryptovirus;* type species: *Human herpesvirus 4* or Epstein-Barr virus

G2: *Rhadinovirus;* type species: *Human herpesvirus 8*

G3: *Macavirus;* ; type species: *Alcelaphine herpesvirus 1*

G4: *Percavirus;* type species: *Equid herpesvirus 2*

Unassigned

Genus: *Cercopithecine;* type species: *Cercopithecine herpesvirus 1*

Table 10.3 presented below shows classification of *Herpesviridae* & the diseases caused by the virus species in humans & animals.

Herpesvirus Clinical manifestations in Humans and Animals

Almost all herpesviruses are capable of establishing latent infections; during latency only a small part of the viral genome is expressed, & are reactivated on various stresses & shed the virus, which forms a focus of infection to other susceptible hosts. Some of the herpesvirus species that infect eukaryotic hosts are cell-associated among which some are oncogenic. But several herpesvirus infections are silent or mild in natural hosts but serious in other hosts, e.g. pseudorabies, which has a broad host range & causes fatal encephalitis in a wide variety of animal species but not in its natural host, the adult pig. Herpesviruses are widespread, are readily cultivated in cell cultures; some producing pocks on the CAM. Herpesviruses causing significant human diseases are mentioned in brief but important animal diseases have been discussed in detail.

Table 10.1 : Classification of *Herpesviridae* & diseases caused by member viruses in humans & animals (Order: *Herpesvirale*: Family: *Herpesviridae*: 3 Subfamilies: SF 1: *Alphaherpesvirinae;* SF 2: *Betaherpesvirinae;* SF 3: *Gammaherpesvirinae).*

Herpesvirus species	Type	Diseases caused	Disease features: means of transmission (Tr); primary target cells (TC); Latency (L); others
A.HUMAN HERPESVIRUS (HHV) INFECTIONS.			
SF1: *Alphaherpesvrinae: G 1: Simplexvirus*			
Human herpesvirus 1 (Herpes simplex virus 1)/HSV 1	HHV 1	Oral & or genital, other infections, cold sores, genital herpes, encepha litis; predominantly orofacial.	Tr: close contact. TC: mucoepithelium; L: neuron.
Human herpesvirus 2 (Herpes simplex virus 2)/HSV 2	HHV 2	Oral & genital, & other herpes simplex infections; predominantly genital.	Tr: close contact & STD; TC: mucoepithelium; L: neuron.
G 2: Varicellovirus			
Human herpesvirus 3 (Vricella zoster virus 3)/ VZV 3	HHV 3	Chickenpox & Shingles.	Tr: close contact & respiratory; TC: mucoepithelium; L: neuron.

SF2: Betaherpesvirinae: G 1: Cytomegalovirus			
Human hrpesvirus 5	HHV 5	Infectious mononucleosis (IM)-like syndrome, retinitis, etc.	Tr: saliva; TC: monocytes, lymphocytes & epithelial cells.
G 3:*Roseolavirus*			
Human hrpesvirus 6	HHV 6	Roseola infantum or exanthem subitum	Tr: close contact, respiratory;TC: T cells; L: T cells.
Human hrpesvirus 7 (Herpes lymphotropic virus)	HHV 7	Roseola infantum or exanthem subitum & pityriasis rosea.	Tr : unknown; TC: T cells; L: T cells.
SF3: Gammaherpesvirinae G 1: Lymphocryptovirus			
Human hrpesvirus 4	HHV 4	IM; Burkitt's lymphoma; Hodgkin's disease; CNS lymphoma in AIDS patients; Nasopharyngeal carcinoma, HIV-associated hairy leukoplakia; (PTLD).	Tr: close contact, transfusion, tisuue transplant & congenital; TC: B cells & epith cells; L: B cells.
G 2: *Rhadinovirus*			
Human hrpesvirus 8	HHV 8	Kaposi's sarcoma; primary effusion lymphoma; some types of multicentric Castlesman's disease.	Tr: close contact, sexual, saliva; TC: lymphocytes & other cells.
B. ZOONOTIC INFECTIONS			
G: *Simpexvirus*			
Cercopithecine herpesirus (CeHV)1Mmonkey B virus	CeHV 1	Herpes simplex-like disease in Asian macaque monkeys.	Transmitted to humans causing 16 deaths of 25 cases with encephalomyelitis/ survivors showed neurological impairment.
SF: *Gammaherpesvirinae*			
G:*Rhadinovirus*			
Murine gammaherpesvirus 68	MuHV 4	Herpes infection in mice with zoonotic value.	Transmitted to humans; infects 4.5% of persons mainly laboratory workers handling infected mice.
C. ANIMAL INFECTIONS			
SF: *Alphaherpesvirinae*: G1: *Simplexvirus*			
Bovine herpesvirus 2 (Bovine mammilitis virus)	BHV 2	Bovine ulcerative mammilitis, & pseudolumpy- skin disease	BHV-2 causes bovine ulcerative mammitis characterized by severe ulceration in the teats of dairy cows. Hosts: Dairy cattle

		(Allerton strain).	worldwide. Tr: By skin abrasions, milers, milking machine, biting insects, & in Africa wild animals act as carriers. TC: teat & udder epith; Infn via skin/ SC tissues > replication at lower temp in mammary & teat epith > vesicles & ulceration. BHV-2 also causes pseudolumpy- skin disease by Allerton strain in subtropical & tropical countries characterized by generalized mild skin lesions; no vaccine exists, control by milking.
G 2: *Varicellovirus*			
Bovine herpesvirus1 (Infectious bovine rhinotracheitis virus/IBRV)	BHV 1	Infectious bovine rhinotracheitis (IBR), vaginitis, balanoposthitis & abortion in cattle.	IBRV, 2 subtypes of BHV are-1.1 respiratory subtype, causes abortion, & rarely encephalitis, & subtype 1.2 genital subtype. Again, BHV - 1.2a causes abortion & vulvovaginitis balan posthitis. BHV- 1.2b causes no abortion but vulvovaginitis, balan- oposthitis. Tr: By resp & genital secretion. TC: mm of URT/ genital mucosa, virus replication > local nerve endings > trigeminal/sacral ganglia. Latency > reactivated & virus back to entry site, transmitted to new ones. Mod live vac used in pregnants by IM or IN route.
Bovine herpesvirus 5 (Bovine encephalitis virus)	BHV 5	Meningoencephalitis in cattle 7 month – 3 yr age in S Am, in some European countries	BHV-5/ bovine encephalitis virus causes meningoencephalitis in cattle 7 mth – 3 yr age in South America & in some European countries. Tr: Via nose & olfactory nerve, henceaffects frontal sinus; latent infection, reactivated by stresses.
Equid herpesvirus 1 (Equine abortion virus)	EqHV 1	Equine abortion in horses worldwide	Equine abortion virus (EqHV-1) causes equine abortion in horses worldwide. Tr: Direct/ indirect contact & droplets. TC: Predilect- ion for vascular epith > vasculitis & thrombosis > local infection, viremia >infection of placenta, fetus, & rarely CNS > abortion. Latency in regional nerve ganglia > reactivated under stress, & corticosteroid. Modified live vac or inactivated vac used in pregnant at 5,7, 9 mths.

Equid herpesvirus 3 (Equine coital exanthema virus)	EqHV 3	Equine coital exanthema in horses worldwide	EqHV-3 causes equine coital exanthema in horses worldwide. Tr: Via coitus, flies on vaginal discharges, recovered acting as life-long carriers. TC: Mucosa of keratinized epith, vulva, vagina, penis & prepuce, virus is temp sensitive, no viremia or abortion. L: reported> reactivation, virus shed >Tr to new ones.
Equid herpesvirus 4 (Equine rhinopneumonitis virus)	EqHV 4	Rhinopneumonitis in horses worldwide up to 2 yrs age	EqHV-4 causes rhinopneumonitis in horses worldwide up to 2 yrs age. Tr: contact, resp route, aerosols & fomites. TC: resp epith & local lymph nodes. L: trigeminal ganglia > reactivation, virus shed & infects
Equid herpesvirus 4 (Equine rhinopneumonitis virus)	EqHV 4	Rhinopneumonitis in horses worldwide up to 2 yrs age	EqHV-4 causes rhinopneumonitis in horses worldwide up to 2 yrs age. Tr: contact, resp route, aerosols & fomites. TC: resp epith & local lymph nodes. L: trigeminal ganglia > reactivation, virus shed & infects foals.
Canid herpesvirus 1 (Canid herpesvirus 1)	CaHV 1	Severe haemorrhagic disease in puppies @ 1 wk old in domestic & wild dogs	CaHV-1 causes severe hemorrhagic disease in puppies @ 1 wk old in domestic & wild dogs. Tr: contact with oral, nasal, vaginal secretion during & after parturition, infc in utero also; inability to regulate temp at @ 1 wk age, don't grow above 36 C. TC: Nasal mucosa, tonsil & pharynx > virus repl > viremia in neonates with subnormal temp, also vaginitis & tracheobronchitis. L: trigeminal ganglia. No vac.
Felid herpesvirus1 (Feline rhinotracheitis virus)	FeHV 1	Feline viral rhinotracheitis & keratitis in cats 3-8 mth age, endemic worldwide	FeHV-1 causes feline viral rhino-tracheitis & keratitis in cats 3-8 mth age, endemic worldwide. Tr: direct/ indirect contact, inhalation, recovered act as carriers; TC: mm of oropharynx & conjunctiva, upper res tract >repl but no viremia > generalized in vey young kittens, in inclusion. Attenuated & killed vac (pregants) used.
Suid herpesvirus1 (Porcine herpesvirus 1/ /Pseudorabies virus)	SuHV 1	Pseudorabies / Aujeszky's disease in pigs (natural hosts), cattle, sheep,	SuHV-1 causes Pseudorabies / Aujeszky's disease in pigs (natural hosts), cattle, sheep, dogs, cats, other dead end hosts.

		dogs, cats, other dead end hosts	Tr : contact, aerosols, fomites, virus shed in secretion- oro-nasal, milk, urine, semen & transplacental. TC: nasopharynx & tonsil epith >repl in alveolar macropha ges> regional LN via axon of cranial nerve > CNS; L: nasopharynx, trigeminal nerve; reactivation.
G 3: Mardivirus			
Gallid herpesvirus 2 (Marek's disease virus type 1)	GaHV 2/ MDV 1	Marek's disease in domestic fowl, turkey, quail, mostly in 8-12 day-old chickens	Gallid herpesvirus 2/ (Marek's diseasevirus type 1) MDV-1: causes Marek's disease in domestic fowl, turkey, quail, mostly in 8-12 days old chickens. 3 serotypes of MDV are MDV-1, -2 -3 of which; types 1 & 2 occur in chickens & type 3 in turkeys. MDV-1 is oncogenic but types 2 & 3 are not. Tr: contact, via resp route, contaminated airborne dust. TC: B cells of bursa, spleen & thymus infected, then T cells, mostly CD4+ cells, spread via cell-associated viremia, T cells are transformed (T cells latency); infiltration in gonads, kidney, liver, skin, muscle, eye, periheral nerve> secondary cytolytic infection in feather follicle epith with cell free virus shed in feather danders & debris. Vaccin day-old chick or 18 day old ovum with MDV3.
Gallid herpesvirus 3 (Marek's disease virus type 2)	GaHV 3/ MDV 2	*Marek's disease*	
Meleagid herpesvirus 1(Tturkey herpesvirus/THV/ MDV3)	MeHV-1	*Turkey herpesvirus infection*	
G 4: Iltovirus			
Gallid herpesvirus 1 (Infectious laryngotracheitis virus)	GaHV 1/ ILTV	Infectious laryngotracheitis in chickens & pheasants	*Gallid herpesvirus 1* (GaHV-1)/ Infectious laryngotracheitis virus (ILTV) causes I LT in chickens & pheasants. Tr: direct/ indirect contact; TC: virus repl in URT epith, larynx & trachea >virus travels via sensory nerve >latent in trigeminal ganglia, I/N inclusions; Grow in CAM; modified live vacc used that don't prevent reactivation.
SF: Gammaherpesviriae G 2: Rhadinovirus			
Alcelaphine herpesvirus 1	AlHV 1	Malignant catarrhal fever (MCF) in cattle, deer & other ruminants in Africa	*Alcelaphine herpesvirus 1(AlHV1)* causes Malignant catarrhal fever (MCF) in cattle, deer & other ruminants in Africa (natural host

Alcelaphine herpesvirus 2	AlHV 2	MCF in antelope & hartebeest to cattle	wildebeest with life-long inappaent infn, Tr: mother to offspring), transmit MCFV to cattle, deer, & other ruminants in Africa. *Alcelaphine herpesvirus 2* (AlHV2) causes MCF in antelope & hartebeest to cattle (natural host hartebeest). *Ovine herpesvirus 2*/ Sheep-associated MCF (OvHV 2) transmit MCF in cattle, deer, bison, water buffaloes & pigs inrest of world (natural host sheep & goats with subclinical infection) > shed virus during lambing, TC: Affects blood vessels in multiple organs, hence confusion with BT, BVD, FMD.
Ovine herpesvirus 2 (Sheep-associated MCF)	OvHV 2	MCF in cattle, deer & other ruminants in rest of world	
Unassigned genus in Herpesviridae			
Anatid herpesvirus 1 (Duck plague/ Duck viral enteritis herpesvirus)	AnHV 1	Duck plague/ duck viral hepatitis in ducks, geese & waterfowls in Asia, Europe & N. America	*Anatid herpesvirus 1* (AnHV-1)/ Duck plague/Duck viral enteritis herpesvirus) causes Duck plague/ duck viral hepatictis in ducks, geese, waterfowls in Asia, Europe & N. America. Tr: direct/ indirect contact viacontaminated feces & carriers that shedvirus for many yrs, traced to Infectionin water fowls. TC: resp , liver, kidney, intestine etc. Modified live vac used.
Suid herpesvirus (Inclusion body rhinitis virus)	SuHV	Inclusion body rhinitis in pigs up to 2 wk old.	*Swuid herpesvirus* (SuHV) /Inclusionbody rhinitis virus Tr: direct/ indirectcontact, aerosols, virus in nasal secretions. Symptoms include atophic rhinitis, & IN inclusions. No vaccine is available.

Abbreviaton: Epith = epithelial cells; Infc = infection; IM = intramuscular; IN = intranuclear; macro= macrophages; LN = lymph nodes; mth= month; N host = natural host; pred = predilection; repl = replication; resp = respiratory route; SC = subcutaneous; STD= sexually transmitted disease; temp = temperature; wk= week; vac = vaccine; yr= year

Herpesvirus Clinical Infections in Humans

SF:*Alphaherpesvirinae*:

Genus: *Simplexvirus:*

HHV-1 /HSV-1 causes oral & or genital herpes infections-mainly orofacial.

HHV-2/HSV-2 causes oral & or genital herpes infections-mainly genital.

Genus: *Varicellovirus*:

HHV-3/VZV causes chickenpox & Shingles in man.

SF: *Betaherpesvirinae*

Genus: *Cytomegalovirus*

HHV-5/CMV causes infectious mononucleosis (IM)-like syndrome, retinitis, etc. in humans.

Genus: *Roseolavirus*:

HHV-6 causes 6th disease or Roseola infantum or exanthem subitum in humans.

HHV-7 causes Roseola infantum or exanthem subitum & pityriasis rosea in humans.

SF: *Gammaherpesvirinae*

Genus: *Lymphocryptovirus*:

HHV-4 /causes IM; Burkitt's lymphoma; Hodgkin's disease; CNS lymphoma in AIDS patients; Nasopharyngeal carcinoma, HIV associated hairy leukoplakia; post- transplant lymphoproliferative syndrome (PTLD) in humans.

Genus: *Rhadinovirus*:

HHV-8 causes Kaposi's sarcoma; primary effusion lymphoma; some types of multicentric Castlesman's disease in humans.

Herpesviral Clinical Infections in Animals & Birds

Alphaherpesvirinae

Genus: *Simplexvirus*

Bovine Ulcerative Mammitis

Bovine ulcerative mammitis is characterized by severe ulceration in the teats & udder skin of dairy cows, may occur sporadically or in outbreaks and often results in marked loss of milk production as well as high incidence of secondary mastitis. The lesions begins as one or more thickened, edematous plaques of varying size on the skin of one or more teats, vesicles develop and rapidly rupture, leaving a raw, ulcerated area that becomes covered with a dark-colored scab. The scabs tend to crack and bleed, especially if milking is attempted. Teats are painful and affected cows resist milking, leading to development of mastitis. Severe lesions may take several weeks to heal.

Etiology: Bovine ulcerative mammitis in dairy cattle is caused by *Bovine herpesvirus 2* (BHV-2). BHV-2 also causes **pseudo- lumpy-skin disease by Allerton strain** in tropical & subtropical regions. Pseudo-lumpy- skin disease is characterized by generalized mild skin lesions. No vaccine exists, & the disease is controlled by proper milking.

Occurrence

Bovine ulcerative mammitis occurs in dairy cattle worldwide, but particularly in N. America, Australia, Europe, & Africa. Bovine ulcerative mammitis was first isolated from cattle in Africa in 1957. The highest incidence is seen in first-lactation cows, but unexposed cows of any age are susceptible. It is a relatively uncommon condition but it can spread rapidly in herds which are affected for the first time and cause significant pain and discomfort. It tends to occur most commonly in early winter. The morbidity rate varies within 18%- 96% but mortality rate is none.

Hosts susceptible

Dairy cattle with the highest incidence are seen in first-lactation cows, occur as an outbreak in cows, mainly heifers within 2 months after calving, and followed by persistent infection. But unexposed cows of any age are susceptible to the virus.

Transmission

By skin abrasions, milers, milking machine, biting insects, & in Africa wild animals act as carriers.

Pathogenesis

After infection by via skin/ subcutaneous tissues, virus replication occurs at lower temperature in mammary & teat epithelium, but there is no viremia & spread occurs by local extension. As compared to poxvirus lumpy skin disease, the lesions in bovine ulcerative mammillitis is more severe. The severity of lesions after calving is probably due to the immunosuppression during parturition & peripaturient udder edema.

Clinical symptoms & lesions

The **incubation periodvaries** between **5-10** days. The clinical signs vary from small irregular fluid-filled blisters to larger areas of ulcers and scabs.Early lesions begin as one or more thickened, edematous plaques of varying size on the skin of one or more teats. The vesicles develop and may rapidly rupture; leaving a raw, ulcerated area that becomes covered with a dark-colored scab. The scabs tend to crack and bleed, especially if milking is attempted. The lesions are of variable size and can include much of the teat wall and orifice. Teats are generally painful and affected cows often resist milking, leading to development of mastitis. Severe lesions may take several weeks to heal, but mild lesions heal in about 10 days.

Diagnosis

Presumptive diagnosis: A presumptive diagnosis is made on the basis of clinical signs and confirmed by histopathology.

Virus isolation: The virus from early lesions can be isolated in cell cultures of bovine origin, but grows best at reduced temperature. The virus produces large, **characteristic syncytia** in cultured cells. Scrapings of blistered skin will contain virus which can be seen under the electron microscope.

Serology: Identification is accomplished by serum neutralization and fluorescent antibody tests. Serological test using paired samples with 4 fold increase in titer, or titer of 1:16 in BHV-2 is confirmative.

Treatment & prevention

No specific treatment is available, but is aimed at supportive care, speeding the healing of the skin and preventing spread to other cattle. The affected cows are separated and are milked at the end. The use of iodophore-containing teat dips with added emollients may help to inactivate the virus. It is important to isolate affected cows and to use separate milking equipment. Furthermore, separate paper towels and clean gloves for milking personnel help to prevent spread of the virus to susceptible animals. Check regularly to ensure that skin damage hasn't resulted in mastitis.

Once cows in a farm contract ulcerative mammillitis, it is difficult to eliminate it. Before buying in dairy cows, ensure that they are not having ulcerative mammillitis. Check the teats and udder of all cows before you purchase them. This will significantly reduce, but not eliminate, the risk of buying cattle with ulcerative mammillitis. Once ulcerative mammillitis is established on a farm, it will be most commonly seen in first lactation heifers during winter housing. Pay particular attention to this group and separate and treat affected heifers as soon as signs of disease appear. Good parlor hygiene and controlling biting flies can significantly reduce the impact of this disease.

Genus: *Varicellovirus*

Infectious Bovine Rhinotracheitis

Infectious bovine rhinotracheitis (IBR) is a highly contagious, infectious disease caused by *Bovine herrpesvirus-1* (BHV-1) capable of attacking many different tissues in the body leading to a variety of clinical diseases in cattle; namely infectious bovine rhinotracheitis (IBR), infectious pustular vulvovaginitis (IPV), balanoposthitis, conjunctivitis, abortion, encephalomyelitis, and mastitis. The clinical diseases caused by BHV-1 are grouped into: **respiratory tract infections, eye infections, abortions, genital infections, brain infections, & generalized infections of newborn calves.**

Etiology: IBR is caused by BHV-1 with two subtypes-BHV-1.1 is respiratory subtype (it is also associated with abortion and very rarely with encephalitis), & BHV-1.2 is genital subtype of which BHV-1.2a causes abortion, vulvovaginitis, & balanoposthitis, & BHV-1.2b causes no abortion but vulvovaginitis & balanoposthitis. Abortions caused by IBR can be caused by exposure to a natural disease strain or exposure of non-protected pregnant cows or their calves with modified live IBR vaccine.

Occurrence

IBR occurs worldwide, and very few countries- Austria, Denmark, Finland, Sweden, & Switzerland have eradicated the disease. Many Pacific countries or territories reported serological evidence without clinical cases (Fiji, Guam, Niue, Samoa, Solomon Islands, Tonga, Vanuatu), & New Caledonia identified clinical cases; it could be absent from other countries.

Hosts susceptible

Both domestic and wild bovines are susceptible. Experimental infection occurs in goats, sheep and pigs.

Transmission

Infection occurs via the respiratory and genital routes. After infection, the virus is shed from nasal and ocular discharges detected for 10-14 days. Virus is also present in amniotic liquid, placenta, foetus and semen of infected bulls. Transmission occurs through aerosols, direct or indirect contact (over short period of time) and via infected bulls by coitus and artificial insemination. Frozen semen is an optimal condition for virus survival. IBR/ IPV may be introduced by importation of the infected animals and semen.

Pathogenesis

After infection, IBRV replicates in the mucous membrane of the upper respiratory tract/genital mucosa and virus is shed in nasal/genital secretions. Semen may be contaminated during the ejaculation. Local nerve cell endings are infected and the virus is **transported to trigeminal/sacral ganglia** where it establishes a lifelong latent infection. Once infected, the animals become

lifelong carriers of the virus. The latent infection may be reactivated on various stresses periodically, with or without clinical signs; the virus is transported back to the site of entry and is shed with potential transmission to other animals.

While the virus replicates in the respiratory tract and circulates in the blood, it crosses the placenta into the fetus. The virus begins to multiply in the fetus causing death 1-3 days after replication begins. Abortion occurs 2-7 days after death of the fetus. The time from infection of the cow to abortion can range from **18 days to 3 months,** abortions occur during the 6th to 9th month of pregnancy. In the second case, modified viruses replicate in non-protected pregnant cows and pass through the placenta into the fetus causing infection and death.

The **genital form, caused by type 1-2a & 1-2b of IBR** is seen in mature cows and bulls and is called infectious pustular vulvovaginitis (IPV). The time course of the infection is 2-3 weeks and respiratory symptoms and abortions do not occur.

Clinical symptoms & lesions

Respiratory form, which is most common form, exhibits the symptoms namely: sudden onset of fever up to 42°C & anorexia, severe hyperaemia of the nasal mucosa (Red nose) with numerous clusters of grayish foci of necrosis on the mucous membranes, abundant serous discharge from the nose and the eyes, conjunctivitis, & hypersalivation. There is dramatic drop in milk yield. The affected animals show tachypnea and tachycardia, & sometimes short explosive cough. Rarely, the affected animals may die due to obstructive bronchiolitis, or secondary bronchopneumonia. An abortion form can complicate the respiratory form with late abortion between the 5th and 8ht month of pregnancy and placenta retention. It can be the only manifestation.

The genital form, pustular vulvovaginitis and balanoposthitis, is characterized by inflammation of the genital mucosa and development of small pustules that coalesce and ulcerate. Infections may be mild or subclinical. Abortion or stillbirths, which are infrequent, may occur 1 - 3 months postinfection.

In the genital form of the disease, the disease runs for 2 to 3 weeks and symptoms include: a thick white-brown colored vulvular discharge, swollen, reddened vulva, small pus-filled pimple in the lining of the vulva and vagina, loss of the desire to mate, excessive tail switching, & frequent urination. Males exhibit a balanoposthitis with pustules and discharge are observed on the bull's penis and prepuce.

The conjunctivitis form is common with occasional involvement of the cornea, and a panophthalmitis.

In the young calf, less than 6 months old, the disease is more severe with symptoms of encephalitis-incoordination, hyperexitation and depression, & salivation, blindness & high mortality rate.

In new born calves the symptoms are: fever and lack of appetite, salivation, inflammation of the nasal mucosa, conjunctivitis, and erosions of the mouth mucous membranes covered with mucopurulent exudate, respiratory distress is common due to swelling of the larynx and pneumonia, & some calves may develop diarrhoea.

PM lesions are usually restricted to the upper respiratory tract and include: swelling and congestion of mucosa, sometimes with necrotic foci, petechiae, & profuse and fibrinopurulent exudate in severe case.

Diagnosis

Collection of specimens for various tests include: for virus isolation blood on EDTA, nasal, pharyngeal, conjunctival, swabs, aborted fetus, placenta, vaginal swab, prepuce washing fluid and semen, & paired sera, plasma or milk for antibodies.

1. *Presumptive diagnosis*: A presumptive diagnosis is based on the clinical signs and lesions. A definitive diagnosis requires demonstration of viral infected cells by immunofluorescence, isolation, and identification of the virus.
2. *Virus isolation*: IBRV is isolated from clinical specimens by the inoculation of cell cultures of bovine origin. The virus produces CPE in tissue culture.
3. *Antigen detection*: Immunofluorescence is used because the virus is often nonviable due to advanced autolysis of fetal tissues. Neutralization or antigen detection methods using monospecific antisera or monoclonal antibodies, PCR are also used for detection of antigen on semen.
4. *Antibody detection*: The demonstration of antibody in serum, plasma & milk is performed by virus neutralization test and ELISA; significant increase in IBR antibody levels between acute and convalescent serum samples is confirmatory. ELISA test is also available to detect antibodies in milk.

Treatment & prevention

There is no direct treatment for the infection. Antibiotic treatment of secondary infections may be necessary. Once IBR is introduced, it is difficult and expensive to eradicate IBR/IPV because animals tend to become inapparent carriers. Systematic testing and elimination of positives has been successful in some countries.

Vaccination

Different types of **modified or inactivated vaccines** are available for IBR. Officially IBR free countries restrict the use of them. Modified live and killed vaccines are usually used in combination with other bacterial and viral antigens. **VISTA ONCE SQ**-INTERVET (IBR, BVD1 & 2, BPI3 & BRSV) is modified live vaccine vaccinated to 3 month old calves & older non pregnant cattle. Inject 2.0 ml SC to healthy cattle 3 months of age or older. Annual revaccination is recommended. **Bovi-Shield Gold FP5L5**-Pfizer (IBR, BVD, BPI3, BRSV live modified & *C. fetus*+ L. Canicola, L. Grippotyphosa, Hardjo, Pomana Bacterin) covers most of the cattle respiratory diseases. Administer a single 2-ml dose IM to all breeding cows and heifers approximately 1 month prior to breeding or being added to the herd & revaccinate annually. **Bovi-Shield Gold FP5**-Pfizer does not contain leptospra serotypes. **Bovilis IBR Marker live** (Intervet) is a marker vaccine for IBR. A single dose of 2 ml reconstituted vaccine per animal for intranasal or IM administration is used. From the age of 3 months onward: intranasal or IM at an age between 2 weeks and 3 months: intranasal (1 ml in each nostril); when the first vaccination is given between the age of 2 weeks and 3 months, the animals should be revaccinated with a single dose at the age of 3-4 months. To maintain immunity, revaccinate every 6 months.

Two types of modified live vaccines are used, **one vaccine is given IM and the second vaccine is given intranasally (IN)**. The IN vaccine is recommended for pregnant cows as it is safe for the fetus. **For eradication programs of IBR, deletion mutant vaccines or marker vaccines** (Bovilis IBR Marker-Intervet) is live or inactivated vaccine that is used to differentiate between vaccinal and natural antibodies using ELISA procedures.

Bovine Meningoencephalitis

Bovine meningoencephalitis in calves in South America & in some European countries is characterized by meningoencephalitis, a fatal disease of different degrees of severity of neurological disease depending on both viral and host factors & highly prevalent in South America. Clinical signs of BHV-5-associated neurological disease include tremors, circling, bruxism, incoordination, nystagmus, & recumbency followed by convulsions, paddling and inevitably death.

Etiology: Meningoencephalitis in calves is caused by *Bovine herpesviru-5* (BHV-5), which is closely related to BHV-1. BHV-1 may be occasionally neuroinvasive but rarely causes encephalitis, whereas **BHV-5 has a marked neurotropism**, frequently leading to fatal disease.

Occurrence

BHV-5 has a limited geographic distribution, with a high incidence of neurologic disease in South American countries, mainly Argentina and Brazil, & sporadically in USA, Australia, Germany and Hungary. The occurrence of BHV-5–associated neurologic disease has been only sporadically reported in other parts of the world. In Brazil and Argentina, many outbreaks occur annually, & most outbreaks are seen in **cattle seven months to three years of age**; occurrence in younger cattle is infrequent, although single case in cattle up to six years of age has been reported. Up to 30% of animals in a herd may be affected.

Hosts susceptible

BHV-5 causes menmigoencephalitis and respiratory disease in young cattle and sheep. Disease is most common in calves up to **ten months of age**. As with all herpesviruses, latent infection can occur, with reactivation at times of stressed and/or immunosuppression. Sites of latency include the CNS and mucosae of the nose and trachea. Young cattle & lambs are naturally susceptible to BHV-5 infection.

Transmission

BHV-5 infection occurs via nose & olfactory nerve, hence affects frontal sinus. Latent infection is reactivated by stresses. Both BHV-1 and BHV-5 are neurotropic viruses that establish latency in the trigeminal ganglion (TG) following intranasal and/or conjunctival inoculation. Animals that recover from BHV-5 infection or become infected following BHV-1 infection become latent carriers.

Clinical signs & lesions

Signs of respiratory disease include tachycardia and tachypnea with pyrexia, dyspnea, mucoid nasal discharge, hypersalivation and abnormal lung sounds. Systemic signs such as lethargy and anorexia are seen.

Neurological signs are normally acute. These signs include opisthotonus, hyperaesthesia, abnormal behaviour, ataxia, head pressing, blindness, proprioceptive deficits, coma and seizures. Sudden death occurs in neonates. Subacute disease is almost always fatal, causing depression, anorexia, ataxia and a pronounced dyspnea. The course is usually 4-7 days but may be as long as 15 days.

Animals that recover from BHV-5 infection or become infected following BHV-1 infection become latent carriers.

Diagnosis

Collection of clinical samples includes; whole brain or portions from cerebrum, cerebellum and brain stem.

Presumptive diagnosis: It rests on the basis of clinical symptoms (meningoencephalitis, blindness, head pressing and deep depression), & characteristic histopathologic lesions in the brain including malacia of the cerebral cortex and encephalitis and meningitis involving mainly the cerebrum and to a lesser extent the brain stem and cerebellum. Inclusion bodies in astrocytes and neurons are often seen.

Virus isolation: The virus can be isolated from the brain and distinguished from IBR isolates.

Virus antigen detection: Diagnosis of BHV-5 infection rests on the virus identification using specific monoclonal antibodies, PCR or ELISA.

Treatment & prevention

There is currently no treatment or specific vaccine for BHV-5, but BHV-1 vaccines seem to provide some cross-protection.

Equine Abortion and Equine Rhinopneumonitis

EqHV-1 is unique in its ability to **target three separate organ systems of the horse-respiratory, reproductive, and central nervous systems** (CNS signs are due to thrombotic lesions, not infection of neural tissue) giving rise to large-scale outbreaks with any of respiratory tract disease, abortion, neonatal mortality, and a paralytic neurological disease.

Etiology: Equine abortion is caused by *Equid herpesvirus 1* (EqHV-1) / Equine abortion virus. EHV-1 causes respiratory infection, abortion and neurologic disease. Equine rhinopneumonitisis caused by*Equid herpesvirus 4* (EqHV-4)/Equine rhinopneumonitis virus that causes respiratory disease, only rarely causes neurologic or abortion disease. They are two distinct species of *Varicellovirus*.

Occurrence

Equine abortion in horses occurs worldwide. EqHV-1 & EqHV-4 are deeply entrenched within the world's horse population as inapparent, latent infections or silent carriers. The capacity of EHV-1 to persist in the body of the horse in a dormant, but reactivatable state after recovery from a primary infection provides an inexhaustible and global biological reservoir of the virus for continuous transmission of infection among adult horses and to new generations of young horses. EHV-1 and EHV-4 are remarkably ubiquitous in the world horse population and are primary respiratory pathogens that can cause respiratory tract disease without major predisposing factors. Evidence suggests that the two herpesviruses circulate and are transmitted year round. While respiratory infections of horses with EHV-1 and EHV-4 are often subclinical, both viruses have the potential for causing widespread outbreaks of severe upper respiratory tract (URT) disease. The two equine herpesviruses is one of continuously repetitive cycles of three consecutive events that amplify and maintain the virus reservoir: 1. vertical transmission of the viruses from latently infected dam to foal; 2. postinfection establishment of viral latency in affected foals; and, 3. periodic reactivation and shedding of latent herpesvirus to result in horizontal horse-to-horse virus transmission.

Hosts susceptible

EHV-1 causes respiratory infection in all ages, but the disease is more severe in younger animals. EHV-4 causes respiratory disease, only rarely neurologic or abortion disease. EHV-1 and EHV-4 are among the most important respiratory pathogens capable of causing clinically significant upper respiratory tract disease (URTD) in the domestic horses. The greatest burden of herpesvirus respiratory disease is borne by young horses, with the highest risk for infection **between weaning and two years of age.**

Transmission

Respiratory infection is acquired by close physical contact with another horse that is actively shedding infectious virus into its respiratory secretions. Virus-laden droplets generated by forced, high velocity expirations through the airways produce infective aerosols capable of traveling over short distances between box stalls, fenced paddocks, etc. Horses infected for the first time may shed the viruses for prolonged periods up to 14 days. Indirect virus transmission occurs through contamination of human hands, feed and water utensils, endoscopes, & other fomites are also possible. The greatest burden of URTD caused by EHV-4 is borne by foals during their first year of life; i.e., as sucklings and weanlings between 4 and 12 months of age. EHV-4 is thus a major etiologic agent for the commonly observed but ordinarily mild upper respiratory disease in foals. The occurrence of overt EHV-1 or EHV-4 respiratory tract disease in foals younger than three months of age is uncommon (particularly in foals from vaccinated dams), presumably because of maternally derived passive antibody. Most mares of breeding age are clinically immune to respiratory disease but not to abortigenic infection. Spread of EHV-1 through a herd occurs most commonly without clinical signs. The virus can **persist in the trigeminal ganglia** and can recrudesce in latent carriers. Stressing pregnant mares may trigger abortion.

Pathogenesis

EHV-1 enters the host through the respiratory tract, and the respiratory mucosal epithelium is the primary target tissue for infection. Respiratory infection is acquired by close physical contact with another horse that is actively shedding infectious virus into its respiratory secretions or via inhalation of infective aerosols capable of traveling over short distances between box stalls, fenced paddocks, etc. Indirect virus transmission occurs through contamination of human hands, feed and water utensils, endoscopes, and other fomites.

The pathogenesis of herpesvirus URTD is characterized by focal, cytolytic destruction and exfoliation of the nasopharyngeal respiratory epithelium down to the basal layer, an outpouring of respiratory glandular secretions, and a concomitant vigorous inflammatory response that includes infiltration of mononuclear cells into the lamina propria underlying the destroyed epithelium. Respiratory signs of EHV-1 or EHV-4 infection like nasal discharge and fever are initiated by the direct viral cytopathic destruction of airway epithelium. Mild pulmonary lesions develop in some foals. Quickly following replication in the upper respiratory tract epithelium, the virus is carried by migratory dendritic cells and macrophages into the draining lymph nodes. Infection of mononuclear leukocytes within draining lymph nodes results in a leukocyte-associated viremia, which may persist for several days. With EHV-1 in particular, viremic viral spread to other viscera is common and often results in widespread infection of vascular endothelial cells. Such an EHV-1 vasculitis in blood vessels of the central nervous system or gravid uterus forms the pathogenetic basis for the post-respiratory sequelae of EHV-1 abortion or neurological disease.

Clinical symptoms & lesions

Upper respiratory tract infection

The **incubation period** for the herpesviruses ranges from **2 to 5 days.** Uncomplicated URTD occurring in horses as a result of infection by EHV-1 presents as an acute rhinitis and pharyngitis with the potential for extension into the more distal airways to cause tracheobronchitis, bronchiolitis and/or pneumonitis. Its clinical presentation is highly variable among individual horses and can range from inapparent illness to a life-threatening, primary viral pneumonia. The most constant clinical manifestation of EHV URTD is bilateral nasal discharge. In the early stages of infection, the nasal discharge is watery, free-trickling, inconspicuous and frequently goes unnoticed by attending personnel. The clear serous secretions are laden with high titers of infectious virus. As infection progresses, the character of the discharge changes rapidly by the second or third day from watery to that of a thicker, mucilaginous state, whitish in color, with the addition of inflammatory leukocytes and desquamated respiratory epithelial cells. The viscous nasal secretions often dry to form more easily recognizable encrustations in and around the nostrils of the affected horse. As secondary bacterial infection ensues by 4 - 5 days after clinical onset, the character of the nasal efflux advances further to become thicker, more opaque and yellowish (mucopurulent).

Abortion

Mares infected with EHV-1 abort with no impending signs, and evidence of the previous respiratory tract infection is usually not observed. Typically there is a **sudden abortion without milk or udder development**. The fetus is delivered in a fresh condition, and may even be born alive and die soon after. The placenta is expelled along with the fetus that is often still enveloped in its amniotic membrane. At the time of abortion, the fetus has usually just died from asphyxia associated with sudden separation of the placenta from the endometrium that precedes fetal expulsion. The aborted fetus possesses high levels of virus and extensive histopathological evidence of **multi-organ infection**. Almost all EHV-1 abortions occur during the last **four months of gestation**. Most abortion with EHV-1 infection involves only one or two mares in a group. However, epidemic abortigenic disease (abortion storms) claiming high percentages of the potential foal crop also occurs. Once a mare has aborted, her **future reproductive potential is not compromised;** most mares conceive successfully shortly after abortion and foal normally the following year.

Neurological disease

Clinically, the most important feature is the dreaded neurological disease. Once regarded as a rare and sporadic occurrence, the malady has in recent years been observed with increasing and alarming frequency. Common to all horses with EHV-1 associated central nervous system disease are a **weakness and paralysis of the muscles of the hind limbs** that give rise to incoordination, gait abnormalities and, in many cases, the inability to rise from the sitting position. The neurologic deficits result from a thrombotic, ischemic inflammation of small blood vessels in the spinal cord and/or brain. The interval between initial EHV-1 infection of the respiratory tract and the subsequent onset of neurological signs is 8 to 12 days. The neurological deficits appear suddenly and reach their peak intensity within 48 hours. The disease is resistant to vaccination, the clinical attack rate is high, and large numbers of fatalities are the rule. The prognosis for non-recumbent horses is favorable, but is poor for animals that remain down for longer than 24 hours.

A major advance in understanding the mechanistic basis of EHV-1 paralytic disease was the recent discovery that a single gene alteration, a mutated version of the viral gene that encodes its replicative polymerase, endows such mutant virus strains with enhanced virulence for the horse. This discovery that a single gene of EHV-1 plays such a prominent role in the viral attribute of hypervirulence has led to a genetic test for identifying latent equine carriers of mutant, neuropathogenic strains of EHV-1.

Neonatal foal death

Fetuses infected with EHV-1 during late gestation may be born alive at term but sick either at birth or within one to two days of parturition. The foals are weak, fail to nurse, become lethargic, pyrexic, lymphopenic, hypoxemic, and exhibit severe respiratory distress. Clinical deterioration in such foals infected in utero with EHV-1 occurs rapidly, and the prognosis is always grave. Mortality in congenitally infected foals approaches 100%, as a viral pneumonia leads to respiratory failure within a few days. The foals are highly susceptible to secondary bacterial disease. Congenital EHV-1 infection can be epizootic and may occur in association with an outbreak of EHV-1 abortion. Rarely, EHV-4 may also cause neonatal foal disease resembling that caused by EHV-1.

Diagnosis

Collection of clinical samples for various tests include: lung, fetal liver and thymus, both frozen and in formalin, & nasal swabs, whole blood, cerebrospinal fluid, acute and convalescent sera, brain, & spinal cord from horses with CNS symptoms.

1. *Presumptive diagnosis*: A first hand diagnosis is based on clinical symptoms, gross lesions & histopathology of the fetus in case of abortion. Fetal lesions include serous pleural and peritoneal fluid, hemorrhages of the entire respiratory tract, petechiae of the oral mucosa and conjunctiva, focal hepatic necrosis with intranuclear inclusion bodies in liver and lung, intranuclear inclusions in fetal tissues and a necrotic and friable thymus. The histopathologic finding of vasculitis in central nervous system tissue is suggestive. But diagnosis should be confirmed by virus isolation or PCR.
2. *Virus isolation*: Virus isolation is done in cell cultures of horse and rabbit (RK-13 cell line) origin. EHV 1 grows in cell cultures of non equine origin, but HV 4 only grows in equine cells. An ELISA test differentiates the two viruses.

3. *Antigen detection*: It is done by demonstration of viral antigens in infected cells by immunofluorescence examination of cryostat sections of affected tissue or byPCR.

4. *Serology*: Serology of the mare is of no value because of the time period which has lapsed between maternal infection or viremia and abortion. But a significant increase in specific antibody can be demonstrated between acute and convalescent sera.

Treatment & prevention

The two therapeutic mainstays for uncomplicated equine rhinopneumonitis are: (1) antipyretics for fever reduction, and (2) non-steroidal anti-inflammatory agents for reduction of respiratory tract inflammation. These two requirements can be conveniently provided by administration of phenylbutazone at 3 mg/kg, 12 h to 24 h or flunixin meglumine at 1.1 mg/kg, IM, 12 h to 24 h. Bacterial rhinopharyngitis commonly occurs when the equine respiratory epithelium is injured by replicating EHV-1 or EHV-4 and, consequently, often becomes the eventual focus of the treatment strategy for herpesvirus URTD. A preparation of trimethoprim/sulfadiazine (30 mg/kg, PO, 24 h) administered for 7 - 10 days is an excellent and popular first choice for broad-spectrum antibacterial therapy because of its capacity for once-a-day, oral administration. In congenitally infected neonatal foals or in young horses in which clinical signs of bacterial infection are severe, progressive or involve the lower airways, optional antimicrobials for treatment include amikacin (20 mg/kg, IM, 24 h), procaine penicillin G (20,000 U/kg, IM, q 12 h), ceftiofur (2.2 mg/kg, IM, q 12 h), ticarcillin (44 mg/kg, IV, 8 h), and ceftazidine (25 mg/kg, IV, 8 h).

Vaccination

The two means for minimizing the economic losses and equine welfare burden caused by infection with EHV-1 & EHV 4 are prophylactic vaccination and careful attention to sound herd-management practices. Vaccination against EHV-1 is recommended as part of the preventive, herd-health program for all horses at risk for acquiring infection.

More than a dozen commercially manufactured both inactivated and attenuated-live vaccines are currently used for controlling abortion and respiratory disease caused by EHV-1. No current vaccine has been demonstrated to protect against the neurological manifestation of EHV-1 infection. Mosly the inactivated product is labeled as a prophylaxis for abortion. It is usually given at 5, 7 and 9 months of pregnancy, & other horses on the premises are also vaccinated. **Pneumabort K-1B** is a killed vaccine (for pregnant mares; 2 ml dose is given IM at the fifth, seventh, and ninth months of pregnancy. In regard to abortion, Pneumabort K-1B is the only rhinopneumonitis vaccine with federal approval for the prevention of abortion in mares due to equine herpsevirus-1 (EHV-1). The EHV-4 initial vaccination is followed by a second dose in four to six weeks, boostered every three to four months for horses that are showing heavily. The vaccine provides protection for up to three months. **Rhino/flu combination vaccine** is a vaccine containing influenza strains and rhinopneumonitis EHV-4. This combination vaccine is excellent for show horses, race horses, or horses in a high-exposure situation (such as medium to large boarding stables) that need rhino/flu vaccines every three to four months.

When used as an adjunct to sound management practices, vaccination can be effective in modulating the severity of EHV-1 respiratory disease in young stock and in limiting the occurrence and severity of abortion storms in broodmares. Annual reboosting with multiple doses of the vaccines is required for optimal results.

Equine Coital Exanthema

Equine coital exanthema (ECE) is a highly contagious, infectious, venereally transmitted mucocutaneous disease of mares and stallions (pustules & ulceration of the vagina, penis, prepuce & perineum.) caused by *Equid herpesvirus* 3 (EqHV-3). The disease is characterized by the development of superficial pock-like eruptions and erosions or ulcers on the external genital organs. The virus is highly contagious but is **noninvasive and relatively benign,** & usually does not result in systemic illness, and neither infertility nor abortion occurs as a result of infection.

Etiology: ECE is caused by *Equid herpesvirus* 3 (EqHV-3), a member of the *Herpesviridae*family & in the Alphaherpesvirinae subfamily. EqHV-3 is antigenically, genetically, and pathogenetically distinct fromEqHV-1, EqHV-2, EqHV-4, and EqHV-5. As with other herpesviruses, the virus remains latent in the host for life.

Occurrence

ECE is endemic in most horse breeding areas worlwide. Maternally derived antibody to EHV-3 is present in new-born foals but **decays to undetectable levels by four months of age**. The seroprevalence of infection is low in young and in unmated horses, but increases slowly with age in breeding animals.

Hosts susceptible

Equine coital exanthema is a benign venereal disease of horses that affects **both sexes**. The only known biological reservoir for the virus of ECE is the

latently infected horses. From latently infected carrier animals, EHV-3 is periodically reactivated and transmitted to others.

Transmission

The disease is spread through direct and sexual contact and possibly through flies carrying infected vaginal discharge. The primary method of virus transmission is **through direct skin-to-skin contact by coitus** with an actively infected, virus-shedding horse. Source of virus in an outbreak of ECE is either a mare brought onto the stud farm for breeding or virus reactivated from a member of the resident stallion or mare population. Subclinically infected horses without visibly noticeable lesions can also transmit the virus to their breeding animals. Iatrogenic transmission of infection can occur by virus-contaminated objects, such as buckets, instruments, tools and examination sleeves, used for the purposes of breeding, grooming, rectal palpation, or gynaecological examination. Reports of ECE lesions on the lips and nostrils of some horses indicate that non-coital transmission of infection by the genito-nasal contact associated with behavioural nuzzling/sniffing may be possible. The likelihood of mechanical transmission by stable flies has also been suggested.

Pathogenesis

Infection by EHV-3 occurs via direct cutaneous contact either during the act of coitus or by the transfer of virus-containing secretions from contaminated objects, such as hands, gloves, instruments, palpation sleeves, sponges and the lips or nose of a horse. The virus is easily transmitted by simple contact with the skin; the epidermal surface need not be damaged for infection to be established.

Viral replication is limited to the stratified epithelium of epidermal tissue present within the skin or at mucocutaneous margins; the virus is **temperature sensitive**. Destruction of epithelium by the lytic virus infection elicits a vigorous, localized inflammatory response that gives rise to the formation of the characteristic cutaneous lesions of ECE. Viral invasion of tissue within blood vessels or the stroma of the dermis underlying the epithelial lesion does not occur, and systemic dissemination of EHV-3 has not been reported. Secondary bacterial infection with *Streptococcus equi zooepidemicus* is common and influences the character, severity, and duration of the epithelial lesions. Recovery from ECE is complete in a matter of two to three weeks and occurs without permanent sequelae.

The horse responds to infection by EHV-3 with the production of serum complement-fixing (CF) and virus-neutralizing (VN) antibodies that reach maximal levels 14 to 21 days after infection. In comparison to the equine humoral immune response mounted against the systemically infecting herpesviruses of the horse, peak antibody titres against EHV-3 are relatively low. Complement fixation titres decline rapidly after infection (six to eight weeks), whereas VN activity declines more slowly with detectable levels persisting for a year or more. Post-exposure immunity to reinfection by EHV-3 is short-lived, and both stallions and mares have been observed to develop the disease in consecutive breeding seasons.

Clinical symptoms & lesions

EHV-3 has an **incubation period** as little as **two days**. The clinical symptoms of ECE are characterized by the presence of superficial lesions on the skin of the external genitalia of mares or stallions. The lesions appear initially as a small (1-3 mm) raised papule, then progresses sequentially to a vesicle, a pustule, and, after epidermal sloughing of the necrotic dome of the pustule, to a shallow, raw or encrusted erosion or ulcer. The progression to fully developed lesions is rapid, occurring over the period of only a few days. Initially, the individual erosions and ulcers are discrete and uniform in size (5 to 10 mm) and distinctly pock-like with raised borders and sunken centres. As they develop in size, the lesions may coalesce to form extensive epidermal erosions or ulcers. Localized inflammation is invariably present and gives rise to tissue congestion and erythema, & in the mare, edema of the vulvar labia, perineum and inner thighs. In the stallion, edema of the prepuce and sheath may occur and extend laterally onto the ventral abdominal wall and scrotum. Lesions infected secondarily with bacteria may exude a whitish discharge. The lesions may be few or many in number and may be at different clinical stages. Both the severity and duration of the disease varies considerably among individuals. Lesions may also be seen on the lips and teats.

Diagnosis

Collection of clinical specimens for laboratory tests for ECE include: clinical material collected from the edges of fresh, active lesions by firm swabbing or scraping, and two clotted blood samples without anticoagulant, one taken during the acute illness and the other three to four weeks later. Specimens for virus isolation should be submitted in 2-3 ml of tissue culture medium containing antibiotics and antimycotics on ice to a competent laboratory.

1. *Presumptive diagnosis*: The genital lesions of ECE in both mares and stallions are characteristic for a clinical diagnosis to be made with reasonable certainty. Carrier animals can sometimes be **identified by spots of pigment loss on black skin in the genital region.** A presumptive diagnosis can be confirmed in the laboratory by PCR, by isolation of the

virus or by demonstration of either seroconversion or a four-fold or greater rise in antibody titre in paired serum samples.

2. *Virus isolation*: EHV-3 isolation is done by inoculation of samples into equine-derived cell cultures; e.g. equine dermal foetal equine kidney or equine embryonic lung. Cytopathic effect by EHV-3 is generally evident by one to two days after inoculation of cell monolayers.

Treatment & prevention

Prevention is based on giving sexual rest to allow healing of ulcers and prevent the spread of the disease. Antibiotic ointments are used to prevent secondary bacterial infections. The affected horses should be isolated until all lesions have healed, and disposable equipment should be used for examinations. During the acute phase of the disease mares should be bred only by artificial insemination. All animals should be examined carefully before they are allowed to breed, keeping in mind that the incubation period is up to 10 days. No vaccine is available.

Fatal Haemorrhagic Disease in Puppies

Fatal haemorrhagic disease, caused by *Canine herpesvirus-1* (CaHV-1) is a severe, often fatal, viral infection of puppies worldwide, usually associated with upper respiratory tract infection or a vesicular vaginitis or posthitis in adult dogs. In puppies about 1 week old in domestic & wild dogs, the disease is characterized by crying, weakness, depression, and discharge from the nose, soft, yellow feces, and a loss of the suckling reflex. **CaHV-1 causes a necrotizing vasculitis that result in hemorrhages around the blood vessels.** Eye lesions include keratitis, uuveitis, optic neuritis, retinitis & retinal dysplasia. There is a high mortality rate, approaching 80 percent in puppies less than one week old, and death usually occurs in one to two days.

Etiology: Fatal hemorrhagic disease in puppies is caused by *Canine herpesvirus-1* (CaHV-1) in the genus *Varicellovirus.*

Occurrence

Fatal haemorrhagic disease in puppies occurs in USA, Canada, Australia, Japan, UK & Germany. In contrast with published results from other parts of the world, *Canine herpes virus-1* infection was shown to be common among the domestic dog population of England. CaHV-1 is very common, about one out of two or one out of three dogs have been exposed and carry this virus in their bodies. Show, kennels and large breeding kennels can not avoid this virus.

Hosts susceptible

Fatal hemorrhagic disease occurs in puppies and in wild *Canidae* less than **two to three weeks old.** In mature dogs and puppies over 3-4 weeks of age, the virus causes a mild respiratory disease, & the dogs recovers, but all recovered dogs carry a few of the virus for life in a latent form & shed the virus on reactivation under stresses.

Transmission

Most dogs become infected with CaHV-1 by inhaling or sniffing virus-containing sneezes and any liquid or moist secretions from an infected or virus-shedding dog. Some dogs get infected at a dog show or kennel or, groomer, or animal shelter or at any place where large numbers of dogs gather at one time. If more dogs are kept together or live in close proximity, it is more likely the virus is to be present. In some kennels, 100% of the dogs show evidence that they harbor CHV-1. A carrier dog relapsed due to a stressful situation sheds the virus.

CaHV-1 is transmitted to puppies in the birth canal, and by contact with infected oral and nasal secretions, vaginal secretion during & after parturition from the mother or other infected dogs. In adult dogs, the virus infects the reproductive tract, which allows it to be sexually transmitted or passed to puppies during birth. Like other herpesviruses, previously infected dogs can from time to time release the virus in vaginal secretions, penile secretions, and discharge from the nose. A stud can transmit CaHV-1 to bitch or vice versa. When a stud is shedding, the virus is present in his semen. When a bitch is shedding, the virus is present in her vaginal secretions. CaHV-1 does not last long in the environment, & in sunlight, common disinfectants and bleach kill the virus rapidly. Hence just passing the dog through an area that has CHV-1 positive dogs is not a problem.

Pathogenesis

One week- old puppies are unable to regulate temp, & hence virus don't grow above 36 C. Hence the virus replicates in the surface cells of the nasal mucosa, tonsils, and pharynx. Low body temperature allows the virus to spread and infect the rest of the body.

In puppies 3-5 week old dogs, the disease is less severe due to their ability to properly maintain body temperature and mount a febrile response. More puppies survive, but they can develop a latent infection. Some dogs later develop neurological disease and show symptoms like difficult walking and blindness. Reactivation of a latent infection may be caused by stress or immunosuppressive drugs such as corticosteroids. The site of **latency is the**

trigeminal ganglion and possibly the lumbosacral ganglion. In adult dogs, the virus infects the reproductive tract, which allows it to be sexually transmitted or passed to puppies during birth. The disease can cause abortion, stillbirth, and infertility.

Clinical symptoms & lesions

The incubation period of CaHV-1 is six to ten days. CaHV-1 infected breeding bitches show a drop in fertility, in case of a single female, the most likely thing to happen is a tie with no puppies at whelping time. If bitch show a rise in virus numbers near the end of her pregnancy without a sufficient rise in her antibody level, all or some of the puppies would die during their first three weeks of life. This may happen that the bitches may have first exposure with the CHV-1 virus, or a relapse due to the stress of pregnancy and other factors, usually the latter. When infection occurs while the puppies are still in her uterus, they may be stillborn, re-absorbed or aborted before they reach term.

When a puppy under 3-4 weeks of age becomes infected with CaHV-1, the disease takes an entirely different course. Puppies up to 3-4 weeks old do not regulate their body temperature well and because the immune systems of these puppies are not sufficiently developed yet, & herpes viruses do notstimulate good immunity. If the mother dog has adequate immunity herself, she will pass it along in her first milk (colostrums) in the form of anti-herpes antibody and immune cells that protect her puppies.

Infected, susceptible puppies usually **die within their first 3 weeks.** But their mothers continue to look fine. If some puppies survive, they are often poor performers & suffer from multiple health problems including heart and nerve damage. **In breeding dogs**, there is lack of breeding success and star-crossed puppies are the most common signs of a canine herpes virus problem. Late term abortions or re-absorption of the puppies is also common. The most common hint of the presence of CaHV-1 in adult animals is **transient, mild, upper respiratory tract problems**. Less commonly, **ulcers** similar to cold sores and inflammation occur on the animal's vagina, or on the prepuce and base of the penis. Problem periods often follow an increase in dog numbers or changes in your husbandry practices. But the majority of infected dogs show absolutely no signs that they are sick.

Puppy may be infected any time from late pregnancy through the first three weeks after birth. Whenever it occurs, it takes 3-7 days from the time the virus first entered the puppy for it to begin its destruction. If the puppies are born alive, the first sign of infection is often a lack of interest in nursing. The puppies whine continuously and appear uncomfortable, they may appear to be in pain due to tender tummies, often have fast, shallow breathing, & they may vomit. They may pass yellowish green stools. Nose and eye discharges are common. Less common signs are an increased tendency to bleed and seizures. Infected puppies sometimes have **pin-point hemorrhages on their gums.**

Young puppies are not capable of running a fever. The virus reproduces much more rapidly at the puppy's lower body temperature than in dogs that can mount a fever. As the disease progresses, the puppy's temperature drops to subnormal (below 98F, 36.7C). The disease progresses very rapidly and the puppies usually die in 1-3 days. If the puppies are lost during their first week, they were probably infected while still in the womb.

If the puppy is three weeks old, its defenses and temperature regulation are better and it will usually not die from CaHV-1. Exact outcomes vary as not every puppy in a litter with this problem may die nor will they all necessarily have the virus. Deaths due to CaHV infection usually occur in puppies 1-3 week old, occasionally in puppies up to 1 month old, and rarely in pups as old as 6 months. Disease onset is sudden, and death occurs after an illness of =24 hour. Older dogs exposed to or experimentally inoculaed with CaHV-1 may develop a mild rhinitis or a vesicular vaginitis or posthitis. In utero infections may be associated with abortions, stillbirths, and infertility. In susceptible populations of domesticdogs, CaHV-1 may be associated with outbreaks of highly contagious ocular infection in the absence of systemic disease. Conjunctivitis was the most frequent ocular lesion detected. Ulcerative andnon-ulcerative keratitis were less prevalent and of variable clinical appearance. Dendritic ulcerative keratitis, a classic and relatively specific ocular lesion associated with alphaherpesvirus infection, was detected in < 20% of dogs.

Gross lesions consist of disseminated focal necrosis and hemorrhages. The most pronounced lesions are seen in the lungs, cortical portion of the kidneys, adrenal glands, liver, and GI tract. All lymph nodes are enlarged and hyperemic, and the spleen is swollen. Lesions may also be found in the CNS. The histologic lesion is necrosis with hemorrhage in the adjacent parenchyma. Most often there is no inflammatory reaction. Single, small, basophilic, **intranuclear inclusion bodies are most common in areas of necrosis in the lung, liver, and kidneys;** occasionally, they are seen as faintly acidophilic bodies located within the nuclear space.

Diagnosis

1. *Presumptive diagnosis*: Diagnosis of the disease in puppies is best accomplished by PM lesions. The most important evidence of CaHV-1 is

extensive hemorrhage in the liver, lungs and kidneys. This occurs because the herpesvirus destroys the puppy's blood-clotting platelets. Damage and bleeding into the spleen, lymph nodes and adrenal glands are also characteristic of puppy death due to herpes virus as are fluid leakage into the chest and abdominal cavities.

2. *Serology*: To ascertain if the dog is shedding the virus, blood samples need to be collected two weeks apart. If the antibody level in the second sample is **3-4 times** as high as in the first sample, the dog is likely in a virus-shedding period and should not be bred. However, a steady, low antibody level or no antibody at all is no guarantee that a female that carries CHV-1 will not begin to shed virus during or after her pregnancy.
3. *Virus antigen detection*: A method in use is to have mouth and vaginal swabs tested for living herpesvirus or virus-related protein by FA test or PCR test.

Treatment & prevention

At dog shows and other community areas with many dogs, keep paper towels and a spray bottle of dilute antiseptic close at hand. Disinfect your hands before touching other dogs or allowing your dog to be handled by others. Keep your dog on a short lead. Keep its head up and do not let it sniff the floor and objects. Spray and wipe off it paws with alcohol. Do not share items, food or water between dogs. Spray and wipe down kennels before between animals. Keep your dogs as isolated from other dogs as possible.

Good disinfectants for herpes are 70% isopropyl alcohol mixed 50-50 with water, 0.5% Lysol, Listerine mixed 50-50 with water and household bleach diluted 7 tables poons-full in 1 quart of water (2000ppm).

Vaccination

The Merial Pharmaceutical Company has developed a vaccine, called Eurican herpes 205, a purified sub-unit vaccine containing glycoproteins of canine herpes virus (CHV) **that boosts immunity to CaHV-1 for about 60 days and makes it less likely that a bitch will be shedding virus during pregnancy,** delivery and nursing. It also makes it more likely that the bitch will pass on her herpes-immunity to her puppies through her first milk (colostrum). Dose: Two 1-ml doses of vaccine, administered by SC route, according to the following schedule: First injection: Either during heat or 7 - 10 days after the presumed date of mating. Second injection: 1 to 2 weeks before the expected date of whelping. Revaccination: during each pregnancy, according to the same schedule. The process must be repeated every time the dog is bred since the immunity it gives is temporary. It is a good insurance for first-time breeders and repeat problem breeders.

Feline Viral Rhinotrachetis and Keratitis

Feline viral rhinotracheitis & keratitis (FHR), also called "feline viral rhinotracheitis" feline herpes (FVR) is very contagious, an acute upper respiratory disease of cats caused by the *Feline herpesvirus type 1* (FeHV-1). The disease is characterized by coughing, sneezing, nasal discharge, conjunctivitis, and sometimes fever up to 106^{0}F and loss of appetite. Frontal sinusitis & emphysema can also result. Secondary bacterial infections can cause the persistence of clinical signs for weeks. FHV-1 also has a predilection for corneal epithelium, causing corneal ulcers, often pinpoint or dendritic in shape. Other ocular signs of FHV-1 infection include conjunctiviis, keratitis, keratoconjunctivitis, and corneal seqestra. Infection of the nasolacrimal duct can result in chronic epiphoa (excess tearing). Ulcerative skin disease can also result from FHV-1 infection. FeHV-1 can also cause abortion in pregnant queens, usually at the sixth week of gestation.

Etiology: Feline viral rhinotracheitis & keratitis (FHR) is caused by*Feline herpesvirus 1*(FeHV-1) under the genus *Varicellovirus.*

Occurrence

FVR causes one-half of all the respiratory diseases in cats, it is the **most important of these diseases** and is found worldwide. The other important cause of feline respiratory disease is *Feline calicivirus.*

Hosts susceptible

Cats specially 3-8 month of age & all members of the Felidae family are susceptible to FVR; in fact, FeHV-1 has caused fatal encephalitis in lions in Germany. The disease is more common in kittens, cats in stressed/overcrowded environments such as animal shelters & multi cat households. Kittens & older cats are more at risk than healthy adults, and are also at greater risk of dying. **Once the cat becomes infected with the FeHV-1, it will remain inapparently infected for life.** FVR is very contagious and can cause severe disease, including death from pneumonia in young kittens.

Transmission

It replicates in the nasal and nasopharyngeal tissues and the tonsils. Viremia is rare. The virus is shed in saliva and eye and nasal secretions, and can also be spread by fomites. The virus is shed for one to three weeks post infection. Latently infected cats (carriers) will **shed FeHV-1 intermittently**

for life, with the virus persisting within the **trigeminal ganglion**. Stress and use of corticosteroid precipitate virus shedding. On stresses, asymptomatic carriers may shed the virus, & they are actively shedding the virus & other cats can become infected.

During the active phase, the virus interferes with the cell's normal metabolism, causing the symptoms associated with the disease. The virus is shed & other cats can become infected. FeHV1 is transmitted by direct contact via oral and respiratory secretions, which are actively shedding the virus. FHV1 is transmitted through indirect contact via contact with infected food bowls, litter trays, bedding etc., which have been in contact with an infected cat shedding the virus. In utero infection occurs for FeHV to be passed onto unborn kittens via the mother.

Pathogenesis

The virus infects & grows in nose, eyes, sinus, throat, mouth & tonsils of a cat which causes inflammation & fever. Due to the nasal discharge, the cat's sense of smell is severely diminished, causing it's appetite to wane. While loss of appetite is dangerous in all cats, it is especially so in kittens where anorexia & dehydration can quickly take hold. Due to the damage caused to the tissues, it is possible for a secondary bacterial infection to take hold. If a pregnant cat catches herpes, it may lead to abortion of the kittens.

Clinical signs & lesions

FVR has **two to five day incubation period**. FVR cause an upper respiratory tract disease infecting the area of the eyes, nose, throat and sinus areas. The clinical symptoms include: sneezing, ocular (eye) & nasal discharge, conjunctivitis which sometimes lead to corneal ulcers, fever, loss of appetite, depression, ulceration of the mouth & tongue, & pneumonia. In chronic nasal and sinus disease of cats, FeHV-1 may play more of an initiating role than an ongoing cause. Infection at an early age may permanently damage nasal and sinus tissue, causing a disruption of ciliary clearance of mucus and bacteria, and predispose these cats to chronic bacterial infections.

Diagnosis

1. *Presumptive diagnosis*: Diagnosis of FVR is usually by clinical signs, especially **corneal ulceration**. Definitive diagnosis can be done by direct immunofluorescence or virus isolation. However, many healthy cats are subclinical carriers of FeHV-1, so a positive test for FHV-1 does not necessarily indicate that signs of an upper respiratory tract infection are due to FVR. Early in the course of the disease, histopathological analysis

of cells from the tonsils, nasal tissue, or nictitating membrane (third eyelid) may show inclusion body within the nucleus of infected cells.

Treatment & prevention

Antibiotics are commonly used to prevent secondary bacterial infections. More recent research has indicated that **systemic famciclovir** is effective at treating this infection in cats without the side effects reported with other anti-viral agents. More severe cases may require supportive care such as IV fluid therapy, oxygen therapy, or even a feeding tube. Conjunctivitis and corneal ulcers are treated with topical antibiotics for secondary bacterial infection. **L-Lysine** has been recommended anecdotally to suppress viral replication, & L-lysine is also used for treatment of ocular signs of FHV-1 infection.

Vaccination

There is a **vaccine** for FeHV-1 available plus various combinations of vaccines, but although it limits the severity of the disease and may reduce viral shedding, it does not prevent infection with FVR. Studies have shown that duration of **immunity of this vaccine is at least three years. ECLIPSE 3**-Intervet (feline rhinotracheitis +feline calicivirus + feline panleukopenia) is a modified live vaccine; inject one dose (1 ml) SC or IM at 9 weeks of age or older and repeat with a second dose 3 to 4 weeks later. Annual revaccination with one dose is recommended. **NOVIVAC TRICAT-Intervet** (feline rhinotracheitis +feline calicivirus + feline panleukopenia) is a live vaccine; the first inoculation is given from the age of 8-9 weeks and the second inoculation from the age of 12 weeks. Revaccination against feline calicivirus and feline herpesvirus type 1 must be given every year & against feline panleucopenia virus can be given every three years (with strain MW-1 as in Nobivac Tricat Trio, where available). **ECLIPSE 4** in addition also includes feline leukemia virus. Inject one dose/1 ml SC or IM at 9 weeks of age or older and repeat with a second dose 3 to 4 weeks later. Annual revaccination with one dose is recommended. **Felocell 3 or Felocell CVR**-Pfizer is a similar vaccine.

The use of serology to demonstrate circulating antibodies to FeHV-1 has been shown to have a positive predictive value for indicating protection from this disease. Most household disinfectants will inactivate FeHV-1. The virus can survive up to 18 hours in a damp environment, but less in a dry environment and only shortly as an aerosol.

Pseudorabies or Aujeszky's Disease

Pseudorabies or Aujeszky's disease is a contagious viral disease that affects pigs (natural hosts), & cattle, sheep, dogs, cats, other dead end hosts. Swine are usually asymptomatic, but can cause abortion, high mortality in piglets with coughing, sneezing, fever, constipation, depression, seizures, ataxia, circling, and excess salivation in piglets and mature pigs. Mortality in piglets less than one month of age is up to 100% , but less than 10% in pigs between one and six months of age. Pregnant swine can reabsorb their litters; deliver mummified, stillborn, or weakened piglets. In cattle, symptoms include intense itching followed by neurological signs and death. In dogs, symptoms include intense itching, jaw and pharyngeal paralysis, howling, and death. In cats, the disease is so rapidly fatal that there are usually no symptoms. Any infected secondary host usually lives only for two to three days. Pseudorabies is considered to be the most economically important viral disease of swine in areas after eradication of hog cholera.

Etiology: Pseudorabies or Aujeszky's disease is caused by*Suid herpesvirus 1* (SuHV-1)/Porcine herpesvirus 1/ Pseudorabies virus ((PRV), and is also known in cattle as **mad itch** under the genus *Varicellovirus*. The virus may potentially survive for seven hours in humid air and spread up to two kilometers. Furthermore, it may survive on well water for up to seven hours, in green grass, soil, and feces for up to two days, in contaminated feed for up to three days, and in straw bedding for up to four days.

Occurrence

Pseudorabies is endemic in most parts of the world. PRV is considered to be the most economically important viral disease of swine in areas after eradication of hog cholera. The disease is usually fatal in hosts such as cattle, sheep, goats, cats. dogs, and raccoons. In 1902 a Hungarian veterinarian, Aladar Aujeszky, isolated PRV from a dog, ox, and cat and showed that it caused the same disease in swine and rabbits. The name pseudorabies came from the symptoms similar to rabies that it caused in rabbits.

Hosts susceptible

Populations of wild boars or feral hogs in the U.S. commonly contract and spread the virus throughout their range. **Healthy male adults (boars) are typically latent carriers**, that is, they harbor and transmit the virus without displaying symptoms. Other domestic and wild mammals, such as cattle, sheep, goats, cats, dogs, and raccoons are susceptible. The disease is usually fatal in these hosts. Pseudorabies has been reported in other mammals, including brown bears, and black bears, Florida panther, raccoons, coyotes, and whitetail deer. In most cases, contact with pigs or pig products was either known or suspected. Outbreaks in farm fur species in Europe (mink and foxes) have been associated with feeding infected pig products. Many other species can be experimentally infected. Humans are not potential hosts.

Transmission

Pseudorabies is highly contagious. In most cases, this disease is transmitted through nose-to-nose contact, which is the most common type of transmission because pseudorabies is mostly present in nasal and oral areas. Movement of carrier pigs is additional means of virus transmission. Transmission of disease between herds occurs by airborne route, at least 3 km, from feral (wild) pigs, birds may spread the virus, & contaminated carcasses. Virus spread occurs mechanically on clothing, boots, vehicles and equipment, or through infected semen via AI or a carrier boar, & from infected slurry.

Pathogenesis

After oronasal infection, PRV first replicates in the **epithelial tissues,** the mucous membrane of the nasopharynx and in the tonsils, & spread it to the regional lymph nodes. In the acute disease, a viremia follows introduction of the virus with rapid dissemination throughout the body. The virus enters to the CNS via axons of the cranial nerves, and may also directly enter nerve endings of sensory neurons in the nasopharynx. After a first round of replication in the epithelia, progeny virus is abundantly produced leading to an increased infection of primary neurons. In virtually all infected animals that survive acute infection, the virus establishes a **latent infection in tonsils and trigeminal ganglia**.

Transplacental infection of the fetus is common. As for BHV-1, the latent infection is the major means for virus survival and transmission in nature, as it may be periodically reactivated. Major sites of **PRV latency are the trigeminal ganglion** (TG), the **olfactory bulb, and the tonsil**. In these organs, viral DNA can be detected in the absence of infectious virus production, and LAT transcription could also be demonstrated by highly sensitive **methods such as RT-PCR**. Interestingly, there appears to be a correlation between precolonisation of trigeminal ganglia with PRV and failure of a super infecting strain to become latent itself. This indicates that the number of neurons in which latency will be established is limited and that, probably, an already "occupied"neuron resists superinfection. It may, however, be deduced that attenuated live vaccine strains with a high potential for establishment of latency may prevent superinfecting wild type virulent strains from becoming latent. Recently, the proteins which are required for neuroinvasion of PRV were detected; one of the key proteins in neuroinvasion is **glycoprotein E.** Deletion of this protein strongly attenuates PRV. Absence of gE does not impair primary viral replication in the nasal epithelium after intranasal infection of mice or pigs. It is also not required for the virus to enter primary neurons. Transsynaptic transfer to second order neurons is severely inhibited, resulting in a dramatic restriction in neuroinvasion. gE, and to a lesser extent gI, are the predominant non essential glycoproteins exhibiting this dramatic phenotype. Other proteins which are required for cell-to-cell spread in culture are also essential for neuronal spread in the animal. These include gB and gH. As in cell culture, gD is not required for transsynaptic transfer but is essential for entry into primary target cells. Thus, phenotypically gD-complemented gD- PRV invades the central nervous system after primary replication, and is virulent in mice.

Clinical symptoms & lesions

Swine are usually asymptomatic, but PRV can cause abortion in sows, high mortality in piglets, and coughing, sneezing, fever, constipation, depression, seizures, ataxia, circling, and excess salivation in piglets and mature pigs. Mortality in piglets less than one month of age is close to 100 percent, but it is less than 10 percent in pigs between one and six months of age. Pregnant swine can reabsorb their litters; deliver mummified, stillborn, or weakened piglets. In cattle, symptoms include intense itching followed by neurological signs and death. In dogs, symptoms include intense itching, jaw and pharyngeal paralysis, howling, and death. In cats, the disease is so rapidly fatal that there are usually no symptoms. Any infected secondary host generally lives two to three days.

Clinical signs of pyrexia, depression, frequent swallowing, facial fasciculations, chorea, excessive salivation, mild tympanites, labored breathing and focal pruritus were followed by death.

Macroscopic lesions were severe focal facial trauma, petechiae in cervicothoracic ganglia and dilated esophagus. The medulla oblongata and the trigeminal, cranial cervical, cervicothoracic and parabronchial ganglia contained pseudorabies virus and pronounced nonsuppurative inflammatory changes. The neural distribution of lesions and virus suggests that the virus **travelled from the respiratory mucosa to the central and sympathetic nervous system by two routes: 1) in the vagus and glossopharyngeal nerves to the medulla oblongata and 2) in the postganglionic fibers to the sympathetic ganglia.** The presence of virus in the nasal mucus indicated that horizontal transmission of pseudorabies virus may occur among sheep.

Diagnosis

Collection of clinical samples include: tonsil, brain, lungs, spleen, kidney, liver, and serum, & pieces of the subcutaneous tissue is taken from the site of pruritis and spinal cord in animals other than pigs.

1. *Presumtive diagnosis*: PM lesions include small focal areas of necrosis may be seen in the liver and spleen of aborted fetuses and piglets. Histologically, these tissues reveal the presence of intranuclear inclusions

typical of herpesvirus. A nonsuppurative meningoencephalitis is the most common microscopic finding in pigs experiencing CNS signs.

For rapid diagnosis, fluorescent antibody tests on frozen sections of tissue from tonsils in carcasses are often used. This is reliable and results are available in few hours. PCR has provided a sensitive, specific and rapid mean to detect DNA sequences in infected swine tissues.

2. *Virus isolation*: For virus isolation, tissues are taken from the lung and tonsils; the virus grows on the CAM of chicken embryos, and in pig kidney and other cell cultures; the virus produces cytopathic changes in about 16 hours. The virus can also be identified by virus neutralization and fluorescent antibody tests.
3. *Serology*: Serum neutralization, latex agglutination, and ELISA tests are used for the detection of antibody. ELISA tests for serum antibody detection are used widely on recovered pigs and in herd diagnosis. Other tests are available to distinguish wild and vaccine type infections.

Treatment & prevention

There is no specific treatment for acute infection with pseudorabies virus.

Vaccination

Vaccination can alleviate clinical signs in pigs of certain ages. Typically, mass vaccination of all pigs on the farm with a **modified live virus vaccine** is recommended. **Intranasal vaccination of sows and neonatal piglets 1-7 days old,** followed by **IM vaccination of all other swine on the premises,** helps reduce viral shedding and improve survival. The modified live virus replicates at the site of injection and in regional lymph nodes. Vaccine virus is shed in such low levels that mucous transmission to other animals is minimal.

PORCILIS AD BEGONIA-Intervet is a freeze dried live attenuated vaccine with strain NIA-3 (tk- and gE-) immunized to pigs in Dluvac Forte. gE deletion allows natural infections to be differentiated from vaccine response. Each dose contains active component $105.^{5}$ $TCID_{50}$ of ADV strain Begonia. The vaccine is dissolved in Diluvac Forte. After reconstituted, when maternally derived antibodies (MDA) are not present, piglets can be vaccinated 2 ml IM as early as 1 week of age without any problems. Immunity after a single injection will last the whole of the fattening period, or at least until 6 months of age. When MDA are present, piglets can be given a single dose at 14 weeks of age. Protection will last the whole of the fattening period. When there is a risk of early infection, pigs carrying varying levels of MDA can be vaccinated from 10 weeks of age onwards and should be re-vaccinated at 14 weeks of age, but no earlier than 4 weeks after the first dose. For eradication, vaccinate at 4 month intervals, three times per year as a herd vaccination programme. Control: end of each pregnancy, not later than 2 weeks before farrowing. **Marker vaccines (Suvaxyn Aujeszky)** –Fort Dodge is a live attenuated Aujeszky's disease virus, strain NIA3- 783: ≥ 105.2 CCID50 per dose. The vaccine has been developed by deleting gE and thymidine kinase (TK). The gE deletion makes it possible to differentiate between vaccinated and field infected animals. TK deletion ensures a safe non virulent vaccine strain, & thus, the virus cannot infect and replicate in neurons. It is recommended that breeding herds be vaccinated IM quarterly, and that finisher pigs be vaccinated after levels of maternal antibody decrease. **PRV/MARKER GOLD**-Intervet is vaccinated to pigs at 3 days of age or older that prevents pseudorabies as well as respiratory form of the disease. Dose 2 ml IM or intranasally. Regular vaccination results in excellent control of the disease. Concurrent antibiotic therapy via feed and IM injection is recommended for controlling secondary bacterial pathogens.

Gammaherpesvinae

Genus: *Rhadinovirus*

Malignant Catarrhal Fever (MCF)

Malignant catarrhal fever (MCF) is a lethal lymphoproliferative disease of cattle, characterized by vasculitis, necrosis, and accumulation of activated, dysregulated cytotoxic lymphocytes in various tissues. MCF is a frequently fatal disease syndrome of ruminant species-cattle, bison, deer characterized by inflammation, ulceration, and exudation of the oral and upper respiratory mucous membranes, and sometimes eye lesions and nervous system disturbances. The causative viruses exist in nature as subclinical infections in sheep, goats that serve as carriers. Lymphocytes are the main target of the virus. MCF **causes inapparent infection in their reservoir hosts, sheep with OvHV-2, wildebeest with *Alcelaphine herpesvirus* 1(AlHV1) but are usually fatal in cattle and other ungulates like deer, antelope & buffaloes.** The important clinical symptoms are the head and eye form, including fever, depression, discharge from the eyes and nose, lesions of the buccal cavity and muzzle, swelling of the lymph nodes, opacity of the cornea leading to blindness, inappetance and diarrhea. Some cases develop neurologic signs, such as ataxia, nystagnus & head pressing. **Peracute, alimentary and cutaneous forms** of the clinical disease occur. Death usually occurs within ten days. The mortality rate in symptomatic animals is 90 to 100 percent. MCF is an important disease where reservoir and susceptible animals mix.

Etiology: Two major epidemiologic types of MCF exist, defined by the reservoir ruminant species from which the causative virus arises. One is commonly known as the **African form,** wildebeest-associated MCF (WA-MCF) caused by *Alcelaphine herpesvirus-1* (AlHV-1), which causes MCF in cattle, deer & other ruminants **in Africa** (natural host wildebeest with life-long inappaent infection). The other is referred to as sheep-associated MCF (SA-MCF) caused by *Ovine herpesvirus* 2 (OvHV-2), which affects cattle, deer, bison & others. Virtually all cases of MCF in the U.S. are SA-MCF, caused by the sheep virus or which exists as a ubiquitous subclinical infection in domestic sheep. Two clinical diseases in nature have been reported, one in white-tailed deer (MCFV-WTD), was found causing the classic MCF syndrome in white-tailed deer in North America. The other, called caprine herpesvirus 2 (CpHV-2), is endemic in domestic goats and was associated with alopecia, chronic weight loss and dermatitis in two species of deer.

Occurrence

Disease of domestic and captive species of Artiodactyla, & disease distribution is world-wide.

Hosts susceptible

Disease outbreaks in cattle are usually **sporadic** although infection of up to 40% of a herd has been reported. Some species appear to be particularly susceptible, for example **Pére Davids deer, Bali cattle and bison,** with many deer dying within 48 hours of the appearance of the first symptoms and bison within three days. In contrast, post infection cattle will usually survive a week or more. AHV-1/OHV-2 can also cause problems in zoo animals, where inapparently infected hosts (wildebeest and sheep) and susceptible hosts are often kept in close proximity. Feedlot bison in North America not in contact with sheep have also been diagnosed with a form of MCF. OHV-2 has been recently documented to infect herds of up to 5 km away from the nearest lambs, with the levels of infected animals proportional to the distance away from the closest herds of sheep.

Transmission

In Africa, wildebeests carry a lifelong infection of AlHV-1; the virus is passed from mother to offspring and shed mostly in the **nasal secretions of wildebeest calves under one year old**. The virus is **transmitted from wildebeest calves to cattle following the wildebeest calving period**. Cattle of all ages are susceptible to the disease, with a higher infection rate in adults, particularly in peripartuent females. Cattle are infected by contact with the secretions, but do not spread the disease to other cattle.

Throughout the rest of the world, cattle and deer contract BMCF by close contact with reservoir hosts, sheep or goats during lambing. The natural host reservoirs for Ovine herpesvirus 2 are the sheep and goats whilst MCF affected animals are from the families *Bovidae*, *Cervidae* and *Suidae*. Susceptibility to OHV-2 varies by species, with domestic cattle and zebu somewhat resistant, water buffalo and most deer somewhat susceptible, and bison, Bali cattle, and pere Davis deer very susceptible. OHV-2 viral DNA has been detected in the alimentary, respiratory and urinogenital tracts of sheep all of which could be possible transmission routes. Antibody from sheep and from cattle with BMCF is cross reactive with AlHV-1

The incubation period of BMCF is not known, however intranasal challenge with AHV-1 induced MCF in one hundred percent of challenged cattle between 2.5 and 6 weeks.

Pathogenesis

Pathogenesis of experimentally produced sheep-associated malignant catarrhal fever (MCF) in rabbits was studied. The principal change was a proliferation of lymphoid cells which began as soon as three days and became quite pronounced by 13 days after inoculation. The appendix, mesenteric lymph node and spleen were most obviously affected. The reason for this was a progressive increase in T-lymphocytes, which appeared to be a hyperplasia rather than neoplasia in T-dependent areas of these organs. Lymphoid cells also accumulated in interstitial spaces of non-lymphoid organs. The use of cyclosporin-A suppressed the lymphoid proliferation but rabbits still developed clinical MCF after a similar incubation period. It is suggested that the agent of MCF might produce its effect by infecting and causing a dysfunction of lymphoregulatory cells, resulting in benign polyclonal T-lymphocyte proliferation. Terminal necrosis could be due to natural killer cell activity.

Clinical symptoms & lesions

Incubation periods in natural cases are not known. Experimentally in wildebeest-associated MCF, the incubation period has varied from **9 to over 70 days.** The most common form of the disease is the **head and eye form.**

Peracute form: In this form, severe inflammation of the oral and nasal mucosa and haemorrhagic gastroenteritis occur with a course of 1-3 days.

Intestinal form: There is pyrexia, diarrhea, hyperaemia of oral and nasal mucosa with accompanying discharges, and lymphadenopathy with a clinical course of 4-9 days is descriptive of this form.

Head-and-eye form: This is the typical syndrome of MCF with pyrexia, nasal, and ocular discharges, progressing from serous to mucopurulent. Encrustation of the muzzle and nares occurs in later stages, causing obstruction of the nostrils and dyspnoea, open-mouthed breathing, and drooling. There is intense hyperaemia and multifocal or diffuse necrosis of the oral mucosa, usually on the lips, gums, hard and soft palate, and buccal papillae, leaving them reddened and blunted. Necrotic skin lesions occasionally are seen, and horn as well as hoof wall may be loosened or sloughed. The course of the head-and-eye form is usually 7-18 days.

Mild-form: This form is usually not fatal. Clinical signs in exotic ruminants are usually manifested by conjunctivitis, photophobia, moderate corneal clouding that may be unilateral, fever, depression, variable lymphadenopathy, occasionally diarrhea, and usually mild serous nasal discharge. Death in some species may be sudden, following a brief course of hemorrhagic diarrhea.

PM lesions: Animals that die peracutely may have few lesions other than hemorrhagic enterocolitis. In the more protracted intestinal and head-and-eye forms, the carcass may be normal, dehydrated, or emaciated. The muzzle is often encrusted and raw. Cutaneous lesions sometimes occur as generalized exanthema with exudation of lymph, crusting, and matting of the hair. Hyperemia is apparent in unpigmented skin. These lesions are frequently seen in the ventral thorax and abdomen, inguinal region, perineum and loins, and sometimes on the head. Generalized lymphadenopathy is common. **Lymphoproliferative changes in the internal organs including CNS are highly suggestive of MCF**. Typical herpesvirus inclusion bodies are not present.

Diagnosis

Collection of clinical samples for antibody testing by cELISA may be done with either serum or plasma. Antemortem detection of viral DNA by PCR may be done on whole blood in EDTA. Preferred postmortem samples for detection of viral DNA by PCR are lymph node or spleen, but other tissues include lung, kidney, and intestine.

Diagnosis of BMCF depends on a combination of history and symptoms, histopathology and detection in the blood or tissues of viral antibodies by ELISA or of viral DNA by PCR. The similarity of MCF clinical signs to other enteric diseases, for example blue tongue, mucosal disease and foot and mouth make laboratory diagnosis of MCF important. The world organization for animal health recognizes histopathology as the definitive diagnostic test, but laboratories have adopted other approaches with recent developments in molecular virology.

Although generally infected early in life, viral DNA is detected by PCR in leukocytes 1-4 weeks post infection. Epidemiologically, most infected lambs and kids do not become PCR positive until about 3 months of age. Therefore, if MCF testing is being done to confirm that lambs or kid are not infected, it is necessary to test after they are at least 4 months of age. Although false negatives may occur, PCR for viral DNA in leukocytes is the optimal test for determining infection status in animals between 3 and 12 months of age.

Treatment & prevention

There is no effective treatment available. Treatment is supportive only. The recent availability of derivatives of **acyclovir compounds that inhibit replication of herpesviruses shows promise in potential treatment regimens**. A report of inhibition of the replication of the alcelaphine herpesvirus by using recombinant interferons could be considered in development of a treatment regimen for valuable animals.

Unfortunately a vaccine for MCF has not yet been developed, because the **virus will not grow in cell culture.** Researchers at the Agriculture Research Service (ARS) found that the **virus undergoes changes within the animal's body, a process known as "cell tropism switching."** In cell tropism switching, the virus targets different cells at different points in its life cycle. This phenomenon explains why it has been impossible to grow the virus on any one particular cell culture.

Because the virus is transmitted from sheep to bison and cattle, researchers are first focusing on the viral life cycle in sheep. The viral life cycle is outlined in three stages: entry, maintenance, and shedding. Entry occurs through the sheep's nasal cavity and enters into the lungs where it replicates. The virus undergoes a tropic change and infects lymphocyte, which play a role in the sheep's immune system. In the maintenance stage, the virus remains on the sheep's lymphocytes and circulates in the body. Finally, during the shedding stage, the virus undergoes another change and **shifts its target cells from lymphocytes to nasal cavity cells**, where it is then shed through nasal secretions. ARS researchers are looking into alternative methods to develop a vaccine. Researchers are experimenting with the MCF virus that infects tofi (an African antelope) because it will grow in cell culture and does not infect cattle. Researchers hope that inserting genes from the sheep MCF virus into the tofi MCF virus will ultimately be an effective MCF vaccine for cattle and bison.

Inclusion Body Rhinitis

Inclusion body rhinitis virus is slow-replicating; cell lysis doesn't occur until several days after infection & associated with chronic infections that may last several months before clinical recovery. The infected cells are often enlarged (cytomegaly), & cytomegaloviruses are maintained in latent form in secretory glands and lymphoreticular cells associated with continuous viral excretion. Inclusion body rhinitis is a viral infection usually manifested in nursing or newly-weaned piglets as a rhinitis and conjunctivitis accompanied by sneezing and nasal discharge. Infection of pregnant, naïve sows may lead to delivery of dead, mummified, stillborn or weak piglets. Piglets may be born dead, die without clinical signs or be pale, anemic and edematous in the generalized form of the disease. A reduction in growth rate frequently occurs.

Etiology: Inclusion body rhinitis is caused by *Suid herpesvirus* (SuHV) / Inclusion body rhinitis virus which can only be cultured with difficulty and which is most easily isolated by the culture of **alveolar macrophages from 3-5 week old pigs**. It can be cultivated in vitro in these or porcine testis or fallopian tube cell lines. There are usually no signs that reveal Inclusion body rhinitis. In alveolar macrophage cultures infected cells enlarge and form **basophilic intranuclear inclusions** which may be demonstrated by immunofluorescence or Giemsa stain. Isolates appear to belong to one antigenic type, although serological differences have been found amongst recent isolates. It is caused by porcine cytomegalovirus.

Occurrence

IBR occurs worldwide in the major swine-raising countries. Infection is common but often is inapparent when herd immunity is present or in pigs over six weeks old.

Hosts susceptible

Inclusion body rhinitis (IBR) occurs in all **age groups** of previously uninfected swine, including developing fetuses. But the disease occurs in **pigs up to 2-week old**. Clinical signs include inappetence and fever in pigs of more than 3 weeks of age in enzootic herds. In non- immune pigs or herds, pigs may be infected in utero or within 2 weeks of birth and may develop rhinitis; sneezing and respiratory distress with mortality rate in affected litter may reach 25%. IBR occurs only in pigs although similar infections with related viruses occur in many other species, including people.

Transmission

Infection can spread by direct contact with urine or respiratory secretions or by aerosol. Virus is shed in nasal secretions mostly between 3 and 8 weeks of age. Infection may occur even up to slaughter weight and may be reactivated by stress and mixing which should be avoided. Boars can excrete virus in urine and nasal secretions. Serum antibody responses develop but low levels of antibody may not prevent infection of the production of conception. Severe disease in adults has been recorded when infection enters non-immune herds.

Pathogenesis

Replication of the virus takes place in the **nasal mucous glands in non-immune piglets following oronasal infection,** in white blood cells (neutrophils) in the blood 14-16 days after infection and finally in epithelial sites such as the nasal mucosa, testicular cells and kidney tubules at 3 weeks of age. The primary site of virus replication is in the nasal mucous glands or the lachrymal or Harderian glands. Destruction of these cells results in a marked rhinitis and conjunctivitis. Viremia follows replication. The virus localizes in epithelial and endothelial cells at many sites as well as within macrophages and reticuloendothelial cells. The intracellular virus causes marked enlargement and destruction of many infected cells but persists and is tolerated by other cells. Regeneration can occur in some simple glands by proliferation and differentiation of ductal cells. **Endothelial cell damage and necrosis is believed to be responsible for the petechial hemorrhages and edema that accompany IBR.** Bone marrow damage is suspected of causing anemia in neonates. Widespread damage caused by the virus or by secondary infections can lead to death.

Where individual sows or whole herds are non-immune, pigs may be infected in utero or within 2 weeks of birth and may develop rhinitis, sneezing and respiratory distress. Mortality in an affected litter may reach 25%. Piglets may be born dead, die without clinical signs or be pale, anemic and oedematous in the generalized form of the disease. Virus may cross the placenta and infect the fetus during the viremic stage at 14-21 days after infection in non-immune sows. Embryonic death occurs in **early gestation**. Fetuses exposed late in gestation are born seronegative.

Clinical signs & lesions

The disease usually is observed in **one to five week old pigs**. In suckling pigs, especially pigs less than three weeks old, signs include mucopurulent rhinitis accompanied by violent sneezing, respiratory distress, conjunctivitis, shivering, perhaps mouth breathing, and a variable death loss. Although unusual, mortality can be high in pigs born to naïve gilts or sows, or if IBR is complicated by other diseases.

Infected **neonatal piglets** appear weak, anemic or stunted and there may be edema around the throat and tarsal joints. Signs in older pigs or dams with viremia may include listlessness and mild anorexia or may be inapparent.

Fetal mummification, stillbirths, neonatal deaths and failure of piglets to thrive have been associated with infection of naive, pregnant sows. Evidence that IBR caused these has been accumulated through field observations and is supported by related research.

PM lesions: In nursing piglets, the most commonly recognized gross lesion is mucopurulent exudate in, and perhaps obstruction of nasal passages. Complications sometimes include sinusitis, otitis media or pneumonia. In neonatal pigs, petechial hemorrhages and subcutaneous edema can occur. Effusions in the thorax, abdomen and pericardial sac and edema of the lungs often are present. Microscopically, **intranuclear inclusions** usually can be found in nasal mucous glands, Harderian glands and lachrymal glands of nursing pigs. They may be present in renal glomeruli and tubular epithelium, liver, capillary endothelium, choroid plexus, glial cells and in various epithelial type cells. **Focal gliosis** is common throughout the central nervous system (CNS). Inclusions sometimes can be found at several sites in fetuses

Diagnosis

1. *Presumptive diagnosis*: The disease usually is diagnosed after finding microscopic, **basophilic intranuclear inclusions in tissues of a typical, infected piglet**. Inclusion body rhinitis is usually suspected when piglets within 2 weeks of birth develop rhinitis, sneezing and respiratory distress. Mortality in an affected litter may reach 25%. Piglets may be born dead, die without clinical signs or be pale, anemic and edematous in the generalized form of the disease.

2. *Serology*: Serum antibody can be detected by indirect immuno-fluorescence or ELISA tests that confirm the presence of IBR in a herd.

If reproductive problems have occurred in a herd, IBR will need to be differentiated from other reproductive diseases, especially parvoviral infection, pseudorabies (PRV) and porcine reproductive and respiratory syndrome (PRRS).

Treatment & prevention

Because the disease seldom is recognized as a cause of severe loss, control measures often are ignored. Growing pigs usually are protected from large losses by antibodies provided by their immune dams. As piglets grow, they are exposed to virus in the environment and respond by producing their own antibodies.

Environmental conditions, if poor, should be improved. Herd immunity via acclimatization of breeding stock is commonly practiced. There is no known effective treatment or medication. Antibiotics may be useful to control concurrent diseases or secondary bacterial infections.

Marek's Disease

Marek's disease (M D) is a highly contagious viral lymphoproliferative disease of chicken caused by *Gallid herpesvirus* 2 (GaHV-2)/ Mark's disease virus 1 (MDV-1) and is characterized by multiple T-cell lymphoma formation in visceral organs (tumors on the liver, kidneys, testes, ova, spleen and lungs), muscles, skin & lesions in peripheral nerves. Clinical signs of MD vary from mild depression followed by ataxia and paralysis, skin nodular lesions, stunting and mortality. MDV infection causes five syndromes: **classical Marek's disease** or **neurolymphomatosis, acute Marek's disease, ocular lymphomatosis, cutaneous Marek's disease, atherosclerosis, & immunosuppression.**

Etiology: Marek's disease is caused by *Gallid herpesvirus* 2 (GaHV-2)/ Marek's disease virus 1 (MDV-) in the genus *Mardivirus*. There are 3 serotypes, *Gallid herpesvirus* 2 (GaHV-2)/ Marek's disease virus type 1(MDV-1) causes Marek's disease in domestic fowl, turkey, quail, mostly in 8-12 day-old chickens. Currently, **virulent MDV-I** serotype 1 strains are further divided into pathotypes, which are often referred to as **mild (m), virulent (v), very virulent (vv), and very virulent plus (vv+) Marek's disease virus strains.** Three serotypes of MDV are MDV-1, -2 -3 of which; types 1 & 2 occur in chickens & type 3 in turkeys. MDV-1 is oncogenic but types 2 & 3 are not. MDV-2 strains are non oncogenic and are widely used as vaccinesagainst Marek's disease in combination with other strains. The related Herpesvirus of Turkeys (HVT), causes no apparent disease in turkeys and continues to be used as a vaccine strain for prevention of Marek's disease.

From the 1980s and 1990s emergence of highly virulent strains has become a problem in North America and Europe. The virus survives at ambient temperature for a long time (65 weeks) when cell associated and is resistant to some disinfectants (quaternary ammonium and phenol). It is inactivated rapidly when frozen and thawed.

Occurrence

Marek's disease is a ubiquitous avian infection, & occurs in chicken flocks worldwide.

Hosts susceptible

Generally, chickens between **8-16 weeks of age** are most often affected. **Quail** can be naturally infected and turkeys can be infected experimentally. However, severe clinical outbreaks of Marek's disease in commercial turkey flocks, with mortality from tumors reaching 40-80% between 8-17 wk of age, were reported recently in France, Israel, and Germany.

Transmission

The route of infection is usually **respiratory** and the disease is highly contagious being spread by **infective chicken dander from feather follicles contain the virus & spreads the disease,** & through fomites, etc. The virus also is excreted in the saliva, and the virus enters the body through the respiratory system. The infected birds with GaHV-2 remain viremic for life & can be carriers and **shedders of the virus for life**. Infection in the older, vaccinated bird is also becoming more frequent. Vertical transmission is not considered to be important. Marek's lies dormant and doesn't show up in birds most of the time. It is usually triggered by stress. A high parasite load or a change in housing, bullying, feeding or management methods can trigger the disease. Point of laying birds seem to be particularly vulnerable.

Pathogenesis

Initial infection of the respiratory tract occurs via inhalation of infectious dust. Three to five days postinfection, B lymphocytes of the bursa of Fabricius, spleen and thymus become infected.

The virus subsequently infects T lymphocytes of mostly the **$CD4^+$ phenotype**; infection becomes latent and the virus spreads throughout the host by a cell-associated viremia. MDV-1 infection has 4 arbitrary phases in vivo: 1) early productive-restrictive virus infection causing primarily degenerative changes, 2) latent infection, 3) a second phase of cytolytic, productive-restrictive infection coincident with permanent immunosuppression, and 4) a proliferative phase involving non productively infected lymphoid cells that may or may not progress to the point of lymphoma formation. Productive infection may occur transiently in B lymphocytes within a few days after infection with serotype 1 strains and is characterized by antigen production, which leads to cell death.

Productive infection also occurs in the feather follicle epithelium, in which enveloped virions are produced. Latent infection of activated **$CD4^+$ T cells and probably $CD8^+$ cells is responsible for the long term carrier state**. No antigens are expressed, but virus can be recovered from lymphocytes by co-cultivation with susceptible cells in tissue cultures. Some T cells, latently infected with oncogenic serotype 1 strains, undergo neoplastic transformation, leading to lesions of lymphomatosis in visceral organs. These transformed cells, provided they escape the immune system of the host, may multiply to form characteristic lymphoid neoplasms. Cell-mediated and humoral immune responses are both directed against viral antigens, with cell-mediated immunity probably being the most important. There is a secondarycy tolytic infection of the feather follicle epithelium from which cell-free virus is produced and shed in feather dander and debris.

Clinical signs & lesions

There are five syndromes that may overlap, & occur after infection with Marek's disease; these syndromes include: **classical Marek's disease or neurolymphomatosis, acute Marek's disease, ocular lymphomatosis, cutaneous Marek's disease, artherosclerosis, & immunosuppression.**

Classical Marek's disease or neurolymphomatosis: causes asymmetric paralysis of one or more limbs; paralysed birds on the floor show with one leg forward and one leg back. There is **vagus nerve involvement**, difficulty in breathing or dilation of the crop may occur. Besides lesions in the peripheral nerves, there are frequently lymphomatous infiltration/ tumours in the skin, skeletal muscle, & visceral organs. Organs that are commonly affected include the ovary, spleen, liver, kidneys, lungs, heart, proventriculus and adrenals.

Acute Marek's disease: is an epidemic in a previously uninfected or unvaccinated flock, causing depression, paralysis, and death in a large number of birds up to 80%. The age of onset is much earlier than the classic form; birds are **four to eight weeks old** when affected. Lymphomatous infiltration into multiple organs/ tissue is observed.

Ocular lymphomatosis: causes lymphocyte infiltration of the iris, making the iris turn grey, anisocria, and blindness.

Cutaneous Marek's disease: causes round, firm lesions at the feather follicles.

Atherosclerosis: is induced in experimentally infected chickens.

Immunosuppression: Impairment of the T-lymphocytes prevent competent immunological response against pathogenic challenge and the affected birds become more susceptible to disease conditions such as coccidiosis and E. *coli* infection. Furthermore, without stimulation by cell-mediated immunity, the humoral immunity conferred by the B-cell lines from the Bursa of Fabricius also shuts down, thus resulting in birds that are totally immunocompromised. Although clinical disease is not always apparent in infected flocks, a subclinical decrease in growth rate and egg production may be economically important.

PM lesions include Grey-white foci of neoplastic tissue in liver, spleen, kidney, lung, gonads, heart, and skeletal muscle. There is thickening of nerve trunks and loss of striation. Microscopically-lymphoid infiltration is polymorphic.

Diagnosis

The demonstration of nerve enlargement, especially with the schiatic nerve along with suggestive clinical signs in a bird that is around three to four months old is highly suggestive of Marek's Disease. The presence of nodules on the internal organs may also suggest Marek's disease but further testing is required for confirmation. This is done through histological demonstration of lymphomatous infiltration into the affected tissue. A range of leukocytes can be involved, including lymphocytic cell lines such as large lymphocyte, lymphoblast, primitive reticular cells and occasional plasma cells as well as macrophage and plasma cells. The T-cells are involved in the malignancy, showing neoplastic changes with evidence of mitosis.

The lymphomatous infiltrates need to be differentiated with another condition that affects poultry known as Lymphoid leukosis as well as an inflammatory event associated with hyperplastic changes of the affected tissue. Marek's disease can develop in chickens as young as 3 weeks of age, whereas lymphoid leukosis typically is seen in chickens older than14 week of age.

Treatment & prevention

There is no treatment for Marek's disease. Sanitation & resistant breeding is recommended.

Vaccination

Vaccination is the only known method to prevent the development of T lymphoid tumors when chickens are infected with the virus. However, administration of vaccines does not prevent transmission of the virus; i.e., the vaccine is non-sterilizing, but it does reduce the amount of virus shed in the dander and hence reduce horizontal spread of the disease. Marek's disease does not spread vertically. The vaccine was introduced in 1970 by Dr. Benjamin Roy Burmester. Before that, Marek's disease caused substantial revenue loss in the poultry industries of the United States and the United Kingdom. The vaccine can be administered to **one day old chicks** through SC inoculation or by in-ovo vaccination when the eggs are transferred from the incubator to the hatcher. In-ovo vaccination is the preferred method, as it does not require handling of the chicks and can be done rapidly by automated methods. Immunity develops within two weeks.

The vaccine originally contained the antigenically similar turkey herpesvirus, which is serotype 3 of MDV. Because vaccination does not prevent infection with the virus, the Marek's disease virus has evolved increased virulence and resistance to this vaccine. As a result, **current vaccines** use`a combination of vaccines consisting of HVT and gallid herpesvirus type 3 or an attenuated MDV strain, CVI988-Rispens. **Salsbury MD-Vac,** a vaccine of chick-embryo tissue culture is recommended. Vaccination at one day of age usually protects birds through their lifetime. **NOBILIS RISMAVAC**-Intervet frozen vaccine contains live MDV strain cv1988: >= 3.0 log^{10} $TCID_{50;}$ dose is .2 ml SC. The vaccine is recommended for use in day-old chicks, and is also indicated where very virulent strains of MDV (vvMDV) are prevalent. **NOBILIS RISMAVAC+CA126** contains live Turkey herpes virus strain FC126 = 3.0 log^{10} PFU and live Chicken herpes virus strain CVI-988 = 3.0 log_{10} PFU. Dose is .2 ml SC in one day chicks or in ovo vaccination.

Bivalent vaccines consisting of HVT and either the SB1 (**MAREXINE CA126+SB1**) or 301B/1 strains of serotype 2 MD virus have been used to provide additional protection against challenge with virulent serotype 1 isolates. Attenuated serotype 1 MD vaccines are also available, e.g., the CV1988/Rispens strain appears particularly effective. A synergistic effect occurs between serotype 2 and 3 strains, has prompted the empirical use of other virus mixtures. Vaccines are also effective when administered to **embryos at the 18th day of incubation by automated technology** and is widely used for vaccination of commercial boiler chickens. Cell-associated vaccines are generally more effective than cell-free vaccines because they are neutralized less by maternal antibodies. Under typical conditions, vaccine efficacy is usually more than 90%, & losses from MD have been reduced dramatically in broiler and layer flocks.

Herpesvirus of turkeys as vectors-**VaxxitekHVT+IBD**-Merial is frozen live recombinant chimera vaccine expressing VP2 of IBD on HTV virus, experimental recombinant vaccines have been shown to be effective against challenge with virulent Marek's disease virus. Each dose of vaccine (0.2 ml) contains at least 3.0 log^{10} PFU of the live vHVT013-69 recombinant virus. It must be administered by means of a single SC injection. The indication is for the active immunization of day-old chickens as follows: To prevent mortality, to reduce clinical signs and lesions of IBD. The onset of protection is from 2 weeks and the protection extends to 9 weeks. A single vaccination is sufficient to provide protection. Vaxxitek HVT + IBD does not show any interference by MDA, hence can be given to day-old chickens.

Genus: *Iltovirus*:

Infectious Laryngotracheitis

Infectious laryngotracheitis, one of the most contagious viral diseases that affects the poultry industry, is a viral infection of the respiratory tract of chickens, pheasants and peafowl exhibiting signs of wet irritated eyes, sneezing, gasping, nasal discharge, failure to thrive, decreased growth, and decreased egg production. As ILT progresses, the clinical signs at later stage become worse including difficulty in breathing, bloody discharge from the nose and mouth, gasping, coughing, and expectoration of bloody mucus. Birds will shake their heads to clear the mucus from their nose and mouth, which results in blood stained mucus on the feathers of many birds in the flock.

Etiology: Infectious laryngotracheitis is caused by *Gallid herpesvirus 1* (GaHV-1) in the genus *Iltovirus*. Different types of ILT virus strains are available in nature which varies in their virulence. The manifestation of virulence among strains varies from mild/ inapparent infection to high morbidity and mortality. Strains have been differentiated on the basis of virulence for chickens or chicks, plaque size and morphology in cell cultures and pock size on the chorioallantoic membranes (CAMs) of chicken embryos. Strains have been differentiated by restriction endonuclease analysis of viral DNA, and the use of the PCR and restriction fragment length polymorphism (RFLP) has enabled differentiation of field and attenuated vaccine-type strains.

Occurrence

ILT was originally recognized as a disease of chickens in the United States in 1926. ILT has now been identified in most countries around the world and remains a threat to the intensive poultry industry. Outbreaks of mild to moderate forms of ILT are common in commercial layer flocks while sporadic outbreaks of ILT in broiler flocks have also been recognized as an emerging problem in several countries. Prevalence of infectious laryngotracheitis was restricted to Peru and Panama (period 2005-2009), then outbreak of ILT has taken place in India for the first time in 1997. Morbidity due to this disease is almost 100% and mortality ranges between 10-70%, depending upon the virulence of the virus strain. **Trigeminal ganglion in chicken is the main site of latency** of Infectious laryngotracheitis virus.

Hosts susceptible

Infectious laryngotracheitis occurs in chickens, pheasants and peafowl.

Transmission

The sources of ILTV are: a) clinically affected fowls, b) fowls which are latent 'carriers' of infection, & c) fomites and poultry farm personnel contaminated with ILTV. Natural portals of entry for laryngotracheitis virus are through upper respiratory tract, ocular route and oral ingestion. GaHV-1 is shed in respiratory secretions and transmitted by droplet inhalation. Transmission occurs more readily from acutely infected birds than through contact with clinically recovered birds. The coughed-up mucosa and blood of the infected bird are the medium through which this disease spreads. Feathers, shed dust, feed trucks, human beings, contaminated equipment and litter are the ideal transporting agents. There is no vertical transmission of the virus from breeders to chicks. ILT is not transmissible to human beings.

Pathogenesis

A study of the pathogenesis of ILT in birds revealed that the **epithelium of the conjunctiva and respiratory tract** are the tissues actively infected by natural routes of infection. The virus propagated at the sites of initial exposure but there was no evidence of spread by viremia. Viral antigen was detected 2-7 days post-exposure and rarely thereafter. Birds infected intratracheally showed intense infection in the nasal turbinates, suggesting that high concentrations of virus were expelled as an aerosol from infected tracheas. Virus applied to the dorsal lip of the vent by drop or brush was rapidly transferred mechanically to the bursa of Fabricius; the epithelial lining between follicles and between follicular cortex and medulla was positive in FA tests 48-72 hours postexposure.

ILTV infection of the upper respiratory tract of susceptible chickens is followed by intense viral replication. Infectious virus usually is present in tracheal tissues and secretions for 6-8 days PI. The virus may remain at very low levels up to 10 days p.i. No clear evidence exists for a viremic phase of infections.

Clinically inapparent - ILTV infection of the respiratory tract is a major feature of ILTV persistence. Studies demonstrated that collecting laryngeal and tracheal swabs from recovered infected birds and then inoculating susceptible chickens, indicated a "field" carrier rate of approximately 2% up to 16 months after a disease outbreak. Other studies with tracheal organ cultures explanted from chickens experimentally infected with Australian wild-type ILTV and vaccine strains have showed latent tracheal infections for similar periods in 50% or more of infected chickens.

Clinical symptoms & lesions

The **incubation period** is two to eight days. In case of an outbreak, there is a spiking mortality among the flock. Severity of the disease and mortality rate varies widely among outbreaks and depends on the following factors: age of the birds, immune status of the flock, virulence of the virus strain & viral load on the farm, concurrent infection with other respiratory pathogens; and harsh environmental factors that adversely affect the respiratory system.

Clinical symptoms noticed during different forms of severity of the disease are as follows:

Peracute form: Infected birds are lethargic, have swollen eye-lids followed by ocular discharge. Birds exhibit mouth breathing, coughing & emit respiratory noises. Some birds stretch out their neck while trying to breathe & cough-up blood stained mucus. Mortality may be as high as 70%.

Acute form: There are less severe respiratory rales & coughing with expulsion of caseous material, mucoid nasal discharge, gasping and swollen eyelids. Mortality may range from 10-30%.

Chronic form: The birds are drowsy with signs of conjunctivitis, squinting eyes and cough. Morbidity is as low as 5%. There is often a concurrent infection with coryza. Egg production may drop to 10%.

PM lesions: Lesions in the per-acute form consist of **hemorrhagic tracheitis with blood clots.** Lumen of the trachea is blocked by mucoid blood clots or sometimes by yellow caseous exudate (cheesy plug). In the acute form, lesions consist of mucoid exudate with or without blood in the trachea. Yellow caseous diphtheritic membranes may be found adherent to the larynx and upper tracheal mucosa. In both acute and sub-acute form, death is due to **suffocation.** In the chronic form, false membrane is found in the upper respiratory tract and causes death.

Diagnosis

1. *Presumptive diagnosis* A presumptive diagnosis of the disease is based on clinical signs and post-mortem lesions.
2. *Virus isolation*: Confirmatory test is done through embryo inoculation method. Suspected virus material collected from tracheal swab of infected birds is inoculated in chick embryos of 11 to 12 day of age through chorioallantoic membrane (CAM). Three days post inoculation, plaques can be observed on CAM. These plaques have opaque edges and depressed central area of necrosis. The size of surviving embryo also gets reduced.
3. *Virus detection*: Agar gel immunodiffusion (AGID) using a hyperimmune serum to ILTV is tested in macerated tracheal and laryngeal tissue from the affected bird, it differentiating ILT from the diphtheritic form of fowlpox. Among the more rapid methods for detecting ILTV are IF or immunoperoxidase (IP), an antigen capture ELISA, EM, DNA hybridisation techniques and the PCR.
4. *Antibody detection*: Monitoring of antibodies to ILTV in chicken serum is done by AGID, VN, indirect immunofluorescence (IIF) and ELISA.

Differentiation of wild-type and modified-live vaccine viruses may be accomplished by restriction endonuclease cleavage of viral DNA and electrophoretic separation of DNA fragments. This method has been used extensively in epidemiological studies of field outbreaks to identify wild-type and vaccine viruses.

Treatment & prevention

There is no treatment for ILT. Prevention and control of ILT rest on (a) sound biosecurity and sanitation, & (b) effective vaccination of parents and progeny.

ILT virus can survive for 10 days or more in droppings and up to 70 days in carcasses at ambient temperature of 13°C to 23°C. The virus lasts longer in winter. It appears that the virus may survive up to 80 days in tracheal mucus on non-conductive material such as wood. However, the disease keeps perpetuating on the farm because of healthy carriers. To get rid off ILT virus from a poultry farm, it is necessary to practice following after cleaning the empty shed: Sunlight, heat and drying (virus gets inactivated at 38°C within 48 hours).

A mist created by 5% hydrogen peroxide in the shed, Cresol 3% or lye 1% solution- apply on floors and walls. Apart from this, biosecurity should also include restricted entries, cleaning up of surfaces, disposal of carcasses, rodent control, insect and pest control, personnel hygiene, disinfection of vehicles, egg trays etc.

Vaccination

The maternal antibodies have no protective role in case of Infectious laryngotracheitis. It is therefore, necessary to confer active immunity to all birds of all ages by proper vaccination schedule:

Although live vaccines are available, the disadvantages of using live vaccines are: the reversion of virulence is seen with all the available live vaccines. These viruses become latent in the trigeminal ganglion and get activated when birds are under stress and perpetuate Infectious laryngotracheitis virus in susceptible poultry flocks. Vaccination is best done with **modified strains of low virulence** applied to the **conjunctiva by eye drop**. Results are less consistent with mass methods of vaccination such as spray or drinking water administration. Broiler flocks in some areas where the disease is endemic must be vaccinated when young, but this is unlikely to be effective if done at less than 4 week of age. Some vaccine producers recommend revaccination when birds are to be held to maturity. Three types of vaccines are available. Tissue culture origin (TCO) vaccines have a relatively low level of infectiousness and are administered by an eye drop. A disadvantage of TCO vaccines is that the level of immunity is limited; the advantage of this is that it causes a less severe reaction and the birds do not shed the virus. Chicken embryo origin (CEO) vaccines can be administered through an eye drop or mass vaccination, such as spray or water. While these CEO vaccines result in a better immunity, it can cause severe clinical signs and disease due to the increased level of infectiousness-hence its use is negligible. Recombinant ILT vaccines have been developed. These recombinant ILT vaccines can be administered as a single dose, by subcutaneous injection, on day 1 or in older bird. It is reported to provide ILT immunity for up to 60 weeks. The recombinant vaccine does not cause shedding of the virus; therefore unvaccinated birds are not placed at risk. It has also limited level of immunity and birds may develop mild clinical signs of ILT. These vaccines are also more expensive.

TRACHIVAX-Intervet is freeze-dried, modified live, ILT virus- $10^{2.8}$ EID_{50} per dose preserved with gentamicin, administered in drinking water. Used in healthy fowls to prevent infectious fowl laryngotracheitis through revaccination of breeders and layers by drinking water administration at 10 weeks of age or older where a longer immunity is desired. **NOBILIS ILT**-Intervet is a live vaccine for immunization of chickens against ILT. Intraocular vaccination of susceptible birds at the age of 4 to 6 weeks and re-vaccination at 14-16 weeks of age is recommended. In emergency, the birds may be vaccinated earlier, but should then always be re-vaccinated one month before the onset of lay, by the intraocular route. In case of an outbreak, emergency vaccination in all unvaccinated chickens will stop transmission of the disease, limiting ILT related losses **BroilerT RakeM/ LT-IVAX**- Intervet are modified live vaccines against ILT for vaccination at 4 weeks of age through immunization by the eye drop method. Initial vaccination is at 4 weeks of age followed by revaccination at 10 weeks of age or older. **Laryngo Vac**-Pfizer is a modified live vaccine for prophylaxis against laryngotracheitis. Vaccinate birds-1 drop intraoculary when they are 4 weeks old or, if conditions dictate, birds may be vaccinated as early as 10 days of age. Revaccinate replacement birds at 16 to 20 weeks of age. Should an outbreak of laryngotracheitis occur on the premises, immediately institute a program of vaccination of birds farthest from the infected birds and work towards the diseased birds.

Inactivated Vaccines

Inactivated vaccines have been used to control Infectious laryngotracheitis. This is a safe method of control. These vaccines have shown to stimulate the desired immune response in chicken.

Unassiged viruses

Duck Plague/Duck Viral Enteritis

Duck plague/duck viral hepatitis is a highly fatal contagious disease of young ducklings, 1-28 days of age & occurs in ducks, geese & waterfowls in Asia, Europe & N. America, & is caused by *Anatid herpesvirus 1* **(AnHV-1)/**

Duck plague/ Duck viral enteritis herpesvirus 1. The disease is characterized by high mortality in flocks of ducks. Symptoms include loss of appetite, decreased egg production, nasal discharge, increased thirst, diarrhea, ataxia, tremors **& drooped-wing appearance**. Most ducks that show symptoms eventually die; mortality may reach 90 percent. Due to the formation of **diptheroid plaques** on the **eyelids** and the mucosae of the respiratory system and gastrointestinal system, the bird may show opthalmic signs and refuse to drink.

Etiology: Duck plague/ duck viral hepatitis is caused by *Anatid herpesvirus 1***(AnHV-1)/** Duck plague/ Duck viral enteritis herpesvirus 1.

Occurrence

Duck plague (also known as duck viral enteritis-1) is a worldwide disease caused by *duck herpesvirus 1* (*Anatid herpesvirus 1*) of the family *Herpesviridae* that causes high mortality in flocks of ducks. Duck plague / duck viral enteritis occurs in North America, Europe, & Asia. It affects ducks, geese and swans of all ages. A herpesvirus infection of ducks and geese was diagnosed in the UK in 1972, mostly in ornamental collections, in USA since 1967, & also the Netherlands and other countries.

Hosts susceptible

Ducklings are most susceptible at the younger ages and gradually become more resistant as they grow older. The disease is rarely seen in ducklings over 4 weeks of age. Duck virus enteritis is an acute, contagious, highly fatal disease of waterfowl caused by a herpes virus. This disease is most likely to affect mature ducks, but is also seen in young ducks.

Ducks or geese and swans of all ages are susceptible to the duck virus enteritis. All waterfowl are susceptible and the Barbary duck is more susceptible than the Pekin.

Transmission

It is spread through contaminated water and direct contact. Migratory waterfowls are a major source in the spread of this disease. DVE is transmitted from bird to bird, by bloodsucking arthropods, or by contact with contaminated water or environment. Transmission is by infected birds, fomites and arthropods. Recovered birds may carry the virus for a year.

Pathogenesis

There is rapid dissemination and active replication of virulent DVE in multiple systemic organs at the early phase of acute infection & accelerate the progression of disease. The relatively high levels of DVE in bursa and small intestine tissues of dead ducklings most likely reflect the abundance of target epithelial and lymphoid cells in these tissues, which therefore play a key role in the pathogenesis of acute DVE and manifest as severe tissue lesions on the bursa and small intestine. The virus replicated in **hepatic macrophages, hepatocytes, and bile duct epithelium.** There were necrosis and degeneration of stratified squamous epithelium of the esophagus and cloaca, epithelium of intestinal crypt and esophageal submucosal glands, macrophages in the lamina propria, and submucosal fibrocytes and lymphocytes. Submucosal hemorrhages occurred after degeneration and necrosis of lymphocytes, macrophages, fibrocytes and epithelial cells. Viral antigens were detected in all these cells by use of fluorescein-labeled antibodies. With the electron microscope, nucleocapsids were seen in the nuclei, budding through the inner nuclear membrane; enveloped virions were present in cytoplasmic vacuoles of macrophages, epithelial cells and fibrocytes. In lymphocytes, nucleocapsids were also in the nuclei, but karyorrhexis and cytolysis occurred before viral maturation was completed. Necrosis of lymphocytes occurred in the bursa of Fabricius, thymus, splenic periarteriolar lymphoid sheath (T lymphocytes), and splenic germinal centers (B lymphocytes). Viral nucleocapsids were present in the karyoplasm of lymphocytes, but these cells necrotized before virions were formed. Periarteriolar reticular sheath cells and sinusoidal lining cells in the spleen, epithelial cells in Hassall's corpuscle of the thymus, epithelial cells between the cortex and medulla of the follicles in the bursa of Fabricius, and macrophages in all 3 tissues contained nucleocapsids in the nuclei and virions in cytoplasmic vacuoles before necrosis occurred.

Clinical symptoms & lesions

The **incubation period is 3-7 days.** The onset of the disease is very rapid, it spreads quickly throughout the flock and may cause up to 90% mortality. Sick ducklings develop spasmodic contractions of their legs and die within an hour in a typical "arched-backward" position. The liver is enlarged and shows hemorrhagic spots.

Duck virus enteritis is an acute, contagious, highly fatal disease of waterfowl caused by a herpes virus. This disease is most likely to affect mature ducks, but is also seen in young ducks. Affected birds show sluggishness, ruffled feathers, greenish-yellow diarrhea that is sometime blood-stained. Dead birds often have blood-stained feathers around the vent and blood dripping from the nostrils. Hemorrhages may be found in tissues throughout the body. **Eruptive lesions of the mucous lining of the esophagus and intestine are characteristic signs of the disease**. Necrotic plaques may be observed in the cloaca. Regular immunization of breeder ducks with an attenuated live duck virus enteritis vaccine provides adequate protection.

Signs of DVE include sudden, persistent high mortality and a drop in egg production (25-40%). Photophobia can occur as half-closed, pasted eyelids. Inappetence, extreme thirst, droopiness, ataxia, ruffled feathers, nasal discharge, watery diarrhea and soiled vents may also be evident. Birds may be unable to stand, have droopy wings outstretched, and head down. Tremors of the head, neck and body, loss of weight, blue beaks, blood stained guy, and mortality (5-100%) may be seen.

Lesions include vascular damage (tissue hemorrhages) and free blood in the body cavity. Eruption in the GI tract and degeneration of lymphoid organs (thymus and bursa) may be seen. Petechial hemorrhage may be seen on the myocardium, on liver, pancreas, intestine, lungs and kidney. Surface hemorrhages and crusty yellow-white plaques on the mucosa of the oral cavity, esophagus, ceca and cloaca may be evident.

Diagnosis

1. *Presumptive diagnosis*: Clinical signs and gross lesions, petechial hemorrhage in the conjnctivae, mucus membrane, trachea, syrinx and intestine are pathognomonic for DVE in all age ducks. It Simulates influenza, fowl cholera and duck viral hepatitis.

Virus isolation: When inoculated in Duck CAMs of 12 day embryos, embryos die in 4 days, perform HA, & intranuclear inclusions are seen. Differentiate from Duck hepatitis, oesophagitis, vent gleet, pasteurellosis, & coccidiosis. A live attenuated vaccine can be administered to ducklings and breeders.

Treatment & prevention

Once DVE is present, depopulation, relocation and intensive disinfection are required to overcome an outbreak. Management practices such as **preventing exposure to wild waterfowl and contaminated water** and screening of new stock should be performed to prevent disease. To prevent this disease, keep age groups isolated.

Vaccination

Vaccinate breeder ducks with attenuated live virus duck hepatitis. Solid natural immunity develops in recovered birds. Healthy appearing birds were subcutaneously vaccinated with a **modified live duck plague vaccine** (Intervet, **Boxmeer, NL**) that stopped losses and resulted in seroconversion in most of the vaccinated birds. Vaccination in face of outbreak is of value, probably through interference. **NOBILIS-DUCK PLAGUE**-Intervet is a live vaccine for the immunization of ducks against duck plague virus enteritis.

This duck plague vaccine is a modified live virus prepared from the chorioallantoic fluid, membrane and embryo of infected chicken embryo and is freeze dried. The vaccine is supplied with diluent. Dose: one ampoule contains 200 doses. One ampoule is diluted in 100 ml diluent and 0.5 ml is given SC. Immunity: one year. Schedule of Vaccination: In healthy atmosphere first vaccination is given at the 7th week and a booster dose is given in the 4th month. (Immunity develops in one week and last for a year). In the face of an outbreak first vaccination can be done from the 3rd week of age followed by a second vaccination after 4 weeks and booster after 4 months.

□□□

Chapter 11

Characteristics and Disease Caused by the Members of Group I Double-Stranded DNA Poxviruses (Family *Poxyviridae*)

Contents

Characteristics of Poxviruses

Poxviruses (L. pock= pustules, ulcers) that belongs to family *Poxviridae* are very large having complex structure & infect both vertebrate & invertebrate hosts. The viruses are **brick- shaped, biconcave or ovoid measuring 220-450 nm x 140-26o nm wide**. Poxviruses are of two types, **intracellular mature virion** (IMV) & **extracellular enveloped virion** (EEV) & both are infectious (Fig 11-1). While IMV bears an internal core, an inner membrane & an outer membrane bearing surface tubules or filaments, & IMV are released on cell lysis as such. When IMV acquires a second outer membrane from trans Golgi while budding, it is called exrtracellular enveloped virion (EEV). Thus EEV consists of an extra outer membrane bearing surface filaments as compared to IMV. The **core** consists of 3 structures; a biconcave axis, a lateral body on each side of the concavity & DNA lying within the core. In case of *Parapoxvirus*, a single long thread coils round the virion. Viral genome contains a single molecule of linear ds DNA 130000–375000 nucleotides long. Capsid symmetry of poxviruses is complex. Virus envelope is derived from host cell membrane & as such contains host cell lipids & virus encoded proteins including hemagglutinin (HA) which is separable & produced by the species of only *Orthopoxvirus.*

Poxviruses can infect humans, animals, birds & insects. Recently, there has been a concern that smallpox may be used as an agent in bioterrorism. Vaccinia virus is used as an effective vaccinal tool for expression of foreign protein to elicit strong host immune response.

Poxviruses are stable at room temp but sensitive to heat, detergents, oxidizing agents & formaldehyde but genera differ in ether sensitivity.

The virus genome

Poxviral genome is not segmented & contains a single molecule of linear double-stranded **DNA of about 130-375kb**. The guanine + cytosine content of the genome are 35–64 % or 20 % (for Entomopoxviruses). The genome termini have redundant sequences; these terminal redundant sequences have reiterated inverted terminal sequences which are tandemly repeated. These sequences are repeated at both ends. DNA is covalently cross-linked at both ends. The viral genome encodes both non-structural proteins & structural proteins. There are more than 40 structural proteins including **DNA dependent RNA polymerase or RNA transcriptase that helps in uncoating the virus.** There are more than 10 antigens including NP antigen. Genetic recombination occurs within genera. Non genetic reactivation (activation of heat inactivated virion by a viable one) occurs within & among genera of vertebrate poxviruses. There are more than 10 antigens including NP antigen. Genetic recombination occurs within genera. Non genetic reactivation (activation of heat inactivated virion by a viable one) occurs within & among genera of vertebrate poxviruses.

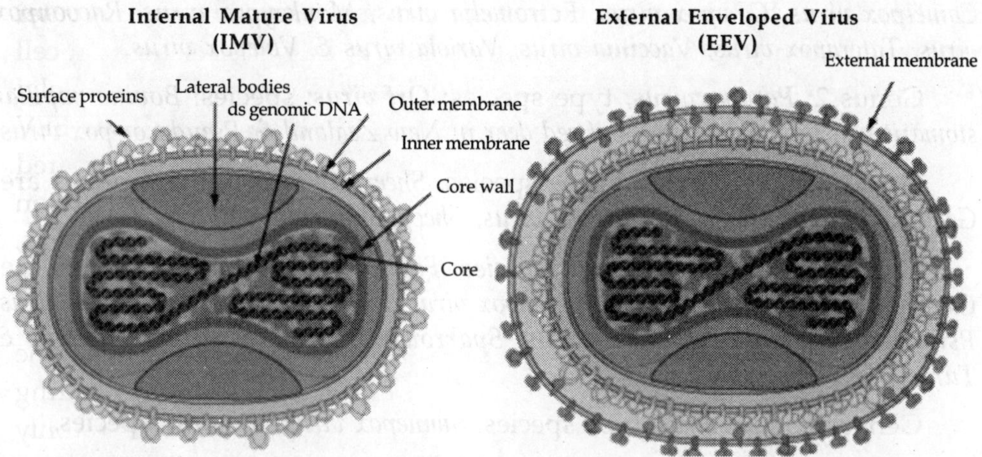

Figure 11.1 : Morphology of Poxvirus

Virus replication

Poxviral replication occurs in the **cytoplasm of host cells** & includes 3 phases: **Early phase, intermediate phase & late phase**. The virus binds to glycosaminoglycans (GAGs) receptors on the host cell surface or components of the extracellular matrix. After binding to the receptor, the virus enters the cell where it is uncoated; firstly the outer membrane is removed while entering the cell, & secondly the virus particle is uncoated further to release the core into the cytoplasm. The **early phase** transcribes early genes in the cytoplasm by viral RNA polymerase. **Early genes** encode the non-structural proteins including proteins necessary for replication of the viral genome. In the **intermediate phase** intermediate genes are expressed which initiates genomic DNA replication. In the **Late phase** late genes are expressed & produce all structural proteins to make the virus particles. The assembly of the virus particle occurs in the cytoskeleton of the cell probably in association with internal membranes of the infected cell to produce a spherical immature particle that matures into brick-shaped intracellular mature virion (IMV). Either IMV virion is released after cell lysis, or may acquire a second double membrane from *trans*-Golgi and bud as external enveloped virion. The virus replication is quick & takes about 12 hrs when the host cell dies by the release of viruses.

Virus classification

Group: Group I dsDNA virus

Family: *Poxviridae*

Subfamily 1: *Chordopoxvirinae*

Genus 1: *Orthopoxvirus;* type species: *Vaccinia virus;* other species are: *Camelpox virus, Cowpox virus, Ectromelia virus, Monkeypox virus, Racoonpox virus, Taterapox virus, Vaccinia virus, Variola virus & Volepox virus.*

Genus 2: *Parapoxvirus;* type species: *Orf virus;* species: *Bovine papular stomatitis virus, Parapoxvirus of red deer in New Zealand & Pseudocowpox virus.*

Genus 3: *Capripoxvirus;* type species: *Sheeppox virus;* other species are: *Goatpox virus, Lumpy skin disease virus, Sheeppox virus.*

Genus 4: *Avipoxvirus; type species: Fowlpox virus;* other species are: *Canarypox virus, fowlpox virus, Juncopox virus, Mynapox virus, Pigeonpox virus, Psitacinepox virus, Quailpox virus, Sparrowpox virus, Starlingpox virus & Turkeypox virus.*

Genus 5: *Suipoxvirus;* type species: *Swinepox virus,* the only species.

Genus 6: *Leporipoxvirus;* type species: *Myxoma virus;* other species are: *Hare fibroma virus, Myxoma virus, Rabbit fibroma virus, Squirrel fibroma virus.*

Genus 7: *Molluscipoxvirus;* type species: *Molluscum contagiosum virus,* the only species.

Genus 8: *Yatapoxvirus;* type species: *Yaba money tumor virus;* other species ae: *Tanapoxvirus, Yaba money tumor virus.*

Genus 9: *Cervidpoxvirus;* type species: *Deerpox virus W-848-83,* the only species.

Genus *Unassigned;* species: *Squirrelpox virus.*

Subfamily 2: Entomopxvirinae - Viruses of insects.

Poxvirus Clinical Manifestations in Humans & Animals

Poxviruses can infect humans, animals & birds; infect the epidermis and produce focal lesions. In general, poxviruses lesions develop as papule, vesicle, pustule, and finally scabs or crusts that frequently become proliferative and later necrotic. Rarely generalized infections can be fatal. Poxviruses occur naturally in most veterinary species, **except the dog**. Recovery from poxvirus infection usually is followed by long-term immunity. Many poxviruses can be cultivated on the chorioallantoic membrane of chicken embryos producing focal lesions or "**pocks**" and most can be grown in cell cultures.

Four genera of poxviruses namely, *Orthopoxvirus, Parapoxvirus, Yatapoxvirus & Molluscipoxvirus* may infect humans while others can infect animals & birds. Smallpox and Molluscum contagiosum are specific to humans. The other viruses cause rare zoonotic infections in humans. Vaccinia virus, which has been used for vaccination against smallpox, can also infect humans. In 1977, the last outbreak of smallpox occurred in Somalia, and the World Health Organization (WHO) certified eradication of smallpox in 1980. Data presented in Table 11-1 describes classification of *Poxviridae*& diseases caused by the member species.

Table 11.1 : Classification of *Poxviridae* & diseases caused by the member viruses in humans & animals.

Chordapoxvirinae	Species	Serotypes	Diseases caused
G1. *Orthopoxvirus*			
	Vaccinia virus: TS	VACV-AMK, COP-WR	*Vaccinia virus* (**VACV**) infects sheep, water buffaloes, rabbits, cattle, horses, humans, & acts as vaccine vectors. The oral rabies vaccine for foxes is a recomb inant poxvirus expressing glycoprotein G (gG) of rabies virus. Poxviruses are also being considered as vectors for other viral protein. VACV infections were transmited from the vesicular lesion on the vaccinee to domestic animals, mainly cattle that in turn, infected VACV to susceptible people. This VACV was called Araçatuba virus & was similar to VACV-Western Reserve (VACV-WR) strain.
	Buffalopox virus	BPXV	Buffalopox (**BPXV**) is a disease of water buffaloes, the virus is identical or closely related to vaccinia virus. The disease is similar to cowpox, & severe outbreaks have been reported from Southeast Asia.

Rabbitpox virus	RPXV	Rabbitpox
Camelpox virus	CMLV-CMS, -GRI	Camelpox (CMLV) causes camelpox in Asia, & Africa, Middle East, Asia producing a systemic infection with pox-like lesions, which are severe in young camels. The symptoms are-pustules around the nose, lips and hairless areas. Disease in young camels may be severe with mortality as high as 25%; but the disease is usually mild with a course of 2 - 3 weeks. The infection is rarely spread to the hands of camel drivers. An attenuated vaccinia virus is used as a vaccine.
Cowpox virus	CPXV-BR, -GRI	Cowpox (CPXV) occurs in cattle, domestic & zoo cats (feline cowpox) & zoo animals, anteaters, & rodents, the latter are the natural reservoir hosts with skin lesions & rarely cause teat lesions in cow, & can be transmitted to humans. After eradication of smallpox, other orthopoxviruses, such as monkeypox virus, vaccinia virus in Brazil, & cowpox virus (CPXV) in Europe still infect humans. Wild rodents act as its natural reservoir. Human CPXV infections are reported from diseased domestic cats, from rats or domesticated house mice.
Horsepox virus		Horsepox also called contagious pustular stomatitis, grease-heel, is a rare disease that occurs sporadically in Europe, is transmitted by contact and fomites such as combs,

		saddles, harness, etc. Symptoms include- papules, vesicles, and pustules on the skin of lips, nares and oral mm; nasal discharge, fever & salivation, the course varies from 10 days to a month. Also seen are infection of the pastern and fetlock region with pustules & crusts; can be transmitted to humans.
Feline poxvirus		Feline poxvirus infection is a frequent disease that occurs in Europe and Asia, the virus has a wide host range- domestic cats, zoo cats-lions, cheetahs, pumas, etc. while wild rodents are the natural reservoir of the virus. Most cats get infections from another cat & occasionally from contact with wild rodents. Symptoms are seen commonly as a chronic form but an acuteform occurs particularly in non-domestic cats with multiple skin lesions- papules, vesicles, & pustules randomly distributed over the body. Severe cases show anorexia, lose condition and develop pneumonia, conjunctivitis and diarrhea & recover within two months.
Ectromelia virus	ECTV-MOS	Mousepox
Monkeypox virus	MPXV-ZAI	Monkeypox **(MPXV)** affects monkeys & humans, is prevalent in central and West Africa, an outbreak occurred in USA in 2003. Human monkeypox is a zoonotic viral disease reported in remote villages of Central and West

		Africa, is transmitted to humans from rodents, pets, and primates through contact with the animal's blood or a bite.
Racoonpox virus	RCNPXV	Racconpox
Taterapox virus	TATV	Taterapox
Variola virus	Variola major virus/ VARV-BSH, -IND	Smallpox major
	Variola virus minor/ VARV-GARD	Smallpox minor
Volepox virus	VPXV	Volepox
T: *Skunkpox virus*	SKPV	Skunkpox
T: *Uasin Gishu disease virus*	UGDV	Usin Gishu disease (UGDV) is a rare disease of horses reported from Kenya & adjacent African countries, causes papilloma-like lesions on skin.
G 2: *Parapoxvirus*		
TS: *Orf virus*	ORFV-SAOO, -NZ2	Orf **(ORFV)** is a highly contagious ecthy ma, widely occurring disease also called contagious pustular dermatitis, infectious labial dermatitis, ecthyma contagiosum, thistle disease & scabby mouth, mainly affects lambs & goats, produces prolifer ative lesions on the muzzle & lips. Orf is transmitted by direct contact, fomites & insects may act as mechanical vectors. Symptoms include the development of pox-like lesions on the lips and nose; and, less often, in other parts of the mouth & on the udder,

		teats, vulva, and coronet of the feet. The affected animals may show bad foot condition and weight loss.
Bovine papular stomatitis virus	BPSV	Bovine papular stomatitis **(BPSV)** affects cattle, produces mild papular lesions on the muzzles & oral cavity of young cattle of 2yrs, there may be proliferative, reddish,raised papules that may ulcerate on the epith of the mouth, muzzle and in the nostrils, & the lesions may also be present in the esophagus, abomasum, and rumen. There is hyperplasia of the mucosa of the affected organ with IC inclusions. The virus is transmitted to humans.
Parapoxvirus of red deer in New Zealand	PVNZ	Red deer pox in NZ
Pseudocowpox virus	PCPV	Pseudocowpox/ milkers nodules **(PCPV)** occur in cows commonly with teat lesions in milking cows. Spread is by milker's hands, teat cup liners and other fomites. Symptoms are the formation of bright red papules, vesicles, scabs, & nodules on the udder &d teats of cows in several weeks but theentire herd become affected. The milker's nodule is of zoonotic value & is transmited tohumans. Farmers, milkers and their close contacts with milking cows develope lesions on the hands, forearms, legs & face with several systemic symptoms.

Squirrel parapoxvirus	SPPV	Parapox of squirrel
G 3: *Capripoxvirus*		
Sheeppox virus	SPPV-A, NIS,-99	Sheeppox is endemic in Asia, Africa & in Southestern Europe, affects sheep & goats causing generalized infection with unique skin lesions & variable mortality. Some differences exist between the viruses causing sheeppox and goatpox but are nearly similar in the clinical aspects. The disease is transmited by direct contact and fomites. Symptoms of sheeppox (goatpox) are the most severe pox disease of domestic animals with generalized infection, and mortality rate may go up to 50% in young lambs and kids. The pox lesions are seen on the skin, & mm of the respiratory and digestive tracts. In severe cases, the affected animals may develop pneumonia.
Goatpox virus	GTPV-G20	Goatpox
Lumpy skin disease virus	LSDV-NI, -NW	Lumpy skin disease occurs in cattle but buffaloes, giraffes, and impalas of all ages are susceptible, the disease is endemic in Africa. In unvaccinated cattle the disease occurs in epidemic form every 5 - 6 years. The virus is transmitted mechanically by biting flies. Symptoms begin after 2 to 4 weeks. Some animals are subclinically infected or only show a mild febrile response with few skin lesions showing fever, lacrimation, &nd nasal discharge. Morbidity is up to 20% but mortality is low.

G 4: *Suipoxvirus*			
	Swinepox virus	SWPV	Swinepox occurs in pigs worldwide, causes mild skin lesions & is transmitted mechanically by the pig louse, *Haematopinus suis*, by contact. Disease morbidity is usually high in young pigs. Symptoms include transient fever & thereafter typical pox lesions-papule, vesicle, pustule, and scab appear on the skin of abdomen, back, and side, on the lower abdomen, lesions with hemorrhagic dark centers are seen. The disease passes through the clinical course without serious effects. But in some cases, congenital infections may occur with typical lesions on the skull and in the oral cavity of newborns.
G 5: *Avipoxvirus*			
	Fowlpox virus: TS	FPV	Fowlpox occurs in chickens, turkeys, grouse, quail, pheasants, canaries, pigeons, sparrow, starlings & other avian species. Fowlpox is highly contagious and occurs worldwide; transmitted by direct contact, fomites commonly contaminated by litter & entrs the skin through abrasions or by the bite of mosquitoes, or via the oral or nasal mm, aerosol droplets leading to the diphtheric form of fowlpox. Mostly adult & young chickens & turkeys are affected with low mortality but may be as high as 50% with the diphtheric form. Lesions are present on the comb, wattles, around eyelids, and

			on other featherless areas, birds recovering within 1 month. The diphtheric form is severe associated with secondary bacterial infection. Lesions are present in the mouth, pharynx, trachea, orbit, and sinuses.
	Canarypox virus	CNPV	Canarypox
	Juncopox virus	JNPV	Juncopox
	Mynahpox virus	MYPV	Mynahpox
	Pigeonpox virus	PGPV	Pigeonpox
	Psittacinepox virus	PSPV	Psittacinepox
	Quailpox virus	QUPV	Quailpox
	Sparrowpox virus	SRPV	Sparrowpox
	Starlingpox virus	SLPV	Starlingpox
	Turkeypox virus	TKPV	Turkeypox
	Crowpox virus	CRPV	Crowpox
	Peacockpox virus	PKPV	Peacockpox
	Penguinpox virus	PEPV	Penguinpox
G 6: *Leporipoxvirus*			
	Myxoma virus	MYXV-LAU	Myxomatosis (MYXV) is endemic in wild rabbits (*Sylvilagus*) in North and South America and in some wild rabbit species of the genus *Oryctolagus*, in Europe, S. America, & Australia.The virus is transmitted by direct contact and mechanically by biting insects. In*Sylvilagus*, rabbits the virus causes localized skin tumors, but inthe European rabbits, *Oryctolqgus cunicuus*, it produces a severe generalized infn with high mortality up to 90%.
	Hare fibroma virus	FIBV	Hare fibroma
	Rabbit fibroma virus	RFV	Rabbit fibroma
	Squirrel fibroma virus	SQFV	Squirrel fibroma
G 7:*Molluscipoxvirus*			
	Molluscum contagiosum virus	MOCV	Molluscum contagiosum affects only humans mainly

			children; symptoms are flesh-colored, dome-shaped, and pearly. 1–5 mm in diameter, not painful, but may itch or become irritated, & 10% cases develop into eczema, often complicated by secondary bacterial infections. It is limited to a localized area on the top most layer of the epidermis. By auto-inoculation, the virus may spread to neighboring skin areas especially in children, and may often show clusters of lesions.
G 8: *Yatapoxvirus*	*Yaba monkey tumor virus*	YMTV	Yaba monkey tumor
	Tanapox virus	TAPV	Tanapox was first seen in persons in the flood plain of the Tana river in Kenya epidemics in 1952 & 1962 with mild fever that lasts 3–4 days, severe headaches and backaches, & often itching at the site where the skin lesion develops. Initially, a small nodule develop, soon becomes papular, become 15 mm by the end of the 2nd week of infn, the draining lymph nodes are enlarged, lesion remains nodular but ulcerates during the third week and then gradually heals within 5 to 6 weeks, leaving a scar. The lesions are always solitary on the upper arm, face, neck, and truck. But in Zaire, 22% of patients had aving lesions on the upper limbs, trunk, and head.
	Yaba-like disease virus	YLDV	Yaba-like disease
G 9: *Cervidpoxvirus*			
Genus unassigned	*Squirrelpox virus*		

Poxvirus Clinical Infections in Humans

Genus: *Molluscipoxvirus:*

Monkeypox **(MPXV)** infects monkeys & humans, is prevalent in central and West Africa, but an outbreak occurred in USA in 2003. Human monkeypox is a zoonotic viral disease reported in remote villages of Central and West Africa. The virus is transmitted to humans from rodents, pets, and primates through contact with the animal's blood or a bite.

Molluscum contagiosum **(MOCV)** affects only humans particularly children. The symptoms are lesions of flesh-colored, dome-shaped, and pearly. 1–5 mm in diameter, not painful, but may itch or become irritated & 10% of the cases develop into eczema, often complicated by secondary bacterial infections. It is limited to a localized area on the top most layer of the epidermis, by autoinoculation, the virus may spread to neighboring skin areas especially in children, and may often show clusters of lesions.

Tanapox **(TAPV)** was first seen in persons in the flood plain of the Tana River in Kenya epidemics in 1952 & 1962 with mild fever that lasted 3–4 days with severe headaches and backaches, and often itching at the site where the skin lesion develops. Initially a small nodule develops, soon becomes papular, become 15 mm by the end of the second week of infection, the draining lymph nodes are enlarged, lesion remains nodular but ulcerates during the third week and then gradually heals within 5 to 6 weeks, leaving a scar. The lesions are always solitary on the upper arm, face, neck, and truck. But in Zaire, 22% of patients had multiple lesions, usually two or three & up to ten found on the lower limbs with a couple of patients having lesions on the upper limbs, trunk, and head.

Poxvirus Clinical Infections in Animals

Genus: *Vacciniavirus:*

Vaccinia Virus Infections

Vaccinia virus **(VACV)** causes mild infections in sheep, water buffaloes, rabbits, cattle, horses, humans, & acts as vaccine vectors. The oral rabies vaccine for foxes is a recombinant poxvirus virus expressing the glycoprotein G (gG) of rabies virus. Vaccinia viruses are also being considered as vectors for other viral proteins. Multiple strains of vaccinia virus exist with varying levels of virulence for humans and animals. Depending on the strain used, vaccinia virus presents varying levels of health risk to animals & laboratory personnel. Strains that are highly attenuated are typically unable to replicate or replicate poorly in human cells. On the other hand, non-highly attenuated strains of vaccinia have the ability to replicate in human cells and thus pose a risk to humans. Risks include localized skin infections and more severe, disseminated reactions to immunocompromized individuals.

Recently in Brazil, several exanthematic **vaccinia virus outbreaks occurred in dairy cattle and rural workers since 1999**. VACV, the prototype of the genus *Orthopoxvirus*, shows serologic cross-reactivity with other Orthopoxvirus species and was used as vaccine during the smallpox eradication campaign. Bovine vaccinial infection causes economic losses and affects public health services in Brazil. VACV reservoirs and the role of wild life in outbreaks remain unidentified; probably VACV strains circulate in rodents in forests in Brazil. Using molecular methods, it was confirmed that monkeys had exposure of to VACV. Studies provided evidence of high prevalence of orthopoxviruses among capuchin and black-howling **monkeys in the Brazilian Amazon**. The relationship between infected monkeys and emergence of VACV in rural regions of Brazil is unknown. From June through November 2005, outbreaks of exanthematic disease among humans and cattle were reported in poor and undeveloped populations living in the rural countryside of Brazil. A zoonotic case of vaccinia virus infection occurred in a 30-year-old patient who became infected after handling sick dairy cattle. The patient had inflamed lesions and systemic symptoms. The Advisory Committee on Immunization Practices (ACIP) recommends smallpox vaccination for laboratory workers who handle non-highly attenuated VACV strains or other orthopoxviruses e.g., monkeypox, cowpox, or variola. On March 1, 2010, a case of contact transmission of vaccinia virus occurred from sexual contact with a member of the military personnel who had been vaccinated against smallpox. Vaccinia virus infection after sexual contact has been reported previously.

VACV infection in animals was contracted when the animals came in contact with people during smallpox vaccination. VACV infections were transmitted from the vesicular lesion on the vaccinee to domestic animals, mainly cattle that in turn, infected VACV to susceptible people. This VACV was called Araçatuba virus & was similar to VACV-Western Reserve (VACV-WR) strain & Araçatuba virus was very similar to Cantagalo virus. These points to the ubiquity of VACV circulating in the wild in Brazil as well as to the public health problems.

Cowpox

Cowpox **(CPXV)** occurs in cattle, domestic & zoo cats (feline cowpox) & zoo animals, anteaters, and rodents, the latter are the natural reservoir hosts. Cowpox virus belongs to the genus *Orthpoxvirus* in the family *Poxviridae.* Cowpox virus & *Buffalpox virus* are antigeically identical. CPXV causes skin lesions, rarely teat lesions in cows & skin lesions in cats & can be transmitted to humans.

Occurrence

Infection with cow pox virus is endemic in wild rodents like voles in UK, Europe, & western Asia; rodents act as reservoir of the virus. Cowpox exists in the wild in Europe and Asia, where it is carried by rats and other animals and is often reported in veterinarians and zoo workers. Cowpox is a rare disease, largely confined to small mammals on the European continent and in Great Britain, with occasional transmission to humans. Historically, most human cases have been reported in Great Britain, with a smaller number from Germany, Belgium, the Netherlands, France, Sweden, Finland, Norway, and Russia. In 2001, 60 cases of possible cowpox were reported in Egypt.

Hosts susceptible

Cowpox occurs in cats, cattle, domestic & zoo cats (feline cowpox), zoo animals, & anteaters. Infection in cattle is rare & is incidental hosts. After eradication of smallpox, other orthopoxviruses, such as monkeypox virus, vaccinia virus in Brazil, and cowpox virus (CPXV) in Europe still infect humans among which CPXV has been restricted to the Old World with wild rodents acting as its natural reservoir.

Transmission

Domestic cats are infected from hunting of rodents. Cattle are the incidental hosts. Transmission from cow to cow occurs through milker's hand or teat cup. Transmission from herd to herd occurs by introduction of the infected animals, milker's hand or by biting insects. The virus gains access to the tissues through injury to teat skin. Human gets CPXV infection from infected cats & cows, from rats or domesticated house mice. Cowpox most commonly is spread through direct contact with an infected ulcer on a cow's teat. It can also be transmitted through direct contact with an infected cat.

The virus is found in wild rodents, most commonly in bank voles, wood mice, and field voles, although transmission from these animals to humans is rare. There has been one proven case of rodent-to-human transmission. Other animals that can transmit cowpox include animals in zoos and circuses. A laboratory worker at the University of Illinois in 2010, is the first person in the USA to become infected with cowpox from lab contamination.

Pathogenesis

In milking cows, the lesions (erythema, papules, vesiculation, pustules & crusts) are confined to teats. In cats, after infection, small papules appear on the head or forelimbs, vesicles appear that ulcerate & finally form scab. The complete resolution occurs in 6 weeks. But in some cats, secondary skin lesions appear. Some animals show signs of coryza, conjunctivitis & rarely pneumonia.

Poxviruses use numerous strategies to evade the host immune system. These include production of homologues of mammalian tumor necrosis factor receptor, interleukin-1beta receptor, interleukin 18-binding protein, interferon-alpha/beta receptor, and interferon-gamma receptor, as well as a complement-binding protein and a caspase inhibitor. These proteins are thought to neutralize the host's antiviral response by binding to cytokines and complement proteins and inhibiting their function. In addition, cowpox virus has been shown to inhibit intracellular transport of major histocompatibility class I molecules, allowing it to evade cytotoxic T cells.

Clinical signs & lesions

The most common symptom in cows is a rash that develops where the skin touched the infected ulcer. This rash looks like one or more blisters, which then fill with pus, then form an ulcer, and eventually scab over with a thick black crust. Eventually, the rash will heal and scars will form. The rash does not spread. Skin lesion in cats appear on the face, neck, forelimbs, and paws, and less commonly upper respiratory tract infection.

After incubation period of 9 to 10 days, symptoms can begin. In humans, most cases exhibit small number of vesicopustular lesions on the hands or face that subsequently ulcerate and develop a black scar before spontaneously resolving. Rarely, cutaneous dissemination and even death may occur. So far about 150 human cases have been reported. Young people, younger than 18 years are at greater risk because of a chance for close contact with animals, such as cats, or because of their not having been vaccinated for smallpox, which may confer some protection against cowpox. Human infections remain localized and self-limiting but can be fatal in immunocompromized patients. Other symptoms of cowpox can include: swelling of lymph nodes, red streaks from infected area to the armpit, throbbing pain along the affected area, fever, chills, loss of appetite, muscle aches & headache.

Diagnosis

Diagnosis of cowpox depends on current symptoms of cowpox, recent exposure to animals & the cowpox rash.

Treatment & prevention

There are currently no treatments that can kill the cowpox virus, & treatments focus on providing relief of symptoms as the body fights the cowpox virus. This is called supportive care that includes: medications aimed to control fever or pain, & antibiotics and wound care taken to prevent secondary infections caused by bacteria.

Buffalopox

Buffalopox is the most contagious disease of water buffaloess caused by Buffalopox virus (BPXV), an **Orthopoxvirus** that is identical or closely related to vaccinia virus. The disease is analogous to cowpox and severe outbreaks have been reported from Southeast Asia. In the **mild form**, the main form, lesions occur localized on the udder, teats, and inguinal region, over the parotid, and the base and inner surface of the ear and eyes. In the **severe form**, the lesions are generalized. The end result is high morbidity and productivity loss. When the virus infects milk animals, it causes mastitis which reduces milk yield and the working capacity of draft animals. The mastitis occurs in approximately fifty percent of the infected animals, in severe cases the reduction in milk production can be permanent.

Occurrence

Buffalopox first occurred in India in 1934, since then many outbreaks have occurred in many parts of the world including Pakistan, Egypt, Nepal, and Bangladesh. Singh and Singh were able to isolate and characterize the virus. An outbreak of buffalopox in domestic buffaloes, with high morbidity and significant production loss, was recorded in the Aurangabad district of Maharashtra State in India in November 2003. The disease was also associated with several cases of human infection, particularly in milkers working with the affected herds. Between 2006 and 2008, there were four outbreaks in domestic buffaloes in India. There was a reduction of milk yield of about 30-35% which was followed by mastitis that was a consequence of a secondary bacterial infection. There is also some evidence of milk attendants spreading the virus between buffaloes and from buffalo to cows.

Hosts susceptible

The incubation time in animals is about 2-4 days and in humans it is 3-19 days. In buffaloes the disease is mainly reported in the **young and old animals**. The main people in danger of contracting the disease are veterinarians, milk attendants, and other people that are in close proximity of the infected animals. There have also been recent reports of nosocomial infections in burn patients and paramedical staff. The milk attendants developed lesions on their chest, lower abdomen, fingers, hands, forearms, legs, scapular region, feet, and forehead and also presented with a fever, lymphadenopathy, and general malaise.

Transmission

BPXV can be spread by sand flies and midges, and transmission studies showed that in addition to infecting buffaloes and cows, the virus can also infect guinea pigs and suckling mice.

Clinical symptoms & lesions

Buffalopox mainly occurs in the **mild form**, &lesions occur localized on the udder, teats, and inguinal region, over the parotid, and the base and inner surface of the ear and eyes. In the **severe form**, the lesions are **generalized.** The buffaloes presented with lesions on the udder, teats, limbs, around the ear, and hind quarters which was indicative of a generalized infection. The severe form is now rare, and the disease is mainly mild. The end result is high morbidity and productivity loss. When the virus infects milk animals it causes mastitis which reduces milk yield and the working capacity of draft animals. The mastitis occurs in approximately fifty percent of the infected animals, in severe cases the reduction in milk production can be permanent.

In **humans** the virus causes lesions that are mainly confined to the hands, forehead, face, buttocks, and legs, and occasionally lymphadenopathy. Human to human transmission has not been reported. Milking of infected animals is one of the major modes of spread. This being the case, the main people in danger of contracting the disease are veterinarians, milk attendants, and other people that are in close proximity of the infected animals. There have also been recent reports of nosocomial infections in burn patients and paramedical staff. Detection of antibodies in young individuals in Maharastra, from endemic area, who were neither vaccinated for smallpox nor had any contact with buffaloes or history of any poxvirus disease, is suggestive of occurrence of subclinical infection. A few children who had no contact with infected animals also showed clinical manifestations with disseminated lesions on the face, arm and buttocks, and thus suspected to have acquired infection through their infected parents or other family members indicating a possible man to man transmission. Therefore, in the light of discontinuation of smallpox vaccination, buffalopox outbreaks need to be monitored carefully as this may emerge as a serious zoonotic disease in India.

Diagnosis

Collection of clinical specimens include: vesicular fluid, scabs, and scrapings from lesions, & serum samples.

1. *Presumpive diagnosis*: A presumptive diagnosis is based on clinical symptoms, lesions & histopathology. Preliminary screening of the scab and serum samples was carried out using counterimmunoelectrophoresis (CIE).
2. *Virus isolation:* Scab samples & milk samples were inoculated onto Vero cell monolayers & were observed daily for the cytopathic effect (CPE). PCR detected Viral DNA isolated from clinical material or cell culture fluid.

3. Direct immunofluorescent staining of scab or biopsy material is probably the most reliable and practical. The crust from skin lesions can be used for detection of orthopoxvirus DNA by PCR.
4. Antibody detection: Serum neutralization test using serum samples collected from both clinically affected and in-contact animals were subjected to a serum neutralization test for detecting antibodies against BPXV.

Treatment & prevention

The lessons heal by themselves in the normal course and the adoption of special measures is not called for; only the usual rules of hygiene need to be observed. The lesions should be cleaned with a 1:1,000 solution of potassium permanganate followed by the application of an antiseptic ointment such as 1:110 boric acids. The affected animals should be isolated and milked by separate milkers. Milk from affected animals should be boiled before use. If the disease assumes serious proportions, vaccination may be undertaken by scarification in the perineum with calf lymph or with material collected from lesions from the infected animal.

Feline Poxvirus Infection

Feline poxvirus infection is a frequent disease that occurs in Europe and Asia; virus has a wide host range-domestic cats, zoo cats-lions, cheetahs, pumas, etc. while **wild rodents are the natural reservoir of the virus**. Most cats get infections from another cat and occasionally from contact with wild rodents. .Symptoms are seen commonly as a chronic form but an acute form occurs particularly in non-domestic cats with multiple skin lesions- papules, vesicles, & pustules randomly distributed over the body. Severe cases show anorexia, lose condition and develop pneumonia, conjunctivitis and diarrhea, & recover within two months.

Etiology: *Feline poxvirus* is closely related to *Cowpox virus*.

Occurrence

Feline poxvirus infection occurs throughout western countries in Europe, including Austria, Belgium, France, Germany, The Netherlands, and Norway and western states in the former Soviet Union. In the UK infection is most commonly seen from July to November when rodents are most common. Infection may also be reported throughout the remainder of the year.

Hosts susceptible

Feline poxvirus has a wide host range that includes domestic cats, & zoo cats (lions, cheetahs, pumas, etc. Immunosuppression caused by feline leukemia or feline immuodeficiency virus infection can greatly increase susceptibility to the cowpox virus.

Transmission

Wild rodents are the natural **reservoir** of the virus & cats get infected by preying on rodents. Cowpox is not a common source for the feline disease. Most feline infections are derived from another cat and occasionally from contact with wild rodents.

Clinical symptoms & lesions

The virus enters the skin through a **bite wound** from a rodent usually on the cat's head, neck or limb. The viral infection becomes apparent after a few days as a small nodule with ulceration. This may be followed by secondary bacterial infection, producing cellulitis and an abscess may form. Once inside the cat's body the virus will multiply in the lungs, nasal passages and various lymphoid tissues for about five days producing a transient systemic virus infection or viremia. The mouth, nasal passages, lungs and gut may be affected with oral and gastrointestinal ulceration, nasal discharge, pneumonia and diarrhea. Usually the signs of viremia are mild and include serous to mucopurulent discharge, pyrexia, depression and a poor appetite.

After initial infection, 10 days to several weeks later, there appear numerous skin lesions, circular ulcerated papules and plaques up to 1 cm in size. Pruritus is not a major feature of this disease and this may help to distinguish it from other conditions. The plaques are usually covered with crust material which will separate as the infection resolves. There may be residual scarring and hair loss. These lesions may be observed on any part of the body.

Infection usually resolves itself over six to eight weeks. Concurrent infection with FIV or FeLV may affect the rate of recovery from cowpox virus infection.

Most of the cowpox virus infections in humans are acquired from cats. As mentioned for cowpox virus, the human infection usually involves a single lesion on the hand or face and serious systemic disease has been reported in immunosuppressed individuals.

Diagnosis

Collection of clinical specimens include: Vesicular fluid, scabs, and scrapings from lesions.

1. *Presumptive diagnosis*: A presumptive diagnosis is based on clinical symptoms, lesions & histopathology.

2. *Virus isolation* is expensive and time consuming. Electron microscopy is done using unfixed scabs or biopsies for the presence of the morphologically characteristic virus.

3. *Direct immunofluorescent staining of scab* or biopsy material is probably the most reliable and practical. The crust from skin lesions can be used for detection of orthopoxvirus DNA by PCR.

4. *Antibody detection*: Serological tests include indirect immunofluorescence and ELISA that detect antibodies. They are not ordinarily used for diagnosis.

Treatment & prevention

Cats that are not eating may require intravenous fluid therapy. Broad-spectrum antibiotics are used to control secondary bacterial infections. Prevent scratching with a collar or by bandaging paws. As a precaution, cats with suspected cowpox infection, where possible, should be isolated from other cats and handled by people not at risk of infection, wearing gloves and avoiding contact between infected material and skin wounds or the eyes. The virus can survive for months to years at room temperature and is resistant to many disinfectants, although hypochlorite-based products should be effective.

Horsepox

Horsepox, also called **contagious pustular stomatitis, grease-heel,** is a rare disease that occurs sporadically in Europe, as a skin eruption on the pasterns, the posterior surface of the joints being chiefly affected. The skin becomes swollen and red; the inflammation extends some distance up the limb, form vesicles or small blisters, followed by pustules that discharge a viscid fluid. A similar eruption appears sometimes in the nose and lips, and also on the mucous membrane of the mouth and nostrils. Horse-pox is a benign infection terminating in recovery without treatment in a few weeks. Experimental and accidental inoculations are said to produce in man an eruption similar to that following the introduction of the vaccine virus, and it is asserted that the disease so conveyed protects the individual from small-pox. Symptoms include- papules, vesicles, and pustules occurring on the skin of lips, nares and oral mucous membranes; nasal discharge, fever and salivation. The course varies from 10 days to a month. Also seen are infection of the pastern and fetlock region with pustules and crusts; can be transmitted to humans.

Etiology: Horsepox is caused by *Horsepox virus* in the genus *Orthopoxvirus.*

Occurrence

Horsepox is a rare disease occurring sporadically in Europe.

Transmission

Horsepox is spread by contact and fomites such as combs, saddles, harness, etc. Transmission to humans has been reported.

Clinical symptoms & lesions

Papules, vesicles, and pustules occur on the skin of lips, nares and oral mucous membranes. Also seen are characteristic nasal discharge, fever and salivation. The clinical course varies from about 10 days to a month. An infection of the pastern and fetlock region with pustules and crusts may be due to horsepox virus, although this is not yet certain.

Diagnosis

Collection of clinical samples includes vesicular fluid, scabs, and scrapings from lesions.

A presumptive diagnosis is made by clinical symptoms & confirmatory diagnosis is attained by electron microscopic demonstration of poxvirus particles in distilled water lysates of lesion material.

The disease is so infrequent that control measures are not required.

Camelpox

Camelpox is a disease of young camels characterized by fever, local or generalised pox lesions on the skin and in the mucous membranes of the mouth, respiratory and digestive tracts. The clinical manifestations range from inapparent infection to mild, moderate and, less commonly, severe systemic infection and death. The disease occurs more frequently and more severely in young animals. Camelpox virus is very host specific and does not infect other animals. Only one suspected case of human camelpox involving mild skin lesions has been described, underlining that camelpox is of no public health importance.

Etiology: Camelpox is caused by *Camelpox virus* in the genus *Orthopoxvirus*. Based on sequence analysis, it has been determined that the camelpox virus is the most closely related to *Variola virus*, the aetiological agent for small pox. Camels have been successfully vaccinated against camelpox with vaccinia virus strains. Poxviruses are susceptible to various disinfectants including 1% sodium hypochlorite, 1% sodium hydroxide, 1% peracetic acid, formaldehyde, 0.5-1% formalin and 0.5% quaternary ammonium compounds. The virus can be destroyed by autoclaving, boiling for 10 minutes, and is killed by ultraviolet rays (245 nm wave length) in a few minutes.

Occurrence

Camelpox occurs in almost every country where camel husbandry is practiced apart from the introduced dromedary camel in Australia and tylopods (llama and related species) in South America. Outbreaks have been reported in the Middle East- in Bahrain, Iran, Iraq, Oman, Saudi Arabia, United Arab Emirates and Yemen; in Asia Afghanistan and Pakistan; in Africa-Algeria, Egypt, Ethiopia, Kenya, Mauritania, Morocco, Niger, Somalia and Sudan and in the southern parts of Russia and India. The disease is endemic in these countries and a pattern of sporadic outbreaks occurs with a rise in the seasonal incidence usually during the rainy season. The morbidity rate of camelpox is variable and depends on whether the virus is circulating in the herd. Serological surveys taken in several countries reveal a high prevalence of antibodies to camelpox. The incidence of disease is higher in males than females, and the mortality rate is greater in young animals than in adults. The mortality rate in adult animals is between 5% and 28% and in young animals between 25% and 100%.

Hosts susceptible

Young camels are more susceptible along with its relatives dromedary camel in Australia and tylopods (llama and related species) in South America. Camelpox virus is very host specificand does not infect other animals. Only one suspected case of human camelpox involving mild skin lesions has been described, underlining that camelpox is of no public health importance.

Transmission

Transmission is by either direct contact between infected and susceptible animals or indirect infection via a contaminated environment. The infection is usually achieved by inhalation or through skin abrasions. Virus is secreted in milk, saliva, and ocular and nasal discharges. Dried scabs shed from the pox lesions may contain live virus for at least 4 months and contaminate the environment. The role of an arthropod vector in the transmission of the disease has been suspected. The role of insects in transmission has been suspected because the disease is often observed after rainfall.

Clinical symptoms & lesions

The incubation period is usually 9–13 days. Clinical manifestations of camelpox range from inapparent and mild local infections, confined to the skin, to moderate and severe systemic infections, possibly reflecting differences between the strains of camelpox. The disease is characterized by fever, enlarged lymph nodes and skin lesions.

Skin lesions appear 1–3 days after the onset of fever, starting as erythematous macules, developing into papules and vesicles, and later turning into pustules. Crusts develop on the ruptured pustules. These lesions first appear on the head, eyelids, nostrils and the margins of the ears. In **severe cases** the whole head may be swollen. Later, skin lesions may extend to the neck, limbs, genitalia, mammary glands and perineum. In the **generalised form**, pox lesions may cover the entire body. Skin lesions may take up to 4–6 weeks to heal. In the **systemic form** of the disease, pox lesions can be found in the mucous membranes of the mouth, respiratory and digestive tracts.

The animals may show salivation, lacrimation and a mucopurulent nasal discharge. Diarrhoea and anorexia may occur in the systemic form of the disease. Pregnant females may abort. Death is usually due to secondary infections and septicaemia.

The PM lesions in camels that die following severe infection with camelpox are multiple pox-like lesions on the mucous membranes of the mouth, respiratory and digestive tract. The size of the lesions in the lungs may vary in diameter between 0.5 and 1.3 cm, occasionally up to 4–5 cm. Smaller lesions may have a hemorrhagic centre. The lung lesions are characterized by hydropic degeneration, proliferation of bronchial epithelial cells, and infiltration of the affected areas by macrophages, necrosis and fibrosis.

Histopathological examination of the early skin nodules reveals characteristic cytoplasmic swelling, vacuolation and ballooning of the keratinocytes of the outer stratum spinosum. The rupture of these cells produces vesicles and localised oedema. Perivascular infiltration of mononuclear cells and variable infiltration of neutrophils and eosinophils occurs. Marked epithelial hyperplasia may occur in the borders of the skin lesions.

Diagnosis

Transmission electron microscopy (TEM) is a rapid method to demonstrate camelpox virus in scabs or tissue samples in which a relatively high concentration of virus in the sample is required. However, currently, TEM is the best method for distinguishing clinical cases of camelpox and orf caused by camelpox and parapox viruses respectively, although the viruses can be differentiated by serological techniques and by PCR.

Camelpox virus grows in following cell lines: Vero, MA-104 and MS monkey kidney, and baby hamster kidney (BHK) and the following primary cell cultures: lamb testis, lamb kidney, camel embryonic kidney, calf kidney, and chicken embryo fibroblast.

Camelpox virus can be isolated on the **CAM** of 11–13-day old embryonating chicken eggs. The eggs should be incubated at 37°C degrees and after 5 days, the eggs containing living embryos are opened and the CAM examined for the presence of characteristic pock lesions: dense, grayish white pocks.

Treatment & prevention

A **live attenuated vaccine, Ducapox**, is manufactured by Highveld Biologicals, Onderstepoort, South Africa and an inactivated vaccine by Biopharma, Rabat, Morocco. A live attenuated vaccine gives long-term protection against camelpox. However, a booster vaccination is recommended for young animals vaccinated before the age of 6–9 months. When inactivated vaccine is used, the animals must be vaccinated annually.

Monkeypox

Monkeypox is a rare viral disease that is found mostly in the rainforest countries of central and west Africa, & was first discovered in laboratory monkeys in 1958. Serological tests of animals in Africa later found evidence of monkeypox infection in various rodent species, was recovered from an African squirrel, which may be the natural host, & the virus could also infect rats, mice, and rabbits. During the first few days, symptoms are nonspecific and include fever, nausea, and malaise. After about 4-7 days, lesions (pustules, papules) develop on the face and trunk that ulcerate, crust over, and begin to clear up after about 14-21 days and lymph nodes enlarge; there may be some scarring.

Etiology: The disease is caused by *Monkeypox virus*, which belongs to the genus *Orthopoxvirus*.

Occurrence

In 1970, monkeypox was identified as the cause of a rash illness in humans in remote African locations. In early June 2003, monkeypox was reported among several residents in the United States who became ill after having contact with sick pet prairie dogs. This is the first evidence of community-acquired monkeypox in the United States.

Transmission

People can get monkeypox from an infected animal through a bite or direct contact with the infected animal's blood, body fluids, or lesions. The disease also can be spread from person to person, but it is much less infectious than smallpox. The virus is thought to be transmitted by large respiratory droplets during direct and prolonged face-to-face contact. In addition, monkeypox can be spread by direct contact with body fluids of an infected person or with virus-contaminated objects, such as bedding or clothing.

Clinical symptoms & lesions

The **incubation period** for monkeypox is about **12 days**. In humans, the signs and symptoms of monkeypox are similar to those of smallpox, but usually milder. Monkeypox causes swollen lymph nodes. The illness begins with fever, headache, muscle aches, backache, swollen lymph nodes, a general feeling of discomfort, and exhaustion. Within 1 to 3 days after onset of fever, the patient develops a papular rash that forms pustules, often first on the face but sometimes initially on other parts of the body. The lesions usually develop through several stages before crusting and falling off. The illness typically lasts for 2 to 4 weeks. In Africa, monkeypox is fatal in as many as 10% of people who get the disease; the case fatality ratio for smallpox was about 30% before the disease was eradicated.

Diagnosis

The presumptive diagnosis of monkeypox is made in Africa by the patient's history and the exam that shows the pox lesions. But, a definitive diagnosis is made by PCR, ELISA, or Western blotting tests that are usually done by the CDC or some state labs. Definitive diagnosis is important to rule out other possible infectious agents like smallpox.

Treatment and Prevention

There is no safe treatment for monkeypox. Smallpox vaccine has been reported to reduce the risk of monkeypox among previously vaccinated persons in Africa. CDC is recommending that persons investigating monkeypox outbreaks and involved in caring for infected individuals or animals should receive a smallpox vaccination to protect against monkeypox. Persons who have had close or intimate contact with individuals or animals confirmed to have monkeypox should also be vaccinated. These persons can be vaccinated up to 14 days after exposure. CDC is not recommending preexposure vaccination for unexposed veterinarians, veterinary staff, or animal control officers, unless such persons are involved in field investigations.

Genus: *Parapoxvirus:*

Orf or Contagious Ecthyma

Orf **(ORFV)** is a highly contagious zoonotic, viral skin disease, also called contagious pustular dermatitis, infectious labial dermatitis, ecthyma contagiosum, thistle disease & scabby mouth mainly affects lambs & goats, and some other domesticated and wild ruminants. The skin lesions are painful and often occur on the mouth and muzzle, where they can cause anorexia or starvation. Lesions on the udder may result in the abandonment of offspring, and foot lesions can cause transient lameness. Secondary bacterial infections can occur and, in rare cases, the lesions may extend into the internal organs. Severe generalized infections have been described in Boer and Boer cross goats. Although contagious ecthyma usually resolves spontaneously and the mortality rate is generally low, fatality rates up to 10% have been reported. ORFV is of zoonotic value as it infects humans, causes a purulent-papule locally and generally no systemic symptoms are seen. Infected site include the finger, hand, arm, face and even the penis. Most infections in humans are localized and heal spontaneously; however large poorly healing lesions can occur in people who are immunosuppressed.

Etiology: Contagious ecthyma is caused *Orf virus*, a member of the genus *Parapoxvirus* in the family *Poxviridae.*

Occurrence

Contagious ecthyma has been found worldwide in all countries where sheep are raised, including those in Europe, the Middle East, the United States, Africa, Asia, Alaska, South America, Canada, New Zealand and Australia. In the U.S.A, this disease is seen most often in the Western states.

Hosts susceptible

Contagious ecthyma occurs in sheep, goats, alpacas, camels, reindeer, musk oxen, bighorn sheep, deer, pronghorn antelope and wapiti. Rare cases have been reported in dogs that ate infected carcasses.

Transmission

The orf virus is found in skin lesions and scabs, & enters the skin through cuts and abrasions. This virus can be carried by clinically normal sheep as well as sick animals. It can be transmitted by direct contact or on fomites. Orf is transmitted by direct contact, fomites, & insects may act as mechanical vectors. Contagious ecthyma is highly communicable. The orf virus is present in the skin lesions and crusts. It can also remain viable on the wool and hides for approximately one month after the lesions have healed. It is very resistant to inactivation in the environment and has been recovered from dried crusts after 12 years. Contagious ecthyma vaccines contain live virus and can infect humans. Recently vaccinated animals can also transmit infections to humans.

Pathogenesis

Skin damage is needed for the establishment of orf virus infection and the development of typical lesions. However, analysis of the pathogenesis of experimental lesions induced by viral challenge of mildly abraded skin, indicated that the virus does not establish in the damaged epidermis, but replicates in the cells of an underlying replacement epidermal layer derived from the walls of the wool follicles. The skin reaction consists of a cellular response with necrosis and sloughing of the affected epidermis and underlying stratum papillare of the dermis. Healing is then completed by the formation of a third epidermis derived from the deeper portions of the wool follicles. Previous cutaneous infection did not prevent reintroduction of the disease, even on the same area of skin although the lesions were less severe and persisted for a shorter period.

Orf virus (ORFV) has evolved novel strategies (proteins and/or mechanisms of action) to modulate host cell responses regulated by the nuclear factor-B (NF-B) signaling pathway. Here, we present data indicating that ORFV *ORFV121*, a gene unique to parapoxviruses, encodes a novel viral NF-B inhibitor that binds to and inhibits the phosphorylation and nuclear translocation of NF-B-p65. The infection of cells with an *ORFV121* deletion mutant virus (OV-IA82_121) resulted in increased NF-B-mediated gene transcription, and the expression of ORFV121 in cell cultures significantly suppressed NF-B-regulated reporter gene expression. ORFV ORFV121 physically interacts with NF-B-p65 in the cell cytoplasm, thus providing a mechanism for the inhibition of NF-B-p65 phosphorylation and nuclear translocation. Notably, the deletion of *ORFV121* from the viral genome markedly decreased ORFV virulence and disease pathogenesis in sheep, indicating that **ORFV121 is a virulence determinant for ORFV in the natural host**.

Orf virus infection provokes a vigorous skin immune response. However, the virus has acquired a range of immuno-modulatory/pathogenesis-related genes that function to limit (at least transiently) the effectiveness of host immunity. With the advent of the orf virus genome sequence, the study of this dynamic process will provide important insights into virus pathogenesis and the host skin immune response to infection.

Clinical symptoms & lesions

The **incubation period** in sheep and goats is 2 to 3 days. The initial signs are papules, pustules and vesicles, found on the lips, nose, ears and/or eyelids, and sometimes on the feet or perineal region. Lesions can also occur inside the mouth, particularly in young lambs. Massive oral lesions have been described in some reindeer. Rarely, the lesions may extend into the esophagus, stomach, intestines or respiratory tract. Nursing lambs can transmit the virus to their dam, resulting in lesions on the teats and udder. The skin lesions eventually develop into thick, brown, rapidly growing scabs over areas of granulation, inflammation and ulceration. The scabs are often friable and bleed easily.

Papillomatous growths sometimes occur. Contagious ecthyma lesions are painful and may result in anorexia or even starvation. Young animals may refuse to nurse, and lesions on the udder of the dam can cause it to abandon its offspring. Foot lesions can cause lameness. Uncomplicated infections usually resolve in 1 to 4 weeks. Secondary bacterial infections and maggot infestations can occur. Contagious ecthyma may predispose animals to bacterial mastitis.

More severe infections have been described in **Boer and Boer cross goats.** In these animals, the disease consisted of multifocal, severe proliferative dermatitis accompanied by chronic pneumonia, arthritis and moderate to severe lymphadenopathy. The disease persisted for three months. Mortality is rare, but may occur in young lambs because of difficulty in feeding.

The papule persist for 7 to 10 weeks and spontaneously resolves, but can be contagious & passed from one human to another. Although orf is a benign self-limiting illness, it may become progressive and even life-threatening in the immunocompromised host.

In humans, contagious ecthyma usually occurs as a single skin lesion or a few lesions. The initial lesion is a small, firm, red to blue papule at the site of virus penetration, most often a finger, hand or other exposed part of the body. The papule develops into a hemorrhagic pustule or bulla, which may contain a central crust and bleeds easily. In the later stages, the lesion develops into a nodule, which may weep fluid and is sometimes covered by a thin crust. It eventually becomes covered by a thick crust. The skin lesion(s) may be accompanied by a low grade fever that usually lasts only a few days, or by mild lymphadenopathy. In uncomplicated disease, the lesion heals spontaneously in 3 to 6 weeks without scarring. Secondary infections can occur.

Large lesions refractory to treatment can occur in people who are immunosuppressed. Unusually large lesions have also been reported in people with atopic dermatitis. Rare cases involving the eye, as well as a generalized vesiculopapular rash on the skin and mucosa, have also been reported. Possible complications include toxic erythema, erythema multiforme and bullous pemphigoid.

Diagnosis

Contagious ecthyma can be confirmed by electron microscopy of the crust, a small biopsy or fluid from the lesion; however, this technique cannot distinguish the orf virus from other parapoxviruses. PCR assays can give a definitive diagnosis. Histopathology can also be helpful. Virus isolation can be attempted but the orf virus grows slowly and cannot always be isolated. Animal inoculation into lambs has been reported. Serology and the detection of viral antigens can be used in research, but are not ordinarily used for diagnosis.

Treatment & prevention

In immunocompetent humans, contagious ecthyma is usually self-limiting. Treatment is supportive and typically consists of moist dressings, local antiseptics, finger immobilization and/or antibiotics to treat secondary bacterial infections. Large lesions can be removed by surgery, and curettage and electrodesiccation may be used for persistent lesions. Cryotherapy has been reported to hasten recovery.

Abraded or cut skin should not be allowed to contact infected animals, scabs and crusts, wool or hides. Nonporous gloves (rubber or latex) should be used when asymptomatic sheep, goats or other susceptible ruminants including deer are handled. This precaution may be particularly advisable when handling an animal's mouth.

Vaccination

Sheep that have recovered from natural infection are highly resistant to reinfection. The presently used commercial single-strain vaccines have produced fair immunity in all parts of the USA. Vaccine breaks appear to be due to the virulence of the infecting strain rather than to differences in antigenicity of the vaccine.

Vaccines should be used cautiously to avoid contaminating uninfected premises, and vaccinated animals should be segregated from unprotected stock until the scabs have fallen off. A small amount of the vaccine is brushed over light scarifications of the skin, usually on the inside of the thigh. Lambs should be vaccinated when ~1 month old. For best results, a second vaccination ~2-3 month later is suggested. Non-immunized lambs should be vaccinated before entering infected feedlots. Experimental work suggests that parenteral administration of virulent vaccine induces better immunity than does the current procedure.

The contagious ecthyma vaccines are pathogenic for humans, and gloves should also be used when vaccinating animals. Any skin that has been exposed should be washed with soap and water. Some sources suggest additional disinfection with 70% isopropyl alcohol after washing. People who are immunosuppressed should avoid contact with infected animals.

Pseudocowpos/Milker's Nodule

Pseudocowpox/ milkers nodule (PCPV) is a viral, most common cause of skin disease that causes mild sores on the teats and udders of milking cows. This virus can also infect humans and the condition is commonly referred to as milker's nodule. Because immunity is short-lived, cows can get infected fairly soon in often less than 6 months after recovering from the disease. Many herds have a chronic recurring problem with pseudocowpox with up to 100% of the herd affected, although only 5% are affected at any one time. The milker's nodule is of **zoonotic value** & is transmitted to humans, farmers & milkers having close contacts with milking cows developing lesions on the hands, forearms, legs and face.

Etiology: Pseudocowpox is caused by *Pseudocowpox virus* (PCPV)/Milkers nodule virus in the genus *Parapoxvirus*. It should not be confused with true cowpox, which is a rare disease of little current importance.

Occurrence

PCP is frequently occurring disease of cows, & has been reported from worldwide.

Hosts susceptible

Cattle are the main species that are affected by the pseudocowpox virus. Milkers, farmers & other persons handling affected cows also contract the infection.

Transmission

The virus spread is by milker's hands, teat cup liners and other fomites. Pseudocowpox can spread from cattle to man by contact. Skin infection in man is known as milker's nodules, and is a painful localised infection.

Clinical signs & lesions

Initially infection causes a small area of swelling and reddening on the teat. This is painful and makes the cow difficult to milk. Over the next two days, the affected area is elevated into an orange papule, which then scabs over. Tissue developing under the scab pushes it up further. Once the lesion has scabbed over, it becomes much less painful and milking is no longer so difficult. Seven to ten days after first signs the scabs start dropping off. This often leaves **a horse-shoe or ring shaped area,** which is very characteristic of pseudocowpox. Affected areas may grow together leading to scabs covering the entire length of the teat. Damaged teats are usually healed around a month after first signs. Most pseudocowpox is found on the teat. However up to 10% of affected cows may have lesions on the udder skin.

Milkers and farm workers caring for dairy cattle (direct contact) and less commonly, slaughterhouse workers and veterinarians get infected. Small, red, raised, flattened spots appear one to two weeks after exposure on the fingers, hands, and arms of the infected person. Within a week, the sores will become lumps that are red-blue, firm, and slightly tender. The disease is usually mild and generally the sores disappear after several weeks. Unlike cows, immunity after infection develops that protects against reinfection.

Diagnosis

A presumptive diagnosis can be made on the basis of clinical signs, & it is easy to diagnose pseudocowpox. However other disease, particularly herpes mammilitis can occur at the same time, so if you are unsure get confirmatory test performed. If signs alone are not sufficient, the virus can be isolated from the teat skin.

Treatment & prevention

Removal of the scabs followed by the application of an astringent disinfectant has been suggested for severely affected individual cases. Locally applied teat ointments appear to have little effect. Emollient teat sprays and dips can have a beneficial effect by reducing the numbers of bacteria and viruses on the teat skin and by aiding the healing of damaged skin.

Control of the infection of cows within a herd is difficult. Sound milking hygiene practices such as effective teat dipping and disinfection of milking units between cows can slow the spread of the virus. Cow to cow spread may also be limited by wearing gloves and disinfecting the milker's hands between cows.

It is important to wear gloves when milking or handling the teats and udders of infected cows. Other sources of exposure are calf muzzles and contaminated milking equipment. In addition to wearing gloves, you should minimize contact with infected animals and thoroughly wash your hands and arms if contact occurs. Prevent introduction of infected cows in the herd. Quarantine cows for at least 14 days before they enter the milking herd. For pseudocowpox, effective teat dipping with an iodophor teat dip is probably the most effective means of control. Improving parlour hygiene by using disinfectable gloves, disposable towels and teat cup disinfection may reduce disease spread.

Bovine Papular Stomatitis

Bovine papular stomatitis (BPSV) affects cattle, produces mild papular lesions on the muzzles & oral cavity of young cattle of 2 years age, there may be proliferative, reddish, raised papules that may ulcerate on the epithelium of the mouth, muzzle and in the nostrils, & the lesions may also be present in the esophagus, abomasum, and rumen. There is hyperplasia of the mucosa of the affected organ with intracytoplasmic inclusions. Reinfection is possible because of the short duration of immunity. Clinically, the disease is mild, but its importance lies in the need to differentiate it from FMD. The virus is transmitted to humans.

Etilogy: Bovine papular stomatitis is caused by *Bovine papular stomatitis virus* (BPSV) in the genus *Parapoxvirus.*

Occurrence

It occurs worldwide in cattle, specially reported from North America, Africa and Europe, causing bovine papular stomatitis.

Hosts susceptible

BPS usually occurs in cattle before the age of two years. There have been reports of both lesions on the hands of milkers and similar infections in sheep and goats, as well as humans.

Transmission

The virus is spread by direct contact with infected cattle or the saliva from an infected animal. People become infected by handling the lesions in an infected animal without gloves, allowing the virus to enter through broken skin or an abrasion.

Clinical symptoms & lesions

Bovine papular stomatitis virus (BPSV), a member of the genus *Parapoxvirus,* causes **proliferative dermatitis** in cattle and humans. Other species of the genus cause similar lesions, the nature of which has been attributed, at least in part, to a **viral-encoded vascular endothelial growth factor** (VEGF) that induces vascularization and dermal edema through VEGF receptor-2 (VEGFR-2). The results of this study showed that BPSV strain V660 encodes a novel VEGF and that the predicted BPSV protein showed only 33–52% amino acid identity to VEGFs encoded by the other species of the genus.

Single or multiple raised red, circular, ulcerated lesions appear on the mouth, lips, muzzle and tongue of cattle. Calves are commonly affected and recover in 2 - 3 weeks.

Skin lesions on hands in humans are raised, red, and painful and then progress to a scabby lesion of variable size, and tend to heal slowly over 1 -2 months.

Diagnosis

Collection of clinical specimens includes scrapings from lesions. The major importance of bovine papular stomatitis is its resemblance to FMD and vesicular stomatitis from which it should be differentiated.

Diagnosis is usually based on **gross and microscopic lesions**. A rapid laboratory confirmation can be obtained by the electron microscopic examination of distilled water lysates of lesion material.

The virus replicates in a variety of bovine cell cultures producing cytopathic changes, including cytoplasmic inclusions.

Treatment & prevention

Prevention includes hygienic milking practices. Since infection of milker's hands with lesions similar to those caused by bovine papular stomatitis virus occurs, it necessitates using gloves while handling sick animal.

Genus: *Capripoxvirus:*

Sheepox and Goatpox

Sheeppox (SPPV) & goatpox are endemic in Asia, Africa & in Southeastern Europe, affect sheep & goats. In sheep and goats, the clinical signs vary from **mild to severe** clinical disease, normally beginning with the onset of fever followed by erythematous macules that develop into papules. Lesions may also develop on the mucous membrane and on internal organs, causing **systemic signs** like respiratory signs, diarrhoea, depression, emaciation, abortion and sometimes death. Some differences exist between the viruses causing sheeppox and goatpox but are nearly similar in the clinical aspects.

Etiology: Sheep pox and goat pox is a contagious viral disease of small ruminants, which result from infection by *Sheeppox virus* (SPV) or *Goatpox virus* (GPV). The two viruses belong to the *Capripoxvirus* genus, *Poxviridae* family, which includes a third virus, causing lumpy skin disease (LSD) in cattle. SPV and GPV cannot be distinguished from each other with serological techniques, including viral neutralization.

Occurrence

Sheep pox virus and goat pox virus are similar in terms of their geographical distribution. During the past 50 years, the geographical range of sheep pox and goat pox has been restricted mainly to Asia and Africa, extending from North Africa to the Equator, from West Africa to East Asia, including Turkey, the Middle East and the Southern regions of the former Soviet Union.

Sheep pox and goat pox recently extended its distribution into Uganda (2000) in the south, for Africa and into Vietnam (2005, to be declared as endemic in 2008), Republic of Korea (2007) and Chinese Taipei (2008) in the east for Asia. The disease reoccurred recently in three countries after years of absence. These are Kenya that notified the reoccurrence of sheep pox and goat pox in 2003 while the previous occurrence was in 1989 (14 years ago); Mongolia , after 30 years of absence, the disease reoccurred in 2006, and remained present since that time and Azerbaijan that notified the reoccurrence of the disease in 2009 after 13 years of absence. In southern Europe, Greece reported several introductions, with the last in 2007 from Turkey. Some European countries, namely Belarus, Belgium, Estonia, Finland, Iceland, Greenland, Latvia, Lithuania, Malta, Slovenia Switzerland and Ukraine have **never reported the disease**. Some other European countries have succeeded in **eradicating it**: Ireland in 1850, the United Kingdom in 1866, Denmark in 1879, Norway in 1882 and the Netherlands in 1893, Germany in 1920, Albania and Sweden in 1934, former Czechoslovakia and Poland in 1950, Andorra in 1952, Austria in 1954, former Republic of Yugoslavia (Bosnia and Herzegovina, Croatia, Montenegro, Serbia) in 1955, Hungary and Romania in 1957, France in 1964, Spain in 1968, Portugal in 1970, Italy in 1983, Armenia in 1987, Cyprus in 1989, Moldavia in 1994, Bulgaria in 1996 and Georgia in 1997. The disease has never been reported in the Americas, in Oceania (Australia, Fiji, French Polynesia, New Caledonia, New Zealand, Philippines, Vanuatu) and in southern Africa (Angola, Botswana, Lesotho, Madagascar, Malawi, Reunion Island (France), South Africa, Swaziland and Zimbabwe.

Sensitivity, morbidity and mortality differ according to the animal, its age, its condition and health, and its own immunity, and the strain of the virus, as some natural mild viruses have been isolated. In endemic areas, the morbidity rate varies and the mortality rate is usually less than 10%. Nevertheless, case-fatality rates of nearly 100% have been reported in young animals. In **naive animals**, it is more severe and the mortality and morbidity rates may reach 100%.

Hosts susceptible

Most isolates are host specific, SPV mainly affecting sheep and GPV goats. However, some strains can affect both species. Moreover, recombination can occur between the two viruses. The susceptible species are **domestic small ruminants**. In 2008, Sudan reported 30 cases of sheep and goat pox disease in **Bohor Reedbuck, an antelope belonging to the family Bovidae.** This infection has never previously been reported in wild ungulates. These findings would therefore constitute the first report of the disease **in wild ungulates.** However, there is no wild reservoir species for the virus.

Sensitivity differs among individuals depending on several factors: Breed: some breeds are more resistant to capripoxvirus than others; Sex: probably linked to their physiology, females are more sensitive than males; Age: young animals are more sensitive than adults; Husbandry conditions: parasitism, malnutrition, exhaustion, and transhumance. In 2003, half of the outbreaks in Algeria occurred in Naama Wilaya, on the transhumance route for sheep flocks. Most animals were likely unvaccinated; & the animal population density: in many countries, sheep pox and goat pox are present in areas with a high density of small ruminants but usually absent in isolated areas where there is less contact between animals.

Transmission

In areas where sheep pox and goat pox are endemic, the disease is commonly first reported in **young animals,** whereas when the disease occurs in previously free areas usually as a result of the introduction of new animals from infected areas, animals of **all age groups** tend to be affected simultaneously.

Transmission of the disease between animals is mainly by direct contact and inhalation. Indirect transmission by contaminated vehicles or products (litter, fodder) or by insects (mechanical transmission) has been established but seems to play a minor role. Transmissions via intradermal or subcutaneous inoculation as well as respiratory, transcutaneous and transmucosal routes have been reported.

The virus can be excreted by sick and recovered animals for several weeks and it **can survive for many years in dried scabs at ambient temperatures.** Virus remains viable in wool for 2 months and in premises for as long as 6 months.

Human infections with sheep and goat pox viruses during the handling of infected animals are rarely seen but have been reported based on clinical signs.

Pathogenesis

After entry, the virus replicates locally in the skin or in the lungs followed by spread to regional lymph nodes & viremia. The virus is then disseminated to various internal organs. Appearance of typical skin lesions occurs on 7 days PI. In lungs, there are areas of consolidation & hemorrhages. Multiple virus-encoded factors are produced during infection, which influence pathogenesis and disease. Lesions are found in the epidermis and include congestion, haemorrhage, oedema, vasculitis and necrosis. All layers of the epidermis, dermis and sometimes musculature are involved. Typical pox lesions are also found in the respiratory and gastrointestinal tracts, as well as in other internal organs including lymph nodes, liver and kidneys.

Clinical symptoms & lesions

The **incubation period** varies from **4 to 21 days**, but it is usually 1 to 2 weeks. Clinical signs generally appear sooner when the virus is inoculated by insects than when it is transmitted in aerosols. After experimental inoculation into the dermis, primary lesions can develop at the site within 2 to 4 days.

The clinical signs vary from **inapparent, mild to severe**, depending on the animal's age, breed, immunity and other factors.

In affected animals, an **initial fever** is usually followed in one to five days by the characteristic skin lesions, which begin as erythematous macules, and develop into 0.5-1.5 cm hard papules. In the common, **papulovesicular form of the disease,** the centers of the papules become depressed, whitish gray and necrotic, and are surrounded by an area of hyperemia. Dark, hard, sharply demarcated scabs eventually form over the necrotic areas. Vesicles might be seen during the intermediate stage, but are uncommon. In the uncommon, **nodular form** of the disease ('stonepox'), the papules develop into nodules. These nodules can be found in the epidermis, dermis and subcutaneous tissues. They become necrotic and slough, leaving a hairless scar. Some European breeds of goats may develop a **flat hemorrhagic form of goatpox**. In this form, the papules seem to coalesce over the body, and the animal invariably dies. Capripox lesions have a **predilection for areas of sparsely wooled/ haired skin such as the axillae, muzzle, eyelids, ears, mammary gland and inguinal area,** but in more **severe cases, they may cover the body**. In animals with heavy wool, the lesions can be easier to find by palpation than visual inspection. Mild infections can easily be missed; only a few lesions may be present, often around the ears or the tail. All **superficial lymph nodes usually become enlarged** within a day of the appearance of generalized papules; the prescapular lymph nodes are particularly noticeable.

Lesions can also develop on the **mucous membranes and internal organs,** causing **systemic signs**. In some cases, these symptoms may precede the onset of skin lesions by a day or two. Lesions in the mouth, nares, eyes or eyelids can cause salivation or inappetence, as well as rhinitis, conjunctivitis or blepharitis with mucopurulent discharges. Affected mucous membranes may become necrotic and ulcerate or slough. Animals with lung lesions may have respiratory signs including coughing, nasal discharge and dyspnea. Nodules in the intestines can cause diarrhea. Depression and emaciation may be seen in some animals. **Abortions** can occur but are not common. Some breeds of sheep can die of acute disease before the characteristic skin lesions appear. Capripox lesions can take several weeks to heal, and may leave permanent scars on the skin. During healing, they are susceptible to fly strike. Secondary bacterial infections, including pneumonia, are common, and death can occur at any stage of the disease. Recovery can be slow if the animal was severely affected.

PM lesions: Skin lesions contain macules, papules and/or necrotic lesions and scabs with congestion, hemorrhage, edema, vasculitis and necrosis. **All the layers of epidermis, dermis and sometimes musculature are involved.** Lymph nodes draining infected areas are enlarged up to eight times the normal size, lymphoid proliferation, edema, congestion, & hemorrhages are seen. There are pox lesions on the mucous membranes of the eyes, mouth, nose, pharynx, epiglottis, trachea, on the rumenal and abomasal mucosae, and on the muzzle, nares, in the vulva, prepuce, testicles, udder, and teats. Lesions may coalesce in severe cases. Lung lesions include severe and extensive pox lesions, focal and uniformly distributed throughout the lungs; congestion, edema, focal areas of proliferation with necrosis & lobular atelectasis. Besides the above, there is enlargement, congestion, edema and hemorrhages of mediastinal lymph nodes.

Diagnosis

Collection of clinical samples includes tissues from active lesion, scabs, liquid & sera samles.

1. *Presumptive diagnosis*: It is based on clinical symptoms and lesions. Confirmatory test is made by the electron microscopic demonstration of poxvirus in lysates of lesion tissues. The virions are like other orthopoxviruses, brick-shaped as opposed to the virions of contagious ecthyma (a parapoxvirus), which are ovoid in appearance. Eosinophylic **intracytoplasmic inclusions** are seen in skin cells. Transmission electron microscopy rapidly identifies typical capripox virions.

2. *Virus isolation*: The virus is isolated in cell culture-primary lamb testis or lamb kidney: the appearance of CPE may take 4–12 days, intracytoplasmic inclusions are clearly seen by hematoxylin and eosin staining, and antigen can be detected by immunoperoxidase or immunofluorescence staining techniques.

   Agar gel immunodiffusion test from lymph gland biopsy material taken from an early case of capripox is confirmatory; it cross-reacts with parapoxviruses. Capripoxvirus antigen and inclusion bodies may also be seen in stained cryostat or paraffin sections of biopsy or post-mortem lesion material.

3. *Antigen detection*: Antigens from clinical specimens is detected by ELISA. Viral genome is detected by PCR using capripoxvirus-specific primers for the attachment protein gene.
4. *Antibody detection*: Virus neutralization test is the most specific serological test, but it is not sufficiently sensitive since immunity to capripox infection is predominantly cell mediated; infected animals may only produce undetectable low levels of neutralizing antibody. Indirect fluorescent antibody test & AGIO tests cross react with other poxviruses.

Western blotting uses P32 antigen of capripoxvirus for reaction with test sera; it is sensitive and specific, but is expensive and difficult to carry out. Genome detection is done by PCR using capripoxvirus-specific primers for the attachment protein gene.

ELISA using P32 antigen or another appropriate antigen expressed by a suitable vector could be used to develop an acceptable and standardized serological test.

Treatment & prevention

There is currently no treatment for sheeppox & goatpox. Additional methods of prevention include: restrictions on movement of sheep and goats between infected and noninfected areas, & restrictions on movement of animal products: meat, hair, wool, hides, & decontamination of animal products before allowing entry into nonendemic areas.

Vaccination

The most relevant strategy for controlling sheeppox and goatpox in endemic areas is mass immunisation of the susceptible population. All strains of capripoxvirus of ovine, caprine or bovine origin, such as sheep and goat pox and LSD for cattle, **share a major neutralising site,** so that animals recovered from infection with one strain are resistant to infection with any other strain.

Nowadays, **live vaccines** are preferred as a single dose of vaccine that can generate long-lasting immunity and protection from all capripoxvirus field strains. In contrast, **inactivated vaccines** are able to generate only short-term immunity. Several strains of live vaccines are used in endemic areas, such as **0240 Kenya strain in sheep and goats**, the **Romanian and RM-65 strains in sheep and in cattle**, and the **Mysore and Gorgan strains used in goats**. Most of them can be used in multiple species, **except for 0240 Kenya** which should not be administered to cattle.

It is recommended to vaccinate annually all sheep and goats regardless of their age. Although some young animals will have maternal derived antibodies, other will not, depending on the immune status of their mother, and considering the low cost of vaccines **all young animals should be vaccinated to ensure optimal protection coverage.** Those that did not generate immunity due to maternal antibodies will be vaccinated the following year. Immunity to virulent field virus following vaccination of sheep or goats with the 0240 strain lasts over 1 year, and protection against generalised infection following intradermal challenge lasts at least 3 years and is effective lifelong. The protective dose depends on the vaccine strain used. Immunity in sheep and goats against capripox following vaccination with the 0240 strain lasts over a year, and will probably provide lifelong protection against lethal challenge. Similarly the Romanian strain gave protection for at least 30 months. The 0240 strain should not be used in *Bos taurus* breeds of cattle. The **Romanian strain has been used for many years and is the most widely used.** The Kenya O 180 strain is thought to have the best safety record and highest efficacy.

Lumpy Skin Disease

Lumpy skin disease (LSDV) is an infectious, eruptive, occasionally fatal disease of cattle characterized by nodules, necrotic lesions on the skin, on mucous membranes of the eye, nose, mouth, pharynx and genitalia, enlarged lymph nodes and swelling of one or more legs with initial fever, discharge from the eyes and nose. Disease occurs in mainly in cattle, but buffaloes, giraffes, and impalas of all ages are susceptible, & the disease is endemic in Africa.

Etiology: Lumpy skin disease (LSD) is caused by *Lumpy skin disease virus* (LSDV)/Neethling poxvirus in the genus *Capripoxvirus* of the family *Poxviridae*. Lumpy skin disease virus is closely related antigenically to sheep and goat poxviruses. Although these three viruses are distinct, they cannot be differentiated with routine serological tests.

Occurrence

Lumpy skin disease is confined to Africa; till 1980s, this disease was only found south of the Sahara desert and in Madagascar, but in 1988, it spread into Egypt. It may also occur in other Middle Eastern countries. In 1989, an outbreak in Israel was eradicated by slaughter and vaccination policy.

LSD can occur as **sporadic cases or in epizootics.** The incidence of disease is highest in wet, warm weather, and decreases during the dry season. New foci of disease can appear at distant sites; in these cases, the virus is thought to be carried by insects. The morbidity rate varies widely, depending on the presence of insect vectors, & host susceptibility, and ranges from 3% to 85%. The disease signs can vary widely among the cattle in a group, with **some animals having inapparent infections and others developing severe disease**. The mortality rate is low in most cases (1–3%), but has been as high as 20% in some outbreaks. Unusually high mortality rates of 75–85% have been reported but remain unexplained.

Hosts susceptible

LSD is primarily a disease of cattle, *Bos taurus* breeds, particularly **Jersey, Guernsey and Ayrshire, are more susceptible** to clinical disease than zebu cattle (*Bos indicus*). A few cases have been reported in Asian water buffalo (*Bubalus bubalis*). More severe disease is seen in *Bos taurus*, particularly Channel Island breeds, than zebu cattle. **Calves and lactating cows seem to be most susceptible to disease.** Wild animals are not thought to play an important role in the spread or maintenance of LSDV.

Transmission

LSDV is transmitted primarily **by biting insects**. This virus has been found in mosquitoes in the genera ***Aedes* and *Culex*** during some outbreaks. Experimentally infected *Aedes aegypti* are infectious for 6 days and can transmit LSDV mechanically during this time. Flies (e.g. *Stomoxys calcitrans*) and other insects might also be involved in transmission, but this remains unproven.

Direct contact is a minor source of infection. LSDV is present in cutaneous lesions, saliva, respiratory secretions, milk and semen. Shedding in semen may be prolonged; viral DNA has been found in the semen of some bulls for at least 5 months after infection. Animals can be infected experimentally by inoculation with material from cutaneous nodules or blood, or by ingestion of feed and water contaminated with saliva. Although direct animal-to-animal transfer of the disease is ineffective, transfer could occur when sick and healthy animals use the same watering troughs. Suckling calves can get the disease from drinking contaminated milk. On the other hand, a calf can be protected up to the age of 6 months if it gets enough colostrum from a cow that has been vaccinated.

LSDV is very resistant to inactivation, surviving in desiccated crusts for up to 35 days, and can remain viable for long periods in the environment.

Pathogenesis

After generalized disease, a viremia occurs with a fever & virus localization occurs in the, skin & inflammatory nodules develop. Experimentally, after ID infection, local lesions develop at the site of inoculation, but here is neither viremia nor generalization of the disease.

Clinical symptoms & lesions

The incubation period in the field is 2-5 weeks, but experimentally infected animals, fever can develop in 6 to 9 days and lesions first appear at the inoculation site in 4 to 20 days.

The clinical signs range from inapparent to severe disease. Host susceptibility, dose and route of virus inoculation affect the severity of disease. *Bos taurus* is more susceptible than *Bos indicus*, and young calves often have more severe disease than adults.

Fever is the initial sign, followed within two days by the development of nodules on the skin and mucous membranes. These nodules vary from 1 cm to 7 cm and penetrate the full thickness of the skin. They are particularly common **on the head, neck, udder, genitalia, perineum and legs.** Although the nodules may exude serum initially, they develop a characteristic inverted conical zone of necrosis, which penetrates the epidermis and dermis, subcutaneous tissue, and sometimes the underlying muscle. These cores of necrotic material become separated from the adjacent skin and are called **sit-fasts.** Secondary bacterial infections are common within the necrotic cores. Some nodules, particularly those on the mucous membranes and udder, ulcerate rapidly. The superficial lymph nodes become enlarged and edematous. Nodules can also occur in the gastrointestinal tract, trachea and lungs; the latter may result in primary or secondary pneumonia. Mastitis could also occur as a result, with heavy losses because of permanent damage to the tissue of the udder.

Feed intake decreases in affected cattle, milk yield can drop markedly, and animals may become emaciated. Rhinitis, conjunctivitis and keratitis can also be seen; ocular and nasal discharges are initially serous but become mucopurulent. Inflammation and necrosis of the tendons, or severe edema of the brisket and legs, can result in lameness. Secondary bacterial infections can cause permanent damage to the tendons, joints, teats and mammary gland. Abortions and temporary or permanent sterility may occur in both bulls and cows.

A few animals die, but the majority slowly recovers. Recovery can take several months, and some skin lesions may take a year or two to resolve. Deep holes or scars are often left in the skin.

PM lesions: can be extensive & comprise characteristic greyish-pink deep nodules with necrotic centers in the skin; these nodules often extend into the subcutis and underlying skeletal muscle, and the adjacent tissue exhibits congestion, hemorrhages and edema. The regional lymph nodes are typically enlarged.

Flat or ulcerative lesions may occur in the mucous membranes of the oral and nasal cavities, pharynx, epiglottis and trachea. Nodules or other lesions can occur in the gastrointestinal tract, particularly the abomasum, udder, urinary bladder, lungs, kidneys, uterus and testes. In the lungs, the lesions appear as focal areas of atelectasis and edema. The mediastinal lymph nodes are enlarged in severe cases, and pleuritis may be seen. Some animals may have synovitis and tendosynovitis with fibrin in the synovial fluid.

Aborted fetuses do not always have the characteristic external lesions, but some may be covered with nodules.

Diagnosis

Collection of clinical specimens includes biopsies from lesions, & sera samples.

1. *Presumptive diagnosis*: LSD should be suspected when the characteristic skin nodules, fever and enlarged superficial lymph nodes, along with gross and microscopic findings are suggestive. Transmission electron microscopy on biopsy material or desiccated crusts is confirmatory.
2. *Virus isolation*: Virus grows in primary cell culture of lamb or calf testis or bovine dermis cells. Microscopic examination reveals characteristic cytopathic effect. Haematoxylin and eosin staining reveals intracytoplasmic inclusion bodies, direct immunofluorescent or immunoperoxidase staining detects the virus, virus neutralization using specific antisera can be done.
3. *Antigen detection*: Capripox antigen detection ELISA detects virus antigen on biopsy suspension or tissue culture fluid. Virus genome is detected by capripoxvirus PCR on EDTA blood, semen, biopsy, or tissue culture samples. It is highly sensitive and specific. **Strains can be identified by sequence and phylogenetic analysis.**
4. *Antibody detection*: Virus neutralization if done cross reacts with all capripoxviruses. Indirect fluorescent antibody test also cross reacts with parapoxviruses. Capripox antibody ELISA is also used. **Western blot is highly sensitive and specific** but expensive and difficult to perform.

Treatment & prevention

No specific treatment exists. Strong antibiotic therapy may control secondary infection. Because biting insects most probably play a role in the transfer, cattle could be sprayed with insecticides during the risk period.Free countries use import restrictions on livestock, carcasses, hides, skins and semen.

Infected countries adapt strict quarantine to avoid introduction of the infected animals into safe herds, in cases of outbreaks, isolation and prohibition of animal movements is practiced, slaughtering of all sick and infected animals, proper disposal of dead animals, e.g. incineration, cleaning and disinfection of premises and implements, & vector control in premises and on animals. With the exception of vaccination, control measures are usually not effective. Vector control in ships and aircraft is highly recommended.

Vaccination

A better method of disease prevention is immunizing by means of vaccination. Calves of mothers that have not been vaccinated or cows that have never been exposed to the disease could be **vaccinated at any age.** Calves of cows that have been vaccinated should only be vaccinated after 6 months of age. After that vaccination should be done annually.

Genus: *Suipoxvirus:*

Swinpox

Swinepox is a mild to severe vesicular disease seen on any part of the body but are common along the flanks, abdomens and occasionally the ears, firstly small circular red areas 10-20mm in diameter commence with a papules, vesicles containing straw-coloured fluid in the centre which after two to three days, ruptures, and a scab is formed which gradually turns black. Often the hooves go crusty due to the animal's water content in its body being used for fighting the infection, & serious swinepox cases can cause malformed hoofs and damage the ability for the pig to walk properly. In some extremely rare cases, the genetics of the animal can be changed by this disease but go unnoticed in terms of physical symptoms; & the disease, if contracted by breeding pigs is very threatening for the potential baby piglets to be born. Piglets born from parents that both have the severest strain of the disease will be born frequently with disfigurements such as a tail that is bulbous, and crooked snouts. The inside of the animal is also affected by the genetic strain by making the muscles and fat of the animal pus filled and also weakens the piglets organs overtime resulting in death.

Etiology: Swinepox is a worldwide disease of pigs caused by a *Swinepox virus* of the family *Poxviridae* and the genus *Suipoxvirus.*

Occcurrence

Swine pox occurs worldwide in the major swine-raising countries. It occurs more often where **insect vectors, the hog louse (*Haematopinus suis*)** of swinepox virus are not controlled. Modern swine raised free of lice rarely exhibit the disease. Swine pox was first reported in Europe in 1842 and in the United States in 1929. The disease persisted and was relatively common, perhaps because it caused little obvious economic loss to swine producers. Outbreaks once were caused by two viruses: vaccinia virus, and swine pox virus. Vaccinia virus is no longer used to vaccinate people against small pox;

hence it`no longer spreads to pigs. Only swine pox virus now causes pox in swine.

Hosts susceptible

Swine pox occurs only in swine. All age groups are susceptible but most outbreaks are encountered in young growing pigs. It occasionally occurs congenitally and in neonates.

Transmission

Persistence of virus within **desquamated scabs** can be transmitted to other pigs when introduced into skin abrasions. The virus can also spread horizontally from nasal and oral secretions from the infected pigs. Once a few virus-containing lesions appear, the virus can be transmitted mechanically by the bites of vectors that have recently fed in pox lesion areas. Common vectors include the hog louse (*Haematopinus suis*), mosquitoes, and biting flies. Once introduced, infected swine or virus-carrying biting insects can initiate outbreaks in susceptible herds. There is evidence of transplacental infection of neonatal pigs.

Pathogenesis

The virus enters locally via skin abrasions and multiplies there or attacks the skin after viremia. Virus introduced into abrasions replicates in cells of the stratum spinosum causing typical skin lesions to develop. The lesions go through the stages of **macules, papules, vesicles, pustules and crusts.** All but the vesicle stage are easily identified. As lesions mature and heal, crusts containing virus desquamate and leave white macules.

A viremic stage of the disease has not been demonstrated. However, it must occur in some animals since transplacental infection of neonatal piglets has been reported. Antibody to swinepox virus is formed as a consequence of infection and immunity is long lasting.

Clinical symptoms & lesions

The incubation period is 3-6 days but may be up to 14 days and the lesions persist for 1-3 weeks. Slight fever, 40 ° C may accompany the appearance of the lesions. Red 1cm papules (spots) appear on the **ventral abdomen and rapidly form circular red brown scabs**, which soon blacken. In young piglets the bursting of the vesicular stage on the face may lead to wetting, scab formation and conjunctivitis. Slight inappetence may accompany the development of the lesions. Affected pigs appear hairy and growth may be depressed. A large percentage of successive litters of sucking and recently-weaned pigs may be affected but the disease is rare in adults.

Systemic clinical signs of disease seldom are observed but the skin lesions are easily seen. Initial lesions usually are along the ventral aspect of the abdomen, inside the legs and in inguinal areas, **all favorite feeding sites of hog lice**. However, lesions have been observed at many cutaneous sites so most of the skin appears susceptible. Initially, there are small vesicles that largely are unnoticed. The papules that result are seen as 1-3 mm circular red spots. As lesions mature, crusts form that eventually heal uneventfully. In **severe infections**, lesions may occur in upper respiratory and digestive tracts. This is particularly true of congenitally-acquired swinepox where piglets are born with or develop lesions over the entire body shortly after birth. Exudative epidermitis (greasy pig disease) and secondary bacterial dermatitis occasionally occur as a sequel to swine pox. Swine pox does not appear to cause a pruritic response in the affected pigs.

Diagnosis

1. *Presumptive diagnosis*: Swine pox is easily diagnosed by identifying the lesions. Lesions are round to oval, usually less than 1.0 cm in diameter. The brown to black crusts are easily seen but the vesicle stage seldom can be identified grossly. If confirmation is needed, histologic diagnosis can be made by identifying typical, large, **intracytoplasmic inclusion** bodies in cutaneous lesions. Pox lesions should be differentiated from those of other vesiculating viral diseases, pityriasis rosea, dermatosis vegetans, streptococcal dermatitis, ringworm and greasy pig disease.

2. *Virus isolation*: Swine pox virus grows in pig kidney cell lines or on the chorioallantoic membranes of eggs to cause recognizable changes (CPE) and intracytoplasmic inclusions.

Treatment & prevention

Treatment or control are rarely attempted because of the mildness of the disease, but the use of insecticide to eliminate lice and flies which transmit the disease on a farm and the thorough cleaning and disinfection of pens in which outbreaks of the disease have occurred to help reduce the incidence. Control of swine pox relies on herd immunity and prevention of transmission. Swinepox seldom is a problem if the usual vectors of virus, especially hog lice, are controlled by insecticides or elimination. Congenital swine pox is generally a sporadic, self-limiting event. There are no treatments. These viruses are extremely resistant to drying and may persist for years in exudates in which they can resist temperatures of 100° C for 10 minutes.

Genus: *Avipoxvirus*

Fowlpox

Fowlpox **(FPV)** is a highly contagious, slow-spreading viral infection of chickens and turkeys characterized by proliferative lesions in the skin (cutaneous form/dry form) that progress to thick scabs, and by lesions in the upper gastrointestinal tract and respiratory tracts (diphtheritic form/wet form). There are **two forms** of the disease, **cutaneous or dry form**, & **diphtheritic form**. The **cutaneous form** is spread by biting insects (especially mosquitoes) and wound contamination and causes nodular lesions on the comb, wattles, around eyelids and beak. Birds affected by this form usually recover within a few weeks. The second **diphtheritic** form is more severe, is spread by inhalation of the virus and causes a diphtheritic membrane to form in the mouth, pharynx, orbit, sinuses larynx, and sometimes the trachea. The prognosis for this form is poor.

Etiology: Fowlpox is a worldwide disease of poultry caused by *Fowl pox virus* of the family *Poxviridae* and the genus *Avipoxvirus*. The viruses causing fowlpox are distinct from one another but antigenically similar, possible hosts including chickens, turkeys, quail, canaries, pigeons, and many other species of birds.

Occurrnce

Fowlpox is highly contagious and occurs worldwide in chickens, turkeys, grouse, quail, pheasants, canaries, pigeons, sparrow, starlings & other avian species.

Hosts sustible

Chickens, turkeys, grouse, quail, pheasants, canaries, pigeons, sparrow, starlings & other avian species are susceptible. Mostly adult and young chickens and turkeys are affected, but the disease may occur in any age of bird, at any time with low mortality but may be as high as 50% with the diphtheric form.

Transmission

Fowl pox can be transmitted by direct or by insects & by fomites.The virus is present in the lesions and is generally transmitted by contact through **abrasions** of the skin. Skin lesions (scabs) containing the virus shed from the recovering birds in poultry houses are highly resistant in dried scabs and under certain conditions, may survive for months on contaminated premises, & act as a source of aerosol infection. Disease may be transmitted by a number of species of **mosquitoes**. Mosquitoes can harbor infective virus for a month or more after feeding on affected birds. Mosquitoes and other **biting insects** may serve as mechanical vectors. Transmission within flocks is rapid when mosquitos are plentiful. After the infection is introduced, it spreads within the flock by mosquitoes as well as direct and indirect contact. Recovered birds do not remain carriers. Since fowl pox usually spreads slowly, a flock may be affected for several months. In some affected birds, the disease may be reactivated by stress (eg, moulting) or by immunosuppression due to other infections. The disease tends to persist for extended periods in multiple-age poultry complexes.

Pathogenesis

In intradermally (id) infected chickens, the virus was first detected in the skin at the inoculation site on day 2 and in lungs on day 4 followed by viremia on the day 5 post-infection (p.i.). Subsequently, the virus was recovered from liver, spleen, kidney and brain, but not from the heart. The chickens infected by intratracheal (i.t.) route showed an almost similar outcome with minor differences as the virus was first demonstrated in the lungs on day 2 p. i., & viraemia occurred on day 4 p. i. Initiation of pocks at the inoculation site in i.d. infected birds was observed on days 3 to 4 p.i., generalized cutaneous pock lesions appeared from 7 to 8 days p.i.

Clinical symptoms & lesions

Cuaneous or dry pox starts as small whitish foci that develop into wart-like nodules on various parts of the **unfeathered skin** of chickens and on the **head** and upper neck of turkeys. Lesions are most commonly seen on the **comb, wattles, ear lobes, eyes, and sometimes the feet**. At one time only a few birds develop lesions. Lesions are prominent in some birds and may reduce flock performance. Lesion may be **generalized on feathered skin**. In some cases, lesions are limited chiefly to the feet and legs. The lesion is initially a raised, blanched, nodular area that enlarges, becomes yellowish, and progresses to a thick, dark scab. Multiple lesions usually develop and often coalesce. Lesions in various stages of development may be found on the same bird. Localization around the **nostrils** may cause nasal discharge. Cutaneous lesions on the eyelids may cause complete closure of one or both eyes. The nodules eventually are sloughed and scab formation precedes final healing. Cutaneous infections usually cause low or moderate mortality, and these flocks generally return to normal production after recovery.

Diphtheritic or wet pox is associated with the **oral cavity and the upper respiratory tract**, particularly the **larynx and trachea**. The lesions are diphtheritic in character and involve the **mucous membranes** to such a degree that when removed, an ulcerated or eroded area is left. In wet form, lesions develop on the mucous membranes of the **mouth, esophagus, pharynx, larynx, and trachea**. Occasionally, lesions are seen almost exclusively in one or more of these sites. Caseous patches firmly adherent to the mucosa of the larynx and mouth or proliferative masses may develop. Mouth lesions interfere with feeding. Tracheal lesions cause difficulty in respiration and may simulate infectious laryngotracheitis in chickens. Laryngeal and tracheal lesions in chickens must be differentiated from those of laryngotracheitis.

Course of the disease in a flock is usually protracted. Extensive infection in a layer flock results in decreased egg producttion. Mortality is usually high in the generalized or diphthertic form.

PM lesions include papules progressing to vesicles then pustules and scabs on sites as mentioned above. In the diphtheritic form, there may be caseous plaques in mouth, pharynx, trachea and/or nasal cavities. Microscopically, **intra-cytoplasmic inclusions (Bollinger bodies)** with **elementary bodies (Borrel bodies)** are seen.

Diagnosis

1. *Presumptive diagnosis*: Cutaneous form produces characteristic gross lesions on comb, wattles, around eye & legs. Microscopic lesions on exam & staining with H & E reveal IC eosinophilic inclusion bodies. IC inclusions may also be detectable by fluorescent antibody and immunohistochemical methods. Negative-staining electron microscopy & ultrathin sections of the lesions detect viral particles with typical poxvirus morphology.
2. *Virus isolation*: The virus can be isolated by inoculating **CAM of 9-12 days old chicken embryo,** susceptible birds, or cell cultures of avian origin.
3. *Antigen detection*: Restriction endonuclease analysis of viral genomes differentiates field isolates and vaccine strains of fowlpox virus. Nucleic acid probes derived from cloned genomic fragments of fowlpox virus can also be used for diagnosis. This procedure is especially useful for differentiation of the diphtheritic form of fowlpox (involving the trachea) from infectious laryngotracheitis.

PCR is used to amplify genomic DNA sequences of various sizes using specific primers. This procedure is useful when an extremely small amount of viral DNA is present in the sample. PCR has been used effectively to differentiate field and vaccine strains of fowlpox virus. **Monoclonal antibodies** that recognize different fowlpox virus antigens have been developed. These monoclonal antibodies can be used for strain differentiation by **immunoblotting**. The complete sequence of the fowlpox virus genome has been identified recently and is useful in comparing the sequences of selected genes of other avian poxviruses.

Treatment & prevention

There is no treatment for fowl pox. If there is evidence of secondary bacterial infection, broad-spectrum antibiotics may be of some benefit.

Mosquito control procedures is beneficial in limiting spread in poultry confined in houses.

Vaccination

Vaccinttion is done through vaccination of replacement birds. Where preventative vaccination is used, all replacement chickens are vaccinated when the **birds are six to ten weeks of age.**

Fowlox is best prevented through vaccination of chickens and turkeys with **live-embryo or cell-culture-propagated vaccines**. The most widely used vaccines are **attenuated fowlpox virus and pigeonpox virus isolates of high immunogenicity and low pathogenicity**. Pigeonpox virus vaccine is highly immunogenic & is of low pathogenicity for chickens, it is propagated in embryonated eggs and administered by the wing-web stick method or by brushing defeathered follicles. **A turkeypox vaccine** has been developed to control pox in turkey flocks in which fowlpox vaccine has been ineffective. In high-risk areas, vaccination is done with an **attenuated vaccine of cell-culture origin in the first few weeks of life and revaccination at 12-16 week is often sufficient**. Since fowlpox spreads slowly, vaccination is often useful in limiting spread in affected flocks if administered when less than 20% of the birds have lesions. Because passive immunity may interfere with multiplication of vaccine virus, progeny from recently vaccinated or recently infected flocks should be vaccinated only after passive immunity has declined. Vaccinated birds should be examined **1 week later for swelling and scab formation** ("take") at the site of vaccination, absence of "take" indicates lack of potency of vaccine, passive or acquired immunity, or improper vaccination. Revaccination with another serial lot of vaccine may be indicated.

Naturally infected or vaccinated birds develop humoral as well as cell-mediated immune responses. One application of fowl pox vaccine results in permanent immunity.

Vaccination of broilers is not usually required unless the mosquito population is high or infections have occurred previously. The chicks may be vaccinated as young as one day of age. During outbreaks, flocks and individuals still unaffected may be vaccinated.

Commercially available live fowlpox vaccine, **AVA-POX-CE**-Intervet is live virus Fowl pox vaccine of chicken embryo origin for vaccination of healthy chickens and turkeys between 8 and 18 weeks of age applied by the wing web method in chickens and thigh application in turkeys. This pox vaccine is the one of choice for vaccinating birds to be kept for laying purposes. **AE+POX** is a live vaccine against Avian Encephalomyelitis (*Tremovirus, Picornaviridae*) and Fowlpox in chickens and turkeys. It contains live AE virus strain Calnek: >= 2.5 $\log^{10}$ EID_{50} and live Fowlpox virus strain Gibbs: >= 2.8 $\log^{10}$ EID_{50} for the active immunization of layer replacement pullets and breeder replacement pullets and turkeys. Chickens should be vaccinated by Wing web method between 8 and 16 weeks of age. Turkeys should be vaccinated between 18 and 26 weeks of age.

Genus: *Leporipoxvirus:*

Myxomatosis

The *Myxoma virus* causes a serious, life threatening, systemic viral disease (myxomatosis) in its aberrant host, in the **European rabbits, *Oryctologus cuniculus.*** Typical skin lesions that are associated with disease in the domestic rabbit include edema of the eyelids, ears, nose, anus, and genitals; blepharoconjunctivitis; hemorrhage; and nodules on the ears, head, body, and legs at the site of infection that may become congested or necrotic". The **tumorous swellings called myxomata** later appear over the entire body. Myxomata are **connective tissue tumors that consist of large star-like cells "myxoma cells"**. In the European rabbits, *Oryctolagus cuniculus* produces a severe generalized infection with high mortality up to 90%. The virus was introduced into Europe, Australia & Chile with upto 90% mortality to control rabbit population damaging agricultural crops but the disease ultimately became endemic with a low fatality rate.

However, it only causes a mild cutaneous fibroma in its natural wild hosts: the jungle rabbit, ***Sylvilagus brasilensis*-Tapeti**(Mexico or Argentina) and ***Sylvilagusbachmani –Bush rabbit***(California). Myxomatosis (MYXV) is endemic in wild rabbits (*Sylvilagus*) in North and South America and in some wild rabbit species of the genus *Oryctulugus*, in Europc, South America, and Australia.

Etiology: Myxomatsis is caused by *Rabbit myxoma virus, a* poxvirus of the genus *Leporipoxvirus* (includes *Rabbit fibroma virus* and *Squirrel and hare fibroma viruses*). Nearly 100 strains are known; some, e.g.,"standard laboratory" and California, are highly virulent for *Oryctolagus cuniculus,* (mortality up to 99%).

Occurrence

Myxomatosis is caused by the myxoma virus, a type of pox virus that only affects rabbits. It was first discovered in 1896 in Uruguay and was imported to Australia in 1951 to control its large rabbit populations - initially having the desired devastating effect. The disease was illegally introduced to France in 1952 and it appeared in Britain the following year. It quickly spread to both wild and domestic rabbit populations and within a few years had spread throughout Europe. Myxomatosis has been a threat to wild and domestic rabbits ever since.

Hosts susceptibility

All rabbits, whether wild or domestic are at risk of myxomatosis.

Transmission

Myxomatosis is typically spread by **blood sucking insects** and in particular the **rabbit flea,** *Spilopsyllus cuniculi*. This flea is frequently found on wild rabbits and transmission in the absence of bites is unusual. All breeds of domestic rabbit can be affected, with little to suggest that one breed is more susceptible than another, and whatever the lifestyle of rabbit, there is a potential risk of this disease.Transmission rarely may also occur by direct contact with infected rabbits or inhalation.

Pathogenesis

The myxoma virus is usually transmitted passively by arthropods- often the mosquito or rabbit flea feeding on the rabbit. There is no replication of the virus within the vector. Replication occurs at the inoculation site within the epidermis and dermis. In the natural *Sylvilagus* host, there is no systemic phase of infection. However, in *Oryctologus cuniculus,* the virus then **spreads within leucocytes to the regional lymph node** where it undergoes more replication and attains a high titre. Often a skin lesion will develop four to five days post inoculation and then enlarge to 3 cm by ten days post inoculation. Viral replication in the regional lymph node results in cell associated **viraemia** and generalised infection with dissemination to the **skin** away from the inoculation site, **spleen, mucosal surfaces like conjunctiva, other lymph nodes, testes, liver and lungs**. The replication occurs within the **lymphoid system.**

By day 9 there is eyelid swelling, the eyes may be completely closed and secondary conjunctivitis with semipurulent ocular discharge. Secondary lesions occur throughout the body especially on the lips, nares, & eyelids. Purulent swollen lesions develop on the mucocutaneous junctions and the base of the ears. Although the virus may be shed in discharges, actual transmission by close contact is thought to be very unusual.

Virulent disease in farmed colonies often leads to spread by inhalation and thus a primary pulmonary site of infection. This results in pneumonia and a secondary pasteurellosis at seven to twenty days instead of the characteristic skin masses. Myxomatosis in colonies may also exhibit rhinitis and ocular discharge. Transmission of the virus by aerosol is much more likely to give the affected animal respiratory signs than transmission by insect.

Clinical symptoms & lesions

The **incubation period** varies depending on the strain and its virulence and is typically at least **five days.** There are bulging eyes associated with myxomatosis, are localised swellings around the head, face, ears, lips, anus and genitalia. Severe swellings can lead to blindness and distortion around the face within a day or so of the onset of symptoms, leading to difficulty with feeding and drinking. Bacterial respiratory infection often complicates the disease resulting in a fatal pneumonia. Progress of the disease may be slower in well cared for pet rabbits and recovery is sometimes possible with intensive care. However, myxomatosis can be a very protracted and profoundly unpleasant disease and euthanasia is generally recommended. Recovery in the wild occasionally occurs but for animals with severe signs death usually occurs about 12 days after initial infection.

Diagnosis

Signs and lesions usually are sufficient for presumptive diagnosis although California strain disease can lack distinctive characteristics. Other methods include **virus isolation** (chick embryo and various cell lines) and identification and animal inoculation. Myxoma virus causes disease similar to fibromatosis in young *Sylvilagus* spp but severe in young *O. cuniculus*.

Treatment & control

Good barrier technique and **vector control** is practised. **A vaccine has been developed**, but is not needed if vector control is adequate.

Vaccination: There is one licensed **rabbit vaccine** to immunise against myxomatosis available in the UK. It is a live vaccine containing the *Shope fibroma virus*, which is closely related to myxomatosis but does not cause disease in the European domestic rabbit. The only clinical sign that may occasionally be seen is a slight temporary lump, or nodule, at the vaccination site. A **single dose of vaccine is given to all rabbits over six weeks of age who are healthy and not pregnant.**

□□□

Chapter 12

Characteristics and Diseases Caused by Group I Double-Stranded DNA Papillomaviruses (Family *Papillomaviridae*)

Contents

Characteristics of Papillomaviruses

Papillomaviruses (L. papilli=pustule, oma=tumours) infect many vertebrates including humans & animals and produce **benign epithelial growths, called papillomas or warts** in humans, monkeys, cattle, buffaloes, dogs, horses, sheep, & goats. Papillomaviruses are non-enveloped & contains **circular capsid** with 40-55 nm diameter having **icosahedral symmetry** made of 72 star-shaped (Fig 12-1) capsomers (T=7). The virion surface appears rough and the surface projections are small. **L1 protein is needed for the formation of viral capsid & is responsible for producing neutralizing antibodies**. Capsid also contains abundant L2 protein, which is not needed for capsid structure but performs other functions like packaging of nascent virions & entry of virus into new host cells. The genome of papillomavirus is not segmented and made of a single molecule of **circular**, **superoiled**, double-stranded DNA about 5300-8000 nucleotides long. Papillomaviruses multiply in the **nucleus of basal cells of squamous surface epithelium**; some infect skin, or mucosal epithelia of the genitalia, anus, mouth or respiratory tract. The viruses are highly host specific & there is rarely inter-species transmission. But inter-species transmission occurs in case of bovine papillomavirus (BPV) type 1 which in its natural host, cattle, induces large fibrous skin warts but BPV-1 infects horses, which are an incidental host for the virus, causing benign tumors called **sarcoids**.

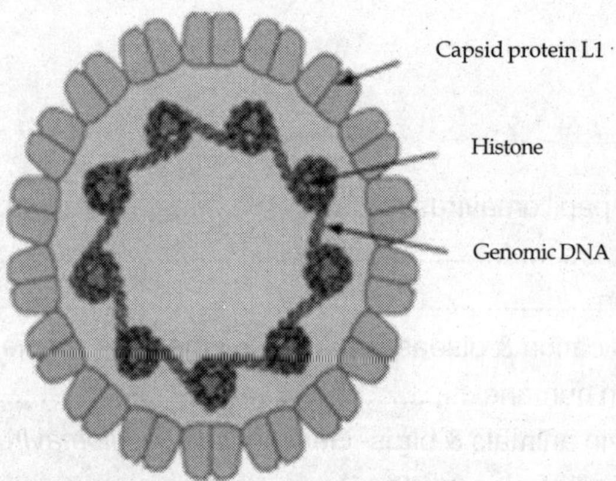

Figure 12.1 : Morphology of a Papillomavirus

The virus genome

The genome is a single molecule of circular, superoiled, double-stranded DNA about 5.3-8 kbp long. The viral genome has a guanine + cytosine content of 40-50 %. dsDNA is associated with cellular histones in a chromatin-like complex.

Papillomavirus genome expression is complex because there are multiple promoters, alternative splicing ways and a link between differentiation and gene expression. Only one strand of the genome is transcribed and divided into **early region** contains two large (E1 & E2) & 4 smaller (E4-E7) open reading frames & a **late region** containing two large genes (L1 & L2). **Early region genes** produce early proteins which are non-structural regulatory proteins (E1-E7). **Late region genes** produce the structural proteins, L1 and

L2 that code for capsid protein. Although all viruses have tropism for squamous epithelial cells infecting the basal cells of the dermal layer, early genes are expressed in these cells but late gene expression, expression of structural proteins and vegetative DNA synthesis is restricted to terminally differentiated cells, keratinocytes of the epidermis.

Papillomaviruses are relatively resistant and remain viable for long periods of time on contaminated premises. Virus transmission occurs mainly by direct contact and fomites. These viruses target squamous epithelial cells of the skin and mucous membrane & produce koilocytotic or vacuolated cells while replicating. The many papillomatoses are common and occur worldwide. The immune response to papillomaviruses concurs with the spontaneous regression of warts and is mediated by both cellular and humoral immune responses.

Virus replication

Papillomaviruses multiply in the nucleus of basal cells of squamous surface epithelia Replication is divided in **two distinct steps that are linked to the differentiation state of the host epithelial cell:** a) The **plasmid replication in the basal squamous epithelial cells** & b) the **vegetative replication in differentiated keratinocytes.**

a) **The plasmid replication** occurs in the basal squamous epithelial cells & corresponds to viral DNA replication in synchrony with the host cell chromosome in order to ensure an average of one viral genome per basal cell.

Virus attaches to host cell receptors, viral L1 protein and sulfated sugars on the cell surface promote attachment of the virus. The virus then enters inside the cell via interaction with a specific receptor, **the alpha-6 beta-4 integrin,** and transported to endosomes. The capsid protein L2 disrupts the membrane of the endosome, allowing the viral genome to escape and traffic with L2 to the cell nucleus in the basal squamous epithelial cell where uncoating of the viral DNA occurs. Firstly, early-region transcription and translation of the early proteins occur followed by steady-state viral DNA nuclear replication. DNA replication requires the origin of DNA replication in cis and the viral E1 and E2 proteins in trans. Virus can persist for decades after infection by the following mechanism. The virus expresses E1 and E2 proteins, which are for replicating and maintaining the viral DNA as a circular episome, the **viral oncogenes E6 and E7 promote cell growth by inactivating the tumor suppressor proteins p53 and pRb proteins, which act as tumor suppressors.** When tumor suppressor proteins are inactivated, tumor growth proceeds unchecked. Then keratinocyte stem cells in the epithelial basement layer can maintain papillomavirus genomes for decades.

b) *The vegetative replication* occurs in differentiated keratinocytes. There is a burst of viral DNA synthesis with active production of virions. It includes vegetative viral DNA synthesis, transcription of the late region & capsid proteins L1 and L2 synthesis. Thereafter, assembly of the virion particles ensues, nucleus breaks down and the virus is released.

The functions of each gene are as follows;

E1– Replication and replication repression;

E2– Activates transcription in HPV types 6, 11 and 16, represses transcription and binds to long control region.

E3– No known product or function.

E4– Cytoplasmic protein in HPV-1-induced warts; E5– Transformation in HPV-6.

E6– Transformation in cooperation with E7 in HPV-16 and HPV-18;

E7– Transformation in cooperation with

E8– No known product or function;

L1– Major capsid protein.

L2– Minor capsid protein

Cell transformation

The transformation process is very complex & depends largely on the early gene products, E1 & E2, & the transferring proteins appear to vary from one virus type to another. The general principle is that two or more early proteins cooperate to give a transforming phenotype. The most confusing thing is that in most cases, all or part of the papillomavirus genome including the transforming genes is maintained in the tumour cells, while in other cases, the virus DNA may be lost after transformation. BPV-4 is an example of one such "hit-and-run" mechanism.

In case of Human Papillomaviruses (HPVs), E2 binds to the early promoter and decreases expression of E6/E7. The loss of E2 is thus the first stage of transformation. E6 then binds to p53 via a cellular protein, p100, and targets it for degradation via the ubiquitin pathway. E7 binds pRB and prevents phosphorylation. This would normally result in apoptosis but both E6 and E7 interact with a number of cellular proteins which influence the outcome of infection. **Oncogenic potential of HPV-16, 18 is due to subsequent increased**

expression of E6 & E7. Some papillomavirus types can cause cancer in the epithelial tissues they inhabit, but the development of papillomavirus-induced cancers occurs over the course of many years.

Virus classification

Group: Group I ds DNA

Family: *Papillomaviridae*

Genera

G 1: *Alphapapillomavirus*; type species: *Human papillomavirus 32*

G 2: *Betapapillomavirus*; type species: *Human papillomavirus 5*

G 3: *Gammapapillomavirus*; type species: *Human papillomavirus 4*

G 4: *Deltapapillomavirus*; type species: *European elk papillomavirus*, Others are *Bovine papillomavirus 1, 2*

G 5: *Epsilonpapillomavirus*; type species: *Bovine papillomavirus 5*

G 6: *Etapapillomavirus*; type species: *Frinzilla coelebs papillomavirus*

G 7: *Iotapapillomavirus*; type species: *Mastomys natalensis papillomavirus*

G 8: *Kappapapillomavirus*; type species: *Cottontail rabbit papillomavirus*

G 9: *Lambdapapillomavirus*; type species: *Canine oral papillomavirus*

G 10: *Mupapillomavirus*; type species: *Human papillomavirus 1*

G 11: *Nupapillomavirus*; type species: *Human papillomavirus 41*

G 12: *Omikronpapillomavirus*; type species: *Phocoena spinipinnis papillomavirus*

G 13: *Pipapapillomavirus*; type species: *Hamster oral papillomavirus*

G 14: *Thetapapillomavirus*; type species: *Psittacus erithacus timmeh papillomavirus*

G 15: *Xipapillomavirus*; type species: *Bovine papillomavirus 3*

G 16: *Zetapapillomavirus*; type species: TS: *Equine papillomavirus 1*

Table 12.1 presented below classify *Papillomaviridae* & shows diseases caused by the member virus species.

Table 12.1 : Classification of family *Papillomaviridae* & diseases caused by the member viruses in humans & animals.

F. *Papillomaviridae*	Species	Serotypes	Diseasescaused
G 1: *Alphapapillomavirus*	*Human papillomavirus 2*	HPV-2, 57	*Members infect oral or anogenital mucosa in humans & primates. *HPV-2, 10: can also cause cutaneous lesions. *HPV-16, 18: are high risk tumor producers associated with human uterine cancers; induce in-vitro cell transformation. *HPV-53, 26, 34: cause malignant or benign tumors. *HPV-61, 7, 6, 54, 90, 71: are low risk tumor producers; cause benign lesions.
	Human papillomavirus 6	HPV-6, 11, 13, 44, 55, 74	
	Human papillomavirus 7	HPV-7, 40, 43, 91	
	Human papillomavirus 10	HPV-10, 3, 28, 29, 77, 78, 94	
	Human papillomavirus 16	HPV-16, 31, 33, 35, 52, 58, 67	
	Human papillomavirus 18	HPV-18, 39, 45, 59, 68, 70, 85	
	Human papillomavirus 26	HPV-26, 51, 69, 82	
	TS: *Human papillomavirus 32*	HPV-32, 42	
	Humun papillomavirus 34	IIPV-34, 73	
	Human papillomavirus 53	HPV-53, 30, 56, 66	
	Human papillomavirus 54	HPV-54	
	Human papillomavirus 61	HPV-61, 72, 81, 83, 84, 62, 86, 87, 89	
	Human papillomavirus 71	HPV-71	
	Human papillomavirus 90	HPV-90	
G 2: *Betapapillomavirus*	TS: *Human papillomavirus 5*	HPV-5, 8, 12, 14, 19, 20, 21, 25, 36, 47	* HPV-8,12,14,19,2,21, 25, 36,47 mainly infect skin of humans (latent) & activated in immune-suppressed. *HPV-5, 9, 49: cause EV (Epidermodysplasia verruciformis in the hosts.
	Human papillomavirus 9	HPV-9, 15, 17, 22, 23, 37, 38, 80	

	Human papillomavirus 49	HPV-49, 75, 76	
	Human papillomavirus 92	HPV-92	
	Human papillomavirus 96	HPV-96	
G 3: *Gammapapillomavirus*	TS: *Human papillomavirus 4*	HPV-4, 65, 95	*HPV-4,65,95,48, 50, 60,88 Members cause cutaneous lesions in the hosts & produce species specific I/C inclusions.
	Human papillomavirus 48	HPV-48	
	Human papillomavirus 50	HPV-50	
	Human papillomavirus 60	HPV-60	
	Human papillomavirus 88	HPV-88	
G 4: *Deltapapillomavirus*	*Bovine papillomavirus1*	BPV-1, 2	*Produce fibropapilloma in ungulates; after transspecies transmission induces sarcoids, cutaneous tumour in horses. *ORFs has transforming act
	Deer papillomavirus	DPV	
	TS: *European elk papillomavirus*	*EEPV*	
	Ovine papillomavirus 1	*OPV-1, 2*	
G 5: *Epsilonpapillomavirus*	TS: *Bovine papillomavirus 5*	BPV-5	*BPV-5 causes cutaneous papillomas in cattle.
G 6: Zetapapillomavirus	TS: *Equus caballus papillomavirus 1/Equine papillomavirus 1*	EcPV-1	*Causes cutaneous lesions in horses.
G 7: *Etapapillomavirus*	TS: *Frinzilla coelebs papillomavirus*	FcPV	*Causes cutaneous lesions in avian hosts.
G 8: *Thetapapillomaviruss*	TS: *Psittacus erithacus timmeh papillomavirus*	PePV	*Causes cutaneous les ions in avian hosts.
G 9: *Iotapapillomavirus*	TS: *Mastomys natalensis papillomavirus*	MNPV	*Causes cutaneous lesions in rodents.
G 10: Kappa*papillomavirus*	TS: *Cottontail rabbitpapillomavirus*	CRPV	*Causes cutaneous & mucosal lesions in rabbits.
	Rabbit oral papillomavirus	ROPV	

G 11: *Lambdapapillomavirus*	TS: *Canine oral papillomavirus*	COPV	*Infects cats & dogs & cause cutaneous & mucosal lesions.
	Feline papillomavirus	FDPV	
G 12: *Mupapapillomavirus*	TS: *Human papillomavirus 1*	HPV-1, 63	*HPV-1, 63 causes cutaneous lesions in humans with species specific I/C inclusions.
G 13: *Nupapapillomavirus*	TS: *Human papillomavirus 41*	HPV-41	*HPV-41 causes benign & malignant cutaneous lesions in the hosts.
G 14: *Xipapapillomavirus*	*Bovine papillomavirus 3*	BPV-3, 4, 6	*BPV 3, 4, 6 cause true papillomas on cutaneous or mucosal surfaces; BPV-3 infects skin, BPV-4 upper alimentary tract, also cause squamous cell carcinoma; BPV-6 produce udder & teat papillomas of cattle.
G 15: *Omikronpapillomavirus*	TS: *Phocoena spinipinnis papillomavirus*	PsPV	*Causes genital warts in cetaceans.
G 16: *Pipapapillomavirus*	TS: *Hamster oral papillomavirus*	HaOPV	*Causes mucosal lesions in hamsters.

Abbreviation: TS– type species

Papillomavirus

Clinical manifestations in humans and Animals

Human Infections

Human papillomas viruses (HPV) contain more than 100 types that produce wart/ lesions but the appearance of lesions & specific tissues infected depend on specific types. For example, HPV1, 2, 3, 4 infect keratinized epithelia of hands & feet; HPV 6, 11, 16, 18, 31, 33 & 45 infect mucosal epithelia of orogenital & oropharymgeal cavity, while HPV2 & 57 infect both skin & genital mucosa. Some HPV types have oncogenic potential. HPV types are grouped as **low, intermediate or high risks oncogenicity based on the growth of abnormal tissue or cells on body skin** & over 60 such types have been identified. **HPV-16, 18: are high risk tumor producers associated with human uterine cancers & induce in-vitro cell transformation**, HPV-53, 26, 34 cause malignant or benign tumors & HPV-61, 7, 6, 54, 90, 71: are low risk tumor producers. HPV can cause abnormal tissue changes on the vocal cords, mouth, hands, feet and genital organs. Each type of HPV infects certain parts of the body, e.g. HPV1 infects soles of the feet while HPV-2 infects palm of the hand and some types of the virus causes growth of abnormal tissues that can lead to cancer of the female organs.

Cancerous growth caused by HPVs include: 1. **Cutaneous squamous cell carcinoma** (SCC) results from malignant proliferation of epidermal keratinocytes, SCC is dependent upon exposure to risk factors like ultraviolet light, and patient age, skin type, and ethnicity. 2. **Invasive cervical cancer** is related to age, with a mean age of 47 years in USA. 3. Penile carcinoma is rare in USA & Europe, but much higher in parts of South America, Africa, and Asia. 4. Vulvar cancer in USA is 2.5 per 100,000 women, most common in postmenopausal women with mean age of 65, & risk factors include cigarette smoking, vulvar dystrophy, vulvar or cervical intraepithelial neoplasia, human papillomavirus (HPV) infection, immunodeficiency syndromes, a prior history of cervical cancer, and northern European ancestry.

Genus: *Alphapapillomavirus:*

Members infect oral or anogenital mucosa in humans & primates.

HPV-2, 10: can also cause cutaneous lesions.

HPV-16, 18: are high risk tumor producers; associated with human uterine cancers, induce in-vitro cell transformation.

HPV-53, 26, 34: cause malignant or benign tumors.

HPV-61, 7, 6, 54, 90, 71: are low risk tumor producers; cause benign lesions

Genus: *Betapapillomavirus:*

HPV-8, 12, 14, 19, 20, 21, 25, 36, 47 mainly infect skin of humans (latent) & activated in immunosuppressed.

HPV-5, 9, 49: cause EV (Epidermodysplasia verruciformis) in the hosts.

Genus: *Gammapapillomavirus:*

HPV-4, 65, 95, 48, 50, 60, 88 members cause cutaneous lesions in the hosts & produce species specific I/C inclusions.

Genus: *Mupapapillomavirus:*

HPV-1, 63 causes cutaneous lesions in humans with species specific I/C inclusions.

Genus:*Nipapapillomavirus*

*HPV-41 causes benign & malignant cutaneous lesions in the hosts.

Clinical Infectins in Animals

Genus: *Deltapapillomavirus:*

BPV-1 infects paragenital areas, penis, teats & udders.

BPV-2 infects skin, alimentary tract & urinary bladder. Both produce carcinomas when grazing land is infested with braken.

Genus: *Epsilonpapillomavirus:*

BPV-5 causes cutaneous papillomas in cattle.

Genus: *Xipapapillomavirus:*

BPV 3, 4, 6 cause true papillomas on cutaneous or mucosal surfaces; BPV-3 infects skin, BPV-4 upper alimentary tract, also cause squamous cell carcinoma; BPV-6 produce udder & teat papillomas of cattle.

Cottantail rabbit papillomavirus (CRPV) can cause protuberant warts in its native host, the North American rabbit of genus *Sylvilagus.*

Bovine Papillomatosis

Bovine papillomatosis is a common viral disease of the skin, mostly of young cattle, manifested as benign tumours or warts, caused by *Bovine papillomavirus* (BPV) that has six serotypes. These cutaneous warts most often regress spontaneously, occasionally persist, and, in the presence of additional critical genetic or environmental factors, can progress to cancer. Papillomavirus infection in cattle could be connected with serious disorders of the metabolism (mainly mineral, energetic and nitrous) probably caused by damage of the liver and kidney with mutagenic, carcinogenic and immunosuppressive cadmium, arsenic and lead, observed in the serum of tested animals. Infection by BPV occurs as a result of the virus exposure to single or multiple lesions of the epithelium. Papillomaviral infection, transformation and multiplication of basal cells, lead to wart formation, but most warts are benign and do not proliferate indefinitely.

Etiology: Bovine papillomatosis is caused by *Bovine papillmavirus; BPV* types 1 through types 6 belonging to 3 different genera:

Genus: *Deltapapillomavirus* (fibropapillomaviruses or formerly subgroup A):

This genus includes BPV-1 & BPV- 2. & DPV, EEPV, OPV 1, 2 are also found in this group. These papillomaviruses infect only keratinocytes (epithelial cells); however, unlike other papillomaviruses, they cause proliferation of both keratinocytes and fibroblasts, causing **benign fibropapillomas involving both the epithelium and the underlying dermis.** The specificity of the types differs:

BPV-1 infects paragenital areas, including penis, teats and udders.

BPV-2 infects skin, alimentary canal and urinary bladder causes cauliflower-like fibropapillma of anogenital & ventral abdominal skin; & is also associated with bladder cancer in cattle.

Genus: *Epsiloallomavirus:*

BPV-5 infects teats and udders, and can cause pure papillomas and fibropapillomas, causes "rice-grain type" papillomas of the teat.

Genus: *Xipapillomavirus* (epitheliotropic BPVs or formerly subgroup B)

This genus includes BPV types 3, 4 and 6, and is unique among papillomaviruses in lacking the E6 oncoprotein. They infect keratinocytes (epithelial cells), causing pure papillomas involving only the epithelium. The specificity of the types differs:

BPV-3 infects skin

BPV-4 infects the upper alimentary tract; malignant transformation associated with concomitant bracken fern ingestion has been reported.

BPV-6 infects teats and udders; causes flattened (frond-like) papillomas of the teat.

Occurrence

Bovine papillomatosis occurs worldwide, mainly affecting young cattle.

Hosts susceptible

Calves are most susceptible, but few cases of warts have been seen in cattle over 2 years of age. Occasionally, warts are found on the teats of lactating dairy cows.

Transmission

Calves are easily infected with the papillomaviruses entering the cut or abraded skin. All too frequently calves are inadvertently infected when tattooed or ear tagged for identification. In fact, it is not unusual to find an entire tattoo overgrown with a mass of warts. Warts will appear 1 to 6 months after inoculation with the virus. Warts often spread from the ear to other sites on the head and neck. *Papillomavirus*is widely distributed in cattle. Cattle are the main source and natural reservoir of infection by the virus; but, halters, ropes, and instruments can serve as a potential source of infection. Not all animals carrying the virus will have warts. It can be transmitted from the inapparent carrier to the susceptible calf.

Clinical symptoms & lesions

Warts can occur anywhere on the body but are most commonly seen in the head and neck area. Less common but often more important sites include teats and scrotum. Warts vary greatly in shape from almost flat pea-sized lumps to large orange-sized balls on stalks. Cattle are usually otherwise healthy; there are normally no systemic effects.

BPV is highly prevalent, with around 50% of cattle being estimated to bear lesions. Cutaneous warts are most common in younger animals (under 2 years) and usually spontaneously regress due to the animal's immune response without significant scarring. The duration of infection is very variable from one month to over a year) and recurrence is possible.

Warts caused by the *Xipapillomavirus* group have a cauliflower-like appearance and can attain the size of a fist; most common on the head, neck and shoulders, they may also occur in other locations. Cutaneous fibropapillomas caused by *Deltapapillomavirus* group have a nodular appearancc. Although unsightly, most skin warts rarely cause problems except in show animals. However, large warts may bleed, potentially leading to secondary infections, and florid warts of the teat can cause mastitis and interfere with suckling and milking. Fibropapillomas can be troublesome when present in the genital area, causing pain and sometimes loss of reproductive functions as well as interfering with calving. Chronically immunosuppressed animals may develop extensive papillomatosis in the upper gastrointestinal tract, which can cause difficulties with eating and breathing

Bovine papilloma virus (BPV)-4 under the genus *Xipapillomavirus* causes squamous cell carcinomas of the alimentary tract. BPV-1, 2 causes carcinomas and haemangioendotheliomas of the urinary bladder. Both carcinomas occur if animals have fed on bracken or when grazing land is infested with bracken like western Scottish Highlands, southern Italy and the Nasampoli Valley in Kenya. Bracken contains several immunosuppressant and mutagens, including quercetin and ptaquiloside. Cows feeding on bracken are at risk of developing BPV-associated cancers. Bracken-associated tumours form a model for some types of human oesophageal cancer in which HPV DNA has been detected in around 18% of cases, and there is an association between exposure to or consumption of bracken being used as a foodstuff and herbal remedy in South America, China, Japan, Korea and other countries and is a risk of developing oesophageal cancer.

Diagnosis

Diagnosis is based on the basis of clinical signs, histopathological findings, and detection of the papillomavirus by transmission electron microscopy. Grossly, tumour tissue was composed of hyperplastic epidermis supported by thin, inconspicuous dermal stalks. In both cases histopathology revealed fibropapillomatosis with acanthosis, hyperkeratosis and down-growth of rete ridges. The virus appears to infect the basal cells of the epithelium, causing hyperplasia with hydropic ballooning of their cytoplasms, large eosinophilic keratohyaline granules and vesicular nuclei. Some cells degenerated, while others were stimulated to excessive growth and formation of warts.

Treatment & prevention

Treatment is not usually required, as most warts eventually regress spontaneously. Surgical removal is possible but may lead to recurrence. Disinfection with formaldehyde of stalls, fence posts and other environmental virus reservoirs can prevent transmission.

In Crotia, the animals were treated successfully by autogenous vaccine and a parammunity inducer / immunomodulator (Baypamun®, Bayer Pharma, Leverkusen, Germany). Regression of papillomas in both cases occurred about 3 weeks after the beginning of treatment, and within 6 weeks all warts spontaneously disappeared and animals completely recovered. No recurrence of papillomas has been observed in treated cows.

Vaccination

Vaccines against BPV types 1, 2 and 4 have been developed that can be used as prophylactic or therapeutic vaccination.

Prophylactic vaccination is done with whole virus like formalin-killed wart tissue suspension, virus like particles (L1 or L1+L2), L1 protein (for BPV-4) or L2 protein confers long-lasting protection against challenge with the same BPV type, but is generally ineffective against existing warts. Protection appears to be mediated via type-specific neutralizing antibodies. Vaccination of calves as early as 4–6 weeks might be necessary to prevent infection.

Vaccination

Therapeutic vaccination with BPV-4 E7 or BPV-2 L2 induces early regression of warts. Wart rejection involves a cell-mediated immune response with infiltration of the site by large numbers of lymphocytes and macrophages.

These vaccine systems have served as models for the successful development of prophylactic vaccines against the human papillomavirus types associated with cervical and anal cancers. Both **Gardsil** (a quadrivalent prophylactic HPV vaccine licensed in 2006) and **Cervarix** (a bivalent prophylactic vaccine license in the EU in 2007 and USA in 2009) contain virus-like particles assembled from L1 protein, an approach successful against BPV, and both vaccines induce sustained immunity. Various therapeutic HPV vaccines based on E6, E7 and L2 are currently in early-stage of clinical trials.

Bovine Alimentary Tract Papillomas-Carcinoma

Bovine papillomavirus type 4 (BPV-4) under the genus *Xipapillomavirus* is the etiological agent of epithelial papillomas of the upper alimentary canal in cattle. These benign tumours can undergo transformation to squamous cell carcinomas in animals feeding on bracken fern. Strong epidemiological evidence suggests that the progression to malignancy is due to the interplay between BPV-4 and mutagenic and immunosuppressing chemicals present in the fern. The carcinomas of the upper alimentary canal are often accompanied by adenomas and adenocarcinomas of the lower intestine and bracken-grazing animals are also heavily immunosuppressed. Florid persistent papillomatosis of the upper alimentary canal was reproduced in animals infected with BPV-4 and immunosuppressed either by a diet of bracken or by treatment with azathioprine; cancer of the upper alimentary tract or of the lower intestine developed only in animals infected with virus and fed on bracken fern. As in field cases, BPV-4 DNA was detected in papillomas but not in cancers. Thus immunosuppression is necessary for persistence and spread of viral papillomas, the fern mutagens are responsible for neoplastic conversion of papilloma cells, and continuous expression of viral functions is not required for the maintenance of the malignant state.

The gross and histological changes observed were predominantly in the upper gastrointestinal tract, consisting of inflammation and neoplastic changes in the mucosa of the abomasum and omasum. In one calf, the omasal and abomasal mucosa exhibited acute infiltration, necrosis, and ulceration in combination with malignant neoplastic changes of the epithelial cell lining. These changes may have altered the mucosal permeability, allowing bacteria and/or toxins to flow into the bloodstream, inducing changes in other organs.

It has previously been shown that **quercetin**, a well characterized and potent mutagen found in BF, causes cell cycle arrest of primary bovine cells, but that a single exposure to quercetin can cause full oncogenic transformation of primary bovine cells partially transformed by BPV-4. Cell cycle arrest correlates with an increase in p53 protein levels and transcriptional activity. However, in cells transformed but non-tumorigenic, p53 protein is elevated and transcriptionally activated in response to quercetin or other DNA damaging stimuli, but the cells bypass quercetin-induced G_1 arrest likely due to E7 expression. In transformed tumorigenic cells, p53 is elevated in response to quercetin but its transcriptional activity is inhibited due to mutation, and the cells fail to stop in G_1 in the presence of quercetin.

Equine Papillomatosis

Equine warts or equine viral papillomatosis are common in horses, usually in **young horses,** are small lumps on the skin caused by *Equine papillomavirus 1*(EqPV-1) in the genus *Zetapapillomavirus*. These viruses affect the skin, particularly on the muzzle and lower part of the head of young horses from the age of **six months to five years old**. Congenital form occurs in newborn foals; usually single or few but can be extensive. Warts are contagious, although some horses appear more susceptible than others. Most cases occur in young weanlings or yearlings during their first season at grass, hence colloquial terms - Grass warts, milk warts. Several different syndromes may relate to different variants of the virus or to different related and unrelated viruses. Aural plaques (Pinnal acanthosis) is a common but poorly understood variant that is probably caused by a different virus and transmitted by the biting flies and especially *Simulium* spp (Black Fly). Initial development in older horses is much less inclined to spontaneous remission. Recently, the complete nucleotide sequence of *Equus caballus papillomavirus type 1* (EcPV-1), obtained from an equine cutaneous papillomas has been done. Evidence for a causal link between PV and disease is limited. It is hypothesized that 2 different types of equine PVs (EPVs) cause viral papillomatosis (warts); **an ear papillomas (aural plaques),** and a 3rd EPV may be associated with **penile papillomas.** Equine papilloma virus has an **incubation period of about 60 days**. The warts reach maturity after a growth period of four to eight weeks and usually disappear spontaneously about three to four months later. In this respect, they resemble human warts in that one day they can be extremely unpleasant, and then the next will suddenly vanish. They affect **various cutaneous sites, as well as oral, ocular, and genital mucous membranes**, and can cause problems because of physical location and esthetics. Spontaneous remission is common within 1 to 9 months. Occasional cases can be severe. **Pinnal acanthosis lesions are common in horses over 4 years of age.** They may progress slowly or rapidly or remain static for many years; very few cases resolve spontaneously although many become static and settle down markedly. Equine warts development in older horses is much less inclined to spontaneous remission. **Aural plaques** occur in horses of all ages, manifesting as well-demarcated raised, depigmented, hyperkeratotic plaques 1 to 3 cm in diameter on the inner surface of the ear pinnae. They rarely, if ever, spontaneously resolve and are susceptible to fly bites and secondary infection. Immunohistochemical (IHC) testing and electron microscopy have implicated *Papillomavirus* (PV) as the etiologic agent for equine papillomas and aural plaques.

Treatment is usually unnecessary and, provided that the warts are neither infected nor causing pain, they should go away on their own, given time. If they are causing a significant problem, then only they should be excised.

Prognosis in case of congenital viral papilloma can be persistent but the lesions are usually amenable to surgical excision. In a few cases, the severity precludes surgical excision. **Cryonecrosis (cryotherapy)** may also be effective. Excellent with the caveat that a few lesions persist and that this is commoner in primary infection in older horses, and especially in the groin region of the latter group. The prognosis for cure of pinnal acanthosis is very poor; most cases persist for many years or even for life. Good responses occur in the common grass/milk wart conditions. Poor or negative responses are seen in adult onset viral papilloma and in congenital and pinnal acanthosis forms.

Equine Sarcoids

Sarcoid is a **tumor of the skin of horses, donkeys and mules** caused by *Bovine papilloma virus*-1, 2 infection, characterized by proliferation of neoplastic fibroblasts and thickening and/or ulceration of the skin. The appearance of sarcoids varies from small, sessile or pedunculated growths that have a warty appearance to firm, freely moveable, nodular dermal masses.Sarcoids are locally invasive and frequently recur after surgical excision, but do not metastasize. These tumors may be single or multiple and, although they occur most frequently on the head, limbs and abdomen, they can occur anywhere on the body including sites of trauma and healed wounds. It is the **most frequently diagnosed tumor in horses** with the prevalence of sarcoid at 20% of all equine neoplasms and 36% of all skin tumors. Sarcoids occur **at any age but are more common in young adult horses 3 to 6-years-old being the most common age group** and males being slightly more prone to developing disease. Even though all breeds are affected, a generic predisposition to sarcoid development may exist. Quarter horses, Appaloosas and Arabians may be at greater risk and Standard breeds at lower risk to develop sarcoids. There is no gender, coat color, seasonal or geographic predilection for the occurrence of the sarcoids.Sarcoids are also more prevalent in certain familial lines, suggesting that there may be a heritable component. There is an association between the presence of *Bovine papillomavirus-1,2* and associated viral growth proteins in skin cells with sarcoid formation, but the exact mechanism that controls or induces epidermal proliferation remains unknown. However, high viral loads within cells are strongly correlated with more severe clinical signs and aggressive lesions.

Clinical Symptoms & lesions

The appearance and number of sarcoids can vary with some horses having single or multiple lesions, usually on the head, legs, ventrum and genitalia or around a wound. The distribution pattern suggests that **flies** are important factor in the formation of sarcoids. Sarcoids may resemble **warts (verrucous form), small nodules (nodular form), oval hairless or scaly plaques (occult form)** or very rarely, **large ulcerated masses (fibroblastic form)**. The occult form is usually seen on skin around the mouth, eyes or neck, while nodular and verrucous sarcoids are common on the groin, sheath or face. Fibroblastic sarcoids have a predilection for the legs, groin, eyelid and sites of previous injury. Multiple forms may also be present on an individual horse (mixed form).

Histolgically, **sarcoids are composed of fibroblasts** (collagen producing cells) that invade and proliferate within the epidermis, dermis, and sometimes the subcutaneous tissue but do not readily metastasize to other organs. Surgical biopsy can definitively diagnose sarcoids, but there is a significant risk of making sarcoids worse. Therefore, diagnosis is based solely on clinical signs, fine-needle aspiration or complete excisional biopsy is safer choice.

Treatment of sarcoids

While sarcoids may spontaneously regress regardless of treatment in some instances, course and duration of disease is highly unpredictable and should be considered on a case-by-case basis taking into account cost of the treatment and severity of clinical signs. The traditional treatments of sarcoids includebanding with rubber rings, surgical excision, cryotherapy, immunotherapy or injection with Bacillus Calmette-Guérin as an immunomodulator, radiotherapy, laser therapy, hyperthermia, topical chemotheraphy, & intratumoral chemotherapy. Sarcoids are locally invasive and frequently recur after surgical excision, but do not metastasize. Surgical removal alone is not effective; with recurrence occurring in 50 to 64% of cases, but removal is often done in conjunction with other treatments. Topical treatment with products containing **bloodroot extract** from the plant *Sanguinaria canadensis* for 7 to 10 days has been reported to be effective in removing small sarcoids. **Sarcoid Cleaning Salve from Balanced Eco**

solutions is an all natural remedy that eliminates the Sarcoid and unlike the treatments mentioned earlier draws the virus from the blood stream. Sarcoid Salve does not burn but is extremely soothing and promotes hair growth in the affected area unlike Blood-root products mentioned earlier. **Freezing sarcoids** with liquid nitrogen (cryotherapy) is another affordable method, but may result in scarring or depigmentation. Topical application of the **anti-metabolite 5-fluorouracil** has also obtained favorable results, but it usually takes 30 to 90 days of repeated application before any effect can be realized. Injections of small sarcoids (usually around the eyes) with the chemotherapeutic agent cisplatin and the immunomodulator BCG have also achieved some success. In one trial, BCG was 69% effective in treating nodular and small fibroblastic sarcoids around the eye when repeatedly injected into the lesion and injection with cisplatin was 33% effective overall (mostly in horses with nodular sarcoids). However, BCG treatment carries a risk of allergic reaction in some horses and cisplatin has a tendency to leak out of sarcoids during repeated dosing. External beam radiation can also be used on small sarcoids, but is often impractical. The sad part is on any of these treatments mentioned so far, the Bovine Papilloma virus, will travel to other points in the body and return more aggressively. These treatments only address a symptom rather than the cause.

There is a chance of sarcoid recurrence for all modalities even after apparently successful treatment. While sarcoids are not fatal, large aggressive tumors that destroy surrounding tissue & can cause discomfort, loss of function and be resistant to treatment, making euthanasia a viable option in some instances. Sarcoid diagnosis is based on the characteristic microscopic arrangement of fibroblasts and collagen fibers and their orientation to the overlying epidermis.

Canine Oral Papillomatosis

Canine papillomatosis is a contagious viral disease, characterized by the formation of **benign tumors** that affect the skin and oral mucosa. Viral warts in dogs tend to possess frond-like structures creating more of a sea anemone or cauliflower-like appearance, though they can be smooth as well. The classical canine viral wart patient is a **young dog** with warts in or around the mouth or eyes. In such cases where warts have a classic appearance in a classic patient, diagnosis may be obvious but in older patients with warts in locations other than the face, other types of growths become more likely. Because growths can appear harmless but behave malignantly, removal and biopsy are often recommended. In dogs, we do not call these growths "warts;" we use the more formal term "viral papillomas.

Papillomas are usually seen in **young animals**, they are benign tumors caused by *Canine oral papillomavirus* (COPV). The virus is transmitted by direct or indirect contact. The infection begins with small bumps, which grow as warts. These can appear on lips, tongue, gums, oral mucosa and sometimes on all of them. Oral papillomatosis may disappear spontaneously within weeks.

The infection is transmitted via direct contact with the papillomas on an infected dog or with the virus in the pet's environment. The **incubation period is 1-2 months.** This virus can only be spread among dogs. To become infected, the dog generally needs an immature immune system, thus this infection is primarily one of **young dogs and puppies**. Beyond this, transmission details are sketchy. It is not known whether the infected dog must actually show visible lesions to be contagious, nor how long after regression of lesions contagion is still of concern.

Papillomas usually appear on young dogs and have a preference for certain body parts such as the lips, tongue, mouth, eye lids and between the toes. All areas of the oral mucosa of young dogs are susceptible to infection with the virus. While the virus as mentioned does not affect humans, it is capable of transmitting mainly between dogs. The dogs most prone to the virus are those with an underdeveloped immune system, therefore explaining why it **affects mainly puppies and young dogs**. In a few instances papillomas developed in the skin around the nose and mouth and at the muco-cutaneous junction of the eyelid. Most old dogs were resistant to infection with this virus, presumably as a result of a previous natural infection. Dogs whose papillomas had regressed resist a second challenge inoculation of virus into the oral mucosa. The virus-neutralizing antibody titer of the serum of five dogs whose tumors had regressed ranged from <1:10 to 1:500.

The **incubation period** between exposure to a dog affected by papilloma virus and the time the dog is infected is between **1-2 months.** Sometimes the growths may become infected requiring antibiotics and there have been instances, even though rare, of papillomas turning malignant. There is also another variety of papilloma that affects senior dogs which is known as "cutaneous pappilloma". In this case, the warts are more likely to appear in various locations on the body on the contrary to those affecting young dogs affecting the oral cavity.

When there is no spontaneous disappearance of warts, treatments such as surgery or the use of drugs such as **interferon or azithromycin** have been recommended and were not always successful. Most cases of papilloma go away on their own as the puppy's or **young dog's immune system grows stronger and fights against the virus.** Puppies usually are able to fight off the virus within 2-3 months. Recently in May, 2008 a study was published by a veterinary research group in Turkey who found that a **10 day course of the antibiotic azithromycin was able to remove all lesions within 15 days with no recurrences during an 8 month follow up period.** This therapy is readily available in the U.S. and is likely to become treatment of choice. Eight months old, a German Bulldog German, which presented a widespread oral papillomatosis, was treated, but it didn't improve after two months of conventional treatment. Then, the dog was treated with **Mic-Five Immuno, one every twelve hours; after 20 days, was added a capsule of Mico-Corio per day.** Papillomas began to shrink and one month and a half later they had disappeared completely. A Bulldog of the same owner was treated with the same result. After 6 months there has been no recurrence.

□□□

Chapter 13

Characteristics and Diseases Caused by Group I DS DNA Polyomaviruses (Family *Polyomaviridae*)

Contents

Characteristics of Polyomaviruses

Polyomaviruses belong to the family *polyomaviridae*, are naked having an icosahedra symmetry with 72 capsomers (T = 7) & a diameter of about 45 nm. The viral genome has circular, **monopartite, double-stranded DNA that exists in a** supercoiled structure **in the virion and is** associated with histones H2a, H2b, H3, and H4 **derived from the host. Both DNA strands code for proteins. The length of polyomavirus genomes is about 5 kilobases. Polyomaviruses have five to seven proteins, including** three capsid proteins, VP1, VP2, and VP3 **(Fig 13-1),** and two proteins, T and t, which are involved in viral DNA replication & a agnoprotein. Polyomaviruses were previously included in the family *Papovaviridae* with the papillomaviruses but now a day papillomaviruses was separated in the family *Papillomaviridae* as discussed above & polyomaviruses belong to the family *Polyomaviridae*. Polyomaviruses (G. poly= several, oma= tumor) refers to the viruses' ability to produce multiple tumors in mouse & other species. These viruses often **persist as latent infections in a host without causing disease**, but may produce tumors in a host of a different species, or a host with an ineffective immune system. *Polyomavirus* is the only genus of the family *Polyomaviridae* with type species *African green monkey polyomavirus.* First of all, murine polyomavirus was discovered by Ludwik Gross in 1953 & subsequently, many polyomaviruses have been detected to infect mammals & birds. In the past polyomaviruses were studied as tumor viruses in humans and animals, which led to basic understanding of carcinogenesis, DNA replication and protein processing.

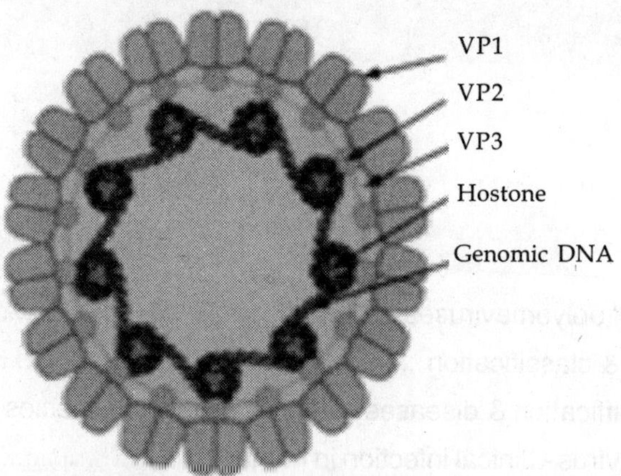

Figure 13.1: Morphology of a Polyomavirus

Polyomaviruses have been divided into **three major clades** or **genetically-related groups:** they include:

1. SV40 clade,
2. An avian clade &
3. Murine polyomavirus clade.

The SV40 clade includes many members; i. *Simian virus 40* (SV-40), ii. *JC polyomavirus* (JCPyV), iii *BK polyomavirus* (BKPLV), & iv. *Simian virus 12* (SV12).

The avian clade includes 2 members namely, i. *Avian polyomavirus* (BFDPyV) that causes Budgerigar Fledgling disease & ii. *Goose hemorrhagic polyomavirus.*

The murine polyomavirus clade includes 3 members, namely, i. *California sea lion polyomavirus* 1, ii. *Murine pneumotropic virus* & iii.*Squirrel monkey polyomavirus.*

The viral genome

The virus genome is circular, made of double stranded DNA of about 5 kilobase pairs in length and contains six genes that comprise: large T, small t, viral protein 1 (VP1), viral protein 2 (VP2), and viral protein 3 (VP3) and agnoprotein. Of these, VP1-3 forms the viral capsid. Transcription is characterized by **2 phases of gene expression, early phase** produces proteins involved in replication (though there is no viral polymerase) and **late phase** encodes proteins involved in capsid formation. Varied transcripts are produced through splicing. Replication and virion assembly occur in the nucleus, and virions are released by destruction of the nuclear and cell membranes.

Virus replication

Virus replication takes place in the cell nucleus but unlike papillomaviruses, **polyomaviruses grow in culture in vitro often causing malignant transformation in cells from heterologous species**. First of all, virion attaches with VP1 to cell receptors- sialic acid residues of gangliosides. Polyomavirus virions are then endocytosed and transported first to the endoplasmatic reticulum where a conformational change occurs revealing Vp2 & then the virus is exported to the nucleus. Polyomaviruses while replicating in the nucleus use the host's machinery because of homologous genomic structure to that of the mammalian host. Viral replication occurs in phases; **early gene expression, genome replication and late gene expression. Early gene** expression is responsible for the synthesis of non-structural proteins that regulate the cellular mechanisms. Enhancer elements lie close to the N terminal which induces activation and transcription of a molecule known as the T-antigen. Early mRNAs are produced by host RNA polymerase II. T-antigen autoregulates early mRNAs. Due to elevated levels of T-antigen, early gene expression is repressed, triggering the late phase of viral infection to begin.

Thereafter genome replication occurs that separate the early and late phase gene expression. The duplicated viral genome is synthesized and processed as if it were cellular DNA, exploiting the host's machinery. As the daughter viral DNAs are synthesized, they associate with cellular nucleosomes to form structures that are often referred to as "minichromosomes". In this manner the DNA is packaged more efficiently.

After genome replication, production of the structural proteins, responsible for the viral particle composition occurs. Like the early gene expression products, late gene expression generates an array of proteins as a result of alternative splicing. Within each viral protein are 'nuclear localization signals' which cause the viral proteins to amass in the nucleus. Assembly of new virus particles then occurs within the nucleus of the host cell.

Release of newly synthesized polyomaviruses occurs; the viruses exit the infected cell by one of two mechanisms. **Less commonly**, they are transported in cytoplasmic vacuoles to the plasma membrane & bud. **More frequently**, the virus particles are released after the cell lysis caused by the cytotoxicity of virus particles present in the infected cell.

The Polyoma large and small T-Antigen

The **large T-antigen** plays a key role in regulating the viral life cycle by binding to the viral origin of DNA replication where it promotes DNA synthesis. Also as the polyomavirus relies on the host cell machinery to replicate, the host cell needs to be in S-phase for this to begin. Due to this, large T-antigen also modulates cellular signaling pathways to stimulate progression of the cell cycle by binding to a number of cellular control proteins. This is achieved by a two prong attack of **inhibiting tumor suppressing genes p53** and members of the **retinoblastoma (pRB)** family, and stimulating cell growth pathways by binding cellular DNA, ATPase-helicase, DNA polymerase α association, and binding of transcription preinitiation complex factors. This abnormal stimulation of the cell cycle is a powerful force for oncogenic transformation.

The **small t-antigen** protein is also able to activate several cellular pathways which stimulate cell proliferation such as the mitogen-activated protein kinasc (MAPK) pathway, and the stress-activated protein kinase (SAPK) pathway.

The Polyoma Middle T-Antigen

The Polyoma Middle T-Antigen is used in animal breast cancer model system like the PYMT system where it is coupled to the MMTV promoter. There it functions as an oncogene while the tissue where the tumor develops is determined by the MMTV promoter.

Virus classification

Group: Group I dsDNA

Family: *Polyomaviridae*

Genus: *Orthopolyomavirus:*TSSV 40

Species Name	Abbreviation
B-lymphotropic polyomavirus (formerly known as African green monkey polyomavirus, AGMPyV)	LPyV
Baboon polyomavirus 1 (formerly known as Simian Agent 12)	SA12
Bat polyomavirus (formerly known as Myotis polyomavirus, MyPyV)	BatPyV
BK polyomavirus	BKPyV
Bornean orang-utan polyomavirus	OraPyV1
Bovine polyomavirus	BPyV
California sea lion polyomavirus	SLPyV
Hamster polyomavirus	HaPyV
JC polyomavirus	JCPyV
Merkel Cell polyomavirus	MCPyV
Murine pneumotropic virus (formerly known as Kilham strain of Polyomavirus, Kilham virus, K virus)	MPtV
Murine polyomavirus	MPyV
Simian virus 40 (formerly known as Simian vacuolating virus 40)	SV40
Squirrel monkey polyomavirus	SqPyV
Sumatran orang-utan polyomavirus	OraPyV2
Trichodysplasia spinuolsa-associated polyomavirus	TSPyV

Other related virus that may be a member of the genus Orthopolyomavirus but has not been approved as a species:

ChPyV: Chimpanzee polyomavirus

Genus Wukipolyomavirus (type species KI polyomavirus)

Species Name	Abbreviation
Human polyomavirus 6	HPyV6
Human polyomavirus 7	HPyV7
KI polyomavirus (formerly known as Karolinska Institute polyomavirus)	KIPyV
WU polyomavirus (formerly known as Washington University polyomavirus)	WUPyV

Genus Avipolyomavirus (type species Avian polyomavirus)

Species Name	Abbreviation
Avian polyomavirus (formerly known as Budgerigar Fledgling disease Polyomavirus, BFPyV)	APyV
Canary polyomavirus	CaPyV
Crow polyomavirus	CPyV
Finch polyomavirus	FPyV
Goose hemorrhagic polyomavirus	GHPyV

Table 13-1 briefly classifies the family *Polyomaviridae* & mentions the diseases caused by the virus species.

Table 13.1 : Classification of the family *Polyomaviridae* & the diseases caused by the member viruses in humans & animals.

G 1: *Orthopolyomavirus/Species*	Serotypes	Diseases caused
B-lymphotropic polyomavirus *(African green monkey polyomavirus)*	LPyV(AGMPyV)	
Baboon polyomavirus 1 (Simian Agent 12))	BPYV-1	
BK polyomavirus	BKPyV	Causes mild respiratory tract infection in children & in young adult humans.
Hamster polyomavirus	HaPyV	
JC *polyomavirus*	JCPyV	Infects resp system, affects kidney & brain in young humans, sometimes with fatality. In immunecompromized humans, JCV is reactivated in the brain causing progressive multifocal leuco encephalopathy (PML).
Merkel cell polyomavirus	MCPyV	Cause most cases of Merkel skin carcinoma in humans.
Murine pneumotropic virus	MPtV	
Murine polyomavirus	MPyV	
Rabbit kidney vacuolating virus	RKV	
Simian virus 12	SV-12	

TS: Simian virus 40	SV-40	
Trichodysplasia spinuolsa-associated polyomavirus	TSPyV	
G2:*Wukipolyomavirus (type species KI polyomavirus)*		
Human polyomavirus 6	HPyV6	
Human polyomavirus 7	HPyV7	
KI polyomavirus	KIPyV	Isolated from respiratory secretions, causes widespread mild infection in younger humans.
WU polyomavirus (Washington University polyomaviru)	WUPyV	Do
G3: *Avipolyomavirus*		
Avian polyomavirus(Budgerian fledgling disease polyomavirus)	APyV	Causes acute, often fatal generalized infection in young budgerigars.
Canary polyomavirus	CaPyV	
Crow polyomavirus	CPyV	
Finch polyomavirus	FPyV	
Goose Hemorrhagic polyomavirus	GHPyV	

Polyomaviral Clinical Manifestations in Humans

All the polyomaviruses in humans are common childhood and young adult infections causing little or no symptoms but are probably **life-long persistent among almost all adults.** HPyVs cause human infections which are common among persons immunosuppressed by AIDS, old age or after transplantation and include Merkel cell carcinoma, PML and BK nephropathy.

JC polyomavirus (JCPyV) infects respiratory tract, kidney & brain; about 80% of adults worldwide are positive for JCV infection; majority showing no clinical symptoms & people are infected in childhood. JCPyV remains latent in the lymphocytes, urogenital tract, and brain of its host and may reactivate to cause disease in immunocompromised hosts causing **multifocal leukoencephalopathy (PML)**, a degenerative disease affecting the oligodendroglial cells in the brain. PML is characterized by development of impaired memory, confusion, disorientation, ataxia, hemiparesis, incoordination, seizures, and/or visual abnormalities. Death usually occurs within 3 to 6 months of onset of symptoms.

BK polyomavirus (BKPyV); about 80% of adults worldwide are seropositive for BKPyV but causes no disease in the immunocompetent population. BKV remains latent in the lymphocytes, urogenital tract, and brain of its host but may be reactivated if the host becomes immunocompromised.

Karolinska Institute polyomavirus (KI PyV) and Washington University virus (WUPyV) are related and isolated from respiratory secretions. In 2010, two additional viruses related to KI and WU were identified in human skin secretions; they cause widespread mild infection in younger humans.

Merkel cell polyomavirus (MCPyV) discovered in 2008 causes the majority of cases of Merkel cell carcinoma, a rare but aggressive form of skin cancer.

Trichodysplasia spinulosa-associated polyomavirus (TSV) discovered in 2010, was detected in the proliferative skin lesion from immunosuppressed patients.

HPyV9 discovered in 2011 is related to a monkey lymphotropic virus (LPV) was isolated in culture from the blood of immunosuppressed patients.

Clinical infections in animals & birds

Simian virus 40 (SV-40) among animal polyomaviruses was isolated as contaminant of Sabin polio virus, replicates in the kidneys of monkeys without causing disease but causes sarcomas in hamasters. The tumor suppressor protein p53 was discovered as a cellular protein bound by the major oncoprotein T antigen made by *Simian vacuolating virus 40*. There was concern that SV40 could cause tumors in humans but studies failed to demonstrate an association between SV40 and human tumors. However, the presence of SV40 antigen sequences in certain rare human tumors has renewed interest in SV40 virus.

Avian Polyomavirus / Budgerigar Fledgling Disease

The avian polyomavirus also called as the *Budgerigar fledgling disease polyomavirus* (BFDPyV) (APyV) causes an acute, frequently fatal, generalized infection in young budgerigars. Neonates develop disease normally when 10-15 day old, then suddenly die with no clinical signs. Mortality is highest in Budgerigars less than 15 days old. Mortality rates vary from 30 to 100%. There is decreased hatchability, embryonic death, abdominal distension in hatchlings, subcutaneous hemorrhages, tremors of head and neck, ataxia, reduced feather down and contour feathers. Symmetrical feather abnormalities in survivors include: dystrophic primary and tail feathers, lack of down feathers on back and abdomen, & lack of filoplumes on head and neck.

Etiology : *Avian polyomavirus* / Budgerigar fledgling disease (BFD) is caused by the virus *Budgerigar fledgling disease polyomavirus APyV*/(BFDPyV).

Occurrence

Budgerigar fledgling disease (BFD) was first reported as a clinical syndrome in 1976 and was first reported as a disease affecting budgerigars (*Melopsittacus undulatus*) in the United States and Canada in 1981. Since its initial recognition as an etiologic agent of disease in psittacine birds, BFD virus has spread throughout aviaries and the pet trade & now a day, it is a leading cause of death in psittacine birds. Avian polyomavirus is distributed worldwide, but there are some apparent regional differences in the clinical changes associated with infections in budgerigars. For example, in Europe a more chronic form of the disease is common in budgerigars, while in the United States and Canada an acute form of disease with high mortality is typical.

Hosts susceptible

Avian polyomaviruses appear to infect a wide variety of Psittaciformes (parrots), Passeriformes (weaver finches, canaries) and gallinaceous birds (chickens and turkeys). In an aviary with BFD, nestling budgerigars, 1-3 weeks of age suffer the highest mortality. A striking finding in these birds is the almost total lack of downy feather development, which is prominent even in budgerigars that survive up to 28 days of age. Normal baby budgerigars are hatched without feathers, but down begins to cover the skin by about 12 days of age; plumage development is complete at a little more than 1 month of age.

Transmission

BFDV is capable of both vertical and horizontal transmission as a result of contact with infected body secretion or feather dander. Birds infected by vertical transmission may have normal development for the first 2 weeks but mortality rates are 30-100% within this time. It is highly contagious and can be transmitted through the egg, regurgitation of crop milk to neonates, contaminated respiratory secretions in the air, feather dander and excrement. Stress associated with changes in weather, diet, breeding or concomitant disease may cause **persistently infected budgerigars to shed virus resulting in outbreaks of disease. Persistence of virus in the kidneys of budgerigars, with subsequent excretion in the urine, has been proposed as a method of virus transmission.** In polyomavirus outbreaks at 23 different budgerigar aviaries, the onset of disease could be traced to the addition of new, clinically normal breeders. Persistently infected budgerigars shed virus resulting in outbreaks of disease. Unvaccinated susceptible psittacine birds may be exposed to polyomavirus through exposure to virus-contaminated feces, feather dust, urates and respiratory secretions. The potential for intraspecies transmission of polyomavirus may be a particular problem for pet retailers that maintain both budgerigars and non budgerigar psittacine birds. In one environmental study, it was found that polyomavirus nucleic acid could be detected using DNA amplification and detection techniques in all of 5 samples collected from 3 different pet shops which housed budgerigars. Budgerigars should be considered the primary reservoir of polyomavirus. 'The potential for budgerigars to continue to spread this environmentally stable virus among unvaccinated psittacine birds is cause for action.

Pathogenesis

Transmission & pathogenesis of BFD have not been fully described. Virus particles have been demonstrated in epithelia of feather follicles, esophagus, crop, lung, and kidney, thus implicating several possible routes of transmission. Feather dust, regurgitated food fed to nestlings, respiratory secretions, and/ or urinary excretions could all contain infectious virus and serve as a source of infection. Vertical transmission of the virus through the egg also has been considered. Inclusion bodies have been demonstrated in the internal organs and skin of 1-day-old budgerigars, and eggs from breeding pairs producing affected young will result in diseased birds when fostered by pairs whose own young are normal.

Clnical symptoms & lesions

The type of clinical disease induced by BFV in budgerigars seems to be influenced by the **age and condition of a budgerigar when it is exposed to the virus**. Budgerigar neonates from infected flocks may develop normally for 10 to 15 days and then die suddenly without premonitory signs. Other infected hatchings may develop clinical signs, including **abdominal distention, hemorrhage under the skin and reduced formation of down and contour feathers**. Some infected budgerigars have been reported to develop neurologic signs characterized by **ataxia** (incoordination) and tremors of the head and neck several days before dying. Infected budgerigars that die shortly after hatching routinely develop more severe and widespread lesions than do birds in which the morbid state is more prolonged. The mortality rate associated with naturally acquired avian polyomavirus infections in young budgerigars may range from 25% to 100%, depending on the age of the birds. **Older birds are relatively resistant to disease**, while at the peak of viral activity, up to 100% of exposed budgerigars less than 15 days of age may die. The mortality rate reported for older (greater than 3 weeks of age) juveniles ranges from 30% to 80%. Although mortality rates vary with the age of the exposed birds, polyomavirus infections in young budgerigars usually are rapidly fatal once clinical signs develop. In most aviary outbreaks, the incidence of clinically recognized disease will progressively increase during a period of several months, with peak virus activity occurring during the most active portion of the breeding season. In one particularly aggressive outbreak of avian polyomavirus, 90% of young budgerigars were affected within a 2-to 3-week period.

Reports vary on the effect of avian polyomavirus on egg and embryonic development. Findings from the first report suggest that avian polyomavirus can cause embryonic deaths and decreased hatchability, while findings from the second study suggest that avian polyomavirus infections do not cause problems in embryonic development. It is possible that both findings are correct and the effect of the virus may depend on as yet unidentified factors. Like mammals, **budgerigars that recover from polyomavirus infections are thought to remain persistently infected.** Evidence suggests that these **persistently infected budgerigars** are responsible for the spread of this virus through budgerigar flocks and within the avicultural industry.

Polyomavirus **inclusion bodies frequently can be detected in feathers, feather follicles, spleen, liver and Kidney from persistently infected, clinically normal adult budgerigars.** Viral inclusion bodies are common in the **renal tubular epithelium.** Persistence of virus in the kidneys of budgerigars, with subsequent excretion in the urine, has been proposed as a method of virus transmission. Viral nucleic acid has been detected in the excrement, feathers and oral mucosa of clinically normal budgerigars.

Histological lesions varied among birds, essentially similar changes were present in all. The most consistent finding was cells with **karyomegaly**. In these cells, the nucleus was enlarged, had marginated chromatin, and often contained a large slightly basophilic to amphophilic inclusion. These cells were **most prominent in feather follicles,** which often were severely affected, although not all follicles were involved. Focal to confluent ballooning degeneration with karyomegaly was prominent in follicular epithelial cells, barb ridges, and cells within the pulp. Karyomegalic cells also were in scattered foci in renal tubular epithelium, glomeruli, brain, spleen, liver, myocardium, pancreas, intestine, lung, skeletal muscle, and bone marrow. In many hepatic periportal zones, there was minimal necrosis with a minimal to moderate number of heterophils. Occasional small foci of coagulation necrosis with heterophils were randomly scattered in the parenchyma. Splenic white pulp was hypercellular with small foci of karyomegalic cells present. The walls of many small arteries and sheathed capillaries also were prominent because of hypertrophy and karyomegaly of the surrounding cells.

Diagnosis

Death at 10-28 days of age with a significant lack of feather development should hint the possibility of BFD. The combination of typical gross necropsy findings like stunted growth, abnormal feather development, and microscopic lesions, including pronounced karyomegaly with **intranuclear inclusions,** leads to a presumptive diagnosis of BFD.

Serologic testing has shown that viral antibodies remain elevated for the lifetime of a persistently infected (carrier) bird. Persistently infected female birds can raise serologically negative uninfected chicks and immunocompetent adult birds can be caged with persistently infected birds and will remain uninfected.

The diagnosis should be substantiated by virus isolation or by identification of the virus via specific immunofluorescence. DNA amplification via the polymerase chain reaction can also be used to detect BFD virus.

Treatment & prevention

In budgerigars, which are known to develop persistent polyomavirus infections, the detection of polyomavirus neutralizing antibodies can be used to screen for infected budgerigars which should be considered a risk for transmitting the virus. Testing budgerigars for the presence of virus-neutralizing antibodies and culling positive birds has been suggested as a method to establish flocks of polyomavirus-free budgerigars. Additionally, depopulation of budgerigar aviaries experiencing outbreaks, followed by restocking with seronegative birds has been suggested as a method of controlling enzootic infections in this species. By using a serologic assay to establish "polyomavirus-free" budgerigars followed by vaccination to protect the budgerigars from subsequent infection, it should be possible to prevent polyomavirus-induced disease in the budgerigar aviary and reduce the role that budgerigars play as a reservoir for polyomavirus in the pet trade.

Vaccination

In non budgerigar psittacine birds, polyomavirus can be controlled using an **inactivated avian polyomavirus vaccine.** Controlling polyomavirus infections in budgerigars presents a different set of problems. It is important for the avicultural industry to control polyomavirus in budgerigars because this group of birds is serving as a reservoir for the virus. A vaccine was developed by identifying a virus isolate which, when administered intramuscularly, will cause an immune response without inducing virus shedding or detectable persistence of the virus. None of the vaccinates had any clinically recognizable adverse reactions following vaccination. The results of this study indicated that the experimental budgerigar polyomavirus vaccine induced a detectable virus-neutralizing antibody response when injected **intramuscularly,** considered an unnatural route of exposure. Serum was tested for virus-neutralizing antibodies on day 0 (which was also the day of vaccination) and approximately 1 month later. None of the vaccinated birds had any clinically recognizable adverse reactions. These safety and immunogenicity trials suggest that the experimental budgerigar vaccine will induce an immune response, as detected by a significant increase in virus-neutralizing antibodies, when injected intramuscularly and that vaccinates do not shed a sufficient quantity of viable virus to be a risk for infecting birds with which they are in direct contact.

□□□

Chapter 14

Characteristics and Diseases Caused by Group II Single-Stranded DNA Parvoviruses (Family *Parvoviridae*)

Contents

Characteristics of Parvoviruses

Parvoviruses (L. parvus= small) belongs to *Parvoviridae* family, are among the **smallest, simplest eukaryotic viruses**, each virion measuring 20-25 nm in diameter. The virus is naked & contains an **icosahedral capsid symmetry** made of 60 capsomers (Fig 14-1).

The genome contains an infectious single stranded DNA of only **5 kilobases.** These viruses are **one of the most environmentally resistant viruses**. Parvoviruses of veterinary importance were discovered in the 1960s while human parvovirus infections were only recognized in the 1980s and affect both vertebrates & insects. Some members of *Parvovirus* agglutinate RBCs (hemagglutination), a feature used in some diagnostic tests; these hemagglutinating viruses have an erythrocyte attachment protein (hemagglutinin) on their surface.

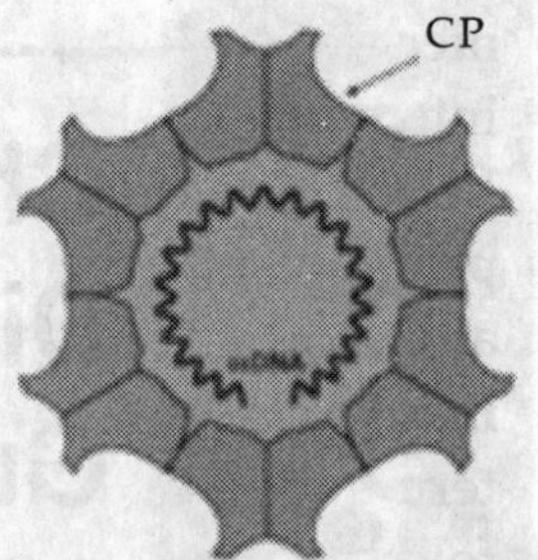

Fig. 14.1 : Morphology of parvovirus

The *Parvoviridae* may be small, but they are mighty & stable in the environment. These viruses are very stable, surviving temperatures of up to **60^0 C** at a **pH 3-9.** Parvoviruses are resistant to lipid solvents, pH 3-9, heating at 56^{0}C, but are killed by formalin, β propiolactone, sodium hypochlorite & oxidizing agents. Parvoviruses of vertebrates agglutinate erythrocytes except *Aleutian mink disease virus & Goose parvovirus.*

The viral genome

The virus genome is not segmented and contains a single molecule of **linear, negative-sense, single-stranded DNA in most cases,** or of linear, **negative-sense and positive-sense single-stranded DNA in up to 50% in some members.** The genome has terminally redundant sequences repeated at both ends and 5000 nucleotides long. Nucleuotide sequences at the 3'-terminus are complementary to similar regions on the 5' end, or unrelated to the 5'-terminus. The 5'-terminus sequence has palindromic repeats, forming a hairpin structure; terminal repeats at the 5'-end are 200-242 nucleotides long. The 3'-terminus has conserved nucleotide sequences of 115-116 nucleotides in length. In species of same genus; sequence has hairpin structure. Populations of mature viruses contain particles with equivalent numbers of positive and negative sense ssDNA. The complementary DNA strands usually form dsDNA upon extraction. The genome has **two open reading frames** (ORF), a right handed ORF encodes the two capsid proteins, VP1 and VP 2, which are transcribed from alternatively spliced mRNA. **The left-handed ORF encodes at least one of the nonstructural proteins (NS1).** Its small genome size allows it very limited coding potential, and prohibits it from inducing replication in host cells. Hence, they are only able to **replicate in dividing cells such as marrow, gut and the developing fetus cells.**

Virus replication

The parvoviruses replicate in the nucleus of **dividing cells** with the use of cellular enzymes. The genome is replicated through **rolling-hairpin**

mechanism. Gene expression requires host proteins to transcribe the genomes into mRNAs. Depending on the virus, there can be one (Erythrovirus and Iteravirus), two (Densovirus and Brevidensovirus) or three (Dependovirus) promoters for mRNA transcription. Some mRNAs are spliced allowing alternative forms of the protein to be produced. The viruses have **unique mechanism of DNA replication.** All parvovirus genomes contain long terminal palindromic sequences, which enable each end of the molecule to fold back on itself to form a **hairpin** structure that is useful during replication. The **palindromic sequence serves as a self-primer for initiation of synthesis of plus sense DNA.** In this type of mechanism of viral replication, the growing strand replicates back on itself, producing a tetramic form from which two plus strands and two minus strands are generated by endonuclease cleavage. All **replication takes place in the nucleus** and occurs only in **dividing cells** with the use of cellular enzymes.

Virus first penetrates into the host cell followed by uncoating, and release of the viral genomic ssDNA into the nucleus. The ssDNA is converted into replicative form of dsDNA by cellular proteins. Viral mRNAs are transcribed when host cell enters **S- phase** and translated to produce viral proteins. Virus replication occurs through rolling-hairpin mechanism, with NS1 nickase binding covalently to the 5′ genomic end. Individual ssDNA genomes are excised from replication concatemers by means of junction resolution. The newly synthesized ssDNA can either: be converted to dsDNA and serve as a template for transcription/replication, or be encapsidated to form new virions that can bud out of the host cell.

Virus classification

Group: Group II ssDNA

Family: *Parvoviridae*

Subfamilies: SF 1: *Parvovirinae* & SF 2: *Densovirinae*

Subfamily 1: *Parvovirinae*

Genus 1: *Parvovirus*; type species: *Murine minute virus*

Genus 2: *Erythrovirus*; type species: B 19 virus

Genus 3: *Dependovirus*; type species: *Adeno-associated virus 2*

Genus 4: *Amdovirus*; type species: *Aleutian mink disease virus*

Genus 5: *Bocavirus*; type species: *Bovine parvovirus*

Subfamily 2: *Densovirinae*

Genus 1: *Densovirus;* type species: *Junonia coeniadensovirus*

Genus 2: *Iteravirus;* type species: *Bombyx moridensovirus*

Genus 3: *Brevidensovirus;* type species: *Aedes aegyptidensovirus*

Genus 4: *Pefudensovirus;* type species: *Periplanta fuliginosadensovirus*

Clinical manifestations

Among the two subfamilies- *Parvovirinae* which includes viruses of vertebrates & *Densovirinae* whose members infects arthropods, only the genus *Parvovirus* species cause many serious diseases in several species of animals & one species infects humans. Among the *Human parvoviruses, B19* is associated with very common **exanthemous** disease of children with **hydrops fetalis** and **aplastic crises** in patients with chronic hemolytic anemia. *Human bocavirus causes* lower respiratory tract infection & is also associated with gastroenteritis.

Among animals infections, *Feline panleukopenia virus* causes panleucopenia in young kittens, *Canine parvovirus* 2 causes very serious enteric disease in young pups with depression, vomting, dysentery & immunosuppression, *Mink enteritis virus* causes enteritis in minks like panleukopenia, *Porcine parvovirus* causes stillbirth, mummified fetuses, embryonic death & reproductive failure in sows, & *Aleutian mink disease virus causes* progressive wasting disease with high mortality in Aleutian minks. *Duck parovirus* causes Derzy's disease/ hepatitis, myositis & myocarditis in gosling & Muscovy ducks.

Table 14-1 presented below shows classification of the family *Parvoviridae* & diseases caused by the member viruses.

Table 14.1 : Classification of the family *Parvoviridae* & diseases caused by the member viruses in humans & animals.

Genera	Species	Serotypes	Diseases caused
G1: *Parvovirus*	*Feline panleukopenia virus*	FPV	Feline panleukopenia (FPV) or feline infectious enterit is, feline distemperis a widespread, common, highly contagious disease of domestic and wild cats of 3-5 months old. Disease is characterized by sudden onset, fever, anorexia, depression, diarrhea, vomiting, nasal discharge,

		dehydration and high mortality with severe and prolonged leucopenia. Infected cats may die in three days after onset with mortality rate up to 90%. Virus main targets cells are lymphoid tissues associated with the oropharynx, after viraemia, the secondary targets are lymph nodes, spleen, thymus, bone marrow and intestinal crypts. Infection of the fetus may lead to embryonic or fetal death, resorption or abortion but late infection leads to cerebellar infection, leading to hypoplasia and ataxia. FPV is transmitted via nasal secretions, feces and urine in which virus is present. Cats get infected by ingestion and transmission is by direct and indirect contact like fomites.
Canine parvovirus	CPV	*Canine parvoviruss*-2 (CPV-2) is a highly contagious disease of dogs less than 6 months old with severe diarrhoea, vomition, leucopenia, immunosupression & often death; intrauterine or perinatal infection causes myocarditis in pups. Dogs become infected with CPV2 via feces, infected soil, or fomites carrying the virus. After ingestion, the virus replicates in the lymphoid tissue in the throat, viremia follows, and the virus then attacks rapidly dividing cells, like those in the lymph nodes, intestinal crysts &

		bone marrow with depletion of lymphocytes in lymph nodes, necrosis & destruction of the intestinal crypts & secondary bacterial infection. After 3-4 days of infection, the virus is shed in the feces for up to three weeks, & the puppies become asymptomatic carrier and shed the virus periodically. The disease is deadly if the host is concurrently infested with worms or other intestinal parasites. If puppies are infected in the uterus or shortly after birth till 8 weeks of age, the virus attacks the heart muscle and the puppy often dies suddenly or after a brief period of breathing difficulty.
		CPV-2
Mink enteritis virus	MEV	Causes enteritis in mink.
Racoon parvovirus	RPV	Causes enteritis in racoons.
HB parvovirus	HBPV	
H-1parvovirus	H-1PV	
Kilhan rat virus	KRV	
Lapine parvovirus	LPV	
LuIII virus	LuIIIV	
TS: *Minute virus of mice*	MVMc	
Mouse parvovirus 1	MPV-1	
Porcine parvovirus	PPV-kr	*Porcine parvovirus* (PPV) infection is the most important cause of infectious infertility. The virus multiplies in the pig intestine without causing clinical signs & is worldwide in its distribution. The virus has no effect on the female but

			only on the fetus. In pregnant sows infected before 35 days of gestation, there are small litters size associated with embryo loss, mummified fetuses of varying size, increased numbers of stillbirths & delay in the farrowing mechanism due to the presence of the mummified piglet; abortions are uncommon, & there may be an increase in low birth weight piglets but neonatal deaths are not seen. If the viruses crosses the placenta in the last trimester, neonatal death may occur, or the birth of healthy piglets with a protective pre-colostral immunity. **SMEDI** indicates stillbirth, mummification, embryonic death, and infertility, is a reproductive disease of swine caused by PPV and *porcine enterovirus.*
	RT parvovirus	RTPV	
	Tumor virus x	TVx	
	Hamster parvovirus	HaPV	
	Rat minute virus 1	RMV-1	
	Rat parvovirus1	RPV-1	
G 2: *Erythrovirus*	TS: *Human parvovirus 19*	B19V	*Human parvovirus 19* **(B19V)** causes childhood rash called exanthema, erythema infectiosum or aplastic anemia (slapped rash symptoms on cheeck).
	Pig tailed macaque parvovirus	PMPV	
	Simian parvovirus	SPV	
	T. *Bovine parvovirus 3*	BPV-3	
G 3: *Dependovirus*	*TS: Adeno-associatd virus 2*	AAV-2	

	Duck parvovirus	BDPV, MDPV	*Duck parvovirus* (**BDPV/ MDPV** causes Derzy's disease/ hepatitis in Muscovy ducks worldwide. Clinical symptoms are like goslings infection & include huddling together, inability to walk, dragging of legs behind the duckling, and enteric signs with no feather loss (unlike goose parvovirus), & the main finding is hepatopathology.
	Goose parvovirus	GPV	*Goose parvovirus* (**GPV**) causes goose viral hepatitis, infection is a highly contagious and fatal disease of goslings and Muscovy ducklings that has been reported from Europe and the Far East where the disease is of serious economic significance.
	Bovine parvovirus 2	BPV-2	
G 4: *Amdovirus*	TS: *Aleutian mink disease virus*	AMDV	Aleutian mink disease (**AMDV**) or Mink plasmacytosis is a highly contagious parvovirus infection of mustelids, causing spontaneous abortion & death in minks & ferrets. AMDV is transmitted via ferret's bodily fluids, & remain dormant in dried urine or on an owner's clothes and shoes for up to two years until stress or injury. AMDV itself causes little or no harm to the host, but the virus produces large antibodies causing systemic vasculitis with renal failure, bone marrow suppression and death. The symptoms are chronic, progressive weight loss, lethargy,

			splenomegaly, anemia, rear leg weakness, seizures and black tarry stool. Then the disease progresses rapidly, usually to death within a few months.
G 5: *Bocavirus*	TS: *Bovine parvovirus*	BPV	*Bovine parvovirus* under the genus *Bocavirus* **(BPV)** causes subclinical infection in cattle & sporadic outbreaks with enteritis & diarrhea in calves.
	Human bocavirus	HBoV	*Human bocavirus* **(HBoV)** was reported in Sweden from clinical samples from infants and children with respiratory tract illness. The role of HBoV in respiratory tract illnesses is unknown but may cause mild lower respiratory tract infection & gastroenteritis.

Parvovirus Clinical Manifestions in Humans

Human Infections
Genus: *Erythrovirus*

Human parvovirus 19 **(B19V)** causes childhood **rash called exanthema, erythema infectiosum or aplastic anemia** (slapped rash symptoms on cheeck).
Genus: *Bocavius:*

Human bocavirus **(HBoV)** was reported in Sweden from clinical samples from infants and children with respiratory tract illness. The genome of HBoV is closely related to canine minute virus and bovine parvovirus, which are members of the genus *Bocavirus*. The role of HBoV in respiratory tract illnesses is unknown but may cause mild lower respiratory tract infection & gastroenteritis.

Parvovirus Clinical Infections in Animals

SF : *Parvovirinae*
Genus: *Parvovirus:*

Feline Panleukopenia

Feline panleukopenia (FP) also known as feline infectious enteritis, feline distemper, feline ataxia, or cat plague, is a widespread, common, highly contagious disease of domestic and wild cats of 3-5 month age with reduced maternal antibodies. The disease is characterized by sudden onset, fever, anorexia, depression, diarrhea, vomiting, nasal discharge, dehydration and high mortality with severe and prolonged leucopenia. Infected cats may die in three days after onset with mortality rate up to 90%. **Virus main targets cells are lymphoid** tissues associated with the oropharynx, after viremia, the secondary targets are **lymph nodes, spleen, thymus, bone marrow and intestinal crypts**. Infection of the fetus may lead to embryonic or fetal death, resorption or abortion but late infection causes cerebellar infection, leading to hypoplasia and ataxia. Subclinical infections are also common, & asymptomatic infections occur in older cats.

Etiology: Feline panleukopenia is caused by *Feline panleukopenia virus* (FPV) in the genus *Parvovirus*.The name, panleukopenia, is derived from the **low white blood cell count** exhibited by the affected animals. Feline panleukopenia and canine parvovirus are extremely closely related, and viruses can be transmitted between dogs and cats.

Occurrence

Although the virus can affect cats of all ages, feline panleukopenia is primarily a **disease of kittens**. The characteristics of the disease may vary considerably from population to population and from outbreak to outbreak. In susceptible populations, the disease may affect nearly 100 percent of individuals; in other populations, only a few animals may be affected. There is a seasonal occurrence of panleukopenia that usually coincides with the production of new populations of susceptible kittens. This seasonal effect may vary according to geographic location. In the northeastern United States, most cases of panleukopenia are seen during the summer and early fall. However, outbreaks of panleukopenia may occur at any time of the year. Among affected kittens, those of two months or less of age, 5% die regardless of treatment. Kittens that are more than two months old have a 60-70% mortality rate with treatment and a nearly 100% mortality rate if not treated. Adult cats have a 10-20% mortality rate if treated, and an 85% mortality rate if not treated. Elderly cats have a 20-30% mortality rate if treated and a 90% mortality rate if not treated. Panleukopenia rarely occurs in populations in which vaccination is routinely practiced.

Hosts susceptible

Domestic and wild cats of 3-5 month age with reduced maternal antibodies are particularly more susceptible. Areas with large populations of unvaccinated cats, such as feral colonies or homes of cat collectors, are particularly susceptible to panleukopenia outbreaks.

Transmission

The feline panleukopenia virus (FVP) is extremely hardy and may survive for months, and even years. FPV is transmitted via **nasal secretions, feces and urine carrying the virus.** Cats get infected by ingestion and transmission is by direct and indirect contact like fomites. It is easily transmitted through contact, either cat-to-cat, or by human-to-cat. The common source of disease spread is through shared food and water bowls, litter pans, & bedding, mutual grooming, by fleas during the active stage, *in utero* from an infected queen, human handling can transfer the FVP virus from one cat to another, & by contact through hands, clothing, and shoes.

Pathogenesis

The virus usually enters orally, with infection occurring primarily in the lymphoid tissues of the oropharynx (tonsillar area) and intestine. Within twenty-four hours of infection, virus is present in the blood, which distributes it throughout the body. Within two days of infection, nearly every body tissue contains significant amounts of virus. As circulating antibodies appear, the amount of virus present gradually decreases. Small quantities of virus may persist for up to one year in certain tissues, but the strong immune response of the host usually neutralizes the virus as it is shed, so that **most persistently infected kittens are not infectious.**

The most severely damaged tissues in the infected newborn cat are those undergoing **rapid cell division -the thymus, lymphoid organ in the chest, and the cerebellum.** Cells of the small intestine in neonates are not damaged, although the virus is present within them. In older kittens, the development of the disease also depends on the reproductive activity of the various tissues within the body. Lymphoid tissues, bone marrow, and the surface cells of the intestine are the most severely affected.

The virus main targets cells are **lymphoid tissues associated with the oropharynx, & after viremia, the secondary targets are** lymph nodes, spleen, thymus, bone marrow and intestinal crypts. The virus primarily attacks the lining of the gastroentstinal tract, causing **internal ulceration and, ultimately, total sloughing of the intestinal epithelium.** This results in profuse and usually **bloody diarrhea**, severe dehydratin, malnuritin, anemia, and often death. It causes a decrease in the cat's WBCs, thus compromising its immune system. Typically, it also causes a decrease in hematocrit and platelet counts on a blood count. This is often key in diagnosing panleukopenia. Terminal cases are hypothermic and may develop septic shock and disseminated intravascular coagulation. Most panleukopenia deaths are due to secondary infections or dehydration resulting from diarrhea. This is because the virus affects the infected cat's immune system, leaving it vulnerable to secondary infection.

If a cat is exposed during pregnancy, the virus can cause cerebellar hypolasia in her offspring. This is why administering modified live feline panleukopenia vaccine during pregnancy is discouraged.

Clinical symptoms & lesions

The **incubation period is usually from 4 - 10 days.** The initial symptoms are: vomiting, diarrhea, depression, disinterest in food and water, appearance of the third eyelid, or haw, in the inner corner of the eye, lack of grooming evidenced by dull & rough coat, evidence of abdominal pain, & a "hunched over" postural appearance. The severity of the clinical signs exhibited can vary tremendously from case to case. Many cats undergo a subclinical infection and do not show signs at all; others may experience a very mild clinical infection, in which a mildly elevated temperature, slight inappetence, and a borderline drop in the white blood cell count are observed. In the **typical case** of panleukopenia, clinical signs develop suddenly. The animal may have a rectal temperature of 104°F or greater and may be severely depressed and not eating. Vomiting usually occurs, and severe diarrhea may develop in 24-48 hours. If vomiting and diarrhea continue, severe dehydration and electrolyte imbalances occur.

Affected cats often assume a typical **hunched posture with the head between the forepaws.** Sometimes the head will hang over a water bowl or food dish. They often act as though they would like to drink and may even take a lap or two of milk or water, but they are unable or reluctant to swallow. The hair coat becomes rough and dull and there is a loss of elasticity of the skin due to the dehydration. The third eyelid (the haw in the corner of the eye toward the nose) often appears. The abdomen is painful, and on touching it will elicit a pain response. The lymph nodes in the abdomen are enlarged, and the digestive tract contains excessive amounts of gas and liquid. Cats that are not going to survive develop a subnormal temperature, with coma and death following in a few hours.

The mortality rate in an outbreak of panleukopenia may vary from 25 to 75 percent. Acute deaths may occur, with kittens showing no warning signs, often causing the owner to suspect poisoning. More commonly, deaths occur within the first five days of illness in uncomplicated cases, or later in cases subsequently complicated by other problems. If a cat survives the first five days of illness, and secondary complications such as bacterial infections or dehydration do not develop, then recovery should follow fairly rapidly. It usually requires several weeks, however, for the animal to regain its lost weight and condition.

Signs in kittens infected *in utero* or just after birth go unnoticed before sudden death, or until the development of ataxia at about two weeks of age when the kittens begin ambulating. The incoordination is exemplified by rolling or tumbling as the cat attempts to walk, by an involuntary twitching of the head, or by swaying of the body. If they are coordinated enough to obtain food, the kittens will survive; however, the ataxia will persist throughout life with little, if any, improvement or compensation as they grow older.

Diagnosis

Collection of clinical specimens for various test include small intestine, mesenteric lymph nodes, and spleen, & paired serum

1. *Presumptive diagnosis* : Diagnosis of feline panleukopenia can be made on the basis of the history, the clinical signs, and the presence of leukopenia. The common necropsy finding is hemorrhagic enteritis often involving the entire intestinal tract. Grossly, the intestine is often dilated and has a "ground glass" appearance. Microscopically, there is **necrosis of the epithelium and dilation of crypts. A leukopenia as low as 2 x 10^9/liter, occurs in FPL.**

The diagnosis can be confirmed by **HI test, widely used for as screening test, virus isolation** (growth of the virus in cells in the laboratory), identification of the virus in infected tissues, or by **demonstration of an increase in circulating antibodies** by testing paired samples-acute and convalescent serum samples taken several weeks apart. The increase in antibodies indicates recent infection.

Treatment & prevention

Feline panleukopenia requires aggressive treatment if the cat is to survive, as this disease can kill cats in less than 24 hours. Treatment involves **whole blood transfusion** to improve pancytopenia, **intravenous fluids** as most cats are dehydrated, injections of **Vitamin A, B, and C, IV antibiotics to prevent septicemia**, which develops in most cats with feline panleukopenia.

Since the FPV virus is hardy, and can persist in the environment for months or years, a thorough disinfection of the entire premises needs to be made after an outbreak of feline panleukopenia in a home shared by cats. The only disinfectant presently acknowledged is a **dilute bleach solution, of 1:9** (one part bleach to nine parts water.). Although feline panleukopenia is considered a "dread disease" of cats, with routine vaccinations, isolation of cats new to the household until they have been tested and vaccinated, and routine sanitary precautions, the average multi-cat household should remain safe from this disease.

Vaccination

When born to a queen with FPV antibodies, kittens will have a natural immunity for the first eight to ten weeks. After that period, vaccination should be started. Protection is offered by commercial feline distemper vaccine (ATCvet codes: Q106AA0 2 for the inactivated viral vaccine and Q106AD01 for the live vaccine). A number of combination live modified vaccines exist. **ECLIPSE 3**-Intervet (feline rhinotracheitis +feline calicivirus + feline panleukopenia) is a modified live vaccine; inject one dose (1 ml) SC or IM at 9 weeks of age or older and repeat with a second dose 3 to 4 weeks later. Annual revaccination with one dose is recommended. **NOVIVAC TRICAT**-Intervet (feline rhinotracheitis + feline calicivirus + feline panleukopenia) is a live vaccine; the first inoculation is given from the age of 8-9 weeks and the second inoculation from the age of 12 weeks. Revaccination against feline calicivirus and feline herpesvirus type 1 must be given every year & against feline panleucopenia virus can be given every three years (with strain MW-1 as in Nobivac Tricat Trio, where available). **ECLIPSE 4** in addition also includes feline leukemia virus. Inject one dose/1 ml SC or IM at 9 weeks of age or older and repeat with a second dose 3 to 4 weeks later. Annual revaccination with one dose is recommended. Similar vaccines are prepared by Pfizer like Felocell 4 or felocell CVR C (feline rhinotracheitis+ Calicivirus+ Panleukopnia + Chlamydia) is a modified live freeze dried vaccine. Rehydrate the freeze-dried vaccine with the sterile diluent provided, shake well, and administer 1 ml IM or SC. For primary vaccination, healthy cats 12 weeks of age or older should receive 2 doses, 3 4 weeks apart. Cats vaccinated at less than 12 weeks of age should be revaccinated at 12 weeks of age. Annual revaccination with a single dose is recommended.

The FPV vaccine is not recommended for kittens under eight weeks of age, since their natural immunity may interfere with the efficacy of the FPV vaccine. An FVP antiserum can be used to immunize kittens less than eight weeks, which have been exposed to the FPV virus, and also for older, unprotected cats who have been exposed.

Canine Parvovirus-2 Infection

Canine parvovirus-2 (CPV-2) causing canine parvovirus infection is a highly contagious disease of dogs **less than 6 month old** with severe diarrhoea, vomition, leucopenia, immunosupression & often death. Intrauterine or perinatal infection causes myocarditis in pups. After ingestion, the virus replicates in the lymphoid tissue in the throat, viraemia follows, and the virus then attacks rapidly dividing cells, like those in the lymph nodes, intestinal crysts & bone marrow with depletion of lymphocytes in lymph nodes, necrosis & destruction of the intestinal crypts & secondary bacterial infection. After 3-

4 days of infection, **the virus is shed in the feces for up to three weeks, become asymptomatic carrier and shed the virus periodically**. The disease is deadly if the host is concurrently infested with bacteria or other intestinal parasites. If puppies are infected in the uterus or shortly after birth till 8 weeks of age, the virus attacks the heart muscle and the puppy often dies suddenly or after a brief period of breathing difficulty.

Etiology: Canine parvovirus is caused by *Canine parvovirus-2* (CPV-2). Three strains- CPV-2a, - CPV-2b, & - CPV-2c have been detected so far. CPV2b (strain FP84) has been shown to cause disease in a small percentage of domestic cats, although vaccination for FPV seems to be protective. CPV2, however, does not cause disease in cats and does so only mildly in mink and raccoons, and is a virus almost exclusively affecting canines. CPV2a and CPV2b were identified in 1979 and 1984 respectively. The antigenic patterns of 2a and 2b are quite similar to the original CPV type 2. Most cases of canine parvovirus infection are believed to be caused by these two strains. CPV-2c differs from CPV-2a and CPV-2b at only one point on the DNA strand. Canine parvovirus type 2c (CPV-2c) is a variant of canine parvovirus. It was first detected in Italy in 2000, and has also been reported in Western Europe, Asia, and South America. Outbreaks of canine parvovirus associated with CPV-2c in the United States were confirmed in 2006 and 2007.

Occurrence

Parvovirus CPV2 is a relatively new disease that appeared in the late 1970s. It was first recognized in 1978 and spread worldwide in one to two years. The virus is very similar to feline panleukopenia; they are 98% identical, differing only in two amino acids in the viral capsid protein VP2. It is also highly similar to mink enteritis, and the parvoviruses of racoons and foxes. The early belief was that the feline panleukopenia mutated into CPV2. It is possible that CPV2 is a mutant of an unidentified parvovirus FPV of some wild carnivore. There are three variants of CPV type 2 called CPV-2a, CPV-2b and CPV-2c. Canine parvovirus type 2b (CPV-2b) is the most common variant of the canine parvovirus in the United States, but CPV-2c is becoming the second most common variant. Variant 2c however has a unique pattern of antigenicity. This has led to claims of ineffective vaccination of dogs, but studies have shown that the existing CPV vaccines based on CPV type 2b, provide adequate levels of protection against CPV type 2c.

Hosts susceptible

CPV2 affects dogs, wolves, foxes, and other canids. CPV2a and CPV2b have been isolated from a small percentage of symptomatic cats and is more common than feline panleukopenia in big cats. Previously it has been thought that the virus does not undergo cross species infection. However studies in Vietnam have shown that CPV2 can undergo minor antigenic shift and natural mutation to infect felids. Analyses of feline parvovirus (FPV) isolates in Vietnam and Taiwan revealed that more than 80% of the isolates were of the canine parvovirus type, rather than feline panleukopenia virus (FPLV).

Generally, dog of any age and sex can be affected by CPV-2 infection. Some breeds including Doberman Pinschers, Rottweilers, American Pit Bull Terriers and German Shepherds are more predisposed to the disease than other dogs. But most severe form of the disease is observed in puppies of **less than three months of age**. Adult dogs are comparatively resistant to CPV-2 infection and develop only mild syndrome.

Transmission

The CPV-2 is very stable in environment and resistant to most of common disinfectants. The virus is transmitted to susceptible dogs by direct contact with the infected dog. Virus is also transmitted indirectly through contamination of the fomites, food, & by feces of infected dogs. The virus can also contaminate kennel surfaces, food and water bowls, collars and leashes, and the hands and clothing of people who handle infected dogs. The virus is shed in feces by infected dogs for at least three weeks after infection.

Pathogenesis

CPV-2 has affinity **towards actively dividing cells in host body**. So, virus attacks the actively dividing cells of the body which includes **bone marrow, lymphoid tissue, intestinal epithelium and myocardial cells in puppies less than three months of age**. Virus was first isolated from mesenteric lymph nodes on day 2 after exposure, tonsil on day 3 and small intestine on day 3. Viraemia occurred subsequently and was present in most dogs on days 4 and 5 after exposure. CPV-2 could be isolated from all tissues during viraemia. Relative pyrexia, lymphopenia and neutropenia occurred on days 5, 6 and 7 after exposure, respectively. Virus excretion in feces began in most dogs on day 4 and continued despite the appearance of neutralizing serum antibody. Specific serum antibody detected in some dogs as early as day 3 and in all dogs by day 7 after exposure, eliminated viraemia and inhibited virus isolation from tissues in cell culture. Lymphoid necrosis and depletion of lymphocytes from lymphoid tissues were most notable on days 5 and 6 after exposure. Lymphocyte hyperplasia occurred following day 7. Epithelial cell changes in segments of the small intestine were more severe on days 6 to 9 after exposure in areas associated with Peyer's patches and in the upper segments of the small intestine. The lymphocyte was the primary infected cell. Virus infected cryptal epithelial cells were not detected until 24 hours after the identification of infected cells in lymphoid tissues on day 4 after exposure. The majority of virus infected epithelial cells were found in crypts intimately associated with or adjacent to Peyer's patches in the upper segments of the small intestine.

There are two forms of CPV2: **intestinal and cardiac**. Along with age and breed, factors such as a stressful environment, concurrent infections with bacteria, parasites, and canine coronavirus increase a dog's risk of severe infection. Dogs that catch parvovirus usually die from the dehydration it causes or secondary infection rather than the virus itself.

Intestinal form

Dogs become infected through oral contact with CPV2 in feces, infected soil, or fomites that carry the virus. Following ingestion, the virus replicates in the lymphoid tissue in the throat, and then spreads to the bloodstream. From there, the virus attacks rapidly dividing cells, notably those in the lymph nodes, intestinal crypts, and the bone marrow. There is depletion of lymphocytes in lymph nodes and necrosis and destruction of the intestinal crypts. **Anaerobic bacteria that normally reside in the intestines can then cross into the bloodstream, a process known as translocation, and cause sepsis.** The most common bacteria involved in severe cases are *Clostridia, Campylobacter* and *Salmonella* species. This can lead to a syndrome known as systemic inflammatory response syndrome (SIRS). SIRS leads to a range of complications such as **hypercoagulability of the blood, endotoxaemia and acute respiratory distress syndrome** (ARDS). Bacterial myocarditis has also been reported secondarily to sepsis. Dogs with CPV are at risk of **intussusceptions**, a condition where part of the intestine prolapses into another part. Three to four days following infection, **the virus is shed in the feces for up to three weeks,** and the dog may remain an asymptomatic carrier and shed the virus periodically.

Cardiac form

This form is less common and affects puppies infected in the uterus or shortly after birth until about 8 weeks of age. The virus attacks the heart muscle and the puppy often dies suddenly or after a brief period of breathing difficulty. Microscopically, there are many points of necrosis of the heart muscle that are associated with mononuclear cellular infiltration. The formation of excess fibrous tissue-fibrosis is often evident in surviving dogs. Myofibrils are the site of viral replication within cells. The disease may or may not be accompanied with the signs and symptoms of the intestinal form. However, this form is now **rarely seen** due to widespread vaccination of breeding dogs.

Even less frequently, the disease may also lead to a generalized infection in neonates and cause lesions and viral replication and attack in other tissues other than the gastrointestinal tissues and heart, but also in brain, liver, lungs, kidneys, and adrenal cortex. The lining of the blood vessels are also severely affected, which lead the lesions in this region to hemorrhage.

Infection of the fetus

This type of infection can occur when a pregnant female dog is infected with CPV2. The adult may develop immunity with little or no clinical signs of disease. The virus may have already crossed the placenta to infect the fetus. This can lead to several abnormalities. In mild to moderate cases the pups can be born with neurological abnormalities such as cerebellar hypoplasia.

Clinical symptoms & lesions

CPV-2 has affinity **towards actively dividing cells in host body**. So, virus attacks the actively dividing cells of the body which includes **bone marrow, lymphoid tissue, intestinal epithelium and myocardial cells in puppies less than three months of age**. Affected dogs show dullness, anorexia, fever, vomiting and diarrhoea. The gastroenteritis is more severe in young pups below 20 weeks of age. The clinical disease is exaggerated by concurrent infection with opportunistic intestinal pathogens like *Salmonella, Clostridium perfringens, E. coli, Campylobacter, Coronavirus* or worms.

The feces are loose and may contain mucus or in severe cases blood. Fluid loss causes rapid dehydration and electrolyte and acid-base imbalance in young dogs. Affection of bone marrow causes reduction in white blood cells of body which might further increase susceptibility of dogs to a number of other infections. If appropriate treatment and care is provided, chances of recovery and survival increase.

Occasionally affection of myocardium by virus may lead to congestive heart failure and pulmonary edema in pups less than three months old, finally culminating in death.

PM lesions include a small amount of fecal staining noted on the tail and the hairs around the anus of most of the pups. The contents of the small intestine were liquid, and the colonic contents varied from liquid to pasty soft and pale to bright yellow. The myocardium in some cases had large tan to pale gray streaks and irregular areas deep within the myocardium. **Histologically**, puppies showed **large intranuclear epithelial inclusions at the tips of the villi in the jejunum.** These inclusions were eosinophilic and often appeared to fill the nuclei. Other intestinal changes noted included **crypt epithelial hyperplasia and single-cell necrosis of crypt epithelial cells.**

These changes also appeared to be limited to the duodenum and jejunum. The other pathologic feature common to all of the cases was moderate to marked depletion and/or necrosis of the lymphoid cells of Peyer's patches.

Diagnosis

Collection of clinical specimens for various tests include: fresh feces, intestine, spleen, and heart, & sera.

1. *Presumptive diagnosis*: History, clinical signs, necropsy findings, & histopathologic lesions are characteristic indicating parvovirus gastroenteritis. Blood tinged diarrhoea and vomiting in unvaccinated but dewormed dogs give suspicion about CPV- 2 infection. Complete blood count and biochemical parameters will further tell about physical condition as well as outcome of the disease.
2. *Virus isolation*: The virus isolation is done in cell cultures of canine and feline origin.
3. *Antigen detection*: Haemagglutination test using porcine or Rhesus monkey RBC (greater than 1:32 in fecal emulsions), & ELISA to detect parvovirus antigens in fecal sample of dogs are most commonly used for diagnosis of CPV-2 infection in dogs. Commercially available fecal tests are able to detect all variants of CPV-2, including CPV-2c.

Treatment & prevention

In severe cases with signs of circulatory collapse, **blood transfusion or plasma expanders** are indicated. Before transfusion of blood, compatibility testing should be done with donor blood. But most commonly, **fluid and electrolyte therapy** remains as a mainstay of treatment of CPV-2 infection. **Lactated Ringers solution and Dextrose** is given intravenously to compensate fluid and electrolyte losses. There is now a licensed treatment for CPV in the UK in the form of the **veterinary interferon omega (rFeIFN-ω)** which has been demonstrated by multiple studies to be an effective treatment. Treatment ideally also consists of crystalloid IV fluids and/or colloids, antinausea injections such as metoclopramide, dolasetron, ondasetron and prochlorpeazine, and antibiotic injections such as cefxitin, metronidazole, timentin, or enroflxacin. IV fluids are administered and antinausea and antibiotic injections are given subcutaneously, intramuscularly, or intravenously. The fluids are typically a mix of a sterile, balanced electrolyte solution, with an appropriate amount of B-complex vitamins, dextrose and potassium chloride. Analgesic medications such as buprenorphine are also used to counteract the intestinal discomfort caused by frequent bouts of diarrhea. In addition to fluids given to achieve adequate rehydration, each time the puppy vomits or has diarrhea in a significant quantity; an equal amount of fluid is administered intravenously. The fluid requirements of a patient are determined by the animal's body weight, weight changes over time, degree of dehydration at presentation and surface area.

A blood plasma transfusion from a donor dog that has already survived CPV is sometimes used to provide passive immunity to the sick dog. Some veterinarians keep these dogs on site, or have frozen serum available. There have been no controlled studies regarding this treatment. Additionally, fresh frozen plasma and human albumin transfusions can help replace the extreme protein losses seen in severe cases and help assure adequate tissue healing. As affected dog is immunosuppressed, **broad spectrum antibiotic with bactericidal drug** is given to check any secondary bacterial infection that might otherwise further aggravate the condition. Feeding and watering is commonly withheld till subsidence of vomition. While recovering, dog should be offered with bland diet containing rice, cottage cheese or commercially available prescription diet with gradual inclusion of normal diet should be given based on the speed of recovery.

Premises of dogs should be kept clean with disinfectants like household bleach (1:30 dilution), formalin, gluteraldehyde, etc.

Vaccination

Canine Parvovirus infection of dogs can be prevented totally by vaccinating dog against CPV-2 infection at right time; sometimes maternal antibodies which provide passive protection against CPV-2 infection may interfere with development of post vaccination immunity. The exact time of disappearance of maternal antibodies from pup is not known. So, vaccination of pups should be started at age of **6-8 weeks and continued at interval of four weeks till 14-16 weeks of age**. This will help in inducing very good level of active immunity in pups against CPV-2 infection. Thereafter **every year annual booster vaccination should be given.** The duration of immunity of vaccines for CPV2 has been tested for all major vaccine manufacturers in the USA and has been found to be at least **three years after the initial puppy series and a booster 1 year later.** Until pups attend the age of 16 weeks with history of complete vaccination against CPV-2, care should be taken to prevent contact with feces of other puppies or dogs during taking your dogs for walks in parks and gardens. **Modified live virus vaccines are most commonly available in the market for CPV-2 infections.** Several combination freeze dried modified live vaccines are available. A combination modified live vaccine containing canine distemper, adenovirus type 1 & 2, canine parvo vaccine & canine parainfluenza virus (**Galaxy DA2PPV**-Intervet) is given to puppies within the first months of life. Give 1 ml dose IM or SC, with a second dose in

2-4 weeks. Annual revaccination is recommended thereafter. Some young dogs may require a third dose, depending on their age when the first vaccination was given. This vaccine also combines with coronavirus and leptospirosis designated as **Galaxy DA2PPV+CV** (CD + Adenovius 2+ Parvovirus+ canine PI3+ Coronavirus) 1ml SC or IM at 6 weeks of age or older. Repeat at 2 to 4 week intervals until the dog is 12 weeks of age. A minimum of two doses is required for primary immunization. Annual revaccination with one dose is recommended. **Galaxy DA$_2$PPVL** modified live virus vaccine which is combined with inactivated *Leptospira canicola* and *L. icterohaemorrhagiae* bacterin. Dose & schedule as above. **Vanguard plus 5, Vanguard plus 5/CV & Vanguard Plus 5L4**-Pfizer are similar vaccines. **RECOMBITEK Canine Parvo**-Merial is recommended for the vaccination of healthy dogs 6 weeks of age and older for prevention of disease due to canine parvovirus. Inject 1 ml (1 dose) SC or IM to dogs. For primary vaccination, revaccinate with a second 1 ml dose 2 to 3 weeks later. Dogs younger than 12 weeks of age should be revaccinated with a single 1 ml dose every 2 to 3 weeks, the last dose given at or over 12 weeks of age. Revaccinate annually with a single 1 ml dose.

Porcine Parvovirus Infection

Porcine parvovirus (PPV) infection is the **most important cause of infectious infertility in swine.** The virus multiplies in the pig intestine without causing clinical signs & is worldwide in distribution.**The virus has no effect on the female but only on the fetus.** If pregnant sows are infected **before 35 days of gestation**, there are small litters size associated with embryo loss, mummified fetuses of varying size, increased numbers of stillbirths & delay in the farrowing due to the presence of the mummified piglet, abortions are uncommon, & there may be an increase in low birth weight piglets but neonatal deaths are not affected. There are no other signs of ill health in the breeding female or in individual affected animals. If the viruses crosses the placenta in the last trimester, neonatal death may occur, or the birth of healthy piglets with a protective pre-colostral immunity. **SMEDI** indicates stillbirth, mummification, embryonic death, and infertility, is a reproductive disease of swine caused by PPV and *porcine enterovirus.*

Etiology: The disease is caused by*Porcine parvovirus* (PPV) in the genus *Parvovirus.* Where as most viruses do not survive outside the host for any great period of time, PPV is unusual in that it can persist outside the pig for many months and it is resistant to most disinfectants. This perhaps explains why it is so widespread and so difficult to remove from the pig environment.

Occurrence

Porcine parvovirus (PPV) is widespread in swine of the United States, Canada, South America and some countries in Europe. Porcine parvovirus is a fairly tough virus that multiplies normally in the intestine of the pig without causing clinical signs. It is world-wide in its distribution. **Pig breeding herd may be in one of three phases:i. Serologically negative herd,**when all females are highly susceptible to infection and reproductive failure can occur occasionally in small herds, from which the virus can die out, & if PPV infects, there is a massive outbreak of reproductive disease: repeats, mummifications, not in pig and possibly a few abortions. Such herds should be vaccinated immediately. **ii. Endemic infection,**when PPV is continually circulating and 50-90% of animals are immune in large herd. PPV infection can take place in the early to mid pregnancy period in any negative animals, & intermittent outbreaks of disease occur, particularly in gilts and second parity females. **iii. Disease in replacement gilts** is common because at least 50% of gilts at point of mating may not have met PPV and therefore are susceptible. Up to a third of such animals may become infected in the first half of pregnancy resulting in reproductive failure.

Hosts susceptible

The porcine parvovirus (PPV) is widespread in swine population. The virus is present in pig herd unless the herd is less than 100 sows when it might have died out. It is therefore an infection you have to live with and manage. The virus is widespread throughout all pig populations, but it may disappear in small herds. Infection is endemic in most pig units.

Transmission

Disease transmission occurs by ingestion and occurs mainly by contact with water and food containing feces and other infectious discharges. Clinically normal but latently infected boars may transmit the virus to sows through semen. In small herds the virus may die out and sows become susceptible. In large herds, pockets of naive breeding females, particularly gilts, can maintain the disease. A naive herd often < 100 sows is at risk. The virus may be present in the semen.

Pathogenesis

Pathogenesis depends on the **age of the animal affected and the efficiency of its immune system.** Colostral protection lasts up **to 5 months of age,** after which it decreases to an all-time low to increase yet again at about 12 months of age.

IF prenatal infection occurs, virus travels from infected mother to fetus via the placenta. In this case, the time of gestation determines the result of the infection.

i. If the fetus is **infected in the first 30 days of fetal life**, death and absorption of all, or some of the fetuses may occur. In this case, some immunotolerant healthy piglets may be born.

ii. If the **infection occurs at 40 days**, death and mummification may occur. Also in this case, some or all the fetuses are involved, i.e. some of the fetuses can be born healthy and immunotolerant, or else become carriers of the disease.

iii. If the **viruses crosses the placenta in the last trimester**, neonatal death may occur, or the birth of healthy piglets having a protective pre-colostral immunity.

iv. Postnatal infection in **pigs up to 1 year of age occurs oro-nasally**, followed by a **viremia** associated with transitory leucopenia.

v. **Infection in adults over 1 year of age** would have an active, protective immune system which protects them from future exposures (e.g. mating with an infected male).

Therefore, it is important to note that the virus is particularly dangerous for the sow in her first gestation, which would be at 7–8 months of age, as she would have a particularly low antibody count at this age and could easily contract the virus via copulation.

Histopathological changes without immunofluorescence were evident in fetuses which had passed the stage of immunocompetence, whilst less obvious histopathological changes with significant antigen fluorescence were present in foetuses which had not reached immunocompetence. Such fluorescence was evident in the parenchyma of lung, liver and kidney, and in neurons and vascular endothelium of the cerebrum. Histopathological changes consisted of **vasculitis, perivascular infiltrations and meningitis of the brain, interstitial hepatitis, interstitial nephritis and placentitis with calcification.**

Clinical symptoms & lesions

The virus has no effect on the female but affect only the foetus. Small litters are associated with embryo loss if infection occurs before 35 days of pregnancy. There are mummified fetuses of varying size, (30-160mm), increased numbers of stillbirths, & these are associated with the delay in the farrowing mechanism, which occurs because of the presence of the mummified fetuses. Abortions associated with PPV infection are uncommon. There may be an increase in low birth weight piglets but neonatal deaths do not occur. The major signs are therefore small litter sizes, mummified pigs of different sizes, and increases in pseudo-pregnancies and no effect in pigs. The acute disease episode often lasts for up to 8 weeks, and then wanes for 4-6 weeks, followed by smaller bouts of mummified pigs for a further 4-6 weeks. The virus can take up to 4 months to infect all sows in a susceptible previously uninfected herd. Sporadic disease is seen in individual females which are infected for the first time. It is usually confined to gilts. There are no other signs of ill health in the breeding female or in individual affected animals. Reproductive problems may appear every 3-4 years in a herd if vaccination is not carried out.

Diagnosis

Collection of clinical specimens includes mummified or aborted fetuses, placenta, fluids and skin lesions.

1. *Presumptive diagnosis*: In the absence of any other signs of illness in the breeding females, PPV disease can be suspected by increases in **variable sized mummified pigs and small litter sizes.** The important features are disease and death in the embryo and foetus from approximately 15-70 days of pregnancy.

2. *Virus isolation*: PPV is propagated in cell cultures of swine testis and kidney, although several subcultures may be required before cytopathic changes are evident. Examination of fetal fluids for hemagglutinating activity is also useful.

3. *Detection of antigen*: The mummified pigs can be examined by fluorescent antibody staining of cryostat sections of fetal liver and lung. Diagnosis is most easily accomplished by fluorescent antibody. The virus agglutinates guinea pig erythrocytes.

4. *Serology* will not help because many sows are positive and normal.

Treatment & prevention

PPV infection results in high antibody levels in the serum which persist for long periods. Neutralizing antibody titer of 1:2 will be equally as protective as a titer of 1:80,000. Blood sampling all the sows in a herd on one occasion only indicates the percentage of animals that have been exposed to parvovirus at some previous period which gives you an idea of the overall breeding herd immunity or susceptibility. **Once an animal has been exposed to PPV, it remains immune for the rest of its life.**

Vaccination

A single injection of **Suvaxyn Parvo ST**-Pfizer is a vaccine for the active immunization of sows and gilts to reduce transplacental infection of progeny with porcine parvovirus. Administer 1dose- 2 ml IM. Primary vaccination to gilts of 6 months of age or older: A single dose, administered at least 14 days prior to mating. Revaccination: A single dose during each lactation period. The recommended interval between vaccination and mating is 14 days. Onset of immunity: 8 weeks after primary vaccination. Duration of immunity: 4 months after primary vaccination. Several commercially prepared inactivated vaccines are available. **PORCILIS PARVO is an inactivated adjuvanted one shot vaccine against Porcine parvovirus (PPV) infection in pigs based on the PPV strain 014, in an aqueous adjuvant Diluvac Forte.** It is used for the active immunization of sows and gilts to protect their embryos and foetuses against PPV infection. Gilts should be vaccinated 2ml IM once between 8 and 2 weeks before first mating but sows should be vaccinated once at least 2 weeks before mating. Annual re-vaccination is recommended. **PORCILIS ERY & PARVO** for the immunization of gilts & sows for the protection of embryos & fetuses against porcine parvovirus & *E. rhusiopathie*. is an inactivated vaccine containing at least 1 ppd *Erysipelothrix rhusiopathiae* antigen, strain M2 (serotype 2) and Porcine parvovirus (PPV) strain 014 inducing at least 7.4 $\log_2$ HI units per dose in an aqueous adjuvant. The vaccine contains 0.05% formaldehyde as a preservative and 150 mg dl-á tocopherol per dose. The dose is 2 ml per pig, given by deep IM route behind the ear not less than 2 weeks before mating; Sows should be revaccinated against erysipelas during each lactation period (i.e. at no more than 6 month intervals) and against parvovirus annually. **Farrowsure Gold B**-Pfizer is a killed vaccine providing protection against abortion caused by swine parvovirus, leptospirosis & *E. rhusiopathiae* also includes Parvovirus, Bratislava-Canicola-Grippotyphosa-Hardjo- Icterohaemorrhagie-Pomona Bacterin & *E. rhusiopathiae*. It contains gentamicn as preservative. Shake well & aseptically administer 2 ml IM. Primary vaccination: healthy swine should receive 2 doses 3-5 weeks apart with the second dose administered 2-4 weeks prior to breeding. Healthy gilts, however, should receive the second dose as near as possible to 14 days prior to breeding. *Revaccination:* Revaccination with a single dose is recommended prior to subsequent breedings. Boars should be revaccinated semiannually.

Genus: Dependovirus

Duck Parvovirus Infection

Duck parvovirus/ Muscovy duck parvovirus **(BDPV/MDPV)** causes **hepatitis in Muscovy ducks worldwide.** Clinical symptoms are like goslings infection & include huddling together, inability to walk, dragging of legs behind the duckling, and enteric signs with no feather loss (unlike goose parvovirus), & the main finding is **hepatopathology**.

Etiology : Duck parvovirus infection is caused by *Duck parvovirus /Muscovy duck parvovirus* (BDPV/ MDPV), a parvovirus distinct from goose parvovirus.

Occurrence

Derzy's disease/ hepatitis in Muscovy ducks occurs worldwide. Mortality is up to 80%.

Hosts susceptible

Muscovy ducks (*Cairina moschata*) domesticated or wild; greatest in youngest ducklings infected in hatchery. Ducklings older than five weeks old seroconvert but do not show clinical signs.

Transmission

Transmissionis by horizontal route; also vertical in ducks infected while in lay or if latent infection reactivates.

Clinical symptoms & lesions

Ducklings are found huddling together, unable to walk, dragging of legs behind the duckling, and show enteric signs. There is no feather loss (unlike goose parvovirus). The main pathological lesion is hepatopathy. Liver is enlarged and congested, there is hepatitis and focal hepatic necrosis; hepatocyte degeneration with vacuolation, & **intranuclear inclusion bodies in hepatocytes.**

Diagnosis

A presumptive diagnosis is based on clinical signs, & gross and histological lesions. Confirmatory diagnosis requires **isolation of virus in muscovy duck embryos or muscovy cell culture.**

It is differentiated from GPV by cross-neutralization tests, serology or molecular methods. DPV antigen in tissues can be detected by a chemoluminescent dot blot assay using a non-radioactive, digoxigenin-labelled DPV DNA probe, but this also detects some GPV strains (B32.37.w6). PCR-RFLP (polymerase chain reaction-restriction enzyme fragment length polymorphism) analysis can be used to differentiate from Muscovy duck parvovirus from goose parvovirus. Goose parvovirus infection (GPV) is differentiated by cross-neutralization tests or by PCR. Muscovy duck reovirus infection is differentiated by absence of exudative pericarditis, tenosinovitis, & splenic lymphoid hyperplasia.

Treatment & prevention

Immunize breeders with two inoculations using **oil-emulsion vaccine** to provide ducklings with maternally-derived antibodies. Duck or goose embryo or duck cell culture attenuated vaccine given to female ducks or goose transferred protection via egg yolk to progeny or vaccinated to gosling proved effective in affording protection against the challenge virus. Vaccinate day-old ducklings with inactivated, aqueous vaccine. Application of good biosecurity prevents the disease entering susceptible flocks.

Goose Parvovirus Infection

Goose parvovirus (GPV) causes **goose viral hepatitis**, also called **Derzsy's disease, goose hepatitis, infectious myocarditis or goose/gosling plague**; a highly contagious and fatal disease of goslings and Muscovy ducklings that has been reported from Europe and the Far East where the disease is of serious economic significance. The disease is characterized by prostration and death in acutely affected goslings, reduced feed intake, excessive water intake, swollen eyelids and eye and nasal discharge, profuse white diarrhea, membrane covering tongue, **loss of down**, & reddening of skin.

Etiology: Goose parvovirus infection is caused by *Goose parvovirus*, a parvovirus distinct from *Duck parvovirus*.

Occurrence

The disease has been reported from all major goose farming countries in Europe including Hungary, Poland, France, Germany and Denmark, and the former Soviet Union, Israel, China, Viet Nam and Japan. **100 per cent mortality occurs in goslings less than seven days old and negligible losses by four to six weeks of age.** The severity of disease in neonatal birds will depend on levels of maternally derived antibody. An outbreak of goose parvovirus (GPV) infection on a Swedish goose farm in the spring of 2004 increased the mortality rates from 2% in the early unaffected hatches to 90% and 99% respectively in the two hatches following virus introduction and 40% in goslings hatched later in the same breeding season.

Hosts susceptible

Goose parvovirus (GPV) infection is a contagious disease of goslings and Muscovy ducklings only. There is species and age-dependent decreasing susceptibility with age. Disease seen in goslings less than four weeks old, and in muscovy (*Cairina moschata*) ducklings. Other ducks appear resistant. Older goslings and those with some maternal antibody may develop subacute rather than acute disease. GPV infects only Muscovy ducks. The younger the bird affected the more acute the condition and the higher the mortality. Losses are negligible in birds over 5 weeks of age.

Transmission

Infected birds excrete large amounts of **virus in their feces** resulting in a rapid spread of infection by direct and indirect contact. Older geese can become subclinically infected, a latent infection is established, & such birds can act as carriers and transmit the virus through their eggs. This results in infertility and hatchability problems and the transmission of infection to other goslings at hatching. Vertical transmission occurs through egg yolk, & from virus on egg shell, horizontal from in-contact goslings and their feces. Survivors of clinical disease and **goslings infected at more than 4 weeks old may become persistent carrier**. Outbreaks usually occur in susceptible goslings following transmission of the virus via eggs laid by **infected breeder geese.** Infected eggs become the source of the virus when outbreaks of *Goose parvovirus* occur in countries or geographic locations formerly free of the disease. No other avian or biologic vectors have been identified. GPV is very resistant to chemical and physical inactivation.

Clinical symptoms & lesions

Three clinical forms are observed: acute disease, subacute & chonic forms. Acute disease is seen in young goslings, sometimes with longer course, and chronic form also seen in survivors.

Acute form runs a short course showing listlessness, anorexia, prostration, & deaths in 2-5 days.

Subacute is a longer course showing anorexia, polydypsia, weakness, reluctance to move, oculonasal discharge and associated head shaking, red, swollen uropygial glands and eyelids, profuse white droppings, & sometimes fibrinous pseudomembrane over oral cavity and tongue.

Chronic form shows severe growth retardation, distended abdomen (ascites) and associated 'penguin' posture, leg weakness, loss of back and neck down (later abnormal feathering) and associated skin reddening, & swollen uropygial gland. Stunting and poor feathering may be seen in survivors.

PM lesions: **In acute cases** lesions include: liver: enlarged and congested, heart: pale and rounded at apex, spleen and pancreas: sometimes swollen and congested, & viscera: may have petechiae.

Subacute cases shows the following features: abdomen: ascites, liver: swollen, copper-coloured, friable and petechiated, sero-fibrinous perihepatitis, gall bladder large and bile-filled, heart: variably dilated, sero-fibrinous pericarditis, & also variably focal pancreatic necrosis, pulmonary oedema, catarrhal enteritis, occasionally hemorrhages in thigh muscles and pectoral muscles. **In muscovy ducks**: there are nephritis, non-suppurative polioencephalomyelitis and myopathy.

Histopathologically, liver shows hepatitis and focal hepatic necrosis; hepatocyte degeneration with vacuolation & intranuclear inclusion bodies in hepatocytes. Heart shows focal myocardial necrosis, degeneration of myocardial cells with loss of striation, fatty infiltration and scattered Cowdry type A intranuclear inclusions.

Diagnosis

Collection of clinical samples includes sick or recently dead birds.

1. *Presumptive diagnosis*: It is based on clinical signs, age incidence & gross and histological lesions.
2. *Virus isolation*: Isolation of virus is made from heart or liver of affected birds in embryonated goose or Muscovy eggs (inoculate at 10-15 days of incubation to produce embryo mortality with haemorrhages and ochre-coloured livers by 5-10 days post inoculation; isolation is done in goose or muscovy cell tissue cultures, & the virus inoculated when cultures become confluent: cytopathic effect is seen at 3-5 days post inoculation. Haematoxylin and eosin (H&E) preparations show Cowdry type A intranuclear inclusions and often syncytium formation. Confirm virus by electron-microscopy.
3. *Virus antigen detection*: Electron microscopic exam detects the virus in the infected culture or may be confirmed by neutralization with specific goose parvovirus antiserum. Serologic tests for goose parvovirus include virus neutralization, agar gel precipitation, and ELISA.

   Direct detection of antigen or virus in tissues from infected birds is done by immunofluorescence, or by the use of PCR.
4. *Antibody detection: Serology*: a) for detection of goose parvovirus neutralizing antibodies use a virus neutralization test in embryonated goose or muscovy eggs or in goose cell primary tissue culture; or b) agar gel diffusion test. ELISA detects viral antigen (antigen capture or double antibody sandwich); blocking ELISA detects antibody.

Detection of antibody in the yolk of eggs can be used to identify individuals or flocks which have been exposed to infection.

Differentiation from Muscovy parvovirus is done by cross-neutralization tests & also by PCR.

Goose parvovirus causes disease in **both geese and Muscovy ducks**, but **Muscovy ducks** are also infected with *Duck parvovirus*, which causes serious disease in Muscovy ducklings **but not in goslings**. Differential diagnoses should also include duck viral enteritis (duck plague) that affects all types of waterfowl. Duck viral hepatitis causes a fatal disease in ducklings but is not pathogenic for goslings or Muscovy ducklings. PCR-RFLP (polymerase chain reaction-restriction enzyme fragment length polymorphism) analysis can be used to differentiate from muscovy duck parvovirus from goose parvovirus. Goose Parvovirus infection (GPV) is differentiated by cross-neutralization tests or by PCR. Muscovy duck reovirus infection is differentiated by absence of exudative pericarditis, tenosinovitis, & splenic lymphoid hyperplasia.

Treatment & prevention

There is no specific treatment. Antibiotics may reduce losses from secondary bacterial infections. Control relies upon good biosecurity, hygiene and eliminating carrier birds. If a **GPV outbreak occurs, it is not advisable to retain recovered or in-contact goslings for breeding, as the birds are potential carriers of the virus** and may transmit GPV via their eggs. Suspect carriers should be reared away from other geese and Muscovy ducks. On breeding units, only eggs from known GPV-free flocks should be incubated together and good hatchery hygiene should be maintained. In the event of an outbreak, in-contact breeding geese that have not been GPV-vaccinated can be monitored serologically for infection. Consideration should then be given to culling sero-positive birds.

Administration of immune serum has been shown to be effective but may require two doses- on day old and around 3 weeks. It is time-consuming.

Vaccination

The preferred approach is to immunize breeding birds with an **attenuated live vaccine**. Vaccinate **breeders 3 to six weeks before egg laying starts.** Active immunization of breeders with an attenuated strain of virus by **IM inoculation** provides maternally-transmitted immunity, it is effective and is more cost-effective than passive immunization. Attenuated vaccines may also be used in goslings. **Only inactivated vaccines should be used in flocks where the infection has not been diagnosed.**

Genus: *Amdovirus*

Aleutian Mink Disease

Aleutian mink disease (AMD) or Mink plasmacytosis is a highly contagious parvovirus infection of mustelids, & the disease is characterized by chronic, progressive weight loss, lethargy, splenomegaly, anemia, rear leg weakness, seizures and black tarry stool. Once symptoms appear, the disease progresses rapidly, usually to death within a few months.

Etiology: Aleutian mink disease is caused by *Aleutian mink disease virus* (AMDV) in the genus *Amdovirus.* Currently, there are at least **five strains of AMDV** that can infect mink, & there are also multiple strains of AMDV that can affect ferrets. Among the several strains of AMDV, the most common strains are **AMDV-Utah,** the original strain discovered which is most virulent in mink, AMDV-F-a ferret-specific strain, and AMDV-G-a non-virulent strain used for laboratory study. The AMDV-F strain is thought to be a mutated form of the original mink AMDV and is only pathogenic in ferrets.

Occurrence

Aleutian mink disease was first recognized in farm-raised mink in 1956. The disease was so named because it was first found in minks that were homozygous for the Aleutian (blue) gene were most severely affected by the illness. It was assumed that the disease was a result of poor genetics, but it was later found that minks of all coat colors were susceptible to the disease - but tend to have a lower mortality compared with Aleutian Mink. The disease spread from minks to ferrets, as the two were raised on the same farms.

Hosts susceptible

AMDprimarily affects all breeds of wild and farmed mink, & ferrets, and can infect related animals such as raccoons, weasels, fishers, martens, and striped skunks. The disease is common in mink farms all over the world, causing high economic losses.

Transmission

Transmission can be **direct via feces, urine, saliva or blood, serum, bone marrow of infected animals and also through the placenta from a jill (dam)** to her kits. Air transmission is also possible, as is transmission through contact with contaminated surfaces. ADV is highly contagious. It is transferred through a ferret's bodily fluids, and it can lie dormant in dried urine or on an owner's clothes and shoes for up to two years. Known cases of AMDV positive ferrets should not be taken to places where they may come in contact with other ferrets. They also should not be allowed to run on floors or other areas where uninfected ferrets or their owners may come in contact with residual traces of the virus from the infected animals.

Pathogenesis

In adult mink, AMD has been classified into three categories: **1) progressive infection, 2) persistent nonprogressive infection, and 3) nonpersistent nonprogressive infection** with clearance of the virus. Thus far ADV infection in ferrets has been similar to that in mink. In adults, the virus **targets macrophages and dendritic cells for replication and sequestration.** The greatest amount of viral antigen is usually found in phagocytic cells of the **liver and lymphoid organs.** Once the ferret becomes infected with AMDV, a strong antibody response and associated hypergammaglobulinemia results from the antiviral immune response. Antibodies are directed against both structural and nonstructural proteins, but **are unable to clear the virus from the body.** Long term infection with AMDV subsequently **causes immune complex disease.** The **deposition of the immune complexes** in various organs including the kidneys, liver, arteries, and nervous tissue accounts for the clinical signs and pathological abnormalities observed. It is possible for ferrets to be infected for years with AMDV before any clinical signs are observed.

In newborn mink kits, AMDV replicates rapidly in type II alveolar cells of the lung causing an interstitial pneumonitis. This disease is more typical of other parvoviral infections including feline panleukopenia, canine parvoviral enteritis, and mink enteritis. It is unknown why these cells are targeted by AMDV in young ferrets and not in adults, but viral infection appears to be more severe in young ferrets than in adults. Little investigation has been done into the disease process in mink kits, but some studies have shown that natural or passive immunity to the virus in kits can prevent fulminate infection. It is interesting that the same immune response in adults is the major contributor to progressive disease.

Currently, there is little information concerning shedding of the virus. It is **suspected that the virus is shed only during times of replication.** One case report from The University of Georgia detected viral DNA in the blood, urine, and feces of one asymptomatic ferret that exhibited persistently high antibody titers. Since asymptomatic carriers of the disease have been identified, control and management of AMDV infection through routine testing has become even more important.

The virus is unusual in that it elicits a strong immune response (production of antibodies) from the animal, but the antibodies produced do not neutralize the virus. Instead, antibodies are produced in massive amounts, which can form immune complexes that are deposited in tissues, producing inflammation that is ultimately responsible for the progression of the disease. In addition, certain immune system cells like plasmacytes and lymphocytes accumulate in tissues. It is actually the immune response to the virus that causes the symptoms rather than the virus directly. This is why vaccination isn't feasible at this point, because it could elicit a similar immune response.

Clinical symptoms & lesions

AMD has often been described as a "wasting disease" characterized by chronic (long term) weight loss. A common manifestation is weakness or paralysis due to spinal cord damage, which progresses from the hind end up to the front legs. Other signs include lethargy, tarry stools (due to blood in the stool), and tremors. Occasionally the disease may cause sudden death. Organs commonly affected include the **kidneys and liver.**

The clinical signs of AMDV infection in most ferrets are compatible with chronic wasting and include progressive weight loss, weakness, ataxia, and posterior paresis. The infected animals also may present with fecal and urinary incontinence as well as severe coughing and dyspnea. **Clinical signs seen in AMD are not specific for the disease but usually are related to the organ system affected by the immune complex deposition.** Clinical signs related to renal failure, liver failure, or intestinal involvement (melena) may be observed. Abnormalities that may be noted on physical examination include **hepatomegaly and splenomegaly**. Central nervous system signs with ADV infection can include tremors, convulsions, and paralysis. There also are instances where ferrets die suddenly without apparent clinical signs. The immune response to AMDV varies from animal to animal. This may be related to the variable pathogenicity of different AMDV strains coupled with the specific immune response by the host against the virus.

Clinicopathologic features of AMD include a hypergammaglobulinemia, in most ferrets, globulins comprised greater than 20% of the overall protein concentration. Thus, hyperglobulinemia in any ferret should warrant further laboratory investigation with the aid of serum protein electrophoresis. Anemia also can be seen and is usually related to chronic inflammation. Clinical pathologic findings suggestive of specific organ damage can include azotemia and increased activity of liver enzymes. Hypoalbuminemia may be present secondary to decreased albumin production by the liver or increased renal loss in the urine.

PM gross lesions can be seen in many organ systems on post mortem examination. The **kidneys** can appear pale and enlarged or small and shrunken, depending upon the chronicity of the disease. The **liver** is usually enlarged and pale with scattered white nodules. Lesions in the **small intestine** include scattered mucosal ecchymoses with intraluminal melena. Mild to moderate enlargement of the spleen and lymph nodes may be observed. Lesions involving the respiratory system may include diffuse pulmonary congestion, serosanguineous pleural effusion, pulmonary edema, pulmonary ecchymoses, and lung lobe consolidation and collapse. Gross lesions usually are not seen in subclinical infections with AMD.

The most common **histological finding** in ferrets with AMDV infection include **lymphoplasmacytic infiltration of numerous organ systems including the brain, spinal cord, heart, lungs, digestive tract, liver, pancreas, and kidneys.** More specific lesions in the liver included periportal cholangiohepatitis with infiltrates of lymphocytes, plasma cells, and neutrophils; bile ductular hyperplasia; and periportal fibrosis. Renal lesions may include multifocal lymphoplasmacytic interstitial infiltrates and mild membranous glomerulopathy. Lymphoplasmacytic perivascular cuffing in the brain and spinal cord may be observed along with a lymphoplasmacytic meningitis.

Diagnosis

Presumptive diagnosis is based on patient history, clinical signs, the presence of hypergammaglobulinemia, & histologic observation of lymphoplasmacytic infiltrates in various tissues and organs.

But definitive disease diagnosis is made through tests such as counter immunoelectrophoresis (CIEP), ELISA, PCR, and DNA *in situ* hybridization. The current standard of testing and screening used is the CIEP for detection of AMDV antibodies; but this test is no longer commercially available. The NP1 ELISA test will only detect viral infections when viral replication is taking place and is not sensitive or specific enough to stand alone. **The new VP1/ VP2 ELISA test** developed at The University of Georgia is more sensitive in that these viral structural proteins are present in active and latent AMDV infections. This test is more specific than the NP1 ELISA; however, false negative test results can occur if the host only produces antibodies to the non-structural AMDV proteins. For this reason, it is recommended that **both ELISAs be used concurrently to detect structural and nonstructural AMDV proteins** (antigens). DNA *in situ* hybridization can be used to detect the presence of the ADV in formalin fixed, paraffin embedded biopsy or necropsy tissues. PCR, along with the results of the ELISA tests and DNA *in situ* hybridization, can help characterize patients as to whether AMDV infection is recent, persistent and progressive, persistent and nonprogressive, or nonpersistent with impending recovery.

Treatment & prevention

Definitive treatment for ADV currently does not exist. Supportive therapy may include administration of fluids, electrolyte supplementation, anti-inflammatory drugs, and antibiotics to prevent secondary infections. Treatment with immunosuppressive drugs has been tried to help decrease the deleterious effects of the immune response. These treatments have shown short-term improvements in clinical signs; however, mortality rates remain high in ferrets with clinical signs of AD.

Levamisole, cyclophosphamide, and interferon inducer have been tested in mink to decrease the hypergammaglobulinemia and immune complex deposits. These therapeutic agents have shown variable response in mink and are currently of limited benefit in ferrets due to their unknown effectiveness. Treatment with gamma globulin-containing anti-AMDV antibody has been shown to decrease mortality rates in mink kits, but has not shown any beneficial effects in adult animals.

Currently, a commercial vaccine does not exist to protect ferrets against the AMDV infection. Some experimental vaccines have been shown to decrease disease severity upon challenge with virulent ADV; however, much more work is needed to document the actual efficacy of these vaccines and reveal any potential side effects.

The **disease is best controlled through prevention.** Mink farms currently use the CIEP test for screening and removal of individuals suspected of having ADV infection. This practice has helped to manage and control outbreaks of ADV in mink colonies, but has not eradicated the disease. Although a test and removal program is helpful in commercial mink colonies, it is not an ideal solution for pet ferret owners. Until effective vaccines and anti-viral treatments are developed, management of AMD will need to be carried out through proper hygiene and quarantine protocols.

Genus: *Bocavirus*

Bovine Parvovirus Infection

Bovine parvovirus under the genus *Bocavirus* (BPV) causes subclinical infection in cattle & sporadic outbreaks with enteritis & diarrhea in calves. *Bovine parvovirus* is now thought to have three species: BPV1, 2 and 3. BPVs are best known for **causing diarrhea in neonatal calves and also respiratory and reproductive disease in adult cattle**. This virus is very resistant to chemical and physical challenges. Anaerobic microbial digestion in manure appears to inactivate the virus.

Occurrence

Bovine parvoviruses have been found in every country where cattle herds have been screened.

Hosts susceptible

Only cattle are naturally infected. Pigs can develop antibodies after ingestion of BPV but develop no clinical signs.

Transmission

BPVs are very efficiently transmitted transplacentally. They are also spread via the fecal-oral route.

Clinical symptoms

Diarrhea is the main clinical sign and often occurs alone. **Abortion and birth of weak or stillborn calves** is the manifestation of reproductive BPV. **Foetuses in the first trimester are most susceptible**. Cough, dyspnoea and nasal discharge may develop. Lymphopaenia is common on haematology. BPV is made worse by concurrent GI infections such as **coccidiosis.**

Diagnosis

Fluorescent antibody test and PCR are commercially available for diagnosis of BPV. BPV can be **isolated in cell cultures,** and confirmed via haemagglutination, **ELISA and electron microscopy.**

Foetuses aborted due to BPV infection are **oedematous** and have increased pleural and peritoneal fluid. **Intranuclear inclusion bodies** are seen in the cells of the small intestine, lymph nodes, liver and cerebellum. Virus can be detected in foetal adrenals, lungs, spleen, heart and thymus by immunofluorescence.

On **PM examination** of infected calves, **intestinal villous atrophy and fusion and crypt degeneration** are visible histologically. There is also lymphoid tissue necrosis associated with the intestinal tract and thymus. Small intestine and caecum appear to be preferential sites for BPV infection and replication.

Treatment & prevention

Control can be achieved using organic acid based disinfectants.

Vaccination

Disease is controlled usually by vaccination of dams during gestation. A vaccine is available against BPV, combined with other gastrointestinal pathogens. It is given in two doses; the **first dose is given 6-8 weeks prior to parturition followed by another 4-5 week prior to calving.**

□□□

Chapter 15

Characteristics and Diseases Caused by Group II Single-Stranded DNA Circoviruses (Family *Circoviridae*)

Contents

Characteristics of Circoviruses

Cirocoviruses, recently included under the famly *Circoviridae,* are non-enveloped, small measuring 17-22 nm in diameter with **icosahedral** symmetry. The genome is unsegmented that have a single molecule of **DNA forming a circle**, & the ends are closed by covalent bonds (Fig 15-1). The genome is about 1.8 to 3.8 kb nucleotides long. These viruses cause disease in vertebrate animals & insects. The *Circoviridae* includes two genera: Genus 1: *Circovirus;* type species: *Porcine circovirus type 1 and 2,* & other species is *Beak and feather disease virus* (BFDV), & Genus 2: *Gyrovirus;*

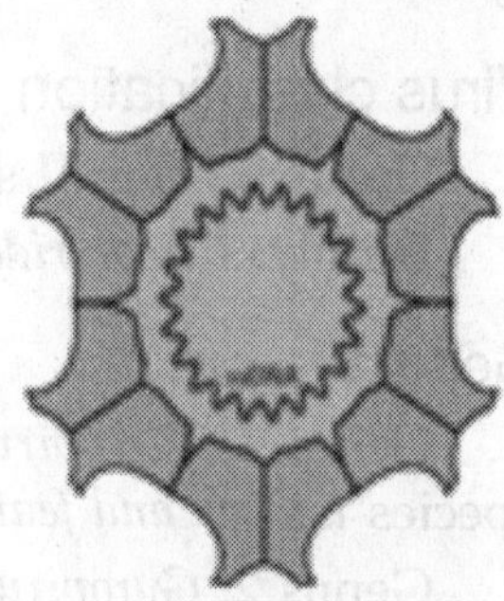

Fig. 15.1 : Morphology of a Circovirus

type species: *Chicken anaemia virus*. *Porcine circovirus type 1* (PCV1) is not linked with a disease, while porcine circovirus type 2 (PCV2) is the etiological agent of **Postweaning Multisystemic Wasting Syndrome (PMWS), a new emerging** Circoviruses are stable at pH 3-9 & resist heating at 60^{0}C for 30 minutes & resistant to some disinfectants, including detergents.

The virus genome

The virus genome is unsegmented that have a single molecule of DNA forming a circle, & the ends are closed by covalent bonds. The genome is about 1.8 to 3.8 kb nucleotides long. The genome encodes only **two major open reading frames**. The gene products- Rep, Rep' and Cap are involved in viral replication, regulation of transcription and capsid formation. Due to their highly limited coding capacity, circoviruses rely on the host's machinery for synthesis of macromolecules.

Virus replication

The virus replicates in the nucleus of dividing cells probably during S phase. The genome is replicated through double-stranded intermediates. The replication (Rep) protein initiates **rolling-circle replication**. During gene expression one or two mRNAs encode for the Rep, capsid, and possibly others proteins. Some mRNAs can be spliced.

The virus first attaches to & enters into the host cell. Ciroviruses are uncoated and the viral genomic is released & ssDNA enters into the nucleus. The ssDNA is converted into dsDNA with the participation of cellular factors. Viral mRNAs are transcribed and translated to produce viral proteins. Replication may be mediated by a Rep protein, and would occur by rolling circle producing ssDNA genomes.

These newly synthesized ssDNA can either i) be converted to dsDNA and serve as a template for transcription or replication, or ii) be encapsidated by capsid protein and form virions which are released from the cell by budding.

Virus classification

Group: Group II ssDNA

Family: *Circoviridae*

Genera

Genus 1: *Circovirus;* type species: *Porcine circovirus* Type 1 and 2, other species is *Beak and feather disease virus* (BFDV)

Genus 2: *Gyrovirus;* type species: *Chicken anaemia virus*

Unassigned Genus 3: *Anellovirus* includes human virus such as Transfusion transmitted virus or *Torque teno virus.*

Table 15.1 : Classification of the family *Circoviridae* & diseases caused by the member viruses in humans & animals.

Genera	Species	Serotypes	Diseases caused
G1: *Circovirus*	TS: *Porcine circovirus 1*	PCV-1, PCV-2	*Porcine circovirus* 2 (PCV-2) first identified in 1997 infects pigs less than 6 week old, under stress or concurrent infection. PCV2 infection is widespread & essentially all pig herds are infected with PCV-2 but relatively few show PCV2-associated disease (PCVAD). PCVAD includes: **i.** postweaning multisystemic wasting syndrome (PMWs), **ii.** Porcine dermatitis and nephropathy syndrome (PDNS), **iii.** Porcine respiratory disease complex (PRDC), **iv.** PCV2-associated reproductive failure, **v.** congenital tremors (CT) type AII, & **vi.** PCV2 associated enteritis. In many cases, different co-factors (infectious and non-infectious) are required, along with PCV2, to reproduce clinical signs and lesions in these pigs.
	Beak and feather disease virus	BFDV	*Beak and feather disease virus* (BFDV) **affects all psittacine species,** but parrots are most affected; Macaws African Grey Parrots, Ring-neck parakeets, Eclectus parrots & Lovebirds are also affected. **BFDV causes fatal infections in young birds,** while older birds overcome the disease & **become virus carriers shedding the virus.** BFDV **attacks the feather follicles and the beak and claws-growing cells of the bird,** affect the liver, brain, and immune system causing reduced resistance to infections with premature death from secondary bacterial, fungal, parasitic, or viral infections.

			Symptoms include irreversible loss of feathers, shedding of developing feathers, development of abnormal feathers, new pinched feathers, and loss of powder down, & overgrown or abnormal beak, symmetrical lesions on the beak and occasionally nails. Immunosuppression, rapid weight loss, and depression are seen in later stages of the disease.
	Canary *circovirus*	CaCV	
	Goose circovirus	GoCV	
	Pigeoncircovirus	PiCV	
	T. Duck circovirus	DuCV	
	T. Finch circovirus	FiCV	
G 2: *Gyrovirus*	TS: *Chicken anemia virus*	CAV	*Chicken anemia virus* (CAV) chicken anaenia, also called **Blue wing disease** (BWD), Anemia dermatitis syndrome, Chicken/ Avian infectious anaemia, Hemorrhagic aplastic anaemia syndrome, Infectious chicken anaemia, Chicken infectious anaemia (CIA), Chicken anaemia agent (CAA) affects poultry, mainly young chicks worldwide in commercial flocks or broilers. CAV infection causes anaemia, bone marrow atrophy, and severe immunosuppresson in poultry as the virus affects the production of RBC, WBC and platelets. Symptoms **include:** chicks are anorectic, lethargic, depressed, and pale. PCV is low, anemic, leukopenia, or pancytopenia, blood is watery and clot slowly. Mortality rate is variable but goes high with secondary infections. Organs are pale; the thymus is atrophied, and the bursa of Fabricius is small, bone marrow

is pale or yellow & hemorrhage may be present in or under the skin, muscle, and other organs. Lymphoid cells are depleted in primary and secondary lymphoid organs & granulocytic and erythrocytes in the bone marrow are atrophic or hypoplastic.

Circovirus
Clinical Infections in Animals & Birds
Genus: *Circovirus*
Porcine Circovirus Infection

Porcine circovirus 2 (PCV-2) first identified in 1997 infects pigs less than 6 weeks old, under stress or concurrent infection. PCV2 infection is widespread & essentially all pig herds are infected with PCV-2 but relatively few show PCV2-associated disease (PCVAD). PCVAD includes: **i. postweaning multisystemic wasting disease (PMWD)**, **ii.** Porcine dermatitis and nephropathy syndrome (PDNS), iii. Porcine respiratory disease complex (PRDC), **iv.** PCV2-associated reproductive failure, **vi.** Congenital tremors (CT) type AII, & **v.** PCV2 associated enteritis. In many cases, different co-factors (infectious and non-infectious) are required, along with PCV2, to reproduce clinical signs and lesions in these pigs. An effective vaccination is now available. Fort Dodge Animal Health (Wyeth) launched the first USDA approved vaccine in 2006, containing an inactivated virus (ATCvet code: QI09AA07).

Etiology: There are two serotypes, PCV-1 & PCV-2; PCV-1 was first identified in 1974 readily infects pigs, but does not cause disease in swine. PCV type 2 first isolated in 1997 has caused problems in recent years with the increasing occurrence of PMWD, which over time results in significant depletion of lymphocytes; PM examination of diseased animals reveals enlarged lymph nodes and abnormal lung tissue.

Occurrence

Most of the clinical conditions associated with PCV-2 have been reported from majority of the countries in the world.

Hosts susceptible

Domestic pig and the wild boar are susceptible, but is frequently occurring disease of pigs about **six weeks of ag**e & other ages according to clinical conditions. No other species are susceptible to the PCV2 infection. At least there has not been any PCV1 or PCV2 infection detected in dog, cat, goat, horse, bovine, rabbit, rat, mouse, chicken or human. PMWS occurs worldwide, & various **stresses or concurrent infection with other agents**, including porcine parvovirus or porcine reproductive and respiratory syndrome virus have a synergistic effect.

Transmission

The virus has been detected in various excretions, including nasal secretions, saliva, tonsils, tracheal mucus, urine, feces, semen and ocular secretions. PMWS cases not only present a significantly higher viral load in serum, they also excrete a significantly higher quantity of the virus. Probably the most probable route of PCV2 transmission is the **oronasal tract**, which would indicate that horizontal transmission (sow-piglet or piglet-piglet) is a frequent or very frequent occurrence. The most recent important fact is the demonstration that PCV2 is not only transmissible, but it can also transmit porcine circovirus from a sick pig to a healthy one. In some of documented transmission models, there is nearly always the co-infection of some other pathogen; this is what usually happens under field conditions. It is also known that PCV2 can be detected in semen; however, it remains unknown whether or not this is sufficient to cause an intrauterine infection with pathological consequences-embryonic death, fetal death, or the subsequent development of porcine circovirus in the infected fetuses.

Pathogenesis

Pathogenesis of PCV2-infections in embryos, fetuses and piglets was studied. It was shown that embryos are protected against PCV2 as long as they are inside their zona pellucia. After hatching, PCV2 infects embryos and kills them, leading to return to oestrus of the sows.

The outcome of the PCV2 infection in fetuses is lethal when the fetus is infected **during the first two months of gestation**. In immunocompetent fetuses, the virus can be controlled leading to the birth of either still- and weak-born or completely normal piglets. **The target cells of PCV2 change during gestation**. Early in gestation the virus replicates in cardiomyocytes, hepatocytes, lymphocytes and monocytes/macrophages. At the end of gestation and shortly after birth, PCV2 replicates mainly in lymphocytes and monocytes/ macrophages in the first two weeks of infection and in monocytes/ macrophages in a later stage.

In piglets, PCV2 replication takes place **for two weeks before the immunity gets activated**. Afterwards, the immunity eliminates virus and infected cells. The stimulation of the lymphoid tissues during infection by vaccination and co-infections clearly activates virus replication. **Main target**

cells are lymphoblasts and cells of the monocytic cell lineage. Why PCV2 evades from immunity and leads to PMWS in some piglets is not fully elucidated. It have been demonstrated that absence of neutralizing antibodies may explain part of the story.

Study on the pathogenesis of PCV2 infection, suggests that PCV2 **initially replicates in the tonsil.** In *Porcine parvovirus* (PPV) and PCV2 coinfected pigs, PPV antigen predominates in the tissues of the pigs killed between 3 and 14 DPI with a maximum observed between 6 and 14 DPI. PCV2 antigen was first observed in minimal amounts in mesenteric lymph nodes at 10 DPI with increasing density and distribution of PCV2 antigen at 14, 17, 21, and 26 DPI (Allan et al., 2000b). **Large numbers of PCV2 antigen or nucleic acids are detected in the cytoplasm of macrophages and dendritic cells.** A recent study found that **antigen presenting cells** in general, and not only macrophages stained positive by IHC for PCV2 antigen, & PCV2 antigen in lymphocytes was only sporadically detected. In thymus, PCV2 was only detected in few histiocytic cells in the medulla suggesting that thymocytes and T cells might be more resistant to PCV2 infection. To a lesser extent, PCV2 antigen is also found in **epithelial cells in lungs and kidneys, in smooth muscle cells, and in endothelial cells** in several tissues in pigs experimentally-infected with PCV2 as well as in pigs with naturally occurring PCV2-associated PMWS. PCV2-antigen was seen in infiltrating macrophages in the tunica albuginea, in interstitial macrophages and in germinal epithelial cells in the testes, and in infiltrating macrophages in the epidiymides of boars 24 to 29 days after they had been coinfected with PCV2 and PPV at 3 days of age. PCV2 was also found in the parenchyma of the secondary sex glands in a naturally infected boar. **PCV2 targets mainly cardiomyocytes, hepatocytes, and macrophages during fetal life, and mainly monocytes in early post-natal life.**

Clinical symptoms & lesions

Postweaning multisystemic wasting syndrome (PMWS)

PMWS was first recognized in high health Canadian herds in 1991 and is seen in almost every country now. Morbidity is usually 100%, mortality can approach 5-50%. This syndrome most often **affects pigs 4-12 weeks of age** and is diagnosed by meeting all of the following three criteria:

i. Clinical signs and gross lesions include: wasting, slowed growth, enlargement of inguinal lymph nodes and frequently dyspnea, noncollapsed and mottled lungs and occasionally jaundice.

ii. Characteristic histological lesions include: lymphocyte depletion in secondary lymphoid tissues, granulomatous inflammation in numerous organs, interstitial pneumonia and often basophilic cytoplasmic inclusion bodies in macrophages.

iii. Demonstration of PCV2 within lymphoid tissue lesions by IHC, PCR or *in situ* hybridization; virus isolation is also offered by some laboratories.

It was demonstrated that disease could be reproduced in cesarean-derived, colostrum-deprived (CDCD) pigs with PCV2 producing clinical signs of PMWS. Similar work has been performed using an infectious genomic clone of PCV2 in specific pathogen free (SPF) pigs to produce the gross and microscopic lymphoid lesions of PMWS. Although PCV2 has been shown to induce PMWS lesions in CDCD and SPF pigs, the presence of additional factors are required.

It has been suggested that immune stimulation may play an integral role in the development of PMWS in PCV2 infected pigs caused by management or environmental stress, coinfection with another pathogen or administration of vaccines and adjuvants. Coinfection with *Porcine parvovirus* (PPV) has shown to potentiate the replication and tissue distribution of PCV2 and increase the severity of clinical signs and lesions of PMWS. Recent work has demonstrated that **oil-in-water adjuvants may contribute to PCV2 induced disease** more than other types of adjuvants.

There is no proven treatment or prevention for PMWS, but administration of corticosteroids appears to be beneficial in an acute outbreak to reduce the severity of the disease and death loss.

Porcine dermatitis and nephropathy syndrome (PDNS)

PDNS was first described in 1993 in the United Kingdom, but presently has a worldwide distribution. Although PCV2 is often found in cases of PDNS, the current diagnostic criteria for PDNS include two criteria:

i. **Necrotizing skin lesions** mainly on rear legs and perineal region and/ or swollen and pale kidneys with generalized cortical petechiae.

ii. Systemic **necrotizing vasculitis and necrotizing and fibrinous glomerulonephritis**.

Currently, PDNS is considered to be a type III hypersensitivity reaction, although the antigen associated with this immune-complex disease is not definitively known.

Porcine respiratory disease complex (PRDC):

PCV2 associated pneumonia is the **most common symptom of PCV2 associated disease**. PCV2 is most often associated with **lung lesions in pigs**

coinfected with PRRSV or *Mycoplasma hyopneumoniae*. But there have been uncomplicated PCV2 pneumonia cases reported in western Canada. PCV2 is determined to be associated with PRDC when PCV2 antigen is associated with characteristic lung lesions. The lesions include **necrotizing and ulcerative bronchiolitis, granulomatous inflammation in the alveolar septa and mixed inflammation and fibroplasias in the lamina propria and peribronchiolar areas.** It is often difficult to differentiate between cases of PMWS and PCV2 associated pneumonia.

PRRSV infection increases PCV2 replication in experimentally dually inoculated pigs and synergism between these two viruses is also commonly observed in the field. Like PPV, PRRSV and PCV2 all replicate in macrophages and can produce immune cell dysfunction. This may be an important factor in the enhanced replication of PCV2 following PPV or PRRSV infection. Although *M. hyopneumoniae* infects different target cells, PCV2 and *M. hyopneumoniae* coinfected pigs show more severe clinical respiratory disease and lung lesions, poorer growth performance, longer PCV2 viremia and greater amounts of PCV2 antigen in serum, lymphoid and lung tissues than pigs infected with only one pathogen. The peribronchial lymphoid hyperplasia induced by *M. hyopneumoniae* seems to provide an important site for PCV2 replication in a lung.

Congenital tremors (CT) type AII

Currently, the association between PCV2 and CT type AII is controversial. A study conducted at Purdue demonstrated by PCR, IHC and *in situ* hybridization showed that PCV2 was present in CNS and liver tissues from both CT pigs and clinically normal pigs; however, there were more PCV2 infected cells in the CNS of CT pigs than normal pigs. Another study conducted in Europe, however, did not demonstrate an association between PCV2 and CT type AII.

Reproductive failure

PCV2 has been associated with reproductive failure, particularly late-term abortions and increased numbers of mummified fetuses, stillborns and weak pigs. The phenomenon of "stair-step" mummies has been observed in which all the fetuses appear to have died during different stages of gestation. The fetuses may have some cardiac hypertrophy and hepatic congestion, but there are not many specific gross lesions observed. There are some characteristic fetal histological lesions, which include **severe myocarditis, cardiomyocyte loss, fibrosis and intranuclear inclusion bodies in cardiomyocytes**, as well as passive hepatic congestion. PCV2 can be detected by IHC in the myocardial lesions. Although it is not always certain how PCV2 is transmitted, it has been proven to be shed in semen of infected boars. It is shed sporadically in **semen for at least 47 days post-inoculation.**

PCV-2 associated enteritis

PCV2-associated enteritis occurred in 6 weaned pigs without PMWS as confirmed by histopathology, virus isolation, and in situ hybridization. The most unique lesions were granulomatous inflammation affecting Peyer's patches, characterized by infiltrates of epithelioid macrophages and giant multinucleated cells. Large, multiple, basophilic or amphophilic, grape-like intracytoplasmic inclusion bodies were often seen in the cytoplasm of histiocytic cells and giant multinucleated cells. No microscopic lesions were observed in the lymphoid tissue, such as lymph node, spleen, and tonsil. A strong hybridization signal for PCV2 was detected in the cytoplasm of histiocytes and giant multinucleated cells in Peyer's patches. PCV-2 was isolated from homogenates of the small and large intestines in 2 weaned pigs. The presence of diarrhea and granulomatous enteritis, and abundant PCV2 DNA associated with the microscopic lesions is suggestive of PCV2-associated enteritis. Thus, PCV2-associated enteritis could be a distinct clinical manifestation.

PCV2 obviously plays a diverse role in the swine industry and the incidence of PCV2 associated disease is on the rise throughout the world. It is known that PCV2 is present on clinically normal farms as well as farms with reported PCV2 associated disease, but the seroprofile of both types of farms is the same. Currently, control of PCV2 associated disease, particularly PMWS and PCV2 associated pneumonia, is based on implementing management practices that minimize stress, eliminating or minimizing the effect of coinfections and eliminating potential triggering factors that induce immune stimulation.

PCV2 is currently a significant research topic around the world and, hopefully, these research efforts will help to unravel much of the mystery surrounding this somewhat elusive pathogen.

Diagnosis

Collection of clinical samples for various tests requires preferably a whole pig, lungs, liver and kidney.

1. *Presumptive diagnosis*: It is based on age susceptibility, clinical signs and lesions. But a confirmatory diagnosis is done by fluorescent antibody staining of the virus in infected tissues. Immunofluorescence assay and ELISA are used to detect antibodies although the presence of specific antibody alone is not diagnostic.

The virus can be cultivated in cells, but virus isolation is not usually attempted for diagnosis since many swine cells used for virus isolation are contaminated with PCV, which may results in false diagnosis.

Treatment & prevention

Vaccination

Vaccine concepts relies on two major approaches to controlling PCV2 infections in pigs, the first one is to vaccinate the sows and allowing maternally derived antibodies to protect the piglets and allow them to build up their own immunity naturally from natural virus exposure. The alternative is to vaccinate the piglets directly and early, before the virus has had a chance to multiply significantly, and thereby stimulate a more complete immune response. An overview of the four vaccines- Merial's vaccine Circovac® (for use in sows) in gilts: one 2 ml injection, followed 3 to 4 weeks later by a second 2 ml injection, at least 2 weeks before mating. One further 2 ml injection must be given a minimum of 2 weeks before farrowing. In sows one 2 ml injection, followed 3 to 4 weeks later by a second 2 ml injection, at least 2 weeks before farrowing. Boehringer Ingelheim's Ingelvac CircoFlex® inactivated when injected 1 ml dose of Ingelvac CircoFLEX protects piglets from 3 weeks through finishing. Option of vaccinating at weaning. Vaccinating at the youngest possible age (3 weeks) protects during early (nursery) and late (grow-finish) forms of disease. Intervet/Schering-Plough's Circumvent PCV® use a plant baculovirus with the ORF2 component inserted into it. Shake well & inject a 2.0 ml dose IM into healthy pigs, 3 weeks of age or older, & inject a 2.0 ml booster dose 3 weeks later. Animals retained for breeding purposes should be given a booster dose semiannually. Fort Dodge's Suvaxyn® PCV2 One Dose is a killed virus & uses PCV1, which is not pathogenic in pigs, with ORF2 inserted to produce a chimeric virus. Dosage: 2 ml IM to swine 4 weeks of age or older. Postera PCV-Pfizer is a chimera killed vaccine containing PCV1 & PCV2. Fostera PCV when vaccinated to pigs three weeks of age and older provides four months of immunity against PCV in a single 2-ml dose. Porcilis –PCV2-Intervet is inactivated baculavirus PCV 2 ORF 2 protein & adjuvanted subunit vaccine. Administer one dose of 2 ml by IM injection in the neck, the first injection (2 ml) can be given from an age of 3 days, with the second injection (2 ml) 2-3 weeks later. Table 15.2 depicts commercial vaccines available to control PCV-2 infection.

Beak and Feather Disease

Beak and feather disease virus (BFDV) **affects all psittacine species,** but parrots are most affected; Macaws African Grey Parrots, Ring-neck parakeets, Eclectus parrots & Lovebirds are also affected. **BFDV causes fatal infections in young birds,** while older birds overcome the disease & **become virus**

carriers shedding the virus. BFDV attacks the **feather follicles and the beak and claws-growing cells of the bird**, affect the liver, brain, and immune system causing reduced resistance to infections with premature death from secondary bacterial, fungal, parasitic, or viral infections. Symptoms include irreversible loss of feathers, shedding of developing feathers, development of abnormal feathers, new pinched feathers, and loss of powder down, & overgrown or abnormal beak, symmetrical lesions on the beak and occasionally nails. Immunosuppression, rapid weight loss, and depression are seen in later stages of the disease.

Table 15.2 : Commercial vaccines available to control PCV 2 infection

Company	Product	Sow/piglet	Type of vaccine	Adjuvant	No of injections
Merial	Circovac®	Sow	killed	Mineral oil	2+bosters each gestation
Boehringer Ingelheim	Ingelvac CircoFlex	Piglet 2 wks +	PCV 2 capsid polymer	Aqueous	1
Fort Dodge	Suvaxyn PCV2 one dose	Piglets 4 wks +	Killed–SL-CD Chimeric PCV 1 & 2	Aqueous	1
Intervet/SP	Circumvent ®	Piglet 3wks +	PCV2 capsid Tocophorol	Diluvac	2

Etiology: Beak and feather disease (BFD) is caused by *Beak and feather disease virus* (BFDV), which belongs to the genus *Circovirus*.

Occurrence

Psittacine beak and feather disease (BFD) was first recognized and described thoroughly in 1975 by Dr Ross Perry, a veterinary practitioner in Sydney. Numbers of birds showing feather and beak abnormalities were identified, initially in private collections and in wild flocks in Australia, but subsequently spread rapidly around the world. Initial theory regarding its cause included genetic or deficiency problems. It has since been recognized as a most significant disease of psittacine birds worldwide.

Hosts susceptible

BFD is a viral disease which affects not only parrots, but other birds too. The viral infection can be seen in cockatoos, African grey parrots, Eclectus parrots, lorikeets, lovebirds, and parrot species of Asian, Australian and African origin. Generally, PBFD affects **young birds, & is seldom seen in birds older than three years of age.**

Transmission

BFD is spread from infected birds to healthy birds by direct contact, usually from the **dust of feathers, dander or feces**; the disease is sometimes transmitted from contact with an **infected nest box**. Infected birds excrete the viruses by their droppings. Their plumage dust and the content of their crops are infectious. Usually chicks and fledglings get infected by their parents in the nest. Often the parents only carry the virus but are not obviously ill. But older birds, too, can be infected by breathing in infectious dust. Infected birds can also pass on the virus to their young. Thus in BFDV, both horizontal & placental transmission occurs. The virus is then transmitted from one bird to another via direct contact, inhalation or ingestion of aerosols, crop-feeding, infected fecal material, and feather dust or via contaminated surfaces such as bird carriers, feeding formula, utensils, food dishes, clothing, and nesting materials. Since the virus can survive outside the bird's body for years and cannot be killed by disinfectants, it can be spread easily and is difficult to control.

Pathogenesis

The incubation period and clinical signs produced by this virus are very variable, depending on the infective dose, and the age of the parrot and the stage of feather development at the time of infection. Nestlings often sicken within three or four weeks whereas elder birds take several months to years until the first symptoms of PBFD appear. As the immune system develops, birds become more resistant to infection, and the signs become less severe. In general, birds over 3 years old are rarely susceptible, but cases can and do occur in older birds if heavily challenged, or may be latent carriers become clinical following an episode of stress. In juvenile birds with an undeveloped immune system, the incubation period between infection and development of disease may be as short as 14-28 days, and illness will be severe. In older birds, incubation can be many months, and clinical signs are insidious and chronic. The course of the disease is very variable and carrier birds shedding the virus are common. It is therefore difficult to eliminate the virus from an infected population, and many collections of birds are positive.

Clinical symptoms & lesions

PBFD is easily recognized by its primary symptoms in the infected birds. There will be general feather loss, which cannot be attributed to bird's self plucking. Other symptoms include: sharp feathers, clubbed feathers, abnormally short feathers (pin feathers), loss of pigment in colored feathers, loss of powder down & bloody shafts in the feathers. As the infection progresses, the bird will become depressed for days, and will then die suddenly. Basically, it is essential that an infection with avian circoviruses causes dysfunctions in growth of beak, feathers and claws.

BFD runs **peracute, an acute, chronic course & carrier state of disease.** In peracute case, there is sudden death with no previous signs of illness in newly hatched chicks, most commonly cockatoos and African grey parrots. The **acute course** is seen in mainly **young birds-chicks & fledglings** that suffer from this and die quite fast. This results from the common appearance of the plumage dysfunction, low immunity, diarrhea, vomitus, and great lassitude.

Older birds usually show **chronic course** which means a creeping aggravation of their constitution. The plumage constitution of infected animals gets worse every molt until these animals show a plumage that might make you guess the bird was a feather picker. Furthermore the beak is growing faster than usual and often even askew or deformed. This are hints for a layman that the bird might be infected with BFD. If the chronic disease is quite advanced, most of the birds are **completely naked.** They also lose the head plumage which is a secure sign they did not pick their unreachable feathers themselves. After a little time the skin gets white and scabbed facings. These are centres of inflammation as the naked skin is very sensible and even smallest injuries can make bacteria as staphylococcus infect the bird. Exceeding claws are quite common in chronic BFD. When elder birds are affected, after an outbreak the disease usually leads to death after one or two years.

In carrier state, the birds show no clinical signs of the disease, but are actively infected and shedding the virus to infect other birds. This usually occurs in mature birds, and commonly in budgerigars, cockatoos and cockatiels.

Diagnosis

Collection of clinical samples includes whole birds and infected feathers.

1. *Presumptive diagnosis*: Clinical signs in the chronic form & histopathologic examination of affected tissues are highly suggestive while most birds suffering acute PBFD have a severe leucopenia. Intranuclear and intracytoplasmic inclusion bodies are commonly found in feathers, beak, and Bursa of Fabricius.

2. Virus antigen detection: Proof of positive birds is obtained by identifying the presence of the virus in the bird, and currently this is best achieved by a PCR test that detects the virus DNA in diseased and asymptomatic birds. This is the best method available for detecting the presence of PBFD virus in the bird's blood when beak or feather lesions are not apparent. This test is accurate and highly sensitive, since minute amounts of virus DNA will be detected. Diagnosis of BFD is made through a DNA probe which is extremely accurate as there is specific DNA present in the BFD Virus.

The virus has not so far been successfully propagated in embryonated eggs or cell cultures.

Treatment & prevention

There is no effective treatment for this viral infection. The infected bird with BFD should be immediately quarantined, & euthanasia is recommended to prevent the spread and stop the bird's suffering. To prevent BFD, strict hygiene should be followed in bird colonies, especially controlling the dust & regularly screening for PBFD. Consequently, if any bird is found infected, quarantine the bird and burn its nest box to prevent the disease from spreading. A well-balanced nutrition for improving the immune system is strongly required.

Vaccination

Fortunately a killed virus vaccine has been developed for prophylactic vaccination. The vaccine is given at the age of 14 days & a booster dose is given one month later. The vaccine induces immune response to the BFDV. The birds are examined until three years of age.

Genus: *Gyrovirus*

Chicken Anemia

Chicken anemia (CA), also called Blue wing disease (BWD), Anemia dermatitis syndrome, Chicken/Avian infectious anaemia, Hemorrhagic aplastic anaemia syndrome, Infectious chicken anaemia, Chicken infectious anaemia (CIA), Chicken anaemia agent (CAA), affects poultry, mainly young chicks worldwide in commercial flocks or broilers. CAV infection causes anaemia, bone marrow atrophy, and severe immunosuppresson in poultry as the **virus affects the production of RBC, WBC and platelets**. Symptoms observed are that chicks are anorectic, lethargic, depressed, and pale. PCV is low, anemic, leukopenia, or pancytopenia, blood is watery and clot slowly. Mortality rate is variable but goes high with secondary infections. Organs are pale; the thymus is atrophied, and the bursa of Fabricius is small, bone marrow is pale or yellow & hemorrhage may be present in or under the skin, muscle, and other organs. Lymphoid cells are depleted in primary and secondary lymphoid organs & granulocytic and erythrocytes in the bone marrow are atrophic or hypoplastic. The disease is under control due to widespread use of vaccinating breeders. But the subclinical form of the disease is ubiquitous.

Etiology: Chicken anemia (CA) is caused by *Chicken anemia virus* (CAV) in the genus *Gyrovirus* & the family*Circoviridae.*

The CA virus is very resistant in the environment, making disease elimination very difficult.

Occurrence

CAV was first described in Japan in 1979 by Yuasa et al. and appears to be ubiquitous in all major chicken producing countries of the world. CAV occurs in poultry, mainly in young chicks worldwide in commercial flocks or broilers.

Hosts susceptible

Chickens of all ages can be infected, but mainly affects young chicks in commercial flocks or broilers. CAV infection predominantly occurs in **young chicks** due to vertical transmission from the breeder hens whose maternal antibodies have not yet formed following virus exposure. Susceptibility to disease rapidly decreases after the first 2- 3 weeks of life. Concurrent infections with immunosuppresive viruses such as Marek's disease virus, Reticuloendotheliosis virus or Infectious bursal disease virus causes a delay in the development of age resistance and cause increased morbidity and mortality amongst the infected birds.

Transmission

CAV is transmitted **horizontally** by the fecal-oral route and by the respiratory route. **Vertical** transmission occurs in seronegative hens until neutralizing antibodies develop; chicks hatched from these eggs are viremic, then CAV is spread from these chicks to susceptible, maternal antibody-negative hatchmates. Roosters shedding CAV in the semen are another source of vertical transmission. Vaccination of seronegative flocks is used to prevent vertical transmission. The virus also can be transmitted mechanically from farm to farm by people, equipment and vehicles. The presence of the infection in some specific-pathogen-free flocks, used for vaccine production, may partially explain the worldwide incidence of the disease.

Pathogenesis

The **bone marrow and thymus are the most important target organs** in the pathogenesis of CAV infection. The destruction of haemocytoblasts in bone marrow results in a severe depletion of erythroid and myeloid cells and produces anaemia. The destruction of T-lymphocyte progenitor cells in the thymus results in depletion of mature cytotoxic and helper T cells and induces severe atrophy.

Disease usually occurs during the **first 3 weeks of life resulting from vertical transmission** or contact exposure close to hatch. CAV can be transmitted between chickens by both the horizontal and vertical routes. Horizontal spread usually occurs via the oral-fecal route, but infection via the respiratory route has also been demonstrated in experimentally infected birds. Vertical spread through hatched chickens is considered to be the most important means of dissemination of the virus.

The virus causes anemia, lymphoid atrophy and increased mortality after infection of day-old susceptible chickens. Infection of older birds with CAV results in subclinical disease and reduced resistance to other pathogens. Dual infection of chickens with other immunosuppressive viruses increases the severity of CAV signs and decreases the resistance of older birds to infection.

Clinical symptoms & lesions

The extent of loss in an infected flock depends on the age at which the chickens are infected, the level of their maternal antibody protection against the CAV and whether they are concurrently infected with other immunosuppressive viruses, such as IBD or Marek's disease virus. CAV infection **in young,** susceptible chickens results in increased mortality of chickens 12 to 28 days of age. Affected birds generally have a depressed, pale (anemic) and anorexic appearance. In uncomplicated cases, surviving chicks recover from the depression and anemia; however, **their body weights remain low**. Lesions can lead to **atrophy of the bone marrow and thymus.** The bone marrow becomes fatty and yellowish. Atrophy and aplasia of the blood-forming tissues can be seen microscopically, as well as replacement by adipose tissue and nonfunctional supportive tissue. The thymus may completely atrophy and become reddish brown. Microscopically, severe **lymphoid depletion** is visible throughout the gland. Gross lesions in the bursa of Fabricius are minimal and may be difficult to detect. In many cases, the liver may be swollen and mottled, and **massive hemorrhages may be observed in the proventricular mucosa** and in subcutaneous tissue and muscle, particularly in the **wing**.

Co-infection with the CAV and other immunosuppressive viruses increases the severity of disease due to the CAV, reduces the protective effect of maternal antibodies against the CAV and decreases age-related resistance to CAA. High levels of mortality associated with CAV infection are also commonly due to secondary bacterial infection. The term ***blue wing*** refers to a CAV infection in which initial skin lesions progress and **become gangrenous because of secondary bacterial infection**. As CAV infection results in immunosuppression, susceptible chicks have reduced ability to respond to vaccinations, resulting in diminished humoral and cell-mediated immune responses. The vertical transmission route has been associated with more severe immunosuppression. Combined infections of CAV and Marek's disease virus result in an enhanced shedding of Marek's disease virus and an increased incidence of Marek's disease tumors.

Diagnosis

Collection of samples includes whole sick chicken, & serum.

1. *Presumptive diagnosis*: It is based on clinical signs, lesions, age dependence, & immunosuppression etc. Laboratory tests for the diagnosis of CAV infections can be divided into those for antigen determination and those for antibody determination.
2. *Viral isolation*: Virus is isolated usually in embryonated specific pathogen free (SPF) eggs after yolk sac inoculation. Virus isolation can also be attempted on MSCC-MSB1 cells culture, a lymphoblastoid cell line established from Marek's disease and Lymphoid leukosis lymphomas. Growth is slow with low titers and at least 7 10 subcultures of inoculated cells are necessary for accurate end points for CAV infective titers. The virus can be isolated from different organs (liver, thymus, lung, heart, Bursa, muscle and bone marrow) but liver and buffy coat preparations are the preferred samples.
3. *Antigen detection*: Immunofluoresence test with fluorescein-conjugated antibodies that attach to the virus when present, for example on MDCC-MSB1 infected cells culture is positive for CAV. *PCR test*: PCR utilizes specific primers which recognize the genome of the virus. The virus can be detected in the same target organs collected for virus isolation.
4. *Antibody detection*: Chicken serum is mixed with CAV growing on embryonated eggs or cell cultures. When the growth of the virus is inhibited, the antibodies in the serum are identified. Usually the ß method is used. This means that known virus is used at a constant concentration and is tested against varying two-fold dilutions of suspect serum. From the serial dilutions the antibody titer is calculated.

A competitive Elisa is also used. The plates are covered with a complex of a monoclonal antibody and CAV. The complex is detected by an enzyme-labeled anti-γ-globulin. After adding an enzyme substrate, a resulting coloured product is measured. This test is useful to confirm the response to field infections and adequate antibody responses to vaccination.

Treatment & prevention

There is no specific treatment for infected birds. Culling of infected birds is normally performed in infected commercial flocks. Appropriate hygiene and biosecurity measures should be employed to control the disease. Birds that have been infected develop immunity to the virus.

Vaccination

Vertical spread of the disease can be controlled by the vaccination of **breeding hens** with both **live attenuated and wild vaccines**. These vaccines reduce the vertical transmission rate.

Breeders are vaccinated during the rearing period between **8-16 weeks of age with a live vaccine**. Care should be taken to ensure that vaccination results in high levels of maternally derived antibodies throughout the production period. Broilers and layer pullets are not commonly vaccinated against CAV in the field. Early protection is achieved by vaccination of the breeders though maternal derived antibodies. Vaccination is the backbone of CAV control strategy & protection against CAV and **only live vaccines** are used. Depending on the manufacturer, live vaccines can be applied **by mass vaccination (e.g., drinking water), otherwise by wing web administration or SC or IM injection**. CAV live vaccines induce **long lasting systemic immunity.**

CAV-VAC® (Intervet/Schering-Plough Animal Health) **is live virus vaccine prepared from a live modified US field isolate of CAV for use in breeder pullets 10 weeks of age and older via the wing web inoculation method.** It is the first **USDA licensed CAV vaccine,** is safe to use in young, antibody-negative chickens, & it induces high levels of protective antibodies for long-term protection of parent flocks and their progeny against CAV. It provides uniform flock protection & does not require addition of diluent. CAV-VAC® is indicated for the vaccination of breeder chickens one time at 10 weeks of age and older for the prevention of chicken anemia in their progeny. Hens should be vaccinated at least 6 weeks before the onset of egg production. The time of administration should be determined by the degree of chicken infectious anemia exposure, type of chicken being vaccinated, and the current management procedures. CAV-VAC is approved for use via wing web application.

□□□

Chapter 16

Characteristics and Diseases Caused by Group III DS DNA Reoviruses (Family *Reoviridae*)

Contents

Characteristics of Reoviruses

The family *Reoviridae* (L. reo; r = respiratory, e = enteric, o = orphan) name is derived from *respiratory enteric orphan viruses,* the term "orphan virus" means that viruses are not associated with any known disease although reoviruses cause various diseases but the original name is still retained. *Reoviridae* is a diverse family of viruses infecting humans, mammals, birds, plants & insects. Reoviruses are spherical, non-enveloped and measure 60-80 nm in diameter with a **double icosahedral capsid structure except for cypoviruses and dinovernaviruses,** which have only the equivalent of the inner capsid. The **outer capsid** measures 75-80 nm in diameter & made of **92 capsomers** (T=13) as in case of *Orthoreovirus,* & the **inner capsid is made of 32 capsomers** (*Orbivirus*) & measures 45 nm in diameter (T =2) (Fig 16-1). Reovirus genome is segmented, linear dsRNA consisting of 10 to 12 segments that code for 10 to 14 proteins. Segments size range from 0.2 to 3.0 kb & genome total size range from 18.2 to 30.5 kb.

Reoviruses differ in case of resistance to environmental conditions. While *Orthoreovirus & Rotavirus* are relatively resistant to wide pH range but *Orbivirus* & *Coltivirus* lose infectivity at low pH.

The virus genome

The reoviruses genome contains segmented, linear ds RNA in **10, 11 or 12 segments** which are placed into three groups as per their size: **L (large), M (medium) and S (small).** These segments range from ~ 3.9 kbp - 1kbp and each segment encodes 1-3 proteins. Proteins encoded by these groups are denoted by the Greek letters, e.g. the L segment encodes for **λ proteins,** the M segment encodes for **μ proteins** and the S segment encodes for **σ proteins.** As regards gene expression, dsRNA genome is never completely uncoated to prevent activation of antiviral state by the cell in response of dsRNA. Viral polymerase synthesizes mRNAs from each dsRNA segment which are translocated to the cell cytoplasm where they are translated. Proteins are produced by alternative initiation and protein processing.

Virus replication

Reoviruses replicate in the cytoplasm of the infected cells often forming IC inclusions. Reoviruses have **three features of virus replication.** First, they are dsRNA viruses which replicate in the cytoplasm & hence they have everything needed for replication and **do not utilize the cell's replication enzymes.** Second, they do not fully uncoat during the process of replication, the coat is resistant to protease digestion & prevent them from destruction by the infected cell. Third, the **mRNA used in translation is synthesized from the negative strand of the dsRNA.** Each negative strand produces many positive strands, and both strands remain in the uncoated core particle. The capped positive strand of RNA found in progeny dsRNA is synthesized from the negative strand template found in the dsRNA within the parental cores. These capped transcripts that result from primary transcription are not polyadenylated. Secondary transcription occurs in the later stage of infection and results in uncapped non-polyadenylated transcripts. The mRNAs leave the core and get translated in the cytoplasm. The segmented genome allows for possible reassortment.

Since these viruses have dsRNA genomes, replication occurs exclusively in the cytoplasm and the virus encodes several proteins which are needed for replication and conversion of the dsRNA genome into (+)-RNAs. The virus via outer capsid ü 1of *Orthoreovirus* or VP4 of rotaviruses attaches to the host cell surface receptor, probably sialic acid and junctional adhesion molecules (JAMs). The virus is partially uncoated by proteases in the endolysosome, where the capsid is partially digested to allow further cell entry. The core particle then enters the cytoplasm by as yet unknown process where the genome remains within the core & RNA is transcribed by RNA-dependent RNA polymerase conservatively causing an excess of (+) sense strands, which are used as mRNA templates to synthesize (-) sense strands. Viral particles begin to assemble in the cytoplasm 6–7 hours after infection. Mature virions are formed in the endoplasmic reticulum & released after cell lysis.

Virus classification

There are15 genera of *Reoviridae* divided in 2009 on the basis of the presence of a "turret" or spike protein on the inner capsid into **two subfamilies; *Sedoreovirinae* containing the non-turreted virus genera & *Spinareovirinae* containing the spiked or turreted viruses in the family.**

Group; Group III ds RNA

Family: *Reoviridae.*

The subfamily 1: *Spinareovirinae* contains 9 genera:

Genus 1: *Aquareovirus;* type species: *Aquareovirus A* (ARV-A)

Genus 2: *Cypovirus;* type species: *Cypovirus 1* (CPV- 1)

Genus 3: Fijivirus; type species: *Fiji disease virus* (FDV)

Genus 4: *Idnoreovirus;* type species: *Hyposeter exiquae reovirus* (HeRV)

Genus 5: *Mycoreovirus;* type species: *Mycoreovirus 1* (MRV-1)

Genus 6: *Orthoreovirus;* type species: *Mammalian orthoreovirus* (MRV)

Genus 7: *Oryzavirus;* type species: *Rice ragged stunt virus* (RRSV)

Genus 8: *Coltivirus;* type species: *Colorado tick fever virus* (CTFV)

Genus 9: *Dinoverna virus;* type species: *Aedes pseudoscutellaris virus*

The subfamily 2: *Sedoreovirinae* contains the 6 genera

Genus 1: *Mimoreovirus;* type species:

Genus 2: *Orbivirus;* type species: *Bluetongue virus* (BTV)

Genus 3: *Phytoreovirus;* type species: *Rice dwarf virus* (RDV)

Genus 4: *Rotavirus*: type species: *Rotavirus A* (RV-A)

Genus 5: *Seadornavirus; type species: Kadipiriro virus (KDV)*

Genus 6: *Cardoreovirus; type species: Eriocheir sinensus reovirus*

Table 16-1 depicted below mentions classification & diseases caused by the virus species.

Table 16.1 : Classification of the family *Reoviridae* & diseases caused by the member viruses in humans & animals.

Genera	Species	Serotypes	Diseases caused
G1: *Orthoreovirus*	Subgroup 1 TS: *Mammalian orthoreovirus*	MRV-1, 2, 3	*Mammalian orthoreovirus 1, 2, 3* **(MRV1,2,3)** cause mild respiratory & enteric infection in **humans & in many animal species.**
	Subgroup 2 *Avian orth-oreovirus*	ARV-s1133 176, SK138a	*Avian orthoreovirus* **(ARV-s1133, 176, SK138a)** cause significant infection; arthritis, tendinitis, gastroenteritis, hepatitis, & myocarditis in commercial flocks in chickens & turkeys, 4-16 wk old.
	Subgroup 3 *Baboon orthoreovirus*	BRV	
	T. Duck reovirus	DRV	
G 2: *Orbivirus*	*African horse sickness virus*	AHSV-1, 2, 3, 4, 5, 6, 7, 8, 9	African horse sickness **(AHSV-1, 2, 3, 4, 5, 6, 7, 8, 9)** affects horses, donkeys, zebras & dogs; elephant, dogs & zebras act as reservoirs; the disease is endemic in Africa, ME, India, Pakistan, Spain & Portugal; Vectors are *Culicoides* species. There are **4 forms** of the disease: the **peracute** or **pulmonary form, the subacute** or **cardiac** form, the **cardiopulmonary** or **mixed form &horse sickness**

		fever. The **acute respiratory form, the cardiac form** is subacute, has an IP of 3-5 days with interlobular edema, & hydropericardium; death in ~1 week, has an IP of 1-2 week.
TS: *Bluetongue virus*	BTV-1through 24	Bluetongue (BTV-1 through 24) or **catarrhal fever** is a **noncontagious, non-zoonotic** *Culicoides species* -borne disease **of ruminants, mainly of sheep** and less frequently cattle, goats, buffaloes, deer, and antelopes. Symptoms follow an IP of 1-12 days with high fever, excessive salivation, swellig of the face and tongue and cyanosis of the tongue; swelling of the lips and tongue gives the tongue its typical blue appearance. Nasal symptoms may be prominent, with nasal discharge and stertorous respiration. Some animals also develop foot lesions with coronitis, with consequent, lameness & in sheep, lead to knee-walking. In cattle, change of position of the feet gives bluetongue the nickname. Vaccines are available.
Epizootic hemorrhagic disease virus	EHDV-1, 2, 3, 4, 5, 5, 6, 7, 8, Ibaraki virus	Epizootic hemorrhagic disease (EHDV-1, 2, 3, 4, 5, 6, 7, 8) like BT occurs in **white tailed & mule deer,** cattle, buffaloes but non-white tailed deer are infected with various types without clinical symptoms; vectors are *Culicoides* species.
Equine encephalosis virus	EEV-1, 2, 3, 4, 5, 6, 7, 8	Equine encephalosis (EEV-1, 2,3, 4, 5, 6, 7, 8) is a peracute illness of horses in South Africa different from EEE, WEE & VEE; vectors are *Culicoides* species.

	Palyam virus	PAV	*Palyam virus* (PAV) infects cattle and sheep, is transmitted by culicine mosquitoes and *Culicoides* gnats. *Palyam virus* has at least 15 viruses in six antigenic complexes.PAV causes fetal lesions & abortion in cattle & sheep.
	Palyam virus (Chuzan disease virus)	PAV-ch	*Palyam virus*(PAV-ch) or Chuzan disease occurs in cattle in SE Asia, Japan; characterized by congenital abnormalities in calves-hydrocephaly or blindness; severity depending on age of the fetus.
G3: *Rotavirus*	TS: *Rotavirus A*	RV-A	*Rotavirus A* (RV-A) causes gastroenteritis with diarrhea in many young animal species up to 8 weeks old; serious in calves, piglets, foals, puppies & kittens mostly of group A. Severity depends on virus virulence, age, colostral uptake & management. Mostly the children become infected with rotavirus by their third birthday; repeated infections occur with different viral strains & most children get episodes of infection in the first years of life. IP is two days. Symptoms include fever, vomition & watery diarrhea, abdominal pain, or profuse watery diarrhea, rarely with dehydration. Symptoms persist for 3-9 days.
	Rotavirus B (Simian rotavirus B)	RV-B	
	Rotavirus C (Porcine rotavirus C)	RV-C	

	Rotavirus D (Chicken rotavirus D)	RV-D	
	Rotavirus E (Porcine rotavirus E)	RV-E	
	T. Rotavirus F (Chicken rotavirus F)	RV-F	
	T. Rotavirus G (Chicken rotavirus G)	RV-G	
G4: Coltivirus	TS: *Colorado tick fever virus*	CTFV, CTFV-56-14-03	Colorado tick fever (CTFV-56-14-03) causes encephalitis & flu-like symptoms in children; it is ticks & mosquitoes- borne; rodents act as virus reservoirs.
G5: *Seadornavirus*	*Banna virus*	BAV-ch	*Seadornavirus* derived its name from South East Asia dodeca RNA virus of which *Banna* (BAV-ch) *virus* causes encephalitis in humans in Japan & Indonesia, & have also been isolated from pigs & cattle.

Reovirus Clinical Manifestations in Humans

Infections in Humans

Among the many genera of *Reoviridae*, 5 genera-*Orthoreovirus, Orbivirus, Coltivirus, Rotavirus & Seadornavirus* infect humans as well as cause many diseases of veterinary importance.

Genus: *Orthoreovirus*

Mammalian orthoreovirus1, 2, 3 (MRV1, 2, 3) cause mild respiratory & enteric infection in humans & in many animal species.

Genus: *Rotavirus*

Rotavirus A (RV-A) is the most common cause of severe diarrhea among infants and children worldwide; most of the children become infected with rotavirus by their third birthday, repeated infections occur with different viral strains & most children get episodes of infection in the first years of life.

Incubation period is two days. Symptoms include fever, vomition, watery diarrhea, abdominal pain, or profuse watery diarrhea, rarely with dehydration. Symptoms persist for 3-9 days.

Genus: *Coltivirus*

Colorado tick fever (CTFV-56-14-03) causes encephalitis & flu-like symptoms in children; it is ticks & mosquitoes- borne; rodents act as virus reservoirs.

Genus: *Seadornavirus*

Seadornavirus derived its name from **S**outh **E**ast **A**sia **do**deca **RNA virus** of which ***Banna* (BAV-ch)** *virus* causes encephalitis in humans in Japan & Indonesia, & have also been isolated from pigs & cattle.

Reovirus Infections in Animals

Genus: *Orbivirus*

African Horse Sickness

African horse sickness (AHSV-1, 2, 3, 4, 5, 6, 7, 8, 9) is a non contagious, infectious, insect-borne viral disease of equids caused by *African horse sickness virus*. The disease is characterized by clinical signs due to damage to the circulatory and respiratory systems resulting in serous effusion and hemorrhages in various organs and tissues. Disease is classified into four forms: the **peracute** or **pulmonary form,** the **subacute or cardiac form,** the **cardiopulmonary** or **mixed form, & horse sickness fever form** (which usually affects only mules, donkeys and partially immune horses). All forms of disease may occur in any one outbreak in susceptible populations of horses, but the **mixed and pulmonary forms predominate,** & mortality rates in these animals are very high. Due to its severity, rapid spread and without apparent warning out of its endemic areas, AHS has been allocated by OIE (Office International des Epizooties) in List A status. The frequency, extent and severity of outbreaks in southern Africa has declined significantly over the last century, coinciding with major decrease in the horse and zebra populations and the introduction of AHS vaccines.

Etiology: *African horse sickness virus* belongs to the genus *Orbivirus* in the family *Reoviridae* and as such is morphologically similar to other orbiviruses like bluetongue virus (BTV) of ruminants and equine encephalosis virus. Nine antigenically distinct serotypes (AHSV-1, 2, 3, 4, 5, 6, 7, 8, 9) have been identified, the last being in 1960. There is some cross relatedness between the serotypes, between AHSV types 1 and 2; 3 and 7; 5 and 8; and 6 and 9, although there is no evidence from the field that there is any intratypic variation. Of the nine serotypes, **types 1 to 8 are typically found only in areas of sub-Saharan Africa while type 9 is more widespread and has been responsible for virtually all epidemics outside Africa,** the only exception being the 1987–1990 Spanish-Portuguese outbreaks which were due to AHSV-4.

The virus is acid sensitive, being readily inactivated at pH below 6.0 but remains relatively stable at more alkaline pH 7.0–8.5. It is resistant to lipid solvents and relatively heat resistant. Infectivity is remarkably stable at 4°C, particularly in the presence of stabilizers such as serum and sodium oxalate, carbolic cid and glycerine. Minimal loss of titer occurs with viruses that have been lyophilized or frozen at –70°C with Parker Davis Medium. But the viruses are fairly labile between –20°C & –30°C.

Occurrence

The disease is endemic in sub-Saharan endemic zone of Africa, ME, India, Pakistan, Spain & Portugal; vectors are *Culicoides* species. During 1965, AHSV-9 spread beyond its sub-Saharan endemic zones and appeared first in Morocco then spreading into Algeria and Tunisia before crossing the Straits of Gibraltar into Cadiz Province, Spain, in October 1966.

Hosts susceptible

AHSV affects horses, donkeys, zebras & dogs; elephant, dogs & zebras act as reservoirs. **Zebras are the natural reservoirs of AHSV, and play a vital role in the persistence of the virus in Africa**. This species rarely exhibits clinical signs of infection. All other equid species and crossbreeds are also susceptible to infection with AHSV. Dogs are susceptible to experimental infection with AHSV and may die, but infection also occurs readily following ingestion of infected horsemeat. Infection in camels is rare and inapparent.

Transmission

AHS is spread by insect vectors; the **biological vector** of the virus is the *Culcoides* (midges) species. However, this disease can also be transmitted by species of mosquito including *Culex*, *Anopheles* and *Aedes*, and species of ticks such as *Hyalomma* and *Rhipicephalus*.

Pathogenesis

After entry into the vertebrate host, virus initially replicates in the regional lymph nodes followed by primary viremia & dissemination throughout the body via the blood and subsequent infection of target organs and cells, namely the lungs, spleen and other lymphoid tissues, and certain endothelial cells.

Virus multiplication in these tissues and organs gives rise to a **secondary viremia,** which is of variable duration. Under natural conditions, the incubation period to the commencement of secondary viremia is less than nine days although experimentally it has been shown to vary between 2 and 21 days. In horses viremia usually lasts for only four to eight days and has not been detected beyond 21 days. In donkeys and zebra the levels of viremia are lower but may extend for up to four weeks. After viremia, **endothelial cells are infected with replication resulting in vascular damage causing increased vascular permeability, hemorrhage and edema.**

In experimentally infected horses, high concentrations of AHSV rapidly accumulate in the spleen, lungs, caecum, pharynx, choroid plexus and most lymph nodes. Subsequently, virus is found in most organs, probably due to their blood content. In the blood, virus is associated with the cellular fraction both **red blood cells and the buffy coat**, while very little is present in the plasma.

In ruminants there is extended viremia, a situation that seems not to occur with AHSV in horses although viremia in the presence of circulating antibody has been reported in zebra. In AHS the onset of viremia usually corresponds with the appearance of fever and persists until it disappears.

Experimentally infected horses with the peracute form of disease, antigen is found primarily in the cardio-vascular and lymphatic systems, and to lesser extent throughout the body. In animals with horse sickness fever, antigen is concentrated in the spleen, with lesser amounts elsewhere. The main locations of antigen were endothelial cells suggesting them to be a primary target of the virus and large cells of the red pulp of the spleen. The presence of antigen in large mononuclear cells, resembling phagocytic cells, and surrounding lymphoid follicles suggests that these cells might also be involved in virus replication and in the transport of viral protein to the lymphoid follicles.

Clinical symptoms

Pulmonary form: This form has an incubation period of **3-5 days**. It is the peracute form of the disease & is characterized by high fever, depression and respiratory symptoms. The clinically affected animal has trouble breathing, starts coughing frothy fluid from nostril and mouth, and shows signs of pulmonary edema within four days. Serious lung congestion causes respiratory failure and results in death within 24 hours. This form of the disease has the highest mortality rate up to 90%.

Cardiac form: This is subacute form of the disease with an incubation period longer than that of the pulmonary form, usually of 1-2 week. Signs of disease start at day 7-12 after infection. **High fever is a common symptom.**

The disease also manifests as conjunctivitis, with abdominal pain and progressive dyspnea. Additionally, edema is present under the skin of the head and neck, most notably in **swelling of the supraorbital fossae,** palpebral, conjunctiva and intermandibular space. Edema is never seen in the lower limbs. The conjunctivae may be congested, petechial haemorrhages may be seen in the eyes and ecchymotic hemorrhages may be seen on the ventral surface of the tongue. Colic is often a feature. Mortality rate is between 50-70% and survivors recover in 7 days.

Mild or horse sickness fever form: Mild to subclinical disease is seen in zebras and African donkeys. Infected animals may have low grade fever and congested mucous membrane. There is only mild to moderate fever and oedema of the supraorbital fossae – there is no mortality. It frequently occurs following infection with less virulent strains of virus or when some degree of immunity exists and is the only form of disease exhibited by the African donkey and zebra. The survival rate is 100%.

Mixed form: Affected horses show signs of both the pulmonary and cardiac forms of AHS. The mixed form is often the **most common form of AHS** and is a combination of the cardiac and pulmonary forms of disease. The mortality rate is approximately 70% and death usually occurs within 3 to 6 days after onset of fever.

PM lesions in the pulmonary from include interlobular edema of the lungs and hydrothorax. The subpleural and interlobular tissues are infiltrated with a yellowish gelatinous exudate and the entire bronchial tree may be filled with a surfactant, & stabilized froth. Ascites can occur in abdominal and thoracic cavities and the mucosa of the stomach may be hyperaemic and oedematous.

In the **cardiac form** the lesions are gelatinous exudate in the subcutaneous, subfacial and intramuscular tissues and lymph nodes. Hydropericardium is seen and hemorrhages are found on the epicardial and/or endocardial surfaces. Petechial haemorrhages and/or cyanosis may also occur on the serosal surfaces of the caecum and colon. In these instances, a distinct demarcation can often be seen between affected and unaffected parts. This may be due to a selective involvement of endothelial cells. As in the pulmonary form, ascites may occur but oedema of the lungs is either slight or absent.

In the **mixed form** of AHS, lesions common to both the pulmonary and cardiac forms of the disease occur.

Diagnosis

Collection of clinical specimens includes freshly collected and refrigerated whole blood, spleen, lung, lymph nodes and salivary glands.

1. *Presumptive diagnosis*: Presumptive diagnosis is made on the basis of clinical signs and pathologic lesions.
2. *Virus isolation*: Virus isolation is conducted in one-day-old mice inoculated intracerebrally, in embryonated eggs or in various cell cultures like Vero cells. The virus is then identified by virus neutralization tests or immunofluorescence.
3. *Virus antigen detection*: Specific virus antigen is detected by ELISA, complement fixation and agar gel immunodiffusion.
4. A RT-PCR is used to detect viral nucleic acid.
5. There are nine serotypes of the virus that are identified by **serum neutralization tests**. Their distribution varies with regions.

Group specific antibody against AHSV can be detected using assays that are directed primarily towards the VP7, including CFT, AGD, immunofluorescence, and ELISA. An indirect ELISA detects antibody against segment 10 (NS3) has now been used for AHSV serotype 4 which is used to distinguish between naturally infected animals and those vaccinated with purified, inactivated vaccine.

Treatment & prevention

There is no specific treatment for animals suffering from AHS apart from rest and good husbandry. Complicating and secondary infections should be treated appropriately during the recovery period.

AHS can only be spread via the bites of infected vector species of *Culicoides*. Protection from vector bite & strict import regulations are measures to prevent introduction of AHS virus into countries free of the disease.

Vaccination

Polyvalent, attenuated vaccines are commercially available from Onderstepoort Biological Products (OPB), which was previously based on virus attenuation by multiple suckling mouse brain passage. But now a day, further attenuation of the vaccine virus strains is done through passage in cell culture. The OPB, AHS vaccines currently used in southern Africa are supplied in two polyvalent vials containing AHSV types 1, 3 and 4, and 2, 6, 7 and 8, respectively. However, these vaccines do not prevent viremia and reversion to virulence of vaccine strains has been reported.

Bluetongue

Bluetongue (BT-1 through 25) or **catarrhal fever** is a non contagious, non-zoonotic *Culicoides species* -borne disease of ruminants, mainly of sheep and less frequently cattle, goats, buffaloes, deer, and antelopes. Symptoms follow an IP of 1-12 days with high fever, excessive salivation, swelling of the face and tongue and cyanosis of the tongue. Swelling of the lips and tongue gives the tongue its typical blue appearance. BT disease is characterized by vascular injury with hemorrhage, edema and tissue necrosis. Inherent, species-specific differences in the susceptibility and responses of endothelial cells may be responsible for the occurrence of BT disease in BTV-infected sheep but not cattle.

Bluetongue disease is emerging globally, and currently is responsible for a massive pandemic amongst ruminants in Europe in cattle, sheep, goats, and non-domestic ruminants including wildlife. There is massive impact of this epidemic on reproductive performance in cattle, with up to 40% fetal losses amongst susceptible cattle. Similarly, additional serotypes of BTV recently have appeared in North America.

Etiology: Blue tongue is caused by *Bluetongue virus* (BTV) of the genus *Orbivirus*, a member of the *Reoviridae* family. There are 25 serotypes of BTV. It is transmitted by a midge, *Culicoides imiicola* and other culicoids.

Occurrence

Bluetongue has been observed in Australia, the USA, Africa, the Middle East, Asia and Europe. BT was first recognized in southern Africa, subsequently in the Middle East, Asia and southern Europe. Now global spread of BT occurs in ruminants and/or vector insects from all continents except Antarctica. As BTV infection of ruminants is not contagious, the global distribution of BTV coincides with the distribution of competent *Culicoides* insect vectors and hot or warm climatic conditions. BT is classified in List A by the Office International des Épizooties (OIE). Concerns over the potential impact of BT on animal production have been heightened by the recent re-emergence of BT in Mediterranean and south-eastern Europe. BTV infection occurs throughout extensive regions of northern and eastern Australia yet outbreaks of BT disease have not yet been described. Similarly, there are very few descriptions of BT amongst ruminants in the Caribbean islands or in Central and South America, despite endemic BTV infection in much of this region.

Recent outbreaks of bluetongue occurred **in August 2006** in the Netherlands, then Belgium, Germany, and Luxembourg. In 2007, the first case of bluetongue in the Czech Republic was detected in one bull near Cheb at the Czech-German border.In September 2007, the UK reported its first case of the disease, in a Highland cow on a rare breed farm near Ipswich, Suffolk. Since then the virus has spread from cattle to sheep in Britain. By October **2007 bluetongue had become a serious threat in Scandinavia and Switzerland** and the first outbreak in Denmark was reported. In **autumn 2008,** several cases were reported in the southern **Swedish** provinces of Småland, Halland, and Skåne as well as in areas of the Netherlands bordering Germany, prompting veterinary authorities in Germany to intensify controls. Norway saw its first report in February 2009, when cows at two farms in Vest-Agder in the south of Norway showed an immune response to bluetongue. Norway has since been declared free of the disease in 2011.

Hosts susceptible

Sheep, & less frequently goats, cattle, buffaloes, deer, dromedaries and non-domestic ruminants including wildlife are susceptible. Selected breeds of sheep and wild ruminant species, e.g. white-tailed deer are most susceptible to BT disease. Sheep that are native to tropical and subtropical regions of the world where BTV is endemic are usually resistant to BT, whereas **fine wooled European breeds such as the Merino are highly susceptible.** Nutritional status, immune status and age also influence the severity of BT in individual sheep, as can environmental stress such as high temperature and ultraviolet radiation.

Transmission

Culicoides insects are **biological vectors** of BTV, & **once infected, they remain infected for lifetime.** The virus replicates within the tissues of each insect after infection from feeding on the blood of a BTV infected ruminant. Vector insects can only transmit BTV to another susceptible ruminant after an extrinsic incubation period of approximately 10 to 14 days, during which time the virus is disseminated from the gut of the insect to its salivary glands. Although venereal and vertical transmission of BTV can occur in ruminants, these routes are unimportant to the maintenance of BTV and the distribution of BTV in the world coincides only with that of competent vector insects. BTV is capable of transplacental infection of the ruminant fetus. Midges will then spread the disease from the calves to other animals, starting a new season of infection. Based on this finding, it is advised to pay special attention to newborn animals in an effort to eradicate the disease.

Pathogenesis

The pathogenesis of BTV infection is similar in sheep and cattle, & most species of ruminants. There are marked differences in the severity of disease that occurs in different ruminant species after BTV infection, except cattle being especially resistant to expression of BT disease. After cutaneous instillation of virus through the bite of a BTV-infected *Culicoides* vector, the virus travels to the regional lymph node, where initial replication occurs. The virus then is disseminated to a variety of tissues throughout the body where **replication occurs principally in mononuclear phagocytes and endothelial cells. Viremia** in BTV-infected ruminants is highly **cell associated**, and viremia is prolonged but not persistent. The virus associates with all blood cells, thus titres of virus in each cell fraction are proportionate to the numbers of each cell type. Specifically, BTV is associated mostly with platelets and erythrocytes and, because of the short lifespan of platelets; virus is mostly associated with erythrocytes late in the course of BTV infection of ruminants. BTV infection of **erythrocytes facilitates both prolonged infection of ruminants** and infection of haematophagous insect vectors that feed on viremic ruminants. Interestingly, BTV nucleic acid may be detected by PCR in the blood of infected cattle and sheep for many months after it no longer can be detected by virus isolation in cell culture or inoculation of susceptible sheep. Furthermore, ruminant blood that contains BTV nucleic acid, but not infectious BTV by virus isolation, is not infectious to vector insects by either intrathoracic inoculation or oral feeding. Ruminant blood that is positive by PCR assays but not by virus isolation is also not infectious to other ruminants.

Ruminants infected with BTV develop a prompt and high titred antibody response to a variety of viral proteins. **Serotype-specific neutralizing antibodies** are directed against **VP2**, and these can be detected by the serum neutralization test. Antibodies directed against core protein VP7, as well as other structural and non-structural proteins, may be detected with serogroup-reactive assays such as the agar gel immunodiffusion and competitive ELISA. A positive serological result confirms only that an animal was previously infected with BTV. Thus, although BTV infection of cattle and sheep often is prolonged, there is no evidence of truly persistent BTV infection of ruminants and the vast majority of seropositive cattle and sheep from BTV-endemic regions are not infected with the virus.

Clinical signs and lesions in BTV-infected sheep possibly reflect virus-mediated endothelial injury, as BTV replicates in **endothelial cells causing cell injury and necrosis**. Similarly, **white-tailed deer**, which are highly susceptible to BT, develop consumptive coagulopathy as a consequence of BTV-induced damage to endothelial cells. Coagulopathy disseminated intravascular coagulation in BTV-infected sheep and deer predisposes to the bleeding tendency that characterizes fulminant BT. Endothelial injury is also probably responsible for increased vascular permeability leading to oedema in tissues, such as the lung-pulmonary oedema, and vascular thrombosis leads to tissue infarction.

As regards foetal infection, it now is increasingly clear that only strains of BTV that have been modified by growth in cell culture, such as modified live virus (MLV) vaccine strains, have the capacity to cross the ruminant placenta. Once MLV BTV strains cross the placenta they cause embryonic or foetal death, and cerebral malformations after infection of older foetuses that survive congenital infection.

BTV enters into insect cells via the viral inner core VP7 protein and in mammalian cells via the external capsid VP2 hemagglutinin, which is the major determinant of BTV serotype and neutralization. BTV replicates in mononuclear phagocytes and endothelial cells where it induces expression of inflammatory cytokines as well as apoptosis. BTV can remain as nonreplicating entities concealed in **erythrocytes for up to five months.** Homologous protection against one BTV serotype involves neutralizing antibodies and T cell responses directed to the external VP2 and VP5 proteins, whereas heterologous protection is supported by T cells directed to the NS1 non structural protein and inner core proteins.

Clinical symptoms

The incubation period is 5–20 days, and all symptoms usually develop within a month. Major signs are high fever, excessive salivation, swelling of the face and tongue and cyanosis of the tongue. Swelling of the lips and tongue gives the tongue its typical blue appearance, though this sign is confined to a minority of the animals. Nasal symptoms may be prominent, with nasal discharge and stertorous respiration. Most BTV-infected sheep develop mild or no obvious disease in BTV-endemic areas. Outbreaks of BT occur either when susceptible sheep are introduced into BTV-endemic regions, or when the virus spreads into immunologically naive sheep populations at the interface of BTV-endemic and non-endemic regions.

The clinical signs of BT in sheep reflect congestion, oedema and hemorrhage as a consequence of virus-mediated vascular injury. Thus, sheep with BT have combination of fever, serous to bloody nasal discharge, oral erosions and ulcers, lameness with hyperaemia of the coronary band, and weakness secondary to muscle necrosis.

PM lesions of affected sheep include hyperemia, hemorrhages, erosion and ulceration of the mucosa of the upper gastrointestinal tract-oral cavity, oesophagus, & forestomachs. Subintimal hemorrhages in the pulmonary artery; pulmonary oedema; pleural and/or pericardial effusion; oedema within the facial planes of the muscles of the abdominal wall; necrosis of skeletal and cardiac muscle, with the papillary muscle of the left ventricle are characteristic.

Diagnosis

Two types of viral antigen are used for BTV testing. All Bluetongue serotypes share a common antigenic determinant called **antigen protein P7,** while the antigen **protein Ps** is variable and is used to determine the specific serotype of a virus.

Collection of clinical specimens includes whole blood, spleen, & serum.

1. *Presumptive diagnosis*: Specific clinical signs and gross PM lesions afford to arrive at presumptive diagnosis.
2. *Virus isolation*: Confirmative diagnosis needs virus isolation from blood of viremic animals by the intravenous inoculation of tissues from spleen, & brain in chicken embryos and subsequently in cell cultures like Vero cell line. BT virus is among the most difficult animal viruses to isolate. Now a day, **PCR test has proven to be very sensitive and specific for BTV RNA.**
3. *The serologic tests* most often used to determine exposure are CFT, the agar gel immunodiffusion (AGID) and a competitive ELISA, which is a sensitive and specific test. Several cattle in the United States have antibodies to BT virus. In such endemic regions paired serum samples and demonstration of **rising titers may be required to demonstrate acute infection**. Antigenically related orbiviruses may cross-react and give false positive results in AGID tests. **Monoclonal antibody detection** is used with ELISA to decrease the chance of cross-reaction. But the detection of BTV antibodies is poorly correlated with BTV viremia.

Treatment & prevention

There is no efficient treatment. Prevention is effected via quarantine, inoculation with live modified virus vaccine and control of the midge vector. Housing livestock during times of maximum midge activity (from dusk to dawn) may lead to significantly reduced biting rates. Similarly, protecting livestock shelters with fine mesh netting or coarser material impregnated with insecticide will reduce contact with the midges. Identifying breeding grounds and breaking the breeding cycle will significantly reduce the local midge population. Dung heaps or slurry pits should be covered or removed, and their perimeters (where most larvae are found) regularly scraped.

Vaccination

Outbreaks in southern Europe have been caused by **serotypes 2 and 4**, and vaccines are available against these serotypes for sheep, & for cattle. However, the disease found in northern Europe (including the UK) in 2006 and 2007 has been caused by **serotype 8**. Vaccine companies Fort Dodge Animal Health (Wyeth), Merial and Intervet were developing vaccines against serotype 8. Fort Dodge Animal Health has vaccine for serotype 4 for sheep, serotype 1 for sheep and cattle and serotype 8 for sheep and cattle. A vaccine for this is now available in the UK, produced by Intervet. Fort Dodge Animal Health has their vaccines available for multiple European countries. **BTVPUR AlSap 8**-Merial is the latest inactivated liquid vaccine containing purified Bluetongue virus serotype 8 antigen in aluminium hydroxide and saponin adjuvants. It is the latest member of Merial's range of bluetongue vaccines, which have been used in different parts of Europe since 2004. **BTVPUR AlSap** 8 is specifically designed to immunize cows and sheep against the bluetongue serotype that is prevalent in the United Kingdom. The I ml vaccine is given SC in sheep from 1 month of age in naïve animals and 2.5 months of age in young animals born to immune sheep. In cattle there are two 1 ml injections, 1 month apart, again from 1 month of age in naïve animals and from 2.5 months of age in young animals born to immune cattle. Onset of immunity is 3 weeks after completion of the primary course. It is recommended that animals are revaccinated at least 2 weeks before each risk period. **BLUETONGUE VACCINE**-Colorado Serum Company is modified live virus, type 10 for sheep & goat. Penicillin and streptomycin are added as preservatives. Inject 2 ml of the rehydrated vaccine IM or SC into each animal. All breeding stock should be protected with BLUETONGUE VACCINE approximately three weeks prior to the breeding season or after lambing. Intervet has also developed **Bluetongue vaccine** against serotype 8 for sheep & cattle. **The Onderstepoort Bluetongue Vaccine**, a modified live virus vaccine is used in sheep in the Republic of South Africa for more than 50 years and they are known to induce effective and long lasting immunity. They are currently produced in cell culture, freeze-dried and subjected to tests to conform to stringent Onderstepoort and international standards. The present **Onderstepoort Bluetongue Vaccine** (Reg. No. G 358 Act No. 36/1947) comprises 3 bottles (Vaccines A, B, and C) and includes the following serotypes of BTV:

Bottle A: BTV serotypes 1, 4, 6, 12 and 14

Bottle B: BTV serotypes 3, 8, 9, 10 and 11

Bottle C: BTV serotypes 2, 5, 7, 13 and 19

The three bluetongue vaccines are administered separately at 3-week intervals. Each vaccine contains 100 doses, and all are in stock.

Epizootic Haemorrhagic Disease

Epizootic hemorrhagic disease virus (EHDV-1, 2, 3, 4, 5, 6, 7, 8, 9, 10) causes epizootic hemorrhagic disease (EHD) an acute, insect-born, infectious, often fatal viral disease of **white tailed deer & some wild ruminants**. This malady, characterized by extensive hemorrhages, has been responsible for significant epizootics in deer in the northern United States and southern Canada. There are 3 forms of the disease, **peracute, acute, and chronic**. The **peracute** cases show only edema of the head, neck, tongue, eyelids, and lungs. The **acute** form animals live longer & show the acute or "classic hemorrhagic" form with edema of the head but also show hemorrhages or congestion in the heart, rumen, abomasum, or intestines with erosions or ulceration on the dental pad, tongue, palate, rumen, omasum, and abomasum. The **chronic** form shows growth interruptions on the hooves and sometimes peeling of hoof walls or ulceration, scarring, and loss of papillae in the rumen.

Etiology: Epizootic hemorrhagic disease is caused by *Epizootic hemorrhagic disease virus* that belongs to the genus *Orbivirus*, family *Reoviridae*. Ten serotypes of EHDV are serotype **1 through 10**. The Ibaraki virus is closely related to EHDV. According to some authors, it is a distinct virus belonging to the EHDV serogroup but others considers the Ibaraki virus and the Australian EHDV serotype 2 are nearly identical topotypes. There is more than one strain of the Ibaraki virus.

Occurrence

Epizootic hemorrhagic disease occurs in North America, Australia, Asia and Africa. Seropositive animals have been found in South America. Among 10 serotypes, only two serotypes, **EHDV-1 and EHDV-2 occur in North America**.

Ibaraki disease in cattle has been reported from Japan, Korea, and Taiwan. Seropositive animals have also been found in Australia and Indonesia.

Hosts susceptible

EHD viruses infect most wild and domestic ruminants. Clinical signs are seen mainly in **white tailed deer,** with mule deer and pronghorn antelope affected to a lesser extent. Other wild animals found to be seropositive include black-tailed deer, red deer, wapiti, fallow deer, and roe deer.

Rare outbreaks of EHD have been reported in cattle. Sheep can be infected experimentally but rarely develop clinical signs, and goats do not seem to be susceptible to infection.

Transmission

The viruses of the EHDV serogroup are transmitted by **biological vectors,** usually biting midges in the genus *Culicoides*. In North America, *C. varipennis* is the major vector. Some species of gnats and mosquitoes can also transmit EHDV. Infected deer can be viremic for up to 2 months.

Pathogenesis, clinical symptoms

Extensive hemorrhages ranging from pinpoint to massive in size involving different tissues and organs in individual animals are characteristic. No organs appear to be exempt from hemorrhages, with the most regularly involved being the heart, liver, spleen, kidney, lung and intestinal tract. Extensive hemorrhaging is the result of **interference with the blood-clotting mechanism together with degeneration of blood vessel walls.** Generalized edema and increased pericardial fluid are consistently found in EHD. These changes also reflect the wide spread interference with normal blood circulation.

Deer: The incubation period for EHD in deer is 5 to 10 days. Three forms of the disease are **peracute, acute, and chronic** may be seen in deer. **Peracute** disease is characterized by high fever, anorexia, weakness, respiratory distress, and severe and rapid edema of the head and neck. Swelling of the tongue and conjunctivae is common. Deer with the peracute form usually die rapidly, typically within 8-36 hours; some animals may be found dead with few clinical signs.

In the **acute form (classical EHD),** the symptoms may be accompanied by extensive hemorrhages in many tissues including the skin, heart, and gastrointestinal tract. There is often excessive salivation and nasal discharge, which may both be blood-tinged. Animals with the acute form can also develop ulcers or erosions of the tongue, dental pad, palate, rumen, and omasum. High mortality rates are common in both the peracute and acute forms.

In the **chronic form**, deer are ill for **several weeks but gradually recover**. After recovery, these deer sometimes develop breaks or rings in the hooves caused by growth interruptions, and may become lame. In severe cases, animals slough the hoof wall or toe; some of these deer may be found crawling on their knees or chest. Deer with the chronic form may also develop ulcers, scars, or erosions in the rumen; extensive damage to the lining of the rumen can cause emaciation even when there is no shortage of food.

Cattle: Ibaraki disease in cattle is characterized by fever, anorexia, and difficulty in swallowing. The swallowing disorders are caused by damage to the striated muscles of the pharynx, larynx, esophagus and tongue, and may lead to dehydration, emaciation, and aspiration pneumonia. Edema, hemorrhages, erosions, and ulcerations may be seen in the mouth, on the lips, and around the coronets. The animals may be stiff and lame, and the skin may be thickened and edematous. **Abortions and stillbirths have also been reported in some epidemics.** Some affected cattle die.

Outside Japan, in Korea and Taiwan, most EHDV infections in cattle appear to be subclinical. Symptomatic infections resemble Ibaraki disease, but tend to be less severe. Typical symptoms include fever, oral ulcers, salivation, lameness associated with coronitis, and weight loss. In pregnant cows, the fetus may be resorbed or develop hydranencephaly if it is infected between 70 and 120 days of gestation. Deaths are uncommon with the North American strains of EHDV; however, some animals may be lame and unthrifty for a prolonged period. EHD has not been reproduced in experimentally infected cattle; although animals become viremic, they remain asymptomatic.

Sheep can be infected by EHDV but rarely develop symptoms. Experimentally infected goats do not become viremic.

PM lesions in deer in the peracute form are severe edema of the head, neck, eyes, and lungs. In the acute form, widespread hemorrhages and edema can be seen in the many parts of the body including the mucous membranes, skin and viscera, particularly the heart and gastrointestinal tract. There may also be erosions and ulcerations in the mouth, rumen, and omasum. Dry, gray-white necrotic lesions can sometimes be found in the hard palate, tongue, dental pads, esophagus, larynx, rumen, and abomasum.

The lesions of the chronic form may include rings or breaks on the hooves, or sloughing of the tips or walls of the hooves. Deer with chronic disease can also develop ulcers, scars, or erosions in the rumen.

Histopathologic lesions may include widespread **vasculitis with thrombosis, endothelial swelling, hemorrhages, degenerative changes, and necrosis in many organs.**

Diagnosis

Collection of samples for various tests include in deer: tissues for virus isolation are spleen, lymph node, and unclotted whole blood in EDTA or heparin, & serum (for serology), liver, and lung. In cattle, blood should be collected into anticoagulant (calcium citrate, EDTA, or heparin) for virus isolation or RT-PCR. Paired serum samples should also be collected if possible.

1. *Presumptive diagnosis*: Swelling of the head and neck, respiratory distress, or excessive blood-tinged salivation, sudden death, particularly when

the animal is found dead near water (an indication of high fever). Chronic disease can be the cause of hoof abnormalities and emaciation.

2. *Virus isolation*: EHDV can be isolated in a variety of cell lines or embryonated chicken eggs. Ibaraki virus can be isolated in eggs or bovine cell cultures, including primary cultures of bovine, sheep or hamster lung origin, and L cells. This virus can also be isolated by intracerebral inoculation of mice.
3. *Antigen detection*: Immunofluorescence is used to identify the virus in frozen tissue sections. RT-PCR tests, dot blot or *in situ* hybridization are used. Viral RNA can sometimes be found in deer tissues for up to 160 days.
4. *Serology*: Serology is less useful than detection of the virus, & ELISA, serum neutralization, and agar gel immunodiffusion (AGID) are employed using paired serum samples.

Treatment & Prevention

Vector controls such as modifying the environment to reduce *Culicoides* breeding areas, spraying with insecticides or larvacides, and using insect repellents could decrease the risk of infection.

There are few practical measures to prevent infection; effective disinfectants for EHDV serogroup viruses include acids, oxidizing agents such as sodium or calcium hypochlorite at 20,000-30,000 ppm (2-3%), alkalis such as sodium hydroxide at 2% (w/v), or glutaraldehyde at 2% (w/v). These viruses are, like most nonenveloped viruses, resistant to lipid solvents. They can be inactivated by heat treatment at 50°C for 3 hours, 60°C for 15 minutes, or 121°C for 15 minutes.

No vaccines are available for most EHDV viruses; however, **a live attenuated Ibaraki disease vaccine is used** in Japan.

Palyam Virus (PAV-CH) or Chuzan Disease

Palyam virus (PAV) infects **cattle & sheep,** is transmitted by culicine mosquitoes and *Culicoides* gnats. *Palyam virus* has at least 15 viruses in six antigenic complexes. Although 11 serotypes have been identified in the serogroup by a cross-neutralization test, the pathogenesis of these viruses was not well understood. Palyam viruses could be divided into three groups: 1. those that cause death, 2. those that cause death only when large amounts of virus were inoculated and 3. those that cause death and deformities. PAV causes fetal lesions & abortion in cattle & sheep. *Palyam virus* (PAV-ch) or Chuzan disease occurs in cattle in SE Asia, Japan; & is characterized by congenital abnormalities in calves-hydrocephaly or blindness; & severity depends on age of the fetus. When infection occurs when the fetus is infected at about four months of age, calves born may be blind and display seizures and opisthotonus. Usually beef cattle are affected more often than dairy cattle. The orbivirus genome contains 10 double-stranded RNA (dsRNA) segments in a double-layered capsid. These dsRNA segments encode seven structural viral proteins (VP1 to VP7) and four nonstructural proteins (NS1 to NS3 and NS3A). The outer layer is composed of the two major proteins, VP2 and VP5. The VP2 protein encoded by RNA segment 2 is a major neutralizing antigen and has a serotype-specific determinant. The VP7 protein encoded by RNA segment 7 is incorporated in the viral inner layer and is a serogroup-specific antigen.

Experimentally, one of the calves which was born to a dam inoculated with Chuzan virus at 120 days of gestation, showed impairment of movement, and the remaining 14 were healthy. Postmortem examination revealed that this calf had hydranencephaly- cerebellar hypoplasia (HCH) syndrome and that the remaining calves were normal. Two of the 15 calves, including the one that had HCH syndrome, had antibody to Chuzan virus in their precolostral sera. These findings provide additional evidence that Chuzan virus is the etiological agent of an epizootic of congenital abnormalities with HCH syndrome of calves in Japan,

Aino, Akabane and Chuzan viruses are arthropod-borne (arbo) viruses transmitted by blood-sucking insects like mosquitoes and Culicoides biting midges. These arbovirus infections are mainly associated with abortion, stillbirth and congenital defects in pregnant cattle, sheep and goats, causing a considerable economic loss in livestock industry. The viruses seem to be widely distributed in Southeast Asia and Australia. As a control strategy, an **inactivated trivalent vaccine against Aino, Akabane and Chuzan virus** was developed by using binary ethylenimine or formalin as an inactivating agent. The immune responses were significantly detected within 2-weeks after second vaccination without any side effects. Since the field application of experimental vaccine also revealed increased antibodies in inoculated cattle, it was demonstrated that these trivalent vaccines could be used as a vaccine to control the arboviral infections in ruminants.

Transmission

Transmission is by *Culicoides oxystoma* & in India by *Culex* species and Culicoides species.

Diagnosis

Diagnosis is based on clinical history, microscopic lesions, and supportive serologic results.

Equine Encephalosis

Equine encephalosis (EEV-1, 2,3, 4, 5, 6, 7, 8) is a peracute, insect-borne, viral disease of horses in South Africa different from EEE, WEE & VEE. This disease is not present in Australia at this time. EEV can cause a severe illness with nervous signs or cardiac failure.

Etiology: Equine encephalosis (EE) is caused by *Equine encephalosis virus* (EEV-1 throgh 8) belonging to the *Orbivirus* genus of the family *Reoviridae*. EEV was originally isolated in 1967 from horses showing central nervous signs and sudden death.

Occurrence

Outbreaks of equine encephalosis in South Africa have occurred at irregular intervals of two or more years. The disease shows a seasonal pattern, occurring during the months of December to June (Northern Hemisphere). Between October 2008 and January 2009, EE virus infection in horses with a febrile illness was observed in dozens of stables across Israel.

Hosts susceptible

All equids-horses, donkeys, zebras, and sometimes elephants are susceptible to infection.

Transmission

The virus is transmitted by vector (biting insects) with *Culicoides imicola* assumed to be the major species responsible.

Clinical signs

The **incubation period varies from 2 -6 days.** The common symptoms are: fluctuating fever that lasts one to five days, varying degrees of listlessness, depressed appetite, increased heart and respiratory rates, & red/brown discoloration of visible mucous membranes.

Most infected horses usually show only mild clinical signs & recover uneventfully. The mortality rate is generally less that 5%. However, less common but more serious signs can include **facial swelling, CNS signs particularly loss of control or co-ordination of the hindquarters, depression, frenzy, excitability sensitivity to sound/noise, convulsions, respiratory**

distress, petechial hemorrhages in eye membranes, clear or blood-tinged nasal discharge, & signs of chronic heart failure. Pregnant mares usually abort.

Outbreaks of EEV infection have furthermore been associated with equine fetal abortion during the first **5-6 months of gestation**. An early undetected abortion could therefore be misdiagnosed as infertility in a mare. Until now, EE has not been recorded in other parts of the world.

PM examination showed that facial swelling and petechial hemorrhages in eye membranes lesions are attributable to severe damage of certain blood vessels. There is no encephalitis. There is venous congestion, fatty degeneration of the liver, brain oedema and highly conspicuous enteritis especially in the small intestine. The heart may have lesions and appear flabby with a grey-white mottled or streaky appearance. In Israel outbreak, the signs included high body temperature for 1-5 days, unrest, decreased appetite, edema of lips and eyelids, accelerated pulse and breathing rates, congested mucosae, abortions, & neurological symptoms.

Diagnosis

Diagnosis is carried out serologically by serum neutralization or ELISA, PCR and virus isolation in tissue culture.

Treatment & prevention

There is no specific treatment besides supportive treatment. 90 percent of affected animals recover without complications. No vaccine is available.

Genus: *Orthoreovirus*

Avian Orthoreovirus Infection

Avianorthoreovirus (ARV-s1133,176,SK138a) causes significant infection; arthritis, tenosinuvitis, gastroenteritis, hepatitis, myocarditis & respiratory disease in commercial flocks in chickens & turkeys, **4-16 weeks old**. Avian orthoreoviruses (ARVs) belong to the family *Reoviridae*, genus *Orthoreovirus*. They infect wild and farm-raised birds and are important fowl pathogens associated with various disease conditions such as **gastrointestinal malabsorption syndrome, tenosynovitis (arthritis), growth retardation, and sudden death.**

Occurrence

Distribution of avian orthoreovirus is **worldwide** and it is present in most poultry flocks.

Hosts susceptible

ARV is more common in **young birds**, because resistance begins to develop from as young as two weeks of age. It is reportedly more common in broilers. ARV has also been isolated from asymptomatic birds.

Transmission

The virus can be transmitted horizontally via the feces or rarely, vertically. It is not a zoonosis.

Clinical symptoms

Lameness is the principle sign of disease, and may be accompanied by **swelling, haemorrhage, skin discoloration** and refusal to move. In severe cases, the **gastronomies may rupture** and birds may become recumbent and struggle to feed. Diarrhoea, **dehydration and anorexia** can also be caused by the virus (malabsorption syndrome). Neurological signs develop in severe cases. Birds appear soiled and ruffled and may huddle together. **Mortality** in the flock increasing and fluid consumption rising may also be indications of disease.

On post-mortem, the digital flexor tendons, metatarsal extensors and tendon sheaths are inflamed, swollen and surrounded by exudate. Cartilage may be eroded and synovial membranes hemorrhagic. Fibrosis and adhesions develop in chronic cases. On histopathology, oedema and synoviocyte hypertrophy and hyperplasia arc cvident. Visceral damage varies greatly due to the differing capacity of viruses to disseminate.

Diagnosis

A presumptive diagnosis can be made based on the observation of clinical signs. Diagnosis is often made from the observation of lameness and swollen hock joints. This can be confirmed using virus isolation, CFT, ELISA, immunodiffusion or histopathology following PM examination.

Virus isolation can be made from the respiratory, enteric and reproductive tracts or from tendons, plasma and blood cells of recently killed birds. Its site of primary replication is the epithelia of the small intestine. The viruses can then be **cultured on chicken eggs and chicken embryo liver cell** cultures. Infection induces formation of **syncytia, degeneration and holes in the monolayer**. Presence of he virus can be confirmed by **electron microscopy and PCR.**

Serology: Agar gel immunodiffusion and ELISA can be used to detect antibodies serologically.

Treatment & prevention

No treatment options exist. Hygiene measures can help control disease.

Vaccination

Vaccines should be used in face of an outbreak. **Live attenuated and inactivated vaccines** are available. Attenuated vaccines are for use in young birds and inactivated for breeding hens which provides maternal protection for chicks. **Nobilis REO 1133** –Intervet is a live attenuated vaccine: In high exosure areas, vaccination should begin at 7 days of age. Revaccination is recommended at 5 to 7 weeks of age and again at 9 to 11 weeks. In areas where there is less exposure, vaccination should be carried out at 5 to 7 weeks of age and again at 9 to 11 weeks. To complete this programme for breeding birds, the administration of an inactivated Reovirus vaccine e.g. **NOBILIS REO INAC**-Intervet is recommended between 16 to 18 weeks of age. Dose is 0.2 ml per bird SC in the back of the neck or IM in the breast muscle or thigh.

NOBILIS REO+IB+G+ND-Intervet is combined inactivated vaccine for immunization against Avian reovirus, IB (Massachusetts), IBD & NDV in chickens in water in oil emulsion. The vaccine is recommended for the booster vaccination of breeding stock for protection against the Massachusetts serotype of Infectious Bronchitis and for protection against Newcastle Disease; and for immunization against Reovirus infection and Infectious bursal disease virus, in order to protect the offspring of the vaccinated birds against Reovirus infections and Gumboro disease by maternal antibodies for at least the first weeks of life. **Nobilis Reo + IB + G + ND** should be given to birds not less than 4 weeks before the expected onset of lay. For an optimal booster effect, the birds must be primed with live vaccine against Infectious bronchitis, Newcastle disease, Avian Reovirus infection and Infectous bursal disease. The best results will be obtained if vaccination with inactivated vaccine takes place 6 or more weeks after the administration of the live primer but in no circumstances should it be carried out earlier than 4 weeks after priming. Dose: each bird: 0.5 ml IM in the thigh or breast muscle or SC in the lower part of the neck.

IBD-Reo vaccine-Pfizer is recommended for the revaccination of healthy chickens against IBD caused by standard and variant IBD strains and avian reovirus infections which cause malabsorption syndrome. Progeny of vaccinates are protected via maternal antibodies. **TENO-VAXIN**-Intervet is a live tenosinovitis vaccine for vaccination of chickens 10-17 weeks old for controlling reovirus-induced tenosinovitis in broiler breeders. ELISAs can be used to monitor efficacy.

Genus: *Rotavirus*

Rotavirus Infection in Animals

Rotavirus A (RV-A) causes **gastroenteritis with diarrhea in many young animal species up to 8 weeks old**; serious in calves, piglets, foals, puppies & kittens mostly of group A; severity depends on virus virulence, age, colostral uptake & management. These rotaviruses are a potential reservoir for genetic exchange with human rotaviruses. There is evidence that animal rotaviruses can infect humans, either by direct transmission of the virus or by contributing one or several RNA segments to reassort with human strains. Rotavirus is a pathogen of livestock and cause economic loss to farmers because of costs of treatment associated with high morbidity and mortality rates.

There are seven serogroups, A through G classified on the basis of differences in the major capsid antigen VP6.

Occurrence

Rotavirus infection in animals occurs in many parts of the world. Rotaviruses occur widely in many animal species and humans, & are endemic in many swine and dairy cattle herds. Rotavirus infection occurs most frequently when the immune status of the piglets or calves is lowered and there is an overwhelming buildup of the virus. The viruses can be recovered frequently from the intestine of many normal calves, pigs and other domestic species.

Hosts susceptible

Rotaviruses infect and cause diarrhoea in young animals- apes, calves, piglets, foals, sheep, rats, cats and dogs, mice, horses, rabbits, chickens and turkeys. Rotavirus infection occurs usually in young animals up to eight weeks of age; mostly after the first week of life.

Transmission

The virus is spread via contact and animals are infected by the oral/fecal route. Rotavirus is present in feces up to three weeks after infection.

Pathogenesis

Rotavirus infects mature epithelial cells of the distal half of the villi of the small intestine. There is selective killing of villous cells leading to villous atrophy, malabsorption, and diarrhea. Lack of colostral antibody contributes to the development of these infections. Enteropathogenic *E. coli* coinfection favours causing diarrhea, after the intestinal mucosa has been rendered vulnerable by necrosis and the loss of epithelial cells.

Clinical symptoms

The incubation period is about 24 hours. Clinical symptoms seen are vomiting, anorexia, depression and a profuse, watery diarrhea of sudden onset, which quickly results in extreme dehydration.

In piglets, Rotaviral infection is widespread worldwide. Rotavirus affects pigs 1 - 4 weeks of age, & the virus is excreted in feces up to three weeks after infection.

In calves, Rotavirus infection occurs in calves 1 - 7 days of age. Coronavirus infects calves from 1 day to 3 weeks of age & thus both viruses can act in concert to produce profuse, watery diarrhea of sudden onset. In poultry, only group D viruses have been implicated in avian infections. In newborn foals, puppies and kittens, infection provokes similar diarrhea.

Diagnosis

Collection of clinical specimens for various tests includes portions of small intestine with fecal content.

Diagnosis is arrived at by fluorescent antibody test of frozen sections of intestine or by electron microscopic examination of feces and intestinal contents.

Treatment & prevention

Treatment includes oral or intravenous electrolyte solutions to prevent dehydration. Broad spectrum antibiotic may be used in case of bacterial infection. It is recommended to keep young animals warm and dry, & adequate supply of colostrum and milk is ensured. Use of disinfection & cleaning of quarters reduces the virus load.

Due to widespread occurrence of rotaviruses with carriers, it is not possible to eradicate the disease.

Vaccination

Both **modified live and killed** vaccines are available. It is advisable to vaccinate pregnant animals. **Calf-Guard** -Pfizer contains modified-live bovine rotavirus- and coronavirus propagated on established cell lines and freeze-dried to preserve stability. Vaccine is rehydrated in a 3-ml dose with sterile diluent. Oral vaccination of healthy newborn calves, or for IM vaçcination of pregnant cows as an aid in passive maternal immunization of their calves against neonatal calf diarrhea (scours) caused by bovine rotavirus and bovine coronavirus.

Scour Guard 4 KC-Pfizer is a combination killed vaccine (Bovine rotavirus+ coronavirus+ *C. perfringens* type C + *E. coli* Bacterin-toxoid) for pregnant animals. Vaccination of healthy, pregnant cows and heifers is recommended. Inject 2 ml IM in the muscular region of the neck. Primary vaccination: Administer 2 IM doses approximately 3 weeks apart to pregnant cows, with the second dose given 3–6 weeks before calving. Revaccination with a single dose 3–6 weeks before each subsequent calving is recommended. **GUARDIAN SCOURS VACCINE**-Intervet (Rotavirus+ *C. perfringens* C & D+ *E. coli*) is for prevention of neonatal calf diarrhea & enterotoxaemia. Administer 2 ml SC, primary dose may be given 12 weeks precalving. Booster is given 3-6 weeks after primary dose. Annual revaccination 60 days preslaughter. Long duration of immunity means 3rd dose is never needed. **BOVILIS LACTOVAC C**-Intervet (rotavirus+ coronavirus +*E. coli*) in Aluminium hydroxide & quil A as adjuvant for vaccination of pregnant cows & heifers to reduce severity of diarrhea in neonatal calves. Each 5 ml dose contains the following: Inactivated bovine rotavirus, strain 1005/78 at least $10^{7.4}$ $TCID_{50}$, inducing ≥ 1 RPU, Inactivated bovine rotavirus, strain Holland at least $10^{7.0}$ $TCID_{50}$, inducing ≥ 1 RPU, inactivated bovine coronavirus, strain 800 at least $10^{5.8}$ $TCID_{50}$, inducing ≥ 1 RPU & Inactivated *E. coli* K99/F41 250 HAU, inducing ≥ 1 RPU, Adjuvants Aluminium hydroxide 60 mg & Saponin / Quil A. Dose 5 ml SC to Heifers & cows. Heifers are given 2 doses, first at 4 -5 weeks & second 2-3 weeks before calving. Cows are given a single booster dose 2- 6 weeks before calving.

□□□

Chapter 17

Characteristics and Diseases Caused by Group III Double-Stranded RNA Birnaviruses (Family *Birnaviridae*)

Contents

Characteristics of Birnaviruses

Birnaviridae (L. bi = two, rna = ribonucleic acid) are so named as these viruses contain **two segments of linear ds RNA**. Birnaviruses are small, naked, & spherical measuring about 70 nm in diameter. Birnaviruses infect animals: vertebrates, insects, molluscs and crustaceans. Among the four genera, only ***Avibirnavirus* with type species *Infectious bursal disease virus* (IBDV) is of major veterinary importance.** The capsid is round and exhibits **icosahedral** symmetry made of **132 capsomers (T=13)**. The capsid is composed of **260 trimers** of **VP2** that form spikes projecting radially from the capsid. Minor amounts of **VP1** are also incorporated in the virion. The T=13 shell of the IBDV capsid is formed by trimers of VP2 (Fig 17-1). VP3 is a multifunctional component lying under the T=13 shell & influence the structural polymorphism of VP2. The virus-encoded RNA-dependent RNA polymerase VP1 is incorporated into the capsid through its association with VP3. VP3 also interacts extensively with the viral dsRNA genome. IBDV genome consists of linear, dsRNA containing **two segments, A (larger) and B (shorter).** The **segment A** (3.2 kb) encodes viral proteins **VP2, VP3, VP4, and VP5**. Among them, **VP2 protein elicits protective immune response** and most of the amino acid (AA) changes between antigenically different IBDVs are clustered in the hypervariable region of VP2 & hence the hypervariable region of VP2 is the target for the molecular techniques applied for IBDV detection and strain variation studies. The smaller **segment B** encodes the 97 kDa **VP1 with RNA polymerase and capping enzyme activities**.

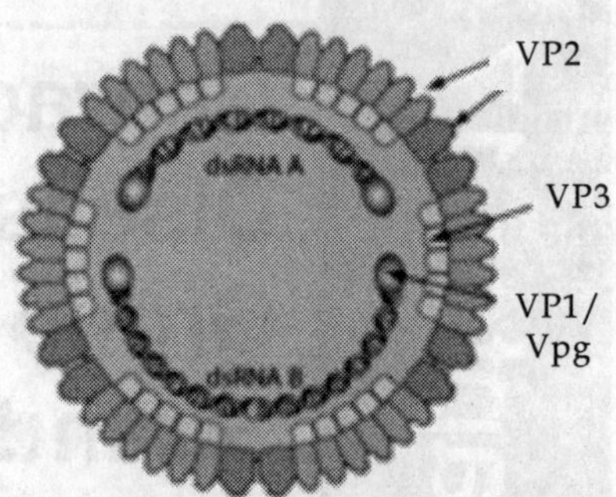

Fig. 17.1 : Morphology of Birnavirus

Viruses are stable at environmental conditions, resist heat and a wide pH range, & it is difficult to eradicate IBDV from poultry farms.

The virus genome

The viral genome is segmented and made of linear double-stranded RNA. The two genomic segments are called segment A (longer) 3100-3200 nucleotides long, & segment B (shorter) is 2750-2850 nucleotides long, total genome being 5880-6400 nucleotides long. Minor amounts of non-genomic nucleic acid are also found in the virions. The genome guanine + cytosine content is 45.5-54.5 %. The 5'-end of the genome has a cap on both segments & genome-linked protein (VPg). The peptides derived from pre-VP2 C-terminal cleavages remain associated within the virion. VP3 forms a ribonucleoprotein complex with the genomic RNA. Minor amounts of VP1 are also incorporated in the virion.

Virus replication

Birnaviruses **replicate in the cytoplasm** when dsRNA serves as a template for the production of mRNA (+) and progeny genomes. Two segments A & B encode for 5-6 proteins. The segment A encodes for a structural polyprotein which is matured in *cis* by VP4. Segment may also encode an alternative ORF translated by ribosomal alternative initiation (VP5). Genomic segment B encodes for VP1 which is found in a free form and covalently attached at the 5′ genomic RNA end (VPg).

For viral replication to occur, the virus penetrates into the cytoplasm helped by pep46 that deforms membranes and induces pores. Transcription of the dsRNA genome occurs by viral polymerase inside the virion, so that dsRNA is never exposed to the cytoplasm. The plus-strand transcript is used as template for translation. Then (+) RNAs are encapsidated in virion particle, inside which they are transcribed to give RNA (-) molecules with which they become base-paired to produce dsRNA genomes. Mature virions bud out from the infected cell.

Virus classification

Group: Group III dsRNA

Family: *Birnaviridae*

Genera:

Genus 1: *Aquabirnavirus;* type species: *Infectious pancreatic necrosis virus*

Genus 2: *Avibirnavirus;* type species: *Infectious bursal disease virus*

Genus 3: *Blosnavirus;* type species: *Blotched snakehead virus*

Genus 4: *Entomobirnavirus;* type species: *Drosophila X virus*

Birnavirus Clinical Infections in Birds

Infectious bursal disease caused by IBDV is a highly contagious disease of young chickens & characterized by immunosuppression and mortality generally at 3 to 6 weeks of age. It is of immense economically important to the poultry industry worldwide due to increased susceptibility to other diseases and interference with effective vaccination against many diseases. Now it has became possible to detect the very virulent infectious bursal disease virus (vvIBDV), differentiate IBDV strains, and study the molecular epidemiology of the virus with the help of reverse transcription polymerase chain reaction (RT-PCR) and restriction fragment length polymorphism (RFLP).

Table 17.1 : Characteristics of *Birnaviridae*

Family	Genus	Species (Italics)	Types	Diseases caused
Birnaviridae	*Birnavirus*	*Infectious bursal disease virus*	*Infectious bursal disease virus-1 &* 2, only serotype IBDV-1 is pathogenic. Classical IBDV, subclinical IBDV & very virulent IBDV exist. There are 6 genotypes of IBDV.	Infectious bursal disease (IBD) is a highly contagious disease of young chickens characterized by immuno-suppression and mortality generally at 3 to 6 weeks of age.

Infectious Bursal Disease or Gumboro Disease

Infectious bursal disease (IBD), also called **Gumboro disease**, is a highly contagious viral infection of chickens distributed worldwide & is characterized by rapid drop in feed and water consumption, mucoid (slimy) diarrhoea with soiling of the vent feathers, ruffled feathers, listless chicks with unsteady gait or sitting in hunched position, picking at own vent and sleeping with beak touching the floor. There is lasting immunosuppression and mortality occurs generally at 3 to 6 weeks of age proving to be economically important to the poultry industry worldwide due to heavy losses caused by clinical infection, increased susceptibility to other diseases and interference with effective vaccination against many diseases.

Etiology: IBD/ Gumboro disease is caused by *Infectous bursal disease virus* (IBDV). IBD was first described in the **USA near the town of Gumboro, Delaware in 1962**. There are **two serotypes of the virus**, IBDV serotypes 1 & 2; & within them, antigenic variation between strains is considerable. **Serotype 2 infects chickens and turkeys but does not cause clinical disease or immunosuppression**, but **only serotype 1 viruses cause clinical disease in poultry. There exist six antigenic subtypes of IBDV serotype 1**, detected by in vitro cross-neutralization assay. These antigenic subtypes are commonly known as **variants**, which were reported to break through high levels of maternal antibodies in commercial flocks, causing up to 60 to 100% mortality in chickens. Variant viruses induce damage in the BF in chickens, even when high and uniform antibody titers are present. Variant strains do not cause obvious clinical disease, but induce severe immunosuppression. The BF of affected chickens undergoes rapid atrophy (lymphocyte depletion) without the inflammatory changes observed early in the infection with the classical IBD viruses. These variants are not from a different serotype, but are antigenically different enough to cause problems. **Very virulent strains of IBDV (vvIBDV) causing severe mortality in chicken up to > 70% have recently emerged in late 1980's in Europe, Latin America, South East Asia, Africa & Middle East countries & India.** Now it has became possible to detect the vvIBDV, differentiate IBDV strains, and study the molecular epidemiology of the virus with the help of reverse transcription polymerase chain reactio (RT-PCR) and restriction fragment length polymorphism (RFLP).

Occurrence

IBDV is frequently occurring, worldwide infection of chickens. At the end of the 1980s, very virulent (vv) IBDV strains in Europe (antigenically similar to the "classical strains") emerged in vaccinated flocks and rapidly spread all over the world causing severe mortality in chicken up to > 70% in Europe, Latin America, South East Asia, Africa & Middle East countries. The disease is not present in New Zealand, & the **Australian field strains of IBD are relatively mild.** Thus there are **3 pathogenic types of IBDV; classic virulent (cvIBDV), subclinical (scIBDV), and very virulent (vvIBDV), & all three IBDVs cause immunosuppression** which leads to secondary infections and a failure to produce an immune response to vaccines. The cvIBDV typically cause a high morbidity and low mortality disease while the scIBDV cause very little morbidity and no mortality, but vvIBDV cause an acute disease in chickens characterized by high morbidity and high mortality.

Susceptible hosts

Young chickens generally at **3 to 8 weeks** of age that have highly active bursa of Fabricius are more susceptible to disease but birds over eight weeks are resistant unless infected by highly virulent strains. Infections before 3 weeks of age are usually subclinical but severe infections have been reported in Leghorn chickens up to 18 week old. **Leghorns are more susceptible than broilers** and brown-egg layers.

Transmission

The virus transmission occurs by direct contact and indirectly by fomites. **IBDV is shed in the feces** that spread the virus between birds or by contact with a contaminated environment. Virus is also possibly spread via air on dust particles. The virus transmission occurs from house to house on **fomites and rodents.** As the virus is **very stable in the environment**, it is difficult to eradicate them from the premises. There is no vertical transmission. Mealworms and litter mites harbour the virus for 8 weeks, and affected birds shed large amounts of virus for about 2 weeks after infection.

Pathogenesis

After ingestion, The main route of infection is oral, less commonly via the conjunctiva and respiratory tract. The virus has predilection for **lymphoid cells** and especially those of **B-lyphocytes.** Since bursa of Fabricius, a lymphoid organ is well developed in young birds 2-8- week old; they are more susceptible to IBDV. After initial infection, the virus is found in Kuppfer cells of the liver; and in macrophages and lymphoid cells of the jejunum, duodenum and cecum. Within 12 hours, cells of the bursa of Fabricius are infected. Following viremia, the thymus, the Harderian gland and spleen are infected. Birds over eight weeks are resistant to infection but can be infected by highly virulent strains. The **virus destroys the lymphoid follicles in the bursa of Fabricius as well as the circulating B-cells in the secondary lyphoid tissues present in gut-associated lymphoid tissue, conjuntiva, bronchial, caecal tonsils & Hardenian gland**, etc. Virus produces necrotizing effect on these host tissues

& causes acute disease, and death is due to the same. The **surviving birds remain immunocompromised** & become more susceptible to other diseases. Vaccination against several other diseases will not be effective.

Passive immunity as well as infection with avirulent strains protects against disease. Hence breeder flocks in broiler farms are immunized against IBD so that they would confer protective antibodies to their progenies to be slaughtered for consumption before their passive immunity wanes.

Clinical signs

Acute form: In clinical infections, onset of the disease is sudden after an incubation of 3-4 days. In the acute form birds are depressed, debilitated and dehydrated producing watery diarrhea and have swollen, blood-stained vent. Signs of the disease can include a rapid drop in feed and water consumption, mucoid (slimy) diarrhoea with soiling of the vent feathers, ruffled feathers, listless chicks with unsteady gait or sitting in hunched position, picking at own vent and sleeping with beak touching the floor. Mortality rates vary according to the virus virulence, the infection dose & the flock's ability to mount an effective immune response.

Less virulent strains do not produce clinical signs but the birds may have fibrotic or cystic bursa of Fabricius that is atropied prematurely before six months of age. Such birds may die of infections by agents that would not usually cause disease in immunocompetent birds. Clinical signs are also not present in very young birds less than 3 week old but the immune system becomes impaired.

Gross lesions are seen as **swelling, oedema and haemorrhages of the bursa of Fabricius**, the main target of IBDV, **haemorrhages in the muscles and kidney changes in the advanced stages**. Lesions in lymphoid tissues show degeneration of lymphocytes in medullary areas. Gross and histologic lesions characteristic of acute vvIBDV included edematous bursas, hemorrhages at the junction of the proventriculus and gizzard as well as hemorrhages on skeletal muscles. Microscopic lesions included severe lymphoid necrosis and inflammation in edematous bursas, lymphoid necrosis in thymus, spleen, Peyer's patches and cecal tonsils. Besides huge economic losses due to the clinical disease, the damage caused to the immune system results in lowered resistance to other infectious agents like *E. coli, Clostridia,* Coccidia & Ranikhet disease and a poor immune response to commonly used vaccines.

Subclinical infections before or at 3 week age are the most important form of the disease due to economic losses and induction of severe, long-lasting immunosuppression due to destruction of immature lymphocytes in the bursa of Fabricius, thymus, and spleen. The humoral B cell immune response is most severely affected but the **cell-mediated T cell immune response is also affected to a lesser extent**. Chickens immunosuppressed by early IBDV infections do not respond well to vaccination and are predisposed to infections with normally nonpathogenic viruses and bacteria. Common diseases are usually exacerbated by IBDV infections. Subclinical infections by the "variant" strains occur in immature birds, and severe long-term immunosuppression and bursal atrophy result from early infections.

Diagnosis

1. *Presumptive diagnosis*: Flocks' history, the clinical signs and PM lesions afford first hand diagnosis. Necropsy examination usually show changes in the bursa of Fabricius such as swelling, oedema, hemorrhage, the presence of a creamy transudate and eventually, atrophy. Pathological changes, especially hemorrhages, may also be seen in the muscle, intestines, kidney and spleen. Confirmation of a diagnosis of clinical IBD can be made at necropsy by examining the BF during the early stages of disease for characteristic gross lesions. During later stages of disease it is difficult to confirm a diagnosis of IBD by examining only shrunken, atrophied BF, as other diseases e.g. Marek's disease, mycotoxicosis produce similar changes. In birds less than 3 weeks of age or in young chickens with maternal antibodies, IBD virus infections are usually subclinical. Thus, typical clinical signs are not present, and diagnosis should be supported by histopathologic study of suspect BF, serologic studies, or by virus isolation. Definitive diagnosis is achieved by the specific detection and/or isolation and characterization of IBDV. Immunofluorescence or immunohistochemistry tests, based on anti-IBDV labeled antibodies, or in-situ hybridization, based on labeled complementary cDNA sequence probe, are useful for the specific detection of IBDV in infected tissues.

2. *Virus isolation*: IBD is normally diagnosed in veterinary laboratory by the isolation of causative virus in eggs and/or cell cultures and demonstration of bursal lesions. However, these procedures can be relatively time consuming and some strains either can not adapt themselves or not show characteristic changes on embryos.

3. *Immunoperoxidase technique*: By this test, IBDV antigens were observed in the macrophages and lymphocytes of the bursa of Fabricius. It was observed that the method is sensitive and specific and it could be used in the diagnosis of this disease. It can be performed very rapidly; a large number of specimens can be processed quickly. Moreover, subclinical infection of IBD may be diagnosed by this technique.

4. Detection and strain identification of IBDV is important because antigenic subtypes found within serotype 1 make it necessary to tailor vaccination programs to the antigenic type found in the bird's environment.
5. Antigen-capture enzyme-linked immunosorbent assay (ELISA) is used in some cases, but commonly used for detecting antibodies, & for monitoring vaccine responses and might be an additional information of infection for unvaccinated flocks.
6. *Molecular assays*: Reverse transcription-polymerase chain reaction (RT-PCR) as compared with antigen-capture ELISA, has greater versatility and are more sensitive and specific. Nucleotide sequencing of the hypervariable region of the VP2 (vVP2) gene segment of the IBDV genome, & nucleotide sequencing of a fragment of the VP1 gene in the segment B genotype is associated with highly pathogenic vvIBDV. Strain identification has been accomplished using a variety of post-RT-PCR assays, including restriction enzyme digestion of the RT-PCR products. The resulting restriction fragment length polymorphisms (RFLP) are used to differentiate viruses into molecular groups that correlate with antigenic and pathogenic types. Recently, two types of real-time RT-PCR have been used to identify and differentiate strains of IBDV. Both methods use distance-dependent interaction between two dye molecules, known as fluorescence resonance energy transfer (FRET). The dye molecules are attached to one or more nucleotide probes that detect specific nucleotide sequences of the virus. It is possible to identify single-nucleotide mutations among IBDV strains. A mutation probe is used in this assay to detect substitution mutations in a region of the viral genome that encodes a neutralizing epitope of the virus-VP2. These assays are accurate, reliable and inexpensive compared with conventional RT-PCR because they do not require RFLP or other labor-intensive post-RT-PCR assays to distinguish viral strains.

Prevention and treatment

No treatment exits for IBD except that supportive therapies namely vitamin and electrolyte supplements are given and antibiotics are used to treat secondary bacterial infections. Since virus is resistant to environmental conditions, even rigorous disinfection of contaminated farms achieves limited success in preventing disease spread.

Vaccination

Prevention of IBD is only achieved through good biosecurity and vaccination including passive protection via Breeder stocks vaccination and vaccination of progeny chicks based on the virus virulence strains and age of the birds. The **antigenic site eliciting neutralising antibodies lie within variable domain of VP2;** this site is also responsible for serotype specificity. **VP3 is a group-specific antigen that is recognized by non-neutralising antibodies,** which may cross-react with both serotypes.

In most countries, **breeders are immunized with a live vaccine at 6-8 weeks of age and then revaccinated with an oil-based inactivated vaccine at 18 weeks.** Recovered birds from a natural infection develop strong immunity.

Chicks are vaccinated with a live vaccine but the immunity may be poor in presence of high maternal antibody at the time of vaccination. Since variation between naturally occurring IBD viruses occur, hence **a number of vaccines are available.** The main method of control relies on vaccination of parent chickens and transmission of maternal antibody to the chicks. Different modified live vaccines (MLVs) have been developed and classified as **"mild", "intermediate", "intermediate plus" IBD vaccines,** depending upon their ability to break through maternally derived antibodies (MDA) that can neutralise the vaccine virus. MLV sometimes are not completely efficacious against vvIBDV, when they are applied in presence of significant MDA titres. Furthermore, they can induce moderate to severe bursal lesions and immunosuppression that can impair a chicken's response to other vaccinations.

Therefore, a new vaccine combining excellent safety and efficacy in the presence of high maternally derived IBDV titres was required. **Vaxxitek HVT+IBD**-Merial is live recombinant chimera vaccine virus expressing VP2 gene of IBD on HVT virus for protection against IBD+ MD for *in ovo* vaccination of 18 to 19 days old embryonated chicken eggs. For *in ovo* vaccination only healthy embryonated eggs should be used. This vaccination is also recommended for SC vaccination of healthy one-day-old chickens. Each dose of vaccine (0.2 ml) contains at least 3.0 log10 PFU of the live vHVT013-69 recombinant virus. It must be administered by means of a single SC injection. The vaccinated chickens synthesize only anti-VP2 antibodies that are protective against all types of IBDV challenges (classic, variant and very virulent strains). Several other commercially vaccines are available: **BURSA-VAC 3**-Intervet is an attenuated live intermediate classic IBD strain vaccine used for vaccination of 1 day old chicks by intraocular (one drop) or 14 day old chickens by drinking water. **Bursal-VAC 51**-Intervet is a live vaccine for vaccination of chickens 2 weeks of age or older for IBD caused by standard & variant IBDV. 10-day-old SPF broilers are vaccinated by eye drop method or 14-day-old chickens are vaccinated via the drinking water. **NOBILIS GUMBORO BROILER**-Intervet is a live vaccine (strain 228TC) for immunization of broiler & pullets & for primary vaccination of future breeding stocks. Dose is at least 3,0 log_{10} $TCID_{50}$ per fowl dose of live Gumboro disease virus strain 228 TC. Inactivated vaccines for vaccination of breeder stocks to protect offspring against IBD include as fllows. **NOBILIS GUMBORO INAC** - Intervets recommended for the booster vaccination of breeding stock previously vaccinated with attenuated live virus. Vaccine should be given to birds not less than 4 weeks before the expected onset of lay; dose is .5ml by IM route. **NOBILIS IB+ G+ ND**-Intervet; each bird should be given 0.5 ml of vaccine IM or SC. **Nobilis Reo+ IB+ G+ ND**-Intervet should be given to birds around 16-20 weeks of age but not less than 4 weeks before the expected onset of lay. Priming with live vaccines for IB, ND and Gumboro disease is necessary unless serological tests indicate otherwise. The interval between priming and boosting should be more than 4 weeks and less than 6 weeks. **NOBILIS IB MULTI+ G+ ND**-Intervet is inactivated combined vaccine for the booster vaccination of future breeders to protect against the chickens against IB (Massachusetts and D207/ strain D274 and related strains), IBD and ND. Each bird is given 0.5 ml IM. **Poulvac maternavac IBD-Reo vaccine**-Pfizer is recommended for the revaccination of healthy chickens against IBD caused by standard and variant IBD strains and avian reovirus infections which cause malabsorption syndrome. Progeny of vaccinates are protected via maternal antibodies. Inject 0.5 ml (0.5 cc) IM or SC for primed birds, a single dose between 16 and 22 weeks (approximately 4 weeks prior to lay) is indicated.

□□□

Chapter 18

Characteristics and Diseases Caused by Group IV Single-Stranded (+) RNA Picornaviruses (Family *Picornaviridae*)

Contents

Characteristics of Picornaviruses

Picornaviruses (L. pico= very small; rna = ribonucleic acid) are so named because they are very small non-envelope RNA viruses measuring 27-30 nm in diameter. These viruses have **icosahedral capsid** that consists of **60 identical subunits** each containing 4 proteins, **VP1, VP2, VP3, & VP4** (Fig. 18-1) and has a diameter of 27-30 nm. Picornaviruses contain unsegmented, linear, ssRNA positive-sense genome of 7.1-8.9 kb long, is polyadenylated & the genome naked + ssRNS is tightly packed into the capsid. The genomic RNA has unique feature having a protein **VPg on the 5' end used as a primer for transcription by RNA polymerase.** The capsid has four unique proteins: VP1, VP 2, VP 3 and VP 4. The VP4 protein lies in the inner surface of the capsid. Picornaviruses are one of the oldest viruses; records of poliovirus dates back to 1400 B. C. & cattle most serious disease virus, Foot-and-mouth virus was one of the first viruses to be recognized in 1898 by Loeffler and Frosch. The viruses of the family *Picornaviridae* are also one of the most diverse viruses containing more than over 200 sereotypes, causing infections in humans like Polio, Hepatitis A, the common flu, & enteroviral gastritis. Animals' infections include **FMD in cattle, Teschen disease in pigs, Avian encephalomyelitis in turkeys, chickens, pheasants & Japanese quail worldwide, & duck hepatitis**.

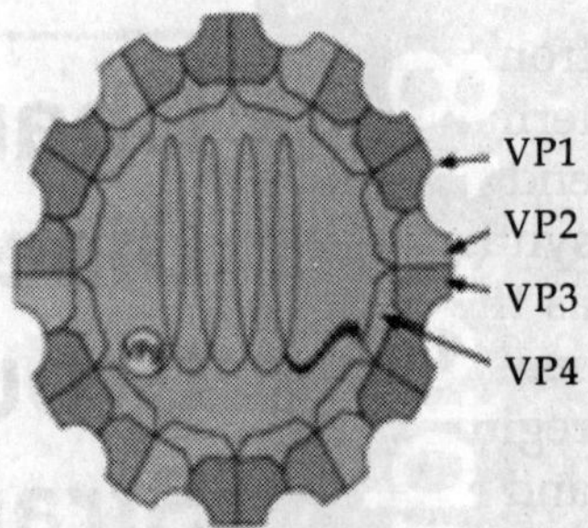

Fig. 18.1 : Morphology of a Picornavirus

Other features of picornaviruses are that most viruses can be propagated in cell culture producing a characteristic and rapid cytopathic effect, except some rhinoviruses, which require a lower temperature and can be cultured in vitro in very few cell types such as human fetal tracheal cells. Majority of picornaviruses are host specific or have limited host range except FMDV & encephalomyocarditis virus.

As regards picornaviruses environmental resistance, these viruses are able to survive in the environment for some time being infectious for several hours to one year, depending upon the conditions. Picornaviruses are resistant to ether, chloroform, and alcohol, & highly resistant to most disinfectants. Enteroviruses grow at 37^0 C & are stable under acid conditions and survive exposure to gastric acid. Rhinoviruses grow better at 33^0 C & are acid-labile being inactivated at low pH and hence rhinovirus infections are restricted to the nose and throat. But these viruses are susceptible to radiation, phenol, and bleaching (chlorination) & 0.2% citric acid & 0.4% sodium carbonate or acid-containing iodophore disinfectants are effective.

The virus genome

The virus genome consists of a single molecule of unsegmented, linear, postitive-sense, single-strand RNA. 7.1-8.9 kb long made of a single ORF encoding a polyprotein. The 5'-end of the genome has a long untranslated region (UTR) of 600-1200 bases long, which plays role in translation, virulence, and possibly encapsidation. The 5'-end UTR has clover leaf like structure called the **Internal Ribosome Entry Site(IRES)**, which distinguishes picornaviruses from other RNA viruses, & is important in translation and replication. The 5'-terminus also has **covalently-attached VPg protein instead of a cap.** The 3′ end has a shorter UTR of 50-100 bases long, which is important in (-) strand synthesis & is polyadenylated. **The viral RNA is infectious and serves both as the genome and viral mRNA because the genome itself is of the same sense as mammalian mRNA, being read 5' to 3'**. The genome contains **3 regions: P1, P2 & P3.** P1 region encodes the structural polypeptides, while P2 and P3 regions encode the nonstructural proteins associated with replication. L is N-terminal leader protein present in some genera that can either be a protease in aphthoviruses & erboviruses or have other functions as in *Kobuvirus* & *Cardiovirus*.

The IRES allows direct translation of the polyprotein, which is then processed by the viral protease(s) into various precursor and mature proteins to yield the structural proteins, replicase, VPg, and a number of proteins that modify the host cell, ultimately leading to cell lysis.

Virus replication

Picornavirus virion replication takes place in cell cytoplasm; the viral RNA is infectious and serves as both as the genome and viral mRNA. Firstly, the virion binds to the cell surface receptors that vary in different genera causing a conformational change in the viral capsid proteins with **release of myristic acids**. Myristic acids form a **pore in the cell membrane aiding RNA to enter** the host cell. While inside the cell, viral RNA uncoating occurs. Firstly the (+) strand RNA genome is replicated through a double-stranded RNA intermediate, which is formed using viral RNA-dependent RNA polymerase. Translation by host cell ribosomes is initiated (not by a 5' G cap) by an IRES (Internal Ribosome Entry Site).VPg is removed from the viral RNA, which is then translated into a processed polyprotein. Viral RNA replication occurs on membrane vesicles derived from the endoplasmic reticulum. A negative-sense complementary ssRNA is synthesized first using the genomic RNA as a template. New genomic RNA is synthesized using the negative-sense RNA as a template & is packaged into preformed procapsids. These **viruses are released through cell lysis except Hepatits A, which is non-lytic and thus creates a more persistent infection**. In enteroviruses, rhinoviruses, and aphtoviruses, shutoff of cellular cap-dependent translation occurs through the cleavage of the translation initiation factor eIF4G by viral protease. Maturation of provirions occurs by host protease.

The viral replication is very rapid & is completed in about 8 hours. Cell protein synthesis declines to almost zero in 30 minutes after infection by shutting off the macromolecular synthesis of cell proteins. Before cell death there is a loss of margination of chromatin & homogeneity in the nucleus and a vacuole appears in the cytoplasm close to the nucleus & the cell plasma membrane becomes permeable & cells die.

Virus classification

On the basis of physical characters, virion density and pH-sensitivity, serological relatedness, & recently based on nucleotide sequence, the ICTV has recognized **thirteen distinct genera** within the family: Group: Group IV ss (+) RNA

Order: *Picornavirales*

Family: *Picornaviridae*

Subfamily: *Picornavirinae*

Genera:

Genus 1: *Enterovirus*, type species: *Poliovirus* (PV)

Genus 2: *Rhinovirus*, type species: *Human rhinovirus A* (HRV-IA)

Genus 3: Cardiovirus , type species: *Encephalomyocarditis virus* (EMCV)

Genus 4: *Aphthovirus*, type species: *Foot-and-mouth disease virus* (FMDV)

Genus 5: Hepatovirus, type species: *Hepatitis A virus* (HAV)

Genus 6: Teschovirus, type species: *Porcine teschovirus 1*(PTV)

Genus 7: *Parechovirus*, type species: *Human parechovirus* (HPeV)

Genus 8: *Erbovirus*, type species: *Equine rhinitis B virus* (ERBV)

Genus 9: *Kobuvirus*, type species: *Aichi virus* (AiV)

Genus 10: *Sapelovirus*, type species; *Porcine Sapelovirus* (PSV)

Genus 11: *Senecavirus*, type species: *Seneca valley virus* (SVV)

Genus 12: *Tremovirus*, type species: *Avian encephalomyelitis virus* (AEV)

Genus 13: Avihepatovirus: type species; *Duck hepatitis A virus* (DHAV)

Plant picornaviruses fall under the family *Secoviridae*

Table 18-1 presented below depicts classification of *Picornaviridae*& diseases caused by the virus species in humans & animals.

Table 18.1 : Classification of *Picornaviridae* & diseases caused by the member viruses in humans & animals.

Genus	Species	Serotypes	Diseases caused
G 1: *Enterovirus*	*Bovine enterovirus*	BEV-1, 2	*Bovine enterovirus* (BEV-1,2) occurs endemically in cattle but are not pathogenic.
	Human enterovirus A (Coxsackie A virus/CV-A)	HE-A 21 include HEV-A+CV-A	* *Human enterovirus A* (CV-A) causes a blister -like rash on hand foot & mouth in children.

Human enterovirus B (Coxsackie B virus/CV-B) (Echovirus/ EV-B) (Swine vesicular disease virus (EV-B5)	HEA-A 59 types, 71 + CV-B+EV-B + SV-B5	* *Human enterovirus B* **(CA-B)** causes mild cold, often myocarditis, pericarditis, meningitis & pancreatitis in humans. *Echovirus **(EB-B)** cause fever, mild rash, URT infection in humans, rarely meningitis (Echo 9); *Human rhinoviruses cause cold, fever, mild rash, URT infection, & favour development of asthma after respiratory infection. * Swine vesicular disease virus **(EV-B5)** causes swine vesicular disease **(SVD)**, a mild disease of pigs that occurs sporadically in some parts of Europe & Asia. There is mild fever, inappetence followed by development of vesicular lesions on feet, coronary band, rarely on lips, tongue & snout with lameness.
TS: *Human enterovirus* C (Coxsackie A virus/ CV-A) (Poliovirus/PV)	HEC-19 types: + CV-A + PV-1,2,3	* *Human enterovirus* C / Poliovirus **(PV-1,2,3)** causes poliomyelitis, which is being controlled globally.
Human enterovirus D	EV-3 types:68, 70, 94	*Human enteroviruses **(EV 71)** causes hand, foot & mouth disease with rash in children, & rarely causes CNS encephalitis.
Porcine enterovirus B	PEV – 9, 10	*Porcine enterovirus B* **(SMEDI** (stillbirth, mummification, embryonic death, and infertility) is a reproductive disease of swine caused by *porcine enterovirus* and *porcine parvovirus;* also causes abortion, neonatal death, and decreased male fertility. It is spread by ingestion of food and

			water contaminated with infected feces or sexual contact and contact with aborted tissue. A vaccine is used to control the disease.
	Simian enterovirus A	SEV-A1	
	Human rhinovirus A	75 types	
	Human rhinovirus B	25 types	
	Human rhinovirus C	> 7 types	
G 2: *Cardiovirus*	TS: *Encephalomyocarditis virus*	EMCV-1	Encephalomyocarditis **(EMCV1) occurs in rodents, the natural host & also affects humans, monkeys & pigs**. Rats & mice are the reservoir hosts excreting virus in feces & urine. Infection in pigs is subclinical but piglets die from heart failure, & reproductive failure may occur. A vaccine is used to control the disease.
	Thelovirus	TMEV-12 types	
G 3: *Aphthovirus*	TS: *Foot-and-mouth disease virus*	FMDV-7 types O, A, C, Asia1, SAT1, SAT2, SAT3	FMD **(FMDV-O, A, C, Asia-1, SAT1, SAT2 & SAT3)** is highly contagious viral disease of cloven footed animals characterized by fever that declines after 2-3 days followed by formation of vesicles inside the mouth causing excessive stingy salivation, and vesicles on the feet that rupture and cause lameness, & myocarditis and death in newborn animals.
	Equine rhinitis A virus	ERAV	*Equine rhinitis A virus* **(ERAV)** infection is widespread, horses get infection at an early age & are associated with acute respiratory disease, but it is a minor respiratory pathogens. Horses under surgery or sternous exercise

			or mixed infection with bacteria contract infection, viremia follows with shedding of virus in urine.
	Bovine rhinitis B virus	BRBV	
G 4: *Hepatovirus*	TS: *Hepatitis A virus*	HAV	Hepatitis A (**HAV**), previously called infectious hepatitis is an acute infectious disease of liver, is spread by the fecal-oral route, & transmitted person-to-person by ingestion of contaminated food or water or through direct contact with an infected person. The IP is 2-6 with an average of 28 days. Symptoms include: fatigue, fever, abdominal pain, nausea, inappetence, jaundice dark amber colour urine & clay coloured feces. Symptoms last less than 2 months, but in some persons may last 6 months. Hepatitis A is prevented by vaccination, good hygiene & sanitation.
G 5: *Parechovirus*	TS: *Human Parechovirus*	HPeV 1 to 14	*Human Parechovirus* (**HPeV**) causes mild respiratory & gastrointestinal illness & also myocarditis. Infection is contracted during early life at 2-5 yrs of age.
	Ljunaan virus	LV-1 to 4	*Ljunaan virus* (**LV-1,4**) occurs in voles but is of zoonotic value as it is associated with diabetes, & intrauterine fetal disease in humans.
G 6: *Erbovirus*	TS: *Equine rhinitis virus*	ERBV-1 to 3	*Equine rhinitis virus* (**ERBV**) causes upper respiratory febrile disease in foals & weanlings.
G 7: *Kobuvirus*	TS: *Aichi virus*	AiV	
	Bovine kobuvirus	BKV	
G 8: *Teschovirus*	TS: *Porcine teschovirus*	PTV-1 to 11	*Porcine teschovirus* (**PTV-1**) causes Teschen disease or Talfan disease

			in pigs by serotype 1 having highly virulent and mildly virulent variants. Symptoms include fever, depression followed by neurological symptoms-weakness & incoordination leading to paraplegia & posterior paralysis & pigs adopt dog-sitting poster. Mortality rate is high but mildly affected pigs recover.
G 9: Sapelovirus	TS: *Porcine sapelovirus*	PSV	
	Simiansapelovirus	SSV 1 to 3	
	Avian sapelovirus	ASV	
G 10: *Senecovirus*	TS: *Seneca valley virus*		Possesses oncolytic activity
G 11: *Tremovirus*	TS: *Avian encephalomyelitis virus*	AEV	Avian encephalomyelitis (AEV-1) occurs in turkeys, chickens, pheasants & Japanese quail world wide with ataxia, tremor of head, neck & limbs in young ducklings. AEV is transmitted for ~1 week via eggs laid by the infected hens, and then infected chicks shed virus & spread to other hatch-mates.
G 12: *Avihepatovirus*	TS: *Duck hepatitis A virus*	DHAV1 to 3	*Duck hepatitis A virus* (DHAV-1) type 1 is more virulent & causes an acute disease of young domestic (Pekin) ducklings, which can inflict very high mortality.

Picornaviral Clinical Manifestations in Humans and Animals

Infections in Humans

Various types of clinical infections are caused by the members of the genera- *Enterovirus, Hepatovirus & Parechovirus*

Genus: *Enterovirus*

Human enterovirus A **(CV-A)** causes a blister -like rash on **hand, foot & mouth in children.** Human enteroviruses **(EV 71)** also cause hand, foot & mouth disease with rash in children, & rarely cause CNS encephalitis.

Human enterovirus B **(CA-B)** causes mild cold, often myocarditis, pericarditis, meningitis & pancreatitis in humans.

Echovirus **(EB-B)** causes fever, mild rash, URT infection in humans, rarely meningitis (Echo 9);

Human rhinoviruses cause cold, fever, mild rash, URT infection, & favour development of asthma after respiratory infection.

Human enterovirus C /Poliovirus **(PV-1, 2, 3)** causes poliomyelitis, which is being controlled globally.

Coxsackievirus A24 and echovirus 70 causes conjunctival infection with subconjunctival hemorrhage, severe pain in the eyes, photophobia, and occasional keratitis.

Rhinoviruses produce the common cold with flue-like symptoms in which most cases show rhinorrhea and nasal obstruction, & the throat is frequently sore or scratchy.

Skeletal muscles infection called **pleurodynia (Bornholm disease)** is also usually caused by coxsackie virus B and is characterized by fever and severe pain in the chest, & in the abdomen if diaphragm is involved. Some individuals develop **myalgic encephalomyelitis (ME)**, but the most important symptoms include fatigue following by even minor physical activity, and depressive psychological illness.

Skin and mucous membranes infections are caused almost entirely by coxsackievirus A with rashes. **Herpangina is an infection of the pharynx with herpes-like features** e.g. vesicles of the soft palate, fauces, uvula & posterior wall of the pharynx which resolves spontaneously in a few days.

Genus: *Hepatovirus*

Hepatitis A **(HAV)** infection, previously called **infectious hepatitis** is an acute infectious disease of liver spread by the fecal-oral route, & transmitted person-to-person by ingestion of contaminated food or water or through direct contact with an infected person. The incubation period is 2-6 weeks with an average of 28 days. Symptoms include: fatigue, fever, abdominal pain, nausea, inappetence, jaundice, dark amber colour urine & clay coloured feces. Symptoms last less than 2 months, but in some persons may be 6 months. Hepatitis A is prevented by vaccination, good hygiene & sanitation.

Genus: *Parechovirus*

HumanParechovirus **(HPeV)** causes mild respiratory & gastrointestinal illness & also myocarditis. Infection is contracted during early life at 2-5 yrs of age

Ljunaan virus **(LV1, 4)** infection occurs in voles but is of zoonotic value as it is associated with diabetes & intrauterine fetal disease in humans.

Picornavirus Clinical Infections in Aanimals & Birds

Various types of clinical infections are caused by the members of the genera- *Enterovirus, Cardiovirus, Aphthovirus, Erboviru, Teschovirus, Tremovirus & Avihepatovirus.*

Genus: *Enterovirus*

Swine Vesicular Disease

Swine vesicular disease (SVD), is a mild disease of pigs characterized by mild fever, inappetence followed by development of vesicular lesions which turns into ulcers on feet, coronary band, rarely on lips, tongue & snout with lameness.

Etiology: Swine vesicular disease is caused by *Swine vesicular disease virus* (EV-B5/SVDV) that belongs to the genus *Enterovirus* in the family *Picornaviridae.* This virus evolved from human coxsackievirus B5 (CV-B5); SVDV is currently classified as a porcine variant of CVB5, with SVDV an accepted synonym for this variant. There is only one serotype and a number of strains of SVDV. Based on genetic and antigenic analyses, these isolates fall into four phylogenetically distinct groups. Two groups contain viruses found before 1981; the other groups contain more recent European isolates.

Occurrence

SVDV occurs sporadically in some parts of Europe & Asia, Hong Kong, Japan & Malta.

Hosts

Pigs are the **only natural hosts** for SVDV, but young animals are more severely affected. One-day old mice can be infected experimentally. Humans have been infected while working with the virus in the laboratory.

Transmission

SVDV transmission occurs directly or indirectly by **infected feces, the infected tissues & refrigerated pork** containing the virus for long period, by shedding of virus before symptoms appear, & by movement of pigs. It is also spread by ingestion of food and water contaminated with infected feces or sexual contact and contact with aborted tissue. Pigs can excrete SVDV in nasal or oral secretions and feces up to 48 hours before clinical signs.

Pathogenesis

In natural outbreaks, infection occurs probably through broken skin or mucous membranes or by ingestion followed by virus replication locally & subsequently through lymphatic to the blood. Viremia occurs for a short period during which the virus disseminates to several organs & tissues. The virus is shed during the first week before clinical symptoms causing infection to other animals through tonsil, gastrointestinal tract & skin abrasion. The virus is present in feces & tissues from the infected pigs for months. The virus has affinity for epithelium of tongue, lips, snout, coronary band & for the myocardium. Lesion is seen histologically in the brain mainly in brainstem without nervous symptoms.

Clinical symptoms

Clinical signs are very similar to those of FMD and other vesicular diseases. The symptoms include: fever, appearance of vesicles in the mouth and on the snout and feet, lameness and an unsteady gait, shivering and jerking-type leg movements. Rupture of vesicles causes ulcers on limbs and feet, and foot pads may be loosened. Young animals are more severely affected. Recovery often occurs within a week. There is no mortality with SVDV.

Swine vesicular disease may be subclinical, mild or severe, depending on the virulence of the strain and the husbandry conditions. More severe lesions are seen when pigs are housed on concrete, particularly damp concrete, than on straw bedding or in grass. In addition, the symptoms are usually more severe in young animals. Most pigs recover completely within 2-3 weeks; however, a dark horizontal line may be seen on the hooves where the growth was temporarily interrupted.

Diagnosis

Swine vesicular disease should be included in the differential diagnosis when vesicles or erosions are found on the mouth and/or feet of pigs but, pigs are the only species affected. However, vesicular diseases are clinically indistinguishable and must be differentiated with laboratory tests.

Clinical specimens for various tests include vesicular fluid, affected skin and mucous membranes, blood with anticoagulant, and serum.

1. Viral antigens in lesion material are detected by ELISA. Immunohistochemistry may also be used. The virus is also identified with RT-PCR even in feces, in clinical samples & when a subclinical infection is suspected.

2. Virus isolation is done by growing suspect tissue preparation on porcine cell cultures including IB-RS-2 cells; & a cytopathic effect is observed.
3. Virus neutralization is definitive test to detect Abs, but takes 2-3 days to perform. ELISAs are used for surveillance. Other serological tests include double immunodiffusion, radial immunodiffusion and counter-immunoelectrophoresis.

Treatment & prevention

There is no vaccine for SVD. Preventive measures for SVDV are similar to those for FMD: controlling animals imported from infected areas, and sanitary disposal of garbage from international aircraft and ships, and thorough cooking of garbage. Infected animals are kept in strict quarantine. Eradication measures for the disease include quarantining infected areas, depopulation and disposal of infected and contact pigs, and cleaning and disinfecting contaminated premises.

Porcine Enterovirus B Infection

Porcine enterovirus B (PEV-B) along with *porcine parvovirus* **causes reproductive disorder in pigs called SMEDI** (stillbirth, mummification, embryonic death, and infertility), & also causes abortion, neonatal death, and decreased male fertility. *Porcine enterovirus B* (PEV-B) consists of a two serotypes: porcine enterovirus 9 (PEV-9) and PEV-10.

Etiology: Porcine enterovirus B infection syndrome SMEDI (stillbirth, mmmificaton, embryonic death, and infertility) is caused by *Porcine enterovirus B* (PEV-B) along with *porcine parvovirus*. Enteroviruses are subdivided into serotypes of which at least 11 are known. Four of these, serotypes 1, 3, 6 and 8, have been implicated in reproductive problems in pigs. Serotype 1 is the teschen/talfan virus which can also cause paralysis in pigs. Usually, each pig herd has an array of different serotypes which circulate in weaned and young growing pigs sub-clinically. The pigs are protected by circulatory antibodies derived from their dam's colostrum. By the time they reach breeding age they are solidly immune. **Reproductive problems only occur when a new serotype, to which the gilts are not immune, enters the herd and multiplies in the breeding females.** This probably does not happen very often. It is interesting to note that since the **introduction of parvovirus vaccine** and the excellent results achieved, the effects from SMEDI viruses would appear to be almost nonexistent, suggesting that this group of viruses is not important as a cause of reproductive failure.

Occurrence

Porcine enteroviruses capable to cause SMEDI are widely distributed in commercial pig herds in many countries; they are pathogenic only for embryos & fetuses.

Hosts: Only pigs are affected. The enteroviruses are prevalent in many swine herds.

Transmission

The disease is spread by ingestion of feces infected food and water and occasionally through sexual contact and contact with aborted tissues.

Pathogenesis

This depends on the age of the animal affected and the efficiency of its immune system. Colostral protection lasts up to 5 months of age, after which it decreases to an all-time low to increase yet again at about 12 months of age. Natural infection of enteroviruses takes place by mouth through the ingestion of infected feces. They multiply in the small and large intestines and in the absence of circulating antibodies escape from the intestine into the blood streams to the uterus. They cross the placenta, to produce the typical symptoms of embryo mortality, mummification and stillbirths. In some cases infertility associated with absorption of embryos also occur. If reproductive failure results there will be increases in embryo mortality, foetal deaths and mummified and stillborn piglets. Infection and disease only occur in non-immune sero-negative animals.

1. *Prenatal infection*: Virus travels from infected mother to fetus via the placenta. In this case, the time of gestation determines the result of the infection.

   If the fetus is infected in the first **30 days of fetal life**, death and absorption of all, or some of the fetuses may occur. In this case, some immunotolerant healthy piglets may be born.

   If the infection occurs at **40 days of fetal life**, death and mummification may occur. Also in this case, some or all the fetuses are involved, i.e. some of the fetuses can be born healthy and immunotolerant, or else carriers of the disease.

   If the viruses crosses the placenta in the **last trimester**, neonatal death may occur, or the birth of healthy piglets with a protective pre-colostral immunity.

2. *Postnatal infection*: Infection in pigs up to 1 yearof age occurs oro-nasally, followed by a viremic period associated with transitory leucopenia.

3. *Infection in adult pigs*: Pigs **over 1 year of age** would have an active, protective immune system which protects them from future exposures e.g. mating with an infected male.

The virus is particularly dangerous **for the sow in her first gestation,** which would be at 7–8 months of age, as she would have a particularly low antibody count at this age and could easily contract the virus via copulation.

Lesions

Histologically, the pregnant sow develops lesions in the myometrium due to the infiltration of monocytes. The fetus shows retarded growth, congestion of superficial vessels which may be associated with hemorrhage and dehydration & results in mummification of the fetus.

Diagnosis

Samples collected for clinical specimens include tissue from fetuses, lungs and stillborn pigs.

1. The viruses are cultivated in primary pig kidney cell cultures with low frequency of isolations because of the absence of viable virus at the time clinical disease becomes apparent.

Treatment & prevention

Vaccination

A vaccine is used to control the disease. Piglets vaccinated with a single oral dose of live porcine enterovirus strain T80 were protected to a highly significant degree against an oral challenge dose of 140 plaque forming units of T80 virus.

Genus: *Cardiovirus*

Encephalomyocarditis

Encephalomyocarditis (EMCV1)virus can cause encephalitis and myocarditis in rodents (rats & mice); they are the reservoir hosts excreting virus in feces & urine. Infection in pigs is subclinical but piglets die from heart failure, & reproductive failure may occur. Severe epidemics have been reported in swine & elephant, & also affect humans, monkeys & zoo animals.

Etiology: EMC is caused by *Encephalomyocarditis virus* (EMCV) of the genus *Cardiovirus* in the family *Picornaviridae.*

Occurrence

EMC has been reported from many parts of the world. Be sides rodents, EMC also affects swine and exotic mammals.

Hosts susceptible

Rodents (rats & mice) are the natural hosts, & the virus is transmitted from rodents to other animals. Severe epidemics have been reported in swine & elephant, & also affect humans, monkeys & zoo animals. These, and presumably other rodent species, shed the viruses in feces and urine, which may contaminate food and water supplies of large mammals. Various exotic mammals have been fatally afflicted with EMC in zoologic parks in the USA, Australia, and other parts of the world, and have included African & Indian elephants, rhinoceroses, hippopotamuses, sloths, llamas, various antelope species, and many types of nonhuman primates (chimpanzees, orangutans, baboons, cynomologous monkeys, lemurs, etc).

Transmission

EMCVs are always associated with rodents, and disease in other mammalian species is transmitted from populations of mice and rats shedding virus in feces & urine that contaminate water supplies for other animals. Ingestion of rodents dead or dying of EMC may be another means of infection. Pigs shed virus in nasal secretions and feces during the first **3 days of experimental infection**. During this short period, the virus may be transmitted to other pigs by contact. Cardioviruses are resistant to adverse environmental influences and may remain infective for weeks to months under favorable conditions. An episode of lion deaths at a zoo in the USA was associated with the feeding of the carcass of an African elephant that had died of EMC, and a spontaneous outbreak of fatal EMC was reported in free-ranging African elephants at Kruger National Park in South Africa in 1995.

Humans appear to be resistant to fatal infections with EMC viruses. Swine may die acutely at any age due to associated myocardial failure or may be affected with near-term abortions, fetal mummification, and apparent reproductive failure.

Serologic studies have revealed that subclinical infections are common in EMC outbreaks; although EMC antibodies are frequently detected, no deaths have been confirmed.

Clinical symptoms and lesions

EMC has predilection for the CNS and cardiovascular systems of mice, and both encephalotropic and cardiotropic strains have been reported. In swine and zoologic species, acute and subacute deaths are due to the destructive effects of the virus on the myocardium, with resultant cardiac insufficiency, pulmonary edema, and frothy transudation in the respiratory tract. Affected animals often appear to have asphyxiated in their own respiratory fluids. Other clinical signs may include fever, **anorexia, listlessness, trembling, staggering, dyspnea, and paralysis.** Mortality approaching 100% has been described in suckling swine but becomes successively lower in older age groups.

EMC viruses cross the placenta in swine and have been recovered from fetuses in cases of reproductive failure due to near-term abortions (107-111 days of gestation), with stillbirths, and mummifications. Reproductive problems often persist in affected herds for 2-3 months and may affect sows.

Diagnosis

1. *Presumptive diagnosis*: Clinical symptoms, lesions-pale necrotic heart muscle lesions are suggestive.

2. *Virus isolation*: Myocardial tissue and spleen are collected from acutely dead animals or fetuses are the specimens of choice for virus isolation. Because EMC viruses are very stable, they may be recovered from frozen tissues.

3. *Serologic diagnosis*: It is made using virus neutralization, hemagglutination-inhibition, or ELISA for which acute and convalescent sera are collected, but the frequency of subclinical EMC infections makes single serum determinations of little value in aborting sows. Detection of antibody against EMC viruses in stillborn or large mummified fetuses is significant for fetal infection, however, because **maternal immunoglobulins are not transferred across the placenta in swine.**

Treatment and Control

There is no specific treatment for EMC, but mortality may be minimized by avoiding stress or excitement in animals at risk. EMC viruses appear to cycle in rodents and are most likely to affect swine and zoo animals when rodent populations are high. **Rodent control is thus important for minimizing exposure of susceptible species.** Prompt and proper disposal of animals that have died of the disease is also recommended. EMC viruses are inactivated by the judicious use of many disinfectants labeled for livestock use.

Vaccination

Killed vaccines for the prevention of myocarditis in weaned swine are available. Pigs are inoculated IM at =4 week of age, revaccinated 2-3 week later, and semiannually thereafter. These vaccines have been used extra-label in susceptible exotic animal species in zoos and amusement parks where EMC has been problematic. Vaccines are available in South Africa for commercial pig vaccine in U.S., experimental elephant vaccines available in U.S. & zoos in endemic areas may vaccinate but further studies are needed.

Genus: *Aphthovirus*

Foot and Mouth Disease (FMD)

Foot-and-mouth disease (FMD), a highly contagious disease of cloven-footed animals caused by *Aphthovirus (Picornaviridae)* is characterized by rapid spread, formation of vesicles on epithelial tissues of feet, mouth, mammary gland & fever with catastrophic economic losses (List A disease in the world). Although FMD does not result in high mortality in adult animals, the disease has debilitating effects, including weight loss, decrease in milk production, and loss of draught power, resulting in a loss in productivity for a considerable amount of time. Mortality, however, can be high in young animals, where the virus can affect the heart. In addition, cattle, sheep, and goats can become carriers, and cattle can harbor the virus for up to 2 to 3 years. Since FMD spreads widely and rapidly and because it has grave economic as well as clinical consequences, FMD is one of the most dredful animal diseases of cattle, water buffaloes, sheep, goats, pigs, antelopes, deer & bison.

Etiology: FMDV belongs to genus *Aphthovirus* of the family *Picornaviridae*, & exists in seven different serotypes: A, O, C, Asia1, and SAT1, SAT2, and SAT3, but more than 64 subtypes have evolved within these serotypes. FMDVs have been divided into genotypes based on VP1 sequence.

FMDV **serotype O** is the most prevalent of the seven serotypes of FMDV & is divided in **11 antigenic subtypes.** Serotype O has eight distinct genetic lineages, which fall into geographically distinct regions. These have been designated topotypes and named Europe South America (Euro-SA), Middle East South Asia (ME-SA), South-East Asia (SEA), Cathay (an ancient and poetic name for China and east Tartary), West Africa (WA), East Africa (EA), Indonesia-1 (ISA-1) and Indonesia-2.

FMDV **serotype A** is most diverse antigenically and contains **33 subtypes;** some of these subtypes seems to be genetically distinct (eg. A22, A24). Comparison about 300 Vp1 sequences has shown that type A viruses can be grouped into three major geographically restricted genotypes, (i) Euro-SA, (ii) Asia, and (iii) Africa.

FMDV **serotype C** has a very limited distribution & is mostly become confined to the Indian sub-continent, & have **5 subtypes. Sequencing of nucleotides of VP1 gene** (VP1), VP2, VP3, VP4 & trace of VP0 Ags) is used to compare different isolates obtained from FMD outbreaks.

FMDV **serotype Asia 1** only occurs in Asia & is antigenically less diverse than those belonging to types O, A or C. Only **five antigenic subtypes** exist. Asia 1 belonged to 6 groups within the Asia 1 serotype. Although two major genotypes could be distinguished, relationships were generally above 85% and all the isolates could be included in a single topotype. It is clear that genetic variation amongst FMD Asia 1 viruses is much lower than that found within other serotypes.

FMDV three serotypes, South African Territories (SAT), SAT-1, SAT-2 & SAT 3 types are endemic to southern Africa, & three SAT types differ from each other on the basis of geographic distribution, infection rates and wildlife involvement in the FMD outbreaks of livestock.

SAT-1 has **7 subtypes** (SAT 1-7), is important due to its extensive distribution throughout sub-Saharan Africa and previous incursion into North Africa and the Middle East. In addition, SAT-1 has the highest seroprevalence rate in the maintenance host, the African buffaloes. Despite the high incidence of SAT-1 type virus in buffalo, it caused only 36% of the SAT-type outbreaks of FMD in cattle in southern Africa. A total number of six SAT 1topotypes have been identified in Africa.

FMDV SAT-2 caused most outbreaks (48%), has only **2 subtypes** (SAT2-3) & occurs throughout sub-Saharan Africa and has made recent incursions into the Middle East from north-east Africa. SAT 2 type viruses from all major regions on the continent has eleven distinct topotypes, & most frequently associated with outbreaks of the disease in livestock in southern and West Africa and with clinical cases of the disease in wildlife. Buffalo are the primary source of infection for other cloven-hoofed species in southern Africa.

SAT-3 accounts for only 16% of outbreaks & has **2 subtypes**- SAT 3-4. SAT 3 has the most restricted distribution with five different topotypes in South Africa, Zimbabwe, Zambia, Namibia, Botswana, Malawi, and Uganda.

Occurrence

FMD is endemic in parts of Asia, Africa, the Middle East, **parts of Europe** and South America. FMD outbreaks have occurred in every livestock-containing region of the world with the exception of New Zealand, and the disease is currently enzootic in all countries **except Australia and North America.** The disease affects domestic cloven-hoofed animals, including cattle, swine, sheep, and goats, as well as more than 70 species of wild animals, including deer. **A pandemic strain of serotype O named "O pan Asia"** caused outbreaks in several countries, first identified in India in 1990, spread to Nepal 1993, Bangladesh 1996, Bhutan 1998, then spread westward in Saudi Arabia 1994, Near East countries, Europe Turkey, Bulgaria, & Greece in 1996, China 1999, & SE Asia, Korea, Japan, Russia, Mongolia & affected many hosts-cattle, buffaloes, pigs, sheep, goats, camels, deer, & antelopes. The recent outbreaks of foot-and-mouth disease (FMD) occurred in a number of FMD-free countries; in Taiwan 1997, the UK in 2001, **China & Korea in** 2005 **(Asia-1)**, UK in August 2007, Japan 2010, & Bulgaria in 2011. These recent FMD outbreaks have significantly increased public awareness of this highly infectious disease of cloven-hoofed livestock. Newzealand, Australia, west European countries, North & Central America & Caribbean countries are free from FMD.

Table : Geographical distribution of serotypes & subtypes of FMD virus.

FMD Serotypes	Subtypes	Distribution
'O'	O-11	Worldwide
'A'	A-33	Worldwide
'C'	C-5	Worldwide
Asia-1	Asia 1-3	Asia
SAT-1	SAT 1 -7	Africa & Asia
SAT-2	SAT 2-3	Africa
SAT-3	SAT 3-4	Africa
O, A, C	South America, Eastern European countries	
O, A, C, SAT1, SAT2 & SAT3	Africa	
O, A, C, Asia1	Asia	

- Each serotype differs antigenically/ immunologically, each has antigenically distinct subtypes & immunity to one FMDV type don't protect against others.
- **Sequencing of nucleotides of VP1 gene** (VP1, VP2, VP3, VP4 & trace of VP0 Ags) is used to compare different isolates obtained from FMD outbreaks.
- Serotypes O & A are more prevalent; prevalence depends largely on meat trade between countries.
- Change of antigenicity & strain adaptation to a animal species do occurs, e.g. **porcinophilic** strains

Hosts susceptible

FMD affects domestic cloven-hoofed animals, including cattle, swine, sheep, and goats, & more than 70 species of wild animals, including deer.

- All cloven footed animals are susceptible of which immature & well fed are more susceptible.
- In cattle susceptibility in ascending order is: indigenous → hill → cross breed → exotic cattle, morbidity up to 100% & mortality in adult @ 2%; & in young stocks 20%.
- Domesticated buffaloes are more susceptible than cattle.
- Sheep are susceptible; some virus strains are more virulent.
- Goats are susceptible; some virus strains are more virulent.
- Pigs are susceptible in which strain adaptation occurs with increased virulence occurred with up to **23% death in 1997.** FMD outbreaks in Taiwan. Pigs are important virus transmitter to other animals.
- Elephants, camels & yaks are susceptible.
- Wildlife African buffaloes, deer, antelopes, deer & hedgehogs are susceptible & they act as virus transmitter.
- Humans are slightly susceptible, & they develop **small vesicles in mouth**/ hands; & **transmit virus to animals**.

Transmission

- Among herds & countries: FMD mode of transmission differs among herds, countries & continents. Transmission between herds: occurs through animal movement, **human nasal mucosa**, inanimate objects, uncooked meat products, milk and infected semen. Transmission in disease -free countries occurs mainly through meat products from pigs, birds, contact with meat & other routes.
- In enzootic areas: Disease transmission occurs through direct contact, aerosols, mechanical carriage, vehicles, humans, movement of animals **across states & at international borders**, nomadic cattle, fomites & animal products.
- In non-enzootic areas: Disease transmission occurs through pigs: Pigs → eat infected meat scrapings → via people, abattoir waste, animals → cattle herds.

- Wind-born transmission: In 1981 FMD outbreak occurred from 250 km in France to UK under proper humidity & low temp. Pigs are potent excretors & **cattle most vulnerable to air transmission.**
- Source of the virus: **All secretions, excretions, urine, feces & semen, & embryos** are infective before symptoms appear.
- *Carriers*: Some **cattle, sheep & goats remain carriers after clinical recovery**. FMDV persists in **vaccinated ones exposed to infection with different subtypes**. FMDV can persist for **3 years in carrier cattle**, for several months in sheep & up to **5 years in Cape buffaloes** (in Africa).
- *Nasopharynx*: **Nasopharynx** is the main site of virus persistence, low virus excretion occurs up to 2 years & mammary tissues secrete virus up to 4 weeks.
- *Reservoirs*: African Cape buffaloes in Sahara (SAT types), small rodents & hedgehogs act as reservoirs for FMFV.
- *Other factors*: Cattle long transportation, animal fair, flood & inundation of areas favour FMDV outbreaks.
- *Cyclic occurrence*: FMD **occurs in 4-6 years cycle**: When immunity wanes, reinfection starts in small foci → to almost all areas → immunity lasts for 1-2 yrs in cattle, shorter in pigs → immunity declines, reinfection → cycle repeated.
- Frequent infections occur in vaccinated ones by other virus types/ subtypes.
- *Environment*: The virus remains viable for 1 yr in the infected premises, 10 wks on clothing, 1 month on hair, 3 days in soil in summer & 28 days in winter; in frozen semen & in uncooked meat. NaOH & formalin kills the virus, high or low pH is detrimental for the virus. Lactic acid in dead animals inactivates the virus but the virus survives in offal.

Pathogenesis

After virus enters through ingestion, contact with broken epithelium, inoculation or insemination, the virus replicates in the mucosal epithelial cells & lymphatic tissues of pharynx. The cells disintegrate; the viruses are released & infect newer more cells. The virus through **efferent lymphatics enters** blood causing **viremia.** The virus is disseminated to epidermal sites of stratified epithelium of mammary gland, other organs, epithelial cells of mouth, muzzle, teats, interdigital space, coronary band involving **deeper layer of stratum spinosum. The lesion starts as foci of** necrosis & death of keratinocytes. There is accumulation of fluid in the space (vesicles) followed by necrosis of overlying keratinocytes that rupture leading to erosions. **Gross lesions are seen in areas prone to mechanical injury** e.g. mouth, feet, teats & mammary gland epithelium (acinar necrosis), & snout of pigs. Virus localization occurs in feet, mouth, & lesions that heal rapidly. But lesions are **aggravated by bacterial infections,** & clinical symptoms of lameness & off feed are seen.

- **Young ones & malignant form:** Lesions develop in heart (rarely skeletal muscle) with necrosis & degeneration. **FMDV don't cross placenta but abortion occurs due to pyrexial reactions.**

Clinical Symptoms

Incubation period is 2-14 days with average 3-6 days & runs a course of 7 days.

- There is fever 104-106 F, anorexia, & **drastic fall in milk 70-90%**. Fever subsides after 1-2 days.
- Acute painful stomatitis is present with **ropy stringy salivation.**
- Vesicles on buccal mucosa, dental pad & tongue appear that rupture within 24 hrș with a raw painful surface with erosion & ulcers; teats lesions are seen with mastitis, as well as nose lesions are seen.
- Concurrently **vesicles on feet: clefts, on coronet**, vesicles rupture & cause acute lameness, & **recumbency** occurs in crossbred.
- Complication by **bacterial infections** involves deep structure of feet, & hoof may slough off in crossbred.
- Young animals are more susceptible with myocardial involvement; & **calves die due to myocarditis.**
- **Mild form & malignant form** of FMD: Sometimes milder form is seen in indigenous cattle. **Malignant form** occurs in adult cattle with typical course but **relapses after 5-6 days** with dyspnea, weak & irregular heart **&death during convulsion due to myocardial failure.**
- Occasionally the virus localizes in **alimentary tract with dysentery/ diarrhea & enteritis.**
- After effects: **'Panting'** (endocrine disturbance) with **dyspnea, anemia, overgrowth of hair & heat intolerance** are the main symptoms.

Sheep & goats

Symptoms are mild & slightly less severe with fewer, lesser lesions but **severely involve all 4 feet.** Young animals are more susceptible. Sometimes symptom like **'panting'** in adult sheep is seen with loss of hooves after bacterial infections. They are important as virus transmitter to cattle.

Pigs

Pigs show mild but protracted symptoms, & foot lesions are more severe with marked lameness. Pigs are the most important virus transmitter to cattle. 1997 Taiwan FMD outbreak was devastating with **large vesicles on snout & 23% mortality.**

Pathological lesions of FMD

- Gross lesions include vesicles, rupture, erosion in the mouth, on feet, on teat & mammary gland with ulcers; & teats & mammary gland with lesions are often swollen.
- Feet lesions are often maggot infested.
- Vesicles occasionally occur in **pharynx, esophagus, fore stomach & intestine.**
- In neonates & malignant form in adult cattle there is involvement of heart.

Histologically, vesicles start as small foci of progressive swelling, necrosis & lysis of keratinocytes, fluid accumulation in the deeper epidermis spinosum, necrosis of overlying keratinocytes, vesicles rupture- erosions with mild leucocytes infiltration.

- Mammary gland shows similar changes with acinar necrosis & interstitial infiltration.
- Heart lesions in young & malignant form in adult cattle: show severe hyaline degeneration, necrosis & rarely calcification of myofibers, mononuclear interstitial infiltration, epicardial hemorrhages, & **'tiger heart'** due to alternate area of hemorrhages & normal tissues.
- **Pancreatic islet degeneration** is seen in some cases.

Diagnosis

FMD is diagnosed by virus isolation, detection of viral antigens or nucleic acids, and serology.

Samples collection for diagnosis includes fresh vesicles with epithelial tissues, oral mucosa, and fresh feet lesions in glycerine saline for diagnosis. Tissues from oral mucosa, skin with vesicles or fresh lesions, heart, infected mammary gland & pancreas are collected for histopathology.

1. *Presumptive diagnosis*: Clinical symptoms & lesions are characteristic; FMD should be differentiated from Blue tongue, **VSIV, VEV & SVDV**.

2. *Virus isolation*: FMDV is usually isolated using primary bovine thyroid cells or primary pig, calf or lamb kidney cells, BHK-21 or IB-RS-2 cells, but cell lines are less sensitive than primary cells.
3. *Virus antigen detection*: FMDV is identified by ELISA, complement fixation or RT-PCR tests. ELISAs identify viral antigens directly in tissues; complement fixation is less specific and sensitive. RT-PCR techniques are also available. **The virus serotype can be determined with either ELISA or RT-PCR.** ELISA detects antibodies to nonstructural proteins (NSP) & diagnoses previous or current infections in vaccinated animals. **Persistently infected animals are not detected by anti-NSP tests but detected by isolating FMDV from the esophageal-pharyngeal fluids, or by RT-PCR test.** Tissue culture, CFT, ELISA, RT-PCR, DNA probe, animal inoculation; plaque reduction neutralization, radial immunoassay & serum neutralization tests are used.
4. *Detection of FMD antibodies*: **ELISAs and virus neutralization tests detect antibodies in previous or current infections in unvaccinated animals, and are serotype specific test.**

Lab animals, guinea pigs: Fresh vesicular fluid inoculated intradermally into plantar pad causes vesicles in foot pads in 1-7 days & in mouth in 1-2 days later.

Treatment & prevention

Treatment includes removal of necrosed tissues & debris, & dressing with mild disinfectant to prevent secondary infections.

Use turpentine oil/ loraxene, himax etc in maggot infested feet lesions, clean mouth with alum solution. IM use of flunixin meglumine is good especially in crossbred cattle. Use broad-spectrum antibiotics in case of crossbred cattle with badly damaged hoof.

Preventive measures include restriction of movement of animals from infected foci. Keep separate attendants for sick & healthy animals. Keep constant monitoring & surveillance in the epidemic area. Inert materials e.g. bedding, feed, feeding utensils, farm machinery, animal products; human clothing, & motor vehicles should be disinfected or burnt. Infected animals should be buried & premises or farms should be disinfected using acid or alkaline (NaOH) preparations. Quarantine of animals coming from border areas is practiced.

Vaccination

FMD eradication by slaughter is impossible in endemic countries, UK FMD in **1967 costed Rs 1200 million**, hence decided to adopt test &

vaccination policy in future. In 1997 Taiwan outbreak, about 22000 pigs were disposed daily. There are seven different types and more than 60 subtypes of FMD virus, and there is no universal vaccine against the disease. Vaccines for FMD must match to the type and subtype present in the affected area. When matched to type and subtype, the vaccine will normally protect animals from developing clinical signs of disease, but will not necessarily protect animals against FMD infection. The vaccine bank is housed at USDA's Foreign Animal Disease Diagnostic Laboratory (FADDL) at the Plum Island Animal Disease Center. It is the only place in the United States where scientists can conduct research and diagnostic work on FMD at a biosafety-3 level, which means that they are designed, constructed, and operated to prevent the escape of microorganisms from the laboratory into the environment. Scientists at FADDL monitor FMD outbreaks around the world and stock the vaccine bank with antigens for the most active serotypes or strains of the virus. If necessary, these scientists can isolate and identify an FMD serotype from a field sample in as little as 4 days. With this information, FADDL scientists would know what vaccine type to order from an overseas supplier, and if it were not in stock, the supplier could use the isolate to create a new vaccine. FADDL scientists also test currently available vaccines. Their testing has helped ensure that FMD vaccines are not contaminated with other microorganisms and that they do not produce adverse reactions following administration.

Currently 3 types of FMD vaccines are used:

1. *Inactivated (killed) vaccines*
   - i. Formalin inactivated FMD vaccine,
   - ii. Acetylethyleamine or binary ethyleneimine (BEI) inactivated FMD vaccine,
   - iii. Inactivated adjuvant vaccine,
   - iv. Inactivated vaccine using FMD isolates from local outbreaks.

   The adjuvant for ruminants is commonly Al $(OH)_3$ with or without saponin, whereas pig vaccines require oil adjuvants.
2. *Attenuated vaccines*
   1. Tissue culture adapted, mice & rabbit adapted & hens egg adapted vaccines have been prepared.
3. *Genetically engineered FMD vaccine*: FMD vaccine genetically engineered. On June 18, 1981, the U.S. government announced the creation of a vaccine targeted against FMD, the world's first genetically engineered vaccine.

Inactivated vaccines: **Inactivated polyvalent FMD vaccine** (O, A, C, Asia1-1) in India or (O, A, C) in western countries: The virus serotypes are grown on BHK cell/ other cell suspensions separately & formalin or acetylethyleamine or BEI inactivated vaccines are in general use. **Immunity appears about 7-20 days** after vaccination. The vaccines give immunity for 6-8 mths & require 6 monthly vaccinations. Some reactions like swelling & gangrene do occur.

Inactivated FMD Vaccine using FMDV isolates from local **outbreaks** affords protection **for 1 year. Inactivated FMD adjuvant vaccine gives protection for 1 yr,** requires yearly vaccination in adults & biannual in young stocks. Reaction due to inactivated vaccine is prevented using emulsifying agents.

Some preparatory FMD vaccines are as floows:

1. **Bovilis FMDV Gel (MVDV O, A, Asia1)**, cell culture, BEI inactivated & concentrated Ags, adsorbed on Aluminium hydroxide+ saponin. Dose: C, B: 2ml SC; S, G:1 ml SC; Calves at 6-8 mths, S, G after 3 mths; booster in calves, S & G-1 to 1& 1/2 mths later; vaccination- 6 mthly
2. **Bovilis FMDV Clovax (MVDV O, A, Asia1),** Cell Culture, BEI inactivated & concentrated, emulsified in **mineral oil adjuvant**.

   Dose: C, B: 2 ml preferably IM; S, G: 1 ml IM; Calves, S, G: after 4 mths, booster after 6 mths; revaccination- annually.
3. **FMD Vaccine (FMDV O, A, Asia1),** Cell Culture, BEI inactivated, concentrated Ags, emulsify in **mineral oil adjuvant for use in epidemic area**.

   Dose: C, B: 2 ml IM; S, G:1 ml IM; Calf, S, G: at 3 mths, 1st booster 4-6 wk later; 2nd 24 wks of 1st booster, revaccination at every 44-48 wks after 2nd booster.
4. **DECIVAC FMD DOE**-Merck is an inactivated oil adjuvant vaccine for immunization of pigs, cattle, buffaloes, sheep & goats. Types included depend on the area where the vaccine is required. Decivac FMD DOE may contain antigens of the FMDV types O, A, C, Asia1 and SAT1, SAT2, SAT3 (monovalent or multivalent). The actual combination of antigens depends on the local situation. Each dose (2 ml) of vaccine contains at least 3 PD50 of the virus types indicated. The FMD viruses are propagated on BHK cells, chemically inactivated and subsequently purified and concentrated. The resulting antigens are stored at ultra low temperature until formulation of the final vaccine. Dose: Cattle, Buffalo, Pigs: 2ml SC or IM but pigs IM. Primary vaccination

from two weeks of age onwards, followed by revaccination 4-6 months later. Young animals with, or suspected of having, maternal antibodies: primary vaccination from 4 months of age onwards, followed by revaccination 4-6 months later. Adult animals: every 6 months. Sheep, Goats: 1ml SC or IM Young animals with, or suspected of having, maternal antibodies: primary vaccination from 2 months of age onwards, followed by revaccination 4-6 months later. Adult animals: every 6 months. In areas where FMD is endemic, a booster vaccination is recommended at 6 weeks after the primary vaccination.

5. **RAKSHA OVAC**- Indian Immunological Ltd: Raksha OVAC contains inactivated tissue culture FMD virus strains O, A, C and Asia-1 adjuvanted with mineral oil. Complete inactivation of the virus is ensured by the use of Aziridine compound. Dose: Cattle, buffaloes, calves & pigs-2ml, IM, primary vaccination at 4 months of age & first Revaccination 9 months after primary vaccination, subsequent revaccination : Annual Sheep & goats: 1 ml IM primary vaccination at 4 months of age, first revaccination 9 months after primary vaccination & subsequent revaccination : Annual. Pigs: Weaners should be vaccinated at two months of age by which time maternal antibodies would have waned. Breeding stock should be revaccinated at six month intervals. All stock should be revaccinated if the risk of infection is high.

Attenuated FMD vaccine

Attenuated FMD vaccineis prepared after serial passage in mice, rabbits, hens egg & tissue culture (TC). **South Africa & Venezuela** controlled FMD using **attenuated vaccines (killed vaccine failed)**. FMD control has been possible in **Russia using attenuated lapinized vaccine**. But **some FMD outbreaks occurred.**

Sheep, goats & pigs vaccination provides better FMD control. Sheep vaccination gives protection for 6 months but sheep may remain **inapparent carrier.**

Pigs: Inactivated adjuvant vaccine protects pigs for 6-12 months.

Genetically engineered FMD vaccine: Uses FMD virus polypeptide VP1 & incorporated into hepatitis B virus or **Synthesized VP1 peptide** vaccine that gives encouraging results but awaits practical application.

Improved killed vaccine is still favored. Instead of mass vaccination, ring vaccination in limited areas of actual FMD outbreak gives better result.

Equine Rhinitis A Virus Infection

Equine rhinitis A virus (ERAV) **infection** is widespread respiratory infection of horses, which get infection at an early age, but it is a minor respiratory pathogens. Horses under surgery or sternous exercise or mixed infection with bacteria contract infection, viremia follows with shedding of virus in urine.

Etiology: *Equine rhinitis A virus* (ERAV) belongs to genus *Aphthovirus* in the family *Picornaviridae*. The clinical symptoms most closely resemble the febrile respiratory tract infections similar to rhinoviruses rather than the systemic disease. However, broad host cell range, viremia and persistent infection are associated with ERAV are not seen with rhinovirus infections but reminiscent of FMDV infection. ERAV also shares unusual features of genome structure and organization with FMDV. The similarities between the two viruses suggest that ERAV may be a useful model system for analyzing the biology of FMDV.

Pathogenesis

The virus shedding with clinical signs of two Australian ERAV isolates was studied in experimentally infected horses. Two ERAV seronegative 8 month old horses were infected intranasally with one of two ERAV isolates. Following infection, the ERAV isolates were reisolated from the nasopharynx and disseminated to distal sites, after a transient viremia. Viremia and shedding of infectious virus from the nasopharynx ceased with the appearance of virus neutralizing antibodies. However, in presence of neutralizing antibody response, ERAV **established a persistent infection in both animals**, with high levels of virus excreted in the **urine on day 37** post infection. Although virus shedding was detected in the nasopharynx and plasma, clinical signs of acute febrile respiratory disease were not observed.

To investigate the chronic urinary shedding of ERAV, 215 urine samples collected from Thoroughbred race horses were tested by RT-qPCR for ERAV. ERAV was detected in 23% of the urine samples tested, and was most prevalent in samples collected from 2 to 4 year old horses. Analysis of the VP1 sequence from five ERAV isolates indicates that variants of a single virus, closely related to an Australian ERAV isolate cultured in 1990, are circulating in the Victorian Thoroughbred horse population.

ERAV persistence and chronic urinary shedding was assessed in 3 inbred mice strains susceptible to ERAV infection and the dissemination of ERAV following the intranasal infection of CBA mice was characterized. ERAV viremia was detected as early as 1 day post infection, and virus shedding in the urine detected until day 7 post infection. Virus-specific neutralizing antibodies were detected as early as day 3 post infection. ERAV replication in the lungs of animals was confirmed using immunohistochemistry and a negative strand-specific RT-qPCR assay. Although, viral RNA was detected in the hearts and bladder of mice, viral antigen positive cells were not detected in sections by immunohistochemistry. Several studies have shown that the antigenic structure of the ERAV capsid is more complex than FMDV. In contrast to the linear immunodominant epitope of FMDV, the equivalent site of ERAV is conformational and formed within the quaternary structure of the capsid. Whole virus or virus-like particles (VLPs) retain this conformational site. The immunogenicity of a plasmid-based DNA vaccine, designed to express as VLPs was assessed in mice. The plasmid construct, pcD.P12A.3C, contained the capsid precursor (P1-2A) and the viral protease 3C, under the transcriptional control of a cytomegalovirus (CMV) promoter. Mature viral capsid proteins and VLPs were detected in vitro in transfected COS7 cells.

Immunization of BALB/c mice with pcD.P12A.3C induced virus neutralizing antibodies and enhanced the virus neutralizing antibody response to an inactivated ERAV trial vaccine. This study further supports the use of DNA vaccines to elicit neutralizing antibodies to complex antigenic proteins.

Genus: *Teschovirus*

Teschen Disease or Talfan Disease in Pigs

Porcine teschovirus **(PTV)** causes Teschen disease or Talfan disease in pigs first reported from Czechoslovakia in 1929. This disease was established in most European countries by 1950 and then in Canada, the United States and Australasia. However, there have been no outbreaks of this disease in any country in recent years. It is an **infection of the motor nerves only and not the sensory nerves.** Disease is characterized by **fever, loss of appetite, lassitude, slight incoordination of movement, & lately irritability, stiffness, muscular tremors or rigidity, and convulsions.** There may also be grinding of the teeth, smacking of the lips and squealing as if in pain. The voice may change or be lost entirely. Teschen disease is used for the most severe form of the disease, while milder outbreaks have usually been called Talfan disease (Talfan is a hill in Wales where an outbreak occurred).

Etiology: PTV belongs to the genus *Teschovirus in* the family *Picornaviridae* & is caused by PTV serotype 1, which has highly virulent strains & mild strains. Highly virulent strains of PTV cause Teschen disease & mildly virulent but widely distributed strain causes Talfan disease (posterior paresis).

Occurrence

The disease was first reported from Czechoslovakia in 1929 & then established in most European countries by 1950 and in Canada, the United States and Australasia. However, there have been no outbreaks of this disease in any country in recent years.

Susceptible hosts

Only pigs are susceptible, but **young pigs in a herd are more susceptible.** Sporadic infection occurs when weaned pigs are mixed to the herd.

Transmission

Transmission occurs by fecal-oral route directly or indirectly. PTV multiplies in the intestines and is shed in large quantities in the feces up to 7 weeks & remains in environment up to 5 months. The virus is relatively resistant, survives outside the body, and is highly infectious requiring only a small dose of infected feces to be ingested to establish infection in the intestines. Hence the disease is easily transmitted between herds on clothes, boots, Lorries, machinery and equipments. It can also spread between herds through the movement of young subclinical carrier pigs. PTVs are found in intestines and oral secretions.

Pathogenesis

After infection, the virus replicates in the tonsils, intestinal & respiratory epithelium & lymph nodes followed by viremia. Viremia may lead to invasion of CNS that depends on the virulence of PTV strains & age of the pigs. The virus can invade the CNS, multiply in the nerves and cause nerve damage when there are no circulating antibodies or when they are at very low level. The virus can then be carried in the blood stream to the CNS. This happens if the mother has never been infected with the virus, if the newborn piglet didn't get enough colostrum, or if the virus enters a naive herd for the first time. Within a herd the virus cycles in the weaner pigs, the virus is prevented from multiplying in the intestines of suckled piglets by the sow's colostral immunity. After the pig has been weaned, the lactogenic immunity is not available and the virus is able to multiply in the intestines but it cannot get to the nervous system (CNS) because whenever the virus escapes from the gut it is neutralized by the sow's colostral antibodies which are still circulating in the pig's blood stream.

Clinical symptoms

Affected pigs develop an ascending paralysis of muscles which may progress to a complete hind end paralysis. The pig partially loses the use of its lower back legs, its thighs and then the rear end of its body. The partial loss may progress to a total paralysis. It is an infection of the motor nerves only and not the sensory nerves. The pig still has sensation and can feel pin pricks. In the beginning the pigs are slightly off its feed, depressed for a day but after that it is otherwise fine with a good appetite and normal temperature. Its only problem is that it can't walk around very well to eat and drink and in severe cases can't rise from a **dog-sitting position**. Since in the severe form of the disease the motor nerves are totally destroyed, the disease is irreversible. The pig never recovers.

When cases occur in **weaned and young growing pigs,** the disease does not often progress to full paralysis probably because the pigs have a level of immunity or because it is a **milder strain of the virus**. It occurs in older growing pigs & in adults. The pigs develop a drunken swaying gait from which many may recover spontaneously. It was thought that the disease occurs in herds set by early weaning or segregated weaning. In natural disease, sporadic cases of encephalomyelitis occur in one or a few litter or small number of weaned pigs. Suckling litters are mildly or transiently ill, but in very young litters morbidity is 100% & almost all die, among litters over 3 week old, only few of them are affected.

Diagnosis

Collection of clinical samples includes brain, spinal cord, and intestine.

1. *Presumptive diagnosis*: The clinical signs are suggestive of Teschen disease. Microscopic examination of the brains and spinal cord of pigs show changes typical of any virus disease but they are not specific for Teschen disease.

2. *Virus isolation*: The viruses can be propagated in cell cultures of swine origin in which they produce cytopathic changes. Identification is done by virus neutralization tests using specific antisera. Animal inoculation is done to determine the pathogenicity of the isolate.
3. *Virus antigen detection*: RT-PCR is used but is not widely available.
4. *Serology tests*: Virus neutralization and ELISA with four-fold rise in PTV-1 titer is diagnostic. Serum samples are taken in paired blood samples from a group of pigs at the start of the disease and 10-14 days later. Tests used are serum neutralization test with 4-fold increase in titre.

Treatment & prevention

There is no effective treatment. The only preventative measure is to ensure that all piglets receive a good amount of colostrum.

Vaccination

Attenuated or inactivated vaccines are used, could be made fairly readily but these are none available commercially because the disease is so uncommon that they would not be cost effective. **Teschen disease vaccine,** inactivated cultural emulgated prepared by AllergenTrade House is used for Teschen disease prophylaxis.

Genus: *Tremovirus*

Avian Encephalomyelitis

Avian encephalomyelitis (AEV-1) occurs in turkeys, chickens, pheasants & Japanese quail world wide with symptoms of **ataxia, tremor of head, neck & limbs in young ducklings**. AEV is transmitted for ~1 wk via eggs laid by the infected hens, and then infected chicks shed virus & spread to other hatch-mates. Symptoms are seen at 7-10 days of age & include unsteadiness, sitting on hocks, paresis, and even complete inability to move, & muscular tremors seen after exercise. About 5% of the flock is affected, but morbidity and mortality are high. The disease in adult birds is inapparent except for a transient drop in egg production. The disease in turkeys is usually milder than in chicks.

Etiology: Avian encephalomyelitis is caused by *Avian encephalomyelitis virus* (AE V-1) is a species in the genus *Tremovirus* in the family *Picornavirus* infecting primarily **young chicks,** but also found in turkeys, pheasants, and guinea fowl. It causes a fatal neuronal degeneration and is transmitted by mechanical contact.

Occurrence

Avian encephalomyelitis (Strain 1143) virus was isolated from the brain of a chicken, showing neurologic symptoms, at the N.Y. College of Veterinary Medicine by Dr. Bruce W. Calnek in 1961. The virus was passaged in chicken embryos by the yolk-sac route and by oral passage in Specific Pathogen Free Chickens. Avian encephalomyelitis is frequently occurring but economically important disease with worldwide distribution. It affects chickens, pheasants, turkeys, and quail.

Hosts susceptible

AEV-1 infects **chickens, Japanese quail, turkeys, pheasants and pigeons but ducklings, partridges and guinea fowl are susceptible to experimental infection**. Avian encephalomyelitis virus normally causes disease in chicks/ poults. The virus primarily affects the nervous system.

Transmission

The virus is **transmitted via the eggs** and by the oral/fecal route. Both vertical & horizontal transmission occurs. Chicks infected in ovo hatch normally but shed virus & infect some of the fellow chicks in the incubator soon after hatching. AEV1 causes enteric infection & shed virus in the feces, which form a source of infection to other chicks. Infected hens lay eggs some of which are infected.

Pathoenesis

The virus is transmitted via the eggs and by the oral/fecal route. Both vertical & horizontal transmission occurs. Chicks infected in ovo hatch normally but shed virus & infect some of the fellow chicks in the incubator soon after hatching. Infected hens lay eggs some of which are infected. In adult birds previously infected as chicks, the virus can cause **iridocyclitis and cataracts and general eye enlargement.** The lens of the eye becomes fragmented and can no longer function properly to focus images.

AEV1 causes enteric infection & shed virus in the feces, which form a source of infection to other chicks. Infection of the intestinal tract followed by viremia, & the virus is transmitted to CNS in absence of neutralizing antibodies. In the brain, the virus damage the neuronal cells.

Clinical symptoms

AEV-1 is a disease of young chicks during the first **six weeks of age**, & the typical clinical disease usually occurs between 1 - 3 weeks of age. Young birds show clinical symptoms of **tremor of the head, incoordination, and leg weakness with loss of condition followed frequently by prostration and death.** Mortality rate is about 20%. In laying birds, clinical signs are not apparent other than a decline in egg production, & reduced hatchability, which last 2 - 3 weeks.

Some infections are **asymptomatic** and are only diagnosed by the finding of brain lesions. The lesions in the brain and spinal cord consist of **loss of neurons and perivascular cuffing that is mainly observed in the cerebellum, medulla, and pons.** Diffuse lymphoid nodular hyperplasia is observed in the proventriculus, spleen, pancreas, and liver.

Diagnosis

Collection of clinical specimens include brain and spinal cord, & sera

1. *Presumptive diagnosis*: Clinical signs provide a presumptive diagnosis, & microscopic lesions are suggestive of AEV- 1 infection.
2. *Virus isolation*: It is made by intracerebral inoculation of day-old susceptible chicks. If virus is present, epidemic tremor develops in 10 - 12 days, and the brains can be harvested for histopathologic examination. Or the virus is inoculated into chicken embryos via the yolk sac; signs of encephalomyelitis are observed after hatching. Or the virus can be cultivated in primary whole embryo cell cultures.

3. *Detection of antibodies*: Antibodies can be detected best by means of neutralization tests in chicken embryos employing an embryo-pathogenic strain of the virus. A commercial ELISA, which is very sensitive, is available for the serologic monitoring of chicken flocks.

Treatment & prevention

Vaccination

A live virus vaccine is used in the drinking water to 10 - 16 week-old birds. Killed vaccines are used by wing -web method to revaccinate breeders with poor antibody response. **AE+POX**-Intervet is a combination live virus vaccine against Avian encephalomyelitis & fowl pox vaccine of chicken embryo origin manufactured from SPF (Specific Pathogen Free) eggs for the prevention of fowl pox and avian encephalomyelitis in chickens. The vaccine contains neomycin as a preservative. This vaccine is for wing-web application to chickens 12 weeks of age and older. It is used in breeder replacements and commercial layers in areas where avian encephalomyelitis and fowl pox are known to exist. Successful vaccination will appear at the point of vaccination from 7 to 10 days after vaccination showing brownish, black scabs found on both the under and upper surfaces of the web of the wing through which the needle vaccinator was thrust. Similar vaccine **Ae Pox Vac**-Pfizer exists.

Genus: *Avihepatovirus*

Duck Hepatitis A Virus Infection

Duck hepatitis A virus (DHAV-1) type 1 is more virulent & causes an acute disease of young domestic (Pekin) ducklings before 6 weeks old, which can inflict very high mortality. The disease is a highly fatal, contagious disease of young ducklings, 1-28 days of age. Ducklings are most susceptible at the younger ages and gradually become more resistant as they grow older. The disease is rarely seen in ducklings over 4 weeks of age. The onset of the disease is very rapid, it spreads quickly through the flock and may cause up to 90% mortality. Sick ducklings develop spasmodic contractions of their legs and die within an hour in a typical "arched-backward" position. The liver is enlarged and shows hemorrhagic spots.

Etiology: Duck hepatitis A infection is caused by *Duck hepatitis A virus* (formerly called DHV-1), belongs to the *Picornaviridae* that causes disease in ducklings before 6 weeks old. The other two viruses are duck astrovirus (formerly known as DHV-2), which causes disease in ducklings between 6 and 10 weeks old and DHV-3 caused by another virus unrelated to DHV-1 and DHV-2 which causes milder disease. DVH is an OIE notifiable disease.

Occurrence

DHAV (formerly DHV-1) is present in Northern America, Europe and Asia, DHV-2 has only been found in the United Kingdom and DHV-3 has only been found in the United States of America.

Susceptible species

Young ducks and geese are susceptible.

Transmission

The disease is very contagious and the virus excreted by feces is transmitted by direct contact between birds or through fomites such as brooders, water, feed, & equipment. Recovered animals can shed the virus for up to 8 weeks. DHAV may be introduced by the importation of live ducks from an infected country. Introduction by duck meat or duck product is possible but at low risk according to the instability of the agents. Rats have been described as a reservoir and control of this pest on arrival should be done.

Clinical symptoms & lesions

DHV-1 causes the most severe disease. The **incubation period** is 1 to 2 days and clinical signs include lethargy, anorexia and sudden death with opisthotonos within a few days. Morbidity is often 100% and mortality reaches 80%. Disease is less severe in ducks older than 7 weeks.

The lesions **are observed in the liver, which is enlarged with hemorrhagic lesions including petechiae, ecchymosis and decolouration. The spleen and kidneys can be augmented.**

Diagnosis

Liver specimens are collected during PM for virus identification.

Serological test is performed using serum neutralization, however due to the short course of the disease serological test is not used for diagnosis on live animals.

Duck hepatitis A infection is differentiated from Duck virus enteritis, Coccidiosis, Mycotoxicosis & *Pasteurella anatipestifera.*

Treatment & prevention

If accidentally introduced, strict isolation and control of rats are necessary measures to control DHV. To prevent this disease, keep age groups isolated and vaccinate breeder ducks with an attenuated live virus duck hepatitis vaccine (to produce maternally immune ducklings).

Vaccination

Live attenuated vaccine against DHAV-1 has efficiently prevented epidemics of DHAV-1 until 2002. Emergence of DHV-3 is also being controlled by the live attenuated virus, AP-04203P100, facilitating the prevention of duck hepatitis caused by DHAV-3 around East Asia including South Korea. A killed vaccine is also available against DHAV-1.

□□□

Chapter 19

Characteristics and Diseases Caused by Group IV Single-Stranded (+) RNA Caliciviruses (Family *Caliciviridae*)

Contents

Characteristics of Calicivirus

The viruses under the family *Caliciviridae* (L. calyx= cup) are so named because these viruses contain **cup like depressions on the surface (Fig 19.1),** they are small, naked & contain icosahedral capsid measuring 35-39 nm in diameter. The viral capsid is hexagonal or sperical having an icosahedral symmetry (T= 3) & is composed of 180 capsid proteins & measure 35-39 nm in diameter. Viral genome is made of unsegmented, linear +ssRNA of about

7.3 to 8.3 kb. 5′ end has a protein (VPg) covalently linked to genome, whereas 3′-end is polyadenylated. The caliciviruses have been reported from humans, cattle, pigs, cats, rabbits, chickens, reptiles, dolphins & amphibians.

Human *Calicivirus* infections usually appear after an incubation period of 2 days, & **symptoms include acute gastroenteritis with vomition and diarrhoea**. These symptoms usually last for 3 days, but is severe in immunocompromised persons who need hospitalization & rehydration therapy.

Animal infections include *Feline calicivirus* (FCV), which is an important pathogen of cats. *Sapovirus, Norovirus, and Vesivirus* have been reported in pigs. The *Norovirus of which* first mouse norovirus, *Murine norovirus 1* (MNV-1) was discovered in 2003 & then many norovirus strains have been identified. *Rabbit hemorrhagic disease virus* (RHDV) causes major problems in rabbits throughout the world where rabbits are reared for food and clothing.

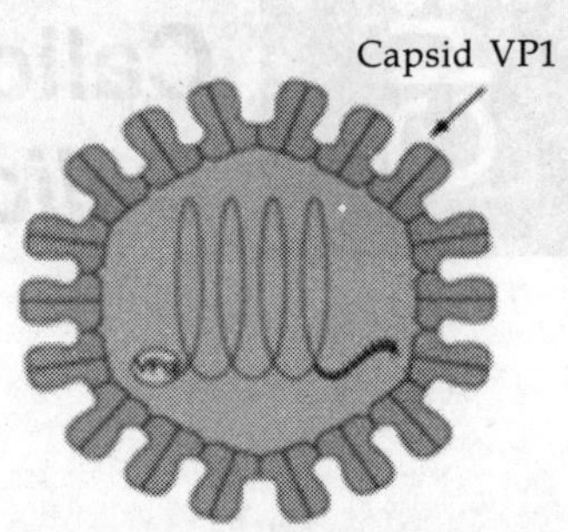

Fig. 19.1 : Morphology of a Calicivirus

The caliciviruses are resistant to ether, chloroform & mild detergents, are relatively resistant to heat but sensitive to pH changes.

The virus genome

Calicivirusgenome consists of unsegmented, linear, single-stranded, positive-sense RNA of 7.3 to 8.3 kb. The virus 5′-end has a virus protein (VPg) covalently linked to the genome. 3′-end of the virus is polyadenylated. The virion RNA is infectious acting both as the genome and as viral mRNA. The viral genomic ORF 1 encodes a polyprotein. One or two smaller ORFs are expressed from a subgenomic RNA. The polyprotein is cleaved by the virus-encoded 3C-like cysteine proteinase yielding the mature nonstructural proteins. **The 3′-end terminal ORF encodes a basic protein as well as the capsid protein.** Vesiviruses are unique because the ORF2 encodes a capsid precursor protein that is proteolytically processed by the viral proteinase to yield the mature capsid protein.

Virus replication

The virus replicates in the cell cytoplasm. The virion RNA is infectious and serves as both the genome and viral mRNA. Virus attaches to host receptors and is internalized, uncoated, and viral genomic RNA is released into the cytoplasm. VPg is removed from the viral RNA followed by its translation into a processed ORF1 polyprotein to yield the mature non-structural proteins involved in RNA transcription.

Firstly, negative-sense complementary ssRNAs are synthesized using the genomic RNAs as a templates & then new genomic RNAs are synthesized using the negative-sense RNAs as templates. Expression of subgenomic RNA yields the basic protein and capsid protein. Thereafter virus particles are assembled and released by cell lysis.

Virus classification

Group: Group IV (+) ssRNA

Family: *Caliciviridae*

Genera:

Genus 1: *Vesivirus*; type species: *Vesicular exanthema of swine virus*

Genus 2: *Lagovirus*; type species: *Rabbit hemorrhagic disease virus*

Genus 3: Norovirus; type species: *Norwalk virus*

Genus 4: *Sappovirus*; type species: *Sapporo virus*

Genus 5: *Nebovirus*; type species: *Newbury-1 virus, the single species under this genus, subtypes are* Bovine enteric calicivirus, Jena virus & Newbury agent 1.

The classification & diseases caused in humans & animals are presented below in Table 19.1.

Table 19.1: Classifiction of *Caliciviridae* and the diseases caused by the member viruses in humans & animals.

Genera	Species	Types	Diseases caused
G1: *Vesivirus*	*Vesicular exanthema of swine virus*	VESV,13 serotypes	Vesicular exanthema (VESV) affects swine, horses & dogs in USA & resemble FMD, vesicular stomatitis & swine vesicular disease in symptoms but is usually benign.
	Feline calicivirus	FCV, several serotypes	*Feline calicivirus* (FCV) infection occurs in cats-kittens 2-6 month old (also in cheetah), is one of the 2 important (other is Feline herpesvirus) respiratory diseases. Different strains vary in mononuclear cells, disease is usually acute with respiratory distress, & fatal coagulative hepatic necrosis; inactivated vaccine is used.
	European brown hare syndrome	EBHDV	European brown hare syndrome (EBHSV) is like RHD, occurs in

	virus		domestic & wild hares in many European countries; causes liver necrosis & high mortality in old hares.
G 2:*Lagovirus*	*Rabbi haemorr-hagic disease virus*	RHDV	RHDV affects domestic & wild rabbits & hare worldwide spread is orofecal, affects mononuclear cells, disease is usually acute with respiratory distress, & total coagulatine hepatic necrosis, inactivated vaccine is used.
G 3:*Norovirus*	*Norwalk virus*	NWV	Norwalk virus (NW V) infection also called "stomach flue" is a common cause of gastroenteritis in humans with nausea, vomition, diarrhoea & stomach cramps; spread is oro-fecal.
G 4:*Sappovirus*	*Sapporo virus*	SV	Sapporo virus (Japan) virus infection is also a common cause of gastroenteritis in humans, mainly in infants & young children but is milder than Norwalk virus infection.
G 5:*Nebovirus*	*Newbury-1 virus*	Bovine enteric calicivirus, Jena virus & Newbury agent 1	Genogroup III noroviruses (NoVs GIII) and neboviruses are associated with enteric disease in cattle.

Caliciviral Clinical Manifestation Humans

Clinical Infections in Humans

Genus: *Norovirus:* Norwalk virus **(NWV)** infection also called **"stomach flue"** is a common cause of gastroenteritis in humans with nausea, vomition, diarrhoea & stomach cramps, spread is orofecal.

Genus: *Sappovirus*: *Sapporo virus* **(SV)** (Japan) infection is also a common cause of gastroenteritis in humans mainly in infants & young children but is milder than Norwalk virus infection.

Calicivirus Clinical Infections in Animals

Genus: Vesivirus:

Vesicular Exanthema of Swine

Vesicular exanthema of swine (VESV) is viral, an acute, highly infectious disease characterized by fever, formation of blisters on the snout, oral mucosa, soles of the feet, the coronary band, and between the toes. VESV affects swine, horses & dogs in USA & resemble FMD, vesicular stomatitis & swine vesicular disease in symptoms but is usually benign.

Etiology: The disease is caused by *Vesicular exanthema of swine virus* (VESV) in the genus *Vesivirus* in the family *Caliciviridae.* VESV **has 13 types from pigs, and 16 types of *San Miguel sea lion virus* (SMSV) from marine sources.**

Occurrence

The disease was reported from United States, & sporadic, isolated outbreaks were recorded in Hawaii and Iceland but the disease has not been reported since 1956.

Hosts susceptible

VESV naturally infects only **pigs of all ages & breeds; horses and dogs** are also susceptible, & hamsters can be infected experimentally. The SMSV has been isolated from throat and rectal swabs from premature and 4-moold California sea lion pups, dead and weanling northern fur seal pups, and nursing northern elephant seal pups. It has also been isolated from vesicular lesions on marine mammals, commercial seal meat produced in Alaska, and perch-like fish collected from tidal pools off the southern California coast.

Transmission

VESV transmission occurs from pig to pig by direct contact. Disease outbreaks start by feeding infected uncooked pork scraps.The infected pigs excrete the virus in saliva & feces. In 1959, the USA was declared free of VES; it has never been reported as a natural infection of pigs in any other part of the world.

Pathogenesis

After infection, virus excretion occurs 48 hours before vesicles appear followed by a viremia for 72-84 hours. The virus localization occurs in the buccal mucosa, & the skin above the hooves. Vesicles appear on the hairless parts on the snout, oral mucosa, and sole of the feet, the coronary band, and between the toes. Mild virus encephalitis occurs in pigs inoculated with VESV. Vesicles break within 24-48 hrs to form erosions.

Clinical symptoms

After an **incubation period of 1-3 days**, there occurs a high fever, followed by development of vesicles on the snout, in the mouth on teats, udder, on coronary skin, the sole, heel bulbs between claws with lassitude & anorexia. Vesicles rupture with eroded skin & the affected feet, & the affected feet become sensitive with severe lameness. The disease is usually benign and runs a course of about two weeks.

The clinical symptoms in pigs are indistinguishable from FMD, VSV, and swine vesicular disease. The disease was confined to California, became widespread in the USA during the 1950s, but a vigorous campaign to eradicate the disease was successful. In 1959, the USA was declared free of VES, & it has never been reported as a natural infection of pigs in any other part of the world.

Diagnosis

Collection of clinical specimens includes vesicular fluid, affected mucous membranes, blood, and the serum.

1. *Presumptive diagnosis:* Clinical symptoms T lesions are suggestive of VES.
2. *Virus isolation:* The virus is cultured in swine embryonic kidney cells, & cytopathic effects are noticed. In virus infected cell cultures, the virus can be identified by neutralization test and viral antigens can be detected by immunofluorescence.
3. *Virus antigen detection:* Virus in the vesicular fluid can be detected by CFT, ELISA and electron microscopy on epithelial tissue, or after passage in swine tissue cultures.

Treatment & prevention

The VES has now been eradicated from the United States, but occurrence of infection from marine mammals may occur. It is a reportable disease and is dealt with by the same strict measures used to control other vesicular diseases.

Feline Calicivirus Infection

Feline calicivirus (FCV) infection occurs in kittens **2-6 moth old** (also in cheetah), characterized by sneezing, nasal discharge, fever, rhinitis, runny eyes, salivation, ulceration of the tongue & palate.

Etilogy: Feline calicivirus infection is caused by *Feline calicivirus* (FCV), a species of the genus *Vesivirus* of the *Caliciviridae* family, and there are several strains which vary in virulence & can infect cats. About 80 - 90% of all feline respiratory disease complexes are caused by either *Feline calicivirus or Feline rhinotracheitis virus* (feline herpesvirus) & even dual infection with both feline calicivirus & feline herpesvirus are common. There is a particularly virulent form of FCV known as **'virulent systemic feline calicivirus' (VS-FCV) with a mortality rate of 67%**. These more virulent strains cause pneumonia.

Occurrence

Feline calicivirus occurs worldwide. Most of the outbreaks of VS-FCV have been reported in the USA, & was originally described in 1998 in Northern California. The prevalence of FCV varies depending on the environment. In private households, FCV is present in about 10 percent of cats either in active or carrier state, while the prevalence in shelters or catteries is 25 to 40 percent.

Hosts susceptible

FCV infects about 50 percent of cats with upper respiratory infection. Cats of all ages are susceptible but kittens **2-6 moth old** or more susceptible, & Cheetahs are the other species of the family *Felidae* who become infected naturally.

Transmission

FCV is transmitted by direct contact; infection being passed from a **sick or carrier cat via eye, nasal & mouth discharges that contain the virus.** FCV can also be transmitted indirectly via contaminated food bowls, bedding etc. Calicivirus is resistant to many disinfectants & can live in the environment for long periods of time. FCV replicates in the oral and respiratory tissues and is secreted in saliva, feces, urine, and respiratory secretions. It can be transmitted through the air, orally, and on fomites. Infected cats usually **shed the virus for two weeks.** Following this period, infected cats never shed the virus again or become latently infected and shed the virus continuously or intermittently. **Some cats remain carriers for years after infection.** Some cats become infected, become sick & recovered, but the virus is still being shed in excretions for years & infects other cats.

Pathogenesis

There are several factors which influence the FCV pathogenesis. Firstly, there are **different strains** of FCV that vary in virulence. **Virulent systemic feline calicivirus** (VS-FCV) or FCV-associated virulent systemic disease (VSD) causes a severe systemic disease in cats. Secondly, FCV has a **high mutation rate** which makes it more adaptable to environmental pressures, makes the development of vaccines difficult as well as allows evolvement of more virulent strains. In persistently infected cats, the gene for the major viral capsid protein evolves through immune-mediated positive selection and **allows the virus to escape detection by the host immune system.**

The disease is caused by direct viral invasion of epithelium and endothelium and secondary host immune response. Initially, virus replicates in the oropharynx & the rapidly disseminated to URT & conjunctiva. There is a transient viremia. FCV replicates in the oral and respiratory tissues and the virus is secreted in saliva, feces, urine, and respiratory secretions.

Clinical symptoms & lesions

The **incubation period is** 2 - 5 days. **Clinical symptoms** in cats infected with FCV may show **acute** or **chronic** symptoms, or **no symptoms at all** depending on the virulence of the infecting virus strains. There are several strains of calicivirus which infect cats, and clinical symptoms differ according to the virulence of the virus causing infection. Some FCV strains cause mild symptoms, while others cause severe symptoms. Latent or subclinical infections usually become symptomatic when the **cat is stressed,** such as at the time of adoption. Coinfection with either *Feline herpesvirus* or *Feline immunodeficiency virus* causes a more severe disease.

Acute symptoms of FCV include **fever, conjunctivitis, nasal discharge, sneezing, and ulceration of the mouth.** Pneumonia may develop with secondary bacterial infections. Some cats may develop a **polyarthritis** via immune-mediated immune complex deposition. Stomatitis and polyarthritis can develop without any upper respiratory infection symptoms, but fever and loss of appetite occur.

Chronic cases due to immune complex deposition cause **glomerulonephritis.**

VS-FCV causes a rapid epidemic with a mortality rate of up to **67 percent.** Main symptoms include **discharge from the eyes and nose, ulceration in the mouth, anorexia, and lethargy, and occur in the first one to five days of kittens. Later symptoms include fever, edema of the limbs and face, jaundice, and multiple organ dysfunction syndrome.**

FCV can also cause **lameness** in cats called as **limping syndrome&** seen in natural infection but also after vaccination. FCV infection can be complicated by secondary bacterial infections, anorexia & dehydration. Feline calicivirus has been observed in the mouths of some cats with gingivitis.

Diagnosis

1. *Presumptive diagnosis:* Clinical signs in the cat furnish a presumptive diagnosis. If oral ulcers are present, it shows feline calicivirus infection, but presence of corneal ulcers shows presence of herpesvirus infection.

2. *Virus isolation:* The virus is easily propagated in cell cultures of feline origin producing cytopathic effect. After observing characteristic CPE, the virus can be identified by virus neutralization with specific antiserum.

Treatment & prevention

There is no specific treatment for FCV but antibiotics are used to control secondary bacterial infections. Immune modulators like **lymphocyte T-cell immune modulator** is used for immune support. Nursing care and rehydration are used for dehydrated and anorectic cats. Corticosteroids or azathioprine may be used for polyarthritis. Antibiotics, corticosteroids, and tooth extractions are used with varying success. FCV is prevented by avoiding overcrowding of feline populations, & reducing stresses.

Vaccination

Feline calicivirus is highly immunogenic, hence both inactivated and attenuated -live vaccine of cell culture origin are used, mostly in combination with other viruses. These **vaccines are administered intranasally or intramuscularly**. Attenuated FCV vaccine may cause mild upper respiratory infection, while the inactivated vaccine does not, but it causes more local inflammation and possibly predisposes the cat to vaccine-associated sarcoma. The vaccine licensed for prevention of FCV is **CaliciVax,** manufactured by Fort Dodge Animal Health, a division of Wyeth. It is given I ml SC to healthy cats 8 to 10 weeks of age or older. The vaccine contains an additional feline calicivirus strain isolated from a hemorrhagic calicivirus outbreak and has been shown by challenge to protect cats against virulent systemic feline calicivirus (VS-FCV). Repeat in 3 to 4 weeks. Annual revaccination with a single dose of vaccine is recommended. **FVR C**-Intervet is modified live vaccine for prevention of feline rhinotracheitis & feline calicivirus infection. Primary vaccination: healthy cats 12 weeks of age or older should receive one 0.5-ml dose IN. Cats vaccinated at less than 12 weeks of age should be revaccinated at 12 weeks of age. Annual revaccination with a single dose is recommended.

Genus: *Lagovirus*: Rabbit Haemorrhagic Disease

Rabbit hemorrhagic disease (RHDV) is a highly infectious and often fatal disease affecting domestic & wild rabbits & hares worldwide & is characterized by **infection of mononuclear cells**, disease is usually acute with respiratory distress & fatal coagulative hepatic necrosis.

*Etiology:*Rabbit hemorrhagic disease (RHD) is caused by the *Rabbit hemorrhagic disease virus* (RHDV), a member of the genus *Lagovirus* and family *Caliciviridae*. Many strains of RHDV circulate in rabbit populations, which have distinct epidemiological and genetic characteristics. But only a single serotype is known with **two major subtypes: RHDV and the antigenic variant RHDVa.** Nonpathogenic strains of RHDV have been detected in wild rabbits.

Occurrence

RHD was first recorded in 1984 in Angora rabbit in China. RHDV probably emerged from a virulent calicivirus spreading asymptomatically in European rabbit populations in Germany. The virus then spread westward and was recorded in Europe in 1988, then in Mexico, Cuba, Australia, New Zealand, the USA & in 1992, & the UK by the late 1990s. RHD has been recorded from forty countries. The United States experienced other outbreaks of RHD in 2001 and 2005.

Hosts susceptible

RHD primarily infects only adult rabbits; rabbits **younger than 8 weeks of age are resistant to the virus.** This disease affects only wild or domesticated rabbits of the species *Oryctolagus cuniculus.*

Transmission

RHD is spread by is direct contact with sick and indirect contact and mechanically by mosquitoes and other insects. The virus is shed in all secretions and excretions. RHD transmission occurs mainly by fecal-oral route & by inhalation or via conjunctiva. Animals may remain infectious for up to a month. **Long-term, persistent or latent infections have recently been recognized in rabbits.**

Pathogenesis

RHDV affects cells of **mononuclear phagocyte lineage.** Disseminated intravascular coagulation occurs in the terminal stages of disease, and results in hemorrhages in many organs and tissues. The trachea is often hyperemic and contains frothy, blood-stained mucus. Congestion and multifocal hemorrhages are seen in the lungs, hemorrhages are also common in the thymus, and petechiae may be found on the serosal membranes or viscera. Infarcts may be seen in most organs. In subacute disease, catarrhal enteritis of the small intestine and jaundice may also be seen. Congestion of the meninges has been reported.

Clinical symptoms

The incubation period for the RHDV is 1 to 3 days, with death following 1 to 2 days after the infection. There is a wide range of RHD symptoms; most rabbits show no signs of symptoms of RHD.

Symptoms of RHD include **fever, squeals, and often coma leading to death within 12 to 36 hours**. In less severe cases, rabbits may display **uneasiness, excitement, anorexia, swollen eyelids, paralysis, ocular**

hemorrhage, and paddling. Convulsions may be seen. A fatal bloody discharge from the nose has been seen along with blood-stained cage floors. Rabbits that have recovered from the less severe symptoms usually develop severe jaundice with weight loss and lethargy. Diarrhea, constipation and abdominal cramping are then seen before death.

RHD causes **rapid formation of blood clot in major organs like the heart, lungs and kidneys. The clots block blood vessels causing heart and respiratory failure.** An infected rabbit that has died from RHD will often have its legs straight out and head over its neck as if trying to catch its breath.

Diagnosis

1. *Presumptive diagnosis:* RHD DIAGNSIS is made when several animals in the herd die showing fever and lethargy. The most important PM lesions are **hepatic necrosis and splenomegaly.** The liver is also usually friable and swollen, & the spleen is black in colour and also swollen with rounded edges, while the kidneys are dark brown in colour. Hemorrhages are seen in many other organs and tissues. The trachea may present a foamy, bloody mucous. Enteritis of the small intestine and swollen meninges may also be seen.
2. *Antigen detection:* Laboratory tests such as RT-PCR, ELISA, Western blotting, negative-staining immunoelectron microscopy may be performed on samples from the liver, blood, spleen or other organs.

Treatment & prevention

RHD free countries may place restrictions on importation of rabbits from endemic countries. RHD being highly infectious requires strict quarantine in face of outbreaks. Depopulation, disinfection, surveillance and quarantines are the only way to eradicate the disease. Good disinfectants include 10% sodium hydroxide, 1-2% formalin, 2% One-Stroke Environ, and 10% household bleach. The RHD virus is resistant to ether or chloroform. Deceased rabbits must be removed immediately and discarded in a safe manner. Surviving rabbits should be quarantined or humanely euthanized. Test rabbits may be used to monitor the virus on vaccinated farms.

Vaccination

An effective, inactivated vaccine, ATCvet is used in various countries, particularly Spain, which gives protection for 5 to 15 months & a booster dose annually. The vaccination is also recommended in areas where the disease is widespread and eradication efforts have been made. **Allergen Trade House supplies Rabbit calicivirus vaccine**, an inactivated, tissue, adsorbed on Aluminium hydroxide for the prophylaxis of Rabbit virus haemorrhagic disease.

European Brown Hare Syndrome

European brown hare syndrome virus (EBHS) affects wild and farmedhares of the species *Lepus europaeus* and *Lepus timidus, &* is like RHD. EBHS is a highly contagious, acute and fatal disease of the European brown hare (*Lepus europaeus*) and mountain hare (*Lepus timidus*). The disease was first described in Sweden, but epidemics have been reported all over Europe: Germany, Belgium, United Kingdom, Croatia, Sweden, Finland, Austria, Spain, Poland, Switzerland, and Slovakia. The infection has become endemic In Italy, following the initial epidemic peak that occurred in the late 1980s. Disease occurs in domestic & wild hares in many European countries with liver necrosis & high mortality in old hares. From 1999 to mid-2003, 97 European brown hares (*Lepus europaeus*) died in Greece & were examined by necropsy, histopathology,and RT-PCR for the presence of EBHS andEBHS virus respectively. Hare losses were sporadic,starting in the cold season and lasting for many months. The most prominent gross lesions were observed in the **liver** and included **swelling and discoloration; congestion andhemorrhages** were present mainly in lungs and tracheal mucosa.Necropsy findings were suggestive of EBHS, which was confirmedby histopathology and RT-PCR.

Thesyndrome, a severe **necrotic hepatitis**, has affected up to 100%of a hare population in which animals usually died within **48–72 hour**. The disease was first reported duringthe 1980s and occurred simultaneously in many European countries. The viral etiology was first demonstratedin 1988 by electron microscopy. Sequencingthe viral genome has demonstrated EBHSV sharinga similar genomic organization to RHDV, but that the two viruses are distinct caliciviruses.

European brown hare syndrome has significant similarities toRHD in its epidemiology, clinical signs, and pathology. Findingsin the two diseases are **characterized by rapid progression,mild nervous symptoms, severe necrotic hepatitis, and circulatorydysfunction in various organs**. Ninety-seven European brown hares found dead or shot throughoutGreece were submitted by hunting federations from 1999 to mid-2003.All hares were adults and in fair or poor body condition. Gross lesions were found in 85 hares.**Edema, congestion, extensive hemorrhages in the lungs, and severecongestion of the tracheal mucosa were observed.** The spleenwas enlarged and dark red-black, and the kidneys were congested.In 83, the liver was swollen, discolored, and friable. Tissuesamples from liver, lungs, spleen, and kidneys from all exceptthe five decomposed hares were fixed in 10% buffered formalinand routinely processed for histopathologic examination. Inaddition, samples of liver and spleen from all hares were collected for RT-PCR analysis. The RNA extractions were carried out using a commercial RNA isolation kit. The RNA samples were subjected to reverse transcription, followed by PCR using the primers HEF 5'-CCGTCCARCATTCGTCCTGTCAC-3'and HEB 5'-CATCACCAGTCCTCCGCACCAC-3', which were designed to amplify a part of the gene encoding the structural polypeptide VP60. The expected size of the RT-PCR product was 265 bp).

Histopathologically, in the 85 hares with gross lesions, **interstitial and alveolar hemorrhages and edema were observed in the lungs; and in the spleen, the red-pulp was congested and edematous.** In 83, **acute hepatic lesions**, characterized by variably sized areas of **periportal and midzonal hepatocellular necrosis,** were the most prominent and consistent histopathologic findings. Acidophilic bodies were occasionally seen around or in the necrotic areas in connection with hepatocyte degeneration and calcium deposits. Three of the seven hares with no gross lesions had a mild periportal inflammatory reaction, prominent periportal fibroplasia, and bile duct proliferation accompanied by periportal degeneration and necrosis of hepatocytes corresponding to chronic hepatitis.

European brown hare syndrome virus RNA was detected in liver and spleen specimens from the 83 hares with acute hepatic lesions,the three hares with chronic hepatitis, and in spleen from the two hares with changes limited to the lung and spleen. On the basis of the morphology of the liver changes, we recognized the two forms of the disease as described by, **an acute and a subacute form.** Furthermore, we found alterations in the liver of three hares corresponding to the chronic form of the disease. Detection of viral RNA in this form of the disease may imply that these animals could play a role in the epidemiology of EBHS by spreading and maintenance of the virus.

□□□

Chapter 20

Characteristics and Diseases Caused by Group IV Single-Stranded (+) RNA Togaviruses (Family *Togaviridae*)

Contents

Characteristics of Togaviruses

Viruses belonging to the family *Togaviridae* (L. toga= cloack or mantle) are small, spherical, enveloped viruses bearing spikes & measure 65-70 nm in diameter. Virus specific glycoproteins, which act as attachment proteins are attached tightly to icosahedral capsid. There are 3 peplomer proteins- **E1, E2 & E3 of which E1 & E2 (Fig. 20.1) are responsible for viral specificity.** The **icosahedral** capsid is made of 240 monomers (T= 4). The viral genome is linear, single-stranded, positive sense RNA made of 10,000-12,000 nucleotides. Like cellular mRNA, viral RNA 5′ end has methylated nucleotide cap & 3′ end contains a polyadenylated tail.

Among the two genera, *Alpphavirus* & *Rubivirus*, **alphaviruses are arthropod-borne being transmitted by mosquitoes**, while the *Rubivirus* with sole member of *Rubella* virus is non arthropod-borne. Within alphaviruses, *Eastern equine encephalitis virus* (EEEV) is maintained in nature in **endemic transmission cycle** in swampy area & involves Passerine birds & mosquitoes-*Culiseta melanura* that inhabits fresh water swamps with high mortality in pheasants. **Epidemic transmisssion cycle** involves mosquitoes, *Aedes sollicitans & other* mosquitoes that **feed both birds & mammals;** while horses & humans are incidental dead-end hosts. VEEV is maintained in **sylvatic cycle** between rodents & mosquito of *Culex spp* in swampy areas & virus mutation causes epizootic cycles. WEEV transmission cycle involves *Culex tarsalis* & indigenous with horses as end hosts. Interactions between viruses, vector species, and vertebrate hosts confine the geographic spread of alphaviruses. Occasionally, a virus may escape its usual ecological niche and cause widespread epizootics e.g. *Venezuelan equine encephalitis virus* or urban epidemics caused by *Chikungunya virus*. Human infections are seasonal and are acquired in endemic areas.

Alphaviruses have been grouped into **seven antigenic complexes** of which four medically important antigenic complexes are *Venezuelan equine encephalitis virus, Eastern equine encephalitis virus, Western equine encephalitis virus,* and *Semliki Forest virus.* The capsid protein induces antibodies but anti-capsid antibodies do not neutralize infectivity or inhibit hemagglutination. The **E2 glycoprotein elicits and is the principal target of neutralizing antibodies**.

Susceptibility to physical & chemical agents show that mature alphaviruses are not stable in the environment being sensitive to pH change, heat, detergents & disinfectants.

The viral genome

The togavirus genome is linear, single-stranded, positive sense RNA 10,000-12,000 nucleotides long. The 5'-end has a methylated nucleotide cap and the 3'-end has a polyadenylated tail like cellular mRNA. The positive sense viralRNA acts as mRNA & synthesize (-) RNA, which acts as template to synthesize (+) genomic RNA as well as a subgenomic 3′ end RNA called 26S. Two-thirds of the RNA on the 5' end is translated into a polyprotein, which is autocleaved into four non-structural proteins (NSP1, 2, 3, 4) that include NSP1-methylation and capping of viral RNA, NSP2- helicase and protease, NSP3-converts RNA replicase to plus strand replicase & NSP4- replicase. The 3' end third of subgenomic RNA in the late phase is translated into another polyprotein which is autocleaved encoding all the stuctural proteins that include **capsid protein, E1, E2, E3 & 6k proteins**. E3 remains virion-associated in *Semliki forest virus* but remain as a soluble protein in most other alphaviruses.

Virus replication

Togaviral replication occurs in the cytoplasm of the host cell. The genomic RNA is infectious and serves as both genome and viral mRNA. The whole genome is translated in a non-structural polyprotein by 5′ two third which is processed by host and viral proteases. Structural polyprotein is encoded through a subgenomic 3′ one third mRNA.

Virus **attaches via E2** to host cell receptors and is endocytosed into vesicles in the host cell, viral membrane & endosomal vesicle membrane are fused & RNA genome is released into the cell cytoplasm. Then the +genomic ssRNA is translated into a polyprotein, which is cleaved into non structural proteins. Virus replication occurs at the surface of ER & initially a negative-sense complementary ssRNA is synthesized using the genomic RNA as a template. New + genomic RNA as well as subgenomic RNA are synthesized using the negative-sense RNA as a template. Subgenomic RNA is translated into structural proteins.

Virus assembly occurs at the endoplasmic reticulum & the virion buds at the endoplasmic reticulum, then transported to the Golgi apparatus, and finally bud from the cell membrane acquiring the envelope. The virus replication cycle is fast & is completed in about 4 hours.

Virus classification

Group: Group IV +ssRNA

Family: *Togaviridae*

Genera

Genus 1: *Alphavirus;* type species: *Sindbis virus* (SINV), other species include, **encephalitis group**like *Eastern equine encephalitis virus* (EEEV), *Western equine encephalitis virus* (WEEV), *Venezuelan equine encephalitis virus* (VEEV), &*Everglades virus (EVEV)*, & **arthritis group** include-*Chikungunya virus* (CHIV), *Getah virus*(GETV), *Ross River Virus* (RRV), *O'nyong'nyong virus* (ONNV), *Semliki forest virus* (SFV) & others.

Genus 2: *Rubivirus;* type species: *Rubella virus* (RUBV) is the sole species.

A classification of *Togaviridae* & diseases caused by the member viuses are presented below in Table 20.1.

Table 20.1: Clssification of *Togaviridae* & diseases caused by the member viruses in humans & animals.

Genera	Species	Types	Diseases caused
G1: *Alphavirus*	*Chikungunya virus*	CHIKV	Acute flue-like onset, pharyngitis, rash, arthritis, minor hemorrhagic manifestation in humans, contracted in jungle by reservoirs in monkeys or via mosquitoes.
	Eastern equine encephalitis virus	EEEV	Causes EEE (more virulent), encephalitis in horses, humans & pheasants in N & S America, & Caribbean islands; virus cycle between birds & mosquitoes.
	Everglades virus	EVEV	Related to EEE & occurs in Florida in USA
	Getah virus	GETV	Causes sporadic disease in horses in East USA, S.E Asia, and Australia with fever, urticaria & edema of limbs & subclinical infection in pigs.
	Mayaro virus	MAYV	In S. America
	O'nyong-nyong virus	ONNV	Like CHIKV but occurs in East Africa
	Ross River virus	RRV	Caused epidemics in Australia & Pacific islands
	Semliki forest virus	SFV	Like Chikungunya, occurs in Africa, M.E & Asia; virus cycle between birds & mosquitoes.
	TS: *Sindbis virus*	SINV	Like Chikugunya in Africa, Asia; virus cycle between birds & mosquitoes.
	Venezuelan equine encephalitis virus	VEEV	Causes VE encephalitis in horses, donkeys, humans & small mammals in Central & S. America; virus cycle between rodents & mosquitoes.
	Westernequine encephalitis virus	WEEV	Causes WEE a milder disease in horses & humans (dead end hosts) in America; virus cycle between birds & mosquitoes.
G2: *Rubivirus*	*Rubella virus*	RUBV	Causes Rubella, an exanthematous disease in humans rarely with arthralgia; fetal infection in pregnant women with congenital malformation.

Alphavirus Clinical Infections in Humans & Animals

Encephalitis group viruses

Everglades virus (EVEV) is a variation of VEEV & is related to EEE & occurs in Florida in USA.

Arthritic group viruses

Chikungunya*virus* (CHIKV) is characterized by sudden onset, fever, and intense arthritic pain lasting 3-7 days. Chikungunya virus has been isolated from humans and mosquitoes in eastern, southern, western, and central Africa and in southeastern Asia, where it has been responsible for illnesses in hundreds to thousands of individuals.

Getah **(GETV)** causes sporadic disease in horses in East USA, S.E Asia, and Australia with fever, urticaria & edema of limbs & subclinical infection in pigs.

O'nyong-nyong *virus* (ONNV) is transmitted by *Anopheles funestus* and *A. gambiae* mosquito. After an incubation period 3-12 days, there is myalgia and severe arthritis & the patients recover after about two weeks. 'O'nyong nyong' means 'weakening of the joints' in the Acholi Uganda dialect. Several million cases were reported from Uganda, Kenya, Tanzania, Malawi and Mozambique during 1959 to 1961.

Ross River*virus* (RRV) causes the disease called **epidemic polyarthritis (EPA)** in Australia, the disease is characterized by arthritic symptoms.

Barmah Forest*virus* (BFV) causes arthritic symptoms similar to that of Ross River virus. The disease occurs throughout eastern Australia, especially in the northern state of Queensland.

Sindbis (SINV) causes coincident onset of fever with rash and arthritic pain. Sindbis is found in Africa, India, and Malasia, and has been observed to reach epidemic proportions in Egypt and South Africa.

Mayaro virus (MAYV) also causes rash, fever and arthritic pain, Mayaro is found in Central and South America. Many epidemics have been reported in the Amazon Basin.

Semliki Forest Virus (SFV) is like Chikungunya, occurs in Africa, M.E & Asia; virus cycle is between birds & mosquitoes.

Rubiviruses infection:

Rubella*virus* (RUBV) is a highly contagious mild infection of early childhood often called as the "German Measles". When infection occurs during

first trimester of pregnancy, the virus is extremely **teratogenic** and often causes congenital rubella syndrome (CRS) resulting in abortions, miscarriages, stillbirths, and severe birth defects. The most common congenital defects observed are cataracts, heart disease, sensorineural deafness, and mental retardation.

Genus : *Alphavirus*

Eastern, Western and Venezuelan Equine Encephalitis

Three equine encephalitides are caused by three serologically distinct species of the genus *Alphavirus* (family *Togaviridae*) called*Eastern equine encephalitis virus* (EEEV), *Western equine encephalitis virus* (WEEV) &*Venezuelan equine encephalitis virus* (VEEV). The three viruses produce similar clinical symptoms. RNA sequence analysis shows that most of the WEEV genome is closely related to the EEEV genome.

Etiology: Eastern equine encephalitis, Western equine encephalitis & Venezuelan equine encephalitis are caused by *Eastern equine encephalitis virus* (EEEV), *Western equine encephalitis virus* (WEEV) & *Venezuelan equine encephalitis virus* (VEEV), respectively.

Occurrence

EEEV is a zoonotic alphavirus present in North, Central and South America and the Caribbean countries. The EEE virus has only one serotype but **two antigenic variants**- North American variant is more virulent, & South & Central American variant is less virulent. **The EEEV is maintained in nature through a bird – mosquito** (*Culisetu melanura* and *Cs. morsitans*) **cycle**. These mosquitoes feed on the blood of birds. Transmission of EEEV to mammals occurs via other mosquitoes; they bring the virus from avian populations to mammalian populations & include *Coquiletidia perturbans, Aedes vexans, Ochlerotatus sollicitans* and *Oc. canadensis*. **Humans, horses and other infected mammals do not circulate enough viruses in their blood to infect additional mosquitoes.** The **reservoir hosts are mainly wild birds and small rodents.** It is estimated that ~10% of the horses infected develop clinical disease. The mortality in horses is up to 90%; & in humans 30 - 50%.

WEEV is transmitted by mosquitoes of the genera *Culex* & *Culiseta &* wild birds. WEEV has six related viruses- WEE, J Highlands, Sindbis, Aura, Fort Morgan & Y62-3 3. The disease occurs in U.S. since 1964 & mainly occurs in states west of the Mississippi River in USA & Canada, & in countries of South America. WEE causes disease in equids and humans. The **reservoir hosts are wild birds**; the avian and mosquito infections are harmless. WEE infection is milder than EEE. The mortality in horses is 20 - 30%; & in humans about 10%. WEEV commonly cause a **subclinical infection**; symptomatic infections are uncommon.

VEEV is transmitted mainly by mosquitoes that bite an infected animal and then bite and feed on another animal or human in South America & Central America. There are **six subtypes of the VEEV:** I- VE E, II- Everglades, III-Mucambo, IV- Pixuna, V-Cabassou & VI-AG0-663. These viruses are divided into **epizootic subtype, & endemic subtype. Endemic subtype** causes diseases endemic to certain areas. Epizootic subtype I has 5 variants of which **virulent subtypes in horses are 1-AB & 1-C. EEEV** are associated with the **rodent-mosquito transmission cycle.** These forms of the virus can cause human illness.

Hosts susceptible

Horses, cattle, pigs, dogs, ratites & humans are accidental hosts. All the 3 species EEEV, WEEV & VEEV are maintained in host-vector relationship as discussed above. Horses are the dead end hosts for EEE & WEE but spread VEE. EEE & WEE occur as sporadic infections but **VEE occurs as epidemics.** The disease is severe in unvaccinated horses, & young foals from nonimmune mares infected with WEE, mortality rate is upto 100%. VEE affects all equine species, such as horses, donkeys & zebras. After infection, equines may suddenly die or show progressive CNS disorders. Humans also can contract this disease, which experience flu-like symptoms, such as high fevers and headaches, but persons with weakened immune systems and the young and the elderly can become severely ill or die from this disease.

Transmission

Mosquitoes of various genera as mentioned above are the principal vectors. These viruses infect and **replicate in mosquitoes for their entire life.** In tropical and subtropical regions the viruses are endemic in swamp habitats in a **bird/rodent-mosquito cycle**. The peak period for these diseases is late summer when number of mosquito is maximum, & incidence is drastically reduced during winter. **VEE** is transmitted primarily by mosquitoes that bite an infected animal and then bite and feed on another animal or human. Epizootic subtypes spread rapidly through large populations, these viruses are highly pathogenic to equines and can also affect human health. **Equines, rather than rodents, are the primary animal species that carry and spread the disease**. Infected equines develop an enormous quantity of **virus in their circulatory system.** When a blood-feeding insect feeds on such animals, it picks up this virus and transmits it to other animals or humans. **Cattle, swine, and dogs, can become infected, but they generally do not show signs of the disease** or contribute to its spread.

Pathogenesis

These viruses after bite of the infected mosquito, replicate near the site of entry, & then travel to the regional lymph nodes near the site of bite via the lymphatics. The viruses **replicate in neutrophils and macrophages followed by viremia** of slight nature or high level viremia with generealized infection throughout the body, in bone marrow & some other tissues in case of VEE. The virus then replicates in other organs. The virus replicates in the **endothelial cells lining the brain vessels & enters the brain.** Transplacental transmission in case of VEE virus occurs from infected at near term pregnant mares. Although the virus is shed in saliva & nasal secretions but natural horizontal transmission does not occur.

The virus invades the CNS when the disease is severe, causes neuronal degeneration & perivascular lymphatic cuffing in the grey matter of cerebral cortex, thalamus & hypothalamus with vasculitis, thrombosis & hemorrhages. The neurological signs develop in less than a week of infection. But in most cases CNS involvement does not occur, the only symptom is fever. All the three encephalitis viruses cause subclinical infections.

Clinical symptoms

After virus exposure, there is an incubation period of about 1 to 3 days in case of EEE is, 2-9 days for WEE & 1-6 days for VEE. Clinical manifestations caused by all the three viruses are similar. Initially at the viremic stage, there are fever, anorexia & depression, **early nervous signs include pharyngeal paralysis, head pressing, incoordination, paralysis of the legs, recumbency and death frequently occurs in 2 - 7 days.** EEEV causes encephalitis & myocarditis in piglets less than 2 months old.

Diagnosis

Collection of clinical specimens for various tests includes whole blood collected at the febrile stage, brain tissue from horses that have died & acute and convalescent sera.

1. *Presumptive diagnosis:* Clinical signs and microscopic brain lesions with inflammatory cells, perivascular cuffing, and congestion and edema of the meninges (EEE and WEE) as well as a neutrophilic inflammatory cell response (VEE) furnish a presumptive diagnosis.

2. *Virus isolation:* It is done in various cell cultures, in young mice inoculated intracerebrally, newly hatched chicks or embryonated eggs.

3. *Antibodies detection:* Tests include virus neutralization, CFT, & HI test or capture ELISA in sera collected at acute and convalescent stage with 4-

fold increase in the antibody titer. **Detection of viral nucleic acid** is done by PCR test in clinical samples.

Treatment & prevention

There is no specific treatment but steroids are given to reduce inflammation as well as general supportive therapy is given. Vector control measure include spraying at vector habitats, destruction of mosquito breeding areas, use of mosquito repellants & construction of insect proof building.

Vaccination

Formalin inactivated univalent, bivalent or trivalent vaccines are available to vaccinate horses with annual revaccination. Live attenuated VEE vaccines are more effective in preventing or controlling epizootic VEE than inactivated multivalent vaccines. **Encevac® T+VEE with Havlogen-**Merckis Encephalomyelitis vaccine- Eastern, Western and Venezuelan killed virus & tetanus toxoid for vaccination of healthy horses, 6 months of age or older, against Eastern, Western and Venezuelan Equine Encephalomyelitis and Tetanus. For primary immunization, inject 1 ml IM and repeat the dose in 3 to 4 weeks. A 1 ml dose should be administered annually and at any time epidemic conditions exist or are reported and exposure is imminent.

Getah Virus Infection

Getah virus infection is transmitted by mosquitoes, causes a highly infectious disease of horses manifested clinically by fever, mucosal exanthema and edema of the limbs. Outbreaks of clinical disease due to Getah virus infection occur infrequently, and only one outbreak, besides Japan in 1978 has been reported outside Japan; this was in India in 1990. Clinical signs of the disease are mild and nonlife-threatening and are characterized by pyrexia, edema of the hind limbs, swelling of the submandibular lymph nodes, and urticarial rash.

Etiology: Getah virus infection is caused by *Getah virus* (GETV), a member of the family *Togaviridae*, genus *Alphavirus*.

Occurrence

Serologic studies suggest that Getah virus is widely distributed from Eurasia-including Siberia and Mongolia to Australasia. Getah virus infection outbreak occurred in race horses in Japan in 1978, then in India in 1990. The infection was mild and characterized by fever, edema of the hind legs, and urticaria. Till January 2006, clinical disease has been reported only in Japan and India.

Species susceptible

Clinical signs have been reported only in **horses & pigs**. Experimentally mice have been infected but serologic studies suggest that asymptomatic Getah virus infections occur in many vertebrates including horses, pigs, cattle, water buffalo, kangaroos, wallabies, birds, reptiles, non-human primates, and humans. Mice, rats, rabbits, hamsters, and guinea pigs can be infected experimentally.

Transmission

Getah virus is maintained in a natural cycle between **mosquitoes and various vertebrate hosts**. This virus seems to be transmitted mainly by various **species of *Aedes* and *Culex*,** but the specific vector varies with the climate and geographic region. The amplifying hosts include horses, pigs, and possibly other species such as rodents. Getah virus is also directly contagious between horses, probably via aerosols or direct contact with nasal secretions. This route is thought to be uncommon; high doses of virus are needed to establish intranasal infections, but only small amounts of virus are found in the nasal secretions of naturally infected horses. Getah virus has not been recovered from the feces or urine of horses; however, it was found in the feces of an experimentally infected piglet with diarrhea. **Vertical transmission has been reported in pigs, as well as in experimentally infected mice,** hamsters, guinea pigs, and rabbits. There is no indication that vertical transmission occurs in horses.

Clinical symptoms & lesions

The **incubation period in both horses and pigs** is short; in horses it is **3 to 4 days** after intranasal infection, & after intramuscular injection, the incubation period is **2 to 6 days**. Experimentally infected pigs become symptomatic **1 to 3 days** post-inoculation.

In horses, Getah virus infection is a **mild, self-limiting illness characterized by fever, hind limb edema mainly in the fetlock, and stiffness.** Swelling of the **submandibular lymph nodes, mild abdominal pain, depression, mild icterus, and scrotal edema have also been reported.** An **urticarial rash** is often seen 3-5 mm papules mainly on the neck from the shoulder to the forearm, and over the hindquarters from the thigh to the gaskin. Serous nasal discharge has been reported in experimentally infected horses but not in natural cases. In some horses, the clinical signs are limited to one or two symptoms such as fever alone, fever and a skin rash, or fever and limb edema. Getah virus does not seem to cause abortions or birth defects in horses; pregnant mares delivered normal foals after an outbreak at a breeding farm in India. Horses recover fully in approximately 1 to 2 weeks.

Getah virus may be pathogenic in swine in which, fetal deaths occurred after natural or experimental infection of sows in few cases. Other symptoms reported in experimentally infected **pigs** include **transient fever, anorexia and, in young piglets, mild depression and diarrhea.**

Experimentally infected neonatal **mice** develop **polymyositis, fetal deaths and decreased litter sizes** have been reported in pregnant mice.

PM lesions: **Generalized lymphadenopathy** was seen in experimentally infected horses; the splenic and inguinal lymph nodes were particularly prominent. Some horses also had a slightly enlarged spleen and/or liver. Moderate glomerular congestion was noted in one horse, while another had congestion and slight turbidity of the piamater in the brain. In horses with a rash, the subcutaneous tissues were moderately edematous due to lymph stasis. These horses had scattered maculae in the dermis; on cut section, the maculae were thickened and circumscribed, with pale reddish foci.

Histopathologically, moderate lymphoid hyperplasia in the submandibular, axillary, splenic, renal and inguinal lymph nodes, as well as in the spleen was seen. The skin lesions contained perivascular or diffuse infiltrates of lymphoid cells and histiocytes, thickened blood vessel walls, and edematous smooth muscle cells. Scattered hemorrhagic foci and eosinophilic infiltrates were seen in some lesions. Perivascular cuffing with mononuclear cells was reported in the cerebrum of two horses.

Diagnosis

Collection of samples for various tests includes in horses, plasma collected at the onset of pyrexia is preferred for virus isolation, the axillary and inguinal lymph nodes have the highest viral titers and seem to contain virus for the longest period. In both species, paired acute and convalescent samples can be collected for serology.

1. *Presumptive diagnosis:* In horses, Getah virus infection is suggested by a fever, hind limb edema, stiffness & a rash or swelling of the submandibular lymph nodes. The diagnosis should be confirmed by laboratory testing. In pigs, Getah virus infection may be a consideration in cases of reproductive disease; however, this link has not been conclusively established.

   The differential diagnosis includes equine viral arteritis and the mild form of African horse sickness (horse sickness fever).

2. *Virus isolation:* Getah virus is isolated in VERO, RK-13, BHK- 21, and many other cell lines as well as by intracerebral inoculation of suckling mice.

3. *Serology:* In horses, serologic tests include serum neutralization, complement fixation, and hemagglutination inhibition. ELISA test has been developed for swine.

Treatment & prevention

Vaccination

An inactivated vaccine is available for the prevention and control of Getah virus infection in horses in Japan.

Equine Getah virus infection inactivated vaccine is prepared by Nisseiken Co Ltd.

□□□

Chapter 21

Characteristics and Diseases Caused by Group IV Single-Stranded (+) RNA Flaviviruses (Family *Flaviviridae*)

Contents

Characteristics of *Flaviviridae*

The viruses under the family *Flaviviridae* (L. *flavus* = yellow) derived its name from *Yellow fever virus,* which cause jaundice with yellowness in the patients. Flaviviruses are a large group, enveloped bearing peplomers, are spherical or pleomorphic & measure 40-60 nm in diameter. Small spikes surrounded by a prominent fringe make up the surface projections. The capsid is round and exhibits an **icosahedral** symmetry measuring 40-50 nm & consists of a single type of capsid protein. Around the viral capsid a spherical shaped envelope is present. The capsid has an inner core protein. The core is measured 20 nm to 30 0nm in diameter, and it is isometric.

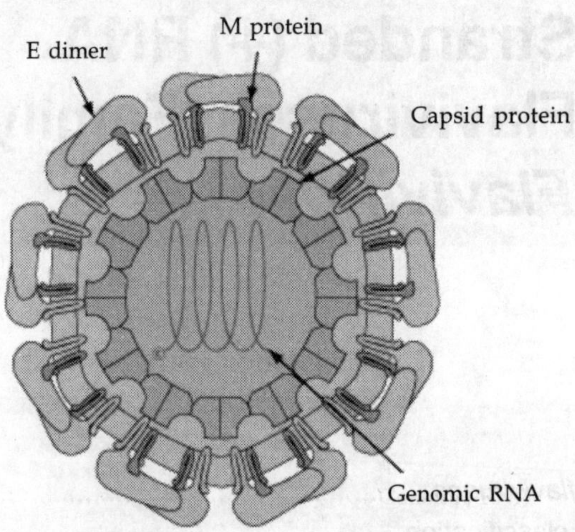

Figure 21.1 : Morphology of a flavivirus

The virus genome consists of single, linear, (+) ssRNA 9.7-12 kb long. The virus 5′ end has a methylated nucleotide cap or a genome-linked protein, VPg but hepaciviruses & pestiviruses members of this family are uncapped and encode an internal ribosome entry site. The 3′ end is not polyadenylated but forms a loop structure. Viruses of the *Flaviviridae* are similar to each other in virion morphology, genome organization, and replication strategy, but lack serological cross-reactivity across the family. Among the 4 genera- *Flavivirus, Hepacivirus, Hepatitis G virus & Pestivirus,* virus species of *Flavivirus* are **transmitted mostly by ticks or mosquitoes as vectors & agglutinate goose red cells**.

The flaviviruses are labile & sensitive to heat, detergents & organic solvents.

The virus genome

Flaviviruses genome contains single, linear, (+) ssRNA of about 9.7-12 kb. The 3′ end is not polyadenylated but forms a loop structure. The 5′ end in ***virus***has a methylated nucleotide cap that allows for translation or a genome-linked protein, VPg but other members of this family are uncapped and encode an internal ribosome entry site. The viral RNA is infectious and serves as both the genome and the viral mRNA. Production of a complementary RNA strand is not necessary for viruses in this family to produce protein.The *Flaviviridae* genome contains only one ORF; & on both ends of ORF there exists non-structural regions of about 100 nucleotides. The viral entire genome is translated in a polyprotein, which is cleaved co- and post-translationally by host and viral proteases. 5′ one third encodes the 3 structural proteins & 3′ two third encodes **7 non structural proteins** that enable the virus to replicate. Seven non structural proteins include NS 1, NS2A, NS2B, NS 3, NS 4A, NS 4B & NS5. NS3 protein contains epitope for T cells. NS 2B & amino terminus of NS 3 together function as serine protease. Non-structural proteins include protease, helicase, replicase and virion maturation. Among the **3 structural proteins, C, M & E (Fig 21-1)**, viral genome is encapsidated by a small capsid protein, C or C/V2, membrane or matrix protein M or M/V1 & envelope & glycoprotein E or E/V3). **E protein** is the major protein of the virus that remains glycosylated, shows hemagglutination activity, **& forms the neutralizing antibodies**. Flavivirus particles assemble by budding through Golgi vesicles & contain prM but mature at cell surface where prM is cleaved by cell enzyme furin to mature into M. But Pestiviruses contain 4 structural proteins-a capsid protein, & 3 envelope glycoproteins called E^{rns}, E1 & E2.

Virus replication

Virus replication takes place in the cell cytoplasm & uses the host cell's RNA dependant RNA polymerase to replicate. The virus first produces complementary, minus strand genomic RNA. This complementary genome then serves as a template strand for further replication; during replication, about ten plus strands accumulate for each negative template strand. Virus first attaches to host cell receptor, and is endocytosed into vesicles followed by fusion of virus membrane with the vesicle membrane releasing RNA genome into the cytoplasm.

The + genomic ssRNA is translated into a polyprotein, which is cleaved into all structural and non structural proteins. Virus replication occurs at the surface of endoplasmic reticulum. A negative-sense complementary ssRNA is synthesized using the genomic RNA as a template. New genomic RNA is synthesized using the negative-sense RNA as a template.

Virus assembly occurs at the endoplasmic reticulum, then the virion buds at the endoplasmic reticulum, is transported to the Golgi apparatus, and then bud from the cell membrane.

Virus classification

Group: Group IV + ssRNA
Family: *Flaviviridae*

Genera

Genus 1: Flavivirus; type species; *Yellow fever virus* (YFV), others include: **tick-borne viruses**: *Kyasanur Foresd disease virus* (KFDV), *Louping ill virus* (*LIV*), *Powassan virus* (POWV), & *Tick-borne encephalitis virus* (TBEV). **Mosquito-borne viruses**: *Dengue virus* (DENV), *Japanese encephalitis virus* (JEV), *Murray valley encephalitis virus* (MVEV), *St. Louis encephalitis virus* (SLEV), & *West Nile virus* (WNV).**Yellow fever group:** *Wesselsbron virus (WESSV) & Yellow fever virus* (YFV).

Genus 2: *Hepacivirus;* type species: *Hepatitis C virus*- the single member

Genus 3: *Hepatitis G Virus* -The GB agent and the hepatitis G virus (HGV)

Genus 4: *Pestivirus;* type species: *Bovine virus diarrhea,* others include classical *Swine fever virus* or hog cholera, & *Border disease virus*-contains viruses infecting non-human mammals.

Flavivirus Clinical Infections in Humans & Animals

The family of the *Flaviviridae* contains 4 genera: 1. *Flavivirus,* 2. *Hepacivirus,* 3. *Hepatitis G virus* & 4. *Pestivirus.* Among them, Flaviviruses contain > 69 human pathogens of which infections like *Yellow fever virus* (YFV), *Dengue fever virus* (DENV), *Japanese encephalitis virus* (JEV) and **Tick-borne encephalitis virus** (TBEV) are emerging world-wide. Three pathogens namely, *Louping ill virus, Wesselsbron virus* & **Japanese encephalitis virus** (JEV) are important animal pathogens. *Hepatitis C virus* (HCV) infection exceeds over 140 million people, four times the number of HIV-positive persons are chronically infected with the HCV. Hepatitis G virus (HGV) has not yet been assigned to a genus & impact of this recently discovered virus is yet to be established. The Pestiviruses include *Bovine viral diarrhea virus* (BVDV), *Classical swine fever virus* (CSFV) and *Border disease virus* (BDV) having a serious impact on livestock. Following are the important diseases caused by these viruses (Table 21.1).

Table 21.1: Classification of *Flaviviridae* & diseases caused by the member viruses in humans & animals.

Genera	Species	Serotypes	Diseases caused
Tick-borne viruses			
G 1: *Flavivirus*	*Kyasanur Forest disease virus*	KFDV	**Kyasanur forest disease** (KFDV) is a tick-borne hemorrhagic fever in humans endemic to South Asia including India .The symptoms are fever, headache, severe muscle pain, cough, dehydration,

		gastrointestinal symptoms and bleeding problems, low blood pressure, and low platelet, red blood cell, and white blood cell counts. Some patients recover but in most patients, the illness is biphasic and the patient develop a second wave of symptoms in the third week with fever and signs of encephalitis.
Louping ill virus	LIV; 5 subtypes	**Louping ill** (LIV) occurs in sheep, often cattle, deer, horses, pigs, red goose, humans & wild rodents in Europe. It is transmitted by *Ixodex ricinus* ticks & the symptoms include a bibhasic fever with CNS involvement.
Omsk hemmo-rhagic fever virus	OHFV	**Omsk hemorrhagic fever** (OHFV) found in Siberia is named for an outbreak in Omsk. The symptoms include chills, headache, pain in the lower and upper extremities, rash on the soft palate, swollen glands in the neck, appearance of blood in the eyes, dehydration, hypotension & gastroi-ntestinal symptoms. Patients may show CNS symptoms. In 1–2 weeks, some patients recover, may show a focal hemorrhage in mucosa of gingival , uterus and lungs, a rash in papules, the soft palate, cervical lymph adenopathy, and occasional neurological involvement. Some patient after 3 weeks show a second wave of symptoms, signs of encephalitis & on recovery they show hearing loss, hair loss, and behavioral or psychological difficulties associated with neurological conditions & some patient will die.
Powassan virus	POWV	**Powassan virus** (POWV) causes tick-borne encephalitis (TBE) related to the classic TBE, was first recognized in the town of Powassan, Ontario, & is transmitted by *Ixodex cookei* among small mammals in Canada and the United States. Powassan encephalitis appears after 1–3 weeks & is severe.
Tick-borne encep-halitis virus	TBEV; 5 subtypes	**Tick-borne encephalitis** (TBEV) has incubation period of 7-14 days and

symptoms are a biphasic febrile illness for 2 to 4 days with the viremic phase, malaise, anorexia, muscle aches, headache, nausea, and/or vomiting. At 8 days, the second phase of the disease occurs in 20 to 30% of patients and involves the central nervous system with symptoms of meningitis or encephalitis or meningoencephalitis. In contrast to RSSE, TBE is more severe in adults than in children.

Group	Virus	Abbreviation	Disease
Mosquito-borne viruses			
	Dengue virus	DENV	**Dengue fever** (DENV-1, 2, 3, 4), also called breakbone fever is not a deadly disease; deadly dengue viruses are **Dengue hemorrhagic fever** (DHF) and **Dengue shock syndrome** (DSS) showing symptoms of fever, headache, muscle & joint pain & skin rashes. In minority cases, the disease develops to life-threatening dengue hemorrhagic fever with bleeding, low platelets and blood plasma leakage, and dengue shock syndrome, when circulatory failure occurs.
	Japanese ence-phalitis virus	JEV	**Japanese encephalitis** (JEV) occurs in Asia in birds (water fowl) & bats, pigs, horses & humans; it is **mosquito-borne, pigs & wild birds act as reservoirs.** Incubation period is 5 to 15 days and the majority of infections are asymptomatic but 1 in 250 infections develop into encephalitis. Vaccines are used to prevent the disease.
	Murray valley encephalitis virus	MVEV	**Murray Valley encephalitis** (MVEV) is of zoonotic importance endemic to northern Australia & Papua New Guinea; in humans can cause permanent neurological disease or death. MVEV is related to *Kunjin virus*. The symptoms in majority of infections are subclinical, some show a mild form of the disease with symptoms such as fever, headaches, nausea and vomiting, and only a very small number of cases develop MVE & one-quarter die from the disease.

	St. Louis encephalitis virus	SLEV	**St. Louis encephalitis** (SLEV) is caused by the *Culex* mosquito, is related to *Japanese encephalitis virus*, occurs in USA, often in Canada & Mexico. Symptoms are mild illness, fever and headache; when severe the patients show headache, high fever, neck stiffness, stupor, disorientation, coma, tremors, occasional convulsions and spastic paralysis, & some aged die with 3-30% fatality.
	West Nile virus	WNV	**West Nile disease** (WNV) is a serious illness in North America; **few people** show high fever, headache, neck stiffness, stupor, disorientation, coma, tremors, convulsions, muscle weakness, vision loss, numbness and paralysis lasting several weeks, and neurological effects may be permanent. Milder symptoms develop in some people & no symptoms occur in most people in 80% cases. Clinical signs of encephalitis in horses and in some other species include a general loss of appetite and depression, in addition to any combination of the following signs: fever, weakness of hind limbs, paralysis of hind limbs, ataxia, weakness, impaired vision, down, trouble rising, head pressing , aimless wandering, convulsions (seizures), inability to swallow, walking in circles, hyperexcitability or coma.
	Israel turkey meningitis virus	ITV	**Israel turkey meningitis** (ITV) occurs in Israel & S. Africa in turkeys with progressive paresis & paralysis.
Yellow fever virus group			
	Wesselsbron virus	WESSV	**Wesselsbron** (WESSV) occurs in sheep, cattle, & humans in Saharan Africa, Thailand; causes generalized infection, hepatitis & abortion in ewes, cows; death of newborn; hairy birth coat in lambs; it is mosquito-borne. Most human cases are subclinical.
	TS: *Yellow fever virus*	YFV	and other species, found in tropical & subtropical areas in S. America and Africa,

			but not in Asia with only hosts are primates and several species of mosquito. Symptoms are fever, nausea, and pain that subside after several days. In some patients, a toxic phase follows, in which liver damage with jaundice occur and leads to death. Because of the increased bleeding tendency, yellow fever belongs to the group of hemorrhagic fevers; around 90% of the infections occur in Africa.
Virus with no arthropod vector	*Dakar bat virus*	DBV	
	Cell fusing agent virus	CFAV	**Cell fusing agent virus** (CFAV) was originally isolated in the laboratory from an *Aedes aegypti* cell line.
G 2: *Hepacivirus*	*Hepatitis C virus*	HCV; 10 genotypes	***Hepatitis C*** (HCV) *virus* causes an acute hepatitis & chronic hepatitis in humans, may also cause certain types of vasculitis & glomerulonephritis.
G 3: *Hepatitis G Virus*	*Hepatitis G virus*/ HGCV		**Hepatitis G virus** (HGC) or **GB virus C** (GBV-C) infects humans, but is not known to cause human disease. HIV patients coinfected with GBV-C can survive longer than those without GBV-C, but the patients may be different in other ways. There is current active research into the virus' effects on the immune system in patients coinfected with GBV-C and HIV. The majority of immunocompetent individuals appears to clear GBV-C viremia within the first few years following infection but may persist for decades in some individuals. About 2% of healthy US blood donors are viremic with GBV-C, and up to 13% of blood donors have antibodies to E2 protein, indicating prior infection. Parenteral, sexual and vertical transmission of GBV-C occurs, and because of shared modes of transmission, individuals infected with HIV are commonly co-infected with GBV-C. Among people with HIV infection, the prevalence of GBV-C viremia ranges from 14 to 43%. Some studies have suggested that

			co-infection with GBV-C will actually slow the progression of HIV disease.
G.4: *Pestivirus*	*Border disease virus*	BDV; 2 subtypes	**Border disease** (BDV-2) occurs worldwide in sheep, kids & rarely in calves; spread directly or indirectly; pregnant ewes abort & show congenital abnormalities in lambs.
	Bovine viral diarrhea virus1	BVDV-1; 4 subtypes	**Bovine viral diarrhea** (BVD-1, 4) occurs worldwide in cattle. Two BVDV biotypes-CP (cytopathic, derived from NCP), & NCP (non cytpathic) are 95% field or classical strains. There are 2 genotypes-BVDV 1 & BVDV 2. If NCP infects 40-140 day pregnant cows, virus crosses placenta, infects fetus, calves born are immunotolerant (dont infected with NCP strains). Cattle are viremic & shed virus to infect others, become persistently infected (PI). If PI cattle are infected with CP biotype, symptoms of acute MD result & cattle die of MD. Mutation of NCP to CP biotype occurred that killed the animal.
	Bovine viral diarrhea virus 2	BVDV-2; 3 subtypes	
	Classical swine fever virus	CSFV	**Classical swine fever** (CSFV) still occurs in S. Africa with neurological signs, abortion in pregnants, still birth, leucopenia, petechial hemorrhages in all serous surfaces, turkey-egg kidney, button ulcer on intestinal mucosa.

Clinical Infections in Humans

Genus : *Flavivirus*

Tick-borne infections

Kyasanur forest disease virus (KFDV) causes a tick-borne hemorrhagic fever in humans endemic to South Asia including India. The symptoms are fever, headache, severe muscle pain, cough, dehydration, gastrointestinal symptoms and bleeding problems, low blood pressure, and low platelet, red blood cell, and white blood cell counts. Some patients recover but in most patients, the illness is biphasic and the patient develop a second wave of symptoms in the third week with fever and signs of encephalitis.

Omsk hemorrhagic fever virus (OHFV) causes Omsk hemorrhagic fever, a tick- borne disease occurring in Siberia & is named for an outbreak in Omsk. The symptoms include chills, headache, pain in the lower and upper extremities, rash on the soft palate, swollen glands in the neck, appearance of blood in the eyes, dehydration, hypotension & gastrointestinal symptoms. Patients may show CNS symptoms. In 1–2 weeks, some patients recover, may show a focal hemorrhage in mucosa of gingival, uterus and lungs, a rash in papules, the soft palate, cervical lymph adenopathy, and occasional neurological involvement. Some patient after 3 weeks show a second wave of symptoms, signs of encephalitis & on recovery they show hearing loss, hair loss, and behavioral or psychological difficulties associated with neurological conditions & some patient will die.

Powassan virus (POWV) causes tick-borne encephalitis (TBE) related to the classic TBE, was firsrt recognized in the town of Powassan, Ontario, is transmitted by *Ixodex cookei* among small mammals in Canada and the United States. Powassan encephalitis appears after 1–3 weeks & is severe.

Tick-borne encephalitis *virus* (TBEV) causes TBE, has incubation period of 7-14 days and symptoms are a biphasic febrile illness for 2 to 4 days with the viremic phase, malaise, anorexia, muscle aches, headache, nausea, and/ or vomiting. At 8 days, the second phase of the disease occurs in 20 to 30% of patients and involves the central nervous system with symptoms of meningitis or encephalitis or meningoencephalitis. In contrast to RSSE, TBE is more severe in adults than in children.

Dengue fever virus (DENV-1, 2, 3, 4), causes Dengu fever, also called breakbone fever is not a deadly disease; **deadly dengue viruses are Dengue hemorrhagic fever (DHF) and Dengue shock syndrome (DSS).** The symptoms are fever, headache, muscle & joint pain & skin rashes. In minority cases, the disease develops to **life-threatening dengue hemorrhagic fever** with bleeding, low platelets and blood plasma leakage, and **dengue shock syndrome**, when circulatory failure occurs.

Murray Valley encephalitis virus (MVEV) is of zoonotic importance endemic to northern Australia & Papua New Guinea; in humans can cause permanent neurological disease or death. MVEV is related to *Kunjin virus.* The symptoms in majority of infections are sub-clinical, some show a mild form of the disease with symptoms such as fever, headaches, nausea and vomiting, and **only a very small number of cases** develop MVE & one-quarter die from the disease. MVEV is a mosquito-borne (*Culex annulirostris*) virus that is maintained in a bird-mosquito-bird cycle. Water birds including herons and cormorants act as the natural reservoir for MVE.

St. Louis encephalitis virus (SLEV) is caused by the *Culex* mosquito, is related to *Japanese encephalitis virus,* & occurs in USA, often in Canada & Mexico. Symptoms are mild illness, fever and headache; when severe the patients show headache, high fever, neck stiffness, stupor, disorientation, coma, tremors, occasional convulsions and spastic paralysis, & some aged die with 3-30% fatality.

West Nile disease *virus* (WNV) is a serious illness in North America **in a few people with** high fever, headache, neck stiffness, stupor, disorientation, coma, tremors, convulsions, muscle weakness, vision loss, numbness and paralysis lasting several weeks, and neurological effects may be permanent. **Milder symptoms develop in some people with** symptoms such as fever, headache, and bodyache, nausea, vomiting, and sometimes swollen lymph glands or a skin rash on the chest, stomach and back & last for a few days. **No symptoms develop in most people in** 80% cases.

Yellow fever virus (YFV) affecting humans is an acute viral hemorrhagic disease transmitted by the bite of female mosquitoes *Aedes aegypti*, and other species, found in tropical & subtropical areas in S. America and Africa, but not in Asia with only hosts are primates and several species of mosquito. Symptoms are fever, nausea, and pain that subside after several days. In some patients, **a toxic phase** follows, in which **liver damage** with jaundice occur and leads to death. Because of the increased bleeding tendency, yellow fever belongs to the group of hemorrhagic fevers; around 90% of the infections occur in Africa.

Genus: *Hepacivirus*:

Hepatitis C virus (HCV) causes an **acute hepatitis & chronic hepatitis** in humans, may also cause certain types of **vasculitis & glomerulonephritis**. Acute hepatitis C encompasses first 6 months after infection; most people suffer no symptoms upon infection but for those who do the main symptoms are generally mild and nonspecific, and rarely lead to a specific diagnosis of hepatitis C. Symptoms of acute HCV infection include decreased appetite, fatigue, abdominal pain, itching, jaundice, and flu-like symptoms. If HCV persist for > 6 months, it is chronic infection that may progress to scarring of the liver or fibrosis, and advanced scarring or cirrhosis, which is generally apparent after many years. In some cases, those with cirrhosis will go on to develop liver failure or other complications of cirrhosis, including liver cancer or life threatening esophageal and gastric varices.

Genus: *Hepatitis G virus*:

Hepatitis G virus (HGC) or GB virus C (GBV-C) infects humans, but is not known to cause human disease. HIV patients coinfected with GBV-C can survive longer than those without GBV-C. There is current research into the virus' effects on the immune system in patients coinfected with GBV-C and HIV. The majority of immunocompetent individuals appears to clear GBV-C viremia within the first few years following infection but may persist for decades in some individuals. About 2% of healthy US blood donors are viremic with GBV-C, and up to 13% of blood donors have antibodies to E2 protein, indicating prior infection. Parenteral, sexual and vertical transmission of GBV-C occurs, and because of shared modes of transmission, individuals infected with HIV are commonly co-infected with GBV-C. Among people with HIV infection, the prevalence of GBV-C viremia ranges from 14 to 43%. Some studies have suggested that co-infection with GBV-C will actually slow the progression of HIV disease.

Flaviviral Clinical Infections in Animals

Genus : *Flavivirus*

Louping Ill

Louping ill(LIV), also called **Ovine encephalomyelitis, Infectious encephalomyelitis of Sheep, Trembling-ill,** is a tick-borne, zoonotic acute viral disease **primarily of sheep** that is characterized by a biphasic fever with CNS involvement, depression, ataxia, muscular incoordination, tremors, posterior paralysis, coma, and death. The name 'louping ill' is derived from Scottish word describing the effect of the disease in sheep whereby meaning they 'loup' or spring into the air. The symptoms include a bibhasic fever.

Etiology: Louping ill is caused by *Louping ill virus* (LIV), a member of the genus *Flavivirus* in the family *Flaviviridae.* This virus is closely related to *Tick-borne encephalitis virus* (TBEV) and is a member of the same viral complex. **Four subtypes** of louping ill virus- the British, Irish, Spanish and Turkish subtypes have been detected but a recent genetic analysis suggests that the Turkish subtype is more closely related to TBEV than *Louping ill virus.*

Occurrence

Louping ill occurs mainly in the British Isles- Scotland, Ireland, northern England, and Wales wherever the tick vector *Ixodes ricinus* is found. Louping ill virus or a close relative causes a very similar disease in Norway, and a Spanish subtype of the virus has been documented in the Basque region of Spain. LI can occur at any time of the year, but the disease is most prevalent during the periods of maximal tick activity between April and June and again in September.

Hosts susceptible

Sheep are the main hosts for louping ill virus, but lambs born to nonimmune ewes getting virus infection may develop a peracute terminal illness with death. Clinical cases have also been recorded in other mammals like cattle, goats, horses, llamas, alpacas, pigs, dogs, deer and European elk. Fatal cases have been reported among grouse-red goose & and their relatives. LIV also infects many small mammals including shrews, wood mice, voles, rats, hares and rabbits. Humans seem to be accidental hosts. **Sheep are the most important reservoir hosts,** & irrespective of clinical symptoms, **sheep consistently develop sufficient viremia to transmit the virus to the tick vector. Red grouse and ptarmigan are** highly susceptible and developed high viremias, succumb, & both may act as amplifying hosts of the virus in endemic areas. Mountain hares (*Lepus timidus*) have been implicated as maintenance hosts via non-viremic transmission between co-feeding ticks. Horses may sometimes develop viremia that is sufficient to amplify this virus. Human infection is accidental infection following tick bite, penetration of the virus through skin wounds, or by aerosol exposure in the laboratory.

Transmission

Louping ill is transmitted mainly by three-host tick, *Ixodes ricinus*. Transstadial transmission occurs. All stages of ticks, larva, nymph, and adult, acquire the virus by feeding on a viremic host. Other species of ticks including *Rhipicephalus appendiculatus, I. persulcatus* and *Haemaphysalis anatolicum* are also capable of transmitting louping ill virus, but they are not important in the epidemiology of this disease. **Only sheep and red grouse** consistently develop viremia sufficient to infect ticks and amplify the virus but Grouse can act as amplifying hosts for a short period, but die very quickly.

Louping ill virus can also be transmitted by other routes. This virus is shed in the milk of goats, and to a lesser extent, sheep; lambs and kids may become infected when they nurse. Red grouse can be infected by eating ticks, and one group of pigs became ill after they ingested raw meat from infected lambs. Iatrogenic spread can occur on needles or surgical instruments. Louping ill virus can also be transmitted to humans via infected tissues or cultures.

Pathogenesis

Following tick bite, LIV replicates in the lymph nodes producing a viremia with a peak at 2-4 days, then declines with the induction of circulating Abs. Viremia allows virus dissemination to other lymphatic organs & often to brain & spinal cord. Invasion of CNS ensues in the early viremic phase in most infected animals but the lesions are small isolated with no clinical neurological symptoms. Clinical CNS symptoms occur if the virus replicates in the brain producing severe inflammatiom in the whole CNS with necrosis in brainstem, & ventral horn neurons. Infected animal that survives LI is due to early evoking of immune response to LIV with high Ab titer in cerebrospinal fluid.

Coinfection with *Ehrlichia* or *Phagocytophilia* -tick-borne fever causes more severe & prolonged viremia & more severe disease.

Clinical symptoms and lesions

The incubation period for louping ill is **6 -18 days** in sheep, & 2 to 8 days in red grouse.

Infection with LI virus may result in subclinical or clinical infection, depending on host range and environmental factors. Clinical symptoms of LI in sheep include initial fever, viremic stage & usually accompanied by depression and anorexia, followed in some cases by neurological signs. The **fever is biphasic, the second rise occursg about the fifth day after the appearance of clinical signs when the virus may invade CNS**; if it does not invade CNS, the animal recover rapidly and develop a durable protective immunity. In endemic areas, many animals develop mild or subclinical infections.

Sheep with encephalitis show muscle tremors and/or rigidity, incoordination, ataxia, hypersensitivity, salivation and nervous nibbling, progressing in some cases to head pressing, posterior paralysis, recumbency, convulsions and/or coma & death. Affected sheep may develop an unusual "louping gait," during which they move both hind legs, then both forelegs, forward in concert. Death is common among animals with neurological signs, often within a few days. Peracute deaths may also occur. Surviving animals may have residual CNS defects. Coinfection with *Anaplasma phagocytophilum* increases the severity of the clinical signs, probably by suppressing the immune system.

Natural infection of **LI in cattle, horses and pigs** produce similar clinical symptoms like in sheep. Evidence of neuromuscular dysfunction is seen. Affected cattle frequently have a staggering gait, hyperexcitability, head-pressing, recumbency, and convulsions and then die. Young piglets infected with LI virus can have a range of nervous signs, including aimless movement, head-pressing, ataxia, muscular spasms, and convulsions. Natural cases or outbreaks of LI in horses are very uncommon, and most cases of infection with the virus are apparently subclinical. The louping gait does not occur in species other than sheep.

The clinical signs in experimentally infected red grouse include depression, anorexia, **regurgitation of the crop contents** during handling, and muscle weakness, followed by death. But even if CNS involvement or neurological signs have not been seen, decreased body weight and poor survival of chicks, as well as deaths in birds of all ages, have been reported among wild populations. Some other species of grouse and ptarmigan also develop fatal disease after experimental inoculation.

With the exception of congestion of meningeal vessels, there is no pathognomonic gross lesion.

Diagnosis

Collection of clinical specimens for various tests includes heparinized blood during acute viremia for virus isolation, unfixed portions of brain and spinal cord in 50 percent glycerol and, paired serum samples, acute and convalescent for serology & half of the brain and portions of spinal cord in 10 percent formalin: fresh and formalin fixed brain tissue.

1. *Presumptive diagnosis:* Clinical signs, history & histologic lesions of meningoencephalomyelitis furnish a presumptive diagnosis.
2. *Virus isolation:* Virus is isolated in young mice inoculated intracerebrally, and in cell cultures.
3. *Antibodies detection:* It is carried out by ELISA, complement fixation, hemagglutination inhibition (virus agglutinates goose red cells), gel diffusion and indirect immunofluorescence.

Treatment & prevention

There is no specific treatment for encephalitic cases of LIV in sheep, but cattle affected with LI respond to good nursing and symptomatic treatment. Animals are dipped with acaricidal dipping or spraying of of sheep, etc. with an aim to control ticks.

Vaccination

A **formalin-inactivated vaccine** is used in endemic areas, with two doses 2 to 8 weeks apart. Vaccination of **pregnant ewes during the last trimester protects lambs for 1 year,** vaccination of **lambs after weaning & the same LI** vaccine is used in cattle with annual revaccination against the disease. **Louping ill vaccine**-MSD is a white oily emulsion vaccine prepared from louping-ill virus grown in tissue culture, inactivated with formalin, concentrated by ultra filtration and emulsified with a mineral oil. It contains liquid paraffin/Montanide as adjuvant and thiomersal as preservative. Vaccine is used for the active immunization of sheep to stimulate a serological response to the Louping III virus. Onset of immunity is within 4 weeks of vaccination and duration as shown by an anamnestic response is at least 18 months. Dose:1 ml SC. Animals should be revaccinated after 2 years, at least 4 weeks prior to the period of greatest infection risk.

Japanese Encephalitis

Japanese encephalitis **(JEV)** occurs in Asia in birds (water fowl), bats, pigs, horses & humans; it is mosquito-borne. Pigs & wild birds act as reservoirs. The majority of infections are asymptomatic but 1 in 250 infections develop into encephalitis.

Etilogy: Japanese encephalitis is caused by *Japanese encephalitis virus* (JEV).

Occurrence

JEV occurs in SE Asia & Far East Asia. Countries which had major epidemics in the past, but which have controlled the disease primarily by vaccination, include China, Korea, Japan, Taiwan and Thailand. Other countries that still have periodic epidemics include Viet Nam, Cambodia, Myanmar, India, Nepal, and Malaysia. Rare outbreaks in U.S. territories in Western Pacific have occurred. Japanese encephalitis has been reported on the Torres Strait Islands and two fatal cases were reported in mainland northern Australia in 1998.

Hosts susceptible

Occurs in Asia in birds (water fowl), bats, pigs, horses & humans; **pigs & wild birds act as reservoirs.** Infection in swine is asymptomatic, except in pregnant sows, when abortion and fetal abnormalities are common sequelae.

Transmission

Transmission occursby the bite of mosquitoes (rice field breeding mosquitoes, mainly the *Culex tritaeniorhynchus* group) infected with the *Japanese encephalitis virus.* Mosquitoes become infected by feeding on domestic pigs and wild birds infected with the J EV. Infected mosquitoes then transmit the *Japanese encephalitis virus* to humans and animals during the feeding process. The Japanese encephalitis virus is amplified in the blood systems of domestic pigs and wild birds. Only **domestic pigs and wild birds are carriers of the JEV**. *Japanese encephalitis virus* is not transmitted from person-to-person. Residents of rural areas in endemic locations, active duty military deployed to endemic areas, and expatriates who visit rural areas get infection. Japanese encephalitis does not usually occur in urban areas. *Culex tritaeniorhynchus* group, which feeds on cattle in preference to humans, it has been proposed that moving swine away from human habitation can divert the mosquito away from humans and swine.

Pathogenesis

Upon entry through mosquito bite, the virus infects **Langerhan's dendritic cells in the skin** and is carried to nearest draining lymph nodes, thereby initiating a round of early immune response. Unfortunately for the host, this is not sufficient to counter the virus and it spreads to secondary lymphoid organs before entering the blood circulation through the efferent lymphatic system. During the ensuing transient viremia, peripheral organs such as kidney, liver and spleen are infected, after which the neurotropic flavivirus spreads to the CNS. Once the virus evades the immune system, it crosses the blood-brain barrier (BBB) to enter the CNS. JEV may cross the BBB by passive transport across the endothelium, by active replication in endothelial cells, or by a 'Trojan horse' mechanism in which the virus is carried into the brain by infected inflammatory cells.

Monocytes and macrophages are thought to be probable carriers of the virus into the CNS as studies has shown that the virus can survive for a prolonged time and replicate within these cells. Due to the impaired functioning of the BBB, peripheral inflammatory cells are recruited to the infected brain at later stages of JE that exacerbates the damage. JEV causes extensive **neuronal damage in the brain,** though in many cases, the virus is probably not directly involved in the destruction of brain tissue but may cause damage indirectly by triggering cell-mediated immune response by activating microglia. Microglial activation is viewed as an adaptive response whereby microglia release neuroprotective factors to facilitate the recovery of injured neurons and they also phagocytose dying or damaged neurons, before they lyse and release toxic agents into surrounding areas. JEV infection has been shown to activate microglia both morphologically and functionally, in vivo, that leads to an elevation of proinflammatory mediators, such as IL-6, TNF-α, RANTES and MCP-1. These proinflammatory mediators and cytotoxins released from activated microglia are instrumental in inducing neuronal death.

Clinical symptoms & lesions

Incubation period **for Japanese encephalitis** is usually 5 to 15 days. Mild infections occur without apparent symptoms other than fever with headache. More severe infection is marked by quick onset, headache, high fever, neck stiffness, stupor, disorientation, coma, tremors, occasional convulsions, especially in infants and spastic (but rarely flaccid) paralysis. Case-fatality rates of Japanese encephalitis range from 0.3% to 60%.

Treatment & prevention

There is no specific therapy. Intensive supportive therapy is indicated. The use of **rosamarinic acid and arctigenin** has been shown to be effective in a mouse model of Japanese encephalitis. **Curcumin** imparts neuroprotection against JEV infection in an in vitro study. Curcumin possibly acts by decreasing cellular reactive oxygen species level, restoration of cellular membrane integrity, decreasing pro-apoptotic signaling molecules, and modulating cellular levels of stress-related proteins. It has also been shown that the production of infective viral particles from previously infected neuroblastoma cells are reduced, which is achieved by the inhibition of ubiquitin-proteasome system. **Minocycline** in mice resulted in marked decreases in the levels of several markers, viral titer, and the level of proinflammatory mediators and also prevents blood brain barrier damage.

A breakthrough in the field of Japanese encephalitis therapeutics is the identification of **macrophage receptor involvement** in the disease severity. A recent report of an Indian group demonstrated the involvement of monocytes and macrophages receptor CLEC5A in severe inflammatory response in JEV infection of brain. This transcriptomic study provides a hypothesis of neuroinflammation and a new lead in development of appropriate therapeutic against Japanese encephalitis.

Vaccination

Vaccines are used to prevent the disease. All current vaccines are based on the genotype III virus. A formalin-inactivated mouse-brain derived vaccine was first produced in Japan in the 1930s and was validated for use in Taiwan in the 1960s and in Thailand in the 1980s. In the UK, JE IXIARO (licensed) is used. **Green Cross requires three doses given at 0, 7–14 and 28–30 days.** The dose is **1 ml for children and adult, and 0.5 ml for infants under 36 months of age.IXIARO, the new vaccine** has been produced by Intercell Biomedical Ltd and requires **only 2 doses**, and is currently licensed in the U.S., Europe (inc UK), Canada and Australia. Use of JE vaccine among travelers and laboratory workers are recommended. **IMOJEV** is a recombinant chimeric virus vaccine, developed using the Yellow fever virus (YFV) vaccine vector YFV17D, by replacing the cDNA encoding the envelope proteins of YFV with that of an attenuated JEV strain SA14-14-2. IMOJEV was found to be safe, highly immunogenic and capable of inducing long-lasting immunity in both preclinical and clinical trials. Moreover, a single dose of IMOJEV was sufficient to induce protective immunity, which was similar to that induced in adults by three doses of JE-VAX, a mouse brain-derived inactivated JE vaccine.

West Nile Disease in Horses

West Nile disease *virus* (WNV), causes West Nile disease in horses characterized by general loss of appetite and depression, in addition to any combination of the following signs: fever, weakness of hind limbs, paralysis of hind limbs, ataxia, impaired vision, down, trouble rising, head pressing , aimless wandering, convulsions (seizures), inability to swallow, walking in circles, hyperexcitability or coma.

Occurrence

West Nile virus has been described in Africa, Europe, , the Middle East, west and central Asia, Oceanic (subtype Kunjin), and most recently, North America. Recent outbreaks of West Nile virus encephalitis in humans have occurred in Algeria (1994), Romania (1996 to 1997), the Czech Republic (1997), Congo (1998), Russia (1999), the United States (1999 to 2009), Canada (1999–2007), Israel (2000) and Greece (2010).

Epizootics of disease in horses occurred in Morocco (1996), Italy (1998), the United States (1999 to 2001), and France (2000). In 2003, West Nile virus was found in horses in Mexico. In 2002, more than 14,000 cases of WNV were reported in horses in the United States. Many of these horses recovered. The majority of these cases were reportedly not vaccinated against WNV. In Pennsylvania, 97 cases were reported in 2002. It is thought that many more horses were infected without showing any clinical symptoms of disease.

Hosts susceptible

Although the vast majority of infections have been identified in birds, WN virus has been shown to infect humans, horses, cats, dogs, bats, chipmunks, skunks, squirrels, and domestic rabbits. A relatively small number of WNV infected dogs and WNV infected cats have been reported to CDC. Dogs and cats become infected when bitten by an infected mosquito. There is also evidence that cats can become infected with the virus after eating experimentally infected mice. The horses become infected by the bite of infectious mosquitoes. The virus is located in the mosquito's salivary glands. In the 1999 New York area epidemic, several crows died, & 200 species of birds found dead in the United States. Horses and birds seem to be the most susceptible to illness from infection.

Transmission

The virus is transmitted through the bite of mosquito vectors, which bite and infect birds. **The birds are amplifying hosts**, developing sufficient viral levels to transmit the infection to other biting mosquitoes which go on to infect other birds (American robin & American crow are the most common carriers) and also humans, horses. The infected mosquito species vary according to geographical area; in the US *Culex pipiens* (Eastern US), *Culex tarsalis* (Midwest and West), and *Culex quinquefaciatus* (Southeast) are the main sources. In mammals the virus does not multiply as readily, does not develop high viraemia during infection), and it is believed that mosquitoes biting infected mammals do not ingest sufficient virus to become infected, making mammals so-called dead-end infections.

Additional routes of human infection were detected during the 2002 West Nile epidemic. In small percentage of cases, WNV transmission occurs through transplanted organs and through blood transfusions. Although transmission of WNV and similar viruses to laboratory workers is not a new phenomenon, two recent cases of WNV infection of laboratory workers have been reported. There is no documented evidence of person-to-person or animal-to-person transmission of West Nile virus.

Pathogenesis

Following peripheral inoculation, initial WNV replication occurs in skin Langerhans dendritic cells, these cells migrate to draining lymph nodes, resulting in a primary viremia and subsequent infection of peripheral tissues such as the spleen and kidney. By the end of the first week, WNV is largely cleared from the serum and peripheral organs and infection of the CNS is observed in a subset of immunocompetent animals. Rodents that succumb to infection develop a CNS pathology similar to that observed in human WNV cases, including infection and injury of brain stem, hippocampal, and spinal cord neurons. WNV infection is not significantly detected in non-neuronal CNS cell populations in humans or animals. In surviving wild-type mice, WNV is cleared from all tissue compartments within 2 to 3 weeks after infection. However, **persistent viral infection in the brains of CD8$^+$ T-cell or perforin-deficient mice and in the brains and kidneys of infected hamsters has been reported**. Persistent infection has also been documented in a WNV-infected immunosuppressed patient in whom viremia was detected for more than 60 days.

The mechanisms by which WNV and other neurotropic flaviviruses cross the blood-brain barrier (BBB) remain largely unknown, although tumor necrosis factor alpha (TNF-α)-mediated changes in endothelial cell permeability may facilitate CNS entry. It is likely that WNV infects the CNS at least in part via hematogenous spread, as an increased viral burden in serum correlates with earlier viral entry into the brain. Additional mechanisms may contribute to WNV CNS infection, including (i) infection or passive transport through the endothelium or choroid plexus epithelial cells, (ii) infection of olfactory neurons and spread to the olfactory bulb, (iii) a "Trojan horse" mechanism in which the virus is transported by infected immune cells that traffic to the CNS, and (iv) direct axonal retrograde transport from infected peripheral neurons. Although the precise mechanisms of WNV CNS entry in humans require additional study, changes in cytokine levels that may modulate BBB permeability and infection of blood monocytes and choroid plexus cells have been documented in animal models.

Clinical symptoms & lesions

Incubation period in humans for West Nile disease is usually **2 to 15 days. Incubation period** in horsesis 7 - 14 days.

Although all horses do not usually develop clinical symptoms of WNV, horses that do become ill may show symptoms ranging from very mild signs to deadly illness. Typical signs include ataxia (incoordination, stumbling, limb weakness) that either appears suddenly or appears gradually and worsens, sleepiness, dullness, listlessness, facial paralysis (droopy eyelids, lower lip), and an inability to rise. Some horses may develop mild fevers, blindness, muscle trembling, seizures, and other signs. Horses cannot spread the disease to humans, but humans are susceptible to the disease if bitten by a carrier mosquito. Clinical symptoms include incoordination, dragging hooves, buckling at knees, difficulty in eating and drinking, stumbling, muscle weakness, dullness, somnolence, paralysis, & inability to rise. Some horses develop mild infection with low fever, muscle trembling and evidence of a less severe disease. Horses that recover from the disease have residual abnormalities such as irregularities of gait, behavioral changes and neurological deficits six months after diagnosis. In horses, the mortality rate in unvaccinated horses with clinical disease is ~33%. Survivors are considered immune for life.

PM lesions in horses are like eastern equine encephalitis (EEE) having perivascular lymphocyte cuffing, gliosis and neuronal degeneration. Unique feature with WNV infection is a poliomyelitis affecting the gray matter of the spinal cord. Mainly the brainstem and midbrain are affected. But in EEE the whole brain is affected with the cerebrum is most affected.

Diagnosis

Collection of clinical specimens include whole blood collected during the febrile stage and brain tissue from horses that have died, & sera from acute and convalescent cases.

1. *Presumptive diagnosis:* Clinical signs and the microscopic brain lesions are suggestive of WNV.
2. *Virus isolation:* The virus is propagated on the chorioallantoic membrane, where it produces plaques, and in various cell cultures.
3. *Serology: A definitive diagnosis can be obtained by demonstrating a significant increase in specific antibody between acute and convalescent sera.*

Treatment & prevention

In horses, steroids are sometimes used to reduce inflammation along with general supportive therapy. The best method of prevention of infection with West Nile Virus for people and animals is to reduce the risk of exposure to the mosquitoes that may carry the virus. Reducing the risk involves eliminating mosquito breeding sites to reduce the number of mosquitoes. Mosquitoes lay eggs and develop in stagnant water, so reduction of these sites involves eliminating stagnant water sources. Strict mosquito control that greatly reduces the chances of exposure, & keeping horses indoors from dusk to dawn when insects are most active; keep lights off during the evening and keep stable areas clear of birds and poultry.

Vaccination

In humans, the current yellow fever vaccine is used as the template for a WNV vaccine when yellow fever vaccine genes are replaced with corresponding WNV genes. A weakened strain of the yellow fever virus is used as the backbone of the vaccine, and the gene that encodes the yellow fever virus's protein coat is replaced with the corresponding gene from the WNV. The yellow fever vaccine used as the basis for this process has been safely and effectively given to millions of people.

The first effective **horse vaccine, West Nile-Innovator** DNA, a DNA vaccine was introduced by Fort Dodge Animal Health (Wyeth). Inject one 2 ml dose IM & a second 2 ml dose 2 to 4 weeks after the first dose. Revaccinate annually with one 2 ml dose. Subsequent revaccinations with one 2 ml dose may be advisable when horses are faced with an outbreak or other conditions which might make exposure likely. Shortly thereafter, a second, one-annual-dose vaccine called **PreveNile**, live flavivirus chimera vaccine was introduced by Intervet/Schering-Plough Animal Health (Merck), one dose is all that's needed for primary immunization. Single dose for horses previously administered other West Nile vaccines. PreveNile prevents viremia, and aids in the prevention of disease and encephalitis caused by West Nile virus infection. A DNA-based vaccine, called **Recombitek Equine WNV (Merial)**, which is Canarypox virus-vectored recombinant vaccine. Recombitek Equine WNV combines rWNV with reliable killed EEE and WEE virus vaccines and tetanus toxoid to help prevent four out of five core diseases in a single annual dose-2ml IM at 4 months & older but unvaccinated horses require a primary two-dose vaccination, four to six weeks apart. In 2009, a new killed virus vaccine was introduced by Boehringer-Ingelheim, a privately held pharmaceutical company, incorporating an equine origin WNV strain (E159), representative of the more recent WNV strains impacting horses.

Wesselsbron Disease

Wesselsbron is a mosquito-borne disease occurring in **sheep, cattle, & humans in Saharan Africa & Thailand;** causes generalized infection, hepatitis & abortion in ewes & cows; death of newborn & hairy birth coat in lambs. Mortality in newborn animals may reach 27% in lambs and 18% in goat kids. Infection in adults is usually subclinical, but disease may be severe in the presence of pre-existing liver pathology. Occasional abortion in ewes, together with congenital malformation of the CNS with arthrogryposis of the ovine fetus and hydrops amnii in ewes, is also seen. In humans, it causes a nonfatal influenza-like disease. Infection is common but clinical disease is infrequent.

Etiology: Wesselsbron disease is caused by *Wesselsbron virus* (WESSV), a mosquito-borne virus in the genus *Flavivirus* of the family *Flaviviridae*.

Occurrence

Wesselsbron virus has been isolated from vertebrates or arthropod vectors in several countries in southern Africa including Cameroon, the Central African Republic, Nigeria, Senegal, South Africa, Uganda, and Zimbabwe. There is serological evidence of its presence in other sub-Saharan countries in Africa including the island of Madagascar. In addition, this virus has been isolated from mosquitoes in Thailand. In cattle, sheep, and goats, the seroprevalence may be as high as 50%. Animals of all ages seem to be susceptible to infection. Outbreaks mainly occur when heavy rains favor the replication of mosquitoes that breed in flood waters. The mortality rate in newborn lambs can be as high as 30%.

Hosts susceptible

Wesselsbron disease is seen **mainly in humans, sheep. Goats, cattle, pigs, and horses** can also be infected; a link with abortions is suspected in cattle and goats. The virus has also been recovered from a **camel** and a fatal infection in a **dog**. The **reservoir host** is unknown, but may include **domestic ruminants, wild birds, wild rodents such as gerbils, or other animals.**

Transmission

Wesselsbron virus is transmitted by mosquitoes in the genus *Aedes* including *A. caballus* and *A. circumluteolus*. A high seroprevalence among domestic herbivores in warm, moist regions suggests that these animals may have a role as viral reservoirs. In ruminants, there seems to be no direct virus transmission between animals. In humans infection occurred by handling the virus or contaminated material; in these cases, transmission was thought to occur by contact or possibly aerosols.

Clinical symptoms & lesions

Most clinical cases are reported in sheep, particularly pregnant ewes and newborn lambs. **Abortions** are the usual symptom in pregnant ewes. They are often accompanied by **neurologic defects in the fetus** and sometimes by hydropsamnii (excessive accumulation of amniotic fluid in the amniotic cavity). Complications of the abortion may lead to the death of the ewe. In newborn lambs, the clinical signs may include fever, anorexia, weakness, and an increased respiratory rate.

Up to 30% of affected lambs may die. In non-pregnant adult sheep, the disease usually is limited to fever; however, during one atypical outbreak in South Africa in 1957, the symptoms also included a nasal discharge, diarrhea, jaundice, and subcutaneous edema of the head. Many of the sheep died in this epidemic.

Infections with Wesselsbron virus in adult goats, cattle, horses, and pigs are usually inapparent and limited to fever. The virus has been associated with abortions in goats in Botswana. It is also suspected as a cause of abortion in cattle. However, the incidence of abortion in this species may be low; in one experiment, infection of 15 pregnant cows resulted in no abortions. A fatal infection has been reported in a dog.

PM lesions: Congenital malformations of the CNS and arthrogryposis have been reported in ovine and bovine fetuses. Necropsy lesions in young lambs may include hepatomegaly with a yellowish to orange-brown liver, and moderate to severe icterus. Petechiae and ecchymoses are common in the abomasal mucosa; the contents of the abomasum may be chocolate-brown from gastrointestinal hemorrhages. Subcutaneous edema has also been reported.

On histopathology, there is usually mild to extensive necrosis of the liver parenchyma, with foci of necrotic hepatocytes. Lesions in adult animals are similar but usually much milder.

Diagnosis

Wesselsbron disease can be diagnosed by virus isolation or serology.

1. *Virus isolation:* The virus is isolated from blood, serum, liver or brain from aborted fetuses, and the spleen or liver from dead lambs by inoculation into suckling mice or chick embryos, or tissue culture in BHK or lamb kidney cells. The identity of the virus can be confirmed by virus neutralization. Immunohistochemistry, using formalin-fixed liver tissues, has been used to confirm the disease in newborn lambs.

2. *Serology:* Antibody can be detected by hemagglutination-inhibition, complement fixation, and virus neutralization. Although there is a high degree of cross-reactivity with other flaviviruses in hemagglutination-inhibition tests, the homologous Wesselsbron titers are usually much higher than the heterologous titers. An ELISA has also been published; this test had greater sensitivity and lower cross-reactivity than the hemagglutination inhibition test.

Treatment & prevention

Treatment is supportive and symptomatic; there is no specific treatment for the virus. People who work with Wesselsbron virus or contaminated tissues should wear gloves and other protective clothing, and avoid techniques that would aerosolize the virus. **Mosquito control measures** such as repellants and mosquito netting also decrease the risk of infection.

Vaccination

Sheep can be immunized with an **attenuated vaccine**. Immunity is life-long. But production of an attenuated vaccine was discontinued shortly before 2000. Incidence of disease is low in sheep, and injudicious use of the vaccine in pregnant ewes resulted in severe economic losses in the past due to abortion and fetal malformations. Attempts to control mosquito vectors are of little value as a preventive measure.

Israel Turkey Meningitis

***Israel turkey meningitis virus* (ITV)** occurs in Israel & S. Africa in turkeys with progressive paresis & paralysis. This disease has been reported only in turkeys and generally is seen only in birds **less than10 week of age**. It has been reported only in **Israel and South Africa**. While the specific vector has not been identified, the seasonal incidence and sporadic occurrence in flocks on the same farms strongly suggest that **it is transmitted by insect vectors, most likely mosquitoes and *Culicoides* spp flies.** Turkeys exhibit **neurologic dysfunction characterized by progressive paresis and paralysis, with variable mortality**. Morbidity and mortality rates generally average 15-30% but may be as high as 80% . Turkey breeder hens exhibit a severe drop in egg production. Gross lesions in affected turkeys include **splenomegaly or atrophy of the spleen, catarrhal enteritis, and myocarditis.** The principal microscopic lesions are **meningoencephalitis characterized by submeningeal and perivascular lymphocytic infiltration and focal myocardial necrosis.**

Genus: *Pestivirus*:

Border Disease

Border disease (BD) in Britain or hairy shaker disease in Australia and New Zealand causes a **congenital disorder of lambs** characterized by **barren ewes, abortion, stillbirth** and **the birth of persistently infected weak lambs with** low birth weight and viability, showing tremor, abnormal body conformation and hairy fleeces, & excessively hairy birth coat in normally smooth-coated breeds. Border disease is a **congenital disease of sheep and goats,** first reported in the Border region of Wales and England. **The economic importance of the disease** is due to reproductive failure, abortions and low survival rate of affected lambs. Kids may also be affected with a similar condition, & often occurs in calves.

Etiology: Border disease is caused by *Border disease virus* (BDV) in the genus *Pestivirus* under the family *Flaviviridae.* BDV is closely related to the viruses of *Bovine viral diarrhea virus* (BVDV-2) & *Classical swine fever virus* (CSFV). Nearly all isolates of BDV are non cytopathogenic in cell culture. There are no defined serotypes but virus isolates exhibit considerable diversity. Three distinct antigenic groups & two separate genotypes have been identified.

Occurrence

Border disease (BD) of sheep and goats was first reported in sheep in 1959 from the border region of England and Wales, and since then has been recorded **worldwide**. Distribution of BDV is world-wide including USA. Prevalence rates vary in sheep from 5% to 50% between countries and from region to region within countries.

Hosts susceptible

BD mainly occurs in **sheep, occasionally in goats & rarely in cattle**. Ruminants and probably pigs can be readily infected by contact with these persistent excretors or with acutely infected sheep. Sheep may acquire infection from persistently infected cattle as sheep and cattle are equally susceptible to all strains of border disease virus.

Transmission

Vertical transmission plays an important role in the epidemiology of the disease. Infection of fetuses with BDV can result in the birth of **persistently infected (PI) lambs**. These PI lambs are viremic, antibody negative and constantly shed virus in their excretions and secretions, including semen. The virus spreads from sheep to sheep, & PI animals are the source of infection. Infection in goats is less common with abortion being the main presenting sign. Ruminants and probably pigs can be readily infected by contact with these persistent excretors or with acutely infected sheep. BDV is present in the placenta & fetal fluids at the birth of persistently infected lambs. The virus is introduced into susceptible flocks by the addition of persistently infected sheep.

Pathogenesis

BDV infection occurs via oro-nasal route. Outcome of **infection with BDV in sheep depends on the age of the animal, age of the fetus in pregnant animal, infecting virus strain & genotpe of the host.**

Infection with BDV in non pregnant sheep results in **viremia & subclinical infection.** Acute infections in immunocompetent animals usually are **transient** and subclinical and result in immunity to challenge with homologous but not heterologous strains of virus.

If BDV infects susceptible pregnant ewes, the **virus crosses the placenta, invades the fetus, causes placentitis 10-30 days after infection and may cause fetal death with expulsion, resorption, or mummification.** Abortion may occur at any stage of pregnancy and may pass unnoticed because there is little maternal discomfort.

Final outcome of fetal infection rests on the age of the fetus. Sheep develop immunocompetence **between 61-80 days of gestation.** When infection with BDV occurs between 45-72 days of pregnancy, the virus becomes widely distributed in fetal tissues, & pathologic changes are most obvious in the skin, skeleton, and CNS, there is fetal death with resorption, abortion or mummification. The surviving fetuses become immunotolerant, **remain persistently infected**, the clinical signs gradually regress, but such animals remain infected and excrete virus for the **remainder of their lives,** exposing their progeny and flock-mates & the lambs at birth show tremors, hairy birthcoat & other congenital defects due to **interference in organogenesis.**

Congenital defects in lambs consist of skeletal growth retardation, hypomyelinogenes, enlarged hair follicles & reduced number of secondary follicles. Infection after 80 days of pregnancy induces immune response, eliminates the virus & gives birth of healthy lambs.

Clinical Symptoms & lesions

Affected flocks are recognized first at lambing time by an increase in the number of barren ewes and in the birth of undersized lambs with excessively hairy and sometimes excessively pigmented fleece. Some lambs exhibit involuntary muscular tremors, particularly of the trunk and hind legs. The tremors are reduced at rest and exacerbated by movement. In others, skeletal defects such as dropped pasterns and mandibular brachygnathia may predominate. Affected lambs have a low survival rate. In survivors, nervous signs gradually disappear within 3-4 months. Outbreaks of BD with low fertility in ewes and poor viability and ill-thrift in lambs are becoming associated more often with border disease virus infection. PM lesions include cavitation of the cerebrum, microscopical lesions in white matter of the CNS show a deficiency of myelin and an increase in interfascicular glial cells, in which myelin-like lipid droplets may accumulate. These changes are most obvious in the newborn and gradually resolve.

Diagnosis

Collection of clinical samples for various tests includes whole blood and serum; & affected lambs for necropsy.

1. *Presumptive diagnosis:* Clinical signs, history & the histological finding of nerve fibers with defective myelin sheaths furnish presumptive diagnosis.
2. *Virus isolation:* BDV is propagated in many cell cultures, from serum or buffy coat cells in cell cultures but without any cytopathic effects. Viral antigen can be demonstrated in infected cell cultures, blood smears, and affected tissues by immunofluorescence.
3. *Virus antigen detection:* Viral antigen can be detection by ELISA using heparinized or EDTA blood. RT-PCR is used for detecting viral RNA in clinical specimens and **for typing BDV**.
4. Virus neutralization and ELISA are used on dam serum samples to determine the degree of flock infection.

Treatment & prevention

There is no effective treatment for BD.

Prevention is best accomplished by maintaining closed flocks, serological screening should be don, & separate persistententy infected lambs. Control of the disease involves regular serological testing by ELISA or virus neutralization of all animals and removal of positive animals; only negative animals are maintain ed in the flock.

Vaccination: An inactivated, adjuvanted vaccine containing BDV and BVDV-1 is used.

Bovine Viral Diarrhea

Bovine viral diarrhea (BVD), is a disease of cattle which reduces productivity, increases death loss, & occurs worldwide in cattle. Clinical signs are **mucosal erosions and diarrhea** which occur in the acute form of BVD & have a significant effect on those animals infected, but more economically important are those animals who become **persistently infected** (PI). PIs fail to reach their genetic potential, exhibit decreased weight gain, increased disease susceptibility, reduced fertility, shed the virus throughout their life-time, causing infection to the other herd mates, & reproductive loss in the unimmunized animals in the herd.

Etiology: Bovine viral diarrhea (BVD) is caused by *Bovine viral diarrhea virus* (BVDV-1, 4). There are 2 BVDV biotypes-**cytopathic (CP) biotype & non cytopathic (NCP) biotype** based on their effect on tissue culture cells. NCP virus biotypes include 95% field or classical strains, can cross the placenta, invade the uterus & cause persistent infection in the fetus, & can cause congenital, enteric & reproductive disorders. **Cytopathic biotype of BVDV is mainly associated with only mucosal disease in persistently infected animals that are infected with NCP biotype of the virus.** If PI cattle are infected with CP biotype, a recombination between CP & NCP occurs & NCP is mutated into CP strains within that animal. If NCP infects 40-140 day pregnant cows, virus crosses placenta, infects fetus, calves born are immunotolerant, cattle are viremic & shed virus to infect others, become **persistently infected (PI)**, & symptoms of acute MD results & cattle die of MD. Mutation of NCP to CP biotype occurred that killed the animal.

There are also 2 genotypes of BVDV-BVDV-1 & BVDV- 2. BVDV-2 Genotype of BVDV causes a **severe, hemorrhagic form of disease found in the USA and Canada**. Clinical signs include haematochezia, haemorrhagic nasal and ocular discharges, epistaxis and clotting dysfunction causing petechiation with high mortalities.

Occurrence

BVDV was first identified in a New York State dairy herd in 1946. BVD affects mainly cattle worldwide but sheep, goats, pigs, water buffaloes and wild ruminants are also susceptible.

Hosts susceptible

BVDV affect cattle of all ages. This disease continues to have a heavy economic impact in the cattle industry. Young & unvaccinated cattle are the most susceptible, while the the persistently infected calves are the major source of the virus.

Transmission

Transmission of the pathogenic virus can occur through secretions from an **acutely infected or a persistently infected animal**. BVDV transmission may occur vertically causing congenital infection of the fetus, which may cause resorption, abortion, stillbirth, or live-birth. Congenitally infected fetuses that survive *in utero* infection may be born as BVDV-infected calves. The BVDV infection in these calves **will persist during the entire life of the calf, and they will shed BVDV continuously in the farm environment;** they are called persistently-infected (PI) animals. Discharges from reproductive tract & aborted fetuses of infected animals of either PI or systemically infected animals contain the virus. Transmission of the virus can occur through **semen of PI bulls**, through **PI females** & through embryo transfer from PI or transient infected animals. Indirect contact with infected fomites or flies can transmit the disease.

Pathogenesis

The BVDV infection occurs through **oronasal route**, the virus initially replicates in the oronasal mucosa. A viremia occurs & the virus is disseminated in the whole body either free in the blood or with leukocytes. The virus affects both **B & T lymphocytes** whose number decreases causing **immunosuppression.** Immunosuppressive effect of the virus predisposes calves to secondary respiratory & enteric infections.

Further, viral pathogenesis depends on several interacting factors but most importantly on host factors-age & gestational status of the fetus, & virus virulence.

BVDV in non-pregnant immunocompetent animals causes usually **mild** and show symptoms of respiratory disease comprising of **conjunctivitis, nasal discharge, lethargy, decreased milk yield in cows, depression and a cough.** In case of acute infection, **calves** show signs of illness exhibiting respiratory or gastrointestinal symptoms.

Many animals may show no symptoms although these animals have inapparent infections; such calves may incur a mild fever, a drop in white blood cell count and recover without significant illness. But cattle with inapparent disease shed the pathogenic virus during their short infection period & show immunosuppression favouring other infections to attack.

Outcome of BVDV infection in the pregnant animals depends on the stage of gestation.

A normal calf could be born to a cow becoming infected during late gestation **>180 days**, when the fetus has a competent immune response in utero, and it would be born without any negative results.

An infection during early pregnancy **<125 days** results in detrimental effects on the fetus; there may be early embryonic death, abortion, fetal mummification **or a calf born with a persistent infection.** A persistent infection describes an animal that carry the infection for the rest of its life. When PI calf is born, it never reach their productive potential, exhibiting **stunted growth, reduced fertility and increased susceptibility to other diseases,** will shed the virus for the rest of its life, acting as a constant source of infection for other cattle in the herd. Fetuses exposed to BVD **at 150 days or more of gestation** usually develops congenital defects including poor brain development, eye abnormalities, structural malformations and stunted growth. Calves born with congenital defects usually have difficulty in standing and walking and may exhibit an early death due to a poor ability to nurse the dam.

When PI animal is infected with CP biotype, BVD virus **mutate within that animal into the cytopathic form of BVD** causing **mucosal disease,** which causes **ulcers, blisters and erosions on the oral mucosa and snout.** Mucosal disease is invariably fatal; death occurs over days or weeks and is usually see n in cattle 6-18 months of age.

Genotype 2 BVD is a **severe, hemorrhagic form of disease found in the USA and Canada.** Clinical signs include haematochezia, hemorrhagic nasal and ocular discharges, epistaxis and clotting dysfunction causing petechiation. Mortalities are high.

Clinical symptoms & lesions

The clinical signs of BVDV infection are highly variable, from few to no signs to very severe signs that kill the animal depending on the genotype of the virus, whether the infection was recently acquired i.e., **acute** or has been acquired for months i.e., **chronic,** whether the animal is pregnant, as well as other factors.

Infection of non pregnant, seronegative cattle with NCP biotype of BVDV may result in a variety of clinical manifestations, ranging from inapparent infections to gastroenteric, respiratory and hemorrhagic syndromes to the severe acute BVD and the fatal mucosal disease. Most cases of BVD **in non-pregnant immunocompetent animals** causes usually **subclinical or inapparent infection or mild** infection showing symptoms of respiratory disease comprising of **conjunctivitis, nasal discharge, lethargy, decreased milk yield in cows, depression and a cough.**

In case of **acute infection,** calves show signs of respiratory or gastrointestinal symptoms. Some of the signs of acute infection are fever, lethargy, loss of appetite, ocular discharge, nasal discharge, oral lesions, diarrhea, and decreasing milk production. Chronic infection may lead to signs of mucosal disease.

A peracute form of BVD, is caused by BVD type II virus causing enteric form, which is highly fatal, occurs in immunocompetent, seronegative cattle, & is caused by virulent isolates of type II virus

An infection during early pregnancy (<125 days) result in early embryonic death, abortion, fetal mummification or a calf born with a persistent infection. Fetuses exposed to BVD at 150 days or more of gestation could be born with congenital defects that include poor brain development, eye abnormalities, structural malformations and stunted growth. Calves born with congenital defects usually have difficulty in standing and walking and may exhibit an early death due to a poor ability to nurse the dam. **Surviving** fetuses from early gestation may be born with congenital anomalies such as ocular defects, alopecia, arthrogryposis, and cerebellar hypoplasia.The signs of cerebellar hypoplasia in newly born calves are ataxia, tremors, wide stance, stumbling, and failure to nurse. The defects are severe enough that compensation will not occur, and the calves may die

There are two sources of PI animals; either transmission of BVDV from a PI cow to her fetus or through acute infection of a pregnant cow during the first 120 to 150 days of gestation.

Mucosal disease occurs in animals that are persistently infected; they are carrying the NCP biotype and become exposed to the CP biotype. Clinical signs of mucosal disease are associated with gastrointestinal symptoms. Affected cattle may exhibit explosive diarrhea and ulcerative lesions throughout the digestive tract. Mortality rates in mucosal disease are extremely high (95-100%). Fever, leukopenia, anorexia, loss of condition, salivation and a thick, stringy nasal discharge may be noticed and shallow erosions on the oral and nasal mucosa are frequent. The skin of the muzzle may be eroded and crusty. PM lesions include erosions and ulcerations of the upper respiratory and digestive tracts; characteristic ulcers are seen in the esophagus and involving Peyer's patches. The virus has an affinity for lymphoid tissues, resulting in suppression of the cell-mediated immune response.

Diagnosis

Collection of samples for various tests includes: nasal discharge, feces, blood, blood smears, spleen, kidney, lymph nodes, turbinates, intestine, lung, acute and convalescent sera, fetal liver and kidney & ear notch.

1. *Presumptive diagnosis:* Characteristic signs, history & lesions are suggestive of the disease.
2. *Virus isolation:* Virus isolation from whole blood & tissues from affected lambs is furnished by growing the virus in bovine & ovine cell lines.

Since most BVDV strains are non cytopathic, the presence of the virus in cultures is confirmed by FA staining.

3. *Antigen detection:* The PCR is used for pooled samples of blood or milk because minute amounts of virus may be identified by PCR.
4. *Antibody detection:* Neutralization test is used to detect a four-fold increase in the level of BVD antibody between acute and convalescent serum samples.
5. The ear notch test is only to identify PI cattle. Ear notches may also be don e using ELISA as a recent adapted test. The immunohistochemistry IHC is suitable for herd screening because samples are collected from cattle of any age, it is easy, the samples are stable during transport and handling, and the test result is not affected by passive antibodies from the dam.

Treatment & prevention

Treatment includes supportive therapy in face of outbreaks of BVD, but not well in case of mucosal disease. Prevention is achieved with a combination of removal of PI cattle by regular testing of herd by the isolation of BVD virus from the serum or by the demonstration of viral infected leukocytes by FA, vaccination, and enhanced biosecurity.

Vaccination

There are two broad categories of BVDV vaccines: 1. Modified live virus (MLV) vaccines and 2. Killed virus (KV) vaccine. MLV BVDV vaccines replicate in the vaccinated animal, increase the virus level and the boost the immunogenic potential, require only one dose during the initial immunization step but are contraindicated in pregnant animals & MLV vaccines also can be reactivated by some chemicals. KV vaccines require more antigens per dose than MLV vaccines, are more expensive, are safe but require more than one dose of KV. Vaccine must usually be given during initial immunization, requiring a herd to be gathered more than once for vaccination. The duration of immunity has been reported to be short from 140 days to as long as 18 months. **Bovilis BVD**-Intervet is an inactivated vaccine containing cytopathogenic BVD virus strain C86 used for protection against infection with Bovine viral diarrhoea virus (BVDV) and protection against foetal infection. Dose is 2 ml IM, two doses, 4 weeks apart are required in the first year, with an annual booster in subsequent years. Vaccination should be completed 4 weeks before mating. Calves can bevaccinated from 4 months of age. Many combination vaccines exist. **Bovi-Shield Gold FP 5-Pfizer** (IBR+BVD+ BPI3+BRSV) is a freeze-dried modified live virus; an adjuvanted sterile diluent is provided to rehydrate the freeze-dried component. Primary Vaccination: a single 2-ml dose to all breeding cows and heifers approximately 1 month prior to breeding or being added to the herd. Annual revaccination with a single dose of Bovi-Shield GOLD FP 5 is recommended. **Cattlemaster Gold FP 5**-Pfizer as above is a modified live & killed virus for vaccination of healthy cattle, including pregnant cows, & contains a unique combination of adjuvants, including Amphigen® to enhance the immune response to its fractions. Primary vaccination: healthy cattle an initial 2 doses 3 weeks apart 2 ml SC. As an aid in preventing IBR-induced abortion and BVD persistently infected calves, administer a 2-ml dose at approximately 5 and 2 weeks prior to breeding. Calves vaccinated before the age of 6 months should be revaccinated after 6 months of age. Annual revaccination with a single dose is recommended. **Bovi Shield Gold FP5L5**-Pfizer in addition contains L. Canicola-Gripotyphosa, Hardjo, Icterohaemorrhagiae, Pomona Bacterin. Give 5 ml SC & repeat in 3 weeks. When used for fetal protection, give at 5 and 2 weeks prior to breeding. Calves vaccinated before 6 months of age should be revaccinated at 6 months of age. Annual booster dose is recommended.

Classical Swine Fever (CSF)

Classical swine fever or hog cholera, is a highly contagious disease of pigs & wild boar characterized by acute, clinical symptoms with high mortality, including neurological symptoms and hemorrhages within the skin caused by highly virulent strains, or subacute or chronic infections in older pigs that may escape detection, while still causing abortions and stillbirths, & is cause by less virulent strains. Infected piglets born to infected but subclinical sows help maintain the disease within a population. Other signs include lethargy, fever, immunosuppression, chronic diarrhea, secondary respiratory infections, abortion in pregnant sows, still birth, leucopenia, and petechial hemorrhages in all serous surfaces, turkey-egg kidney, & button ulcers on intestinal mucosa.

Etiolgy: Classical swine fever (hog cholera) is caused by *Classical swine fever virus* (CSFV) that be longs to the genus *Pestivirus* and family *Flaviviridae*. Only one serotype of CSFV occurs but minor antigenic variability has been demonstrated between viral strains. There are **virulent virus strain that cause acute CSF, & mild virulent strains of CSFV.** CSFV is related to the ruminant pestiviruses that cause bovine virus diarrhea and border disease.

Occurrence

Classical swine fever occurs in many parts of Asia, some Caribbean islands, the African countries of Madagascar and Mauritius, and parts of South and Central America. This disease has been eradicated from the United States, Canada, New Zealand, Australia and most of western and central

Europe. CSFV is endemic in wild boar in parts of Europe; the significance for domesticated pigs is unclear. CSF was eradicated in the UK by 1966, but an outbreak occurred in East Aglia in 2000.

Hosts susceptible

CSF affects domesticated and wild pigs, & all feral and wild pigs, including European wild boar and collared peccaries, are susceptible.

Transmission

Infected pigs are the only reservoir of CSF virus. Blood, secretions and excretions including oronasal and lacrimal secretions, urine, feces and semen and tissues contain infectious virus. Virus is shed **before the onset of clinical signs,** and occurs throughout the course of **acute or subclinical disease.** Chronically or persistently infected pigs can shed virus continuously or intermittently for months.

Transmission between pigs occurs mainly by the oral or oronasal routes, via direct or indirect contact. CSFV is spread by feeding uncooked contaminated garbage. Animals are also infected through the mucus membranes, conjunctiva and skin abrasions. CSFV can be spread by genital transmission or artificial insemination. **Infected carrier sows may give birth to persistently infected pigs.**

The virus can also be spread on fomites, and mechanically spread by insects, birds and other wild or domesticated animals. Airborne transmission seems to be possible over short distances. While aerosol transmission occurred only within a radius of 250 meters, in one study transmission could occur up to 1 km.

CSFV is moderately fragile in the environment; this virus is reported to survive for 3 days at 50ºC and 7 to 15 days at 37ºC. Some studies suggest that virus inactivation occurs within a few days, while others describe survival, under winter conditions, for up to four weeks. CSFV can remain infectious for nearly three months in refrigerated meat and for more than four years in frozen meat. Reported virus survival times in cured and smoked meats vary with the technique, and range from 17 to more than 180 days.

Pathogenesis

After virus entry through oronasal route, the virus multiplies in the **tonsil.** The virus then spreads to regional lymph glands & through lymphatic vessels enters capillaries leading to initial **viremia.** The virus then spreads to spleen, peripheral & visceral lymph nodes, bone marrow & Peyers' patches. The virus exerts its **pathogenic effect on endothelial cells, lymphoreticular cells, macrophages & epithelial cells.** In acute cases, a **B lymphocyte deficiency** is caused due to destruction of germinal centers in the lymphoid tissues that is the due to pathoimmunological result of acute infection.

Most of the lesions result from the hydropic degeneration & **proliferation of vascular endothelium causing occlusion of blood vessels. This results in characteristic lesions of congestion, hemorrhages & infarction due to changes in the arterioles, venules & capillaries.** Thrombosis of small & medium size arteries also results. Vascular changes are marked in lymph nodes, spleen, kidneys & GI tract. Lesions due to effect on endothelial cells are also seen in eyes, adrenals, & CNS. A **leucopenia** at early stage, then leukocytosis, anemia & thrombocytopenia are observed. Disseminated intravascular coagulation is common with microthrombi in small blood vessels of kidneys, liver, lymph nodes, lungs, intestine & intestinal lymph nodes. Non-supurative encephalitis with perivascular cuffing is observed in most infected pigs. Secondary bacterial infections aggravate the lesions & clinical changes.

Outcome of infection in pregnant sows depends on the age of the fetus & the virulence of the infecting virus strains. In case of infection with CSFV during early gestation, the virus invades the fetuses causing fetal death with resorption or abortion. In utero infection can cause stillbirth, weak newborn piglets with congenital tremors & often birth of clinically normal piglets. Piglets with immune tolerance to the virus remain **persistently infected excreting virus continuously**. Piglets born clinically normal may subsequently develop late onset disease.

Clinical symptoms & lesions

Incubation period is 2 to 15 days, depending on the virulence of the strain, the age, & susceptibility of pigs.

The symptoms of classical swine fever vary with the strain of virus, and the age and susceptibility of the pigs. More virulent strains cause **acute disease; less virulent strains cause mostly chronic, mild or asymptomatic infections,** & most epizootics are now caused by **moderately virulent strains.** Older animals are less likely to show severe symptoms than younger pigs. Some breed-specific differences have also been reported.

Acute swine fever

Acute swine fever is the most severe form of the disease showing common symptoms of a **high fever, huddling, weakness, drowsiness, anorexia, conjunctivitis, and constipation followed by diarrhea.** Pigs may be incoordinated or exhibit an unsteady, weaving or staggering gait, which progresses to posterior paresis. Some pigs may vomit yellow, bile-containing fluid, or develop respiratory signs. The abdomen, inner thighs, ears and tail may develop a purple **cyanotic discoloration. Hemorrhages can also occur in the skin**. Severe leukopenia usually occurs soon after disease onset, and convulsions may be seen in the terminal stages. Pigs with acute classical swine fever often die within one to three weeks.

Subacute swine fever

Subacute disease is caused by moderately virulent strains of CSFV & also occurs in older pigs. The subacute form is similar to acute classical swine fever; however, the symptoms are less severe, and the fever may persist for two to three weeks. Some pigs with subacute classical swine fever may survive; others die within a month.

Chronic swine fever

Chronic disease is caused by less virulent strains or in partially immune herds. In the initial stages, chronic disease shows anorexia, depression, elevated temperatures, leukopenia, and periods of constipation or diarrhea. Affected pigs usually improve after several weeks. But when they appear relatively normal, they develop recurrent symptoms that may include intermittent fever, anorexia, periods of constipation or diarrhea, wasting or stunted growth, alopecia and skin lesions. **Immunosuppression may lead to concurrent infections.** The symptoms of chronic infections can wane for weeks to months, and may affect only a few animals in the herd. Affected pigs may survive for one to three months, but chronic infections are always fatal.

In some breeding herds infected with less virulent strains, **poor reproductive performance may be the only sign of disease. Sows may abort or give birth to stillborn, mummified, malformed, weak or dead piglets.** Some piglets may be born with a congenital tremor or congenital malformations of the visceral organs and central nervous system. Other piglets may be asymptomatic at birth, but persistently infected. These animals are persistently viremic and become clinically ill after several months, called late onset disease. The symptoms can include inappetence and depression, as well as stunted growth, dermatitis, diarrhea, conjunctivitis, ataxia or posterior paresis. Although affected pigs usually survive for more than six months, all die within a year. Congenital infections may be limited to a few piglets in the.

PM lesions

The skin may be **discolored purple**, the lymph nodes may be swollen and hemorrhagic, petechial or ecchymotic hemorrhages can often be seen on serosal and mucosal surfaces, particularly on the kidney, urinary bladder, epicardium, larynx, trachea, intestines, subcutaneous tissues, and spleen. Severe tonsillitis, sometimes with necrotic foci, is common. Splenic infarcts are occasionally seen. The lungs may be congested and hemorrhagic. In some acute cases, lesions may be absent or inconspicuous.

The lesions of chronic disease are less severe and may be complicated by secondary infections. In addition, necrotic foci or "button" ulcers may be found in the intestinal mucosa, epiglottis and larynx. In growing pigs that have survived for more than a month, bone lesions can also occur at the costochondral junction of the ribs and the growth plates of the long bones.

In congenitally infected piglets, common lesions include cerebellar hypoplasia, thymic atrophy, ascites, and deformities of the head and legs. Edema and petechial hemorrhages may be seen in the skin and internal organs.

Diagnosis

Collection of clinical specimens for various tests include: kidney, spleen, tonsil, lymph nodes, brain, and blood.

1. *Presumptive diagnosis:* is based on the clinical signs, gross and microscopic lesions.
2. *Virus isolation:* The virus can be cultivated in several cell cultures of swine origin including PK–15 cells but shows no CPE. Cell culture coverslips are stained with specific FA to confirm the presence of virus or immunoperoxidase staining or RT–PCR.
3. *Antigen detection:* Viral antigens are detected by direct immunofluorescence or ELISAs.
4. *Differentiation of pestiviruses:* Virus-specific monoclonal antibodies are used to distinguish the viruses of CSFV, BVDV and BDV.
5. *Serology:* Serology is useful in herds infected 30 or more days previously, & if herds are infected with less virulent strains, viral antigens may be more difficult to find. The virus neutralization tests, the fluorescent antibody and the neutralizing peroxidase–linked assay & various ELISAs, & monoclonal antibodies can differentiate between different pestiviruses and CSFV. The definitive test for differentiation is the **comparative neutralization test.** Congenitally infected pigs are immunotolerant and are negative on serology.

Treatment & prevention

Countries free of CSF apply strict importation and quarantine requirements to prevent entry of the disease. Quarantines, movement control and good surveillance are important in controlling outbreaks. This virus is sensitive to drying and ultraviolet light, stable at pH 5-10, but is inactivated by pH 3 or less, or pH greater than 11. Sodium hypochlorite and phenolic compounds are effective disinfectants. Detergents, organic solvents, quaternary ammonium compounds, and aldehydes (formaldehyde, glutaraldehyde) are also reported to destroy this virus. CSFV can survive for several months in refrigerated meat and years in frozen meat. Hence heating the meat to 65.5°C or greater for 30 minutes, or 71°C for one minute is safe.

Vaccination

Attenuated virus vaccines are used in countries where the virus is endemic but are inappropriate where eradication is being attempted in that the virus may continue to circulate subclinically in vaccinates.Pigs develop protective immunity one week to ten days after vaccination and the immunity lasts **two to three years** (i.e. the lifetime of many sows and boars). Piglets which are suckled by vaccinated sows receive colostral protection which lasts about **6-8 weeks.** During this time they cannot be vaccinated successfully because the maternal antibodies neutralize the vaccine virus before it has had time to stimulate immunity.

There is only one serotype of CSF virus which produces a strong long-lasting immunity. The virus in CSF vaccines was attenuated by frequent passage in rabbits but many vaccines now contain viruses that have been attenuated by continual growth in cell cultures.

In CSF endemic areas, all pigs are vaccinated over two weeks of age initially. Piglets born to vaccinated sows would be vaccinated over **8 week's age.** This policy usually results in elimination of the virus from that region.

A marker vaccine (gene-deleted vaccine) has been developed that doesn't express one of the viral glycoproteins. Thus the vaccinated animals can be differentiated from infected (wild type virus) by the lack of an antibody response to the viral glycoprotein. Marker vaccines are not yet widely used in eradication programs. **Byovac CSF E2-**Bayer Liverkusen is an emulsion vaccine containing as the active component a minimum of 32 ìg of classical swine fever virus (CSFV) E2 antigen (subunit vaccine) per dose of 2 ml. Dose 2 ml IM. The basic vaccination consists of 2 doses, the second dose being given after a 4-6 weeks interval. Revaccination with a single dose is recommended at 6-month intervals. For fattening pigs over the age of 10 weeks and in emergency situations one IM inoculation with one dose is administered for basic immunization. **Porcilis Pesti-**Intervet is a water-in-oil emulsion containing as the active component 120 ELISA Units (EU) of the CSFV E2 antigen (subunit vaccine) per dose of 2 ml with baculovirus expression system.

Active immunization of pigs from the age of 5 weeks onwards is done to prevent mortality and to reduce clinical signs of Classical swine fever, as well as to reduce infection with, and excretion of, CSF field virus. Dose: 2 ml IM to pigs from the age of 5 weeks onwards to prevent mortality and to reduce clinical signs of Classical Swine Fever, as well as to reduce infection with, and excretion of CSF field virus.

□□□

Chapter 22

Characteristics and Diseases Caused by Group IV Single-Stranded (+) Coronaviruses (Family *Coronaviridae*)

Contents

Characteristics of Coronaviruses

Coronaviruses (L. *corona*= crown) are large, enveloped, pleomorphic viruses measuring 75-160 nm in diameter; have club shaped peplomers, about 20 nm long that project from the envelope imparting crown-like appearance to the virus. Coronavirus morphology is unique as large club-shaped surface projections or peplomers, 20 nm long extend from the envelope that encloses a coiled **helical nucleocapsid** structure. It is noteworthy that other single, unsegmented +sense, ssRNA have capsid of icosahedral symmetry except cornaviruses. Virion size ranges from 75 nm to 160 nm in diameter. Toroviruses having tubular nucleocapsid is disc or kidney-shaped or rod -shaped & measure 120-140nm in diameter. The virus genome is made of a single molecule of positive-sense ssRNA about 27-31kb long, **the largest among RNA virus genomes**. 5′ end of the genome is capped & 3′ end is polyadenylated. Viral RNA is infectious & acts both as genome & as mRNA. There are 4 structural proteins-S, M, HE & N. The envelope contains 3 types of glycoproteins, M (E 1), HE (E3) (absent in some coronaviruses), and S (E2). **Fig 22.1** depicts the structure of a coronavirus. **The S (E2) is large & makes up** the club shaped spike or projections, **binds to cellular receptors, causes membrane fusion and induces the production of neutralizing antibodies**. M (El) is a transmembrane protein that performs the role of matrix protein & is located on the inner part of the envelope, HE (hernagglutinin esterase, E3), present in the antigenic group II coronaviruses, binds to erythrocytes of some species and has receptor-destroying (acetylesterase) activity. The helical ribonucleoprotein is made of the genomic RNA and the phosphorylated nucleocapsid protein N. The structural phosphoprotein N constructs the helical symmetry of the nucleocapsid, which encloses the genomic RNA.

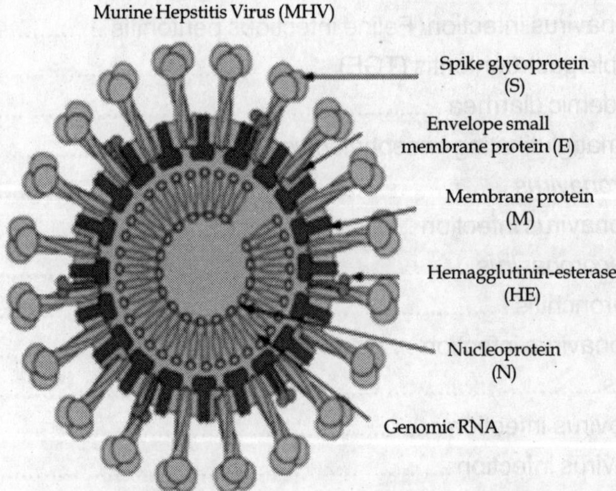

Figure 22.1 : Morphology of Coronavirus

Various members of *Coronavirus* and *Torovirus* cause mild respiratory and enteric infections in humans and other vertebrate animals but also known cause severe infections like SARS (severe acute respiratory syndrome). But coronaviruses are associated with respiratory infections in several animals like pigs, cats, dogs, mice and chickens.

Coronaviruses are sensitive to heat, lipids, formaldehyde, oxidizers & non ionic detergents, but susceptibility to pH is variable, being stable at pH 3.

The Viral Genome

Coronavirus virion genome is made of unsegmented, linear, positive sense, ssRNA genome of 27-32kb in size, being the largest among RNA viruses. 5′ end is capped, and 3′ end is polyadenylated. The leader RNA (65-89 bp) is present at the 5′ end of the genome as well as at the end of each subgenomic RNAs. Coronaviruses RNA is infectious and serves as both the genome and viral mRNA. The genomic RNA encodes for ORF1a, and ORF1b, which are translated by a frameshifting mechanism. The proteins produced are proteins pp1a and pp1ab, are processed into the viral polymerase (RdRp) and other non-structural proteins involved in RNA synthesis. The structural proteins are expressed as subgenomic RNAs. Each RNA either as genomic or subgenomic RNA is translated to yield only the protein encoded by the 5′-most ORF.

Virus Replication

Virus replication occurs in the cell cytoplasm. After viris attachment, & release of the (+) strand genomic RNA in the cytoplasm, an RNA-dependent RNA polymerase is synthesized, which transcribes a full-length (-) strand RNA, from which is synthesized (a) new genomic RNA, (b) an overlapping series of subgenomic mRNAs, and (c) leader RNA. The genomic RNA and mRNAs are capped and polyadenylated and form a "nested set" with common 3' ends and a common leader sequence on the 5' end. Only the unique sequence of the mRNAs toward the 5' end is translated, to produce several nonstructural proteins (NS) and four structural proteins: M (EI), transmembrane glycoprotein; S (E2), peplomer glycoprotein; N, nucleoprotein; and in some coronaviruses HE (E3), hemagglutinin-esterase glycoprotein. Maturation and assembly occur in the rough endoplasmic reticulum and the Golgi, and virions are released by exocytosis.

Virus Classification

Group: Group IV (+) ssRNA

Order: Nidovirales

Family: Coronaviridae

Subfamily: Coronavirinae

Genus 1: Alphacoronavirus: type species: Alphacoronavirus 1, Group 1 coronaviruses include- *Canine coronavirus* (CCoV), *Feline coronavirus* (FCoV), *Human coronavirus* (HCoV229E), *Porcine* epidermal diarrhea virus (PEDV) and *Transmissible gastroenteritis virus* (TGEV).

Genus 2: Betacoronavirus: type species: *Murine coronavirus*, Group 2 coronaviruses include- *Sars coronavirus* (SARS-CoV), Bovine *coronavirus* (BCoV), *Murine* hepatitis virus (MHV) and *Human coronavirus* (HCoV-OC43)

Genus 3: Gammacoronavirus: type species: *Avian coronavirus*, Group 3 coronaviriruses- *Infectious bronchitis virus* (IBV), *Turkey corona virus* (TCoV)
Subfamily: Torovirinae

Genus 1: Bafinivirus: type species: *White bream virus* (fish nidoviruses)

Genus 2: *Torovirus*: type species: Equine torovirus (EToV) include- *Bovine torovirus* (BToV-Breda), TS: *Equine torovirus* (EToV-Berne) & *Porcine torovirus* (PToV).

Coronavirus Clinical Manifestations in Humans and Animals

Clinical Infections in Humans

Genus: *Alphacornavirus*

Human corona virus **(HCoV-229E)** infection in humans is usually mild or subcinical, but in very old or infant, severe lower respiratory tract symptoms are seen as common cold, & rarely involve CNS.

Genus: *Betacoronavirus*

Human corona virus **(HCoV-OC-43)** causes common cold in humans.

Sars corona virus **(SARS CoV)** causes **severe acute respiratory syndrome** (SARS) in humans in S E Asia, was first reported in China in 2003, & subsequently worldwide. The first SARS symptom is a fever of 38°C (100.4°F) or higher, early symptoms include non-specific flu-like symptoms, including chills/rigor, muscle aches, headaches, diarrhea, sore throat, runny nose, malaise, and myalgia lasting 2-7 days. Further symptoms are a dry cough, shortness of breath, and an upper respiratory tract infection. In severe cases, SARS develops into **respiratory failure and acute respiratory distress syndrome (ARDS)**, and in 70-90% of the cases, they develop **lymphopenia**. The incubation period is 2-10 days, & up to 13 days, with the mean being 5 days. The disease progresses in the following way. After 2-10 days, the IgM antibody titrates to the SARS-CoV, then peaks during the acute or early convalescent phase (week 3) and declines by week 12. IgG peaks at week 12.

Table 22.1 : Classification of *Coronaviridae* & diseases caused by the member viuses in humans & animals.

Genera	Species	Serotypes	Diseases caused
	Group 1: coroaviruses		
G 1: *Alphacoronavirus*	*Canine corona virus*	CCoV	***Canine corona virus*** **(CCoV)** infection occurs in dogs of all ages worldwide but is **severe in puppies**, & mild to subclinical in adults; spread is via oro-fecal route, shedding of virus in the feces & carrier dogs. Symptoms are diarrhoea, vomition, enteritis, atrophy of small intestinal villi; the infected dogs shed virus in the feces.
	Feline corona virus (Feline infectious peritonitis virus)	FCoV, FIPV	***Feline corona virus*** **(FCoV-FIPV)** infection is mild in cats, affects enterocytes, produce mild gastroenteritis or inapparent infection in kittens; Feline infectious peritonitis **(FIPV)** (wet & dry forms) is a progressive debilitating disease of *Felidae* of all ages worldwide but severe in **6 month to 2 year** old cat, this mutated strains of FCV becomes tropic to **macrophages.** The disease is spread via contact, carriers, & infected cats. The virus affect intestinal epith & regional lymph nodes. & Ag-Ab complex causes vasculitis, & multifocal granulomatous lesions on various organs.
	Human corona virus	HCoV-229E	**Human corona virus (HCoV-229E)** infection is usually mild or subclinical, but in very old or infant severe lower respiratory tract symptoms are seen as common cold, & rarely involve CNS.
	Porcine epidermal dirrhoea virus	PEDV	***Porcine epidemic diarrhea virus*** **(PEDV)** affects swine of all ages in Asia & Europe; infection occurs via oro-nasal route. There is; watery diarrhea, older pigs are more severely affected but there is less mortality in neonates. There is shortening of small intestinal villi like TGE.
	Transmissible gastroenteritis	TGEV	**Transmissible gastroenteritis virus (TGEV)** affects **newborn pigs**; transmission is via fecal-

	virus		oral route, via virus shedding in feces, nasal secretions & milk. TGEV causes atrophy of small intestine mature villous enterocytes with vomition, diarrhea, dehydration, acidosis & high mortality. Live & attenuated vaccines are used.
G2: *Betacoronavirus*	Group: 2 coronavirus		
	Bovine corona virus	BCoV	***Bovine corona virus*(BCoV)** causes diarrhea in calves & **winter dysentery in adult cattle** worldwide; virus is spread via oro-fecal route & shedding of virus in feces. The virus destroys mature enterocytes in small intestine & colon.
	Human corona virus	HCoV-OC-43	Human corona virus **(HCoV-OC-43)** causes common cold in humans.
	Murine hepatitis virus	MHV	***Murine hepatitis virus* (MHV)** causes enteritis, hepatitis & encephalomyelitis in mice.
	Porcine haema gglutinating encephalomyelitis virus	PEV	*Porcine hemagglutinating encephalomy elitis virus* **(PEV)** or **vomition & wasting disease virus** (1 serotype) infects young pigs in America & Europe. The disease is spread via aerosols with symptoms of vomition & wasting & acute encephalomyelitis. The virus replicates in tonsils & epith cells of URT, peripheral nerve to CNS, vagus sensory ganglion & intramural plexus of stomach damage is responsible for vomition & delayed gastric evacuation.
	Sars corona virus	SARS CoV	***Sars corona virus*** (Severe acute respiratory syndrome/**(SARS CoV)** occurs in humans in SE Asia, first reported in China, & subsequently worldwide. There is initially fever, flu-like symptoms, muscle pain, headache, & 2-10 days later respiratory symptoms, cough, dyspnoea, pneumonia with some mortality.
G3: *Gammacoronavirus*	*Group 3*		
	TS: *Infectious bronchitis virus*	IBV-8 serotypes	***Infectious bronchitis virus*** **(IBV)** causes **infectious bronchitis,** a highly contagious disease that occurs in **young chickens** worldwide which affects respiratory,

			reproductive & renal systems with high mortality. Transmission is by aerosols, & shedding of virus from RT. The common symptoms are coughing, gasping, tracheobronchitis, and stunting, reduced egg production in layers, misshapen & soft shelled egg. Some neurotropic strains cause intestinal nephritis, mild respiratory signs with high mortality. Both live & killed vaccines are used.
	Turkery corona virus	TCoV	*Turkey corona virus* (TCoV) causes **Blue comb disease** or transmissible enteritis that is an acute, highly contagious disease of turkeys, especially young poults, characterized by sudden onset, marked depression, anorexia, diarrhea, dehydration, and weight loss. The disease is spread via direct or indirect contact, or contaminated premises, recovered carrier birds, stresses & secondary infections.
SF2: *Torovirinae:* G: *Torovirus*	*Bovine toro-virus*	BToV-Breda	***Bovine torovirus*** **(BToV-Breda virus)** infection causes diarrhea in newborn calves not fed colostrum.
	TS: *Equine toro-virus*	EToV-Berne	***Equine torovirus*** **(EToV-Berne virus)** infection has been reported from rectal swab with diarrhea in horses.
	Porcine toro-virus	PToV	***Porcine torovirus*** **(PToV)** infection is common in swine shortly after weaning, virus is shed after 4-14 days post weaning & lasts for 1-9 days with normal stool.

Coronavirus Infections in Animal & Birds

Genus: *Alphacoronavirus*

Canine Coronavirus Infection

Canine corona virus (CCoV) causes gastroentestinal infection in dogs of all ages worldwide with mild to subclinical symptoms in adults including anorexia, depression, diarrhea, vomition, enteritis, & atrophy of small intestinal villi but it is **severe in puppies.** *Canine coronavirus* equals *Canine parvovirus* as the leading viral causes of diarrhea in puppies. Clinically, the two infections can be indistinguishable, but *Canine coronavirus* rarely kills the puppy while *Canine parvovirus* often kills.

Etology: Canine coronavirus infection is caused by*Canine coronavirus* (CCoV) which belongs to the genus *Alphacoronavirus* in the family

Coronaviridae. There are slight antigenic differences between coronavirus strains isolated from pups with diarrhea. Hence puppies and dogs immune to a particular strain of Coronavirus may not be immune to other strains of the virus.

Occurrence

The Canine coronavirus is worldwide in distribution. The virus was discovered in 1971 in Germany during an outbreak in watch dogs.

Hosts susceptible

The virus is highly contagious, & affects dogs of all ages, but the disease **is severe in pups.**

Transmission

The disease is highly contagious and the affected dogs **shed the virus for 6-9 days, but sometimes for six months** following infection. Disease is spread through the **feces of infected dogs,** & infection occurs via oro-fecal route by ingestion. Transmission is by direct and indirect contact.

Pathogenesis, Clinical Symptoms & Lesions

The virus invades and replicates in the villi of the small intestine. The virus causes virus-induced apoptosis or programmed cell death of the epithelial mucosa of the small intestine.Within 2-3 days of infection, coronavirus spreads to the upper two-thirds of the pet's small intestine. The **incubation period is only 1-3 days.** In very rare cases the virus may also invade the spleen, liver and brain and lungs. During this period diarrhea begins. Diarrhea usually lasts 2-7 days. The diarrhea is due to **malabsorption of nutrients** and a deficiency in digestive enzymes.

The symptoms of coronavirus in puppies are **watery diarrhea** & not containing much mucous. It differs from the diarrhea produced by parvoviruses in that it rarely contains digested blood. Some pups with the disease **vomit,** others do not. Coronavirus diarrhea is often less violent than parvovirus diarrhea, but coronavirus can not be differentiated from parvovirus by clinical signs alone. Coronavirus diarrhea typically lasts **2-4 days and very few puppies die from it.** If puppies do die, there is usually concurrent infection at the same time, such as parasites, dual infection with parvovirus or malnutrition. There is feeling of gas-filled tender loops of intestine and enlarged mesenteric lymph nodes in their abdomens.

Usually, clinical signs are mild with anorexia, depression, and loose stools, followed by vomiting and diarrhea having a fetid odor. But in majority of cases, there is an asymptomatic infection especially in older dogs. Sicks recover in 1 - 2 weeks and fatal infections in uncomplicated cases are rare. **PM lesions** include nonspecific enteritis; & microscopic lesions consist of atrophy and fusion of intestinal villi.

Diagnosis

Collection of clinical samples includes fresh feces and intestine.

1. *Presumptive diagnosis:* Clinical symptoms & lesions are suggestive of coronavirus infection.Demonstration of coronavirus under electron microscopy of feces or by the fluorescent antibody staining of cryostat sections of intestine is good diagnostic test.
2. *Virus isolation:* Coronavirus can be isolated in cell cultures of canine origin.

Treatment & Prevention

There is no specific treatment for canine coronavirus except for prevention of **vomition** by metoclopramide /Reglan/ Chlorpromazine/Thorazine, and prochlorperazine /Compazine. **Diarrhea** is checked by giving medicines that relax intestinal spasms such as metoclopramide, in severe cases, loperamide, oral opiods or diphenoxylate/ Lomotil. **Dehydration** is corrected in case of all severe diarrheas by giving pedialite, a good oral liquid to them or if the pups are sicker, the fluids are given intravenously or subcutaneously. **Antibiotics** are given to control secondary bacterial infection until its own immune system conquers the virus.

It is ensured that pups are free from intestinal worms, receiving a quality diet, kept under reduced stress environment, avoiding of dog to dog contact or contact with objects that are contaminated with the virus, avoiding new puppy to places that other dogs visit until puppy is vaccinated, avoiding crowding, dirty facilities, grouping large numbers of dogs, & avoid poor sanitation. Quarantine newly-arrived puppies. Enteric Coronaviruses are moderately resistant to heat, acids and disinfectants but not nearly so much as Parvovirus, hence sanitizing the environment with a **1:20 dilution of ordinary household bleach or** sodium hypochlorite helps control the disease in kennels.

Vaccination

Inactivated vaccine is available; puppies are vaccinated against coronavirus at **9 and 12 weeks of age & then annually**. Adult dogs do not require yearly boosters. **Galaxy CV-** Intervet is a killed virus vaccine recommended for the vaccination of healthy dogs as an aid in the prevention of disease caused by canine coronavirus infection. The virus has been chemically inactivated and combined with an adjuvant designed to enhance the immune response. Dose: 1 ml SC or IM to dogs at 6 weeks of age, & a second dose is given 2 to 4 weeks later. A minimum of two doses is required for primary immunization. Annual revaccination with one dose is recommended. **Firstdose CV-**Pfizer is a killed coronavirus vaccine that provides protection against Corona virus infection in dogs which is the second most common cause of viral gastroentritis in dogs. Healthy dogs 6 weeks of age or older should receive 3 doses, each administered 3 weeks apart. Annual revaccination with single dose is recommended. Two combination vaccines include **Vanguard Plus 5/CV-** Pfizer is a live & killed virus vaccine (CD+ ICH+ PI+ Coronavirus+ Parvovirus) for vaccination of healthy dogs 6 weeks of age or older. Dose 1 ml SC or IM 3 doses, each given 3 weeks apart. Annual revaccination with a single dose is recommended. **Vanguard Plus 5 L4 CV-** Pfizeris a live & killed vaccine (CD+ ICH-2+ PI+ Coronavirus+ parvovirus+ L. Canicola+ Grippotyphosa +Haemorrhagiae + Pomona Bacterin). Dose I ml IM or SC to dogs 6 weeks of age or older, 3 doses 3 weeks apart & annual vaccination with a single dose. **Recombitek Corona MLV-**Merial is the only modified-live, canine-origin coronavirus available today, providing early rapid protection against canine coronavirus (CCV). The vaccine prevents intestinal damage, prevents shedding of virulent virus, no virus isolated in over 90% of small intestine samples, rapid, early protection against clinical and asymptomatic forms of CCV & affords proven protection in the face of maternal antibodies. It is recommended for the vaccination of healthy dogs 6 weeks of age and older for prevention of disease due to canine coronavirus. Dose: inject 1 ml (1 dose) SC or IM into healthy dogs; for primary vaccination, revaccinate with a second 1 ml dose 2 to 3 weeks later. Dogs less than 12 weeks of age should be revaccinated with a single 1 ml dose every 2 to 3 weeks, the last dose given at or over 12 weeks of age. Revaccinate annually with a single 1 ml dose.

Feline Coronavirus Infection/ Feline Infectious Peritonitis

Feline corona virus(**FCoV**) infection is mild in cats & ferrets, **affects enterocytes**, & produces mild gastroenteritis or inapparent infection in kittens, some remaining permanent virus excretors. Feline infectious peritonitis virus **(FIPV)**, a mutated form of FCoVis a progressive debilitating disease of *Felidae* of all ages worldwide, which is invariably fatal, & FIPV strains become tropic to macrophages.

Etiology: Feline coronavirus infection / feline infectious peritonitis is caused by *Feline corona virus* (FCoV) that belong to group 1 Coronavirus in the genus *Alphacoronavirus*, which also contains porcine gastroenteritis coronavirus (TGEV), the canine coronavirus (CCoV) and some human coronavirus.

The FCoV that infects cats & ferrets occurs in 2 forms, **Feline enteric coronavirus (FECV) and Feline infectious peritonitis virus (FIPV)** having 2 serotypes along with different antigens resulting in production of different antibodies: The **FCoV serotype I is most frequent; 80% of infections are due to type I FECV that could mutates to FIPV type I.** FCoV serotype I strains are wholly feline. They are difficult to grow in cell culture and cause a slowly developing cytopathic effect. **FCoV serotype II strains** seem to have arisen by recombination between FCoV serotype I and CCoV. They grow more rapidly than serotype I viruses, induce a **lytic cytopathic effect, & the type II cultures are easier to perform, so many studies are being conducted about type II,** though it is less common. FIPV and FECV strains can be serotype I or II serotype. FCoV type II is a recombinant virus type I with spike genes (S protein) replacement from FCoV by the canine enteric coronavirus (CCoV) spikes. In the widely accepted **"in vivo mutation" theory**, FIPV arises by mutation from parental FECV in the gastrointestinal tract of an infected cat, spreads systemically and causes FIP. **An alternative hypothesis is the "circulating virulent/avirulent" theory,** which suggests that both virulent and avirulent strains circulate in cat populations, and susceptible individuals exposed to the virulent strains develop the FIP disease. The relationship between virulence and macrophage/monocyte tropism has been firmly established. While both FIPV and FECV may cause viraemia, **only FIPV replicates in macrophages and causes the FIP disease**. Complex immune reactions between the virus, antiviral antibodies, and complement cause disseminated vasculitis, which is the hallmark of FIP.

Occurrence

Feline coronaviruses (FCoVs) are found throughout the world.

Hosts Susceptible

FCoV infection is extremely common in cat populations. Antibodies against FCoV are found in 20%–60% of pet cats and up to 100% of cats in catteries or multi-cat households. FCoVs are highly infectious and spread predominantly by the fecal-oral route. About 75%–100% of cats in multi-cat environments shed the virus. Young kittens are more susceptible with mild transient diarrhea of several days being generally the only sign.

Transmissions

Virus spread via contact, carriers, & infected cats. Most commonly, kittens are infected between the ages of **6 and 8 weeks**, at a time when maternally derived antibodies wane, mostly through contact with feces from their mothers or other FCoV-excreting cats. FECV virus infects gastrointestinal epithelial cells of cats-enterocytes, brush border, microvilli & villi. FECV infection shows few symptoms, is usually chronic, & the virus is **excreted in the feces of the healthy carrier**. Cats living in groups can contaminate each other during visits to a communal litter tray. Some cats are resistant to the virus and avoid infection or do not become carriers, while others may become carriers of FECV. Carriers may heal spontaneously, but acquired immunity may be short and they may go on to reinfect, usually within a few weeks if they are living in a group with healthy, but become persistent excretory carriers. Some cats never heal and they excrete virus in feces permanently.

Cats living in groups, in overcrowding have increased risk of mutation and conversion from FECV to FIPV causing feline infectious peritonitis (FIP). **FIP develops in cats whose immunity is low such as younger kittens, old cats, immunosuppressed due to viral FIV, FeLV and stress, including the stress of separation and adoption**. Infection of macrophages by FIPV is responsible for development of a fatal **granulomatous vasculitis**, or FIP. Therefore, FIP can occur when 2 factors are present: **virus mutation and health of cat.**

Pathogenesis, Clinical Symptoms & Lesions

After infection, FIPV is found in the tonsils and small intestinal mucosa within 24 hours of ingestion. Viral infection of the cecum, colon, mesenteric lymph nodes, and liver occurs over the next 14 days. Further systemic spread to any body organ or system occurs as the disease progresses.

Feline infectious peritonitis is an **immune complex mediated disease and systemic antibodies are not protective**. Pre-existing circulating coronavirus antibodies accelerate disease symptoms and cats do not die of FIP unless and until they make antibodies to the virus (antibody-dependent enhancement, ADE). In ADE, binding or opsonization of virus-antibody complexes by monocytes or macrophages results in infection of these cells rather than virus neutralization. **Virus-infected phagocytic cells disseminate FIPV infection to distant sites.**

The course of disease appears to be established very quickly following pathogenic FCoV infection. The **development of CMI is the most crucial factor in determining the ultimate outcome of FIPV infection**. Cats that produce humoral antibodies but fail to generate an effective CMI response develop **effusive FIP**. Experimental evidence demonstrates that cats with **non-effusive FIP** often have preceding transient effusive disease. Thus, **none effusive FIP is believed to result from a partially protective CMI response that is unable to wall off and contain the virus.**

Cats that mount a successful and rapid CMI response apparently do not develop active pathogenic FCoV disease although they may harbor latent virus for some period of time. In fact, the presence of low level of viremia apparently maintains their CMI status (premunition immunity). These recovered "immune carriers" are not ill but may have the potential to reactivate their latent infection if immunosuppressed. It is suspected that immune carriers may periodically shed infectious FCoV and may be a source of infection for naive cats. If immune carriers completely clear the FCoV infection, they may lose their CMI. If CMI is lost but humoral immunity is maintained, these cats may then be hypersensitive to challenge-exposure with virulent virus.

FECV infections are usually associated with mild disease, many cases remain asymptomatic, and the kittens show mild transient diarrhea of several days duration is generally the only sign. Vomiting occurs in a smaller proportion of cases and is not usually a prominent feature. However many healthy cats and kittens will also shed FCoV in their feces.

Feline Infectious Peritonitis Virus (FIPV)

There are two major forms of FIP. An **effusive form** characterized by high protein fluid accumulation in body cavities and a **noneffusive form characterized by pyogranulomatous lesions in any body organ or system.** Signs common to both forms of FIP include fluctuating **antibiotic-unresponsive fever,** lethargy, anorexia, and weight loss. Effusive FIP is caused by Arthus-type, immune-complex damage to small blood vessels that permits leakage of serum protein and fluid into body cavities. Cats with effusive FIP usually develop progressive, non painful abdominal distention due to peritoneal fluid accumulation. Pleural fluid is present in up to 25% of cats with effusive FIP. If a sufficient amount of fluid is present in the pleural space, these cats may exhibit exercise intolerance and dyspnea. Pericardial or scrotal fluid accumulation has also been observed in cats with effusive FIP.

In noneffusive FIP, vascular damage may produce mild, subclinical effusion early in the course of disease. The major lesions result from immune recruitment causing localized perivascular infiltrations of inflammatory cells (neutrophils, macrophages, lymphocytes, and plasma cells) in tissue parenchyma. These cellular infiltrates cause local tissue necrosis and disruption of normal organ function.

Because nonspecific signs predominate and any organ or system may be affected alone or in combination, the most consistent clinical feature of noneffusive FIP is its variability. The most common sites for lesions in cats with **noneffusive FIP are the eyes, central nervous system (CNS), and parenchymatous abdominal organs**. Ocular lesions include anterior **uveitis, keratic precipitates, hyphema, hypopyon, chorioretinitis, retinal hemorrhages, and retinal detachment**. Any part of the CNS can be affected and reported signs include seizures, vestibular disorders, ataxia, paresis, behavioral changes, peripheral neuropathies, hyperesthesia, and urinary incontinence. Damage to internal parenchymal organs causes a plethora of signs resulting from the site of the lesions, degree of organ damage, and resultant organ dysfunction.

Diagnosis

Collection of sample for various tests include: abdominal and thoracic fluids, lung, kidney, liver, spleen and brain.

1. *Presumptive diagnosis:* A typical history of FIP cases is acquisition of the cat from a cattery, a fever that waxes and wanes and does not improve with antimicrobial therapy, & kittens being infected between the ages of 6 and 8 weeks. FIP in the "wet" form having considerable amount of intracavitary effusion, pyogranuloma and fibrinous plaques on the serosal surfaces of abdominal organs, dyspnea, mild pyrexia, and muffled heart sounds, ocular involvement- uveitis, keratic precipitations, and changes in the coloration of the iris. In the non-effusive form, lesions commonly occur in eyes and CNS, but granulomas may also be found in the peritoneal cavity.
2. *Rivalta test* is used in order to differentiate a transudate from an exudate. A test tube is filled with distilled water and acetic acid is added. To this mixture one drop of the effusion to be tested is added. If the drop dissipates, the test is negative, indicating a transudate. If the drop precipitates, the test is positive, indicating an exudate. Since this test detects acute phase protein, a positive Rivalta's test may be suggestive of inflammation & FIP.
3. *Antibody detection:* Testing for antibodies by ELISA, indirect immunofluorescence assay to coronavirus is not helpful in the diagnosis of FIP, but is useful in screening healthy cats before introducing them to a coronavirus free cat or group. A positive result only indicates exposure to coronavirus and possible shedding of coronavirus, it does not differentiate between FECV & FIP, but it is claimed by some that high titers are suggestive of FIP.

Treatment & Prevention

There is no treatment for FIP. Some supportive measures include draining excessive fluid build-ups can provide temporary relief. A variety of medications & corticoids designed to reduce the abnormal immune response to the virus or reduce the ability of the virus to reproduce have been tried and may provide some relief from the disease.

Prevention of exposure to coronavirus is the best way to prevent FIP. Keeping cats indoors & introducing only bringing coronavirus-negative cats into the household are the best method of prevention.

Vaccination

A vaccine is available, but its use is controversial. The vaccine is given in the nose, and is designed to produce just a local response to prevent the virus from gaining access to the body. The vaccine is not 100 percent effective, and must be given before natural exposure to coronavirus to be effective. **Primucell FIP**, produced by Pfizer Animal Health, is a temperature-sensitive, modified-live virus vaccine that is given as an intranasal vaccine, and is licensed for use in cats at least 16 weeks of age. Primary vaccination: healthy cats 16 weeks of age or older should receive 2 intranasal doses administered 3-4 weeks apart. Revaccination: annual revaccination with a single dose is recommended. The vaccine appears to be safe, but the risks and benefits of vaccination should be weighed carefully.

Transmissible Gastroenteritis (TGE)

Transmissible gastroenteritis **(TGEV)** is a highly contagious enteric disease of pigs characterized by acute **diarrhea, vomiting, dehydration & death in piglets under 10 days,** but is less severe in older pigs of all ages, & in endemic cases, diarrhea is seen in piglets less than 6 days, weaned pigs & older pigs. There is **villous atrophy in small intestine.**

Etiology: Transmissible gastroenteritis is caused by *Transmissible gastroenteritis virus* (TGEV), a member of the *Coronaviridae*. Since 1984, a new respiratory variant of TGEV called *Porcine respiratory coronavirus* (PRCV) has spread throughout many parts of the world and is now found in most countries except Oceania. A deletion mutant of TGEV, porcine respiratory coronavirus (PRCV) appeared in the 1980s and has become prevalent worldwide, including the United States. PRCV replicates primarily in the respiratory tract and, to a minimal extent, in small intestinal epithelial cells. Usually, no clinical disease is produced or, uncommonly, mild respiratory disease is observed. PRCV does not produce clinical enteric disease. PRCV typically forms an endemic infection in intensely managed swine herds and infected pigs produce neutralizing antibodies which also neutralize TGEV. Therefore, when pigs already affected by PRCV get infected by TGEV, these pigs develop a less severe clinical form of TGE. Occurrences of TGE have become more sporadic now.

Occurrence

The disease has been reported on an occasional basis from parts of Europe, North America and Asia. There exists only one antigenic type, & the virus is serologically related to porcine respiratory coronavirus, canine coronavirus, and feline infectious peritonitis virus. The virus may remain viable on premises for up to three days.

Hosts Susceptible

The disease affects piglets of **10 days to 2 week old,** & pigs over 5 week old have mild clinical signs. Probably wild and domestic carnivores (foxes, dogs, possibly mink) and cats seroconvert to TGEV and are suggested as potential subclinical carriers of TGEV, serving as reservoirs between seasonal (winter) epidemics. But, only virus excretion by TGEV infected dogs has been confirmed as infectious for pigs.

Transmission

The virus is **shed in large numbers in the feces of infected pigs,** & stops within few weeks of recovery. The recovered pigs may contain the **virus in pulmonary & intestinal tissues up to 100 days.** Pig feces, therefore are the major source of transmission either directly through the purchased carrier pig or indirectly through mechanical transmission. Dogs become subclinically infected & shed the virus in their feces for **2 to 3 weeks.** Birds and in particular starlings may transmit the disease. Other sources of infection include contaminated feed, poor pen floors, poor pen hygiene associated with bad drainage, poor hygiene procedures between pens. Environmental contamination from one pen to another i.e. boots, brushes, shovels clothing etc, feeder pipes and feed bins, & continual purchase of naive weaners are source s of infection.

Pathogenesis

The route of transmission of TGEV is fecal-oral. The incubation period for TGEV is from 18 hours to 3 days. Initially, the pig swallows the virus which then travels to the small intestine, binds to receptors and is internalized into absorptive enterocytes. The virus replicates within enterocytes and then lyses them to enter the intestinal lumen, resulting in villous atrophy. Intestinal crypts are spared during TGE and become hyperplastic, therefore, secretion continues. However, absorption is partially impaired by enterocyte lysis and villous atrophy-malabsorption. At the same time, osmolarity in the intestinal lumen increases because of the presence of undigested material-maldigestion, which results from decreased enzymatic activity in the damaged intestinal mucosa. This increased osmolarity causes a pull of fluid into the intestinal lumen. Eventually, malabsorption and maldigestion lead to net increase in intestinal mucosal secretion and diarrhea. The ultimate cause of death is associated with dehydration and metabolic acidosis.

TGEV affects younger pigs more because their enterocytes are not able to be replaced as quickly as those of an older animal. Another reason of the higher morbidity/mortality in younger pigs is that the compensatory fluid absorption takes place in the large intestine of older pigs, compared with younger pigs.

Clinical Symptoms & Lesions

In piglets: In the sucking piglet the disease is very severe. There is acute watery diarrhoea, & almost 100% mortality within 2 to 3 days in piglets under 7 days of age due to severe dehydration and electrolyte imbalance. There is no response to antibiotic therapy. The most striking feature is the **wet and dirty hairy appearance of all the litter** due to the profuse diarrhea.

In weaners & growers; when the virus is introduced into a herd for the first time there is rapidly spreading, vomiting and watery diarrhea, eventually affecting almost all the animals. Disease disappears spontaneously over a 3 to 5 week period. Mortality is usually low. The main effect on the individual growing pig is dehydration which is resolved in about a week. But the disease may increase the slaughter age by 5-10 days.

Chronic or endemic disease occurs in herds less than 300 sows; the virus is usually self eliminating provided there are good all-in-all-out procedures in farrowing houses and grower accommodation. In some herds, the virus persists in the growing herd because piglets at weaning time, still under the influence of the maternal IgA antibody, move into houses where the virus still persists. Once the antibody disappears, the pigs become infected allowing the virus to multiply. The pigs then shed the virus, contaminating the weaner rooms and infecting pigs being weaned after them. TGE can become endemic in herds in a mild form with high morbidity but low mortality.

In sows: In acute outbreaks the most striking feature is the rapidity of spread. There is vomiting, diarrhea, & adult animals show varying degrees of inappetence and usually recover over a 5 to 7 day period.

Diagnosis

Collection of clinical specimens for various tests include: portions of jejunum and ileum with contents.

1. *Presumptive diagnosis:* The clinical signs in acute cases are almost diagnostic. There are no other enteric diseases that spread so rapidly across all pigs.
2. *Virus isolation:* The virus may be cultivated in cell cultures of swine origin with little or no observable cytopathic effects.
3. *Antigen detection:* Using the intestine of a fresh dead pig, fluorescent antibody test detects the viral antigen in cryostat sections or scrapings of affected intestine.

Porcine epidemic diarrhea (PED) could give a similar picture but it would be less acute and with less mortality in sucking pigs.

Treatment & Prevention

There is no specific treatment for TGE. Antibiotic treatment by mouth in individual piglets may reduce secondary infections. Provide water containing electrolyte and an antibiotic such as neomycin. Make this available to the litters twice daily. Improve the nursing and environment of the litter by providing extra heat and deep bedding to reduce the weights of infection from the diarrhea. Apply strict sanitary measures to prevent spread to susceptible swine.

Vaccination

Several manufacturers are licensed to produce TGEV vaccines in the USA: the vaccines include modified live and inactivated vaccines. The modified live vaccines are used for oral administration to pregnant sows (to induce passive immunity) or have also been licensed for oral administration to nursing or weaned pigs (to induce active immunity). Inactivated TGEV vaccines are licensed for parenteral inoculation of pregnant sows by the intramuscular route or for intraperitoneal administration to nursing or weaned pigs. In general, these vaccines induced marginal passive protection against TGEV challenge of nursing piglets when evaluated under controlled experimental conditions or in the field in TGEV/PRCV herds. Although they fail to adequately protect against epizootic TGE, data suggest that these vaccines may provide some efficacy against enzootic TGEV by stimulating an anamnestic antibody response to TGEV in serum and milk Vaccination of sows orally **prior to farrowing** with non attenuated vaccine provides better colostral derived Ig A antibodies to piglets. Recombinant TGE virus **subunit S**

glycoprotein vaccine used SC or IM is used with an aim to produce colostral Ig A antibodies that protects the piglets till weaning. Since stronger and long lasting immunity is achieved via natural infection, one method is to feed infectious intestine and feces to pregnant sows about a month before farrowing. **TP VAC** (Porcine Transmissible Gastroenteritis, Porcine Epidemic Diarrhea)- Komipharm International Co Ltd is a killed vaccine containing strain 175L (PTG) & SM98P (PED) with adjuvant Montanide IMS 1313 NPR is licensed in South Korea. **Nisseiken TGE/PED Vaccine**(Porcine Transmissible Gastroenteritis, Porcine Epidemic Diarrhea)- Nisseiken Co Ltd is a killed vaccine containing strain H-5 (TGE) & P-5V (PED) with no adjuvant & is licensed in Japan.

Porcine Epidemic Diarrohea

Porcine epidemic diarrhea **(PEDV)** affects swine of all ages in Asia & Europe; infection occurs via oro-nasal route. There is; watery diarrhea, **older pigs are more severely affected** but there is less mortality in neonates. There is **shortening of small intestinal villi like TGE.**

Etiology: Porcine epidemic diarrhea is caused by *Porcine epidemic diarrhea virus* (PEDV).

Occurrence

Porcine epidemic diarrhea was first reported in UK in 1971, and the virus was identified during episodes of epizootic diarrhea in pigs in Belgium and in the UK.. The disease has subsequently been reported in Canada, Hungary, Germany, China, Korea, and Japan. However, outbreaks of severe PED are now rare in Europe. Very likely, this is due to the enzootic character of the virus and the presence of lactogenic immunity, which protects suckling pigs. More recently, severe outbreaks of PED with high mortality have been reported in Spain, Japan, and Korea. During late 2007, the PED outbreak appeared first in Nakornpathom province before spreading throughout Thailand. The Asian epizootics are so severe that they cannot be differentiated clinically from acute TGEV outbreaks, and they incur heavy economic losses. Until now, PEDV has not been detected in the United States or South America. Seroprevalence of PEDV has been confirmed in most major swine-producing countries worldwide.

Hosts Susceptible

PEDV causes diarrhea in pigs. Two clinical forms of PED exists, PED type I affects pigs 4-5 days age, while PED type II affects pigs causing diarrhea in pigs of all age groups.

Transmission

Mode of transmission of PEDV is like TGEV, but PEDV tends to persist more easily on infected premises. **Fecal-oral transmission is probably the main or only route of infection.** Most commonly, the introduction of infected pigs into susceptible farms causes outbreaks of PED within 4 to 5 days. Virus may also be introduced through contaminated equipments and other fomites or personnel. After a disease outbreak, PEDV may disappear, or it may become enzootic on farms where there are sufficient litters of pigs to allow the virus to be maintained through infection of consecutive litters that have lost their lactogenic immunity at weaning.

Pathogenesis, Clinical Symptoms & Lesions

PEDV replicates in the cytoplasm of villous enterocytes throughout the small intestine, causing epithelial cell degeneration with subsequent villus shortening. But, the effects of TGE are more intense and severe. Enterocytes along the entire length of villi are susceptible to infection with PEDV. The clinical course in gnotobiotic pigs experimentally infected with PEDV was much milder than that in pigs infected with wt-PEDV. The ca-PEDV was notably less virulent, viral replication was slower, and histopathological changes were less evident. Porcine epidemic diarrhea virus has also been detected in epithelial cells of the colon in conventional grower pigs with both experimental and naturally occurring PED. The cause of sudden death accompanied by acute back muscle necrosis that has been described in finishing and adult pigs with PED is unknown.

The severity of clinical disease caused by PEDV is highly variable, depending largely on the immunological or enzootic status of the pig farm. The main and often only clinical sign is **watery diarrhea**. Diarrheic feces are watery and flocculent, and have a characteristic fetid smell owing to steatorrhea. Affected animals commonly vomit. In susceptible breeding herds, pigs of all ages may be affected, with morbidity approaching 100%. Watery diarrhea, and dehydration and metabolic acidosis causing mortality of 50 to 80%, are the principal features of PED in suckling pigs, whereas infections of feeder and grower pigs are characterized by diarrhea, anorexia, depression, and a high morbidity but low mortality (1 to 3%). In enzootic situations, PEDV may cause persistent diarrhea in recently weaned pigs. Clinical symptom are very similar to TGE, but there is often a slower spread of disease and lower mortality in baby piglets, and more severe disease than with TGEV if infection occurs toward the end of the growing period. Mortality in grower pigs may reach 1 to 3%, and pigs often appear to have abdominal pain and may die acutely during the early stages of diarrhea or even prior to its onset. Recovery occurs after approximately 7 to 10 days.

Diagnosis

Porcine epidemic diarrhea cannot be diagnosed on the basis of clinical findings alone, and acute outbreaks of PED cannot be clinically differentiated from TGE regardless of the age of pigs infected. Laboratory methods are necessary for an etiologic diagnosis.

Virus antigen detection: The direct immunofluorescence test (IFT) for detection of viral antigen and enzyme-linked immunosorbant assays (ELISA) to demonstrate PEDV antigen in feces or antibodies in serum are used. The virus can also be detected by immunohistochemistry (IHC), polymerase chain reaction (PCR), indirect fluorescent antibody test (IFA), in situ hybridization, and electron microscopy (EM). Fluorescent antibody test and IHC test, done on sections of small intestine from pigs with acute diarrhea, are the most sensitive, rapid, and reliable methods. They should be used preferably within 3 days of onset of diarrhea. Electron microscopy is widely used to detect viral particles in fecal material of pigs with diarrhea.

Treatment & Prevention

Symptomatic treatment of diarrhea is recommended, including free access to water to diminish dehydration, and withholding of feed, particularly in growing swine.

Sanitary measures should be taken to prevent introduction of PEDV to the farm. Introduction of persistently infected pigs poses the highest risk, and disease can also be spread by human traffic between affected units. After diagnosis of PED, because of the slow spread of disease, the primary concern should be initiation of preventive measures to temporarily prevent virus entrance into farrowing units. Artificial exposure of pregnant sows to feces from PEDV-infected pigs stimulates lactogenic immunity and helps to postpone infection of these sows' piglets until they are older, resulting in fewer deaths. If persistence of the virus is diagnosed in consecutive litters of weaned piglets after an outbreak has occurred, virus elimination can be attempted by removing pigs immediately after weaning to another site for at least 4 weeks.

Porcine epidemic diarrhea virus is stable between pH 5.0 and 9.0 at 4°C and between pH 6.5 and 7.5 at 37°C. Cell Culture adapted PEDV loses infectivity when heated to 60°C for 30 minutes, but is moderately stable at 50°C. Porcine epidemic diarrhea virus is inactivated by most virucidal disinfectants, including cresol, sodium hydroxide (2%), formalin (1%), sodium carbonate (4% anhydrous or 10% crystalline, with 0.1% detergent), ionic and non-ionic detergents, strong iodophors (1%) in phosphoric acid, and lipid solvents such as chloroform.

Vaccination

Recently, the immunoprophylactic effects of chicken egg yolk immunoglobulin (IgY) against PEDV were investigated in neonatal pigs. Administration of IgY was associated with reduced mortality and increased survival rate in piglets after challenge exposure to PEDV. This suggests that IgY against PEDV might be an alternative prophylactic measure similar to stimulated lactogenic immunity. **Nisseiken PED Live Vaccine** containing strain Live P-5V without adjuvant is licensed in Japan for vaccination of pigs against PED. **TP VAC** (Porcine Transmissible Gastroenteritis, Porcine Epidemic Diarrhea)- Komipharm International Co Ltd is a killed vaccine containing strain 175L (PTG) & SM98P (PED) with adjuvant Montanide IMS 1313 NPR is licensed in South Korea. **Nisseiken TGE/PED Vaccine**(Porcine Transmissible Gastroenteritis, Porcine Epidemic Diarrhea)- Nisseiken Co Ltd is a killed vaccine containing strain H-5 (TGE) & P-5V (PED) with no adjuvant & is licensed in Japan.

Porcine Hemagglutinating Encephalomyelitis

Porcine hemagglutinating encephalomyelitis (PEV) or **vomition & wasting disease** is a viral disease of **young pigs less than 3 weeks of age** characterized by **vomiting, constipation, anorexia, & either rapid death or chronic emaciation. Motor disorders** due to acute encephalomyelitis were also seen during some outbreaks infecting young pigs in America & Europe.

Etology: Porcine hemagglutinating encephalomyelitis (PEV) or vomition & wasting disease is caused by *Porcine hemagglutinating encephalomyelitis virus* (PEV), which comprises a single strain and is the only known neurotropic CoV for pigs. The virus grows in several types of porcine cell cultures, in which it causes syncytia. It agglutinates RBC of several animal species.

Occurrence

PEV was first isolated in Canada in 1958 from the brains of suckling piglets with encephalomyelitis; it was later isolated in England from piglets exhibiting vomiting, anorexia, and depression, where it was named "vomiting and wasting disease" (VWD). Neurologic and digestive characteristics of the disease were experimentally reproduced in pigs by using the same field virus isolate. The infection has been reported in the major pig-raising countries of Europe, Asia, and North America, where it seemed to be endemic with no clinical outbreaks.

Hosts Susceptible

PEV or vomition & wasting disease virus infects young pigs less than 3 weeks of age.

Transmission

Immune sows transfer maternal IgA antibodies to their piglets, which are protected until they have developed an age resistance; thus, clinical outbreaks are rare. However, if the virus enters a susceptible herd with neonatal piglets, morbidity and mortality may be high. The virus is shed from nasal secretions & readily transmitted by aerosols.

Pathogenesis

After entry through aerosols, the virus first **replicates in the epithelial cells of nasal mucosa, tonsils, lungs, and to a very limited extent, in the small intestine**. After local replication, the virus **spreads from the peripheral nervous system to the central nervous system.** The virus then invades defined nuclei of the **medulla oblongata via the peripheral nervous system** and subsequently spreads to the **entire brain stem,** and possibly to the cerebrum and cerebellum. **Vomiting is thought to be caused by viral replication in the vagal sensory ganglion**. Wasting is due to vomiting and delayed emptying of the stomach, which is the result of virus-induced lesions in the intramural plexus. Infection of cerebral and cerebellar neurons may rarely cause motor disorders.

Clinical Symptoms & Lesions

Incubation period is 4-7 days. Affected piglets usually exhibits **listlessness, vomiting, anorexia and depression**; hence the disease was known as "vomiting and wasting disease" (VWD) in the past. In severe cases infected piglets will develop encephalomyelitis. **Neurologic signs** such as abnormal gait, dullness, inability to eat, tremors, and nystagmus are observed in some pigs. **The mortality rate in infected piglets under 3 weeks old is nearly 100%,** but the incidence of infection is small as most piglets are protected by maternal antibodies. However, the risk of PEV outbreaks has increased due to the use of pathogen-free pigs which have no antibodies to the virus.

The affected pigs show cachexia and abdominal distention in chronically affected pigs. Their stomachs are dilated and filled with gas. **Microscopically,** perivascular cuffing, gliosis, and neuronal degeneration are found in the medulla in 70-100% of pigs with nervous signs, and in 20-60% of pigs with VWD. Neuritis of peripheral sensory ganglia, particularly the trigeminal ganglia, is seen regularly. Degeneration of the ganglia of the stomach wall and perivascular cuffing are found in 15-85% of pigs with VWD. The lesions are most pronounced in the pyloric gland area.

Diagnosis

Presumptive diagnosis can be made by clinical signs, age susceptibility, and disease course with histopathologic findings.

Virus can be isolated from the tonsils and respiratory tract during the incubation period, which lasts about 5 days. Isolation of virus may be attempted on tonsil, brain, and lung samples from affected piglets.

Molecular detection by reverse transcription coupled real time PCR enables rapid, sensitive and specific detection of the virus and is useful in identifying and isolating infected pigs.

Treatment & Pevention

There is no treatment, once signs are evident, the disease runs its course. Spontaneous recoveries are rare.

Prevention includes: confirmation of the virus, identification PEV carriers, ensure that animal colonies and populations are free of PEV, early prevention of spread of the virus among animals, minimize human exposure to the virus, & safety monitoring of biological products that derive from animals.

Vaccination

Piglets born from non immune sows during an outbreak can be protected by injecting, at birth, either hyperimmune serum or serum from sows randomly selected at slaughter. However, the time lapse between diagnosis and cessation of the disease is usually too short for this procedure to be effective. Maintaining the virus on the farm leads to naturally induced immunity in the sows that avoids outbreaks in piglets.

Genus : *Betacoronavirus*

Bovine Coronavirus Infection

Bovine coronavirus (BCoV) causes **diarrhea in calves & winter dysentry** and dehydration. In some calves, feces contain flecks of blood. Bovine coronavirus (BCV) is also recognized as the primary etiology of **winter dysentery (WD) of adult cows** characterized by high morbidity (50-100%), but low mortality (1-2%), BCoV can also cause a "respiratory syndrome" that is usually mild or even subclinical and occurs primarily in adult dairy cows, and coronaviral diarrhea in young (3 to 21 days-old) calves. WD is a clinically and economically important disease in many countries including the United States. It has the highest incidence of WD between November and April when cattle are kept in close confinement. Virus is spread via oro-fecal route & shedding of virus occurs in feces.

Etiology: Bovine coronavirus infection is caused by *Bovine coronavirus* (BCoV).

Occurrence

BCoV occurs frequently in the northern USA, Canada, the UK, Europe, Australia, New Zealand, Israel, and Japan. Winter dysentery is common in northern climates where animals are housed indoors for extended periods during the winter months. Mortality rates associated with winter dysentery are generally low (1-2%), but morbidity in affected herds is high, with 20-50% of the animals in a herd exhibiting clinical signs within a few days and close to 100% of animals in the herd exhibiting signs within a week.

Hosts susceptible

Coronaviral diarrhea occurs in young calves between **3 to 21 days-old,** but winter diarrhea occurs in **adult cattle**. Adult lactating cows that have recently calved are most severely affected, but the disease can affect younger or older animals and males. Because mucosal immunity is important in preventing or recovering from BCV infection, calves that do not receive colostrum are especially susceptible to BCoV enteritis. Adult lactating cows that have recently calved are most severely affected, but the disease can affect younger or older animals and males.

Transmission

BCoV is present in the **feces** 1 to 2 days before the onset of diarrhea and for several days after the diarrhea has resolved. BCoV can also be found in **nasal secretions** of calves with BCoV diarrhea. Recovered calves that are apparently immune to disease can still **shed BCV in their nasal secretions or feces.**

BCV is transmitted via the fecal-oral route via ingestion of feed or water contaminated with feces from clinical cases or clinically normal carrier animals. Viral particles present in respiratory secretions of affected animals may further favour transmission. Transmission of disease is promoted by close confinement. Winter dysentery is highly contagious and easily introduced to barns by visitors, carrier animals, and fomites.

Coronaviruses survive best at low temperatures and at low ultraviolet light intensities, which can lead to a buildup of virus in the environment during the colder months. Some degree of immunity to winter dysentery appears to develop because recurrences, if seen in the same herd, are noted at 1- to 5-yr intervals. BCoV can infect respiratory epithelium; hence it may predispose calves to opportunistic bacterial infections. Calves with respiratory

BCoV infection can shed high numbers of virus in their nasal mucus and this virus can cause enteric and/or respiratory disease in other cattle.

Pathogenesis

After virus entry by fecal oral route, the virus is present usually in both enteric tissues & respiratory tract of calves. BCoV infection is endemic in farms & is maintained in clinically infected calves & persistently infected clinically normal calves & cows. BCoV replicates in mature enterocytes in small intestine & colon, & destroys them. This causes malabsorption & diarrhea. Inflammatory mediators that cause hypersecretion in the small intestine and colon contribute to the voluminous diarrhea seen in cattle with winter dysentery. In addition, destruction of epithelial cells in the colonic crypts results in transudation of extracellular fluid and blood, explaining the hemorrhagic nature of the diarrhea in some cases.

Clinical Symptoms

The clinical syndrome is characterized by an acute onset of **fluid diarrhea and a profound decrease in milk production** (25-95% production loss). Feces are liquid and homogenous with little odor, dark green to black, and rarely contain blood or mucus. A sweet, musty, unpleasant odor is reported in barns with large numbers of affected cattle. Nasolacrimal discharge or cough may accompany or precede the diarrhea. Other signs include **mild colic, dehydration, depression, a brief period of anorexia, and some decrease in body condition.** Occasionally, animals exhibit more severe signs such as passage of **feces with variable amounts of blood, severe dehydration, and weakness**. Fatalities are rare. Diarrhea in individual animals has a short course, and feces return to normal in 2-3 days in most animals. Disease in the herd typically subsides in 1-2 wk, but milk production may take weeks to months to return to normal.

Lesions include that the small intestine may be dilated and flaccid. Lesions are primarily seen in the large intestine and consist of cecal and colonic mucosal hyperemia, linear streaks or pinpoint-sized hemorrhages mostly along the colonic mucosal ridges, and blood in the lumen of the large intestine. Histological findings may include widespread **degeneration and necrosis of colonic glandular epithelium.**

Diagnosis

Electron microscopy detects coronavirus particles in feces or intestinal contents. Immunofluorescent microscopy detects coronavirus antigens in infected tissues e.g., small intestine and spiral colon of calves, spiral colon of cows, or trachea and lungs of calves with respiratory syndrome. BCoV antigen can also be detected by ELISA in feces or gut.

Serology can detect sero-conversion or a 4-fold increase in serum immunoglobin levels.

Treatment & Prevention

Most affected cattle recover spontaneously. Fresh water, palatable feed, and free-choice salt should be available at all times. The use of astringents, protectants, and adsorbents is controversial. IV fluid therapy or blood transfusions may be required in severely affected cattle.

There is no vaccine for winter dysentery. Isolation of newly introduced cattle for 2 weeks and isolation of any adult cow with diarrhea is advised to decrease the likelihood of disease introduction into a herd. In an outbreak, access to the premises should be restricted, and all persons in contact with affected cattle should ensure that their footwear and clothing are clean before leaving an affected farm.

Genus : *Gammacoronavirus*

Infectious Bronchitis

Infectious bronchitis (IB) is an acute, highly contagious viral disease that occurs in **young chickens worldwide & affects respiratory, reproductive & renal systems** with high mortality. The common symptoms are coughing, gasping, tracheobronchitis, stunting, reduced egg production in layers, & misshapen & soft shelled eggs. Some **neurotropic strains cause intestinal nephritis**, mild respiratory signs with high mortality. Some strains of the virus cause severe **kidney damage** and may be associated with high mortality. The economic losses of Infectious bronchitis is mainly due to poor growth performance and mortality due to the respiratory disease in broilers, egg production losses in layers and breeders, & losses caused by renal damage in broilers, layers and breeders. The negative effects of an IB infection can be prevented by vaccination and implementing sound biosecurity principles.

Etiology: Infectious bronchitis (IB) is caused by *Infectious bronchitis virus*. The virus has the ability to mutate or change its genetic makeup readily, & hence many serotypes have been identified and have complicated efforts at control through vaccination. IBV strains are classified into different serotypes based largely on **virus-neutralization (VN) tests**, & different serotypes do not always cross-protect. Three common serotypes in North America are the **Massachusetts, Connecticut, and Arkansas 99 IB viruses**. In Europe, various "Holland variants," usually designated using numbers (D-274, D-212) are recognized. Several strains of IB virus have a strong affinity for the kidney

(nephropathogenic strains), which may cause severe renal damage. The most important IBV serotype is the **Massachusetts serotype, & it has the ability to cross-protect against a number of viruses belonging to several different serotypes or genotype.**

Occurrence

IB was first described in 1931 in a flock of young chickens in the USA. Since then, the disease has been identified in broilers, layers and breeder chickens throughout the world. Vaccines to help reduce losses in chickens were first used in the 1950s. IB is considered to be worldwide in distribution. The incidence is not constant throughout the year, being reported more often during the cooler months.

Hosts Susceptible

IB has been reported as a disease only in chickens, & **all ages of chickens** are susceptible to infection, but clinical disease severity varies.

Transmission

IBV is **shed from the respiratory tract** for a week after infection; the virus has been recovered over weeks from **feces** of infected birds. Disease is spread by the **respiratory route** in droplets expelled during coughing or sneezing by infected chickens. Spread of the disease through a flock is very rapid. Transmission from farm to farm is related to movement of contaminated people, equipment, and vehicles. Following infection, **chickens may remain carriers and shed the virus for several weeks.** Egg transmission of the virus does not occur.

Pathogenesis

After entry through respiratory tract, IBV is attached to **ciliated epithelial cells** on respiratory tract, primarily **replicates in the respiratory system.** Then viruses spread into blood vessel in which they cause **viremia.** Viremia occurs in **1-2 days** after infection due to which the virus is **distributed throughout the body- in oviduct, kidneys & bursa of Fabricius.** Virulence of the infecting virus strains determines the severity of symptoms & lesions. **Nephropathogenic strain causes swelling, & urolithiasis in kidney.** Grossly, pale color of kidney could be seen. Microscopically, **uric crystals** could be found in the renal tubule or ureter.

Clinical Signs

Clinical signs in **chicks** include **coughing, sneezing, râles, nasal discharge, and frothy exudate in the eyes.** Affected chicks appear depressed and huddle near a heat source. In an affected flock, all birds will typically develop clinical signs within 36 to 48 hours. Clinical disease will normally **last for 7 days.** Mortality is usually very low, unless complicated by other factors such as *M. gallisepticum*, immunosuppression, & poor air quality.

Clinical signs in **chickens** are coughing, sneezing and râles. A **drop in egg production of 5 to 10% lasting for 10 to 14 days** is commonly seen. In face of complicating factors, production drops may be as high as 50%. Eggs produced following infection may have **thin shells, irregular shells, and thin, & watery albumen.** Loss of pigment in brown-shelled eggs is common. In severe complicated cases, chickens may develop **airsacculitis**. Chickens that experienced a severe vaccination reaction following chick vaccination or field infection during the first two weeks of life may have permanent damage in the oviduct, resulting in hens with poor production.

In recent years, **nephropathogenic stains have become more common in laying flocks**. These strains may cause an elevated mortality during the infection or long after as a result of kidney damage that progress to urolithiasis.

PM lesions associated with IB include a mild to moderate inflammation of the upper respiratory tract. If complicating factors are present, airsacculitis and increased mortality may be noted in younger chickens. **Kidney damage** may be significant following infection with nephropathogenic strains. Kidneys of affected chickens will be pale and swollen. **Urate deposits** may be observed in the kidney tissue and in the ureters, which may be occluded. Laying chickens may have yolk material in the body cavity and developing yolks in the ovary may be flaccid. Infection of very young chicks may result in the development of cystic oviducts.

Diagnosis

Collection of clinical samples for various tests includes trachea, lungs, kidneys & sera samples.

1. *Virus isolation*: Virus isolation is done in specific pathogen-free chicken embryos at 9 to 11 days of incubation by the allantoic sac route of inoculation. Several passages may be needed to observe unique stunting, curling of embryo, crystal urate deposition in the kidney or death.

2. *Serology*: commonly used include ELISA, virus neutralization, and HI tests.

Virus typing has traditionally been performed by neutralization using selected IB antisera. More recently, PCR and restriction fragment length polymorphism (RFLP) have been used to differentiate IBV serotypes.

Treatment & Prevention

Vaccination

The common serotypes used in most vaccination programs are the Massachusetts, Connecticut, and Arkansas serotypes that are available in both **modified live vaccines and inactivated water-in-oil emulsions**. In Europe, various **Holland variants** usually designated by number (e.g. D-274, D-1466) are used. Polyvalent vaccines, which contain multiple strains, are also available. Attenuated vaccine is administered to birds at **1 - 2 weeks of age** via drinking water with revaccination 3 - 4 weeks later, often with a killed vaccine injected subcutaneously. There are many types of virus, & hence the vaccine used should include the prevailing type(s) for a given area. Combined vaccine ND+IBV administered at 2 weeks of age include **Triplevac**-Intervet (B1 Strain, Mass/Conn) given in water/spray; **Trivac-Ark** (B1 Strain, Mass/Ark) given through spray, & **Broilerbrone –HN-79** (LaSota Strain-Mass Type/Holland) administered through water /eyedrop. Combined vaccine ND+IBV administered at 5 weeks of age include **Triplevac**- Intervet (B1 Strain, Mass/Conn) given in water/spray; **Combovac -30** (LaSota Strain, Mass/Conn) given through spray, **Trivac-Ark** (B1 Strain, Mass/Ark) or **Broilerbrone –HN-79** (LaSota Strain-Mass Type/Holland) administered through water /eyedrop. Combined vaccine ND +IBV administered at 15 weeks of age include **Triplevac**- Intervet (B1 Strain, Mass/Conn) given in water/spray; **Combovac -30** (LaSota Strain) given through spray, **Trivac-Ark**(B1 Strain, Mass/Ark) given through spray; **Broilerbrone –HN-79** (LaSota Strain-Mass Type/Holland) administered through water /eyedrop or Polybron N-63 (LaSota Strain, Mass/Conn). Combined vaccine IBD/Reo/ND/IBV administered at 18 weeks of age includes **Breeder Vac-IV-Plus** given through IM/SC injection.

Turkery Coronavirus Infection

Turkery corona virus(**TCoV**) causes **Blue comb disease or enteritis** which is an acute, highly contagious disease of turkeys, especially **young poults**. The disease is characterized by sudden onset, marked depression, anorexia, diarrhea, dehydration, and weight loss. TCoV belongs to group III coronaviruses closely related to infectious bronchitis virus (IBV) of chickens. TCoV cannot be propagated readily in cell culture although at least some isolates can be propagated in turkey embryos.

Occurrence

TCoV occurs in USA, Canada, UK & other countries. TCoV was reported in the USA in the 1990's. Studies in the US showed that the condition led to poor feed conversion, poor weight gain and an increase in the use of medication. TCoV was first confirmed in Britain in 2001. The incidence in 13 day old poults includes 20 per cent showing symptoms of **stunting, unevenness and lameness and a mortality rate of four per cent.**

Hosts Susceptible

The disease was most common in young birds aged between **three and 18 weeks.**

Transmission

The disease is spread via direct or indirect contact, or contaminated premises, recovered virus carriers, stresses & secondary infections.

Pathogenesis & Clinical Signs

The clinical signs of TCoV infection usually appear at **7 to 28 days of age** with symptoms of diarrhea, chirping, litter eating, decreased feed efficiency, decreased weight gain, and uneven flock growth. Other symptoms are anorexia, diarrhea, dehydration, and cyanosis or darkening of head, catarrhal enteritis, & intestinal villous atrophy. The sick birds appear cold, chirp constantly, & seek heat. There is severe drop in egg production, and eggs may have chalky shells.

The morbidity is usually high and mortality may be low; however, mortality over 40 to 50% occasionally occurred in Indiana flocks in 1993. It has shown that turkey poult enteritis can be experimentally induced by gavaging turkey poults with intestinal contents from affected poults. Electron microscopic examination of intestinal contents from affected turkey poults often revealed coronavirus. In addition, intestines were often positive for coronavirus by fluorescent antibody testing. However, attempts to isolate turkey coronavirus using various cell lines have not been successful. Turkey embryos have been used for the isolation, propagation and characterization of turkey coronavirus. Turkey coronavirus from affected intestinal contents filtered at 0.22 microns has been successfully passaged and propagated in turkey embryos. This is the only *in vivo* system available in propagating turkey coronavirus. TCoV has been associated as a cause of high mortality in young turkeys; however under laboratory conditions the virus causes diarrhea and growth depression without significant mortality. High mortality in young turkeys has been experimentally reproduced by dual infection with TCoV and enteropathogenic strains of *E. coli* (EPEC). Turkeys inoculated with only EPEC do not show clinical signs of disease. The infected intestines were often dilated and contained gas and greenish-brown fluid.

Diagnosis

Control of turkey poult enteritis needs continuous monitoring of turkey poult intestines and sera from the field by fluorescent antibody testing, production of monoclonal antibody to coronavirus & ELISA for turkey coronavirus antibody or turkey coronavirus, and application of PCR for the detection of turkey coronavirus are under way. A recombinant TCoV antigen-based ELISA was developed based on the complete nucleocapsid protein of TCoV. This ELISA performed significantly better at detecting antibodies against TCoV in turkey sera than a commercially available IBV ELISA kit. The RT-PCR was sensitive and specific for TCoV; RT-PCR could effectively differentiate between TCoV and IBV. The closely related bovine coronavirus and transmissible gastroenteritis virus of pigs were differentiated from TCoV using the same RT-PCR with slight modifications.

Treatment & Prevention

There is no effective treatment for TCoV infection of turkey poult enteritis; strict biosecurity and use of crumble feed are helpful in reducing the severity of the disease. Preventative measures include removal of any dead birds and good management of the litter as well as controlling contact with vermin and wild birds. Prevention was also aided by monitoring for the conditions and switching from multi-age to single age sites. Vaccines arenot available to control the disease.

Genes : *Torovirus*

Bovine Torovirus (BTOV-Beda Virus) Infection

Bovine torovirus **(BToV-Breda virus)** infection causes **diarrhea in newborn calves not fed colostrum.** The BToV belongs to the *Torovirus* genus within the *Coronaviridae* family. The BToV produces mild to moderate diarrhea in calves under both experimental and field conditions. The BToV has been recognized in diarrheic dairy and **beef calves from a few days through 5–6 months of age**. In addition, calves up to 10 months of age develop diarrhea associated with this virus. After oral or intranasal inoculation of calves with BToV, the virus infects the small and large intestines, resulting in moderate to watery diarrhea by 24–72 hours post inoculation along with depression and anorexia that lasts for 3–5 days. The virus infects the epithelial cells from the middle and lower parts of the villi extending into the crypt cells, inducing cytopathic effects, necrosis, and exfoliation of the enterocytes. In severe cases, calves dehydrate by 24–48 hours after onset, and death may ensue in 48–96 hours

In 1972, a virus was isolated from a horse in Berne, Switzerland, in 1982, & a similar, unclassified virus was isolated from calves in Breda, Iowa & in

1984 particles resembling these viruses were discovered in the feces of humans. This virus has been detected by electron microscopy, immunofluorescence, and ELISA in the United States and in other countries such as Belgium, Canada, Costa Rica, The Netherlands, India, France, Italy, South Africa and Germany. On the basis of the available information on these viruses, BToV was detected at a significantly higher rate in diarrheic samples than in asymptomatic samples, suggesting that BToV may act as a risk factor for diarrhea in Japanese cattle. Epidemiologic studies have shown that bovine torovirus is widespread in **The Netherlands, Germany and Switzerland, the United Kingdom, and the United States, with approximately 90% of dairy cattle being seropositive.** In one study from Belgium, bovine toroviruses were found to play a role in **respiratory, digestive, and reproductive disorders of cattle.** In a recent study from Saskatchewan, Canada, BRV-like particles were detected in 42 of 221 fecal or intestinal specimens of symptomatic calves. The RT-PCR was successfully applied for the diagnosis of torovirus in fecal specimens of calves. It remains impossible to determine whether bovine torovirus was the primary cause of diarrhea in the symptomatic calves or had concomitant infections with other viral agents of enteritis.

Equine Torovirus (ETOV) Infection

Equine torovirus **(EToV-Berne virus)** infection has been reported from rectal swab with diarrhea in horses. Transmission probably takes place via the fecal-oral route. The equine torovirus Berne virus (BEV), induces apoptosis in infected cells at late times post infection. Observation of BEV infected cells by electron microscopy revealed that by 24 hours post infection, some cells exhibited morphological characteristics of apoptotic cells. BEV-induced apoptosis at late times post infection, once viral progeny are produced, could facilitate viral dissemination *in vivo* and contribute to viral pathogenesis.

Porcine Torovirus Infection

Porcine torovvirus **(PToV)** infection is common in swine shortly after weaning, virus is shed after 4-14 days post weaning & lasts for 1-9 days with normal stool. PToV infection occurs soon after weaning. Although the prevalence of infection in suckling piglets varied among the farms, PToV prevalence in 7 and 11-week-old pigs were between 50-67% and 58-75%, respectively, in all farms. Sequencing results indicated that more than one PToV strains were circulating in the studied farms. Present data suggest that PToV was endemic on the farms, and provide new insights on the epidemiology of PToV. Development of a significant antibody response to PToV occurred before 7 weeks of age in about 50% of piglets, and the remaining animals developed the response by weeks 11 or 15.

□□□

1984 particles resembling these viruses were discovered in the feces of humans. This virus has been detected by electron microscopy, immunofluorescence and ELISA in the United States and in other countries such as Belgium, Canada, Costa Rica, The Netherlands, India, France, Italy, South Africa and Germany. On the basis of the available information on these viruses, BToV was detected at a significantly higher rate in diarrheic samples than in asymptomatic samples, suggesting that BToV may act as a risk factor for diarrhea in Japanese cattle. Epidemiologic studies have shown that bovine torovirus is widespread in The Netherlands, Germany and Switzerland, the United Kingdom, and the United States, with approximately 90% of dairy cattle being seropositive. In one study from Belgium, bovine toroviruses were found to play a role in respiratory, digestive, and reproductive disorders of cattle. In a recent study from Saskatchewan, Canada, BRV-like particles were detected in 42 of 221 fecal or intestinal specimens of symptomatic calves. The RT-PCR was successfully applied for the diagnosis of torovirus in fecal specimens of calves. It remains impossible to determine whether bovine torovirus was the primary cause of diarrhea in the symptomatic calves or had concomitant infections with other viral agents of enteritis.

Equine Torovirus (EToV) Infection

Equine torovirus (EToV-Berne virus) infection has been reported from rectal swab with diarrhea in horses. Transmission probably takes place via the fecal-oral route. The equine torovirus Berne virus (BEV) induces apoptosis in infected cells at late times post infection. Observation of BEV infected cells by electron microscopy revealed that by 24 hours post infection, some cells exhibited morphological characteristics of apoptotic cells. BEV-induced apoptosis at late times post infection, once viral progeny are produced, could facilitate viral dissemination *in vivo* and contribute to viral pathogenesis.

Porcine Torovirus Infection

Porcine torovirus (PToV) infection is common in swine shortly after weaning. Virus is shed after 4-14 days post weaning & lasts for 1-9 days with normal stool. PToV infection occurs soon after weaning. Although the prevalence of infection in suckling piglets varied among the farms, PToV prevalence in 7 and 14-week-old pigs were between 60-67% and 58-75%, respectively, in all farms. Sequencing results indicated that more than one PToV strains were circulating in the studied farms. Present data suggest that PToV was endemic on the farms, and provide new insights on the epidemiology of PToV. Development of a significant antibody response to PToV occurred before 7 weeks of age in about 30% of piglets, and the remaining animals developed the response by weeks 14 or 19.

□□□

Chapter 23

Characteristics and Diseases Caused by Group IV Single-Stranded D (+) RNA Arteriviruses (Family *Arteriviridae*)

Contents

Characteristics of Arteriviruses

Arteriviruses under the family *Arteriviridae* derived its name from the disease **Equine arteritis** having the type species *Equine arteritis virus, &* the family *Arteriviridae* was included within the order *Nidovirale* alongwith *Coronaviridae* in 1996. Arteriviruses are small, spherical, enveloped viruses, 40-60 nm in diameter having an **icosahedral core**, 20-30 nm in diameter. Core contains an unsegmented, linear, positive-sense ssRNA genome of 12-16kb long. The family has only **one genus** ***Arteivirus***, which includes type species, *Equine arteitis virus* (EAV), & other viruses namely *Porcine reproductive* *and respiratory syndrome virus* (PRRSV), *Lactate dehdrogenase elevating virus* (LDV) of mice and *Simian haemorrhagic fever virus* (SHFV). The arteriviruses are highly species specific, but share many biological and molecular properties, including virion morphology, a unique set of structural proteins, genome organization and replication strategy, and the ability to **establish prolonged** or **true persistent infection in their natural hosts**.

Arteriviruses are comparatively labile, sensitive to heat, low pH, lipid solvents, detergents, UV light, & various disinfectants.

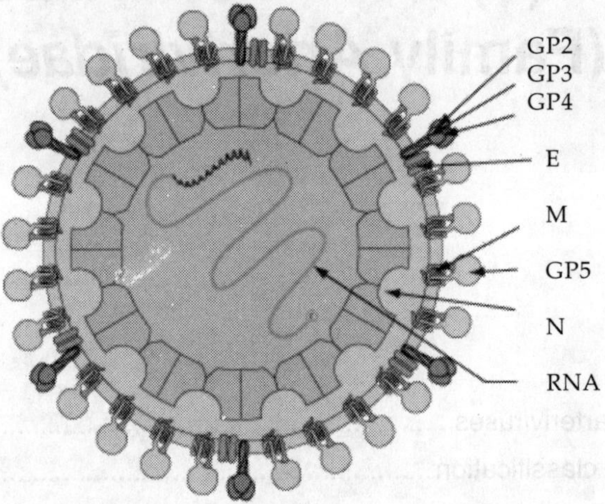

Figure 23.1 : Morphology of an Arterivirus

The Virus Genome

The virion contains unsegmented, linear, positive sense, ssRNA genome of 12-16kb in size, capped, and polyadenylated. 5′ end of the virus has **leader RNA (65-89 bp), which is also present at the 5′ end of each subgenomic RNAs**. The virion RNA is infectious and serves as both genome and viral mRNA. Genomic RNA encodes for ORF1a, and ORF1b which are translated by a frameshifting mechanism. The proteins pp1a and pp1ab are processed into the viral polymerase (RdRp) and other non-structural proteins involved in RNA synthesis. Structural proteins are expressed as subgenomic RNAs. The mRNA2 is bicistronic. The 3′ proximal region of SHFV contains in addition a large insertion that may encode three additional glycoproteins.

Virus Replication

The virus replicates in the cytoplasm of the infected cell. First, the virus attaches to the host cell receptors, endocytosed into vesicles & then the virus membrane & the vesicle membrane fuse releasing ssRNA(+) genome into the cytoplasm.

Synthesis & proteolysis of replicase polyproteins occurs. Replicase first produces the complementary ssRNA(-), which serves as a template for the synthesis of genomic RNA and subgenomic mRNAs.

Synthesis of structural proteins is encoded by the subgenomic mRNAs. Then virus assembly occurs & the viruses bud at membranes of the endoplasmic reticulum, the intermediate compartments, and/or the Golgi complex, & new virions are released.

Virus Classification

Group: Group IV (+) ssRNA

Order: *Nidovirale*

Family: *Arteriviridae*

Genus: *Arterivirus*; type species: *Equine arteritis virus* (EAV), & other species are *Porcine reproductive and respiratory syndrome virus* **(PRRSV),** *Lactate dehdrogenase elevating virus* (LDV) of mice and *Simian haemorrhagic fever virus* (SHFV).

Table 23.1 : Classification of *Arteriviridae* & diseases caused by the member viruses in humans & animals.

Genus	Species	Serotypes	Diseases caused
Arterivirus	TS : *Equine arteritis virus*	EAV	Equine arteritis (EAV) is an acute, contagious & economically important systemic disease ofhorses, donkey & mules worldwide (Japan, Iceland free). The symptoms include fever, depression, conjunctivitis, nasal discharge, pneumonia in foals, edema in dependent part-limbs, abortion, fetal death, & vascular damage. Disease transmission occurs via direct or indirect contact, venereal, nasal discharges, & carrier stallion. Pathogenesis: virus → macrophages → bronchial lymph nodes → whole body endothelium + mesothelium of vessels→ necrotic arteritis, vascular damage in placenta, liver, spleen, lungs, brain in fetus & edema-hypovolemic shock → virus shed. A live modified vaccine is used.
	Lactate dehydrogenase virus	LDEV	*Lactic dehydrogenase elevating virus* (LDEV) does not produce apparent symptoms although mice remain persistently infected (macrophages) for life with a life-long viremia.

Porcine respiratory and reproductive syndrome virus	PRRSV	*Porcine respiratory and reproductive syndrome virus* (PRRSV) infection occurs widely in N. America & Europe in swine; causes a systemic disease; adults show mild & short anorexia & respiratory disease in newborn, pregnant sows abort, & there are stillbirths & mummified fetuses. Transmission occurs via direct indirect contact, fomites, aerosols, & boars shedding virus in semen. Modified live & killed vaccines are used in sows & in 2-3 week old pigs.
Simian hemorrhagic fever virus	SHFV	*Simian hemorrhagic fever virus* (SHFV) causes a systemic disease, is a highly pathogenic virus in monkeys, & causes some death.

Arterivirus Clinical Infections in Animals

Genus: *Arterivirus*

Equine Arteritis

Equine arteritis (EAV) is an acute, contagious & economically important systemic disease of **horses, donkey & mules** worldwide (Japan, Iceland free). The symptoms include **fever, depression, conjunctivitis, nasal discharge and pneumonia in foals, edema in dependent part- limbs, abortion, fetal death, & vascular damage.**

Equine viral arteritis is caused by *Equine arteritis virus* (EAV), an RNA virus in the genus *Arterivirus,* family *Arteriviridae* and order *Nidovirales.* Various isolates vary in their **virulence to induce abortions.** Only one serotype has been recognized. Genetic analysis suggests that EAV strains found among donkeys in South Africa may differ significantly from isolates in North America and Europe.

Occurrence

Antibodies to EAV have been found in most countries; seropositive horses have been reported in North and South America, Europe, Asia, Africa and Australia. Infections are common among horses in continental Europe, but rare in the United Kingdom. This virus appears to be absent from Iceland and Japan.

Hosts susceptible

Equine arteritis virus is found in the ***Equidae.*** Antibodies to this virus have been reported in **horses, ponies, donkeys and zebras.** Illness occurs mainly among horses and ponies, but clinical signs have also been reported in experimentally infected donkeys. EAV may cause disease in South American camelids: polymerase chain reaction assay (PCR) detected viral nucleic acids in an **alpaca** that had aborted.

Transmission

Equine arteritis virus can be transmitted by the respiratory and the venereal routes. Acutely affected horses excrete the virus in respiratory secretions; aerosol transmission is common when horses are gathered at racetracks, sales, shows and other events. This virus has also been found in urine and feces during the acute stage. It occurs in the reproductive tract of acutely infected mares, and both acutely and chronically infected stallions. In mares, EAV can be found in vaginal and uterine secretions, as well as in the ovary and oviduct, for a short period after infection. Mares infected late in pregnancy may give birth to infected foals. **Stallions shed EAV in semen, and can carry the virus for years**. Transmission from stallions can occur by natural service or artificial insemination. Some carriers may eventually clear the infection. True carrier states have not been reported in mares, geldings or sexually immature colts. But, EAV can occasionally be found for up to six months in the reproductive tract of older prepubertal colts.

Equine arteritis virus can be transmitted on fomites including equipment, and may be spread mechanically by humans or animals. This virus is inactivated in 20–30 minutes at 56-58ºC (133-136ºF), but can remain viable for 2 to 3 days at 37-38ºC (99-100ºF) and for up to 75 days at 4-8ºC (39-46ºF). Semen remains infectious after freezing.

Pathogenesis

It was possible to determine the pathogenesis of EAV infection in adult horses and foals by following its distribution of viral antigen and lesions in experimental and natural infections.Twenty-four hours post-infection (PI) or later, the virus invades the respiratory epithelium and alveolar macrophages. Forty-eight hours PI, the virus can be found in the bronchial lymph nodes. Three days PI, the virus replicates in bronchopulmonary lymph nodes, endothelium, and circulating monocytes. Systemic distribution of the virus follows with localization within macrophages and dendritic cells of lymphoid tissue. About 6 to 8 days PI, the virus localizes within endothelium and medial myocytes of blood vessels and mesothelium. At day 10 PI the most severe damage occurs to blood vessels. After 10 days PI, EAV Ag is decreased in all the locations except the tunica media of small muscular arteries. The last site to be invaded is the renal tubular epithelium where the virus may persist for additional two weeks. Infective EAV is no longer detectable in most tissues after day 28 PI, with the exception of the reproductive tract of some colts and stallions. In the pregnant mare EAVAg can be identified within the uterine small blood vessels (endothelium, myocytes and sometimes pericytes), and within the endometrial glandular and surface epithelium. The salpynx epithelium can be also infected. In the infected fetus EAVAg can be identified within the trophoblastic epithelium and mesenchyme, and shortly after, within pneumocytes, alveolar macrophages, within the thymic epithelium and enterocytes. Pathogenesis: virus → macrophages → bronchial lymph nodes → whole body endothelium + mesothelium of vessels→ necrotic arteritis, vascular damage in placenta, liver, spleen, lungs, brain in fetus & edema-hypovolemic shock → virus shed.

Clinical Symptoms & Lesions

The **incubation period varies from 2 days to 2 weeks**. Infections transmitted venereally become apparent in approximately one week.

Most EAV infections, especially those that occur in mares bred to long-term carriers, are asymptomatic. The clinical signs are generally more severe in old or very young animals, and in horses that are immunocompromised or in poor condition.

Severe infections with acute interstitial pneumonia and/ or enteritis can be seen in foals up to a few months of age. Systemic illness also occurs in some adults. In adult horses, the clinical signs may include **fever, depression, anorexia, limb edema in the hindlimbs, and dependent edema of the prepuce, scrotum, mammary gland and/or ventral body wall**. Conjunctivitis, photophobia, periorbital or supraorbital edema and rhinitis can also be seen. Some horses develop urticaria localized to the head or neck, but are sometimes generalized.

Abortions or stillbirths can occur in mares that are pregnant when they are exposed. Abortions are not necessarily preceded by systemic signs. Temporary decreases in fertility, including reduced quality sperm and decreased libido, may be seen in stallions during the acute stage of the disease. The decrease in sperm quality has been attributed to increased scrotal temperature and edema, and can persist for up to 4 months. The quality of the semen is not decreased in carrier stallions. Except in cases of severe disease in foals, deaths are rare.

Outbreaks have not been reported among donkeys or mules, and although antibodies have been found. Fever, sometimes accompanied by mild depression, mild conjunctivitis, a slight oculonasal discharge and/or mild dependent edema were reported in donkeys inoculated with an EAV strain that is moderately virulent for horses. The clinical signs were mild, and could readily have been missed if the animals were not closely monitored. Donkeys inoculated with a South African donkey strain developed mild to more severe clinical signs including fever, depression, serous ocular and nasal discharge, and conjunctivitis. Pregnant donkey mares did not abort, and their foals were clinically normal when born. Horses inoculated with this donkey strain had very mild clinical signs.

PM lesions in acute cases are edema, congestion and hemorrhages of the subcutaneous tissues, visceral organs and lymph nodes. These changes are often found in the subcutaneous tissues of the limbs and abdomen, the thoracic and abdominal lymph nodes, and the small and large intestines (especially the colon and cecum), but may occur throughout the body. Accumulations of clear, yellowish fluid may be found in the peritoneal cavity, pleura and pericardium. Foals may also have pulmonary edema, interstitial pneumonia, emphysema, splenic infarcts and enteritis. In mares that abort, the endometrium may be swollen and congested, and can contain hemorrhages. Aborted fetuses are often partially autolyzed, but may be well preserved. In some fetuses, the only gross lesions may be excess fluid.

Diagnosis

Collection of clinical specimens for various tests include: nasal swabs, ocular swabs, whole blood, semen, fetal tissues, and semen from suspect stallions. Equine viral arteritis can be diagnosed by virus isolation, the detection of viral antigens or nucleic acids, and serology.

1. *Presumptive diagnosis:* Equine viral arteritis should be suspected when the clinical signs include fever, depression, edema, conjunctivitis, nasal discharges and abortions. This disease is difficult to differentiate from other systemic and respiratory illnesses of horses.
2. *Virus isolation:* The virus can be isolated in rabbit, equine and monkey kidney cells or cell lines. **RK-13 (rabbit kidney) cells are the system of choice**. The virus can be confirmed using serum neutralization, reverse-transcription PCR (RT-PCR) assays, immunofluorescence or immunohistochemistry. EAV is not found in the respiratorysecretions, blood or urine of carriers.
3. *Antigen detection:* RT-PCR can also detect viral nucleic acids in clinical samples from live horses or tissues taken at necropsy. Immunohistochemistry can identify viral antigens in necropsy samples, as well as in skin biopsies from acutely infected horses.
4. *Serological tests:* Serological tests include virus neutralization, complement fixation, agar gel immunodiffusion, indirect fluorescent antibody, fluorescent microsphere immunoassay (MIA) and ELISA. A complement-

enhanced micro-neutralization test is often used to detect antibodies to EAV. In acute cases, a **fourfold increase in titer should be seen in serological tests**. Carriers can also be detected by breeding the stallion to seronegative mares, which are checked for seroconversion four weeks after breeding.

Treatment & Prevention

Acutely infected horses should be isolated to prevent transmission in secretions and excretions. Precautions should also be taken to avoid spreading the virus on fomites. EAV is readily inactivated by detergents, common disinfectants and lipid solvents. No specific treatment is available; however, most healthy horses other than young foals recover on their own. Good nursing and symptomatic treatment should be used in severe cases. Excellent hygiene and decontamination of fomites should be practiced when breeding infected horses or collecting semen. Although some experimental methods may be promising, there is no proven method to eliminate carriage in stallions.

Venereal transmission is controlled by good management and vaccination. To protect pregnant mares from abortion, they should be separated from other horses and maintained in small groups according to their predicted foaling dates. Newly acquired horses should be isolated for 3 to 4 weeks.

Vaccination

Immunization prevents uninfected stallions from becoming long term carriers. **Stallions that are not carriers should be vaccinated before the start of the breeding season. Prepubertal colts are given the vaccine when they are 6-12 months old.** Carrier stallions are identified and **bred only to well vaccinated or naturally seropositive mares.** Similarly, semen that contains EAV should be used only in these mares. Because first-time vaccinates may shed field viruses for a short time after exposure, these mares should be isolated from seronegative horses, particularly pregnant mares, for three weeks after breeding. Naturally infected mares and those that are not first-time vaccinates are isolated for 24-48 hours, to protect other horses from the viruses present in semen. **ARVAC Equine Arteritis Vaccine-** Fort Dodge is a dessicated modified Equine Arteritis virus propagated on an equine cell line culture system for the vaccination of healthy non-stressed horses to stimulate the development of protection against viral abortion and respiratory infection due to equine arteritis virus. Aseptically rehydrate to liquid form using the diluent supplied. Administer one 1 ml dose IM. Vaccinate males and young animals at any time, but stallions should be vaccinated not less than 3 weeks prior to breeding. Vaccinate mares preferably as maidens or when open. Mares in foal should not be vaccinated until after foaling and then not less than 3 weeks prior to breeding. Maiden and barren mares may be vaccinated anytime but should be vaccinated not less than 3 weeks prior to breeding. Pregnant mares should not be vaccinated during the last two months of gestation Repeat with annual booster dose.

EAV is sensitive to sunlight and low humidity, and uninfected stallions have been kept near carriers for years without infection.

Porcine Respiratory and Reproductive Syndrome

Porcine respiratory & reproductive syndrome virus (PRRSV) causes **porcine reproductive and respiratory syndrome (PRRS),** which is an infectious viral disease of swine transmitted via **direct contact** to susceptible pigs and **vertically to foetuses**. PRRS is considered the **most economically important viral disease of intensive swine farms in Europe and North America.** It is characterised by **reproductive failure in sows and respiratory distress in piglets and fattening pigs,** which, due to rapid spread, can cause significant production and economic losses. PRRS, also known as Mystery Swine Disease, Blue Ear Disease, Porcine Endemic Abortion and Respiratory Syndrome (PEARS), and Swine Infertility Respiratory Syndrome (SIRS), is not known to be a **zoonosis.**

Etiology: PRRS is caused by *Porcine respiratory & reproductive syndrome virus* (PRRSV), which have currently two major serotypes of the virus; the **European and the American types.** This classification is significant in that vaccines made for one serotype will not completely protect against the other.

Occurrence

PRRS was first detected in **North America in 1987 and in Europe in 1990** and has since then been recorded in most major pig-producing areas throughout the world, but occurs widely in N. America & Europe. Only Australia, New Zealand and Switzerland are free from PRRSV infection. The most recent outbreaks have occurred in **Sweden, South Africa, Russian Federation, Viet Nam and China in 2009.**

Hosts Susceptible

The **pig** (*Sus scrofa*), both domestic and feral, is the **only species** known to be naturally susceptible to PRRS.

Transmission

The virus is **shed in saliva for six weeks, urine for two weeks, semen for six weeks and in mammary gland secretions,** & is very contagious. Transmission occurs via inhalation, ingestion including ingestion of infected meat, coitus, transplacental, artificial insemination, also from vaccinated boars, pig bites and needles and other inanimate objects or water & food. Arthropod transmission has been suggested by some preliminary reports. PRRSV is highly infectious and easily transmitted through direct contact among pen mates. Aerosol transmission is difficult, although it has been experimentally shown for distances of up to 2.5 meters.

PRRSV is unstable outside the pH 5.5-6.5 range. Low concentrations of detergents and solvents such as chloroform and ether rapidly inactivate PRRSV. The virus survives in water for up to 11 days, but drying quickly inactivates it. PRRSV can be isolated from muscle and lymphoid tissues up to 24 hours after slaughter, & even from muscle that had been frozen at –20°C for one month.

Pathogenesis

The PRRS virus replicates mainly in porcine **alveolar macrophages (PAMs) and dendritic cells (DCs) and develops persistent infections, antibody-dependent enhancement (ADE), interstitial pneumonia and immunosuppression.** The syndrome presented, respiratory or reproductive, is dependent on the age of the pigs affected.

The pathogenesis of PRRSV was determined in gnotobiotic pigs by studying the sequential development of virus distribution and replication & microscopic lesions. Infected pigs were **viremic by 12 hours** post exposure (PE) and subsequently developed **pneumonia, lymphadenopathy, vasculitis, myocarditis, and encephalitis**. Lung lesions developed by day 3 PE, persisted through day 21 PE. Affected lungs were characterized by alveolar septa thickening by macrophages, alveolar proteinaceous and karyorrhectic debris, alveolar syncytial cells, and **multifocal type II pneumocyte hypertrophy**. Lymph node lesions varied in distribution and severity and were characterized by germinal center hypertrophy and hyperplasia, lymphocyte necrosis, multiple cystic spaces, and polykaryocytes within the cystic spaces. Heart lesions were a late feature of infection and all infected pigs had **heart lesions on day 21 PE** characterized by subendocardial, **myocardial, and perivascular foci of lymphocytes. Vasculitis** also varied in distribution and severity and affected all sizes of vessels. PRRSV is a multisystem disease characterized initially by viremia with subsequent virus distribution and replication in multiple organs causing interstitial pneumonia, vasculitis, lymphadenopathy, myocarditis, and encephalitis.

Aerosol infection of **non-immune pregnant gilts** to PRRSV in late gestation at 84 days caused clinical disease. Following incubation period of 4-7 days, infected sows became inappetent & listless; some sows showed blue –

colored ear, with abdominal respiration. Sows furrowed at 116-117 days of gestation **giving birth to dead, mummified fetus, & live weak piglets**. Four 4 week old, conventional, PRRSV antibody-negative pigs were intranasally inoculated with PRRSV (ATCC VR-2402) that developedr persistent infection. It provided direct evidence of persistent PRRSV infection and explains field observations of long-term herd infection and transmission via purchase of clinically normal, but PRRSV infected animals.

Clinical Symptoms

The clinical signs of PRRS vary greatly between herds. In general, PRRS is characterized by **reproductive failure of sows and respiratory distress of piglets and growing pigs**. The characteristics of the reproductive failure are **infertility, late foetal mummification, abortions, agalactia, stillbirths, and weak piglets** that usually die shortly after birth due to respiratory disease and secondary bacterial infections, such as *Salmonella cholerasuis, Haemophilus parasuis, Streptococcous suis, Mycoplasmahyopneumonia* and swine influenza virus.

In young piglets, **high mortality** rates will occur and at the peak of an outbreak, mortality may reach 60-70%; 30-50% percent losses are more common.

The disease in **weaned and fattening pigs** is characterized by anorexia, lethargy, cutaneous hyperemia, dyspnea, rough hair coats, failure to thrive and an increase in mortality from secondary infections. Mortality rates are also elevated in the post-weaning period, varying between 4-20 percent. Depressions in post-weaning weight gain of up to 65 percent have been reported.

Older pigs may show mild respiratory signs, which may also be complicated by secondary infections. Finishing pigs, boars, gilts and sows are often found to have sub-clinical infection.

Diagnosis

Collection of clinical samples includes- nasal swabs, blood, serum, lung tissue, and aborted fetuses.

1. *Presumptive diagnosis:* It is based on clinical symptoms, abortion cases & lesions.
2. *Virological isolation:* Isolation of the virus can be done on porcine macrophages, in a continuous cell line derived from African green monkey kidney cell, ascitic fluids or tissue cultures from organs such as lung, tonsil, lymph node and spleen. Virus identification & characterization are done by immunostaining with specific antisera.

For laboratory confirmation, immunohistochemistry and in situ hybridisation on fixed tissues and reverse-transcription PCR (RT-PCR) are used.

3. *Antibody detection:* The detection of antibodies to PRRSV can be done using a wide range of serological tests like the immunoperoxidase assay, the indirect immunofluorescence assay and ELISA.

Treatment & Prevention

The PRRS control and eradication programme rests on early disease detection, rapid laboratory confirmation; quick identification of the infected farms; and control of the infection through different stamping out strategies.

Because PRRS is transmitted by direct contact, control measures are advisable at slaughter plants, meat processing plants and sale yards.

Vaccination

Vaccination is the most effective tools to control PRRS, although it does not prevent PRRSV infection. Vaccines should contain the specific antigenic type to be effective. Vaccination with a homologous strain is more effective than vaccination with a heterologous strain. In the United States there are **approved modified-live virus** (MLV) vaccines for PRRS. **MLV vaccines are used in piglets from three weeks of age or sows and gilts 3-6 weeks prior to breeding**. In Europe and United States, an **inactivated virus vaccine against the reproductive form of PRRS is also available on the market**. One recommended strategy is the vaccination of seronegative replacement breeding stock **60–90 days before introduction.** Animals vaccinated with MLV vaccines shed the vaccine strain virus, which is then transmitted in the field, complicating the problem of detecting infection with wild-type virus, both through virology and serology. **Porcilis PRRS**-intervet is a freeze dried vaccine based on the attenuated European strain DV of PRRS virus containing at least 10^4 $TCID_{50}$ of PRRSV strain DV. The active component is dissolved in Diluvac Forte. Dose is 2 ml IM or .2ml ID injection of the attenuated live PRRSV results in active immunisation against infection with PRRS virus; a single dose is given to fattening pigs from 2 weeks of age onwards. Pigs should be vaccinated at least 2-4 weeks before a PRRSV infection occurs. It is advised to vaccinate all target pigs within a herd. This activity is enhanced by the adjuvant Diluvac Forte. In gilts a revaccination 2-4 weeks before mating is recommended. To maintain a high homologous level of immunity, revaccination at regular intervals is recommended, either before each consecutive gestation or at random at 4 month intervals. Pregnant sows should only be vaccinated after previous exposure to European PRRSV. Newly introduced PRRSV-naive animals (e.g. replacement gilts from PRRSV-negative herds) should be vaccinated prior to pregnancy.

Lactic Dehydrogenase Elevating Virus Infection

Lactic dehydrogenase elevating virus **(LDEV)** doesn't produce apparent symptoms although **mice remain persistently infected** (macrophages) for life with a **life-long viremia**. Since the virus causes persistent viremia, it can be spread by blood-sucking ectoparasites. LDEV has a very high specificity **for peritoneal macrophages,** & consistently yielded the highest virus titers. Further studies have shown that in the first twenty-four hours after infection of a macrophage, there is very rapid virus replication, this rate gradually falls off to a very low level but continues **as long as the macrophage continues to divide**. The viremia arises because **LDV lyses the cell after replication**. The virus is most commonly found in the **liver, spleen, lymph nodes, and skin.** The main effect of the virus on the host cell is to increase the activity of certain plasma enzymes, this increase in activity is not directly related to the level of viral infectivity, but does depend on the balance between rate of entry and rate of clearance and evidence leans more heavily towards the rate of clearance. In the plasma, **LDH consists of five isoenzymes and LDV generally only has an effect on LDH A4**. Another effect only occurs in the C58 and AKR type mice and involves **destruction of lower motor neurons producing age-dependent polioencephalomyelitis**. Other effects of the virus include a temporary fall in the total white blood cell count that lasts for twenty-four hours after infection.

Simian Hemorrhagic Fever

Simian hemorrhagic fever virus **(SHFV)** causes a systemic disease, is highly pathogenic virus in **monkeys** causing some deaths. Simian hemorrhagic fever is an **acute fatal disease of Asian macaques**. It is caused by *Simian hemorrhagic fever virus* (SHFV), an *Arterivirus* in the family *Arteriviridae*, order *Nidovirales*. In contrast to its closest relatives, *Equine arteritis virus, Lactate dehydrogenase-elevating virus,* and *Porcine respiratory and reproductive syndrome virus,* SHFV is almost completely uncharacterized. Thus far, SHFV has never been isolated from wild animals, and all outbreaks have occurred within primate-holding facilities. Recently, scientific interest in simian hemorrhagic fever has increased in the biodefense community because the disease closely **resembles viral hemorrhagic fevers (VHFs) caused by certain arena-, bunya-, flavi-, and filovirids.** SHFV does not cause disease in humans, is not listed as a Select Agent. SHFV may therefore be a valuable tool for developing nonhuman primate models for VHF, which may not only allow for the better characterization of VHF pathogenesis and the testing of general anti-VHF pharmaceuticals, but may also be used as a training tool for new maximum-containment facilities in regards to safety testing of infrastructure and standard operation procedures.

□□□

Chapter 24

Characteristics and Diseases Caused by Group IV Single-Stranded D (+) RNA Astroviruses (Family *Astroviridae*)

Contents

Characteristics of Astroviruses

Astroviruses under the family *Astroviridae* (G, aster= star) derived its name as they contain **unique five- or six-pointed star-like surface structure** under electron microscopy, are 28–35 nm in diameter, non-envelope & have an **icosahedral symmetry**. Astrovirus was first reported in 1975 from cases of an outbreak of diarrhea in humans, and then astroviruses were isolated from many mammalian animal species and were classified as genus *Mammoastrovirus. Astroviruse* were also isolated from avian species such as ducks, chickens, and turkey poults & were classified as a second genus *Avastrovirus*.

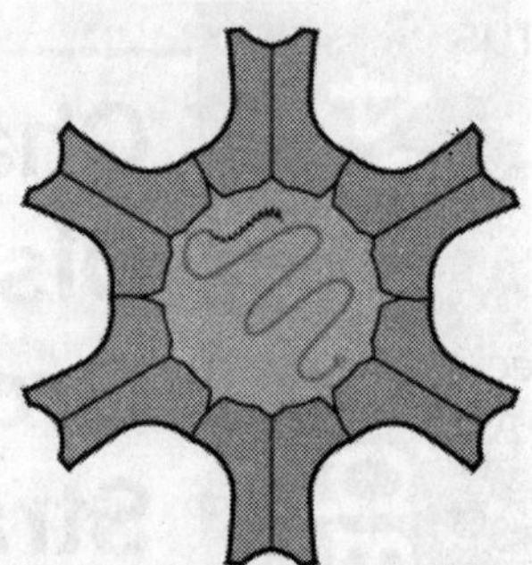

Fig. 24.1 : Morphology of an Astrovirus

The virus contains non-segmented, linear,+ sense ssRNA of about 6.8-7.9 kb long. **Human** astroviruses cause **gastroenteritis in young children** worldwide. Astroviruses also cause **mild gastroenteritis in cattle and other domestic animals**. The diseases associated with astroviruses are usually self-limiting. Members of the *Astroviridae* are species-specific having different antigenic types. Astroviruses are transmitted by contaminated food and water mainly through fecal-oral route. Young children in childcare backgrounds or adults in military barracks are most likely to develop the disease.

These Astroviruses are resistant to low pH, detergents, & heating at 60c for 5 minutes.

The Virus Genome

The virus genome is made of a single strand of positive sense ssRNA nearly 6.8-7.9 kb long. 5′ end of the RNA has no cap & 3′ end has polyadenylated tail. The virus genome has **3 open reading frames** (ORFs) with an overlap of about 70 nucleotides between ORF1a and ORF1b & the third ORF is called ORF2. The virion RNA is infectious and serves as both the genome and viral mRNA. Astroviral nonstructural proteins are translated from the genomic RNA as two large polyproteins, nsP1a and nsP1a/1b via a translational frameshifting mechanism. ORF1a and ORF1b encode the viral protease and polymerase respectively, and probably other proteins involved in genome replication. ORF 2 is expressed as subgenomic RNAs and encodes the capsid protein.

Virus Replication

Virus replicates in the cell cytoplasm. The virus attaches to host receptors, then it is uncoated, and the viral genomic RNA is released into the cytoplasm. Viral RNA is translated into two processed polyproteins.

For replication of viral RNA, a negative-sense complementary ssRNA is synthesized using the + genomic RNA as a template. Then new genomic RNA is synthesized using the negative-sense RNA as a template. Subgenomic RNA translation gives rise to the capsid protein precursor. Lastly maturation of the capsid occurs by proteolytic cleavage & then the virus is released by cell lysis.

Virus Classification

Group: Group IV + ssRNA

Family: *Astroviridae*

Genus 1: *Mamastrovirus;* type species: *Human astrovirus* (HAstV); other species are; *Bovine astrovirus* (BAstV), *Feline astrovirus* (FAstV), *Ovine astrovirus* (OAstV), *Porcine astrovirus* (PAstV), *& Mink astrovirus* (MAstV).

Genus 2: *Avastrovirus;* type species: *Turkey astrovirus* (TAstV); other species are; *Chicken astrovirus* (CAstV), *& Duck astrovirus* (TAstV).

Table 24.1 : Classification of *Astroviridae* & disease caused by the member viruses in humans & animals.

Genera	Species	Serotypes	Diseases caused
G1:*Mamastrovirus*	*Bovine astrovirus*	BAstV-1, 2	*Bovine astrovirus* (BAstV-1, 2) causes mild or subclinical gastroenteritis in bovine.
	Feline astrovirus	FAstV-1	*Feline astrovirus* (FAstV-1) infection is poorly known; only one report suggests that less than 10% cats in the UK have antibody against astroviruses. Sick animals develop green and watery diarrhoea lasting 4-14 days, sometimes accompanied by vomiting, pyrexia and depression.
	TS: *Human astrovirus*	HAstV-1, 8	*Human astrovirus* (HAstV-1, 8) causes self limiting & host restricted, usually watery diarrhea in children & mild or subclinical gastroenteritis in adults. The disease has been reported in USA & Europe.
	Ovine astrovirus	OAstV-1	*Ovine astrovirus* (OAstV-1) causes diarrhea in lambs & calves.
	Porcine astrovirus	PAstV-1	*Porcine astrovirus* (PAstV-1) were isolated in some cases from pigs with acute diarrhea.
	Mink astrovirus	MAstV-1	*Mink astrovirus* (MAstV-1) study revealed infection with astrovirus to be a risk factor for causing mild gastroenteritis in mink.

G 2: *Avastrovirus*	*Chicken astrovirus*	CAstV, AHV-1, 2	*Chicken astrovirus* (CAstV, AHV-1, 2) causes mild gastroenteritis in chickens.
	Duck astrovirus	DAstV-1	*Duck astrovirus* (DAstV-1) causes mild gastroenteritis in ducks that may develop into an acute fatal hepatitis.
	TS: *Turkey astrovirus*	TAstV-1, 2	*Turkey astrovirus* (TAstV-1, 2) causes diarrhea and growth depression in poults; type 2 TAstV is more pathogenic.

Astrovirus Clinical Manifestations in Humans

Clinical Infections in Humans

Genus : *Mamastroovirus*

Human astrovirus (HAstV-I, 8) causes self limiting & host restricted, usually watery diarrhea in children & mild or subclinical gastroenteritis in adults, reported in USA & Europe.

Astrovirus Clinical Infections in Animals

Genus : *Mamastrovirus*

Bovine Astrovirus Infection

***Bovine astrovirus*(BAstV-1, 2)** causes mild or subclinical gastroenteritis in bovine. The isolation of bovine astrovirus was first reported in England in 1978. Astrovirus was considered to be avirulent. In 1984 a U.S. isolate of bovine astrovirus (US1), antigenically related to the isolate in England (UK), was shown to **cause infection and cytopathology of the M cells of the dome epithelium covering the Peyer's patches of the calf ileum.** These gnotobiotic calves also remained clinically normal during the course of infection, although there was a color change of the feces from brown to yellow. Calves infected with BAstV alone did not cause diarrhea. When **astrovirus was mixed with rotavirus or Breda virus 2,** the calves developed severe diarrhea and more extensive astrovirus infection of the dome epithelium. The dome epithelial cells showed degeneration and a few cells showed degeneration with Breda virus 2 infection. The astrovirus infected cell cultures and the epithelial cells of domes in the ileum, and there was cross-immunofluorescence with antiserum to the United Kingdom astrovirus.

Three isolates of BAstV, one from the UK and two from the USA possessed common antigens by immunofluorescence and strain-specific antigens by neutralization and were designated as **two, and probably three, distinct**

serotypes. The isolate US2, despite being a different serotype, possessed the same restrictive cell tropism and cytopathology as previously reported for isolate US1, of the M cells of the dome epithelium of the Peyer's patches. Serotyping of 16 field isolates indicated the presence of more undefined serotypes.

Feline Astrovirus Infection

***Feline astrovirus*(FAstV-1)** infection in cats is poorly known; one report suggests that less than 10% cats in the UK have antibody. Infected cats produce green and watery diarrhoea lasting 4-14 days, sometimes accompanied by vomiting, pyrexia and depression. Feline astroviruses have been identified by electron microscopy in the feces of either asymptomatic or symptomatic cats, and experimental infection with one isolate was shown to induce enteric clinical signs and virus excretion, thus suggesting a possible role as enteric pathogen. In one case a dual infection was reported by *Feline astrovirus* and *Feline panleukopenia virus* in a 4-month-old cat with severe gastroenteritis and panleukopenia. Upon sequence analysis, the *Feline astrovirus* strain was found to be genetically related to astroviruses identified in human. Astroviruses were also detected by electron microscopy in the feces from a 4 month old kitten with diarrhea. The clinical disease manifested by the cat and the observed morphology of the viral particles were consistent with previous reports on astroviruses of other species.

***Ovine astrovirus* (OAstV-I)** causes diarrhea in lambs & calves.

Porcine Astrovirus

(PAstV-I) in some cases was isolated from pigs with acute diarrhea. Hysterectomy-produced, colostrum-deprived, **4-day-old pigs developed mild diarrhea** after oral exposure to porcine astrovirus propagated in the cell culture; and the virus was isolated again from diarrheal stool specimens. The virus showed a **cytopathic effect characterized by an enlargement of cells and the appearance of fine granules in the cytoplasm.**

Genus : *Avastrovirus*

Recent studies identify *Avian nephritis virus* 1, *Avian nephritis virus* 2, *Chicken astrovirus* 1, *Chicken astrovirus* 2, & unclassified Chicken astroviruses within the genus *Avastrovirus.*

Chicken Astrovirus Infection

Chicken astrovirus **(CAstV, AHV-1, 2)** causes **mild gastroenteritis as reported in chickens.** Two genetically different isolates of *Chicken astrovirus* (CAstV), CAstV612 and CAstV11672, which show low levels of antigenic relatedness in cross-indirect immunofluorescence (IIF) tests, have been identified in UK in 2009. CAstV antibodies were detected in 78% (73% CAstV612; 46% CAstV11672) of serum samples from UK broiler flocks and in all 10 flocks tested, indicating that infections were very common. Twenty-three (96%) out of 24 and 26 (93%) out of 28 broiler parent flocks, aged 23 to 26 weeks from three UK organizations, were positive for antibody to CAstV612 and CAstV11672, respectively. Since late 2004, **broilers throughout the USA States were showing cases of a runting and stunting syndrome (RSS) in the winter and spring.** Reoviruses and chicken astroviruses were confirmed as the infectious agents in RSS in broilers. **RSS affects young broilers between one and two weeks of age causing severe weight suppression during the first few weeks of age, lack of flock uniformity, diarrhea, distention of the intestines, a significant increase in the feed conversion ratio, & cystic enteropathy by histopathological examination of small intestine samples.**

Avian astroviruses cause intestinal & extra-intestinal illness in avian species. *Avian nephritis virus* infects chickens & the viral antigens have been detected in liver, spleen, pancreas, kidneys, jejunum & ileum. The virus caused growth retardation, & acute intestinal nephritis.

Duck Astrovirus Infection

Duck astrovirus (DAstV-1) is an important pathogen **causing duck viral hepatitis (DVH),** a highly contagious and fatal disease in young ducklings. Duck astroviruses (DAstVs) causing duck viral hepatitis were reported in a recent outbreak of fatal hepatitis in ducklings **in China in 2006**. Sequence comparisons and phylogenetic analysis showed that DAstV was more closely related to turkey astrovirus (TAstV) type 2, TAstV-3 and TAstV/MN/01 (a possible new TAstV serotype) than to TAstV-1 or other astroviruses. These findings indicate that astroviruses may transmit across ducks and turkeys. DAstV-specific antibodies were detected in 12 (28.6%) of 42 sera samples from a different flock without DVH, indicating a wide distribution of **subclinical infections** caused by DAstV.

Turkey Astrovirus Infection

***Turkey astrovirus* (TAstV-1, 2)** causes diarrhea and growth depression in poults; type 2 TAstV is more pathogenic.Turkey astrovirus is an important pathogen of poult enteritis and mortality syndrome (PEMS), which has caused significant losses to turkey industry in the USA. Turkey astroviruses are found in **turkey poults** which are mainly confined to farms. There are distinct subtypes of turkey astrovirus like **TAstV-1, 2.** Turkey astrovirus **causes growth depression, decreased thymus size and enteric infection in infected turkeys.**

Lab experiment shows that 0.3% formaldehyde, 1.5% Virkon S, 0.1% β-propriolactone, and 90% methanol are the only effective products that can be used for the virus inactivation.

After the turkey has been infected and then consumed by human, it typically cause watery diarrhea which lasts for about 2-4 days. It can also cause although **less commonly, vomiting, headache, fever, abdominal pains, and anorexia in children under 2**, elderly and immunocompromised people. Turkey virus can be isolated in embryonated eggs & then detected by RT-PCR primers specific for virus has been the only accurate way to detect new astrovirus isolates. RT-PCR is one of the tests to detect the Turkey astroviruses in the fecal samples.

□□□

Chapter 25

Characteristics and Diseases Caused by Group V Single-Stranded (-) RNA Orthomyxoviruses (Family *Orthomyxoviridae*)

Contents

Characteristics of Orthomyxoviruses

The viruses under the family *Orthomyxoviridae* (G. *orthos* = straight; *myxa*= mucus) are large, enveloped, peplomer carrying particles, which are spherical or elongated or pleomorphic in shape & the envelope can occur in spherical and filamentous forms measuring 80-120 nm in diameter & 200-300(-3000) nm long. Fig 25-1 depicts morphology & structure of an orthomyxovirus. There are some 500 distinct surface projections from the envelope each projecting 10 to 14 nm from the surface. From the outer surface of the envelope projects 2 types of main glycoprotein spikes called hemagglutinin (HA) (a trimer) is so called as it agglutinates certain species of RBCs, & neuraminidase (NA), a tetramer. Some spikes like **hemagglutinin esterase (HEF)** is densely dispersed over the surface, while main glycoprotein HA is spaced widely apart & is interposed irregularly by **clusters of NA** with a ratio of HA to NA is 4-5 to 1. The inner side of the envelope is lined by the M1 matrix protein. The **M2 protein projects from the envelope & form ion channels allowing pH changes in the endosome. Fusion protein** causes viral envelope & endosomsl membrane to fuse releasing nucleocapsid into the infected cell cytoplasm during virus replication. Matrix protein encloses the nucleocapsid (RNA+N); nucleoproteins of different sizes occur with a loop at each end. NA destroys the HA receptors & help in final release of newly produced virions from the infected cell. The **RNP** have helical nucleocapsids (each RNA segment + NP form a nucleocapsid) are filamentous and vary from 50 to 130 nm long and 9 to 15 nm in diameter. Virus genome of this family contains **6 to 8 segments of linear, (-) sense ssRNA** with total genome length of 12000-15000 nucleotides (nt). Genome has terminal repeated sequences at both ends. Terminal repeats at the 5'-end is 12-13 nucleotides long & at 3'-terminus is identical. 3 polymerase polypeptides, PB1, PB2 & PA **are associated with each end of each segment**. RNA dependent RNA polymeraseis essential for infectivity since virion (-) RNA is translated into mRNA.

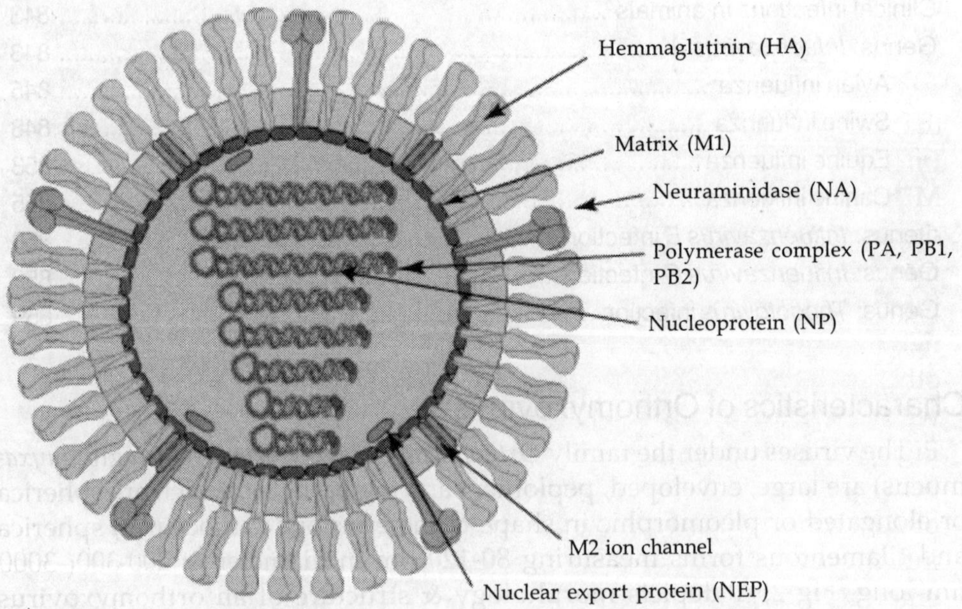

Figure 25.1 : Morphology of an Orthomyxovirus

Orthomyxoviridae includes **five genera**: *Infuenzavirus A, Infuenzavirus B,Infuenzavirus C, Isavirus* and *Thogotovirus, & a* sixth have recently been described. The first three genera contain viruses that cause influenza in vertebrates, including birds, humans, and other mammals. Isaviruses infect salmon, & thogotoviruses infect vertebrates and invertebrates, such as mosquito and sea lice & some mammals. *Influezavirus A, Influezavirus B & Influezavirus* C cause influenza in humans, swine, birds, horses & dogs. Among 3 genera, *Influezavirus A* causes very serious infuenza & pandemic flu in humans, pigs, horses & birds, *Influezavirus B* causes influenza in humans & seals. *Influezavirus* C (carr is only 7 RNA segments) causes influenza in humans & animals. The 3 genera- *Influezavirus A, Influezavirus B & Influezavirus* C are classified on the basis of antigenic properties of NP & M proteins. The antigens on one genus/ type are unique & do not cross-react with other genus/species. Only influenza A viruses are further classified by subtypes on the basis of the two main surface glycoproteins, HA and NA. Sixteen H subtypes (H 1 to H 16) and nine different N subtypes (N1 to N 9) exist in *Infuenza A virus.Influenza A* subtypes and Influenza B viruses are further classified by strains. More than one 100 combinations of HA & NA subtypes of *Influenza A virus* have been identified among possible 144 HA-NA combinations.

Nomenclature of Influenza A viruses as per WHO includes: **Virus type, host of origin, geographical area, strain number & year of isolation** followed by **in parenthesis** HA & NA subtypes. For example, **A / swine / Iowa / 3/ 7 (H1N1)**. But in case of human isolates, host origin is not written. For example, **A/ Scotland/ 42/ 89 (H3N2).**

As regards **epidemiology** of influenza A viruses, it may be mentioned that many **aquatic birds, wild birds & water fowls act as reservoir of various *Influenza A virus* strains** carrying all 16 HA subtypes & 9 NA subtypes. **Migratory water fowls disseminate these viruses across the nations**. Adult ducks remain asymptomatic carriers but young ducks become subclinically infected & shed the virus in the feces from where live bird markets spread infections to the domestic birds. These wild birds are a source of emergence of new *Influenza A virus* subtypes through genetic recombination infecting all other animals. Presence of many avian subtypes favour genetic reassortment with emergence of new subtypes & its **occasional transfer to pigs & humans.** Pigs can be infected with both avian influenza A & human influenza A viruses besides swine influenza virus A strains providing a mixing pot for emergence of **Antigenic Shift.** If a pig is infected with human Influenza virus A & swine influenza virus A strains at the same time, Antigenic Shift occurs resulting in emergence of a new virus having most of human influenza virus A genes but HA & NA of avian strain virus which may infect humans & spread person to person. Infection with certain avian Infuenza A virus type, e.g. H5N7 causes widespread, serious disease in domestic birds & turkeys.

The infuenza viruses resist slow drying at room temperature kept on blankets & glass, survive in dust for 2 weeks, & for several weeks if contained in allantoids fluid or infected tissue kept in glycerin saline, & are preserved for long interval at -70^{0}C. These viruses are inactivated at 56^{0}C for 30 minutes, by 20% ether in the cold, phenol, formaldehyde, heavy metals, detergents, soaps, halogens & other substances.

Antigenic Variation

The internal proteins consist of nucleocapsid protein (NC), some matrix proteins (M1) and three polymerases (PA, PB1 and PB2) of which proteins NC and M1 determine type specificity; these proteins elicit cytotoxic T cells that are important in recovery from infection. The nucleoprotein antigen (A, B, C) determines the virus type. The HA and NA antigens determine subtypes. The HA is an envelope antigen (spike) that can attach to erythrocytes and cause agglutination. The attachment of the virion to cell surface receptors (neuraminic acid, sialic acid) can be blocked by antibody; thus it is very important in protective immunity mediated by neutralizing antibody. A HI titer of 1/40 is regarded to be protective.

A unique feature of influenza A viruses is their ability to undergo high rate of antigenic changes in HA & NA proteins, either produced gradually overtime (**Antigenic Drift**) generating new influenza virus strain or suddenly (**Antigenic Shift**) causing emergence of a new influenza A virus subtype. **Antigenic Drift occurs in all the 3 genera of influenza viruses, while Antigenic Shift occurs only inInfluenza A viruses.** There are approximately **16 H antigens** (H1 - H16) and **9 N antigens (N1 - N9),** which may occur in all possible combinations.

Antigenic Drift occurs all the time through natural point mutation in genes of HA & NA proteins in a known influenza virus strain & causes minor change in HA & NA proteins such that persons to the original strain is not immune to the antigen- drifted strain. Hence Antigenic Drift causes sporadic outbreaks & limited epidemics.

Antigenic Shift occurs suddenly due to genetic recombination between non-human & bird or human & animal *Influenza A virus* subtypes infecting the same cell simultaneously. Antigenic shift can occur either through direct poultry-to-human transmission or through mixing of human influenza A and animal influenza A virus genes resulting in a new human influenza A subtype virus through a process called **genetic reassortment.** When 2 different subtypes of *Influenza A virus* infect the same cell simultaneously, it causes reassortment of RNA segments wherein emergence of a new Infuenza A virus subtype occurs carrying major change in HA & or NA antigens that was not currently circulating. Antigenic Shift occurs because, RNA segments are exposed during virus replication, mRNAs are transcribed, the host cells form new virions that reassort their HA & NA antigens, e.g. H5N2 & H5N7 can form H5N7. The host immune system does not recognize new antigens causing highly dangerous new influenza A subtype leading to pandemics. *Influenzavirus A* has gone 4 Antigenic Shift since 1933 (H0N1); 1941 (H1N1), 1968 (H3N2), 1977 variant of H1N3, & 2009 (H1N1).

The Virus Genome

Orthomyxoviruses genome consists of **6 to 8 segments** of linear negative-sense ssRNA with total genome length of 12000-15000 nucleotides. Genome sequence has terminal repeated sequences; repeated at both ends. Terminal repeats at the 5'-end are 12-13 nucleotides long. Nucleotide sequences of 3'-terminus is identical; the same in genera of same family. Terminal repeats at the 3'-end are 9-11 nucleotides long. Each virion may contain defective interfering copies.

Each of the 8 segments is of different length, encodes 10 different polypeptides with different functions as detailed below:

Segment 1 (2341 nt) encodes polypeptide **PB2 (polymerase basic 2)** that acts as transcriptase, a component of viral polymerase & is cap binding.

Segment 2 (2341 nt) encodes polypeptide **PB1-F2** that acts as transcriptase, fusion protein & is an elongation factor.

Segment 3 (2233 nt) encodes polypeptide **PA** that acts as transcriptase & has protease activity.

Segment 4 (1778 nt) encodes polypeptide **HA** that acts as hemagglutinin, binding to sialic acid residue of epithelial receptors, & is needed for transbility.

Segment 5 (1565 nt) encodes polypeptide **NP** that acts as nucleoprotein, RNA binding, part of transcriptase comples, & nuclear & cytoplasmic transport of vRNA.

Segment 6 (1413 nt) encodes polypeptide **NA** that acts as neuraminidase, causes release of virus, ie allows the virus to escape the cell after it has replicated.

Segment 7 (127 nt) encodes 2 polypeptides, **M1** that acts as Matrix protein: a major component of virion membrane, & **M2** an integral membrane protein - ion channel.

Segment 8 (890 nt) encodes 2 polypeptides, **NS1** that is a non-structural protein: nucleus; effects on cellular RNA transport, splicing, translation & anti-interferon protein, & **NS2**, non-structural protein: nucleus+ cytoplasm, mediates export of vRNA. NS1 & NS2 exist only in infected cells.

Viral RNA polymerase (PB1, PB2 and PA) transcribes one mRNA from each genome segment, before it cap of cellular mRNAS is cleaved by Cap snatching. Then mRNAs are polyadenylated by the viral polymerase stuttering on a poly U track. MP and NS mRNA can be spliced, giving rise to mRNA coding for M2 and NEP proteins. PB1-F2 is translated from the +1 ORF of PB1 mRNA.

Virus Replication

Virus replication takes place in the infected cytoplasm **involving nucleus for RNA replication**. These viruses via HA proteins attach to cellular receptors, N-acetylneuraminic acid / sialic acid found on glycoproteins & glycolipids, is endocytosed in the host cell, followed by endosome acidification, which causes fusion of virus membrane with the vesicle membrane. Then uncoating occurs & nucleocapsids are released into the cell cytoplasm. Nucleocapcid is transported to the nucleus where –viral RNA is released. In the nucleus primary transcription of genomic segments occurs starting from cap snatching by viral PB2. This is then used as the primer for the transcription of the protein PB1, a viral transcriptase. In influenza A and B, ten proteins result from the translation of the eight segments of the genome.

Then eight (+c) RNA strands are made from the eight -RNA segments (in influenza A and B but influenza C has seven segments). From this cRNA, a (-) RNA is produced. Various proteins then help this negative sense RNA transport into the cytoplasm. In the cytoplasm, the hemagglutinin and neuraminidase undergo glycosylation, polymerization and acylation. The hemagglutinin, neuraminidase, and the matrix protein, M2 all travel together to the plasma membrane. There the proteins meet with the other matrix protein (M1), and begin the budding process. At least eight RNA segments come to the site (the mechanism is not completely known), and the virus buds. The NA destroys the sialic acid receptors on the membrane, thus allowing the virus to leave through budding from the cell.

Virus Classification

Group: Group V (-) ssRNA

Order: *Unassigned*

Family: *Orthomyxoviridae*

Genera

Influenzavirus A; type species: *Influenza A virus* - Infects humans, birds, pigs, horses & dogs, seals, whales. The current circulating serotypes in humans are- H1N1, H1N2 & H3N2; in birds are- H5N1, H7N2, H1N7, H7N3, H13N6, H5N9, H11N6, H3N8, H9N2, H5N2, H4N8, H10N7, H2N2, H8N4, H14N5, H6N5, H12N5 and others; in pigs are H1N1(classic swine HlNl), avianlike HlNl, H1N2, H3N1, H3N2 (human- and avianlike H3N2), & H2N3; in horses are- H7N7 & H3N8, & in dogs is- H3N8, which is now endemic in birds, horses and dogs.

Influenzavirus B; type species: *Influenza B virus*- Infects humans & seal

Influenzavirus C; type species: *Influenza C virus*- Infects humans & pigs. *Isavirus*; type species:*Infectious salmon anemia virus*- Infects Atlantic salmons.

Thogotovirus; type species: *Thogoto virus* & other is *Dhori virus*- Infects mosquito & ticks & mammals including humans.

Orthomyxovirus Infections in Humans, Animals & Birds

Genus: *Influenzavirus A:*

Table 25.1 : Classifications of *Orthomyxoviridae* & diseases caused by the member species in humans & animals.

Genus1: *Infuenzavirus A:* Type species: *Influenza A virus*-the only species that mainly infect humans, birds, pigs, horses, dogs, & seal.

Subtype	Species	Diseases caused
	Human Influenza A viruses	**H1N1, H1N2 & H3N2 are influenza A virus subtypes currently circulating among humans.** Humans are infected with influenza A viruses either directly from birds or from the infected pigsor through mutations in existing human influenza A viruses in HA & NA genes. New subtypes of influenza A viruses cause pandemics at about 20 years intervals. But sporadic influenza outbreaks occur due to Antigenic drift resulting in antigenically different strains. All influenza pandemics since last 300 years arose in China / Russia/Asia & next pandemics will also probably arise in this region. Epidemics & Pandemics caused by various *Influenza A virus* subtypes in humans are presented below.
	Avian Influenza A viruses	*Only* influenza A *viruses of all known subtypes can infect birds.* Avian influenza A virus strains are classified into **low pathogenic avian influenza (LPAI)** or **highly pathogenic avian influenza (HPAI)** based on molecular genetic and pathogenesis criteria. Most avian influenza A viruses are LPAI viruses that are usually associated with **mild disease in poultry**, but **HPAI viruses cause severe illness and high mortality in poultry.** LPAI viruses can

change to HPAI viruses. Avian influenza A virus subtypes H5 and H7 like H5N1, H7N7 and H7N3 viruses are HPAI, and human infection with these viruses have ranged from mild (H7N3, H7N7) to severe and fatal disease (H7N7, H5N1). Human infections caused by LPAI viruses include very mild symptoms e.g., conjunctivitis to influenza-like illness by LPAI viruses H7N7, H9N2 and H7N2.

There are genetic differences between the influenza A subtypes that infect birds & those that infect both humans and birds. Three main subtypes of the avian influenza A viruses that are known to infect both birds and people are: Influenza A H5 (HPIA-H5N1), Influenza A H7(LPAI-H7N2) & HPAI (H7N3, H7N7, & H9 that rarely infect humans.

Aquatic birds, mainly ducks are reservoir of all subtypes of HA (H1-H16) & of NA (N1-N9), & provide a pool for genetic reassortment to create new subtypes able to infect mammals. Migratory water fowl being the source of all influenza viruses disseminate the viruses across the various nations. Strains of *Influenza A virus* are transmitted from wild fowl to only domestic birds, pigs, horses, seals, whales and humans; and only between humans and pigs and between humans and domestic fowl; and not other pathways such as domestic fowl to horse except H5N1 epizootics. Occasionally, new subtypes of Infueunza A viruses are generated due to gene ressortment with new antigens that are transmitted from these birds to other species and may then cause devastating outbreaks in domestic poultry or may mutate to give rise to human influenza pandemics. H5N1 was transmitted to tigers, leopards, and domestic cats that were fed uncooked domestic fowl (chickens) with the virus. Laboratory mice have been infected successfully with a variety of avian flu genotypes. Avian influenza A viruses is of concern to humans, who have no immunity against it, infection in birds can mutate to infect humans. Such mutation could start a deadly worldwide pandemic. Avian influenza A viruses include: H5N1, H7N2, H1N7, H7N3, H13N6, H5N9, H11N6, H3N8, H9N2, H5N2, H4N8, H10N7, H2N2, H8N4, H14N5, H6N5, H12N5 and others. Known outbreaks of highly pathogenic flu in poultry 1959-2003 are given below.

H5N1	Chickens	Outbreaks occurred in 1959 in Scotland in chickens.
	Turkeys	H5N1 outbreaks occurred in 1991 in England in turkeys.
	Chickens	H5N1 outbreaks occurred in 1997 in Hong Kong, China in chickens.
	Chickens	H5N1 outbreaks occurred in 2002 in Hong Kong, China in chickens.

H7N3	Turkeys	Outbreaks occurred in 1963 in England in turkeys.
	Chickens	H7N3 outbreaks occurred in 1992 in Victoria, Australia in chickens.
	Chickens	H7N3 outbreaks occurred in 1994 in Queensland, Australia in chickens.
	Chickens	H7N3 outbreaks occurred in 1994 in Hong Kong, China in chickens.
	Chickens	H7N3 outbreaks occurred in 2002 in Chile in chickens.
H5N9	Turkeys	Outbreaks occurred in 1966 in Ontorio, Canada in turkeys.
H7N7	Chicken	Outbreaks occurred in 1976 in Victoria, Australia in chickens.
	Chicken	H7N7 outbreaks occurred in 1979 in Germany in chickens.
	Turkeys	H7N7 outbreaks occurred in 1979 in England in turkeys.
	Chicken	H7N7 outbreaks occurred in 1985 in Victoria, Australia in chickens.
	Chicken	H7N7 outbreaks occurred in Netherland in chickens.
H5N2	Turkeys	Outbreaks occurred in 1983 in Pennsylvania,USA in turkeys.
	Chickens	H5N2 outbreaks occurred in 1994 in Mexico in chickens.
	Turkeys	H5N2 outbreaks occurred in 1997 in Italy in turkeys.
H5N8	Chicken	Outbreaks occurred in 1983 in Ireland in chickens.
H7N4	Chickens	Outbreaks occurred in 1997 in New South Wales, Australia in chickens.
H7N1	Turkeys	Outbreaks occurred in 1999 in Italy in turkeys.
	Swine Infuenza A viruses	**Swine influenza or pig influenza, swine flu, hog flu and pig flu,** is an infection by any one of several types of *swine influenza A virus* & is common in pigs worldwide. *Swine influenza virus* **(SIV)** or **S-OIV (swine-origin influenza virus) is any strain of the influenza viruses that is endemic in pigs.** Pigs can be infected with influenza A viruses from birds, from humans & from pigs providing another pool for genetic reassortment resulting in emerging of a new subtype that can infect humans causing pandemics. Swine inluenza A was first observed in the United States during the catastrophic 1918 to 1919 human influenza pandemic. Swine influenza A viruses subtypes include H1N1(classic swine HlNl), avian-like HlNl, H1N2, H3N1, H3N2 (human- and avian-like H3N2), & H2N3 viruses. **In pigs, three influenza A virus subtypes (H1N1, H1N2, and H3N2) are the most common strains worldwide.** Transmission of the virus

from pigs to humans is not common and does not always lead to human influenza except the production of antibodies in the blood. People with regular exposure to pigs are at increased risk of swine flu infection. The meat of an infected animal poses no risk of infection when properly cooked. During the 20th century, influenza subtypes were identified, & since then, 50 such transmissions have been confirmed. These strains of swine flu rarely pass from human to human. Symptoms of zoonotic swine flu in humans resemble human influenza.

Pigs serve as major reservoirs of HlNl and H3N2 influenza viruses which are frequently involved in interspecies transmission of influenza viruses. Although these strains have shown a limited capacity to spread from pigs to humans, their maintenance in pigs and the frequent introduction of new viruses from other species may be important in the generation of pandemic strains of human influenza.

Equine influenza A viruses	Equine influenza or Horse flu refers to varieties of *Influenza A virus* that affects horses. Horse flu viruses were only isolated in 1956. There are two main subtypes of virus called **H7N7 or equine-1,** which commonly affects horse heart muscle, and **H3N8 or equine-2,** which is usually more severe. The disease has a nearly 100% infection rate in an unvaccinated horses. Equine influenza is not known to affect humans.
Canine flu	Canine influenza or Dog flu refers to varieties of Influenza A virus that affects dogs. The equine influenza virus **H3N8** was found to infect and kill with respiratory illness in greyhound race dogs at a Florida race track in January 2004. **H3N8 is now endemic in birds, horses and dogs.**

Genus 2: *Influenzavirus B*. This genus has only one species, *Influenza B virus* that infects **mostly humans** and is less common than *Influenzavirus A*. The other animals infected are **the seal and the ferrets.** The virus mutates 2–3 times slower than type A and hence is less genetically diverse, with only one influenza B serotype & due to antigenic diversity, a degree of immunity to influenza B is usually acquired at an early age but even these mutations do not enable to induce lasting immunity. Due to reduced antigenic change, its limited host range & lack of antigenic shift, **pandemics of influenza B do not occur.**

Genus 3: *Influenzavirus C*. This genus has one species, *Influenza C virus*, which infects humans, dogs and pigs often causing both severe illness and local epidemics. But influenza C is less common than the other types and usually causes **mild disease in children.**

Genus 4: *Isavirus;* type species *Infectious salmon anemia virus,* the only species in the genus. *Infectious salmon anemia virus* infects Atlantic salmon.

Genus 5: *Thogotovirus;* type species: *Thogoto virus* whose RNA has 6 segments; second species is *Dhori virus* whose RNA has 7 segments. *Thogoto virus* was isolated from ticks in

Africa and southern Europe. *Thogoto virus* infects humans in natural settings. Dhori virus was isolated from India, eastern Russia, Egypt, and southern Portugal & is able to infect humans, causing a febrile illness and encephalitis.

Human Influenza A Viruses Epidemic Outbreaks & Pandemics

H1N1, H1N2 & H3N2 are human influenza A virus subtypes currently circulating among humans. Humans are infected with influenza A viruses either directly from birds or from the infected pigs or through mutations in existing human influenza A viruses in HA & NA genes. Auatic birds & water fowls acting as reservoir of all HA & NA subtypes provide a pool of subtypes & favour genetic reassortment with emergence of new subtypes that can occasionally infect humans & occasionally infect pigs. Pigs are infected with Influenza A viruses from birds & also from humans giving another opportunity for creation of a new subtypes infecting humans. Such new subtypes of influenza A viruses cause pandemics at about 20 years intervals. But sporadic influenza outbreaks occur due to Antigenic drift resulting in antigenically different strains. All influenza pandemics since last 300 years arose in China / Russia/ Asia & next pandemics will also probably arise in this region. Epidemics & Pandemics caused by various *Influenza A virus* subtypes in humans are presented below:

H1N1 1918 pandemicor Spanish flu was of avian origin, spread across the world & even to Arctic & remote Pacific islands killing 50-100 million people. **HINI1976 flu epidemic** caused human flu at Fort Dick killing 13 soldiers. **H1N1 1977 Russian flu pandemics** outbreak occurred in May 1977 in China & spread to Russia & Northern hemisphere. **H1N1 2009 swine-origin flu pandemics** occurred in Feb 2009 in Mexico, later spread to 41 countries with 11034 cases & 85 deaths. Triple assorted swine virus H3N2 reassorted with Eurasian avian like swine viruses causing emergence of **S-OIV H1N1.** Pigs are reservoirs of H1N1 & H3N2 both.

H2N2 1957 Asian flu pandemic arose in China in 1957, spread to Hongkong 1957, Japan 1957, & UK & USA 1957 & killed about 1-15 million people. It was avian flu virus origin, arose through reassortment between human & avian virus segments that introduced avian origin H2 & N2 segments to human population.

H3N2 1968 Hongkong flu pandemic was introduced in Hong Kong in 1968, is endemic in China & Vietnam, caused pandemics in 1969-1970 & spread to USA killing 33800 people & a total of .75 million people. It arose through reassortment between human & avian virus segments which contained H3 gene & PB1gene of avian virus.

H5N1 flu 1997 outbreak was due to a highly pathogenic avian influenza A virus (HPAIA) that occurred in Hong Kong in 1997 infecting 18 humans & killing 6, & was controlled by depopulation of poultry. H5N1 new outbreak started in 2003 & spread to Europe & Africa with 424 human infections & 261 deaths. H5N1 has unusual features that include: i, its lethality to poultry as some H5N1 kill natural reservoir waterfowls, ii, they kill mice, iii. fatally infects a no of mammalian species, iv. fatally infects pigs & v, its increased pathogenicity in ferrets & continued transbility to humans, but sustained human to human infections have not occurred although swine origin H5N1 spread among humas but have caused limited fatal infections. It is presently dominant genotype epidemic in birds in South East. H5N1 mutated through antigenic shift of dozen of pathogenic strains. It is of greatest pandemic threat to humans.

H7N7 2003 influenza flu occurred in Holland where 89 people were infected with H7N7 (highly pathogenic strains) subtype with 1 death following an outbreak in poultry on several farms. H7N7 can infect humans, birds, pigs, seals, and horses in the wild; and has infected mice in laboratory studies. This unusual zoonotic potential represents a pandemic threat.

H1N2 2001-2002 flu **called bird flu virus & currently pandemic in both humans & pigs was identified** during the 2001-2002 flu season in Canada, USA, Ireland, Latvia, France, Romania, Oman, India, Malaysia & Singapore with earliest documented outbreak of the virus occurring in India on May 31, 2001. The virus does not cause more severe illness than other influenza viruses. H1N2 was identified by WHO from cases in the UK, Israel & Egypt. H1N2 Wisconsin strain appears to have resulted from the reassortment of the genes of the currently circulating influenza H1N1 & H3N2 subtypes.

H1N2 2010 – 2011 again caused outbreaks in 6 cities in China, & the virus is spreading further. 19 people have passed away, while tens of thousands are currently sick. HA is similar to that of the currently circulating A(H1N1) viruses and the NA is similar to that of the current H3N2 viruses.

H9N2 1999 outbreak was due to bird flu virus & WHO isolated A(H9N2) subtype in 1999 from Hong Kong. H9N2 has infected humans over the years, caused illness in children between 9 months to 5 yrs in Hong Kong & has potential to cause pandemics. Three lineages have been confirmed.

H7N2 2002 flu was a subtype of *Influenza A virus* (bird flu virus) that infected one person in Virginia in USA in 2002 and one person in New York in USA in 2003 following outbreak in poultry; both persons fully recovered. Again H7N2 outbreak occurred in 2007, an outbreak of H7N2 was confirmed at a poultry farm near Corwen in Wales & 9 people who were associated with the infected or dead poultry and reported flu-like symptoms were tested. Four tested positive for H7N2 and were successfully treated for mild flu.

H7N3 2004 bird flu virus caused outbreak in 2004 at many poultry farms in British Columbia in North America infecting 2 humans with conjunctivitis & flu -like symptom. H7N3 was confirmed in UK in 2006 infecting poultry birds & 1 poultry person. In Sept 2007 H7N3 outbreak occurred in Canada & the virus was confirmed as HPAI H7N3 by genotyping.

H10N7 1979 flu was a subtype of *Influenza A virus* (bird flu virus) & the first reported H10N7 outbreak occurred in Minnesota in USA on two turkey farms in 1979 & on a third in 1980 with a mortality rate as high as 31%, to subclinical infection. The viruses were also isolated from healthy mallards on a pond adjacent to the turkey farms. In 2004 in Egypt, H10N7 was reported for the first time in humans in 2004 in Egypt. It caused illness in two one-year old infants in Ismailia, Egypt; one child's father was a poultry merchant.

Avian Influenza

Avian influenza (AI), also called bird influenza or bird flu is an infectious viral disease of birds (especially wild water fowl such as ducks and geese) often causing no apparent signs of illness but can sometimes spread to domestic poultry and cause large-scale outbreaks of serious disease. Some of these AI viruses have also been reported to cross the species barrier and cause disease or subclinical infections in humans and other mammals.

Only *Avian influenza A virus* of all known subtypes can infect birds. Avian influenza A virus strains are classified into **low pathogenic avian influenza (LPAI)** or **highly pathogenic avian influenza (HPAI)** based on molecular genetics and pathogenesis criteria. Most avian influenza A viruses are LPAI viruses that are usually associated with **mild disease** in poultry, but HPAI viruses cause **severe illness and high mortality** in poultry. Avian influenza A virus subtypes H5 and H7 like H5N1, H7N7 and H7N3 viruses are HPAI, and human infection with these viruses have ranged from mild (H7N3, H7N7) to severe and fatal disease (H7N7, H5N1). Human infections caused by LPAI viruses include **very mild symptoms e.g., conjunctivitis to influenza-like illness by LPAI viruses H7N7, H9N2, and H7N2.** There are genetic differences between the influenza A subtypes that infect birds & those that infect both humans and birds. Three main subtypes of the avian influenza A viruses that are known to infect both birds and people are: Influenza A H5 (HPIA-H5N1), Influenza A H7 (LPAI-H7N2) & HPAI (H7N3, H7N7, & H9 that rarely infect humans.

Aquatic birds, mainly ducks are reservoir of all subtypes of HA (H1-H16) & of NA (N1-N9), & provide a pool for genetic reassortment to create new subtypes able to infect mammals. Migratory water fowl being the source of all influenza viruses disseminate the viruses across the various nations. Strains of *Influenza A virus* are transmitted from wild fowl to domestic birds, pigs, horses, seals, whales and humans. Occasionally, new subtypes of Infuenza A viruses are generated due to gene ressortment with new antigens that are transmitted from these birds to other species and may then cause devastating outbreaks in domestic poultry or may mutate to give rise to human influenza pandemics. H5N1 was transmitted to tigers, leopards, and domestic cats that were fed uncooked domestic fowl (chickens) with the virus. Laboratory mice have been infected successfully with a variety of avian flu genotypes. Avian influenza A viruses is of concern to humans, who have no immunity against it, infection in birds can mutate to infect humans. Such mutation could start a deadly worldwide pandemic. Avian influenza A viruses include: H5N1, H7N2, H1N7, H7N3, H13N6, H5N9, H11N6, H3N8, H9N2, H5N2, H4N8, H10N7, H2N2, H8N4, H14N5, H6N5, H12N5 and others.

Cause

Etiology: Avian influenza A virus. The many strains of virus infecting waterfowl provide sources for new mammalian strains, e.g., strain H5N1 is a highly pathogenic avian influenza with high mortality in humans in Hong Kong. Subtypes H5H7 has caused serious outbreaks of avian influenza in commercial flocks of chickens and turkeys.

Occurrence

The avian influenza occurs widely in chickens, ducks, turkeys, quail, pheasants, other fowl and particularly in waterfowl. Avian influenza has recently caused serious outbreaks in SE Asia, & since 2007, tens of millions of chickens have been destroyed to prevent spread of the virus. About 1.2 million chickens were destroyed in 2005 including death of more than 20 people. Avian influenza occurs periodically in several East coast states of the United States. Migratory waterfowl play important role in the outbreaks.

Transmission

Disease transmission is by droplet infection, direct and indirect contact (fomites) & as avian influenza is highly contagious, it spreads rapidly. It is important to note that migratory **waterfowl with subclinical, enteric infections excrete virus for long periods, & act as source of infection for domestic poultry.**

Clinical Symptoms & Lesions

As stated previously, several strains or subtypes of avian influenza viruses exist, mainly associated with subclinical or mild to moderate respiratory infections characterized by coughing and sneezing. Sinusitis may develop and infected birds often experience decreased egg production. Concurrent bacterial infections exacerbate the disease. Highly pathogenic forms of avian influenza cause severe generalized disease with high mortality in commercial flocks; fatality occurs as early as 24 - 48 hours after the onset of clinical signs with occasional neural involvement. The comb and wattles are cyanotic, there is edema of the head region with coughing, gasping, blood-stained oral and nasal discharges, and diarrhea. **PM** lesions depict hemorrhages and congestion of serous and mucous membranes, consolidation of lungs, and caseation involving the air sacs. Focal necrosis may be noted in the skin and internal organs.

Diagnosis

Collection of clinical samples includes whole birds killed in acute phase or lung, trachea, air sac, kidney, spleen, and serum.

1. *Virus isolation* : Virus sample is inoculated in the embryonated eggs and identified using virus neutralization and hemagglutination inhibition tests with specific antisera. Disease is differentiated from NDV with specific immune sera, & allantoic fluid from infected chicken embryos agglutinates RBCs.

2. *Antibody detection* : Sera are tested for antibody using an agar gel diffusion test and embryonated egg antigen.

Treatment & Prevention

Amantadine hydrochloride is used to reduce the severity of influenza in some avian species, but amantadine-resistant viruses have emerged. Antibiotic therapy may be beneficial in controlling secondary bacterial infections in mild forms of avian influenza.

Vaccination

Inactivated vaccines are used, but emergence of new subtypes complicates immunization. Since the pathogenic avian strain H5N1 causes severe influenza in humans, close contact between large numbers of poultry and people should be avoided. The human flue causing the pandemics of 1918, 1957 and 1968 contained gene segments closely related to those of avian influenza viruses. **NDV-based recombinant live attenuated vaccine against H5N1** completely protects chickens and mice from lethal challenge of homologous and heterologous H5N1 avian influenza viruses. Both a wild-type and a mutated HA open reading frame (ORF) from the HPAIV wild bird isolate, A/Bar-headed goose/Qinghai/3/2005 (H5N1), were inserted into the intergenic region between the P and M genes of the LaSota NDV vaccine strain. The recombinant viruses stably expressing the wild-type and mutant HA genes were found to be innocuous after intracerebral inoculation of 1-day-old chickens. A single dose of the recombinant viruses in chickens induced both NDV- and AIV H5-specific antibodies and completely protected chickens from challenge with a lethal dose of both velogenic NDV and homologous and heterologous H5N1 HPAIV. The European Commission has given authorization to two inactivated, adjuvanted avian influenza vaccines. **Nobilis Influenza H5N2-Intervet and Poulvac FluFend H5N3 RG**-Fort Dodge for administration by injection. Both of the vaccines which have been approved reduce mortality and virus excretion in vaccinated chickens exposed to infection. **Nobilis Influenza H5N2** is for use in chickens- two booster vaccinations, 0.5ml IM/SC are recommended at 4 - 6 weeks and 16 - 18 weeks of age. **Poulvac FluFend H5N3 RG** is for use in both chickens and Pekin ducks.Dose is .5 ml IM or SC 3 weeks of age or older & revaccinate after 3 weeks. The vaccination schedule should be completed at least 4 weeks before the start of laying. In ducks at one day old: 0.2 ml SC in the neck & revaccinate after 3 weeks: 0.5 ml SC in the neck. The vaccination schedule should be completed at least 4 weeks before the start of laying. **TrovacAIV H5**- Merial is a live Fowlpox vectored recombinant vaccines for Avian influenza, the first fowl pox vectored vaccine for AI containing an H5 AIV insert given SC. It provides early protection in both broilers and replacement pullets **having** reputation for reliability and safety. It has been proven to be highly effective in preventing morbidity and mortality due to H5 highly pathogenic AI.Vaccine is easy to use in day-old chicks, can be administered to a large number of birds efficiently at the hatchery, can be administered in a controlled environment, it eliminates the biosecurity risks of on-farm vaccination crews, & it provides early and effective protection. A single administration at 1 day of age and initiates early onset (1 week) of protection, (*b*) easy monitoring of AI infection in vaccinated flocks with agar gel precipitation (AGP) and enzyme-linked immunosorbent assay (ELISA) used as tests to differentiate infected from vaccinated animals (DIVA tests).

Swine Influenza

Swine influenza or pig influenza, swine flu, hog flu and pig flu, is an infection by any one of several types of *swine influenza A virus* & is common in pigs worldwide. *Swine influenza A virus* (**SIV**) or **S-OIV (swine-origin influenza virus)** is any strain of the influenza A viruses that is endemic in pigs. In pigs, influenza infection produces fever, lethargy, sneezing, coughing, difficult breathing and decreased appetite. In some cases the infection can cause abortion. Although mortality is usually low (around 1–4%), the virus can produce weight loss and poor growth, causing economic loss to farmers.

Infected pigs can lose up to 12 pounds of body weight over a 3 to 4 week period.

Etiology: Swine influenza is causd by *Swine influenza A virus*. The phylogenetic origin of the flu virus that caused the 2009 pandemics can be traced before 1918. Around 1918, the ancestral virus of avian origin, crossed the species boundaries and infected humans as human H1N1. The same phenomenon took place soon after in America, where the human virus was infecting pigs; it lead the emergence of the H1N1 swine strain, which later became the classic swine flu. **Swine influenza A virus** subtypes include H1N1 (classic swine HlNl), avianlike HlNl, H1N2, H3N1, H3N2 (human- and avianlike H3N2), & H2N3 viruses. **In pigs, three common influenza A virus subtypes (H1N1, H1N2, and H3N2) are the most common strains currently circulating worldwide.** There are also different strains within these serotypes with differing pathogenicity.

Hosts Susceptible

Pigs of all ages are susceptible. Influenza subtypes & strains from swine may produce serious infections in humans, other mammals, and birds. Young susceptible pigs are continually infected, thereby maintaining the virus.

Occurrence

Swine influenza occurs worldwide.

Transmission

Pigs can be infected with influenza A viruses from birds, from humans & from pigs providing another pool for genetic reassortment resulting in emerging of a new subtype that can infect humans causing pandemics. Influenza is quite common in pigs, with about half of breeding pigs having been exposed to the virus in the US. Antibodies to the virus are also common in pigs in other countries.

The main route of transmission is through direct contact between infected and uninfected pigs. Close contacts are common during animal transport. Aerosol droplets, contact, and fomites are the means of spread. In swine herds where the virus is endemic, young susceptible pigs are continually infected, thereby maintaining the virus. Explosive outbreaks of acute disease occur when the virus is introduced into susceptible, naive herds. Intensive farming increases the risk of transmission, as the pigs are raised in very close proximity to each other. The direct transfer of the virus probably occurs either by pigs touching noses, or through dried mucus. Airborne transmission through the aerosols produced by pigs coughing or sneezing is also an important means of infection. The virus usually spreads quickly through a herd, infecting all the pigs within just a few days. Transmission may also occur through wild animals, such as wild boar, which can spread the disease between farms.

Bird flu viruses, which usually infect the gastrointestinal cells of many bird species, **are shed in bird feces. Pigs can pick these viruses up from the environment and seem to be the major way that bird flu virus RNA segments enter the mammalian flu virus population**. People with regular exposure to pigs are at increased risk of swine flu infection. The meat of an infected animal poses no risk of infection when properly cooked. During the 20th century, influenza subtypes were identified, & since then, 50 such transmissions have been confirmed. These strains of swine flu rarely pass from human to human. Symptoms of zoonotic swine flu in humans resemble human influenza. Pigs serve as major reservoirs of HlNl and H3N2 influenza viruses, which are frequently involved in nterspecies transmission of influenza viruses. Although these strains have shown a limited capacity to spread from pigs to humans, their maintenance in pigs and the frequent introduction of new viruses from other species may be important in the generation of pandemic strains of human influenza.

Clinical Symptoms & Lesions

The **incubation period** is about **three days** followed by an acute onset of respiratory distress with rapid respiration, coughing, anorexia, and prostration. Morbidity is high but the mortality is usually about 2%. Virus infection is mild without secondary bacteria. **The clinical course is usually 2 - 6 days** with rapid recovery in uncomplicated cases. With secondary invaders and particularly *Haemophilus suis* the disease is much more serious and some deaths may occur.

Necropsy in acute cases discloses edematous mediastinal lymph nodes and pneumonic lesions usually limited to the apical and cardiac lobes. Affected areas are firm and purplish in color and there is often a sharp line of demarcation between normal and affected tissue. Exudative bronchitis and interstitial pneumonia are common microscopic findings.

In piglets : The clinical symptoms: Colostrum may prevent infection during the sucking period. There may be coughing, pneumonia & fever.

In sows : The clinical symptoms include: high temperatures which cause abortions, widespread coughing & pneumonia. When the virus first enters the herd two or three animals may be observed sick for the first two days, followed by a rapid explosive outbreak of inappetence and clinically very ill pigs. The effects on the reproductive system follow the sudden onset of a rapid spreading respiratory disease with coughing, pneumonia, fevers and inappetence. Acute respiratory distress persists over a period of 7-10 days (depending on the amount of contact between groups of sows).

At a herd level the following may also be seen: a sudden and rapid onset of acute illness in sows, coughing and pneumonia spreading rapidly, a return to clinical normality over 7-10 days, delayed returns to heat after weaning, increased repeats at 21 days, & increased repeats outside the normal cycle. increased numbers of sows coming through not in-pig, increased numbers of abortions, particularly late term, increased numbers of stillbirth rates and slow farrowings, premature farrowings, occasionally an increase in mummified pigs & during the phases of high temperatures other diseases present in the herd may be triggered off. A typical example would be an increase in abortions associated with leptospira infection.

In weaners & growers: Acute disease : The pigs suddenly become prostrated with breathing heavily & severe coughing. Most of pigs look as if they are going to die but most of them survive without treatment unless the herd already has a respiratory disease problem. SI causes severe pneumonia on its own but when it is combined with other infections such as App, EP and PRRS an intractable chronic respiratory disease syndrome can develop. Severely affected individuals or groups of pigs are therefore best given antibiotic cover to prevent secondary pneumonias developing.

Endemic disease : Here the virus remains in the herd, affecting small groups of pigs often weaners. It may be responsible for continuing respiratory diseases with symptoms as in acute disease but less dramatic.

Diagnosis

Collection of clinical samples includes nasal swabs and lungs, acute and convalescent sera.

1. *Presumptive diagnosis :* It is made on the basis of clinical and pathologic findings. There are no other diseases that are so dramatic in their onset and clinical effects. No other disease affects so many pigs so quickly. In acute disease the spread is so dramatic across all ages that little else can be confused with it. In endemic disease however differentiation from other viral infections can be difficult, but PRRS, PRCV, AD and also erysipelas should be considered. Confirmation is done by demonstration of seroconversion or detection of viral infected cells in frozen sections of lung tissue by immunofluorescence.

2. Virus isolation : Swine influenza virus is readily isolated by the inoculation of embryonated eggs using the allantoic cavity. SIV can be

readily grown from nasal and throat swabs and identified in the laboratory. This is often the best approach to confirm the diagnosis.

3. Serology : Blood samples taken at the time of onset of disease from affected sows and repeated 2-3 weeks later show rising levels of antibody to the specific virus.

Treatment & Prevention

In case the disease is severe, antibiotics may be used to control secondary bacteria. Recovery from swine influenza infection confers immunity, but the duration is probably less than a year.

Vaccination

Present vaccination strategies for SIV control and prevention in swine farms typically include the use of one of several bivalent SIV vaccines commercially available in the United States. Of the 97 recent H3N2 isolates examined, only 41 isolates had strong serologic cross-reactions with antiserum to three commercial SIV vaccines. Since the protective ability of influenza vaccines depends primarily on the closeness of the match between the vaccine virus and the epidemic virus, the presence of nonreactive H3N2 SIV variants suggests current commercial vaccines might not effectively protect pigs from infection with a majority of H3N2 viruses. The United States Department of Agriculture researchers say while pig vaccination keeps pigs from getting sick, it does not block infection or shedding of the virus. **End-FLUence-2-** Intervet is a vaccine for use in healthy swine, 3 weeks of age and older for the prevention of influenza caused by serotype A swine influenza (subtypes H1N1, H1N2, and H3N2). This product has been demonstrated to reduce clinical signs, lung lesions and virus shedding following challenge. This product contains an inactivated US Midwest field isolate of subtype H3N2 and an inactivated subtype H1N1 of swine influenza type A virus in Microsol Diluvac Forte® adjuvant. Following vaccination, Duration of Immunity is at least 10 weeks for H3N2, at least 8 weeks for H1N2, and at least 11 weeks for H1N1. Animals retained for breeding should be given a booster dose semiannually. Inject IM 2.0 ml dose at 3 weeks of age or older, followed by one 2.0 ml dose 3 weeks later. Pigs from SIV seropositive dams should be vaccinated after passive maternal antibody levels have declined to allow active immunization. **MaxivacExcell 3**-Intervet is an inactivated vaccine containing two strains of swine influenza virus type A, subtype H1N1, and swine influenza virus type A, subtype H3N2, in a proprietary dual-acting adjuvant (Emunade®). The vaccine is used in healthy pigs 5 weeks of age or older for the prevention of disease associated with swine influenza virus subtypes H1N1 and H3N2. The vaccine has been demonstrated to reduce pneumonia and lung infection following challenge. Inject 2 ml IM into healthy pigs at 5 weeks of age or older. Revaccinate with 2 ml 2-3 weeks after initial vaccination. Pigs nursing non-immune dams can be safely and effectively vaccinated at weaning. Pigs from immune dams should be vaccinated when maternal antibody levels will allow active immunization. Duration of immunity to H3N2 has been demonstrated by challenge to be at least two months following vaccination. **Maxi Platinum**-Intervet contains in addition *M. hyopneumonia.*

Equine Influenza

Horse influenza / Equine influenza (EI) or horse flu is an acute viral, highly contagious disease of equines (horses, ponies, mules & donkeys) which is the OIE listed disease of equines, & characterized by very high rate of transmission among horses, a relatively short incubation period of 1–5 days, elevated temperature, loss of appetite, harsh dry cough, and nasal discharge which may be watery or thick. EI is very contagious and whole stables can be infected but young stock may be hardest hit and more susceptible to complications. Equine influenza or horse flu refers to varieties of Influenza A virus that affects horses. Horse flu viruses were only isolated in 1956. There are two main subtypes of virus called **H7N7 or equine-1**, which commonly affects horse heart muscle, and **H3N8 or equine-2**, which is usually more severe.

Etiology : Equine Influenza virus A. Subtypes involved are A/equine/ Prague/1/56 (H7N7) or A/equine /Miami/2 /63 (H3N8). These are also referred to as influenza A/equine1 and influenza A/equine 2. They are also referred to as Type 1 or A and Type 2 or A Equi-2 (Miami). New variants resulting from antigenic drift appear to be infrequent. All recent and current outbreaks have been attributed to A Equi-2.

Occurrence

Equine influenza A is frequently occurring highly contagious disease of horses, mules and donkeys with worldwide distribution but Australia, New Zealand and Iceland are free. Variants of A Equi-2 attributed to antigenic drift have been reported. The last outbreak of A Equi-1 was reported in 1980, & 2007. Australia was free of equine influenza until an outbreak in August 2007 occurred, which was controlled and Australia has returned to its equine influenza-free status.

Transmission

Transmission occurs by direct and indirect contact, but droplet infection is the main route of spread. Horses may keep on shedding the virus for 7- 10 days. The most common way of spread is through aerosol route. The virus can be spread by contact between infected and susceptible horses, contaminated equipment, susceptible horses coming in contact with premises or vehicles recently occupied by infected horses, which have not been decontaminated and persons attending the infected animals.

Clinical Symptoms & Lesions

After infection by the respiratory tract, the virus replicates and destroys epithelial cells of the upper respiratory tract. Clinical symptoms appear in about 1 - 3 days. Important symptoms include fever, depression, anorexia, and coughing. The infected horses exhibit ocular discharge and photophobia, and some cases may develop edema of the legs. Pneumonia occasionally occurs if the infection is complicated with secondary bacterial infection. Natural recovery occurs in about 7 - 10 days, although the ability to work is impaired for several weeks. Disease severity depends mainly on immune status and age. Usually young horses are more susceptible.

Diagnosis

Collection of clinical samples includes nasal and ocular swabs during the acute phase, & acute and convalescent sera.

1. *Presumptive diagnosis* : Diagnosis is based on clinical signs, sudden onset, rapid spread, high fever, and coughing.
2. *Virus isolation* : Virus isolation is done in embryonated chicken eggs.
3. *Serology* : A significant rise in specific antibody between acute and convalescent sera using hemagglutination inhibition (HI) tests is confirmatory.

Treatment & Prevention

Animals showing clinical signs should be given symptomatic treatment; broad spectrum antibiotic coverage should be given to the sick animals to avoid secondary bacterial infections. Animal should be given adequate rest for 3-4 weeks. The affected animals should be isolated for 28 days to prevent spread. Premises should be cleaned and disinfected to reduce spread. Maintain strict quarantine and controlled movement of equine influenza infected animals within the state as well as outside the state. Interstate movement of the equines should be minimized and/ or even stopped completely for six weeks. Phenyl (1%), Chloroxylenol (Dettol) (1%), chlorhexidine (1-2%), formalin (0.2-0.5%) when applied for 20 to 30 minutes are effective in inactivating the virus.

Vaccination

Killed vaccines with or without adjuvants are used to prevent the disease. The protection is short and periodic boosters are required. A modified-live virus vaccine protects the horses for six months. A primary course of two injections 21-42 days apart is used. A primary booster 150-215 days after the second injection is given. An annual booster less than 365 days after the third injection is recommended. **Equilis Prequenza Te**-Intervet is an inactivated vaccine containing per dose of 1 ml purified hemagglutinin subunits from equine influenza viruses: 100 AU[1] A/equi-1/ Prague/1/ 56; 50 AU A/equi-2/ Newmarket/1/93; 50 AU A/equi-2/ Newmarket/2/93 and 40 Lf[2] Tetanus toxoid, with an ISCOM-Matrix (375 microgram purified Saponin; 125 microgram Cholesterol; 62.5 microgram Phosphatidylcholine. Inject one dose 1ml by IM route; primary vaccination: first injection from 6 months of age, second injection 4 weeks later. Revaccination- the first revaccination (third dose) against equine influenza is given 5 months after the primary vaccination course. This revaccination results in immunity to equine influenza lasting at least 12 months. The second revaccination is given 12 months after the first revaccination. The alternate use, at 12 months interval, of a suitable vaccine against equine influenza, containing the strains A/equi 1/Prague 56, A/equi 2/Newmarket 1/93 and A/equi 2/Newmarket 2/93, is recommended to maintain immunity levels for the influenza component. For tetanus first revaccination is given not later than 17 months after the primary vaccination course. Thereafter a maximum interval of two years is recommended.

Proteq Flu- /Recombitek- Merial is a Influenza A/equi-2/Ohio/03 [H3N8] & Influenza A/equi-2/Newmarket /2/93 [H3N8] recombinant Canarypox virus (vCP2242) vaccine. Dose is 1ml IM to be given to horses. Horses should receive a primary vaccination, consisting of two injections at 5 - 6 months of age, given 4 - 6 weeks apart. This should be followed by revaccination 5 months later and afterwards by yearly booster vaccinations. In case of increased risk of infection or insufficient intake of colostrums (first milk), an additional initial injection can be given at the age of 4 months, followed by the full vaccination programme (primary vaccination and following revaccinations).

Canine Influenza

Canine influenza or Dog flu is a highly contagious respiratory infection of dogs that is caused by infuenza A virus subtypes. The canine influenza virus is closely related to the virus that causes equine influenza and it is thought that the equine influenza virus mutated to produce the canine influenza virus. Canine influenza is caused by varieties of Influenza A subtypes, such as equine influenza virus H3N8, which in 2004 was discovered to cause disease in dogs.

Because of the lack of previous exposure to this virus, dogs have no natural immunity to this virus. Therefore, the disease is rapidly transmitted between individual dogs. Canine influenza may be endemic in some regional dog populations of the United States. It is a disease with a high morbidity but a low mortality. The equine influenza virus **H3N8** was found to infect and kill with respiratory illness greyhound race dogs at a Florida race track in January 2004. H3N8 is now endemic in birds, horses and dogs.

Etiology : Influenza A virus subtype H3N8. Genome analysis revealed that H3N8 was transferred from horses to dogs and then adapted to dogs through point mutation in the genes. It does not induce a persistent carrier state.

Occurrence

Highly contagious *Equine influenza A virus* subtype H3N8 was found to have been the cause of Greyhound race dog fatalities from a respiratory illness at a Florida racetrack in January 2004. The virus exposure and transfer occurred at horse racing tracks, where dog racing also occurs. This was the first evidence of an influenza A virus causing disease in dogs. However, serum collected from racing Greyhounds between 1984 and 2004 and tested for canine influenza virus (CIV) in 2007 had positive tests going as far back as 1999. It is possible that CIV caused some of the respiratory disease outbreaks at tracks between 1999 and 2003.

Species Susceptible

Canine influenza is a newly emerging disease, hence almost all dogs, regardless of breed or age, are susceptible to infection and have no immunity. Virtually all dogs that are exposed to the virus become infected and nearly 80% show clinical signs of disease. Fortunately, most affected dogs have the mild form.

Transmission

Canine influenza cases occurred in animal shelters, humane societies, rescue groups, pet stores, boarding kennels, and veterinary clinics. Canine influenza virus can be spread via direct contact with respiratory secretions from infected dogs, and by contact with contaminated inanimate objects. H3N8 was also responsible for a major dog flu outbreak in New York State in all breeds of dogs. From January to May 2005, outbreaks occurred at 20 racetracks in 10 states. Till August 2006, dog flu has been confirmed in 22 U.S. states, including pet dogs in Wyoming, California, Connecticut, Delaware, and Hawaii. There are three areas in the United States that may now be considered endemic for CIV due to continuous waves of cases: New York, southern Florida, and northern Colorado/southern Wyoming. There is no evidence that the virus can be transferred to people, horses, cats, or other species.

H5N1 (avian influenza) also caused death in one dog in Thailand, following ingestion of an infected duck.

Clinical Symptoms & Lesions

The **incubation period** is 2-5 days and viral shedding occurs for 7-10 days following the onset of symptoms. Two clinical syndromes have been seen in dogs infected with the canine influenza virus; a mild form of the disease and a more severe form that is accompanied by pneumonia. Majority (80%) of dogs are infected with H3N8 type showing mild symptoms, the rest (20 %) show subclinical infection, and the fatality rate for Greyhounds in early outbreaks was 5 to 8 percent, although the overall fatality rate in the general pet and shelter population is probably less than 1 percent.

Symptoms of the **mild form** include a cough that lasts for ten to thirty days and possibly a **greenish nasal discharge**. Dogs suffering with the mild form of canine influenza develop a **soft, moist cough that persists for 10 to 30 days**. Some dogs have a dry cough similar to the "kennel cough" caused by *Bordetella bronchiseptica*/parainfluenza virus complex. Dogs with the mild form of influenza may also have a thick nasal discharge, which is usually caused by a secondary bacterial infection.

Dogs with the **more severe form** may have a **high fever** (104ºF to 106ºF) **and pneumonia w ith** increased respiratory rates and effort. Pneumonia in these dogs is not caused by the influenza virus, but by secondary bacterial infections. The fatality rate of dogs that develop pneumonia secondary to canine influenza can reach 50 percent if not given proper treatment. Dogs with the severe form of canine influenza develop high fevers and have clinical signs of pneumonia,. Pneumonia may be due to a secondary bacterial infection.

PM lesions in dogs that die from the disease show severe hemorrhagic pneumonia and vasculitis.

Diagnosis

The presence of an upper respiratory tract infection in a dog that has been vaccinated for the other major causes of kennel cough increases suspicion of infection with canine influenza, especially in areas where the disease has been documented. A serum sample from a dog suspected of having canine influenza can be submitted to a laboratory that performs PCR tests for this virus.

Treatment & Prevention

Treatment is largely supportive. Good animal care practices and nutrition assist dogs in mounting an effective immune response. In the milder form of the disease, a thick green nasal discharge, which most likely represents a secondary bacterial infection, usually resolves quickly after treatment with a broad-spectrum bactericidal antimicrobial. In the more severe form of the disease, pneumonia is thought to often be caused by bacterial superinfection, and responds best to hydration (sometimes via intravenous administration of fluids) and a broad-spectrum bactericidal antimicrobial.

Vaccination

U. S. Dept of Agriculture (USDA) under Animal & Plant Health Inspection services (APHIS) approved in June 2009 the first canine influenza vaccine. **NobivacCanine Flu H3N8** -Intervet has been shown to control the spread and minimize the impact of CIV infection and has been proven safe in half a million dogs. Dose is two 1-ml doses given SC 2 to 4 weeks apart. Annual revaccination with one dose is recommended.

Influenzavirus B Infection

Infuenzavirus B genus has only one species, *Influenza B virus* that infects mostly humans and is less common than *Influenzavirus A*. The other animals infected are the seal and the ferrets. The virus mutates 2–3 times slower than type A and hence is less genetically diverse, with only one influenza B serotype & due to antigenic diversity, a degree of immunity to influenza B is usually acquired at an early age. But even these mutations do not enable to induce lasting immunity. Due to reduced antigenic change, its limited host range & lack of antigenic shift, pandemics of influenza B do not occur. The Influenza B virus genome is 14648 nucleotides long and consists of eight segments of linear negative-sense, single-stranded RNA.

Majority of the *Influenza B virus i*n 2004, were similar to a strain called B/Shanghai/361/2002, which is from the so-called B/Yamagata/1688 hemagglutnin lineage. That lineage was not the one that was being used in the vaccine that was current last year. In a minority of the strains that were found during the epidemiological studies were similar to the strain that was in the vaccine for last year, which was B/Hong Kong/330/2001, which belongs to the HA lineage that we represent with the strain B/Victoria/287. New viruses are definitely spreading. The Fujian-like viruses had become widespread around the world and were predominant everywhere, and these B/Shanghai-like strains were predominant not only in North America and the United States, but also in Asia and Europe.

Infuenzavirus C Infection

Influenzavirus C genus has one species, *Influenza C virus,* type species is Influenza C/California/78 (FLUCV) which infects humans, dogs and pigs often causing both severe illness and local epidemics. But influenza C is less common than the other types and usually causes mild disease in children. Genus *Influenzavirus* A and B have 8 RNA segments and encode 11 proteins but *Influenzavirus* C has 7 RNA segments and encodes 9 proteins.The major influenza C virus envelope glycoprotein is called HEF (hemagglutinin-esterase-fusion) because it has the functions of both the HA and the NA as the influenza virion contains 7 RNA segments. Nearly all adults have been infected with influenza C virus, which causes mild upper respiratory tract illness. Lower respiratory tract complications are rare. There is no vaccine against influenza C virus.

Thogotovirus Infection

Thogotovirus can replicate in both tick cells and vertebrate cells and is usually transmitted by ticks. *Thogotovirus has two species: Thogoto virus* RNA has 6 segments. The second species is *Dhori virus* whose RNA has 7 segments. *Thogoto virus* was isolated from ticks in Africa and southern Europe. *Thogoto virus* infects humans in natural settings. *Dhori virus* was isolated from India, eastern Russia, Egypt, and southern Portugal & is able to infect humans, causing a febrile illness and encephalitis.

□□□

Chapter 26

Characteristics and Diseases Caused by Group V Single-Strande (-) RNA Paramyxoviruses (Family *Paramyxoviridae*)

Contents

Characteristics of Paramyxoviruses

The viruses under the order *Mononegavirale* & the family *Paramyxoviridae* (L. para= by the side of; myxa= mucus) are enveloped, peplomer bearing, spherical or filamentous or pleomorphic particles measuring 150-200 nm in diameter & 1000-10000 nm long .

Fusion (F) proteins and **attachment proteins (H/HN/G)** form the spikes on the virion surface. **Matrix proteins (M)** lie inside the envelope & stabilise virus structure. The nucleocapsid **core** is composed of the **genomic RNA, nucleocapsid proteins (NP), phosphoproteins (P) and polymerase proteins**. The nucleocapsid has **helical symmetry** with a diameter of 13-18 nm & 600-800 nm long.The viral genome is **non-segmented**, linear, negative-sense RNA, 15-19 kb in length and contains 6-10 genes. **An ideal structure of a paramyxovurus is shown in Fig 26-1.** Most of the viruses can be propagated in embryonated eggs and in cell cultures with the production of cytopathic effects including syncytia and cytoplasmic inclusions.

Paramyxoviruses cause several important diseases in humans & many diseases of great veterinary importance. Human diseases include **measles, mumps, and human parainfluenza**, which cause bronchitis, croup, and pneumonia in children. Measles and mumps have only one serotype. In 1998, two new virulent paramyxoviruses, the **Hendra and Nipah** viruses, were isolated in Malaysia and Singapore. Diseases of veterinary importance include **canine distemper, rinderpest, Peste des petits ruminants, Phocine distemper**- distemper-like disease in harbor seals, Dolphin distemper, Bovine respiratory syncytial virus infection, & in birds **Newcastle disease & Turkey rhinotracheitis**.

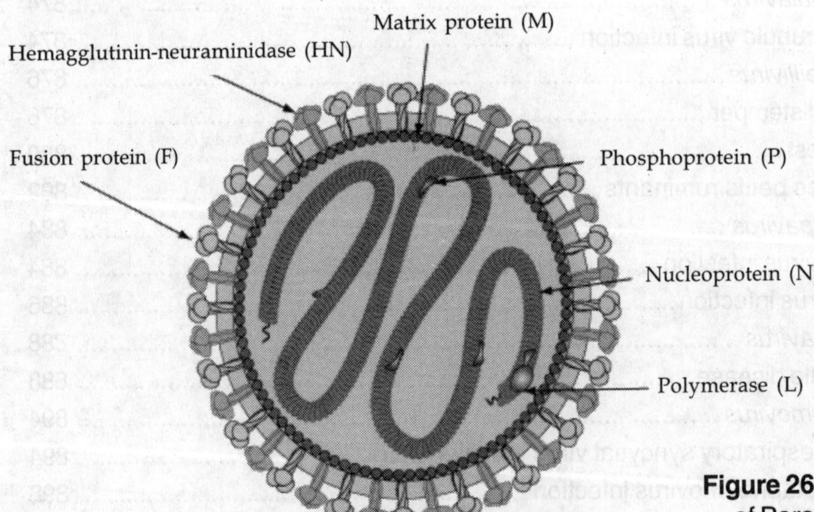

Figure 26.1 : Morphology of Paramyxoviruses

The viruses are generally sensitive to heat, desiccation, drying, lipid solvents and many disinfectants.

The Viral Genome

The viral genome is non-segmented, linear, negative-sense RNA about 15-19 kb in length having 6-10 genes. Extracistronic or non-coding regions include: A 3′ leader sequence of 50 neucleotided (nt) in length which acts as a transcription promoter, a 5′ trailer sequence of 50-161 nt long & intergenomic regions between each gene of three nt long for *Morbillivirus, Respirovirus* and *Henipavirus,* but of variable length (1-56 nucleotides) for *Rubulavirus* and *Pneumovirinae.* Often, virions may contain a positive-sense, single-stranded copy of the genome. The 5'-end of the negative-sense strand does not contain a covalently attached terminal protein, nor a cap & 3′ end has no poly A. Each gene contains transcription start/stop signals at the beginning and end which are transcribed as part of the gene. The viral RNA dependent RNA polymerase binds the genome at the leader region & sequentially transcribes each gene by recognizing start and stop signals flanking viral genes. mRNAs are capped and polyadenylated by the L protein during synthesis. The genome encodes 7-9/9-11, namely three nucleocapsid-associated proteins (N or NP; P and L), three membrane-associated proteins, a matrix protein M and two envelope proteins (F and G, or H, or HN). Viral proteins are described below:

N - The nucleocapsid protein associates with genomic RNA (one molecule per hexamer) and protects the RNA from nuclease digestion.

P - The phosphoprotein binds to the N and L proteins and forms part of the RNA polymerase complex.

M - The matrix protein assembles between the envelope and the nucleocapsid core, it organizes and maintains virion structure.

F - The fusion protein projects from the envelope surface as a trimer, and **mediates cell entry by inducing fusion between the viral envelope and the cell membrane** by class I fusion. One of the defining characteristics of members of the paramyxoviridae family is the requirement for a **neutral pH** for fusogenic activity.

H/HN/G - The cell attachment proteins span the viral envelope and project from the surface as spikes. They bind to proteins on the surface of target cells to facilitate cell entry. Proteins are designated **H (hemagglutinin) for morbilliviruses and henipaviruses, HN** (hemagglutinin -neuraminidse) attachment proteins occur in **respiroviruses, rubulaviruses and avulaviruses.** They possess both haemagglutination and neuraminidase activity which cleaves sialic acid on the cell surface, preventing viral particles from reattaching to previously infected cells. Attachment proteins with neither haemagglutination nor neuraminidase activity are designated **G (glycoproten)** that occur in members of **pneumovirinae.**

L - The large protein is the catalytic subunit of RNA-depedent-RNA polymerase (RDRP).

Accessory proteins - A mechanism known as RNA editing allows multiple proteins to be produced from the P gene. These are not essential for replication but may aid in survival in vitro or may be involved in regulating the switch from mRNA synthesis to antigenome synthesis.

The virion also encodes **6 non structural proteins.** The virus codes for enzymes; besides the polymerase, the virus coded enzymes include a RNA-dependent RNA transcriptase, adenylated transferase, mRNA guanylyl transferase, methyl-transferase, proteinase, and neuraminidase. The non-structural protein is associated with the membrane protein. Others are non-structural proteins are C, NS1, NS2, V, a cystein rich protein having role is zinc binding, SH, a small integral membrane protein, & M2, formerly called 22-kDa with role in transcription processivity factor, which previously was thought to be a second M-like protein.

Virus Replication

Paramyxoviruses replication is like infuenza, but the replication occurs in the cytoplasm. Firstly, the virions via its attachment proteins bind to the surface receptors of host cell, the viral envelope fuses to the cell plasma membrane & the nucleocapsid is released into the cell. The viral genome is transcribed processively from the 3' end by virion-associated enzymes. First of all, negative-sense RNA is transcribed into individual mRNAs, and a positive-sense RNA template, which is used to create negative-sense RNA. Assembly occurs, and new viruses bud from the cell membrane acquiring the envelope. Nucleocapsids are enveloped at sites containing virus capsid proteins. Paramyxoviruses can cause cell-to-cell fusion, creating large multinucleated cells called **syncytia.**

Virus Classification

Groop : group V (-) ss RNA

Order : *Mononegavirales*

Family : *Paramyxoviridae*

Subfamily 1 : Paramyxovirinae

Genus 1 : *Respirovirus;* type species: *Sendai virus* (SeV); others include *Human parainfluenza virus* (HPIV1, 3), *Bovine parainfluenza virus* (BPIV-,3), *Simian virus* (SV-10) & some of the viruses of the common cold.

Genus 2 : *Rubulavirus;* type species: *Mumps virus* (MuV); others include *Human parainfluenza viruses* (HPIV-2, 4), *Simian parainfluenza virus 5* (SPIV-5), *Menangle parainfluenza viruses, Tioman parainfluenza viruses, Tuhoko parainfluenza viruses 1, 2 and 3.*

Genus 3 : *Morbillivirus;* type species: *Measles virus* (MeV); others include *Rinderpest virus* (RPV), *Canine distemper virus* (CDV), *Phocine distemper virus* (PDV), *Peste Des Petits Ruminants virus* (PPRV).

Genus 4 : *Henipavirus;* type species: *Hendra virus* (HeV); others include *Nipah virus* (NiV).

Genus 5 : *Avulavirus:* type species: *Newcastle disease virus* (NDV/APMV1).

Genus 6 : TPMV-like parainfluenza viruses; type species: *Tupaia paramyxovirus.*

Subfamily 2 : Pneumovirinae

Genus 1 : *Pneumovirus;* type species *Human respiratory syncytial virus* (HRSV), others include *Bovine respiratory syncytial virus* (BRSV).

Genus 2 : *Metapneumovirus;* type species *Avian pneumovirus, Human metapneumovirus,* Unassigned viruses

For de Lance virus, Nariva virus, Tupaia paamyxovirus, Salem virus, & j virus.

Table 26.1 : Classification of *Paramyxovirdae* & diseases caused by the virus species in humans & animals.

Species	Serotypes	Diseases caused
SF1 : *Paramyxovirinae*		
G1 : *Respirovirus*		
Bovine parainfluenza virus 3	BPIV-3	*Bovine parainfluenza virus 3* (BPIV-3) is a common cause of mild to subclincal respiratory infection in cattle & sheep serving as an initiator of secondary bacterial infections. Host: Cattle & sheep. Transmission: Direct & indirect contact. Pathogenesis: BPIV-3 damages alveolar macrophags that reduces defence against bacteria mainly *Mannheirnia & P. multocida* causing shiping fever. Diagnosis: Clinical specimens, virus isolation, CPE, 4-fold incease of Ab titre. Teatment: Animicrobial drugs. **Vaccine** : Killed & attenuated BPIV-3 vaccines are used.

Human parainfluenza virus 1	HPIV-1	*Human parainfluenza virus 1* (HPIV-1) is the second most common cause of lower resprratory tract infection in children, is a common cause of croup, & in immunosuprssed people causes severe pneumonia.
Human parainfluenza virus 3	HPIV-3	*Human parainfluenza virus 3* (HPIV-3) is associated with broncholitis & pneumonia in humans.
TS : *Sendai virus*	SeV 3 strains	*Sendai virus* (SeV), also called Murine parainfluenza virus-1 or hemagglutinating virus of Japan (HVJ) causes **respiratory tract infction in mice, G. pigs, rats, & occasionally pigs.** SeV is used in fusion of eukaryotic cells to produce hybridoma.
Simian virus	SV-10	Infects monkeys
G2: *Rubulavirus*		
TS: *Mumps virus*	MuV -5 strains	*Mumps virus* (MuV) causes mumps in children with swelling of the parotid glands and other epithelial tissues causing high morbidity and in some cases more serious complications such as deafness.
Porcine rubula virus	PoRV- 2 strains	*Porcine rubula virus* (PoRV) infection or **blue eye disease** is an emerging disease first seen in La Piedad in 1980 in Mexico & is characterized by encephalitis and respiratory disease in piglets, & reproductive failure in adult pigs, and occasional corneal opacity in all ages.There are 2 strains-La-Piedad-Michoacan-Mexican virus or LPMV & La-Piedad-Michoacan LPMV. **Occurrence**: PoRV infection in swine was first reported in Mexico in 1980 and still occurs there. It has not been reported from outside of Mexico. **Hosts:** Occurs in pigs & ismost severe in pigs younger than three weeks. **Transmission**: PoRV infection occus through direct contact and indirect means like fomites.
Human parainfluenza virus 2	HPIV-2	*Human parainfluenza virus 2* (HPIV- 2) causes croup and other upper and lower respiratory tract illnesses in younger childen.
Human parainfluenza virus 4	HPIV-4	HPIV-4 includes subtypes 4a and 4b.
Mapuera virus	MPRV	MPRV was originally isolated from bats, but its host range remains unknown. It encodes a **V protein** (MPRV/V) that functions as an interferon (IFN) antagonist.

Simian virus SV There are 2 strains SV-5 & SV-41

G3: *Morbillivirus*

Canine distemper virus CDV Canine distemper (CDV) is a viral, contagious, pantropic disease affecting many organs of dogs & other carnivores, & characterized by a diphagic fever, GIT & respiratory symptoms, leukopenia, often neurological symptoms & hard footpad. **Occurrence**: Worldwide. The first case was described in 1905 by French veterinarian Henri Carre. Puppies experience the highest mortality rate. **Hosts**: Animals of family Canidae-dogs, wolves, coyotes & jackal, *Mustelidae*-ferrets, mink & skunk, *Procyonidae*-raccons & coatimundi, & *Vireridae*-binturong. Pupies 3-6 mths are more susceptible. **Transmission**: Aerosols, contact, inhalation, and the infected body fluids.

Phocine distemper virus PDV It is seal distemper virus.

Rinderpest virus. RPV Rinderpest (RPV) also called cattle plague is viral disease of cattle, domestic buffaloes, some species of wildlife & is characterized by fever, oral erosions, diarrhea, lymphoid necrosis & high mortality (roughly 80%) in acute cases. FAO declared in 2011 the global eradication of rinderpest.

Peste des petits ruminants virus PPRV *Peste des petits ruminantsvirus* (PPRV), also called ovine rinderpest, pseudorinderpest of small ruminants, pest of small ruminants, pest of sheep and goats, Kata, stomatitis-pneumoenteritis syndrome, contagious pustular stomatitis, and pneumoenteritis complex, is a highly contagious, an acute or subacute viral disease of goats and sheep characterized by fever, necrotic stomatitis, gastroenteritis and pneumonia.

G4: *Henipavirus*

TS: *Hendra virus* HeV *Hendra virus* (HeV), previously called equine morbilli virus causes an acute viral disease in horses & is characterized by an acute onset, fever, respiratory distress, neurological sign & rapid progression to death. It is of zoonotic importance as humans are also affected in some outbreaks with neurological symptoms. **Occurrence:** HeV was first reported in 1994 in Hendra, Brisbane, Australia killing 14 horses & one trainer, & since 1999, 13

		outbreaks have occurred in horses involving infection of horses, & in 4 outbreaks humans were also infected. Mortality rate is more than 70%. **Hosts:** Horses are susceptible, & no other animals are susceptinble, Humans in close contact become susceptible indirectly. **Transmission: Flyimg foxes are the natural hosts** for HeV. The disease is spread from foxes to horses & foxes to humans, but human-to-human & human to horse spread are not possible. Most human cases probably occurred from bats urine or birthing fluids & to humans remaining in close contact with the sick horses or during autopsies.
Nipah virus	NiV	*Nipah virus* (NiV) causes **'porcine respiratory and neurological syndrome'**, or **'porcine respiratory and encephalitis syndrome'**, or in Malaysia, **'barking pig syndrome'**. The disease is an **emerging zoonotic disease in SE Asia**, a highly contagious viral disease of pigs & other animals also involving humans, & is characterized by **severe respiratory or neurological distress, & encephalitis in humans with high mortality rate. Occurrence**: NiV is an endemic disease in SE Asia- Malaysia, Singapore, Bangla Desh & North India, & was identified in 1998 in pig farms in Malaysia with respiratory distress & neurological disease as well as 15 human deaths in abattoir workers. Other domestic animals like dogs, cats, goats & 1 horse also suffered. **Hosts:** Pigs are the most susceptible, & besides hoseses, goats, sheep, cats, dogs are also susceptible. Fruit bats **(flying foxes)** of the genus *Pteropus*, *P. hypomelanus* & *P. vampyrus* (large flying foxexes) are the reservoir hosts. Humans also suffer from the disease with severe illness showing mainly encephalitis. **Transmission:** Fruit bats (flying foxex).
G5: *Avulavirus*		
New castle disease virus or *Avian parmyxovirus-i* (NDV/APMV-1)	NDV/AP MV-1	*New castle disease virus* or *Avian parmyxovirus-1* (NDV/APMV-1), is a contagious viral disease of birds affecting many domestic and wild avian species characterized by severe respiratoty or nervous signs or diarrhea (Velogenic strains) with rapid spread causing up to 90% mortality or cause coughing, affect egg quality and production and result in up to 10% mortality (Mesogenic strains) or produce mild signs with negligible mortality (Lentogenic strains). **NDV Strains**: There are seven

antigenic varieties, each causing characteristic disease manifestations. These are **five pathotypes** as follows: i. Viscerotropic velogenic NDV causes severe disease in which haemorrhagic lesions are characteristically present in the intestinal tract; ii. Neurotropic velogenic NDV causes respiratory & nervous signs followed by high mortality. iii. Mesogenic NDV causes respiratory & often nervous signs with low mortality; iv. Lentogenic respiratory NDV causes mild or inapparent respiratory infection; v.Asymptomatic enteric NDV causes inapparent enteric infection. APMV-1 isolates are grouped into two clades, called class I and class II, based on the genetic relationship between viruses. The vast majority of APMV-1 strains belong to class II, which is divided into at least nine genotypes (I to IX). Class I isolates have been found mainly in wild waterfowl, and are usually of low pathogenicity.

SF2: *Pneumovirinae*

G1:*Pneumovirus*

Bovine respiratory syncytial virus	BRSV	*Bovine respiratory syncytial virus* (BRSV) causes respiratory disease mainly in young beef and dairy cattle characterized by severe respiratory disease initially but mild to subclinical disease in subsequent infections. BRSV occupies an important place in the bovine respiratory disease complex due to its repeated occurrence, virus predilection for the lower respiratory tract, and predisposition of respiratory tract to secondary bacterial infections. **Occurrence**: BRSV infection occurs throughout the world. In outbreaks, morbidity is high but the mortality is 0-20%. **Hosts:** Cattle, sheep and goats are susceptible to BRSV; it is widely distributed in cattle but mainly in young beef and dairy cattle. Weaned and transported calves are more susceptible.
Human respiratory syncytial virus (TS)	HRSV	*Human respiratory syncytial virus* (HRSV) is the major cause of lower respiratory tract infection during infancy and childhood. Treatment includes supportive care, including oxygen. In temperate climates there is a yearly epidemic during the winter months but in tropical climates, infection is common during the rainy season. Severe HRSV infections have also occrred in elderly patients. There are 3 strains of HRSV.

Murine pneumonia virus/ Pneumonia virus of mice	PVM	*Murine pneumonia virus*/ Pneumonia virus of mice (PVM) is a natural respiratory pathogen of rodent species and an important new model for the study of severe viral bronchiolitis and pneumonia. Even in presence of high virus titers in mouse lung tissue *in vivo*, cell lines *in vitro* are not highly susceptible to PVM infection. Cells induces the synthesis and secretion of proinflammatory cytokines e.g. tumor necrosis factor-α (TNF-α), interferon-β (IFN-β), macrophage inflammatory proteins 1α and 1β (MIP-1α and MIP-1β) and the functional homolog of human IL-8, & mouse macrophage inflammatory peptide-2 (MIP-2). PVM pathophysiology causing bronchiolitis leading to pneumonia and acute respiratory distress syndrome (ARDS) is similar to that of severe respiratory syncytial virus (HRSV) infection in human infants.
Ovine respiratory syncytial virus	ORSV	
G2: *Metapneumovirus*		
Avian metapneumo virus	AMPV	*Avian metapneumovirus* (AMPV) infection causes disease in turkeys and chickens of all ages & is characterized by a upper respiratory frast disease and drops in egg production in layers and breeders with low mortality, but high morbidity primarily in commercial turkeys. **Occurrence**: The disease occurs in most countries in the world. Recently there was an emergence of a virulent type C AMPV in turkeys in Minnesota. **Hosts**: Turkeys & chickens of all ages, pheasants and guinea fowl are susceptible, and antibodies to the virus have been found in wild birds and other domestic species. There are three types of MPV (A, B, C) of which the C type is found only in the United States.
Human metapneumo virus	HMPV	*Human metapnumovirus* (HMPV) causes a repiratory illnesses varying from asymptomatic infection to severe brochiolitis & pneumonia in children as well as in all age groups. HMPV is the second most important cause of pediatric lower respiratory illness, next to RSV. HMPV is ubiquitous worldwide. The clinical symptoms include high fever, myalgia, rhinorrhea, dyspnea, tachypnea, and wheezing. While bronchiolitis, with or without

pneumonia, is the most common symptoms of HMPV illness. Other syndromes include **asthma exacerbation, otitis media, pneumonitis, flu-like illness, community acquired pneumonia, and COPD exacerbation.** The identification of HMPV depends on RT-PCR or the detection of HMPV by nucleic acid using imunofluorescent antibody from nasopharyngeal secretions, staining with **mAbs** or **immunofluorescent assay** to detect HMPV Abs or polyclonal Abs to detect isolation in cultured cells. Treatment: No treatment exists but ribavin is effective in an animal model.

Paramyxovirus Clinical Infections in Humans and Animals

Clinical Infections in Humans

Genus : Respirovirus

Human parainfluenza virus 1 (HPIV-1) is the second most common cause of lower resprratory tract infection in children, is a common cause of croup, & in immunosprssed people, it causes severe pneumonia.

Human parainfluenza virus 3 (HPIV-3) is associated with bronchiolitis & pneumonia in humans.

Genus: Rubulavirus

Mumps virus (MuV) causes mumpsin children with swelling of the parotid glands and other epithelial tissues causing high morbidity and in some cases more serious complications such as deafness.

Human parainfluenza virus 2 (HPIV- 2) causes croup and other upper and lower respiratory tract illnesses in younger childen.

Genus: Pneumovirus

Human respiratory syncytial virus (HRSV) is the **major & most common cause of lower respiratory tract infection during infancy** and childhood. HRSV infects the majority of infants by 2 years of age causing symptoms resembling those of the common cold. In some prematurely born infants or those with chronic lung disease, HRSV can cause life-threatening disease. HRSV infection most commonly occurs in epidemics during the cooler months. The majority of cases are seen in children less than 4 years of age, with the peak of severely ill cases found among children less than 6 months of age, particularly in infants with pre-existing heart and lung disease. Treatment includes supportive care, including oxygen. In temperate climates there is a yearly epidemic during the winter months but in tropical climates, infection is common during the rainy season. Severe RSV infections have also occrred in elderly patients. There are 3 strains of HRSV.

Human metapnumovirus (HMPV) causes a **repiratory illnesses varying from asymptomatic infection to severe brochiolitis & pneumonia in children as well as in all age groups.** HMPV is the second most important cause of pediatric lower respiratory illness, next to HRSV. It was isolated for the first time in 2001 in the Netherlands The clinical symptoms are similar to those seen with HRSV infection and include high **fever, myalgia, rhinorrhea, dyspnea, tachypnea, and wheezing.** While bronchiolitis, with or without pneumonia, is the most common symptoms of HMPV illness, other syndromes include asthma exacerbation, otitis media, pneumonitis, flu-like illness, community acquired pneumonia, and COPD exacerbation. The identification of HMPV depends on RT-PCR or the nucleic acid is detected using imunofluorescent antibody from nasopharyngeal secretions. Other diagnostic tests are staining with monoclonal antibody or immunofluorescent assay to detect HMPV Abs or polyclonal Abs to detect isolation in cultured cells. Treatment: No treatment exists but ribavin is effective in an animal model.

Paramyxovirus Clinical Infections in Animals & Birds

Genus: *Respirovirus*

Bovine Parainfluenza

Bovine parainfluenza-3 is a highly contagious disease commonly causing **mild to subclincal respiratory infection in cattle**. BPI is a respiratory disease present in cattle associated with the bovine respiratory disease complex; it causes only mild disease and is of importance when it results in secondary bacterial infection causing pneumonia.

Etilogy: Bovine parainfluenza is caused by *Bovine parainfuenza virus–3* (BPIV-3) under the genus *Respirovirus* in the family *Paramyxoviridae.*

Occurrence

Bovine parainfluenza virus-3 is common in many countries including Canada and USA. It is highly contagious and prevalent. Nebraska cattle were 86% positive for antibodies. The high number of animals with antibodies suggest that it is the most prevalent and widespread respiratory disease.

Hosts

BPIV-3 infections have been reported in cattle and sheep worldwide.

Transmission

BPIV is transmitted through inhalation of aerosols & through direct & indirect contact.

Pathogenesis

BPIV-3 replicates in macrophages and alveolar epithelium; the mucociliary mechanism is adversely affected. Damage to alveolar macrophages lowers defense against bacteria *Mannheirnia & P. multocida* causing shiping fever & fvours some viral infection.

Clinical Symptoms & Lesions

The clinical signs of BPIV-3 include **pyrexia, cough, serous nasal and lacrimal discharge**, & increased rate of respiration and increased breathing sounds. BPIV-3 favours infections with other viral diseases such as bovine viral diarrhea and infectious bovine rhinotracheitis. The disease worsens when there occurs secondary bacterial pneumonia that causes most of the mortalities. In uncomplicated pneumonia, there is little chance that infection will result in death.

Lesions are more confined to the cranial end of the lungs that include cranioventral lung consolidation, bronchiolitis, and alveolitis with marked congestion and hemorrhage. Inclusion bodies may be identified. Most fatal cases have a concurrent bacterial bronchopneumonia.

Diagnosis

Collection of clinical samples for various tests include nasal and tracheal swabs, transtracheal wash and lung; acute and convalescent sera.

1. *Virus isolation* : Virus isolation in cell cultures of bovine origin is attemted in which the virus produces CPE namely giant cell formation, cell rounding, syncytia and the production of both IC & IN inclusions. **RT-PCR** is also used for detection of bovine parainfluenza virus-3.
2. *Antibody detection* : Disease is detected by antibody detection using ELISA assay for which two samples, one taken at acute stage and the other a week later are taken. There should be 4-fold increase in antibody titre.

Treatment & Prevention

Antimicrobiall drugs are used to control bacterial infections.

Vaccination

Prevention through vaccination is the best way to control the disease. Most vaccines are combined with other respiratory viruses, and are almost always combined with bovine herpesvirus 1 (bovine rhinotracheitis). Both modified live vaccine or inactivated vaccines are usesd through IM route. Temperature sensitive mutant strain vaccine is used through intranasal route. **Bovilis Bovipast RSP/Bovigrip**-Intervet vaccine contains inactivated BRSV (strain EV 908-$10^{5.5}$ $TCID_{50}$) and Parainfluenza-3-Virus (strain SF-4 Reisinger $10^{7.3}$ $TCID_{50}$) as well as inactivated *Mannheimia (Pasteurella) haemolytica* bacteria (serotype A19 x 10^9 cells) propagated under conditions of iron restriction. Aluminium hydroxide and Quil A are included as adjuvants. Sodium timerfonate serves as preservative. Inject 5 ml SC into the side of the neck. Animals from approximately 2 weeks of age should receive two vaccinations separated by an interval of approximately 4 weeks. If booster doses are required, a single dose should be given approximately 2 weeks before each risk period (e.g. transport, introduction into a herd, change of housing). **Bovilis Qarat** - Intervet is an inactivated vaccine for use in cattle as an aid in the control of respiratory disease caused by IBRV, BPI3V, BVDV and BRSV infections. The vaccine contains antigens in an aluminium salt adjuvant. Per 2ml IM dose contains 7.7 log^{10} TCID50 IBRV, 7.7 log^{10} TCID50PI3 virus, 7.4 log^{10} TCID50 BVD virus & BRSV 10^{10} células MDBK PL-4. This vaccine may be given to any animal, pregnant ones included. Calves from vaccinated mothers should only be vaccinated at six months of age. Calves that have been vaccinated before six months, should receive another dose at six months old. Replacement heifers should be vaccinated at eight months with the live vaccine followed by a booster four weeks later. These animals should have a lifelong immunity. Cows may be given the inactivated vaccine annually. **Cattlemaster 4**-Pfizer (IBR, BVD, PI3 and BRSV) vaccination of healthy cattle, including pregnant cows, administer 2 ml IM; for primary vaccination give 2 doses 2-4 weeks apart. Calves vaccinated before the age of 6 months should be revaccinated after 6 months of age. Annual revaccination with a single dose is recommended.

Genus : *Rubulavirus*

Porcine Rubula Virus Infection

Porcine rubula or **"blue eye" disease** is an emerging disease first seen in La Piedad in 1980 in Mexico & is characterized by encephalitis and respiratory disease in piglets, & reproductive failure in adult pigs, and occasional corneal opacity in all ages.

Etiology: There are 2 strains-La-Piedad-Michoacan-Mexican viruses or LPMV & La-Piedad-Michoacan LPMV. Rubulavirus isolates (PAC-4/1993, PAC-6/2001, and PAC-9/2003) showed antigenic differences among the isolates using a hemagglutination inhibition assay.

Occurrence

Porcine rubula or "blue eye" disease is caused by *Porcine rubula virus* (PoRV). PoRV infection in swine was first reported in Mexico in 1980 and still occurs there. It has not been reported from outside of Mexico.

Hosts

Occurs in pigs & is most severe in pigs younger than three weeks.

Transmission

PoRV infection occus through direct contact and indirect means like fomites.

Clinical Symptoms

In PoRV infection, there is sudden onset of fever, depression, and progressive CNS symptoms. The diseased pigs are weak and ataxic, and develop rigidity of the hind legs and tremors. Other symptoms are dilated pupils, nystagmus, and conjunctivitis in some pigs, and about 1 - 10% of pigs develop corneal opacity. The mortality rate may approach 90%. But in older pigs, there are respiratory symptoms like sneezing and coughing, and anorexia and fever. Neurologic signs are often seen in pigs more than 30 days old. The mortality rate is low. Adult swine show subclinical symptoms with often corneal opacity. The pregnant sows show reproductive problems. Boars show orchitis and epididymitis with reproductive failure.

Pathological Lesions

Gross lesions are minimal and nonspecific. Microscopic lesions are those of a nonsuppurative encephalomyelitis and interstitial pneumonitis.

Diagnosis

Collection of clinical samples includes brain, lungs, tonsils and affected eyes.

A presumptive diagnosis is based on clinical symptoms & lesions.

Virus isolation : PoRV is isolated in swine origin cell cultures like PK-15 cells in which syncytial formation is confirmed by virus neutralization.

Antibody detection : Chicken erythrocytes aglulutination test, HI test of paired sera samples & ELIZA test are used for confirmatory diagnosis.

Treatment & Prevention

Prevention includes keeping closed herds, isolation of replacements & regular serological testing.

Vaccination

Inactivated vaccine is available that gives good result.

Genus: *Morbillivirus*

Canine Distemper

Canine distemper **(CDV)** is a contagious, viral pantropic disease affecting many orgns of dogs & other carnivores, & characterized by a **diphasic fever, GIT & respiratory symptoms, leukopenia, often neurologicai symptoms & hard footpad.**

Etiology : Canine distemper is caused by *Canine distemper virus* (CDV) in the genus *Morbillivirus.*

Occurrence

CDV occurs worldwide. The first case was described in 1905 by **French veterinarian, Henri Carre**. CDV now affects all populations of domestic dog and some populations of wildlife. A **vaccine was developed in 1950** but due to limited use, the virus remains prevalent in many populations. The domestic dogs have largely been responsible for introducing canine distemper to previously unexposed wildlife, and now the virus causes a serious conservation threat to many species of carnivores and some species of marsupials. The virus contributed to the near-extinction of the **black-footed ferrets,** & may have played a considerable role in the extinction of the Thylacine (Tasmanian tiger) and recurrently causes mortality among African wild dogs. In 1991, the lion population in Serengeti, Tanzania experienced a 20% decline as a result of the disease. The disease has also mutated to form *Phocine distemper virus* that affects seals.

Hosts

Animals of family Canidae-dogs, wolves, coyotes & jackal, *Mustelidae*-ferrets, mink & skunk, *Procyonidae*-raccons & coatimundi, & *Vireridae*-binturong are susceptible. **Pupies 3-6 months old are more susceptible.**

Transmission

CDV transmission occurs via aerosols, contact, inhalation, the infected body fluids, nasal secretion, tears, urine up to 6-22 days excreting the virus, & the infected food & water.

Pathogenesis

After entry, the virus is first replicates in bronchial lymph nodes and tonsils two days after exposure. Then the virus enters the blood stream on the second or third day. A first round of acute fever begins between **3-8 days after infection**, which is usually accompanied by a low white blood cell count, especially of lymphocytes, as well as low platelet count. These signs may be accompanied by anorexia, a runny nose, and discharge from the eye. The first round of **fever recedes rapidly within 96 hours**. A **second round of fever begins between 11- 12 days and lasts at least a week**. The cell-associated viremia occurs & fever causing infection of all lymphatic tissues, followed by infection of epithelia of respiratory, GI, & urogenital tracts, the CNS and optic nerves with virus replication in these tissues. Lymphoid depletion leads to leucopenia, immunosuppresion & secondary bacterial infection, interstitial pneumonia & encephalitis & hyperketosis of footpad. Gastrointestinal and respiratory problems follow, which may become complicated with secondary bacterial infections. Inflammation of the brain and spinal cord (**encephalomyelitis**) is either associated with this, subsequently follows, or comes completely independent of these problems. A thickening of the footpads sometimes develops, and vesicularpustular lesions on the abdomen usually develop. Neurological symptoms typically are found in the animals with thickened footpads from the virus. About half of sufferers experience **meningoencephalitis**.

Clinical Symptoms and Lesions

Incubation period is 6-22 days, & in severe cases 3-6 days.

Gastrointestinal and respiratory symptoms include a runny nose, vomiting and diarrhea, dehydration, excessive salivation, coughing and/or labored breathing, loss of appetite, and weight loss.

Neurological symptoms within the CNS include a localized **involuntary twitching of muscles or groups of muscles**, seizures often distinguished by salivation, and jaw movements commonly described as **chewing gum fits**, or **distemper myoclonus**. As the condition progresses, the seizures worsen and advance to convulsions, followed by death of the animal. The animal may also show signs of sensitivity to light, incoordination, circling, increased sensitivity to sensory stimuli such as pain or touch, and deterioration of motor capabilities. Less commonly, it may lead to blindness and paralysis. The length of the systemic disease may be as short as 10 days, or the start of neurological symptoms may not come until several weeks or months later. Those dogs that survive usually have a twitch of varying levels of severity. With time, this twitch usually diminishes in its severity.

Chronic distemper encephalitis or old dog encephalitis shows symptoms of ataxia, head pressing or continual pacing, and incoordinated hypermetria in adult dogs.

PM lesions include necrosis of lymphatic tissues, **atrophy of thymus,** a consistent finding in young pups, interstitial pneumonia, and hyperketosis of nose & footpad in dogs with neurological symptoms, & degeneration with IN inclusions in glial body. Bronchopneumonia, enteritis, and skin pustules may also be present. **Histologically**, CDV produces necrosis of lymphatic tissues, interstitial pneumonia, and **cytoplasmic and intranuclear inclusion bodies** in respiratory, urinary, and GI epithelium. Lesions found in the brain of dogs with neurologic complications include neuronal degeneration, gliosis, demyelination, perivascular cuffing, nonsuppurative leptomeningitis, and intranuclear inclusion bodies predominantly within glial cells.

CDV and Paget's disease : CDV have long been suspected as the causative agents of Paget's disease, **a focal destructive disease of bone**. Paget's disease is a chronic condition of bone characterized by disorder of the normal bone remodeling process. As a result, the bone is formed is abnormal, enlarged, not as dense, brittle, and prone to breakage. A virus detection technique, *in situ* RT-PCR, has found CDV in 100% cases of Paget's disease samples.

Diagnosis

Collection of clinical samples includes conjunctival scrapings, blood (buffy coat) smears, lung, urinary bladder, stomach, and brain.

1. *Presumptive diagnosis* : The clinical symptoms- fever, respiratory symptoms with neurological signs, and thickened footpads found in unvaccinated dogs strongly indicate canine distemper. At necropsy, diagnosis is usually confirmed by histologic lesions.
2. *Virus isolation* : Virus isolation by various methods in the dog's conjunctival cells gives a definitive diagnosis.
3. *Brush border slide/smear of the bladder* : The most reliable test to confirm CD is a **brush border slide/smear of the bladder transitional epithelium of the inside lining from the bladder,** stained with Dif-Quick. These infected cells have inclusions which stain a carmine red color, found in the paranuclear cytoplasm readability. About 90% of the bladder cells will be positive for inclusions in the early stages of distemper. This is good for at least the first 21 days from onset of the disease.
4. *Virus antigen detection* : Immunofluorescent assay for viral antigen in tissues; in dogs with multisystemic signs, conjunctival, tracheal, vaginal, or other epithelium, or the buffy coat of the blood can be examined by immunofluorescent assay. These samples are usually negative when the dog is showing only neurologic manifestations or when circulating antibody is present (or both).

5. **Antibody detection:** CD can be diagnosed by serologic demonstration of **virus-specific IgM** or an **increased ratio of CSF to serum virus-specific IgG.**

Treatment & Prevention

Treatment includes palliative, usually antibiotics, electrolyte solutions, parenteral nutrition, dietary supplements, antipyretics, nasal preparations, analgesics, and anticonvulsants.The most successful treatments for CD are **ribavirin and vitamin A**, and **interferon alpha**. Dogs showing neurologic symptoms are treated with with anti-inflammatory drugs.

Infected animals should be quarantined from other dogs for several months due to the length of time the animal may shed the virus. CDV is destroyed in the environment by routine cleaning with disinfectants, detergents, or drying. It does not survive in the environment for more than a few hours at room temperature (20–25 °C), but can survive for a few weeks in shady environments at temperatures slightly above freezing. It can also persist longer in serum and tissue debris.

Vaccination

Several vaccines are available; pups are vaccinated IM with **canine distemper modified live virus (MLV)** in absence of maternal antibody or vaccinated IM with MLV vaccine when **6 week old and at 2- to 4-week intervals until 16 week old** in presence of maternal antibody. **MLV measles vaccine and a combination of MLV measles and MLV canine distemper vaccine are also used**. Pups 6-7 week old should receive the measles or combination vaccine and at least 2 more doses of MLV distemper vaccine when 12-16 week old. MLV vaccines can produce postvaccinal illness in some immunosuppressed dogs. **A recombinant canarypox vector vaccine** expressing distemper virus proteins is available. Annual revaccination has been suggested because of the breaks in neurologic distemper that can occur in stressed, diseased, or immunosuppressed dogs. CDV is destroyed in the environment by disinfectants, detergents or drying.

Glaxy D - Intervet is a modified live virus for **use in dogs only.** Transfer contents of the sterile diluent vial to the Galaxy D vial aseptically. Mix gently until dissolved. Use entire contents immediately after rehydration.

Inject one dose (1 ml) IM or SC, the initial dose is given at 6 weeks of age or older. Repeat at 2 to 4 week intervals until the dog is 12 weeks of age. A minimum of two doses is required for primary immunization. Annual revaccination with one dose is recommended. **Galaxy DA2PPV** (CD+ ICH-1,2+ CPI3 +CPV), **Galaxy CV** (CD+ ICH-1,2+ CPI3 +CPV), **Galaxy DA2PPVL**

(CD+ICH-1, 2+CPI3+CPV+leptospirosis), & **Galaxy DA2PPVL + CL** (CD + ICH-1, 2+parinfluenza PI3+CPV+L. Canicola, L. *icterhaemorhagiae* bacterin & killed +feline enteric coronavirus). **RECOMBITEK® rDistemper** is a recombinant Canarypox vectored vaccine for safe, proven, efficacious protection against canine distemper without the potential risks associated with modified-live distemper vaccines. This vaccine contains DNA sequence of both the HA (hemagglutinin) and F (fusion membrane protein) antigens, show outstanding efficacy even in the face of maternal antibodies & is used throughout North and South America including highly endemic areas of Mexico and Brazil. Dose is 1ml IM. Several other commercial combined vaccines are available.

Rinderpest

Rinderpest (RPV) also called cattle plague is viral disease of cattle, domestic buffaloes, some species of wildlife & is characterized by fever, oral erosions, diarrhea, lymphoid necrosis & high mortality (roughly 80%) in acute cases. **FAO declared in 2011 the global eradication of rinderpest**. RPV is closely related to the viruses of canine distemper, peste des petits ruminants and measles. There is considerable variation in the virulence of virus strains. Experimental infection of cattle with some highly virulent strains is uniformly fatal.

Occurrence

RP occurs in remote parts of Asia and Africa, and for centuries has been the cause of enormous losses of cattle and buffaloes. RPV has been widely distributed throughout Europe and Africa, Asia but has never been reported in North America, Central America, the Caribbean Islands, South America, Australia, or New Zealand. Rinderpest is included in OIE List A.

Hosts

Cattle & buffaloes are mainly susceptible as well as sheep, goats, swine, deer, yak, camels, hippopotamus, warthog, and other wild animals like large antelopes, deer, giraffes, wildebeests and warthogs are also susceptible to RP.

Transmission

RP is transmitted via food, water, and litter contaminated with secretions and excretions from infected animals. Virus is shed in secretions and excretions during the clinical phase of the disease. Infection is by **inhalation of aerosols or ingestion & it could also be transmitted by air.** RP is present in small amounts in nasal secretions 1-2 days before fever, the amount are high in secretions and excretions during the first week of clinical disease and decrease rapidly as animals develop specific antibodies and begin to recover. There is no carrier state; **the virus maintains itself by continual transmission among susceptible animals**. In endemic areas, **young cattle become infected after maternal immunity disappears and before vaccine immunity begins**, with possible auxiliary cycles in sheep, goats, and wild ungulates. In epidemic areas, the virus infects most susceptible animals and tends to limit itself.

Pathogenesis

After inhalation, initial replication occurs in the pharyngeal & mandibular lymph nodes. Viremia follows in three days with infection of the mucous membranes of alimentary and respiratory tracts, and lymphoid tissues. Viraemia occurs in about 3 days dissemonating virus to other lymphoid tissues, mucosa of GIT & RT. The necrosis of lymphoid tissues causes leucopenia & immunosuppression. Virus shedding stops when the affected animals develop normal temperature.

Clinical Symptoms

Incubation period is **3-9 days** followed by anorexia, fever, and acute inflammation of the mm of digestive and upper respiratory tracts & mucosal erosions in the mouth & nasal passage. **Bran like depsits are seen in the mouth.** There is a profuse salivation, mucopurulent nasal discharge, a **watery diarrhea with blood-stained feces**. Severely affected animals die within 12 days. Recoverd animals are convulsant for weeks. During immunosuppression, there are protozoal & bacterial infections. Pregnant animals mostly abort. A **milder disease** may be seen where the disease is **endemic** and less susceptible species are involved.

Characteristic **necropsy lesions** include prominent lesions such as **congestion and hemorrhage of intestinal epithelium** with occasional necrosis of Peyer's 'patches. Mucosal erosions are found in the mouth and upper respiratory tract.

Diagnosis

Clinical specimens for diagnosis include urine, blood, nasal discharge, feces, lymph nodes, and spleen collected in the acute phase of the disease; & serum from surviving animals.

1. *Presmptive diagnosis* : RP is frequently diagnosed by clinical symptoms & unique lesions.
2. *Isolation of the virus* : The virus is grown in cell cultures like primary bovine kidney cell cultures and in the Vero cell line producing CPE, IC & IN inclusions after growth in cell culture.

3. Antigen detection : **The viral aantigen is detected in extracts of tissues by agar gel immunodiffusion, immunofluorescence, and counter immunoelectrophoresis. RT-PCR** test detects RPV & differentiates it from Peste des Petits Ruminants.
4. *Serology* : Virus neutralization tests in cell cultures can be performed on the sera of animals that have survived.

Treatment & Prevention

A global eradication plan was launched by FAO in 1972 using in endemic area by vaccination of domestic cattle & buffaloes, disease monitoring, follow up programmes & cotrol of animal movement. FAO declared in June 2011 global eradication of rinderpest.

Peste des Petits Ruminants

Peste des petits ruminants (PPRV), also called ovine rinderpest, pseudorinderpest of small ruminants, pest of small ruminants, pest of sheep and goats, Kata, stomatitis-pneumoenteritis syndrome, contagious pustular stomatitis, and pneumoenteritis complex, is a highly contagious, an acute or subacute viral disease of goats and seep characterized by fever, necrotic stomatitis, gastroenteritis and pneumonia.

Etiology : A Peste des petits ruminant is caused by *Peste des petits ruminants virus* (PPRV), a *Morbillivirus* under the family *Paramyxoviridae* which is closely related antigenically to RPV.

Occurrence

It was first reported in the Ivory Coast in 1942, is endemc in West Africa, the Middle East, the Indian subcontinent & has recenty been reported from Tibet (2007) & Morocco (2008). African & Asian strains of PPR are different.

Hosts

Sheep & goats are susceptible; **sheep are less susceptible than goats; cattle are only subclinically infected** but humans are not.

Transmission

Close contact, confinement & transportation of sick to the healthy stocks & secretions and excretions of sick animals are sources of infection. There is **no carrier state** but subclinical cases of PPR may spread the infection during the incubation phase. **White-tailed deer are fully susceptible & probably other wild ruminants may play a role in the epidemiology of the disease but not pigs.** Cattle are susceptible but do not exhibit clinical signs or transmit the disease.

Pathogenesis

PPR enters retropharyngeal & lymphoid tissues, there is viremia, damage of lymphoid, alimentary & respiratory systems with leucopenia but **no immunosuppression**, the infected cells beome necrosed & proliferate in respiratory system. Lymphoid necrosis is slight without immune suppression. There is diarrhea & dehydration that lead to death. At later stage, respiratory distress follows that is increased by the concurrent diseases. Pregnant animals may abort.

Clinical Symptoms

Incubation period is about **4 days**. The disease occurs in **acute & subacute forms. Acute form** is seen mainly in **goats**, at 3-4 days PI showing severe respiratory distress, high fever, dullness, sneezing, discharge from eye & nose. Two days later diphtheritic plaques are seen in mouth that extend to the whole oral mucosa & nostrils. Animals are unable to eat, hind legs are sticky with feces, show arched back & difficulty in defecation, & nasal & ocular discharges turn mucopurulent. **Diarrhea is seen 3-4 days** after fever. Later dyspnea, coughing, severe respiratory distress due to secondary bacterial pneumonia develop, & **pregnant animals may abort. Erosion** may occur in vulva & prepuce & death follows 1 week later after illness.

Subacute form is common in **sheep** in which symptoms & lesions are less markd, & sheep mostly recover from illness.

PM lesions : Important pathognmic lesions are present in digestive tracts. Dehydrated carcass, feces soiled hind quarters, crust seen around eyes, lips, erosive necrosis, & ulceration present in the oral mucosa, upper oesophagus extending to abomasums & small intestine. **Hemorrhagic ulcers are seen in ileocecal region, colon & rectum showing zebra stripes**. Regional LN arre enlarged, & spleen may also be enlaged. Interstitial pneumonia may be present. Grossly pneumonia is diffuse. **Microscopic lesions** like RP are seen. At early stage, synsytial cells are seen in oral mucosa & IC inclusion in intestinal crypt epith, rhinotrachietis, bronchitis, bronchopneumonia, & huge glial cells seen showing IN & IC inclusions.

Diagnosis

Collection of clinical samples includes oral lesions, whole blood, spleen, intestine, and acute and convalescent sera.

1. *Presumptive diagnosis :* From clinical symptoms & lesions.
2. *Virus isolation* (unclotted blood, LN, tonsils, spleen, lungs),
3. *Viral Antibody detection :* Antibodies are detected by CFT, or agar gel precipitin test, & virus neutralization. Antibodies with rising titre are diagnostic.

Tretment & Prevention

Treatment includes fluid therapy & antibacterials are administered, cleaning of lesions & hyperimmune sera against RP is used.

RP eradiation method is used.

Vaccination

Attenuated vaccine using embryonic caprine kidney cell culture passage adapted virus is used that protects from PPR for 1 year & RP cell culture vaccine is also used. Some available vaccines against Peste des Petits Ruminants use d in different countries are as follows. **Live PPR-VAC®** (Botswana Vaccine nstitute) containing strain/subtype PPR Nigeria 75/1 (EMVT) without adjuvant licensed in Botswana. **Live freze dried PPR-Vaccine** (Central Veterinary Control & Research Institute) containing strain/ subtype PPR Nigeria 75/1 without adjuvant licensed in Turkey. **Live PESTDOLL-S** (Dollvet) containing strain/subtype PPRV 75/1 (Nigera) without adjuvant licensed in Turkey. **Killed Peste de Petits ruminants Vaccine** (National Veterinary Institute) containing strain-not available without adjuvant licensed in Etiopia. **Live Peste de Petits Ruminants Vaccine** (National Veterinary Research Institute) containing strain-PPRV 75/1 without adjuvant licensed in Nigeria. **Live Peste de Petits Ruminants Vaccine** (Nepal Directorate of Animal Health) containing strain-PPRV 75/1 without adjuvant licensed in Nepal. **Live Pestvac K™** (Vetal Company) containing strain-not available without adjuvant licensed in Turkey. Live PPR-TC attenuated vaccine (Veterinary Serum and Vaccine Research Institute) containing strain-Egypt 87 without adjuvant is licensed in Egypt.

Genus : *Henipavirus*

Hendra Virus Infection

Hendra virus (HeV), previously called equine morbilli virus causes an acute viral disease in horses characterized by an acute onset, fever, respiratory distress, neurological sign & rapid progression to death. It is of **zoonotic importance as humans are also affected** in some outbreaks with neurological symptoms.

Etiology : Hendra vurus infection in horses is caused by*Hendra virus* (HeV) in the genus *Henipavirus.*

Occurrence

HeV was first reported in 1994 in Hendra, Brisbane, Australia killing 14 horses & one trainer. The second outbreak occurred in Mackaya in 1999, &

since 1999, 13 outbreaks have occurred in horses involving infection of horses, & in 4 outbreaks humans were also infected. Mortality rate is more than 70%.

Hosts

Horses are susceptible, & no other animals are susceptinble; humans in close contact become susceptible indirectly.

Transmission

Flyimg foxes are the natural hosts for HeV. The disease is spread from foxes to horses & foxes to humans, but human-to-human & human to horse spread are not possible. Most human cases probably occurred from bats urine or birthing fluids & to humans remaining in close contact with the sick horses or during autopsies.

Pathogenesis

Hendra virus has a predilection for vascular tissues, regardless of route of infection. During initial infection, the vascular lesions range from edema and hemorrhage of vessel walls, fibrinoid degeneration with pyknotic nuclei in endothelial and tunica media cells, to the presence of numerous giant cells in the endothelium and sometimes the tunica media of affected vessels (both venules and arterioles). At later state of disease, there is destruction of alveolar walls, with the appearance of alveolar and intravascular macrophages. The virus becomes more widely distributed in various tissues throughout the body, presumably as a result of a leukocyte-associated viremia. The virus was detected in the vascular endothelium of subarachnoid and cerebral vessels and also affects the vasculature of the renal glomerulus and pelvis, lamina propria of the stomach, spleen, various lymph nodes and myocardium. In addition to its vascular tropism, Hendra virus can also be neurotropic, causing neuronal necrosis and focal gliosis.

Clinical Symptoms

After **incubation period** of 8-11 days in natural cases, affected horses show depression, inappetance, fever, ataxia, trachycardia, huge nasal & hemorrhagic nasal discharge, **swelling of head, severe respiratory distress & death in acute cases. Surviving horses show myoclonic twitches in upper fore-limbs, lower lip, face & upper hind muscles**. Inapparent infections have also occurred in horses. The affected humans show **encephalitis or pneumonitis & respiratory failure.**

PM lesions : Pulmonary edema with hemorrhages & froth in the passage are seen. **Histologically**, interstitial pneumonia, **vascular damage, necrosis of vascular macrophages**, vascular changes like hemorrhages within alveoli, necrosis & thrombosis of alveolar capillaries, syncytial giant cells within lung vessels & other organs are prognostic.

Diagnosis

Collection of clinical samples includes paired sera; lungs, spleen, liver, lymph nodes and brain.

Diagnosis can be made based on clinical symptoms & lesions, immunohistochemical technique, & PCR show virus nucleic acid.

Treatment & Prevention

No specifi treatment exists. No vaccine is available; prevention includes quarantine, restriction of horses movement & slaughter of the infected horses.

Nipah Virus Infection

Nipah virus (NiV) causes **'porcine respiratory and neurological syndrome'**, or **'porcine respiratory and encephalitis syndrome'**, or in Malaysia, **'barking pig syndrome'**. The disease is an emerging zoonotic disease in SE Asia, a highly contagious viral disease of pigs & other animals also involving humans, & is characterized by severe respiratory or neurological distress, & encephalitis in humans with high mortality rate.

Etiology : Nipah virus infection in pigs, other animals & humans is caused by *Nipah virus* (NiV) in the genus *Henipavirus.*

Occurrence

NiV is an endemic disease in SE Asia- Malaysia, Singapore, Bangla Desh & North India, & was identified in 1998 in pig farms in Malaysia with respiratory distress & neurological disease as well as 15 human deaths in abattoir workers. Other domestic animals like dogs, cats, goats & 1 horse also suffered. 12 outbreaks have occurred since 1998 all in Bangla Desh & India involving only humans within the surroundings of its reservoirs. The morbidity rate is about 100%, but the mortality rate is low except in piglets. On one farm, more than 95% of all sows and 90% of the piglets were seropositive.

Hosts

Pigs are the most susceptible, & besides horses, goats, sheep, cats, dogs are also susceptible. Fruit bats (flying foxex) of the genus *Pteropus, P. hypomelanus* & *P. vampyrus* (large flying foxexes) are the reservoir hosts. Humans also suffer from the disease with severe illness showing mainly encephalitis.

Transmission

Fruit bats (flying foxex) of the genus *Pteropus, P. vampyrus & P. hypomelanus* are the reservoir hosts which **shed the virus in urine.** Partly eaten fruits, kidney, fetuses, & birthing are infected. Nipah virus is transmitted from the reservoirs- to- pigs- to humans to other domestic animals. In Banla Desh & North India oubreaks, humans were directly infected by eating fruits-bats infected date palm or palm juice without involving pigs & other domestic animals. Most humans are infect4ed from direct contact with sick pigs, contaminated tissues or via respiratory droplets, contact with throat or nasal secretions from the pigs, or contact with the tissue of a sick animal.

Pathogenesis

The pathogenesis of Nipah infection is associated with its ability to infect blood vessels and extravascular parenchyma in many organs, including the central nervous system.The main histopathological findings included a systemic vasculitis with extensive thrombosis and parenchymal necrosis, particularly in the central nervous system. Endothelial cell damage, necrosis, and syncytial giant cell formation were seen in affected vessels. Characteristic viral inclusions were seen by light and electron microscopy. IHC analysis showed widespread presence of Nipah virus antigens in endothelial and smooth muscle cells of blood vessels. Abundant viral antigens were also seen in various parenchymal cells, particularly in neurons. Infection of endothelial cells and neurons as well as vasculitis and thrombosis seem to be critical to the pathogenesis of this new human disease.

Clinical Symptoms

Incubation period: 4-14 days in pigs & 4-45 days in humans. In pigs, asymptomatic infections are common. Symptomatic infections include acute febrile illnesses, & sudden death also occurs. Mortality rate is low except in young piglets. 1 to 6 mth old pigs, respiratory symptoms seem to be more common than neurologic signs wth fever, nasal discharge, open mouth breathing, rapid and labored respiration and a loud barking cough. Hemoptysis can occur in severe cases.

Neurological signs often seen include trembling, twitching, muscle spasms, myoclonus, weakness in the hind legs, spastic paresis, lameness, uncoordinated gait when driven or hurried, and generalized pain in the hind quarters. Similar symptoms occur in sows and boars, although neurologic disease appears to be more common in sows than younger animals & include agitation, head pressing, and nystagmus, chomping of the mouth, tetanus-like spasms, seizures and apparent pharyngeal muscle paralysis. Some sows may abort, generally during the first trimester. Sudden death may occur.

In piglets, symptoms include open mouth breathing, leg weakness with muscle tremors, and twitching.

PM lesions : In pigs, lesions are seen in the **lungs, brain or both**. Lung lesions can be mild to severe, and include consolidation, petechial or ecchymotic hemorrhages, and emphysema & the interlobular septa may be distended. The bronchi and trachea may contain frothy, sometimes blood strained fluid. In the brain, there is congestion of the cerebral blood vessels and meningeal edema. The kidneys can be congested but are often normal. In humans there is headache, drowsiness, cough, abdominal pain, nausea, vomiting, blurred vision, about 6% sicks become comatosed & need ventilation. In **severe cases relapse encephalitis** is seen. Asymptomatic disease has also been reported in humans.

Diagnosis

1. **Presumptive diagnosis: Cinical symptoms & specific lesions.**
2. *Virus isolation :* Virus is isolated from respiratory secretion, blood, tissues, lungs, spleen in cell lines-Vero, RK-13, BHK, porcine spleen cells & embryonated chicken eggs are used.
3. *Viral antigen detection :* Ags are detected by Immunoperoxidase test or immunofluorescence assay, Serum neutralization test, ELIZA test, & PCR assay.

Tretment & Prevention

There is no specific treatment or vaccine for humans or animals. Supportive treatments are used. Ribavirin in some human cases gave good result. Infected pigs & dometic animals are slautered to prevent spread to humans. Routine cleaning of pig farms with sodium hypochloride or detergents are practiced. Quarantine in case of outbreak, reducing risk of bats to humans or pigs, human-to-human & animal to human transmission is effective.

Genus : *Avulavirus*

New Castle Disease or Avian Paramyxovirus-I Infection

New castle disease virus (NDV) or ***Avian parmyxovirus-1*** (APMV-1) **causes** is a contagious viral disease of birds affecting many domestic and wild avian species especially domestic poultry & is characterized by severe respiratoty or nervous signs or diarrhea (Velogenic strains) with rapid spread causing up to 90% mortality or cause coughing, affect egg quality and production and result in up to 10% mortality (Mesogenic strains) or produce mild signs with negligible mortality (Lentogenic strains).

Etiology : New caslte disease (ND) is caused by *New castle disease virus* or *Avian parmyxovirus-1* (NDV/APMV-1) in the family *Paramyxoviridae*& the genus *Avulavirus*. There are **ten serotypes of avian paramyxoviruses designated APMV-I to APMV-10. ND virus (NDV)/ has been designated APMV-1 that** remains the most important pathogen for poultry while others are known to cause disease in poultry and other types of birds.

NDV has also been categorised into **five pathotypes** based on clinical signs in infected chickens, designated: a) viscerotropic velogenic, b) neurotropic velogenic, c) mesogenic, d) lentogenic or respiratory and e) subclinical enteric. There are **five pathotypes** as follows: i. **Viscerotropic velogenic** NDV causes severe disease in which haemorrhagic lesions are characteristically present in the intestinal tract; ii. **Neurotropic velogenic** NDV causes respiratory & nervous signs followed by high mortality. iii. **Mesogenic** NDV causes respiratory & often nervous signs with low mortality; iv. **Lentogenic respiratory NDV** causes mild or inapparent respiratory infection; v.**Asymptomatic enteric** NDV causes inapparent enteric infection. Velogenic or highly virulent APMV-1 virus has either 1) an intracerebral pathogenicity index (ICPI) of at least 0.7 in day-old chicks, or 2) an amino acid sequence that resembles those seen in highly virulent viruses-multiple basic amino acids at the C-terminus of the F2 protein and phenylalanine at residue 117 of the F1 protein. APMV-1 isolates are grouped into two clades, called class I and class II, based on the genetic relationship between viruses. The **vast majority of APMV-1 strains belong to class II,** which is divided into at least nine genotypes (I to IX). Class I isolates have been found mainly in **wild waterfowl**, and are usually of low pathogenicity.

Occurrence

Newcastle disease was discovered in Newcastle upon Tyne, England in 1926 (Doyle), by Burnet in 1943 in Australia & Ranihket in India. NDV strains are endemic in poultry in Asia, Africa, and some countries of North, Central, and South America. USA and Canada are free of these strains.

Hosts

Chickens are the most and waterfowl the least susceptible of domestic poultry. Young birds are the most susceptible. Humans are often infected, resulting in a mild influenza-like disease with conjunctivitis.

Transmission

Spread of NDV is through direct contact between healthy birds and the discharges of infected birds, through the infected birds' droppings, through secretions from the nose, mouth, and eyes & spreads rapidly in birds kept in confinement namely commercially raised chickens. Infection occurs by aerosols and by ingesting contaminated water or food. **NDV infected birds** shed virus in exhaled air, respiratory discharges, feces, during incubation & the clinical stage, and for short period during convalescence. NDV is '**present in eggs laid during clinical disease** and in the carcass during acute infections. **Cormorants, pigeons, and imported psittacine species** serve as sources of virulent NDV infections of poultry. **Pet birds like Amazon parrots from Latin America are carriers of the disease** without showing symptoms & shed NDV for more than 400 days, hence pose a great risk of introducing NDV into the US. Low virulence NDV is present in poultry and wild birds like waterfowl. NDV is spread mainly from infective feces, by the movement of people and contaminated equipment between poultry flocks. The virus is spread by mechanical means as it is present in birds' bodily discharges that can be picked up on shoes and clothing and carried from an infected flock to a healthy one. NDV can survive for several weeks in a warm and humid environment on birds' feathers, manure, and other materials & survive indefinitely in frozen material. Domestic poultry with low virulence NDV contributes to lower productivity. But, the virus is destroyed rapidly by dehydration and by the ultraviolet rays in sunlight.

Pathogenesis

NDV or avian paramyxovirus-1 is classified into 3 virulence groups by chicken embryo and chicken inoculation as i. Velogenic (virulent), ii. Mesogenic or moderately virulent & iii. Lentoenic or low virulence. Lentogenic strains are used widely as live vaccines in healthy chickens. Clinical manifestations vary from high morbidity and mortality to asymptomatic infections. Disease severity depends on virus virulence, the age, immune status and host susceptibility.

NDV-1 first replicates in the epithelia of respiratory& intestinal tracts, viraemia follows causing haematogenous spread to spleen & bone marrow. Secondary viraemia spreads the virus to other organs like lung, intestine & CNS. Lentogenic strains replicates in respiratory & intestinal epithelia.

Clinical Symptoms

Incubation period is 2-15 days Clinical manifestations depend on whether the infecting virus has a predilection for respiratory, digestive or nervous systems or on the NDV strains, age and the host species.

Disease onset is rapid and symptoms appear in the entire flock within 2-12 days, average 5 days after aerosol infection, but are slower if infection is through fecal-oral route. The affected birds show respiratory signs like **gasping, coughing, & nervous signs** like depression, inappetence, muscular tremors, and drooping wings, twisting of head and neck, circling, complete paralysis, swelling of the tissues around the eyes and neck, greenish, watery diarrhea, and misshapen, rough- or thin-shelled eggs and reduced egg production.

In **acute cases**, the death is very sudden. **Viscerotropic velogenic Newcastle disease (VVND)** shows respiratory signs with depression, watery-greenish diarrhea, and swelling of the tissues of the head and neck although nervous signs may also be seen. Varying degrees of depression and inappetence are observed. A partial or complete cessation of egg production may occur. Eggs may be abnormal in color, shape, or surface, and have watery albumen.

Neurotropic velogenic NDV causes high mortality, usually following respiratory and nervous signs.

Mesosenic NDV causes respiratory signs, occasional nervous signs, but lower mortality.

Lentogenic NDV causes mild or sub-clinical respiratory infection.

Asymtomatic- enteric NDV causes sub-clinical enteric infection.

Mortality is variable but can be as high as 100%. In flocks with good immunity, respiratory and digestive signs are mild and progressive, and are followed after seven days by nervous symptoms, especially twisting of heads. In pigeons nervous symptoms with diarrhea and in cormorants and exotic bird species nervous signs are often seen.

Gross lesions with VVNDV are petechiae on the serous membranes; hemorrhages on the proventricular mucosa and intestinal serosa accompanied by multifocal, necrotic hemorrhagic areas on the mucosal surface of the intestine, especially at lymphoid foci such as cecal tonsils. Splenic necrosis, hemorrhage and edema in the thymus may also be seen. The lesions in birds infected with lower virulence NDV strains include **congestion and mucoid exudates in the respiratory tract with opacity and thickening of the air sacs**. Secondary bacterial infections enhance the severity of the respiratory lesions.

Diagnosis

Collection of clinical samples includes lung, trachea, liver, spleen, brain, and serum.

1. *Presumptive diagnosis :* It is based on the clinical symptoms, & specific lesions.
2. *Virus islation :* Virus culture is made by inoculation of samples in embryonated specific pathogen free (SPF) eggs via the allantoic cavity.

The embryos death varis from more than 100 to less than 50 hours after inoculation. Allantoic fluids containing ND virus agglutinate red cells of chickens, guinea pigs, mice, and humans. The virus can be identified by HI test and virus neutralization tests using specific NDV antiserum.

3. *Virus antigen detection :* Use of specific antiserum in a haemagglutination inhibition (HI) test is confirmatory. Samples are taken by cotton swab from the trachea and the cloaca or the lungs, brain, spleen, liver, and kidneys. Monoclonal antibodies are used for rapid identification of NDV avoiding cross-reactions with other APMV serotypes; mAb is a valuable method for grouping and differentiating isolates of NDV.
4. *Antibody detection :* HI test is most widely used test and detects antibody response to virus glycoprotein (predictor of protection against disease); shows rise in antibodies in paired serum samples. For ELISA test, whole virus is used as antigen, it detects antibody to all of the virus proteins. Commercial ELISA kits are available to assess post-vaccination antibody level.
5. *Pathogenicity index :* Pathogenicity index is determined by intracerebral pathogenicity index (ICPI) in day-old chicks methodology or is determined by molecular basis by correlation of multiple basic amino acids.

   Phylogenetic studies : It allows for the rapid epidemiological assessment of the origins and spread of the viruses responsible for ND outbreaks
6. *Molecular techniques in diagnosis :* Nucleotide sequence analysis detects genetic differences of isolates from different outbreaks and identifies the source of infections; advantage is extremely rapid demonstration of the presence of the virus.

Treatment & Prevention

Vaccinaton

Eight strains of Newcastle disease virus used in live vaccines (FAO, 2002): **Strain Description: F** Lentogenic- Usually used in young chickens but suitable for use as a vaccine in chickens of all ages. **B1** Lentogenic- Slightly more virulent than F, used as a vaccine in chickens of all ages. **La Sota** Lentogenic- Often causes post vaccination respiratory signs, used as a booster vaccine in flocks vaccinated with F or B1. **V4** Avirulent- Used in chickens of all ages.**V4-HR** Avirulent. Heat Resistant V4, thermostable, used in chickens of all ages. **I-2** Avirulent- Thermostable, used in chickens of all ages. **Mukteswar** Mesogenic. An invasive strain, used as a booster vaccine. Can cause adverse reactions (respiratory distress, loss of weight or drop in egg production and even death) if used in partially immune chickens. Usually administered by injection.

Komarov Mesogenic. Less pathogenic than Mukteswar, used as booster vaccine. Usually administered by injection.

Some countries have specified that only lentogenic NDV strains can be used as vaccines. Most live virus vaccines are grown in allantoic cavity of embryonated fowl eggs; some mesogenic strains have been adapted to a variety of tissue culture systems. Live virus vaccines administered to birds by incorporation in the drinking water, delivered as a coarse spray, or by intranasal or conjunctival instillation; some mesogenic strains are given by wing-web intradermal inoculation on day 1-4. But vaccination on the second or third week avoids maternal antibody interference with an active immune response. Concurrent presence of Mycoplasma, some bacteria, and viruses affecting the respiratory tract act synergistically with some vaccines to aggravate the vaccine reaction after spray administration.

Oil-adjuvanted inactivated vaccines are used after live vaccine in breeders and layers and used alone where use of live virus may be contraindicated. In NDV endemic countries, a combination of live virus and inactivated vaccine can be used; a live mesogenic strain vaccine may be used in older birds. The revaccination depends on the risk of exposure and virulence of the field virus challenge. Any birds showing symptoms of ND should be quarantined immediately & new birds should be vaccinated before introduclng to flock. Combined vaccine ND+IBV administerd at 2 weeks of age include **Triplevac**- Intervet (B1 Strain, Mass/Conn) given in water/spray; **Trivac-Ark** (B1 Strain, Mass/Ark) given through spray, & **Broilerbrone –HN-79** (LaSota Strain-Mass Type/Holland) administerd through water /eyedrop. Combined vaccine ND+IBV administerd at 5 weeks of age include **Triplevac**-Intervet (B1 Strain, Mass/Conn) given in water/spray; **Combovac -30** (LaSota Strain, Mass/Conn) given through spray, **Trivac-Ark**(B1 Strain, Mass/Ark) or **Broilerbrone –HN-79** (LaSota Strain-Mass Type/Holland) administerd through water /eyedrop. Combined vaccine ND+IBV administerd at 15 weeks of age include **Triplevac**- Intervet (B1 Strain, Mass/Conn) given in water/spray; **Combovac -30** (LaSota Strain) given through spray, **Trivac-Ark**(B1 Strain, Mass/Ark) given through spray; **Broilerbrone –HN-79** (LaSota Strain-Mass Type/Holland) administerd through water /eyedrop or Polybron N-63 (LaSota Strain, Mass/Conn). Combined vaccine IBD/Reo/ND/IBV administerd at 18 weeks of age include **Breeder Vac-IV-Plus** given through IM/SC injection. **VectormuneFD-ND**-Biomune is a genetically engineered, live fowl pox virus vaccine used for the vaccination of chickens and turkeys as an aid in the prevention of fowl pox and Newcastle disease Fowelpox vetor vaccine. The vaccine recommended for subcutaneous injection of healthy, NDV maternal antibody negative chickens on one day of age or older or by wing web administration to FPV susceptible chickens and nine weeks of age or older. Administer 0.2 ml per chicken or turkey SC in the loose skin on the back of the neck, just below the head. The vaccine may be used SC to turkeys four weeks of age or older. Chickens and turkeys receiving this vaccine must not have been previously exposed to fowl poxvirus either by vaccination or field exposure. Revaccination with **POXIMUNE®** may be necessary after eight weeks of age if VECTORMUNE FP-N is used at day of age. All birds on a farm should be vaccinated at the same time.

Genus : *Pneumovirus*

Bovine Respiratory Syncytial Virus Infection

Bovine respiratory syncytial virus infection (BRSV) causes respiratory disease mainly in young beef and dairy cattle characterized by **severe respiratory disease initially but mild to subclinical disease in subsequent infections.** BRSV occupies an important place in the bovine respiratory disease complex due to its **repeated occurrence,** virus **predilection for the lower respiratory tract,** and **predisposition of respiratory tract to secondary bacterial infections.**

Etiology: BRSV is caused by *Bovine respiratory syncytial virus* in the genus *Pneumovirus.*

Occurrence

BRSV infection occurs throughout the world. In outbreaks, morbidity is high but the mortality is 0-20%.

Hosts

Cattle, sheep and goats are susceptible to BRSV; it is widely distributed in cattle but mainly in young beef and dairy cattle. Weaned and transported calves are more susceptible.

Pathogenesis

In calves infection with BRSV is presumed to occur predominantly via small particle aerosols. Replication of RSV starts with an infection in the upper part of the respiratory tract, peaks around the 4th day post infection (DPI), and is followed by a variable replication in the bronchiolar and alveolar epithelium from 4 DPI peaking around 6 DPI. A major part of the inoculum remains associated with the mucus layer of the URT without reaching the alveoli. BRSV only minimally replicates in alveolar macrophages. Downwards spread of the infection along the bronchiolar and alveolar epithelium is presumably a result of destruction of the ciliated tracheo-bronchial epithelium. Neutrophils are important for the clearance of BRSV excreted into the lumen of the respiratory tract, but these same neutrophils may also contribute to tissue damage by releasing inflammatory products. A peak virus replication in bronchiolar and alveolar epithelial cells of the LRT may coincide with more severe clinical signs: tachypnea, dyspnoea and anorexia [60]. Virus replication in the cells of the respiratory lung epithelium may vary significantly, resulting in no obvious cytopathology, to cytopathology of lung epithelium cells leading to loss of specialized functions such as cilial motility and epithelial destruction. It has been speculated that direct cytopathology due to virus replication plays a minor role in clinical symptoms, whereas the host response to the virus infection (immunity) plays a major role in RSV pathogenesis. The case fatality rate in uncomplicated bRSV infections is usually low, but may increase due to secondary infections. The lungs of animals dying in naturally occurring BRSV outbreaks often show atelectasis, interstitial emphysema or pneumonia, which may be caused by secondary bacterial infection. BRSV enhances bacterial colonization and adherence, and alters specific and non-specific defense mechanisms of the respiratory tract. It has been estimated that 90% of all bacterial pneumonias develop after a previous viral infection. Triggered by infection, a variety of cells (among which mast cells, epithelial cells, dendritic cells, macrophages, other antigen presenting cells, T-cells and B-cells) secrete specific cytokines, the regulatory (key) signals of the immune response. Tumor necrosis factor-α for example has been shown to induce migration of neutrophils and mononuclear cells to the site of infection. Various mediators of inflammation, e.g. degranulation products of mucosal mast cells and eosinophils have been associated with severity of bronchiolitis. Histamine and leukotrienes are major mast cell mediators responsible for constriction of smooth muscle, increased mucus production, and increased vascular permeability . Cellular immune responses are thought to play an important role in clearance of BRSV. Cytolytic T-lymphocytes (CTLs) are likely the principal mediators of resolution of the acute virus infection. However, CTLs probably do not contribute significantly to protection against reinfection, because of the short-lived nature of activated CTLs. Nevertheless, a memory CTL response may be important in limiting the severity of disease. Antibodies appear a principal mediator of resistance to RSV disease and infection. Serum (neutralizing) IgG antibodies protect against lower respiratory tract disease, but do not seem to have a major impact on viral replication in the upper respiratory tract. Humoral immune responses following primary RSV infection initially consist of virus-specific IgM. Virus-specific IgG and IgA antibodies can be detected. Outstanding macroscopic lesions were not seen. Histologically, mild bronchiolitis and alveolitis were observed.

Allergic reactions riggered by natural infection have been described extensively in the literature. Hypersensitivity related to vaccination with formalin-inactivated vaccines is characterized by high fever, pneumonia, abnormal rash, and lymphadenopathy. Also in cattle vaccination with FI-bRSV was shown to predispose calves for enhanced disease upon bRSV challenge infection. It has also been suggested that the altered immune response was a type of delayed hypersensitivity; nonprotective antibody responses elicited by inactivated hRSV immunogens and ultimately associated with the development of enhanced respiratory disease, resulted from lack of affinity maturation due to deficient TLR activation in B cells.

To date, there is still no common understanding of the phenomenon. Vaccine enhanced disease still continues to hamper vaccine development, whereas its pathogenesis has always remained poorly defined.

BRSV induces immunomodulation in the infected host, favouring a Th2 response. IgE responses have been seen to BRSV proteins during infection and particularly in response to vaccination with **formalin-inactivated vaccine in the field and experimentally. Newer vaccine modalities that favor a shift to Th1 cytokine production have provided promising results.** Infection with BRSV is a major contributor to the multi-pathogen disease, bovine respiratory disease complex.

Clinical Signs

Common symptoms are fever (104-108°F [40-42°C]), depression, inapatence, increased respiratory rate, cough, and nasal and lacrimal discharge. Dyspnea with open-mouth breathing is seen in the later stages of the disease. Subcutaneous emphysema may be noticed. BSRV favours secondary bacterial pneumonia. A noticeable obsrevation is **commonly a biphasic disease.**

Gross lesions: There is diffuse interstitial pneumonia associated with subpleural and interstitial emphysema as well as interstitial edema. Bacterial infection causes bronchopneumonia. **Histologically,** there are **syncytial cells** in bronchiolar epithelium and lung parenchyma, IC inclusion bodies, proliferation, degeneration of bronchiolar epithelium, alveolar epithelialization, edema, and hyaline membrane formation are seen.

Dignosis

Collection of clinical samples for varius tests includes slide preparations from nasal and conjunctival scrapings, nasal and conjunctival swabs, lung, and acute and convalescent sera.

A rapid diagnosis is made by the fluorescent antibody (FA) test on cytologic preparations of nasal and conjunctival epithelia collected early in the course of disease. FA or immunoperoxidase staining is used to demonstrate viral infected cells in cryostat sections of lung tissue in animals that have died. Histopathologic lesions are syncytial cells containing cytoplasmic inclusions.

Virus isolation on fresh samples is made in cell cultures of bovine origin in which it produces cytopathic effects consisting of **syncytia and eosinophilic cytoplasmic inclusions.** Enzyme immunoassay also detects BRSV.

Serology: Demonstration of a significant increase 4 -fold in antibody titres between acute and convalescent sera using ELISA or virus neutralization is confirmatory.

Treatment & Prevention

Use of antimicrobial drugs for 3-5 days checks secondary bacterial infections. Supportive therapy as well as fluid therapy to check dehydration is useful. Some resort to antihistamines or Non-steroidal anti-inflammatory drugs (NSAID) which are the drugs of choice. Currently aspirin is the only NSAID that is approved for use in food animals therapy with good result. Most cases recover automatically in several days without any treatment.

Vaccination

Both inactivated and modified live vaccines **are useful and serve to reduce losses associated with the disease. Bovi-Shield BRSV**-Pfizeris a freeze-dried preparation of an attenuated strain of BRSV with the sterile diluent provided for the vaccination of healthy cattle, including pregnant cows, is recommended. After rehydration the, administer 2 ml SC or IM in the neck region. Primary vaccination: administer a single 2-ml dose to healthy cattle to avoid possible maternal antibody interference with active immunization, calves vaccinated before the age of 6 months should be revaccinated after 6 months of age. **Bovi-Shield Gold FP5 L5**-Pfizer (IBR+BVD+BRSV+L.Canicola+L.Gripolyphosa+L.Hardjo+L. Icterohaemorrhagiae +L. Pomona bacterin) combines four respiratory diseases with leptospirosis. **VISTA ONCE SQ**-Intervet is a modified live vaccine for the immunization of cattle, 3 months of age or older, as an aid in the control of disease caused byIBR virus and BVD virus (Types 1 and 2); PI3 and BRSV and *Mannheimia haemolytica* and *Pasteurella multocida.* Inject 2.0 ml SC to healthy non-pregnant cattle, 3 months of age or older. Calves nursing immune-dams should be vaccinated when maternal antibody levels will allow active immunization. Additionally, Vista® Once SQ is for the vaccination of healthy cows and heifers prior to breeding as an aid in the prevention of fetal infection, including persistently infected calves caused by BVD virus Type 1; as an aid in the prevention of persistently infected (PI) calves caused by BVD virus Type 2; and as an aid in the reduction of abortion due to IBR. Annual revaccination is recommended. A revaccination dose can be administered at more frequent intervals based upon individual farm disease risk assessment or any time epidemic conditions exist or are reported. There are many other combination vaccines alongwith PRSV. These include- **VITA 5 SQ**-Intervet (IBR+BVD 1, 2+PI3+BRSV) is a modified life vaccine for immunization of non pregnant cattle.

Genus : *Metapneumovirus*

Avian Metapneumovirus Infection

Avian metapneumovirus (AMPV) infection causes disease in turkeys and chickens of all ages & is characterized by a **respiratory disease in the infected birds and drops in egg production in layers and breeders.** AMPV causes an upper respiratory disease with low mortality, but high morbidity primarily in commercial turkeys.

Etiology: Infection is caused by*Avian metapneumovirus* (AMPV).

Occurrence

The disease occurs in most countries in the world. Recently there was an emergence of a virulent type C AMPV in turkeys in Minnesota.

Hosts

Turkeys & chickens of all ages, pheasants and guinea fowl are susceptible, and antibodies to the virus have been found in wild birds and other domestic species. There are three types of AMPV (A, B, C) of which the C type is found only in the United States.

Clinical Symptoms

AMPV replicates in the respiratory tract and the reproductive tract. The virus initially causes respiratory disease in infected birds and also causes drops in egg production in layers and breeders. Infection in turkeys is commonly referred to as **"Turkey Rhinotracheitis"** and in chickens AMPV infection is commonly associated with **"Swollen Head Syndrome"** (SHS).The economic losses by AMPV is due to poor performance and mortality due to respiratory disease in meat turkeys and broilers & egg production losses in layers and breeders. Experimental infection in tukey poults showed severe clinical signs with copious nasal discharge, swollen sinus, conjunctivitis, and depression from 4 days PI to 12 days PI. **Histopathologic lesions** showed multifocal loss of cilia in nasal turbinate 3 to 11 days PI.

Diagnosis

Diagnosis of AMPV is confirmed by identification of the virus by isolation and identification of the virus using turkey organ cultures or embryonated eggs. Serological tests are used for flock surveys; ELISA is the most satisfactory test.

Tretment & Prevention

Vaccination

The losses due to AMPV infection is minimized or controlled by vaccination with live & attenuated vaccines and implementing biosecurity measures. Nobilis RTV 8544-Intervet is a live freeze dried vaccine for protection against Swollen Head Syndrome involving Avian Metapneumovirus infections in chickens. Each dose contains at least 3.0 log_{10} $TCID_{50}$ of AMPV virus strain BUT 1#8544 grown on chicken embryo fibroblast (CEF) cultures. Vaccine is administered by spray or eye drop. Broilers are vaccinated at day 1 onwards, then Breeders/layers are vaccinated at 10-12 weeks followed by vaccination at 18-20 weeks with Nobilis RT inac. Nobilis RT Inac should be vaccinated @ each bird: 0.5 ml IM in the thigh or breast muscle or SC in the lower part of the neck.

□□□

Chapter 27

Characteristics and Diseases Caused by Group V Single-Stranded (-) RNA Rhabdoviruses (Family *Rhabdoviridae*)

Contents

Characteristics of Rhabdoviruses

Rhabdoviruses (L. rhabdo= rod) are enveloped, peploomer bearing, bullet shaped in vertebrates, 180 nm long and 75 nm wide, are flattened at one end & pointed at the other end. But certain plant rhabdoviruses are bacilliform & almost twice the length. *Rhabdoviridae* has been grouped within the order *Mononegavirale*, which also contains the *Paramyxoviridae, Bornaviridae & Filoviridae* families. The enveloped virion has prominent **spikes, G** on the surface that hemagglutinates RBCs, & inner side is lined by the **matrix protein, M (Fig 27-1).** The inner **helical nucleocapsid is wound helically inside the core** & two non-structural proteins, **L and NS, are associated with the**

nucleocapsid and act in concert as the viral polymerase. The viral genome is unsegmented, linear, negative-sense RNA, about 11-15 kb in size. These viruses do not have a 5' cap or a polyA tail. The virus encodes for 5 to 6 proteins that include: large **RNA-dependent RNA polymerase (L)**, surface **glycoprotein (G), nucleoprotein (N)**, a component of viral polymerase-**phosphoprotein (P)**, and **matrix protein (M)**. **G protein attaches with cell receptors, induces neutralizing antibodies & favours viral endocytosis**. Rhabdoviruses infect a wide host range of animals, including humans, insects, fish & plants. The genus *Vesiculovirus* type species *Vesicular stomatitis virus* is the best studied rhabdovirus & a model system to study the biology of rhabdoviruses, and *Mononegavirales*. The second genus *Lyssavirus* type species *Rabies virus* causes rabies, which contains several strains.

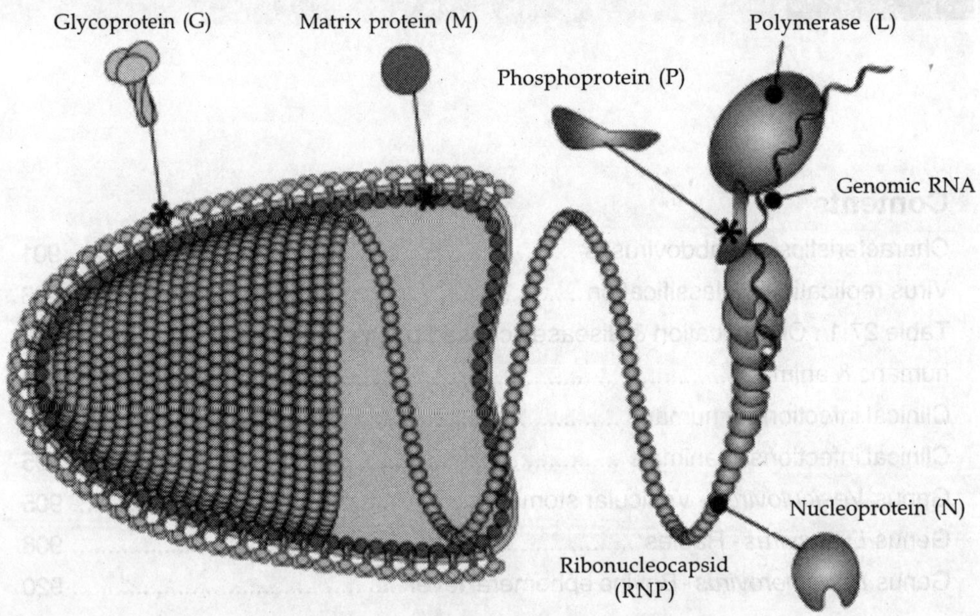

Figure 27.1 : Morphology of a Rhabdovirus

The viral genome

The viral genome is unsegmented, linear, negative-sense RNA, about 11-15 kb in size & encodes for 5 to six proteins. Five sub-genomic transcripts are made and translated, which allows the virus to have differential gene expression. Each sub-genomic transcript makes a distinct amount of the protein it encodes. The viral RNA dependent RNA polymerase binds the encapsidated genome at the leader region, then sequentially transcribes each genes by recognizing start and stop signals flanking viral genes. The mRNAs are capped and polyadenylated by the L protein during virus synthesis.

Virus Replication

Virus replication takes place in the cell cytoplasm. When the rabies virus enters the host, the G protein spikes bind to receptors on the surface of host cells and the viruses enter the cell by endocytosis and fuse with the membrane of the vesicle, mediated by the G protein. Both the L+ P with NS proteins are necessary for transcription, replication occurs in the cytoplasm (several plant viruses replicate in the nucleus.). Five monocistronic mRNAs are produced, capped at the 5' end and polyadenylated at the 3' end and each contains the leader sequence from the 3' end of the vRNA & message at the 5', using the negative sense RNA as a template for transcription of mRNA. After entry into the cell, the virus RNA polymerase synthesizes five mRNAs that code for the viral proteins. These mRNAs are similar to cellular mRNAs and can be translated by cellular ribosomes to produce both structural and non-structural proteins.

Replication requires enough newly synthesized N protein to encapsidate the RNA, neo-synthesized antigenomes and genomes. This occurs during its synthesis and results in the production of a full length anti-genomic copy. This in turn is used to produce more negative-sense genomic RNA. The viral polymerase is required for this process.

Like transcription, the genome is replicated by the L + P polymerase, but additional host cell factors are also required. Replication occurs in an Inclusion body within the cytoplasm/in a portion of the cytoplasm which acts as a **virus 'factory'** and appears as a characteristic cytoplasmic inclusion body- **perinuclear Negri bodies**; from where they bud through various cytoplasmic membranes and the outer membrane of the cell. This process results in the acquisition of the M + G proteins, responsible for the characteristic bullet-shaped morphology of the virus. The virions are assembled around the tightly coiled nucleoprotein core, the ribonucleocapsid interacts with the matrix protein under the plasma membrane M protein and buds from the plasma membrane, releasing the virions, acquiring the M + G proteins.

Virus Classification

Group: Group V (-) ssRNA

Order: *Mononegavirales*

Family: *Rhabdovirdae*

Genera

Genus 1: *Vesiculovirus*; type species: *Vesicular stomatitis Indiana virus* (VSIV)

Genus 2: *Lyssavirus*; type species: *Rabies virus* (RABV)

Genus 3: *Ephemerovirus*; type species: *Bovine ephemeral fever virus* (BEFV)

Genus 4: *Cytorhabdovirus;* type species: *Lettuce necrotic yellow virus* (LNYV)
Genus 5: *Nucleorhabdovirus;* type species: *Potato yellow dwarf virus* (PYDV)
Genus 6: *Novirhabdovirus;* type species: *Infectious haemapoietic virus* (IHV)

Table presented below shows classification *of Rhabdovidae* & diseases caused by each species.

Table 27.1 : Classification of *Rhabdoviridae* & diseases caused by the member viruses in humans & animals.

Species	Serotypes	Diseases caused
F: *Rhabdoviridae*		
G1: *Cytorhabdovirus*		
TS: *Lettuce necrotic yellow virus*	LNYV	Plant viruses
G2: *Vesiculovirus*		
TS: *Vesicular stomatitis Indiana virus*	VSIV	Vesicular stomatitis (VSIV) is a febrile viral disease that affects mainly cattle, horses, pigs and humans & occasionally sheep and goats & is characterized clinically by producing vesicular lesions similar to FMD. VS is of **zoonotic importace as humans are also infected** showing signs of mild influenza-like symptoms & hence it is a notifiable disease.
G3 :*Lyssavirus*		Genus *Lyssavirus* contains the following species divided into 4 serotypes & 7 genotypes as follows: *Rabies virus* (RABV); TS causes rabies & occurs worldwide except Australia & New Zealand. It belongs to genotype 1, serotype 1
		Lagos bat virus (LBV) falls to genotype 2, serotype 2 that occurs in Africa & have also been isolated from insectivorous bats as well as from domestic animals with encephalitis.
		Mokola virus (MOKV) belongs to genotype 3, serotype 3 that occurs in Africa; isolated from shrews & from human infection.
		Duvenhage virus (DUVV) belongs to genotype 4, serotype 4 that occurs in Africa; isolated from humans bitten by insectivorous bats.
		European bat lyssavirus 1(EBLV-1) belongs to genotype 5, occurs in Europe, isolated from insectivorous bats & also from human.
		European bat lyssavirus 2 (EBLV-2) belongs to genotype 6, occurs in Europe, isolated from humans

		with symptoms of rabies, & is present in insectivorous bats. *Australian bat lyssavirus* (ABLS) belongs to genotype 7, occurs in Australia, isolated from fruit & insectivorous bats & also from domestic animals with encephalitis.
Rabies virus	RABV	Rabies (RABV) is a viral disease of all warm- blooded animals & a zoonotic disease being transmitted to humans through the bite of the infected animals. Rabies is characterized by a long & variable incubation period depending on distance of the site of bite to infect brain where the virus travels via peripheral nerve & then to other organs. Rabies shows initial symptoms of malaise, fever, headache, weakness that progress to acute pain, anxiety, violent movement, excitement, partial paralysis, hallucination, hypersalivation, difficulty in swallowing & finally mania, lethargy, coma & death due to respiratory insufficiency. Rabies has been described since 2000 BC but was first reported in the Codex of Eshnunna in about 1930 BC.
G4: *Ephemerovirus*		The envelope glycolprotein G contains type-specific and neutralizing antigenic sites
TS: *Bovine ephemeral fever virus*	BEFV	Bovine ephemeral fever (BEFV) also called 3-Day Sickness is an arthropod vector-borne viral disease of cattle characterized by fever, muscular shivering, stiffness, lameness, nasal & ocular discharges, depression, cessation of rumination & constipation, & enlarged peripheral lymph nodes.
G5: *Novirhabdovirus*		
TS: *Infectious haema-poietic virus*	IHNV	Fish virus
G6: Nucleorhabdovirus		
TS: *Potato yellow dwarf virus*	PYDV	Plant viruses

Rhabdovirus Clinical Infections in Humans & Animals

Genus: *Vesiculovirus*:

Vesicular Stomatitis

Vesicular stomatitis (VSIV) is a febrile viral disease that affects mainly **cattle, horses, pigs and humans** & occasionally **sheep and goats** & is characterized clinically by producing **vesicular lesions** similar to FMD. VS is of **zoonotic importace as humans are also infected** showing signs of mild influenza-like symptoms & hence it is a notifiable diease.

Etiology

Vesicular stomatitis (VS) is caused by *Vesicular stomatitis Indiana virus* (VSIV). Two serotypes & various antigenically related species & subtypes of the virus exit. Two serotypes, *Vesicular stomatitis Indiana virus* (VSIV)-TS &*Vesicular stomatitis New Jersey virus* (VSNJV) occur in North and South America causing major outbreaks. *Vesicular stomatitis Alagoas virus* (VSAV) or Brazil virus (subtype 1 of Indiana virus) occurs in Brazil & *Cocal virus* (COCV) or Argentina virus (subtype 2 of Indiana virus) occurs in Argentina.

Occurrence

VS occurs only in the Western Hemisphere, is an endemic disease in the warmer regions of North, Central, and South America, but outbreaks of the disease in other temperate geographic parts of the Hemisphere occur sporadically. The Southwestern and Western United States have experienced a number of vesicular stomatitis outbreaks in recent years. Outbreaks in the Southwestern United States have usually occurred during the warmer months, often along waterways and in valleys. In some years during outbreaks, only a few premises in a single State were affected. In most years with outbreaks, multiple States and many premises were involved. VS is enzootic in Mexico, Panama & south to Venezuela & Peru & occasionally in USA, Brazil & Argentina where they cause epizootic outbreaks.VS occurs more frequcntly during summer.

Hosts susceptible

VSIV mainly affects cattle, horses, and swine and occasionally sheep, goats, llamas, and alpacas. Humans can also become infected with the disease when handling affected animals. Cattle & horses are more susceptible followed by pigs, camels, humans, & occasionally in sheep & goats. Adult cattle are more susceptible than calves.

Transmission

The virus is transmitted by direct, indirect & mediate means. Virus transmission occurs via contact with the infected animals, skin or mucous membrane abrasions or ingestion of virus infected feeds or water or contaminated pasture or **biologically by black flies for long distance & mechanically by *Culicoides* flies & eye gnats.**

Pathogenesis

After virus entry, there is viremia for 3 to 3 & half days, the virus localizes in the mm of mouth & skin around mouth & coronets followed by development of vesicles (only in 30% cases) at these sites & erosions.

Clinical Signs and Lesions

Incubation period is 3-15 days.

Cattle : There is mild fever, development of vesicles on tongue, dental pads, cheeks, lips, buccal mucosa & their rupture causes ropy salivation & anorexia. Dairy cattle may suffer from teat lesions and subsequent mastitis; a severe drop in milk production usually occurs. Some affected dairy cattle can appear to be normal with no clearly visible symptoms but may only eat about half of their normal feed intake. If there are no complications such as secondary infection, affected animals typically recover in about 2 weeks.

Horses : Clinical symptoms are similar to cattle but in the affected horses there is shallow ulcer, lameness & deformity if coronets are involved. In horses, vesicular lesions generally occur on the upper surface of the tongue, the lips, around nostrils, corners of the mouth, and gums. Lesions in horses may also occur as crusting scabs on the muzzle, lips, or ventral abdomen.

Pigs : Vesicles are seen on snout or on feet with lameness.

Diagnosis

Collection of clinical samples for various tests includes vesicular fluid, saliva, and affected mucous membranes collected at early stage.

1. A rapid **presumptive diagnosis** can be achieved by the electron microscopic demonstration of rhabdovirus in distilled water lysates of the lesion samples. Due to similarity of lesion with FMD, immediate diagnosis is needed. As FMD does not affect horses, it provides a differential diagnosis.
2. *Virus isolation:* The virus is isolated on Vero cell cultures with epithelia from lesions or vesicular fluid or cell cultures from various animal species. Identification is made using serologic procedures, such as ELISA, complement fixation and virus neutralization.
3. *Viral antigen detection:* Viral antigen is detectd by Fluorescet antibody or CFT or ELIZA tests.

Table 27.2 : Differentiation of vesicular diseases in animals.

Disease	Genus/ family	Cattle	Swine	Horse	Guinea pigs
Foot & mouth disease	*Aphthovirus/ Picornaviridae*	+	+	-	+
Vesicular stomatitis	*Vesiculovirus/ Rhabdoviridae*	+	+	+	+
Vesicular exanthema	*Vesivirus/ Calciviridae*	-	+	+	-
Swine vesicular disease	*Enterovirus/ Picornaviridae*	-	+	-	-

Treatment & Prevention

Sometimes non-steroidal anti inflammatory drugs are used. Checks on animal movement & quarantine are used. An **autogenous killed vaccine was used in 1994 outbreaks in USA.**

The following preventive measures are adopted. Separate animals with lesions from healthy animals; as a precautionary measure, do not move animals from premises affected by vesicular stomatitis at least for 21 days after the last lesion has healed. Implement insect control programs that include the elimination or reduction of insect breeding areas and the use of insecticide sprays. Use protective measures when handling affected animals to avoid human exposure to this disease.

Genus: *Lyssavirus*

Rabies

Rabies (RABV) is a viral disease of all **warm- blooded animals**& a zoonotic disease being transmitted to humans through the bite of the infected animals. Rabies is characterized by a **long & variable incubation period** depending on distance of the site of bite to infect brain where the virus travels via peripheral nerve & then to other organs showing initial symptoms of malaise, fever, headache, weakness that progress to acute pain, anxiety, violent movement, excitement, partial paralysis, hallucination, hypersalivation, difficulty in swallowing & finally mania, lethargy, coma & death due to respiratory insufficiency. Rabies has been described since 2000 BC but was first reported in the Codex of Eshnunna in about 1930 BC.

Etiology: Rabies is caused by *Rabies virus* (RABV) type species, under the genus *Lyssavirus.Rabies virus* is designated genotype 1 and serotype 1. Other species are;

Lagos bat virus (LBV) falls to genotype 2, serotype 2 that occurs in Africa & have also been isolated from insectivorous bats as well as from domestic animals with encephalitis.

Mokola virus (MOKV) belongs to genotype 3, serotype 3 that occurs in Africa; isolated from shrews & from human infection.

Duvenhage virus (DUVV) belongs to genotype 4, serotype 4 that occurs in Africa; isolated from humans bitten by insectivorous bats.

European bat lysavirus 1(EBLV-1) belongs to genotype 5, occurs in Europe, isolated from insectivorous bats & also from human.

European bat lyssavirus 2 (EBLV-2) belongs to genotype 6, occurs in Europe, isolated from humans with symptoms of rabies, & is present in insectivorous bats.

Australian bat lyssavirus (ABLS) belongs to genotype 7, occurs in Australia, isolated from fruit & insectivorous bats & also from domestic animals with encephalitis.

Occurrence

RABV is present in animal population in all countries except Australia & New Zealand. Recently, Hawai, & Scandinavian countries have also been free of rabies; & in some countries like Western Europe & Oceania, the virus is present in bat population only. In Asia, Africa & parts of America, dogs are the principal host & their mandatory vaccination is effective in preventing human rabies except in rural areas. There are about 55000 human deaths per annum from rabies, **India having the highest rate followed by Thailand** & other developing countries.

Hosts Susceptible

All warm-blooded animals are susceptible to RABV (birds are only experimentally infected) but the animals that most commonly transmit rabies to other animals include: raccoons, skunks, foxes, coyotes & bats. Most animals can be infected with RABV & can transmit the disease to humans. The infected bats, monkeys, raccoons, foxes, skunks, cattle, wolves, coyotes, dogs, yellow mongoose & cats are the greatest risk to transmit the disease to humans. Infected farm animals, ground hogs, weasels, bears & other wild carnivores are risk to human transmission. Small rodents like squirrels, hamsters, G. pigs, gerbils, rats, chipmunks, mice, rabbits & hare are almost never infected.

Transmission

RABV is present in the nerve & saliva of the symptomatic animals & their bite to humans or animals are the main route of virus transmission.

Other routes namely through broken skins, mucous membranes of the mouth, conjunctiva, anus, genitalia & by aerosol in bat infested caves transmit rabies. Rabies is mainly transmitted by the bite of infected animals, particularly dog bite or skin scratches are the main route of human rabies in Asia & Africa. Different wild lives are the vectors of rabies in different countries. **Vampire bats are the main vectors in South America, foxes in Europe & North America, skunks in in N. America, mongoose in Africa, & raccoon & bats in USA.** Raccoons (37.2%, skunks (30.7%), foxes (5.7%), coyotes, other wild animals- rodents & lagomorphs like rabbits & hare & bats most commonly transmit rabies to other animals. Domestic animals- cats, cattle, dogs, sheep, goats & pigs also get infected. Rarely rabies is transmitted without animal bite through the infected saliva aerosols in heavily populated vats caves. The virus appears in the animal milk but this route is unlikely means of virus spread. Infected domestic animals like cattle are rarely a source if their mouth is manipulated. Consumption of RABV-infected carcasses may infect arctic foxes.

Pathogenesis

After deep bite by the infected animals, the virus enters peripheral nerve endings; rabies virus binds to nicotinic acetylcholine receptors at neuromuscular junctions, multiplies locally in the striated muscles or CT at the site of inoculation and enters the peripheral nerves through the neuromuscular junction. Then the virus spreads to the CNS in the **endoneurium of the Schwann cells.** From the neuroepithelial spindles, the virus enters peripheral nerve, & moves passively within axon to nervous system. Virus may also enter nervous system via motor end plates. The virus through passive movement within axon enters spinal cord & then to brain. RABV pathogenicity is a multigenic trait involving several elements of the RABV genome, the **RABV glycoprotein G plays a major role in rabies pathogenesis by controlling the rate of virus uptake and trans-synaptic virus spread, and by regulating the rate of virus replication.** After entering CNS, there is an ascending wave of neuronal infection & neuronal dysfunction producing primary lesions in CNS.

There are two main symptoms of rabies: **1. Paralytic or dumb form & 2. Furious form.** When **spinal cord** is infected, ascending paralysis of hind quarters is followed by severe signs of mania till death. When the virus invades the **brain, irritation of centres causes mania, excitement & convulsions & death due to respiratory paralysis. Autonomic nervous system** involvement leads to hypersalivation, indigetion, pica, paralysis of bladder & anus. At death there is viral inclusions in almost all the neurons in brain, spinal cord & ganglia. Virus travels to salivary gland & other organs via passage of the virus along olfactory nerve to taste buds & other sensory end organs & oropharynx. Clinical symptoms also vary as per the source of the virus. Virus from bite of Vampire bats causes paralytic form, **fixed rabies** (fixed by serial intercerebral passage) causes furious form while the **street virus** (virus that occurs in nature) commonly causes furious form. The disease is always fatal but rarely infection showing clinical signs have been reported to recover. Recently experimentally infected animals showing symptoms of disease have recovered & similarly two human beings who developed clinical symptoms have recovered.

Clinical Symptoms & Lesions:

Incubation period: 10 days to 7 years, average **3-7 weeks,** depends on host species, virus strains, & amount of inocula at the bite site. The disease begins with the prodromal phase then proceeds to mainly the excitive phase or paralytic phase. There may be overlapping of the latter phases. The prodromal phase involves change in behavior and lasts 2 - 3 days. Anxiety, irritability and unease are characteristic. Some are more alert, restless and sensitive to light and noise. The excitive or furious phase includes signs of restlessness, depraved appetite, hiding, wandering, aggressive biting, excessive salivation, dysphagia, muscle tremors, incoordination and staggering. The paralytic or dumb phase develops in several days with seizures, paralysis, coma and death in 3 - 4 days. In horses and cattle the paralytic phase appears to be predominant.

Cattle: Most commonly observed symptoms in **paralytic form** are abnormal mental behavior, yawning & bellowing, salivation, incordination, reduced sensation in hind quarters, drooling saliva, recumbency & death in 4-7 deaths. **Furious form** occurs in 70% cases & is characterized by hypersensitivity, belligerency followed by paralysis & death.

Sheep: Common symptoms are attacking attitude, wool pulling, sexual excitement, incoordination in gait, salivation, muscle tremor followed by paralysis & death. Most sheep are anorectic.

Goats Show aggressiveness & bleating.

Horses: Common symptoms are depression, ataxia, abnormal posture, lameness, depression, pharyngyeal paralysis & recumbency, loss of anal sphincter tone & death in 4-6 days.

Pigs: Commonly show symptoms of excitement, attacking look, or dullness & incordination. Sows show nose twitching, rapid chewing, salivation & convulsion. Lastly there is paralysis & death.

Carnivores show both paralytic & furious form.

Pathological Lesions

There are no specific lesions & are limited to CNS. There may be congestion of menineal vessels & mild edema. The brain tissues unusually look pink. Perivascular cuffing is seen in CNS with vascular congestion. Neuronophagia & neuronal degeneration & proliferation of capsular cells around ganglionic neurons are seen. **Negri bodies, intracellular inclusions are seen in hippocampal ganglionic cells & Purkinje cells of cerebellum but are present in only 70% cases.**

Diagnosis

Collection of clinical samples includes saliva & skin biopsy for virus isolation; RT-PCR test; serum & spinal fluid for antibodies; postmortem samples include tissues from stem & brain.

1. *Direct fluorescent antibody (DFA) :* For DFA test, tissues from stem or cerebellum are taken, fluorescent labeled antirabies antibodies when incubated with suspect brain tissues, binds to rabies virus antigen, & unbound Ags are washed away. Positive cases are visualized as fluorescent apple green areas under fluorescent microscope. In case of negative DFA test suckling mice are inoculated intracerebrally when mice will die within 7 - 21 days if rabies virus is present.
2. *Histological examination :* In early days biopsy & autopsy samples from brain were sectioned, stained & examined to reveal encephalomyelitis in brain tissues & meninges, & also examined for mononuclear infiltration, perivscular cuffing of lymphocytes or polymorphonuclear lymphoid foci, Babes nodules made of glial cells & Negri bodies.
3. *Immunohistochemistry :* is a sensitive & specific test that detects rabies virus & ultrastructure in formalin fixed tissues using ELIZA test or mAbs.
4. *Electron microscopy :* reveals ultrastructure of the virus & visualizes bullet shaped particles.
5. *Amplifiction methods :* are used when samples are in small quantity. Virus isolation in cell culture, using neuroblastoma cells or BHK cells are used. Alternatively, nucleic acid is amplifieed by biochemical methods, e.g. RNA as DNA copies, using RT-PCR that detects virus in saliva & skin biopsy.

Treatment & Prevention

Treatment: Although a person or animal showing clinical symptoms of rabies die. But on 12.9. 204, Giese, 15 year student at Wisconsin developed rabies after the bite of a vat, & received no vaccine. The patient was kept on induced coma by Dr. Willoughby's to protect herself from her brain, with the hope that she would be survive long enough for her immune system to produce the antibodies to fight off the virus. Giese was given a cocktail of ketamine, midazolan, and phenobarbital to suppress brain activity and the antiviral drugs, ribavirin and amantadine while waiting for her immune system to produce antibodies to attack the virus brought out of the coma after six days. She survived. This treatment was known as Milwaukee protocol. In another attempt, 2 survived out of 25 patients treated under this protocol. Next 10 more patients were treated under the revised protocol omitting ribavirin, & there have been a further 2 survivors.

Vaccination

Surface glycoprotein G induces production of neutralizing antibodies, which are the major immune effectors against a lethal infection. RNP complex Ag is responsible for inducing $CD4^+$ T cells that play a major role in the establishment of immunologic memory and long-lasting immunity.

Antirabies vaccines: Antirabies vaccines include **4 types of vaccine: 1. Animal nerve tissue usually sheep/ rabbit brain adapted vaccine (first used by Pasteur in 1885), 2. Concentrated and purified cell-culture vaccine, 3. Concentrated & purified embryonated egg based rabies vaccines & 4. Recombinant oral vaccine**. Antirabies vaccines derived from animal nerve tissues for post-exposure prophylaxis induce more severe & adverse reactions and are less immunogenic & hence their production and use is not recommended by WHO. **Human diploid cell rabies vaccine** was started in 1967 using **attenuated Pitman –Moore L503 strain** & vaccinated to > 1.5 million humans that contained rabies in Philippine as well as in several countries. In 1979 van Howeling Research Centre of the Silican University Medical centre, Philippine developed a dog vaccine that gave **3 years immunity against rabies** that controlled dog rabies from several countries. Purified Vero Cell culture vaccines & purified chicken embryo cell vaccines used **Wistar strain** of rabies virus. **Embryo adapted vaccines have proved to be safe, cheaper and effective** in preventing rabies. The vaccines are used both for pre-exposure prophylaxis for persons at continual, frequent or increased risk of exposure to the rabies virus namely laboratory workers, veterinarians, animal handlers & cavern explorer. Post-exposure prophylaxis is given to humans or animals soon after bite by rabid animals.

For cell culture vaccines, rabies virus is propagated in cell substrates such as **human diploid cells** (embryonic fibroblast cells), **fetal rhesus diploid cells, Vero cells** (kidney cells from the African green monkey), primary Syrian hamster kidney cells using attenuated Wistar strain of rabies virus. Rabies virus is also adapted in primary chick embryo cells or in embryonated duck eggs. The more recently developed vaccines based on chick embryo cells and Vero cells have safety and efficacy even better than human diploid cell vaccines and are less expensive. After virus growth in the respective cell cultures, the viral harvest is concentrated, purified, inactivated and lyophilized. Some of the vaccines use human albumin or processed gelatin as a stabilizer. Rabies vaccines self life is > 3 years kept at + 7 to 8^{0}C protected from sunlight. Vaccines with a potency of **= 2.5 IU per single IM dose** are supplied in single dose vials for IM injection.

Various manufacturers of antirabies vaccine are: Merial Ltd that prepares **Imran** 1, & Imran 1TF that gives 1 year immunity; Pfizer animal health that prepare **Defensor 1 & Defensor 3** giving 1 & 3 years immunity; Intervet Inc prepares continuous rabis, **continuous DAP-R & continuous DAPP-R** that give 3 years immunity, & **Prorab** for dogs that gives 2 years immunity; Fort Dodge Animal Health prepares **Rabvac 1** (1 year immunity), **Rabvac 3 & Rabvac 3TF** giving 3 year immunity; Pfizer prepares **Rabdomun vaccine,** a cell culture grown inactivated adjuvanted & highly immunogenic vaccine for **beef & dairy cattle, sheep, dogs & cats** & available in liquid form to be stored at 2 to 7 ^{0}C & contains gentamycin as preservative. **Recombinant rabies vaccine V-RG was developed in 1984** by inserting **glycoprotein gene for rabies virus into a vaccinia virus under trade name Raboral V-RG-Merial.** The vaccine is harmless to humans & animals, is stable at higher temperature & can be given orally. The vaccine is given in a bait of fish meal & dropped from helicopter or hand spread where wild lives are abundant. It has successfully controlled wildlife rabies used in Belgium, France, Germany, and the United States to prevent outbreaks of rabies in wildlife & reduced risk to human rabies in several countries.

Pre - exposure vaccine doses : **Humans:** 3 doses regimen: 1 ml or .5 ml IM in deltoid region of arm (not on gluteal region) on day 0, 7, 21 or 28.

Dogs & cats : First at 3 month old or older 1 ml IM or SC, repeat dose 1 year later & revaccination on every 3 years.

Cattle & sheep : First vaccinated 3 month old or older 2 ml, IM, repeat dose 1 year later & revaccination on every 3 years.

Defensor 3-Pfizer is prepared in cell-culture, chemically inactivated rabies virus. The seed virus is a highly immunogenic, fixed strain of rabies virus which originated from Louis Pasteur's original isolate in 1882. The inactivated virus is formulated with a highly purified adjuvant and is packaged in liquid form. Dog & cat: Primary vaccination: a single 1ml dose SC at 3 months of age or older to healthy dogs and cats. A repeat dose should be administered 1 year later. Revaccination every 3 years with a single dose is recommended.

Cattle and Sheep: 2 ml IM. Primary vaccination: a single 2-ml dose at 3 months of age or older to healthy cattle and sheep. A repeat dose should be administered 1 year later. Annual revaccination with a single dose is recommended.

Rabvac 3/Rabvac 3 TF (thimerosal free)-Boehringer Ingelheim Vetmedica, Inc A, is a rabies vaccine recommended for the vaccination of healthy dogs, cats and horses. Vaccine is derived from a cell line culture and chemically inactivated. It meets the 3 year duration of immunity requirements for dogs and cats and 1 year duration for horses. Dosage: Dogs and cats - 1 ml IM or SC at 3 months of age or older. Repeat dose 1 year later, then every 3 years. Horses- 2 ml IM in horses at 3 months of age or older, repeat in 1 year and annually thereafter.

Continuum Rabies -Intervet is an inactivated virus vaccine produced from the highly immunogenic Pasteur rabies virus strain approved for use in cats and dogs. It is approved for 4-year duration of immunity in cats and 3-year duration of immunity in dogs. Dose is 1 ml SC to cats at 12 weeks of age, with a booster injection using 1 year later. Revaccinate every 4 years thereafter with a single dose of Continuum Rabies or Continuum Feline HCP-R.

EquiRab - Intervet horses- 1ml IM at 4 month & then annually.

Rabdomun - Pfizer is a killed rabies vaccine prepared from cell-culture-grown, chemically-inactivated rabies virus. The seed virus is a highly immunogenic, fixed strain of rabies virus which originated from Louis Pasteur's original isolate in 1882. The inactivated virus is formulated with a highly purified adjuvant and is packaged in liquid form for immunization of dogs, cats, cattle & sheep; immunity is 3 years in dogs & cats & 1 yr in cattle & sheep. Dogs & cats: primary vaccination: a single 1 ml dose at 3 months of age or older to healthy dogs and cats. A repeat dose should be administered 1 year later. Revaccination every 3 years with a single dose is recommended. Cattle & sheep: Primary Vaccination: a single 2 ml dose at 3 months of age or older to healthy cattle and sheep. A repeat dose should be administered 1 year later. Annual revaccination with a single dose is recommended.

Imrab 3 -Merial is a killed rabies vaccine for the vaccination of healthy cattle, sheep, horses, dogs, cats and ferrets, 12 wks of age or older. Cattle, sheep, horses - 2 ml IM or SC; revaccinate cattle, sheep and horses annually. Dogs, cats - 1 ml IM or SC; dogs, cats and sheep, repeat in 1 yr, then every 3 years. Ferrets - 1 ml SC & then annually.

Imrab large animals - Merial is a killed rabies virus vaccine for vaccination of cattle, horses & sheep, contains gentamicin as a preservative. Inject 2 ml SC or IM into healthy sheep, cattle, or horses when 3 months of age or older.

Revaccinate cattle and horses annually, and sheep one year after the first vaccination, then every 3 years.

Pure Vax Feline 3/ Rabies - Merial is a combination vaccine containing a nonadjuvanted lyophilized suspension of modified live feline rhinotracheitis, calici, and panleukopenia viruses, & a recombinant canarypox vectored rabies vaccine to produce expression of desired antigens capable of stimulating a protective immune response to rabies. Safety and immunogenicity of this product have been demonstrated by vaccination and challenge studies in susceptible cats. Inject 1 ml (1 dose) SC into healthy cats. For primary vaccination for all antigens except rabies, which requires only 1 dose at 8 weeks of age or older, revaccinate with a second 1 ml dose 3 to 4 weeks later. Cats younger than 12 weeks of age should be revaccinated with a single 1 ml dose every 3 to 4 weeks, the last dose given at or over 12 weeks of age. Revaccinate annually with a single 1 ml dose.

PUREVAX Feline 4/ Rabies - Merial is combination vaccine containing a nonadjuvanted lyophilized suspension of modified live feline rhinotracheitis, calici, and panleukopenia viruses and *Chlamydia psittaci;* recombinant vectored rabies vaccine; plus a sterile water diluent. A canarypox vector has been modified, using recombinant technology, to produce expression of desired antigens capable of stimulating a protective immune response to rabies. For primary vaccination for all antigens except rabies, which requires only 1 dose at 8 weeks of age or older, revaccinate with a second 1 ml dose of 3 to 4 weeks later. Cats younger than 12 weeks of age should be revaccinated with a single 1 ml dose every 3 to 4 weeks, the last dose given at or over 12 weeks of age. Revaccinate annually with a single 1 ml dose.

Continuum Feline HCP-R - Intervet is a modified live virus vaccine containing attenuated strains of FRV, FCV, FPV, and inactivated rabies virus for the vaccination of healthy cats for the prevention of disease caused by FPV, as an aid in the prevention of disease caused by FCV, and as an aid in the control of disease caused by FRV for 3 years following initial and booster vaccinations; for the vaccination of healthy cats as an aid in the prevention of disease caused by rabies for 4 years following initial and booster vaccinations. Administer 1 ml by the SC route, initial vaccination of healthy cats as early as 12 weeks of age, with a booster injection using Continuum Feline HCP-R or Continuum Rabies administered 1 year later. Revaccinate every 3 years with a single dose of Continuum Feline HCP-R or Continuum Rabies.

Continuum DAP-R 3-Year DOI - Merck is a combination modified live virus vaccine containing attenuated Onderstepoort strain of CDV, Manhattan strain of Adenovirus type-2, attenuated CPV Strain 154® of canine origin & and inactivated Pasteur strain of Rabies virus. The vaccine is presented in a

Product name	Produced by	Marketed by	For use in	Dose	Age at primary vaccination*	Booster recommended	Route of vaccination
Monovalent (inactivated)							
Rabvac 1	Boehringer Ingelheim Vetmedica, Inc.† License no. 112	Boehringer Ingelheim Vetmedica, Inc.	Dogs	1mL	3 mos§	Annually	IM or SC
			Cats	1mL	3 mos	Annually	IM or SC
Rabvac 3	Boehringer Ingelheim Vetmedica, Inc. License no. 112	Boehringer Ingelheim Vetmedica, Inc.	Dogs	1mL	3 mos	1 yr later & triennially	IM or SC
			Cats	1mL	3 mos	1 yr later & triennially	IM or SC
			Horses	2mL	3 mos	Annually	IM
Rabvac 3 TF	Boehringer Ingelheim Vetmedica, Inc. License no. 112	Boehringer Ingelheim Vetmedica, Inc.	Dogs	1mL	3 mos	1 yr later & triennially	IM or SC
			Cats	1mL	3 mos	1 yr later & triennially	IM or SC
			Horses	2mL	3 mos	Annually	IM
Continuum Rabies	Intervet, Inc. License no. 165A	Intervet, Inc.	Dogs	1mL	3 mos	1 yr later & triennially	SC
			Cats	1mL	3 mos	1yr later & quadrennially	SC
EquiRab	Intervet, Inc. License no. 165A	Intervet, Inc.	Horses	1mL	4 mos	Annually	IM
Prorab 1	Intervet, Inc. License no. 165A	Intervet, Inc.	Dogs	1mL	3 mos	Annually	IM or SC
			Cats	1mL	3 mos	Annually	IM or SC
			Sheep	2mL	3 mos	Annually	IM
Defensor 1	Pfizer, Inc. License no. 189	Pfizer, Inc.	Dogs	1mL	3 mos	Annually	IM or SC
			Cats	1mL	3 mos	Annually	SC
Defensor 3	Pfizer, Inc. License no. 189	Pfizer, Inc.	Dogs	1mL	3 mos	1 yr later & triennially	IM or SC
			Cats	1mL	3 mos	1 yr later & triennially	SC
			Sheep	2mL	3 mos	Annually	IM
			Cattle	2mL	3 mos	Annually	IM

Rabdomun	Pfizer, Inc. License no. 189	Schering-Plough Animal Health	Dogs	1mL	3 mos	1 yr later & triennially	IM or SC
			Cats	1mL	3 mos	1 yr later & triennially	SC
			Sheep	2mL	3 mos	Annually	IM
			Cattle	2mL	3 mos	Annually	IM
Rabdomun 1	Pfizer, Inc. License no. 189	Schering-Plough Animal Health	Dogs	1mL	3 mos	Annually	IM or SC
			Cats	1mL	3 mos	Annually	SC
Imrab 1	Merial, Inc. License no. 298	Merial, Inc.	Dogs	1mL	3 mos	Annually	SC
			Cats	1mL	3 mos	Annually	SC
Imrab 1 TF	Merial, Inc. License no. 298	Merial, Inc.	Dogs	1mL	3 mos	Annually	SC
			Cats	1mL	3 mos	Annually	SC
Imrab 3	Merial, Inc. License no. 298	Merial, Inc.	Dogs	1mL	3 mos	1 yr later & triennially	IM or SC
			Cats	1mL	3 mos	1 yr later & triennially	IM or SC
			Sheep	2mL	3 mos	1 yr later & triennially	IM or SC
			Cattle	2mL	3 mos	Annually	IM or SC
			Horses	2mL	3 mos	Annually	IM or SC
			Ferrets	1mL	3 mos	Annually	SC
Imrab 3 TF	Merial, Inc. License no. 298	Merial, Inc.	Dogs	1mL	3 mos	1 yr later& triennially	IM or SC
			Cats	1mL	3 mos	1 yr later& triennially	IM or SC
			Ferrets	1mL	3 mos	Annually	SC
Imrab Large Animal	Merial, Inc. License no. 298	Merial, Inc.	Cattle	2mL	3 mos	Annually	IM or SC
			Horses	2mL	3 mos	Annually	IM or SC
			Sheep	2mL	3 mos	1 yr later & triennially	IM or SC
Monovalent (rabies glycoprotein, live canary pox vector)							
PureVax Feline Rabies	Merial, Inc. License no. 298	Merial, Inc.	Cats	1mL	3 mos	Annually	SC
Combination (inactivated rabies)							
Continuum DAP-R	Intervet, Inc. License no. 165A	Intervet, Inc.	Dogs	1mL	3 mos	1 yr later & triennially	SC

Continuum Feline HCP-R	Intervet, Inc. License no. 165A	Intervet, Inc.	Cats	1mL	3 mos	1 yr later & triennially	SC
Equine Potomavac + Imrab	Merial, Inc. License no. 298	Merial, Inc.	Horses	1mL	3 mos	Annually	IM
Combination (rabies glycoprotein, live canary pox vector)							
PureVax Feline 3/ Rabies	Merial, Inc. License no. 298	Merial, Inc.	Cats	1mL	8 wks 3 mos	Every 3 wks until 3 mos & annually 3 wks later and annually	SC
PUREVAX Feline 4/ Rabies	Merial, Inc. License no. 298	Merial, Inc.	Cats	1mL	8 wks 3 mos	Every 3 wks until 3 mos & annually 3 wks later and annually	SC
Oral (rabies glycoprotein, live vaccinia vector): restricted to use in state and federal rabies control programs							
Raboral V-RG	Merial, Inc. License no. 298	Merial, Inc.	Coyotes Raccoons	N/A	N/A	As determined by local authorities	Oral

Abbreviations: IM = intramuscular; N/A = not applicable; SC = subcutaneous; TF = thimerosal free.
* Minimum age (or older) and revaccinated 1 year later.
† Fort Dodge Animal Health was recently acquired by Boehringer Ingelheim Vetmedica, Inc.
§ One month = 28 days.

desiccated form with diluent provided for reconstitution. Dose: 1 ml by the SC route for vaccination of healthy dogs as early as 12 weeks of age, with a booster injection for rabies administered 1 year later. Revaccinate every 3 years with a single dose of vaccine.

Raboral V-RG - Merial is a recombinant oral rabies vaccine for its response in Arctic foxes (*Vulpes lagopus*), it is approved for immunization of raccoons and coyotes, two of the most significant wildlife carriers of rabies in North America. The vaccine, which is currently the only licensed oral rabies vaccine in the United States, induced a strong antibody response and protected foxes against a challenge of 500,000 mouse intracerebral lethal dose 50% of an Arctic rabies virus variant. Raboral V-RG vaccine is efficacious in Arctic foxes. Since 1990, approximately 100 million doses of Raboral V-RG animal vaccine have been distributed in the United States by depositing baits by airplane or by hand in areas with dense populations of target wildlife species (e.g., raccoons in the eastern United States). Human or domestic animal contact with ORV baits has been reported rarely. In 2008, among 16 states where 10,339,969 baits were placed, 291 vaccine-related telephone calls involving human or domestic animal contact (2.8 per 100,000 baits) were reported by public health authorities.

Genus : *Ephemerovirus*

Bovine Ephemeral Fever

Bovine ephemeral fever (BEFV) also called **3-Day Sickness** is an arthropod vector-borne viral disease of cattle characterized by fever, muscular shivering, stiffness, lameness, nasal & ocular discharges, depression, cessation of rumination & constipation, & enlarged peripheral lymph nodes.

Occurrence

BEFV occurs enzootically in tropical & subtropical regions of Africa, most parts of Asia, Middle East & some parts of Australia & Newzealand. Morbidity rate is variable up to 80% & mortality is usually 1-2%.

Hosts

Only cattle of all age groups are susceptible. However calves **less than 6 months are most susceptible**. Water buffaloes are also susceptible. **Inapparent infections can develop in Cape buffaloes, hartebeest, waterbucks, wildebeest, deer, and possibly goats.**

Transmission

Probably mosquitoes of *Aedes* spp & biting midge act as the vectors but *Culex annulirostris* act as biological vector. Direct contact or fomites do not favour transmission, and BEFV does not persist in recovered cattle. The majority of recovered cattle develop a life-long immunity.

Pathogenesis

The pathogenesis of the disease is complex but it appears that the **host inflammatory responses are mediated by the release of cytokines & are responsible for the development of the disease**. Pathogenesis has been studied by IV inoculation of the virus. Initially BEFV multiplies within the **vascular system. A biphasic fever** is seen with peaks at 12-24 hours lasting 2 days & accompanied by increased respiratory rate, dyspnea, limb stiffness & trembling.

A generalized inflammation follows with vasculitis & thrombosis, serofibrinous inflammation in synovial cavities & increased endothelial permeability. BEFV is located in circulating neutrophils, serous & synovial fluid, endothelial cells & synovial membrane. BEFV induces caspase-dependent apoptosis. Sick animals improve in two days after the first symptoms and recover within another one to two days. But lactating cows and animals in good condition take up to a week to recover.

Lesions : Presence of serofibrinous polyserosis in the synovial, pericardial, pleural & peritoneal cavities with neutrophils. Synovial membranes of joints show degenerative changes with increased synovial fluid, congestion of abomasal mucosa & nasal cavities, pulmonary emphysema & bronchiolitis are characteristic features. Presence of petechial hemorrhages or edema may be noted in the lymph nodes. Areas of focal necrosis are common in the major muscle groups.

Clinical Symptoms and Lesions

Incubation period is 2-10 days with mean of 3 to 5 days. Bovine ephemeral is usually mild but severe in bulls and high-producing cows. Subclinical infections are also seen. The classic course begins with a fever, which is often biphasic, triphasic or polyphasic with temperature peaks occur 12 to 18 hours apart. During the first fever peak, milk production often drops, some animals may be depressed, stiff or reluctant to move. On the second peak elevation in temperature is seen & animals usually become inappetent and depressed, with an increased heart rate, tachypnea, and serous or mucoid discharges from the nose. Profuse **salivation, muscle twitching, waves of shivering or a watery ocular discharge can be seen.** Some animals develop submandibular or periorbital edema, or patchy edema on the head. **Shifting lameness, stiffness and joint pain are common;** the joints may or may not be swollen. Pulmonary emphysema and rales may be found in severe cases. Many animals, particularly cows in good condition and bulls, become **recumbent** and are unable to rise. Recumbent animals may be bloated, have ruminal stasis or lose their swallowing reflex. There are leukocytosis, hyperfibrogenesis, hypocalcaemia & increased creatine kinase, which are the characteristic features.

Diagnosis

1. *Presumptive diagnosis* : Clinical symptoms, fever, lameness, temporary paralysis or recumbency, & lesions are suggestive of BEF.
2. *Virus isolation* : Virus is isolated in cell lines of *Aedes albopictus* (mosquito) for the initial isolation or in mice is attempted.
3. *Virus antigen detection* : Fluorescence antibody test detects BEFV, or EELIZA test.
4. *Antibody detection* : A rising titer of BEFV either through virus neutralization or enzyme-linked immunosorbent assay is useful. PCR assays are used for diagnosis in some countries.

Treatment & Prevention

Non-steroidal anti-inflammatory drugs namely phenylbutazone IM @ 8 mg/kg bwt 8 hrly or flunixin meglumine 2.2 mg/kg bwt for 3 days reduces the symptoms. Calcium borogluconate is given to cows.

Vaccination

Attenuated tissue culture vaccine or mouse brain adapted adjuvanted vaccines or oil adjuvant vaccine inducing immunity for 1 year are **vaccinated twice** in some countries that resulted in halting the outbreaks. Formalin killed vaccine using glycoprotein G is not very effective.

□□□

Chapter 28

Characteristics and Diseases Caused by Group V Single-Stranded (-) RNA Bornaviruses (Family *Bornaviridae*)

Contents

Characteristics of Bornaviruses

Bornaviruses are enveloped, spherical viruses with a diameter of 70 to 130 nm; the envelope surrounds the inner matrix protein layer. The virion contains a **helical nucleocapsid**. *Bornaviridae* was so named after the town **Borna in Germany** where it was detected as a neurological diease of horses in 1776. *Bornaviridae* along with *Paramyxoviridae, Rhabdoviridae & Astroviridae* has been placed in the order *Mononegavirales,* but unlike other families of this order, **bornaviruses replicate in the host nucleus** and has overlapping transcriptional units, some of which undergo splicing by the cellular machinery. Bornaviruses are **non-lytic, persistent, neurotropic virus**. *Bornaviridae* has only one genus *Bornavirus* & one member *Borna disease virus. Borna disease virus* has the smallest genome made of unsegmented, linear, minus sense, ssRNA made of 8.9 kilobases. The virus encodes **6 proteins called,**

nucleoprotein, N, Phosphoprotein, P, Matrix protein, M, glycoprotein, G & Polymerase, L. An ideal structure of a bornavirus is shown in **Fig 28-1.**

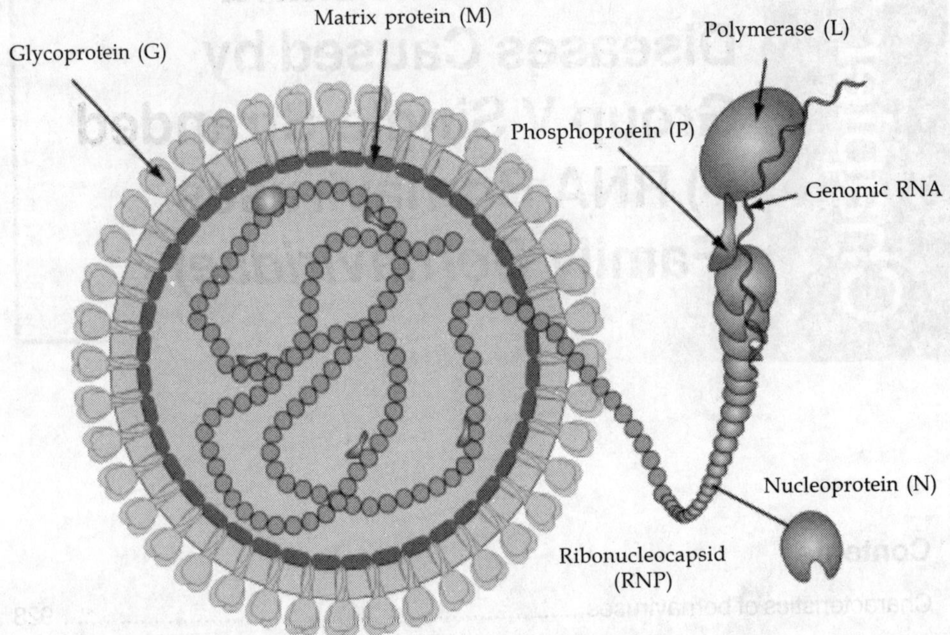

Figure 28.1 : Morphology of Bornavirus

Since 1776 the virus has been recorded in cattle, sheep, dogs and foxes, & **cats suffering from a staggering disease** in Sweden, Japan & Britain. *Borna disease virus* has also been **detected as human infection with neuropsychiatric disorders**. Experimental infection of rats leads to **learning impairments and altered social behavior**. Avian bornaviruses have recently been found to cause **Proventricular Dilatation Disease in pet birds**. Bornavirus nucleoprotein genes have been detected in the genomes of several mammalian species. Based on the molecular biology, the virus has **several unusual features like nuclear localization for replication and transcription,** overlap of open reading frames and transcription units, posttranscriptional modification of subgenomic RNAs, marked conservation of coding sequence across various animal species and tissue culture systems & BDV replication at lower levels than most known viruses, not lytic, and persistence in the nervous system despite a vigorous immune response.

The virus genome

Borna disease virus has the smallest genome made of unsegmented, linear minus sense, ssRNA made of 8.9 kilobases. BDV genome contains at least six open reading frames & has three transcriptional units that encode at least six proteins as named below:

Unit 1: encodes nucleoprotein (N); Unit 2 is overlapping & encodes two proteins- x protein (X) (a negative regulator of the polymerase), & phosphoprotien (P) , Unit 3 is overlapping, & has regulatory splicing encoding 3 protein - matrix protein (M), glycoprotein (G) & polymerase (L). The viral RNA dependent RNA polymerase binds the encapsidated genome at the leader region & sequentially transcribes each gene by recognizing start and stop signals flanking viral genes. mRNAs are capped and polyadenylated by the L protein during synthesis.

Virus replication

Bornaviruses replicate in the nucleus, enter the host by endocytosis that is taken up by endosomes. Virus attaches to host receptors though GP glycoproteins and is endocytosed into vesicles in the host cell, virus membrane fuses with the vesicle membrane; & ribonucleocapsid is released into the cell cytoplasm and then migrates to the nucleus.

Then there is sequential transcription, & viral mRNAs are capped and polyadenylated in the cytoplasm. Virus replication starts when enough nucleoprotein is present to encapsidate neo-synthetized antigenomes and genomes. Bornaviruses negative sense RNA is copied to make a positive sense RNA template that is used to synthesize many copies of the negative sense RNA genome. The nucleocapsid interacts with the matrix protein under the plasma membrane M protein and buds from the plasma membrane, releasing the virion.

Virus classification

Group: Group V ((-) ss RNA

Order: *Mononegavirales*

Family: *Bornaviridae*

Genus: *Bornavirus*

Type species: *Borna disease virus*

Bornavirus Infection in Horses, Other Animals & Humans

Genus : *Bornavirus*

Borna Disease

Borna disease caused by *Borna disease virus* (BDV) under the family *Bornaviridae* is a **subacute meningoencephalitis** in horses, sheep, cattle, rabbits & cats reported from Germany, Sweden & Switzerland, in young ostriches in Isarel, & is common clinical inapparent infections in many species of animals.

The Borna disease is characterized by subacute infection of CNS that takes **weeks to months in development of lesions**, & clinical symptoms in horses include moderate fever, pharyngeal paralysis, lack of food intake, muscle tremors, defects in proprioception, hyperthesia, & at terminal stage by lethargy, somnolence & flaccid paralysis. BDV was first described in 1885 as "heated head disease" of cavalry horses in 1885 in the town Borna in Germany.

Occurrence

The geographic distribution of BDV is unknown but natural infection occurs only in Central Europe, North America, and parts of Asia namely Japan and Israel. However, recently asymptomatic naturally infected animals have been identified meaning that BDV is widespread in many species of animals. Antibodies to BDV have been detected in horses in USA, Japan & Iran. Antibodies to BDV have been reported in humans from North America, Europe & Japan.

Hosts

Borna disease affects **horses, sheep, llamas, ostriches, and cattle, dogs & foxes.** BDV in 1995 was isolated from cats suffering from a staggering disease in Sweden & since then also detected in cats in Japan & Britain. Experimentally, the host range includes possibly all warm-blooded animals. BDV may cause **disease in humans like lymphocytic meningoencephalitis**. Rats can be infected experimentally resulting in impairments and altered social behaviour. BDV has been detected in humans and probably infection is associated with psychiatric disorders.

Transmission

The method of disease transmission is unclear but it is believed to be by **inhalation of saliva or nasal secretions or ingestion**. After infection, animals **may develop Borna disease, or may remain subclinical, possibly acting as a carrier of the virus.** So far no reservoir or the mode of transmission of natural infection is known. But an **olfactory route for transmission occurs** since intranasal infection is efficient, and the olfactory bulbs of naturally infected horses show inflammation and edema early in the course of disease. BDV nucleic acid and proteins in peripheral blood **mononuclear** cells also indicate a potential for hematogenous transmission. Experimental infection of rodents results in virus persistence and is associated with the presence of viral gene products in saliva, urine, and feces; such secreta /excreta may be important in the disease transmission. But natural BDV infection does not occur in rodents; hence their role in BDV transmission to other domesticated animals and humans remains speculative. Vertical transmission of BDV in natural or experimental hosts has not been reported.

Pathogenesis

'After oronasal infection, BDV infects the cells of the CNS, the virus presumably enters to CNS by intra-axonal spread through trigeminal & olfactory nerves & thereafter disseminates throughout the brain. BDV spread within CNS & into the peripheral nerves occurs within axons. **The virus replicates in the nucleus of the cell without damage to the neuron cells.** But the **infected cells express viral antigens on the cell surface inducing CD8⁺ cell mediated immune response that destroy the infected cells.Immunosuppression prevents development of the disease & it takes months to appear lesions.** Non-suppurative encephalitis occurs with perivascular cuffing mostly in **grey matter**. Neuronal degeneration occurs **&IN inclusions called Joest-Degen bodies may be seen in the hippocampus.**

Clinical symptoms and lesions

The disease is subacute involving young horses & it takes months to appear lesions. In natural cases the **incubation period is nearly 4 weeks** to months. The appearance of clinical symptoms depends on the age of animals, virus strains & immunological status of the animals. The clinical symptoms include initially moderate **fever, inappetence, pharyngeal paralysis, muscle tremor & hyperthesia**. In the terminal stage of the disease, there are **lethargy, somnolence, & flaccid paralysis.** Disease runs a course of 3 weeks & mortality rate is 80% to 100%. Horses that survive show **CNS damage & recurrent episodes of neurological symptoms**. Avian bornaviruses cause proventicular dilatation disease in pet birds. Experimentally infected rats show symptoms of impairments and altered social behaviour.

In **humans** BDV is possibly associated with psychiatric disease. In 1990, scientists reported that antibodies to a protein encoded by the Borna virus genome are found in the blood of patients with behavioral disorders. Later studies presented evidence for an association between Borna and human psychiatric disorders. More evidences for a role of Borna virus in psychiatric disorders comes from reports that the drug amantadine, which is used to treat influenza infections, had some success in treating depression and clearing Borna infection.

Diagnosis

Collection of clinical samples includes brain, sera/CSF.

1. *Presumptive diagnosis:* Eosinophilic IN inclusions called **Joest-Degen bodies** are suggestive.
2. *Virus antigen detection:* RT-PCR is used to detect BDV RNA.

3. *Antibody detection:* Complement fixation test, & immunofluorescent tests or ELISA test detect antibodies in serum or cerebrospinal fluid.

Treatment & prevention

No suitable treatment or vaccine is available. Prevention includes separation of affected and seropositive animals from healthy ones.

□□□

Chapter 29

Characteristics and Diseases Caused by Group V Single-Stranded (-) RNA Filoviruses (Family *Filoviridae*)

Contents

Characteristics of Filoviruses

Filoviruses of the family *Filoviridae* under the order *Mononegavirales* are **pleomorphic** that appear in many shapes like long, sometimes **branched filaments & as shorter filaments shaped like a "6", a "U", or a circle measuring up to 14,000 nm in length (Fig 29-1)** with a uniform diameter of 80 nm. Filamentous form is 790 nm long for Marburg virus and 970 nm long for *Ebolavirus* & diameter is about 80 nm. Filoviruses are enveloped having a **helical** nucleocapsid. Filovirus (L. filum= thread-like) was **named from the Latin word filum meaning thread-like appearance** of virus particles in electron microscope. Filoviruses contain one molecule of (-) ssRNA about 19,000 nucleotides in length. Filoviruses cause **viral hemorrhagic fever characterised by coagulation abnormalities** that often lead to fatal bleeding.

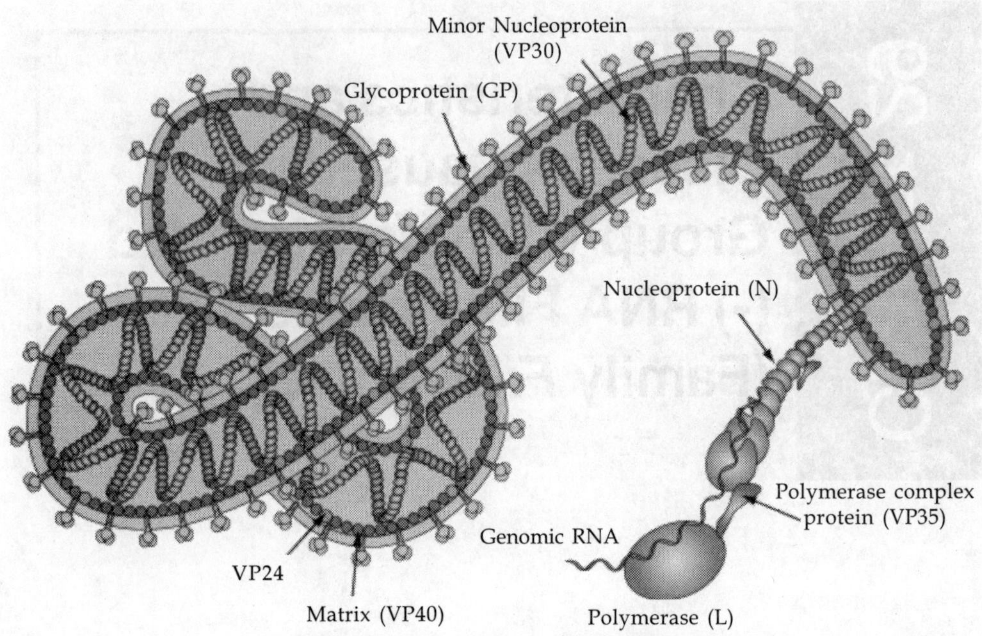

Figure 29.1 : Morphology of Filovirus

The filovirus was first recognized in **1967 in laboratory workers handling tissues from green monkeys in Germany** and Yugoslavia who developed hemorrhagic fever; the virus was named after Marburg, Germany. Ebola virus was first detected in 1976 from outbreaks of Ebola hemorrhagic fever (Ebola HF) in Zaire, Congo and southern Sudan. The outbreaks involved two different species of Ebola virus; *Sudan ebola virus* & *Zaire Ebola virus* & both were named after the nations in which they were discovered. Both viruses showed themselves to be highly lethal, as 90% of the Zairian cases and 50% of the Sudanese cases resulted in death. Filoviruses are estimated to have diverged for less than 10,000 years ago-about the same time scale as the rise of agriculture.

Filoviruses are zoonotic & is transmitted to humans from life cycles in animals other than humans but the natural reservoirs of Ebola and Marburg viruses remain undetected. The first detected cases of Ebola virus outbreaks was in Africa among the dead bodies and carcasses of chimpanzees, gorillas, rodents, duikers and shrews & very soon got transmitted, but they are a natural reservoir for the same. **Birds, arthropods and the plants are considered to be the possible reservoirs of ebola virus** disease. Since the virus replicates in some species of bats native to the areas, bats are presumed to act as carriers. After the virus is transmitted from the natural reservoir to a human, person-to-person transmission involves close personal contact, or their body fluids, and nosocomial transmission.

The viral gnome

Virus genome is made of linear, minus-sense ssRNA, about 18-19 kb in size & encodes for **seven proteins**. The viral genome encodes structural proteins and non-structural proteins. **5 structural protein**(s) are the **envelope protein, GP** form the viral spikes in the form of trimers surface glycoprotein, **nucleocapsid protin (NP)** binds to the genomic RNA, **Nucleocapsid protein VP30, Matrix protein VP40** is a transmembrane protein, or a membrane-associated protein, & **polymerase complex protein (VP 35) & polymerase L.** 3' terminus of the virus is not polyadenylated and the 5' end is not capped. The gene in the virus order is 3' – leader – NP – VP35 – VP40 – GP/sGP – VP30 – VP24 – L – trailer – 5′. The protein-coding genes in the filovirus genomes are having a transcriptional gradient from NP to L protein. Notably, the N-terminal 450 amino acid residues of NP show significant conservation among the *Mononegavirales* and is needed for self-assembly of the nucleoprotein. While expressing viral genes, the viral RNA dependent RNA polymerase binds the encapsidated genome at the leader region, then sequentially transcribes each genes by recognizing start and stop signals flanking viral genes. mRNAs are capped and polyadenylated by the L protein during synthesis.

Virus replication

Replication of the viruses in the cytoplasm needs the host cell machinery and metabolism to produce multiple copies of themselves, and they assemble in the cell.

Filoviruses attach via GP protein to the host cell receptors and are endocytosed into vesicles in the host cell. The virus membrane fuses with the vesicle membrane & nucleocapsid is released into the cytoplasm. mRNAs are transcribed sequentially followed by transcription, & viral mRNAs are capped and polyadenylated in the cytoplasm. Translation of the mRNA into viral proteins occurs using the host cell's machinery. Translation is switched over to replication when viral protein levels rise. The negative-sense RNA is used as a template to create a +cRNA, which is then used to synthesize negative-sense RNA for encapsidation. Viral replication starts when enough nucleoprotein is present to encapsidate neo-synthetized antigenomes and genomes. The ribonucleocapsid interacts with the matrix protein under the plasma membrane, buds from the plasma membrane, releasing the virion.

Virus classification

Group: Group V (-) ssRNA

Order: *Mononegavirales*

Family: *Filoviridae*

Genera

G1: *Ebolavirus*: type species: *Zaire ebola virus* (ZEBOV), others are *Sudan ebolavirus* (SEBOV), *Reston ebolavirus* (REBOV), *Côte d'Ivoire ebolavirus* (CIEBOV) & *Bundibugyo ebolavirus*

G2: *Marburgvirus; type species: Lake Victoria marburgvirus*

Table 29.1: Classification of *Filoviridae* & diseases caused by the member viruses in humans & animals.

Species	Geographical distribution	Reservoir	Transmission	Diseases
G1 *Ebola virus* TS: *Zaire* (ZEBOV)	Congo, Gabon	Not exactly known, probably bat	Direct contact with body fluids, blood, handling organs, & chimpanzee, gorillas, forest antelopes & bats.	Zaire ebola virus **(ZEBOV)** causes ebola hemorrahagic fever (EHF) in humans. The symptoms are fever, headache, myalgia, jaundice, pancreatitis, pharyngitis, delirium, rash, hemorrhages & hypovolemic shock. The virus replicates in macrophages, DC, hepatocytes, & spread to all vital organs, & interstitial endothelial cells. Blood vessel walls are destroyed, the platelets are unable to coagulate, and patients succumb to hypovolemic shock. There is massive lymphocyte apoptosis, multiorgan dysfunction-liver, septic-like syndrome, clotting abnormality, aberrant immunity, many proinflammatory cytokines, & loss of CD4 & CD8 cells. The highest fatality rate is up to 90%. Recombinant VSV with GP protein vaccine is under trial. Diagnosis is by ELIZA, PCR.
Sudan ebola virus (SEBOV)	Sudan, Uganda	Do	Do	*Sudan ebola virus* **(SEBOV)** as above but fatality rate is up to 50%.

Côte d'Ivoire ebolavirus, Tai ebolavirus, Ivory cost ebola virus (CIEBOV)	Congo, Gabon	Do	Do	*Côte d'Ivoire ebolavirus* **(CIEBOV) caused non-fatal disease in human in one case but main cases occur in chimpanzees.**
Reston ebola virus (REBOV)	Reston, Virginia, in nonhu-man primates in Pennsylvania, Texas and Sienna, Italy, Philippine	Do	Handling of *Cyomolgus* monkeys.	*Reston ebola virus* **(REBOV) is non pathogenic to humans; & affects non-human non-human primates. Outbreaks occur several times in monkeys, but can infect humans without serious illness. Recently REBOV has been detected in pigs in Philippines.**
Bundibugyo ebola virus (BDBV)	Uganda	Do		*Bundibugyo ebolavirus* (BEBOV) causes ebola hemorrahagic fever (EHF). Outbreaks occurred in 2007 with fatality rate of 34%.
G2: *Marburgvirus*				
TS: *Lake Victoria marburgvirus*	Africa	Egyptian fruit bat	Via body fluids, blood, excreta, saliva, sperm, & vomition.	Marburg hemorrhagic fever (MHV) occurs in humans & non-human primates. The symptoms include fever, headache, myalgia, jaun-dice, pancreatitis, delirium, rash, haemor-rhages, & hypovolemic shock, Recom-binant VSV with GP protein vaccine is under trial. Diagnosis is by ELIZA & PCR.

Genus: *Ebolavirus*

FilovirusI Clinical Manifestations in Humans & Animals

Genus: Ebolavius

Ebolavirus Infection

Zaire ebolavirus (ZEBOV), named after the **Ebola River in Zaire that causes ebola hemorrahagic fever (EHF) in humans.** The symptoms are fever, headache, myalgia, jaundice, pancreatitis, pharyngitis, delirium, rash, haemorrhages & hypovolemic shock. The virus replicates in macrophages, DC, hepatocytes, & spread to all vital organs, & interstitial endothelial cells. Blood vessel walls are destroyed, the platelets are unable to coagulate, and patients succumb to hypovolemic shock. There is massive lymphocyte apoptosis, multi-organ dysfunction-liver, septic-like syndrome, clotting abnormality, aberrant immunity, many proinflammatory cytokines, & loss of CD4 & CD8 cells. The highest fatality rate is up to 90%. Ebola is transmitted through bodily fluids, conjunctival exposure & use of unsterilized needles. Recombinant VSV with GP protein vaccine is under trial. Diagnosis is by ELIZA & PCR.

Sudan ebolavirus (SEBOV) causes fatality rates from 54% in 1976, 68% in 1979, and 53% in 2000 and 2001. The disease transmission occurs by direct contact with the blood, secretions, organs or other body fluids of infected persons, contact with deceased person, handling of infected chimpanzees, gorillas, and forest antelopes & via contact with sick persons by health care workers.

Reston ebolavirus (REBOV) **causes simian hemorrhagic fever (SHFV)**, which is a highly pathogenic virus in monkeys. EBOV was discovered in 1989 in Reston, Virginia, is non-pathogenic to humans, yet it has been found to affect primates such as monkeys. Subsequently *Ebola Reston virus* outbreaks have occurred in Texas and Italy. **REBOV infection in pigs has been detected very recently with its outbreak in Philippines. Patas are believed to be the natural hosts** as 50% of wild patas monkeys have antibodies for the virus. On July 8, 2009, EBOV was reported in the Philippines, where it infected swine causing concern that infection of swine could both infect the food supply and potentially lead to the emergence of a REBOV variant that affects humans.

Côte d'Ivoire ebolavirus (CIEBOV) or tai ebolavirus, also referred to as *Tai ebolavirus* and, "Ivory Coast", as it was first discovered among chimpanzee from the Tai Forest in Cote d Ivory, Africa, in 1994, where the outbreak of this virus took place for the first time in 1994. The initial outbreak was among the wild African chimpanzees from which it is believed to have got transmitted to humans during necropsy on the dead body of the infected chimpanzees that had contracted the same.

Bundibugyo ebolavirus was identified on November 24, 2007 in Uganda in the Bundibugyo District; National Reference Laboratories and the CDC, the WHO confirmed the presence of the new species. The outbreak had a mortality rate of 34% (39 deaths).

Genus 2: *Marburgvirus*

Lake Victoria marburgvirus (LVMV), the only species in the genus causes the disease **Marburg hemorrhagic fever(MHF)**, also referred to as **Marburg**

virus disease, and previously also known as **green monkey disease** due to its primate origin. Marburg originated in Central and East Africa, and **infects both humans and non-human primates**. The natural reservoir is believed to be the **Egyptian fruit bat which is located in Africa.** The disease is spread through body fluid, blood, excreta, saliva, sperm & vomit. **Incubatin period is 3-9 days**. Early symptoms are non-specific, and include fever, headache and myalgia & after five days, a maculopapular rash appears on the torso. Later-stage Marburg infection is acute and include jaundice, pancreatitis, weight loss, delirium and neuropsychiatric symptoms, hemorrhage, hypovolemic shock, multi-organ dysfunction, with liver failure being the most common. The fatality rate is from 23% to about 50%.

Pathogenesis

Endothelial cells, mononuclear phagocytes, and hepatocytes are the main targets of virus infection. **Ebola replication** overwhelms protein synthesis of infected cells and host immune defenses. **The** blood vessel walls become damaged and destroyed, **the** platelets are unable to coagulate, **and patients succumb to hypovolemic shock. The** incubation period **is generally** 5 to 18 days, mean 2 to 21 days. **Disease is characterized by the rapid onset of fever, malaise, muscle pain, headache, and the inflammation of the pharynx & 6 days following vomiting and bloody diarrhea, individuals may develop** maculopapular rash **with bleeding at needle sites and bodily orifices. In 2005 a vaccine based on attenuated recombinant VSV vector carrying either the Ebola glycoprotein or Marburg glycoprotein successfully protected non-human primates leading to clinical trials in humans. By October the study completed the first human trial giving** three vaccinations over three months showing capability of safely inducing an immune response. **Individuals were followed for a year, and in 2006 a study testing a faster-acting, single shot vaccine began. This study was completed in 2008. In May 2010, a group of scientists from Boston University announced they had developed a drug containing small interfering RNAs packaged into Stable nucleic acid lipid particles (SNALPs) that prevented reproduction of the virus in monkeys.**

❑❑❑

Chapter 30

Characteristics and Diseases Caused by Group V Single-Stranded (-) RNA Arenaviruses (Family *Arenaviridae)*

Contents

Characteristics of Arenaviruses

Arenaviruses (L. arena= sand) are enveloped, pleomorphic, spherical structures with a diameter of 120 nm having **club-shaped surface projections**. Ribosomes are acquired from host cells within the viral envelope giving the virus its characteristic **sandy appearance**. Nucleocapsid structure is helical. Arenaviruses have single stranded, negative sense RNA viruses containing **two RNA segments, one segment is large, L & the second one is short, S**. L segment is about 7,5 kb and S segment 3,5 kb. S segment is more abundant & encodes the nucleoprotein, NP & two glycoproteins GP1 & GP 2. The L segment encodes the viral RNA –dependent RNA polymerase, L at 3′ end & a Zinc binding protein, Z at the 5′ end.

Each arenavirus is associated with a particular rodent host species in which it is maintained. Most arenaviruses cause in rodents, subclinical, **life-long persistent infections with continuous excretion of virus in saliva, urine and feces, which are a source of infection to humans**. Some arenaviruses are **zoonotic viruses** and are transmitted to humans through rodents through mucosal exposure to aerosols, or by direct contact of abraded skin with the infectious materials derived from infected rodents & aersols of rodent dried excreta, especially urine that is dropped in the environment. **None of these viruses is pathogenic for domestic animals.**

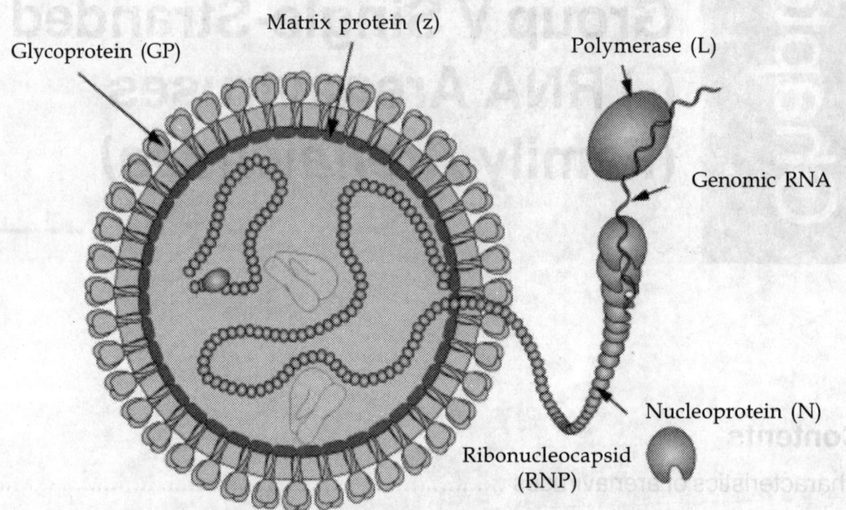

Figure 30.1 : Morphology of an Arenavirus

The prototype of this family is the *Lymphocytic choriomeningitis virus* **(LCMV)**, a virus found to infect wild rodents, mice and occasionally humans. Immunological studies employing LCMV have contributed significantly to our knowledge of tolerance, virus-induced immunopathology, and viral antigen recognition by T lymphocytes, natural killer activation and function. ***Lymphocytic choriomeningitis virus* is a rare cause of aseptic meningitis in humans**. Arenaviruses causing human disease is handled in laboratories under strict containment conditions (Biosafety level 4) to prevent human exposure.

Arenaviruses can be divided into two serogroups, which differ genetically and by geographical distribution.

1. **LCMV-Lassa virus (Old World) complex contains:**

   Ippy virus; Lassa virus; Lujo virus; lymphocytic choriomeningitis virus; Mobala virus & Mopeia virus.

2. **Tacaribe virus (New World) complex the New World viruses have been grouped even more specifically into three lineages based on antigenic data: two groups are pathogenic in humans called A and B, and the third group C is not pathogenic.**

Amapari virus; Chapare virus; Flexal virus; Guanarito virus; Junin virus; Latino virus; Machupo virus chupo virus; Oliveros virus; Paraná virus; Pichinde virus; Pirital virus; Sabia virus; Tacaribe virus; Tamiami virus; Whitewater Arroyo virus.

The viral genome

The virus genome consists of **RNA is in two segments**, called large, **L** and small, **S**; both are circular but the **L strand is negative sense and the S strand is ambisense**. The L strand is 7.2 kb and the S is 3.5 kb. The S strand codes for the **nucleoprotein, NP directly from the ambisense S strand**, and **glycoproteins, GP** are transcribed from a full length template of the genome. The L strand encodes the viral RNA-dependent RNA polymerase & a small RING finger protein, Z, the matrix protein. Both segments are ambisens. The viral RNA dependent RNA polymerase (L) binds to a promoter on each encapsidated segment, and transcribes mRNAs, & is terminated by a strong hairpin sequence at the end of each gene. mRNAs are capped, probably by L protein during synthesis.

Virus replication

The virus replication occurs in the cell cytoplasm & is complex. Virus via GP glycoproteins attaches to host receptors is endocytosed into vesicles in the host cell & the virus membrane & the vesicle membrane fuse releasing ribonucleocapsid in the cytoplasm.

Each of S & L segments uses an ambisense or part positive and part negative nucleotide sequence coding strategy to direct the fusion of two polypeptides in opposite orientation. The S RNA strand codes for the viral glycoprotein (G) and nucleoprotein (NP), the L RNA strand encodes the viral RNA dependent RNA polymerase as well as small RING finger protein Z.

There is sequential transcription of mRNAs, & viral mRNAs are capped in the cytoplasm. Replication presumably starts when enough nucleoprotein is present to encapsidate neo-synthesized antigenomes and genomes. The ribonucleocapsid interacts with the Z protein beneath the plasma membrane and buds, releasing the virion.

Table 30.1: Classification of *Arenaviridae* & diseases caused by the member viruses in humans & animals

Species	Subtypes	Vectors	Geographical distribution	Disease in humans
F. *Arenaviridae* G.. *Arenavirus*				
Lymphocytic choriomeningitis virus	LCMV-4 subtypes	House mouse (*Mus musculus*)	Worldwide	*Lymphocytic choriomeningitis virus* (**LCMV**) **causes Lymphocytic choriomeningitis that infects wild rodents, mice and occasionally humans. There are usually** *influenza -like febrile illness* **and ocassionally cause** *meningitis* **in humans with large numbers of lymphocytes in the CSF. The disease is transmitted by the vector house mouse (***Mus musculus***).**
Lassa virus	LASV-4 subtypes	Natal multi-mammate mouse (*Mastomys natalensis*).	West Africa	*Lassa virus* **(LASV) causes Lassa fever with high fever, severe myalgia, coagulopathy, hemorrhagic skin rash, and occasional visceral hemorrhage as well as necrosis of liver and spleen. The virus can be transmitted person-to -person. LASV also causes inapparent infections particularly among members of hunting tribes. The disease is transmitted by the vector Natal multimammate mouse (***Mastomys natalensis***).**
Junin virus	JUNV-3 subtypes	Drylands Vesper Mouse (*Calomys musculinus*)	Argentina	*Junin virus* **(JUNV) causes Argentine hemorrhagic fever. Most JUNV infections (80%) result in clinical disease of which 3 phases are recognized in Argentine hemorrhagic fever (AHF): prodromal, neurological-**

				hemorrhagic, and convalescence. The disease is transmitted by the vector Drylands Vesper Mouse (*Calomys musculinus*).
Machupo virus	MACV-1 subtype	Large Vesper Mouse (*Calomys callosus*)	Bolivia	*Machupo virus* **(MACV)** causes **Bolivian hemorrhagic fever.** There are fever, malaise, headache and muscular pain. Petechiae on the upper body and bleeding from the nose and gums are seen when the disease progresses to the hemorrhagic phase in 7 days of onset. The disease is transmitted by the vector large Vesper mouse (*Calomys callosus*).
Guanarito virus	GTOV-1 subtype	Short-tailed Cane Mouse (*Zygodontomys brevicauda*)	Venezuela	*Guanarito virus* **(GTOV)** causes **hemorrhagic fever in Venezuelans**. Symptoms include at early stage vomiting, diarrhea and sore throat & then fever, headache, body and muscle aches and abdominal pain. The transmission is by the vector Short-tailed Cane Mouse (*Zygodontomys brevicauda*).
Sabia virus	SABV-1 subtype	Unknown	Brazil	*Sabia virus* **(SABV)** causes **Bolivian hemorrhagic fever.** Symptoms are fever, headache, myalgia, nausea, vomiting, weakness, and pronounced sore throat & conjunctivitis, diarrhea, epigastric pain, and bleeding gums. Leucopenia, thrombocytopenia, and proteinuria are all present in each case. Gastro-intestinal hemorrhage was marked in the index case, though

				generalized hemorrhagic fever has been exhibited in all documented cases. The disease is transmitted by the vector is unknown.
Tacaribe virus	TCRV-4 subtypes	Bat (*Artibeus*)	Trinidad	
Flexal virus	FLEV-1 subtype	Rice rat (*Oryzomys*)	Brazil	*Flexal virus* **(FLEV)** causes **influenza-like illness in humans;** reservoir is Rice rat.
Whitewater Arroyo virus	WHIV-1 subtypes	Woodrat (*Neotoma*)	South western USA	*Whitewater Arroyo virus* **(WHIV)** causes **hemorrhagic fever in humans,** reservoir is woodrat.

Virus classification

Group: Group V (-) ssRNA

Family: *Arenaviridae*

Genus: *Arenavirus*

Group1: **LCMV-Lassa virus (Old World) complex:**

Ippy virus, Lassa virus, Lujo virus, TS: *Lymphocytic choriomeningitis virus, Mobala virus* & *Mopeia virus.*

Group 2: **Tacaribe virus (New World) complex:**

Amapari virus, Chapare virus, Flexal virus, Guanarito virus, Junin virus, Latino virus, Machupo virus, Oliveros virus, Paraná virus, Pichinde virus, Pirital virus, Sabia virus, Tacaribe virus, Tamiami virus & *Whitewater Arroyo virus.*

Arenavirus Clinical Manifestations in Humans and Animals

Clinical Infections in Humans

Lymphocytic choriomeningitis virus **(LCMV)** causes **Lymphocytic choriomeningitis,** with usually influenza -like febrile illness, & *occasionally* cause meningitis in humans with large numbers of lymphocytes in the CSF. House mouse is the vector.

Lassa virus **(LASV)** causes **Lassa fever** with high fever, severe myalgia, coagulopathy, hemorrhagic skin rash, and occasional visceral haemorrhage as well as necrosis of liver and spleen. The virus can be transmitted person-to -person. LASV also causes inapparent infections particularly among members of hunting tribes. The disease is transmitted by the vector Natal multimammate mouse(*Mastomys natalensis*).

Junin virus **(JUNV)** causes **Argentine hemorrhagic fever**. Most JUNV infections (80%) result in clinical disease of which 3 phases are recognized: prodromal, neurological-haemorrhagic, and convalescence. The disease is transmitted by the vector Drylands Vesper Mouse (*Calomys musculinus*).

Machupo virus **(MACV)** causes **Bolivian hemorrhagic fever**. There are fever, malaise, headache and muscular pains. Petechiae on the upper body and bleeding from the nose and gums are seen when the disease progresses to the hemorrhagic phase in 7 days of disease onset. The disease is transmitted by the vector large Vesper mouse (*Calomys callosus*).

Guanarito virus **(GTOV)** causes **hemorrhagic fever in Venezuelan**. Symptoms include at early stage vomiting, diarrhea and sore throat & then fever, headache, body and muscle aches and abdominal pain. The disease transmission by the vector is unknown.

Sabia virus **(SABV)** causes **Bolivian hemorrhagic fever**. Symptoms are fever, headache, myalgia, nausea, vomiting, weakness, and pronounced sore throat & conjunctivitis, diarrhea, epigastric pain, and bleeding gums. Leucopenia, thrombocytopenia, and proteinuria are all present in each case. Gastro-intestinal hemorrhage was marked in the index case, though generalized hemorrhagic fever appears to have been exhibited in all documented cases. The disease is transmitted by the vector large Vesper mouse (*Calomys callosus*).

Flexal virus **(FLEV)** causes influenza-like illness in humans; reservoir is Rice rat.

Whitewater Arroyo virus **(WHIV)** causes hemorrhagic fever in humans; reservoir is woodrat.

□□□

Junin virus (JUNV) causes Argentine hemorrhagic fever. Most JUNV infections (80%) result in clinical disease of which 3 phases are recognized: prodromal, neurological-haemorrhagic, and convalescence. The disease is transmitted by the vector Drylands Vesper Mouse (*Calomys musculinus*).

Machupo virus (MACV) causes Bolivian hemorrhagic fever. There are fever, malaise, headache and muscular pains. Petechiae on the upper body and bleeding from the nose and gums are seen when the disease progresses to the hemorrhagic phase in 7 days of disease onset. The disease is transmitted by the vector large Vesper mouse (*Calomys callosus*).

Guanarito virus (GTOV) causes hemorrhagic fever in Venezuelan. Symptoms include at early stage vomiting, diarrhea and sore throat & then fever, headache, body and muscle aches and abdominal pain. The disease transmission by the vector is unknown.

Sabia virus (SABV) causes Bolivian hemorrhagic fever. Symptoms are fever, headache, myalgia, nausea, vomiting, weakness, and pronounced sore throat & conjunctivitis, diarrhea, epigastric pain, and bleeding gums. Leucopenia, thrombocytopenia, and proteinuria are all present in each case. Gastro-intestinal hemorrhage was marked in the index case, though generalized hemorrhagic fever appears to have been exhibited in all documented cases. The disease is transmitted by the vector large Vesper mouse (*Calomys callosus*).

Flexal virus (FLEV) causes influenza-like illness in humans; reservoir is Rice rat.

Whitewater Arroyo virus (WHIV) causes hemorrhagic fever in humans; reservoir is woodrat.

Chapter 31

Characteristics and Diseases Caused by Group V Single-Stranded (-) RNA Bunyaviruses (Family *Bunyaviridae*)

Contents

Characteristics of Bunyaviruses

Bunyaviruses (Bunyamwera, a place in Uganda where the typee species *Bynyamwera virus* was first isolaed) belong to the **largest family of vertebrate viruses**, are enveloped, the virions are **80-120 nm** in diameter, are covered by surface projections 5-10 nm long spikes which evenly coat the surface & their nucleocapsids are elongated with helical symmetry. The Bunyaviruses genome consists of **three segments of linear negative-sense RNA,** called **Large, L, Medium, M, & Small, S.,** or ambisense, depending on the genus. The L segment is 6300-12000 ntd long and encodes the viral RNA polymerase. The M segment is 3500-6000 ntd and encodes two glycoproteins as a single gene product that is usually co-translationally cleaved. The S segment is 1000-2200 ntd long and encodes the coat protein.

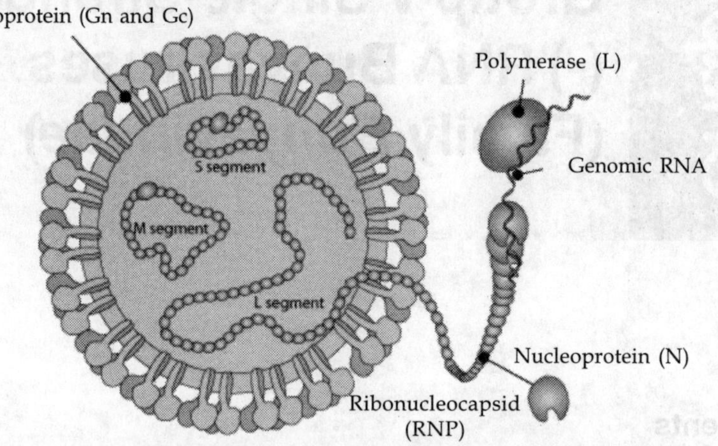

Figure 31.1 : MorpholoGy of a Bunyavirus

The complete genome is 10500-22700 ntd long. Bunyaviruses is the largest family of vertebrate viruses mostly **transmitted by biting arthropods like mosquitoes, tick, or sandfly and with the exception of** Hantaan virus, which are transmitted through contact with deer mice feces. Human infections with certain *Bunyaviridae,* such as Crimean-Congo hemorrhagic fever are associated with high levels of morbidity and mortality; these viruses are handled with a Biosafety level 4 in the laboratory. Akabane disease, Cache valley, Rift valley fever, and Nairobi sheep disease are limited to veterinary importance. Some also cause severe fever with thrombocytopenia. **Tospoviruses infect plants** & are transmitted to plants by minute insects called thrips; the *Tomato spotted wilt virus* causes significant crop losses worldwide.

The virus genome

Bunyaviridae have linear, RNA genome containing **3 segments**, a large, L segment is between 6.8 and 12 kb, medium, M segment is between 3.2 and 4.9 kb, and small, S segment is between 1 and 3 kb & **encodes for four to six proteins.** The terminal sequences of each segment are base-paired due to which, the **RNAs form non-covalently closed circles**. The nucleotide sequences at the 3'-terminus and the 5'-terminus are complimentary, forming panhandle structures. The 5'-terminus is not capped. These RNA segments are single-stranded, and exist in a helical form within the virion. Besides, they exhibit a pseudo-circular structure due to each segment's complementary ends. **The L segment encodes the RNA dependent RNA-polymerase, known as the nucleocapsid-associated L protein** that interacts with the three S, M, and L nucleocapsids. L is necessary for viral RNA replication and mRNA synthesis. **The M segment encodes the viral glycoproteins, Gn & Gc** which project from the viral surface and aid the virus in attaching to and entering the host cell. **The S segment encodes the nucleoprotein protein (N)**. The **L and M segment are negative sense, but the S segment is ambisence** for the genera of *Phlebovirus* and *Tospovirus*. Ambisense means that some of the genes on the RNA strand are negative sense and others are positive sense. The **S segment codes for the viral nucleoprotein (N) in the negative sense and a non-structural (NSs) protein in ambisense**. Total genome size ranges from 10.5 to 22.7 kbp.

Virus replication

The bunyaviruses replicate in the cell cytoplasm, virion attaches to the surface of a host cell through the G1/G2 glycoproteins and is endocytosed. The viral RNA dependent RNA polymerase (L) binds to a promoter on each encapsidated segment, and transcribes a mRNA which is terminated by a strong hairpin sequence at the end of each gene. mRNAs are capped by L protein during synthesis. *Phlebovirus* and *Tospovirus* have ambisens segment (s). The virus membrane fuses with the vesicle membrane through acidification of the endosome and the nucleocapsids are released into the cytoplasm. The RNA-dependent RNA polymerase known as the nucleocapsid-associated L protein interacts with the three S, M, and L nucleocapsids carrying primary transcription and translation. A switch from translation to replication occurs, and full-length cRNA templates are produced, from which full-length genomes are produced and encapsidated. Virions are assembled and bud in the Golgi & are transported to the cell surface in vesicles and are released from the cell.

Virus classification

Group: Group V (-) ss RNA

Family: *Bunyaviridae*

The family *Bunyaviridae* contains 6 genera:

1. Genus *Hantavirus;* type species: *Hantaan virus:* Diseases Hantan virus pulmonary syndrome, Korean hemorrhagic fever
2. Genus *Nairovirus;* type species: *Dugbe virus*
3. Genus *Orthobunyavirus;* type species: *Bunyamwera virus*
4. Genus *Phlebovirus;* type species: *Rift valley fever virus*

5. Genus *Tospovirus*; type species: **Tomato spotted wilt virus- plant virus**
6. Genus *Tenuivirus(unclassified)* plant viruses

Table 31.1 : Geographic distribution, vectors and hosts of *Bunyaviridae* of animal importance and related human diseases.

Species	Serotypes	Geographical distribution	Vectors	Hosts	Animal diseases	Human diseases
G 1. *Phlebovirus*						
Rift Valley fever virus	RVFV-5 subtypes	Africa	Mosquitoes	ruminants, sheep, cattle & goats	Abortion, new-born mortality & hepatitis	Hemorrhagic fever
Sandfly Naples virus Sandfly Sicilian virus Toscona virus	SFNV SFSV TOSV	South Europe north Africa, Balkans, east mediterrar-eans, Iraq, Iran, Pakistan, Afganistan & India	Phleboto-mines *P. papatami*	Humans		Fever, fatigue, abdominal distress, muscle & Joint aches & tachycardia.
Punta toro virus	PTV	Rural Panama	Phleboto-mines	Infction of weaning mice & animals	Animal infection occurs	Fatal hepatic disease like RVFV.
G 2; Nairovirus						
Dugbe virus Nairobi sheep disease virus	NSDV	East Africa, India, Sri Lanka	Ticks	Sheep & goats	Haemorr-hagic gastro enteritis in sheep & goats.	None
Crimean Congo hemorrhagic fever virus	CCHFV-2 types	Africa, Middle East, Asia, southern Europe	Ticks	Ruminants, birds, rodents, hares	None	Hemorrhagic fever
G 3: Ortho*bunyavirus*						
Akabane virus Tinaroo virus	AKAV TINV	Australia, Taipah, Japan, China, Korea, Middle East, Kenya	Mosquitoes, Culicoid flies	Livestock	Congenital malforma-tion arthro-gryposis & hydranencephaly	None
Bunyamwera virus Cache valley virus	CVV	North America	Mosquitoes	Sheep	Teratogenic effect, & congenital malformation	Not documented

California encephalitis virus La Crosse Virus, Snowshoe hare virus Tahyba virus	LACV SSHV TAHV	North America	Mosquitoes	Rodents	Congenital malformation in sheep experimentally	Fever, lethargy, nausea, vomition, abdominal pain, & encephalitis
California encephalitis virus San Angelo virus	SAV	North America	Mosquitoes	Unknown	Congenital malformation in sheep experimentally	Not documented
Main Drain virus	MDV	North America	Mosquitoes	Equine, rodents	Encephalomyelitis, congenital malformation in sheep experimentally	Not documented
Oropouche fever virus	OROV	Central & south America, Amazon region, Caribbeans, Panama	Mosquitoes, biting midges- *C. paraensis*	Sloth, *Callithrix* spp		Next to dengue, dengu-like fever, chills, headache, muscle & joint pain, vomiting or meningitis
Sathuperi virus Douglas virus	DOUV	Old world	Culicoid flies	Animals	Teratogenic effect	None
Shamonda virus Peatom virus	PEAV	Old world				
Aino virus *Shuni* virus	AINOV, SHUNV	Africa	mosquitoes	Animals, humans	Infection in animals	Infection in humans
G 4. *Hantavirus*						
Sin Nombre virus *Bayou virus* *Black creek canal virus* *Newyork virus*	SNV BAYV BCCV NYV	USA	Deer mouse *Peromyscus leucopus* *Oryzomys palustris,* *Sigomdon hispidus,* *Peromyscus leucopus,* *Perompcus maniculatus*	Humans		Hantaan virus Cardiopulmonary syndrome- HCPS, lungs fill up with bloody fluid. Blood pressure drops, some develop serious kidney disease, death

					in 5 days as a result of heart and lung failure.
Puumala virus *Dobrava-Belgrade virus* *Seol virus*	PUUV DOBV SEOV	Scandinavians, Finland, north Europe, Russia, China	Bank vole *Myodes glyreorus* *Brown Norway rat*	Humans	Inhalation of infected dust causes hemorrhagic fever with renal syndrome-HFRS or Nephropathi epidemica.

Bunyavirus Clinical Manifestations in Humans and Animals

Clinical Infections in Humans

Genus : *Phlebovirus*

Rift Valley fever (RVFV) in humans causes several **different disease syndromes.** There is either no symptom or a mild illness associated with fever and liver abnormalities. But, in some cases the illness can progress to **hemorrhagic fever**, which can lead to shock or hemorrhage, encephalitis, or ocular disease. Infected persons show fever, generalized weakness, back pain, dizziness, and extreme weight loss at the onset of the illness & recover within two days to one week of illness with about 1% mortality. Humans contract RVF through bites from the infected mosquitoes and other biting insects, or if exposed to the blood, body fluids, or tissues of infected animals, during slaughter or through veterinary and obstetric procedures or through aerosol in the laboratory environment.

Sandfly Naples virus (SFNV) is a viral infection in humans, & symptoms include headache, fever, conjunctival infection or red eyes, tiredness, nausea and pain in the limbs, back and eyes. The symptoms are self-limiting and can last up to one week. But in some cases recovery may be preceded by **prolonged depression in a small percentage of cases.** SVFV occurs in South Europe, North Africa, Balkans, East Mediterranean, Iraq, Iran, Pakistan, Afghanistan & India. The disease is transmitted by Phlebotomines *P. papatami.*

Punta toro virus* **(PTV) occurs in humans causing fatal hepatic disease like RFFV & has been reported from rural Panama. PTV vectors are infected phlebotomines & hosts are weaning mice & rodents.

Genus : *Nairovirus*

Crimean-Congo hemorrhagic fevervirus (CCHFV) causes severe disease in humans with a fatality rate as high as 30%. CCHFV is endemic in the Balkan

Peninsula, Albania, Kosovo, & Bulgaria & is endemic in Russia and in parts of Asia and Africa. The virus is transmitted to humans by the bite of **ixodid ticks** (*Hyalomma* genus) or by contact with blood or tissues from infected persons or infected livestock. Risk for spread of the virus from person to person is high, which occasionally results in nosocomial outbreaks. After an **incubation period of 3 to 7 days,** the patients develop sudden onset of fever, chills, myalgia, and headache, which rapidly progress to severe illness; a hemorrhagic state follows with bleeding from the mucous membranes and petechiae, associated with thrombocytopenia and leucopenia.

Genus: *Orthobunyavirus*

California encephalitis virus/ La Crosse virus/ Snowshoe hare virus/ Tahyba virus (CEV) occurs in humans after being transmtted by mosquitoes & has been reported from N. America. After an **incubation period of 3-7 days**, a prodromal phase of 1-4 days precedes before encephalitis & includes any or all of the following symptoms: fever, chills, nausea, vomiting, headache or abdominal pain. The **encephalitis symptoms** include fever, somnolence, obtundation, seizures in 50% of children, periodic lateralizing epileptiform discharges (PLEDS) in the temporal lobe, 20% of children develop focal neurologic signs, and 10% of patients develop coma. The total duration of illness lasts 10-14 days. Epilepsy develops in 20% of patients, especially those who had seizures during the acute illness. In adults, infection is asymptomatic or causes a benign febrile illness or aseptic meningitis. Other signs include fever, lethargy, focal neurologic findings, incoordination, focal motor abnormalities & paralysis.

Oropouche fever virus (OROV) occurs in Central & South America, Amazon region, Caribbeans & Panama, & is being transmitted by the bite of infected mosquitoes & biting midges- *C. paraensis* to humans. OROV is next to dengue, there is dengu-like fever, chills, headache, muscle & joint pain, vomiting, or meningitis.

Genus : *Hantavirus*

Sin Nombre virus (SNV) causes **Hantavirus pulmonary syndrome (HPS),** a rare but deadly viral infection being spread by mice and rats. They shed the virus in their urine, droppings and saliva. Tiny droplets with the virus can enter the air. People can get the disease if they breathe infected air or come into contact with rodents or their urine or droppings. Early symptoms of HPS include fatigue, fever, muscle aches, especially in the thighs, hips and back, headaches, chills, dizziness & nausea, vomiting, diarrhea or abdominal pain. Later symptoms include coughing and shortness of breath.

Puumala virus/ Dobrava-Belgrade virus/ Seol virus (PUNV)infection to humans is transmitted by Bank vole *Myodes glyreorus,* Brown Norway rat. Humans get infection after inhalation of the infected dust causing **hemorrhagic fever with renal syndrome-HFRS** or **Nephropathi epidemica**. PUNV infection has been reported from Scandinavians, Finland, north Europe, Russia & China.

Bunyavirus Clinical Infections in Animals

Genus: *Phlebovirus:*

Rift Valley Fever

Rift Valley fever **(RVFV)** is an acute, fever-causing viral disease that affects domestic animals such as cattle, buffaloes, sheep, goats, and camels, and humans. The RVF is **characterized by abortions in sheep, cattle and goats, high mortality in lambs and kids and generalized disease in man.** RVF is most commonly associated with **mosquito-borne** epidemics during heavy rainfall & occurs in Africa.

Occurrence

RVF was originally reported from Kenya in 1950, then from eastern and southern Africa, in sub-Saharan Africa, Madagascar, & in 2000, a RVF outbreak was reported in Saudi Arabia and subsequently Yemen. The RVF epizootic can lead to an epidemic among humans who are exposed to diseased animals. RVF-like fever has also been reported from India.

Hosts

The RVF affects cattle, buffalo, sheep, goats, and camels, and humans. Interactions between animals and humans result in transmission of the RVF virus to humans.

Transmission

An epizootic of RVF is generally observed during heavy rainfall and localized flooding. Transovarian transmission of RVFV occurs in *Aedes* mosquito. The excessive rainfall allows *Aedes* mosquitoes to hatch eggs, and the resulting mosquito's transfer the virus to the livestock on which they feed. Wild & domestic ruminants become infected, they become viremic for 5 days, and other species of mosquitoes can become infected from the animals and can spread the disease to other hosts. Virus can be transmitted by other biting insects. RVFV is present in milk, feces & aborted fetuses.

Humans contract RVF through bites from infected mosquitoes, from infected mouthparts of other biting insects, & if they are exposed to the blood, body fluids, or tissues of infected animals, direct exposure to infected animals during slaughter or through veterinary and obstetric procedures or through aerosol transmission of RVFV in the laboratory environment.

Pathogenesis

After infection with RVFV, the virus **replicates in the hepatocytes in lambs & calves**, age being the main factor in disease progression. Hepatic lesions in very young animas lead to **degeneration & necrosis of hepatocytes, & extensive necrosis throughout the liver**. Such extensive liver lesions result in **liver insuficincy & failure. Encephalomyelitis** is also seen in very young animals.

Clinical symptoms and lesions

After an **incubation period** of less than **3 days**, there is high rate of **abortion at any stage of gestation**, but some show no symptoms. Clinical symptoms in sheep & goats include **abortion rate in sheep from 40 to 100%**, ewe may also retain the placenta & endometritis may develop after aborting the fetus. Symptoms in newborn lambs & kids are most severe in young lambs under 2 weeks old with mortality up to 90% with fever (40-42°C), anorexia & weakness. **Death is due to severe liver necrosis and vascular collapse.** Clinical signs in **cattle** include anorexia, weakness, fetid diarrhea & drop in calving rate.Calves show fever (40-41°C), depression with mortality rate of 10-70% about 2-8 days after the first signs appear. **Adult cattle** show fever (40-41°C), excessive salivation, anorexia, weakness, fetid diarrhea & fall in milk yield. Abortion may reach 85% in the herd. Mortality rate is usually less than 10%.

Lesions include extensive **hepatic necrosis**, venous congestion, & **petechiae in heart, liver & lymph nodes. Microscopically, liver necrosis is focal or diffuse necrosis** usually with acidophilic inclusions.

People infected with RVFV have either no symptoms or a mild illness associated with fever and liver abnormalities, or in some patients the illness progress to hemorrhagic fever, encephalitis, or ocular disease. Patients who become ill usually experience fever, generalized weakness, back pain, dizziness, and extreme weight loss at the onset of the illness but patients recover within two days to one week after onset of illness.

Diagnosis

1. *Presumptive diagnosis:* From clinical symptoms & liver histopathological lesions in lambs which are pathognomonic.
2. *Virus isolation:* It is performed in cell culture, lab animals, & embryonated eggs.

3. *Viral antigens detection:* Antigen in serum is detected by ELISA test or by immunofluorescence test.
4. *Virus antibody detection:* Antibodies in sera are detected by ELISA in paired serum samples, & by hemagglutination inhibition test.

Treatment & prevention

Vector control & quarantine help livestock & humans from RVFV infection.

Vaccination

Vaccination is the best method of disease control. Three types of vaccines are available; **live attenuated vaccine, killed virus vaccine & attenuated vaccine**. Currently, the most commonly used vaccine is a **live-virus vaccine derived from the Smithburn strain**, which was attenuated through serial intracerebral inoculation of mice. One inoculation confers immunity for 3 years and produces protection in 6 to 7 days. The vaccine causes abortion in pregnant ewes. The vaccine also is pathogenic for humans. Immunization of ewes at **70 to 100 days of pregnancy with attenuated MP12-vaccine** induced neutralizing antibodies from 1:80 to 1:320, with no resulting fetus abnormality. Newborn lambs from the immunized ewes did not exhibit neutralizing antibodies against RVFV, and the lambs rapidly acquired neutralizing antibodies (1:80 and more) by having the colostrums of the MP-12-vaccinated ewes. In addition, two-days-old to three-months-old lambs survived the MP-12-vaccination and acquired neutralizing antibodies against RVFV. MP-12 vaccination neither induced virus shedding into milk in lactating cows nor caused abortions in cows during 3-, 5- and 8-month gestations. However, MP-12 vaccination of ewes at the 28th day of gestation induced a low level (4%) of abortion and resulted in teratogenic effects in newborn lambs (14%), which may indicate that the use of MP-12 in early pregnancy could cause some loss of lambs. To test MP-12 as a potential human vaccine, it was initially inoculated into more than 100 human volunteers; it has been shown to be safe and immunogenic when adequate dose is administered. MP-12 is currently undergoing further Phase II clinical evaluation in human. **Inactivated vaccines** also have been developed for use in both animals including pregnant and humans. The animal vaccine has been shown to be safe and effective but requires two inoculations, which has limited its utility in outbreak control. A formalin-inactivated vaccine, derived from a pantropic RVFV strain passaged in baby hamster kidney (BHK) 21 cells, was also used as an animal vaccine. The vaccination significantly reduced the abortion of ewes and mortality of newborn lambs during an outbreak and induced immunity in cattle. The human vaccine is still under investigation, although initial studies suggest that it is safe and provides good long-term immunity. **Mutagen attenuated vaccine:** It is recommended for pregnant animal, young & adult sheep & cattle. **Recombinant RVFV vaccines using vaccinia virus (VACV) as a vector** for use in livestock; the first vaccine, vCOGnGc, was attenuated by the deletion of a VACV gene encoding an IFN-γ binding protein, insertional inactivation of the thymidine kinase gene, and expression of RVFV glycoproteins, Gn and Gc. The second vaccine, vCOGnGc γ, is identical to the first and also expresses the human IFN-γ gene to enhance safety. Both vaccines are extremely safe; neither resulted in weight loss nor death in severe combined immunodeficient mice, and pock lesions were smaller in baboons compared with the controls. Furthermore, both vaccines induced protective levels of antibody titers in vaccinated mice and baboons. Mice were protected from lethal RVFV challenge. Thus, two safe and efficacious recombinant vaccines for RVF have been developed.

Genus : *Nairovirus*

Nairobi Sheep Disease

Nairobi sheep disease virus (NSDV) is a tick transmitted disease characterized by fever, **acute hemorrhagic gastroenteritis, abortion & high mortality.** NSD virus belongs to genus *Nairovirus* underfamily *Bunyaviridae*. Other antigenically related viruses are *Ganjam virus* is in Indian small ruminants, *Dugbe virus* in west Africa & *Crimean –Congo virus hemorrhagic fever virus* in human.

Occurrence

Nairobi sheep disease occurs in East & central Africa, India, Sri Lanka, & is transmitted by tick bite.

Hosts

Sheep and goats can be infected readily by NSDV, and are important as reservoir hosts. A few fatal cases of Nairobi sheep disease have been reported among duikers in zoos or in the wild. The African field rat can be infected experimentally.

Transmission

Nairobi sheep disease virus and Ganjam virus are transmitted through tick bites. *Rhipicephalus appendiculatus* in East Africa, they can transmit the virus for more than two years after they are infected. Other vectors include *R. pulchellus*, *R. simus*, and *Amblyomma variegatum*. Transovarial transmission occurs in *R. appendiculatus* as well as in *R. pulchellus* in Somalia. Transstadial transmission occurs in all host ticks. In Asia, *Haemaphysalis intermedia* is the main tick vector for *Ganjam virus*, & the virus also occurs in *H. wellingtoni* and *R. haemaphysaloides*, & in the mosquito *Culex vishnui*.

The virus is present in urine and feces, but NSDV does not seem to be contagious via contact. However, animals may be infected experimentally with large oral doses (50 cc) of blood or serum, & by injecting blood, serum or organ suspensions.

Pathogenesis

After tick bite, the NSDV replicates in the endothelium, in liver, spleen, lungs & other organs.

Clinical symptoms & lesions

The symptoms are fever, leukopenia, rapid respiration, anorexia and profound depression, followed by fetid diarrhea and a concomitant drop in body temperature. At the onset, the feces are thin followed by profuse and watery diarrhea; later, blood and mucus may appear. Straining and signs of colicky pain may be seen. The superficial prescapular and precrural lymph nodes are often palpable, and some animals have a blood-stained mucopurulent or serosanguineous nasal discharge. Conjunctivitis may also be seen.

Pregnant animals often abort. Many animals die during the early febrile stage of the disease; in some cases within 12 hours of the onset of the fever. Deaths are also seen later, from hemorrhagic diarrhea and dehydration. Goats may have less severe clinical signs than sheep.

Ganjam virus infection in Asia is reported to be similar but less severe. However, at least one outbreak with severe clinical signs has been reported and improved disease diagnosis and investigations are needed to determine whether NSDV and Ganjam virus differ in their ability to cause disease.

Diagnosis

Clinical specimens for various tests include whole blood, spleen, mesenteric lymph nodes, sera from acute cases and convalescent sera.

1. A **presumptive diagnosis** is based on the clinical signs and history of the disease.
2. **Virus isolation** is made by culturing in BHK-21-C13 cells, a baby hamster kidney cell line, & primary hamster or lamb kidney cells. The virus is most easily isolated by the intracerebral inoculation in infant mice.
3. **Detection of antibodies** is done by a significant increase in antibody levels between acute and convalescent sera using indirect fluorescent

antibody test, immunodiffusion, complement fixation, & indirect hemagglutination and ELISA.

Treatment & prevention

Disease is controlled by animal movement control, quarantine and euthanasia of infected animals. NSDV in the premises is decontaminated by hypochlorite, phenolics, 2% glutaraldehyde and other disinfectants that are effective decontaminants for the virus.

Sheep and goats can be protected from tick vectors by dipping and/or spraying with an acaricide. Nairobi sheep disease is a reportable in countries that are disease free.

Vaccination

Experimental vaccines have been developed, and may be available in some regions. These vaccines can be used to protect naive animals entering enzootic areas, or to protect animal populations when the tick vector expands its geographic range. Two types of experimental vaccines have been developed; a modified live virus vaccine attenuated in mouse brain and an inactivated oil adjuvant vaccine. A single dose of the modified live vaccine produces rapid immunity; however, revaccination is necessary to maintain full protection. Two doses of the inactivated vaccine are required to elicit good protection. Neither of these vaccines is produced commercially.

Genus : *Orthobunyavirus*

Akabane Disease

Akabane disease is a viral disease of **ruminants** characterized by **fetal damage,** inapparent infections in adults leading months later to abortions, **still-births and congenital defects in newborns, & death of most affected neonates**. Before vaccines were developed, Akabane disease caused significant economic losses in some countries between 1972 and 1975, this virus resulted in the birth of more than 42,000 abnormal calves in Japan. A few strains of Akabane virus can also cause outbreaks of **encephalomyelitis in calves and adult cattle**.

Etiology

Akabane virus belongs to the genus *Orthobunyavirus* and the Simbu serogroup of the family *Bunyaviridae*. Some closely related viruses including Tinaroo virus, Sabo virus and Yaba-7 virus are now considered to be strains or isolates of Akabane virus. Strains of Akabane virus differ in their virulence, but most isolates only affect unborn ruminants, a few variants like the Iriki strain can cause neurological disease in postnatal cattle. Distinct groups of Akabane viruses circulate in Asia, Oceania and Africa.

Occurrence

Akabane virus/Tinaroo virus **(AKAV)** has been reported from Australia, Taipei, Japan, China, Korea, Middle East, & Kenya. The disease is transmitted by **biting midges (gnats)** in the genus *Culicoides*, as well as by mosquitoes. Where Akabane virus is constantly present, animals usually become infected before their first pregnancy, and clinical signs do not occur in their offspring.

Hosts

Symptomatic infections have been seen only in **cattle, sheep and goats**. Wild ruminants can be infected with Akabane virus; congenital defects might occur in these species, but there are no reported cases. Antibodies to Akabane virus have also been found in horses, donkeys, buffalo, deer and camels. One isolate (NT-14) was reported to be widespread **among pigs in Taiwan**. Mice and hamsters can be infected experimentally.

Transmission

Akabane virus is transmitted by biting midges (gnats) in the genus *Culicoides*, & by mosquitoes. *Culicoides oxystoma* is the main vector in Japan. *Culicoides brevitarsis* in Australia, but the virus has also been found in *C. wadei*. *C. milnei* and *C. imicola* &can transmit Akabane virus in Africa. Experimentally, virus replication has been demonstrated in *C. nubeculosus* and *C. variipennis*. Akabane virus has also been found in mosquitoes including *Aedes vexans* and *Culex tritaeniorhynchus* in Japan, and *Anopheles funestus* in Africa. Outbreaks coincide with movement of vectors or after the introduction of susceptible animals to the endemic areas.

Vertical transmission of Akabane virus occurs **across the placenta to the fetus**, and the primary effect is on the offspring of infected animals. Akabane is not contagious by casual contact; horizontal transmission has only been reported via insect vectors. Ruminants do not become long-term carriers of this virus.

Clinical symptoms and lesions

Most strains of Akabane virus infect **non-pregnant animals subclinically**. A few isolates can cause encephalomyelitis in calves and adult cattle. Neurological signs include tremors, ataxia, lameness, paralysis, nystagmus, opisthotonos and hypersensitivity.

More often, Akabane disease is characterized by **asymptomatic infections in postnatal animals**, but **abortions, stillbirths, premature births and**

congenital defects in fetuses and newborns. Two syndromes can be seen in the fetus: **arthrogryposis and congenital malformations of the brain**. Some calves have only one of the two syndromes, but others may have both. Encephalitis can also be seen in fetuses infected near term. Birth complications, particularly when the fetus is malformed from arthrogryposis, may cause injuries to the dam that result in infertility or death.

Akabane virus has **different effects at each stage of gestation**, particularly evident in cattle, which have a longer gestation period than small ruminants. In cattle, **abortions, stillbirths and premature births** may be the first sign of an Akabane outbreak. Aborted fetuses can appear normal on first examination, but severe hydranencephaly may be found if the skull is opened. In some outbreaks, nonsuppurative encephalomyelitis can be seen in calves that were infected late in gestation. These calves may have a variety of neurological signs including flaccid paralysis, exaggerated movements and hyperexcitability. Many cannot stand, and those that can rise with assistance are ataxic. The next calves to be born, which were infected during an earlier stage of their gestation, usually have **arthrogryposis at birth**. One or more **joints are rigid and fixed in flexion** and the associated muscles are often atrophied. The first calves tend to have less severe defects than calves born later. Torticollis, scoliosis, kyphosis and spina bifida may also be seen occasionally.

Affected **calves** born late in the outbreak, which were affected during an early stage of gestation, have congenital lesions in the brain ranging from small cavitations to severe hydranencephaly. Although these animals can usually stand and walk, they have behavioral abnormalities. **Many are blind, depressed or dull, deaf** and unaware of their environment; they may wander aimlessly. The suckle reflex can be slow or absent. Other neurological signs may also be seen, and the gestation is often extended. A few calves may have both arthrogryposis and CNS defects. Most affected neonates die or must be euthanized soon after being born.

The range of fetal and neonatal defects seen in **sheep and goats** is similar, but there is more overlap. Arthrogryposis and CNS lesions are seen at the same time during the outbreak, and often occur in the same animals. Additional defects including pulmonary hypoplasia are seen in small ruminants.

Diagnosis

Collection of samples includes placenta and fetus.

1. **Presumptive diagnosis:** Clinical signs and gross lesions in affected fetuses give a presumptive diagnosis.

2. **The virus isolation** is made by the intracerebral inoculation of young mice and in various cell cultures.
3. **Antibody detection:** Detection of specific neutralizing antibodies in neonates and aborted calves, lambs and goats is attempted by virus neutralization, ELISA, agar gel immunodiffusion, hemagglutination inhibition and hemolysis inhibition assays.

Treatment & prevention

Vector control is useful.

Vaccination

Vaccination is used to control the disease. **A killed vaccine is used in Japan & Australia.** Nisseiken Co Ltd prepares **live Akabane vaccine** using strain TS-C2 without adjuvant in Japan which is effective. Nisseiken also prepares a **killed Akabane combined vaccine** (Akabane, Chuzan Disease, Aino Virus) using strains OBE-1 (A) K-47 (CD) JaNAr28 (AV) with Aluminum chloride in Japan. Akabane disease is controlled by moving susceptible animals into endemic regions after immunity develops. Changing herd management to avoid infections during the most susceptible period of pregnancy may be helpful.

Cache Valley Virus Infection

Cache Valley virus (CVV), a mosquito-borne virus infection **producing teratogenic effect & congenital malformation in sheep** is widespread in North America, where it circulates between mosquitoes and mammals. It also caused a few cases of human disease, a fatal case of acute encephalitis in the southeastern United States. Cache Valley virus is a potential cause of the birth of abnormal lambs, and that the most dramatic effects of the virus lead to birth defects in lambs, mostly affecting the brain and central nervous system. The virus also affects the skeletal tissue and muscles.Many sheep flock owners in **South Dakota, USA in 2011 reported** an unusual number of lambs born with skeletal and other developmental deformities. Sheep-flock owners have also reported a higher incidence of open ewes and lower lambing rate this winter; lower ewe reproductive efficiency. CVV also can contribute to reduced ewe reproductive efficiency. Most lambs born with these severe defects are stillborn, yet CVV also can cause the birth of lambs that act abnormal. The lambs can be drowsy, weak, or unsteady and typically all lambs within a set of twins or triplets are affected.

□□□

Chapter 32

Charactristics and Diseases Caused by Group VI RNA (+) Retroviruses (Family *Retroviridae*-RT)

Contents

Characteristics of Retroviruses

Retroviridae (L. retro = reverse) has been coined because the viruses contain reverse transcriptase that transcribes DNA from viral RNA template i.e.*Retroviridae* use a DNA intermediate to replicate. Retroviruses are enveloped carrying glycoprotein peplomers, & measure 80-100 nm in diameter. These viruses contain **3 layers**: (a) inner **nucleoprotein** containing ++ viral RNA, reverse transcriptase, protease, integrase with helical nucleocapsid, (b) **icosahedral capsid**, (c) **envelope** carrying glycoprotein peplomers. The surface projections are small or distinctive glycoprotein spikes that cover the surface evenly, are densely dispersed and 8 nm long. *Retroviridae* is a large and diverse family that is defined by common structure, composition, and replicative properties. Retroviruses have a unique mechanism, which upon entering the cell, the ss RNA and reverse transcriptase are released from the virion envelope, reverse transcriptase with the help of host cell RNA polymerase II converts ssRNA to ds DNA, which is incorporated into the host's genome as a **provirus.** Provirus depends on the host-cell machinery for the expression of the viral DNA.

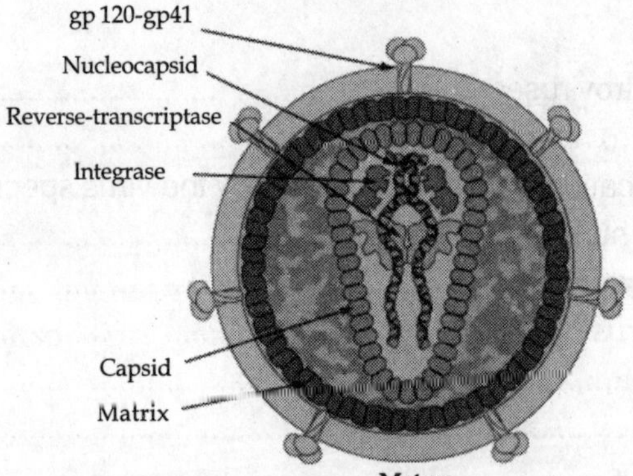

Figure 32.1 : Morphology of Retrovirus

This viral DNA is then transcribed to produce mRNA that is processed and then translated into a long polyprotein, which is cleaved by the protease to yield the individual proteins that make up the virion. The full-length mRNA have two functions – they encode for the gag and pol gene products and they are packaged into the virion particles as the progeny genomic RNA. Retroviruses were discovered in 1908 by Vilhelm Ellermann and Oluf Bang, in the 1960s and 1970s, study focused on the viral replication cycle and pathogenic effects at the cellular level. But current study of retroviruses focuses on the diverse pathogenic effects of these viruses at the cellular and molecular levels, retroviruses are modified for gene therapy, and continue to be used in the majority of gene therapy clinical trials, & lastly scientist believe in RNA theory of evolution.

Retroviruses cause several clinical infections in humans like HTLV-I, HTLV-II, HIV-1 and HIV-2; & several important animal diseases namely, Avian leucosis, Avian sarcoma, Avian myeloblastosis, Rous sarcoma; Mouse mammary tumor, Ovine pulmonary adenocarcinoma, Enzootic nasal tumor virus, Feline leukemia, Feline sarcoma, Avian reticuloendotheliosis, Bovine leukemia, Maedi/Visna Caprine arthritis encephalitis, Equine infectious anemia, Feline immunodeficiency, Bovine immunodeficiency, Human immunodeficiency 1 and 2 & Simian immunodeficiency.

The retroviruses are sensitive to lipid solvents, detergents, heat, but are relatively resistant to ultraviolet light damage.

Virus genome

Viral genome consists of ss (++) RNA duplex, 2 linear RNAs arranged as inverted dimer, each 7-11kb in size with 5′end cap & 3′end poly. **Retroviral genome possesses 5 unusual properties**: 1. ss + RNA is diploid, 2. Viral RNA does not serve as mRNA, 3. RNA is associated with specific tRNA to stimulate replication, 4. It is the only RNA to be synthesized by host cell mRNA processing unit, 5. It is the only virus to encode reverse transcriptase (RT). Retroviruses have the following 4 classes of genes:

1. Retroviral common major genes (*gag*, pro, *pol* & *env* genes) that encode structural proteins.
2. Genes that encode regulatory proteins & control virus expression (*tat, rev & nef* genes).
3. Genes that encode virion maturation (*vif & vru*).
4. Genes that encode transcriptional activator proteins (*vpr*).

Retrovirus genomes contain **three ORFs** that encode for proteins found in the mature virus:

*The *gag* (group-specific antigen) gene encodes internal virion proteins that form the **matrix, the capsid and the nucleoprotein structures.**

* The *pro gene-pro* domain encodes the virion **protease.**

*The *pol* (polymerase) gene encodes precursor polyprotein that is cleaved into **nonstructural proteins essential for virus multiplication**. These proteins include p64 (**reverse transcriptase & RNAse activity**), p51 (**reverse transcriptase**), p10 a **protease** that cleaves gag polyprotein, p32, an integrase (help provirus integration into host cell DNA).

*The *env* (envelope) gene encodes precursor polyprotein (160 Kda) that on cleavage yields envelope gycoproteins, gp120, the external envelope glycoprotein, and gp41 the transmembrane protein.

Simple retroviruses carry the above mentioned regions in their genome, while, complex retroviruses code for additional regulatory non-virion proteins derived from multiply spliced messages. *Deltaretrovirus, Lentivirus* and *Spumavirus* are considered to be complex, the other four are simple retroviruses.

Among the **regulatory genes** (*tat, nef, rev*), *tat* encodes a protein that remain attached to viral RNA and helps transcription, *nef* possibly stimulates cells for virus production and *rev* encodes regulatory protein associated with switching RNA transcripts. These genes and structural genes overlap.

* Two genes (*vif* & *vpu*) encoding proteins **Vif & Vpu** respectively are needed for virus maturation, the *vif* (**the virus infectivity factor**) helps assembly of new viruses. The *vpu* (**virus protein U**) encodes protein needed for virus maturation. **The gene *vpx* is present in HIV-2 in place of *vpu* in HIV-1**. The *vpr* gene encodes protein that is a weak transcriptional activator.

*The viral oncogene **(v onc)** is responsible for rapid malignancy, & is possessed by replication defective, rapidly transforming viruses that need non-defective helper viruses for replication. Since oncogene is acquired into the viral genome in place of some normal viral gene, some part of gene remains defective, usually enve gene (**except *Rous sarcoma virus* having full *gag, pol*&*env* genes**)& hence need non-defective helper viruses for replication. Lentiviruses have other accessory genes.

*The ***tat* gene** that encodes potent transactivator which in association with cellular factors enhance 1000 fold transcription by cellular RNA polymerase.

*The *rev* gene which encodes a protein that helps splicing of viral RNA transcripts & its export to cytoplasm.

*The *nef* gene that is required for replication in macrophages for SIV; Nef protein also down regulates CD4 & IL-2 expression. (8). *vif* gene which encodes viral infectivity factor is required for virus morphogenesis & infectivity.

*The *vpu, vpr & vpx* genes are found in primate lentiviruses. Vpu induces maturation of viral glycoprotein & release of virions. Vpr is a weak transcription activator & Vpx is required for replication in T cells & macrophages.

Genome termini have 5′long terminal repeats (LTR) & 3′LTR are noncoding regions having promoter & enhancer but are important in replication, and internal regions that encode virion proteins for gene expression. The 5' end includes 4 regions- **R, U5, PBS, and L**. R region is a short **repeated sequence at each end** of the genome during the reverse transcription in order to ensure correct end-to-end transfer in growing chain. **U5** is a short **unique sequence** between R and PBS. **PBS (primer binding**

site) consists of 18 bases complementary to 3' end of tRNA primer. L region is an **untranslated leader region that gives signal for packaging of genome RNA.**

The 3' end includes 3 regions-**PPT (polypurine tract), U3**, and **R**. PPT is primer for plus-strand DNA synthesis during reverse transcription. **U3** is a sequence between PPT and R, which **has signal that provirus can use in transcription. R** is the terminal repeated sequence at 3' end.

Retroviruses are divided in 2 ways: A (1) replication competent & (2) replication defective, & B (1) exogenous retroviruses & (2) endogenous retroviruses .

1. The **exogenous retroviruses** are of 2 types;

   i. **Slowly transforming (cis acting), replication competent** &

   ii. **Rapidly transforming, transducing, replication defective. Slowly transforming retroviruses** are transmitted horizontally, contain full genome, do not possess oncogene but induce B cell, T cell & myeloid cell tumours after long incubation. To induce cell transformation, **Provirus** must be integrated with the help of integrase into the host cell DNA near a cellular oncogene (*c-onc*) to interfere with cell division, producing tumours.

   Rapidly transforming, transducing, replication defective retroviruses **do not contain full genome&** hence are replication defective requiring helper virus for replication. **They possess V onc, which induces cell transformation** (sarcoma, leukemia & carcinoma) rapidly. If viral genes are lost during integration, it becomes replication deficient & require helper virus & rarely cause rapidly developing neoplasm. *Bovine leukemia virus* depends on *tax* gene which regulates viral LTR & cellular promoter (transactivation) even if present on a different chromosome. The virus replicates in CD4 T cells only when dividing, so it takes long period to effect T cell production by mitogens, cytokines, Ag stimulation & transactivating protein by certain other viruses. Hence HIV is precipitated by the viruses. HIV ligands on gp 120 peplomers V1, V2, V3, V4 & V5 bind to CD4 T cells. CD4 T cells are also expressed on macrophages lineage, dendritic cells in the skin, lymph node, spleen & astroglia in brains, B cells & other cells.

2. **Endogenous retroviruses** (ERVs) are derived from ancient viral infections of germ cells in humans, mammals and other vertebrates as proviruses,

are passed to the next generation and now remain in the genome. **The endogenous retroviruses** have been acquired through germ line cells, possess provirus genome, & are distributed widely among vertebrates. They are replication competent, are transmitted as provirus through germ cells & are regulated by cellular factors. These viruses do not possess v-once, are not pathogenic but may contribute env gene to produce recombinant feline leukemia virus & can be activated by **irradiation, mutagens & carcinogens.** Many endogenous retroviruses play roles in host biology, e.g. control of gene transcription, cell fusion during placental development in the course of the germination of an embryo, and resistance to exogenous retroviral infection.

Virus classification

The family contains 7 genera.

Group: Group VI ssRNA-RT

Sufamily 1: Orthoretrovirinae

Genera:

G1: *Alpharetrovirus;* type species: *Avian leukosis virus* (ALV), others are: *Rous sarcoma virus,* (RSV), *Avian carcinoma Mill Hill virus* (ACMHV), &*Avian myeloblastosis virus.* (AMV).

G2: *Betaretrovirus;* type species: *Mouse mammary tumor virus* (MMV), *Mason-Pfizer monkey virus* (MFMV) *& Jaagsiekte sheep retrovirus* (JSRV).

G3: *Gammaretrovirus;* type species: *Murine leukemia virus* (MLV), *Feline leukemia virus* (FeLV) *& Porcine Type C oncovirus* (PCOV), *& Reticuloendotheliosis virus* (REV).

G4: *Deltaretrovirus;* type species: *Bovine leukemia virus* (BLV) & *Primate T-lymphotropic virus* (HTLV1, 2, 3).

G5: *Epsilonretrovirus;* type species: It comprises fish tumor viruses-*Walleye dermal sarcoma virus* (WDSV).

(Retroviruses of G1-G5 are called oncogenic retroviruses because they induce neoplastic transformation of cells).

G6: *Lentivirus;* type species: *Human immuno deficiency virus* (HIV-1, 2), *Bovine immunodeficiency virus* (BIV), *Feline immuno deficiency virus* (FeIV), *Equine infectious anemia virus* (EIAV), *Simian immunodeficiency virus* (SIV), *Visna/maedi virus* (VISNA), & *Caprine arthritis encephalitic virus* (CAEV).

Subfamily 2: Spumavirinae

G1: *Spumavirus;* type species: *Simian foamy virus,* contains viruses causing vacuolation of contaminating cultured cells but cause no classical symptoms e.g. *Bovine foamy virus, Feline foamy virus & Equine foamy virus.*

Retroviral Clinical Infections in Humans & Animals

Retroviruses cause several clinical infections in humans like HTLV-I, HTLV-II, HIV-1 and HIV-2; & several important animal diseases namely, Avian leukosis, Avian myeloblastosis, Rous sarcoma; Mouse mammary tumor, Ovine pulmonary adenocarcinoma, Feline leukemia, Feline sarcoma, Bovine leukemia, Maedi/Visna, Caprine arthritis encephalitis, Equine infectious anemia, Feline immunodeficiency, Bovine immunodeficiency, Equine infectious anaemia, Human immunodeficiency 1 and 2, Caprine arthritis encephalis & Visna/maedi. Table 32-1 presented below depicts in short important diseases caused by each virus species.

Table 32.1 : Classification of retroviruses & diseases caused by the member viruses in humans & animals.

Genus	Species	Serotypes	Diseases
Alpharetrovirus			
	Avian leucosis virus: TS	ALV-1, 2, ALV-A1	***Avian leucosis virus***(ALV) produces disturbed blood formation in chickens, induces neoplastic conditions like lymphoid, erythroid, & myeloid leukoses, fibrosarcoma & nephroblastoma. They are distinguished by symptoms like paralysis, tumor formation, leukemia, and eye damage. Incubation period is months to years. Development of neoplasia depends on genetics make up, the age and sex of the host. Within **B**-cells, the provirus induces neoplasia by integrating closely to the **host c-myc oncogene** causing stimulation of the cell to divide when the viral genes are being transcribed. In case of erythroblastosis, virus integration is near the c-erb B gene, with a similar outcome.
	Avian myeloblastosis Virus	AMV	***Avian myeloblastosis virus*** (AMV) induces acute monoblastic leukemia in chickens and transforms only myelomonocytic cells. The long terminal

			repeat (LTR) regulatory region of AMV is unique among the known classes of avian retrovirus LTRs.
	Rous sarcoma virus	RSV	Rous sarcoma is a **spindle-cell sarcoma** of fowls which is transplantable, metastasizes & usually destroys the host bird within a short time, & is caused by the *Rous sarcoma virus*, which occurs in several serotypes and is transferable to rabbits, mice, rats, hamsters and primates as well as chickens. **RSV** was discovered in 1911 by Peyton Rous & Rous was awarded the Novel prize for the significance of his discovery in 1956. RSV has three genes: gag - encodes capsid proteins, pol - encodes reverse transcriptase & src - encodes a tyrosine kinas that attaches phosphate groups to the amino acid tyrosine in host cell proteins, & the env gene was lost during the recombination. The src gene is oncogene triggering uncontrolled mitosis of host cells, providing these cells for fresh infection.
Betaretrovirus			
	Jaagsiekte sheep retrovirus	JSSRV	*Jaagsiekte sheep retrovirus* (JSRV) **causes a contagious lung cancer in sheep called** Jaagsiekte, or **ovine pulmonary adenocarcinoma (OPA)**, which is a slowly progressing neoplastic lung disease of adult sheep being invariably fatal. The disease is characterized by clinical symptoms of **dyspnea, respiratory distress on slight exercise, profuse watery pulmonary discharge, loud fluid sound on auscultation, prolonged clinical course, & progressive emaciation & almost fatal**. The disease was called "Jaagsiekte" based on Afrikans words for Jaag= chase, and siecte= "sickness" to describe the respiratory distress or animal becoming out of breath when being chased. Both exogenous & endogenous form of JSRV viruses occur but only **exogenous virus is infectious**. Endogenous JSRV has several roles in the evolution of the domestic sheep as they are able to block the JSRV replication, play a

		critical role in sheep conceptus, development and placental morphogenesis.
TS:*Mouse mammary tumor virus*	MMTV	*Mouse mammary tumor virus* (MMTV) causes mammary breast cancer, which is a milk transmitted, MMTV can be transferred either through an **exogenous (horizontally) or endogenous (vertical) routes.** If the virus is transferred exogenously, it is passed from the mother mouse to her pups through her milk **via lymphocytes in the milk.** Virus is contained as a DNA provirus integrated in the DNA of milk lymphocytes. The viruses infect **host immune cells-T cells**, become transported through the gastrointestinal tract to the Peyer's where they infect the new host's macrophages, and then to lymphocytes. Endogenous MMTV responds to **glucocorticoid hormones**, mostly progesterone, so when the mouse reaches puberty the virus begins to express its mRNA in the estrogen sensitive tissues. Hence, after puberty all mammary cells will contain the active retrovirus and begin to replicate in the genome and express viral mRNA in all new mammary tissue cells.
Gammaretrovirus		
Feline leukemia virus	FeLV	*Feline leukemia virus* (FeLV) infects cats & causes cancer of the blood cells (lymphocytes) leukemia. FeLV can be transmitted between infected cats via saliva or nasal secretions, if not defeated by the animal's immune systems the virus can be lethal. The disease is characterized by varied signs: loss of appetite, poor coat condition, infection of the skin, bladder and respiratory tract, oral disease, seizers, lymphoadenopathy, skin lesions, fatigue, fever, weight loss, stomatitis, gingivitis, litter box avoidance, pancytopenia, poor grooming, reoccurring bacterial and viral illnesses, anemia, diarrhea, and jaundice.Four subgroups of FeLV exist: A; B; C, and T, but **only subgroup A** is transmissible between cats. The other

		subgroups arise *de novo* and as results of recombination with an endogenous DNA feline sequence.
Deltaretrovirus		
Bovine leukemia virus: TS	BLV	*Bovine leukemia virus* (BLV) causes **B-cell leukemia called enzootic bovine leukosis** in adult cattle, & is characterized by **varied clinical signs**, enlargement of superficial lymph nodes, a digestive form, a cardiac form, a nervous form, & a respiratory form. Many cows remain in **preclinical form for years with** disease appearing in small number of these animals, 5-10% show **peracute case**& die suddenly with involvement of adrenal glands, & rupture of abomasal ulcers or affected spleen. **Subacute to chronic (majority)** cases show loss of appetite, pallor & muscular weakness. BLV is an exogenous type C retrovirus that causes a benign mononucleosis-like disease in cattle, & only some of these animals later develop B-cell leukosis. **BLV** contains *gag, pol* and *env* genes, & also a X region located between the env and the 3' LTR. Occurrence of the disease in cattle is called "leukosis" which was first reported by Leisering who described as early as in 1871 the presence of yellowish nodules in the enlarged spleen of a cow.
Human T-lymphotropic virus	HTLV-1, 2, 3	*Human T-lymphotropic virus* (HTLV-I) virus causes adult T cell leukemia/ lymphoma, or ATL. There are **four kinds of ATL**. Most adults have **acute ATL** with skin lesions that develop very fast, lesions in their bones, & abnormalities in their lungs, stomach and intestines, & have many abnormal lymphocytes circulating throughout their blood stream. Patients die in 6 months after diagnosis. **In chronic ATL,** patients do not have any bone lesions or problems with their stomach or intestines but abnormalities in the lungs and skin of smoldering ATL. The third kind of ATL is **lymphomatous ATL**, in which people have enlarged lymph nodes. HTLV-I also causes

			Tropical Spastic Paraparesis or HTLV-I associated myelopathy/tropical spastic paraparesis or HAM/TSP. The sick persons have muscle spasms, stiff muscles and problems with their bladder. Some patients develop arthritis and an inflammation in their lungs, muscles, skin or eyes. Still others may develop ATL. HTLV-II virus does not cause disease.
Lentivirus			
	Bovine immunodeficiency virus	BIV	*Bovine immunodeficiency virus* (BIV) infections have been shown to be prevalent globally and variably associated with **alterations in animal production, weight loss, secondary disease, diminished milk production and increased incidence of encephalitis.** Although BIV induces dysfunction of monocytes and neutrophils, BIV inoculated calves did not exhibit severe clinical symptoms, and pathogenesis of BIV in cattle remains unclear. BIV is similar to *Human immunodeficiency virus* **(HIV) and infects cattle. Mainly lymphocytes and monocytes/ macrophages are infected.**
	Equine infectious anemia virus	EIAV	**Equine infectious anemia (EIA)** (also calledas **swamp fever**), is a contagious, viral disease of horses that runs in 3 clinical forms: **acute, subacute & chronic forms** characterized by fever, depression, petechiae on mucous membrane & conjunctiva, & rarely severe epistaxis, ventral edema & death, but majority of sick horses recover. After varied period, the disease recurs in recovered animal. In **chronic form**, there are weight loss, anemia, ventral oedema & debilitation leading to death.
	Feline immunodeficiency virus	FeIV	*Feline immunodeficiency virus* (FIV) affects house cats worldwide and causes feline AIDS. FIV is the only non-primate lentivirus to cause an AIDS-like syndrome, but is **not fatal for cats**, as they can live healthily as carriers and transmit the disease for many

years. FIV replicates in **CD4 helper T lymphocytes, macrophases, astroccytes,& microglial cells.** The infected cats remain **persistently viremic.**

FIV was first isolated in 1986 by Pedersen et al. in a colony of cats that had a high prevalence of opportunistic infections with degenerative conditions but has since been identified as an endemic disease in domestic cat populations worldwide. Two subtypes of FIV- **FIV-O & FIV-P** have been detected with varying virulence. A vaccine is available.

Human immunodeficiency virus: TS	HIV-1

Human immunodeficiency virus (HIV-1 and HIV-2) cause **acquired immuno deficiency syndrome (AIDS)** in humans in which progressive failure of the immune system favours life-threatening opportunistic infections & cancers to develop. HIV infection occurs by the transfer of **blood, semen, vaginal fluid, pre-ejaculate or breast milk;** in these HIV is present as both free virus particles and virus within infected immune cells. The four major routes of transmission are **unsafe sex, contaminated needles, breast milk, and transmission from an infected mother to her baby at birth.** The virus affects CD4+ T lymphocytes, which are decreased. They develop fungal infections of histoplasma and coccidioides, the yeast infections of candida and cryptococcus that spread throughout the body, while candida infects the mouth, lungs and esophagus, & viral infections by herpes simplex, *Varicella zoster* or cytomegaloviruses. Herpes attacks their lungs and esophagus, varicella causes a painful skin infection, while the cytomegalovirus infects the eyes. People with AIDS can develop various cancers and brain infections. According to the CDC till 2010, there are approximately 1 million people with HIV in the U.S., and more than 18,000 people die with AIDS every year.

Caprine arthritis encephalitic virus	CAEV	*Caprine arthritis-encephalitis virus* (CAEV) **causes polyarthritis in adult animals, encephalitis in kids between 2 and 6 months of age, a hard udder or mastitis, hypogalactia, chronic interstitial pneumonia, and progressive weight loss & infection resulting in a persistent, lifelong infection.** The CAE virus has a predilection to infect mononuclear cells, specifically tissue macrophages of the lung, CNS, synovium, and mammary gland. Viral transmission usually occurs horizontally through the ingestion of viral-infected goat milk and/or goat colostrum.
Visna/maedi virus	VISNA	Visna virus, (also called as Visna/maedi virus, Maedi-Visna virus or ovine lentivirus) **causes encephalitis and chronic pneumonitis in sheep or ovine progressive pneumonia, or Montana sheep disease.** The disease is characterized by virus replication in mature macrophages, virus dissemination to various organs like lungs, mammary glands, joints and the brain, with **clinical signs of dyspnea, loss of weight, mastitis and arthritis, all related to the location of these lesions.** In these organs, the virus induces slowly progressing inflammatory lesions containing B and T lymphocytes. **VISNA is known as visna when found in the brain, and maedi when infecting the lungs.** Life-long, persistent infections in sheep occur in the **lungs, lymph nodes, spleen, joints, CNS, and mammary glands. Monocytes/ macrophages lineage are the target of Visna virus.**

Lentiviral Infections in Humans

Genus : *Deltaretrovirus*

Human T-lymphotropic virus (HTLV-I) virus causes adult T cell leukemia /lymphoma, or ATL. There are **four kinds of ATL**. Most adults have **acute ATL** with skin lesions that develop very fast, lesions in their bones, & abnormalities in their lungs, stomach and intestines, & have many abnormal lymphocytes circulating throughout their blood stream. Patients die in 6 months after diagnosis. **In chronic ATL**, patients do not have any bone lesions or problems with their stomach or intestines but abnormalities in the lungs and skin of smoldering ATL. The third kind of ATL is **lymphomatous ATL in which** people have enlarged lymph nodes. HTLV-I also causes **Tropical Spastic Paraparesis or HTLV-I associated myelopathy/tropical spastic paraparesis or HAM/TSP.** The sick persons have muscle spasms, stiff muscles and problems with their bladder. Some patients develop arthritis and an inflammation in their lungs, muscles, skin or eyes. Still others may develop ATL. HTLV-II virus does not cause disease.

Genus : *Lentivirus*

Human immunodeficiency virus (HIV-1 and HIV-2) viruses cause **acquired immunodeficiency syndrome (AIDS)** in humans in which progressive failure of the immune system favours life-threatening opportunistic infections & cancers to develop. HIV infection occurs by the transfer of **blood, semen, vaginal fluid, pre-ejaculate or breast milk;** in these HIV is present as both free virus particles and virus within infected immune cells. The four major routes of transmission are **unsafe sex, contaminated needles, breast milk, and transmission from an infected mother to her baby at birth**. The virus affects CD4+ T lymphocytes, which are decreased. They develop fungal infections of histoplasma and coccidioides, the yeast infections of candida and cryptococcus that spread throughout the body, while candida infects the mouth, lungs and esophagus, & viral infections by herpes simplex, *Varicella zoster* or cytomegaloviruses. Herpes attacks the lungs and esophagus, varicella causes a painful skin infection, while the cytomegalovirus infects the eyes. People with AIDS can develop various cancers and brain infections. According to the CDC till 2010, there are approximately 1 million people with HIV in the U.S., and more than 18,000 people die with AIDS every year.

Retrovirus Clinical Infections in Animals

Genus : *Alpharetrovirus*

Avian Leucosis

Avian leucosis(ALV) produces **disturbed blood formation in chickens, induces neoplastic conditions like lymphoid, erythroid, & myeloid leukoses, fibrosarcoma, osteopetrosis, myxosarcomas, nephroblastoma, & other tumours.** They are distinguished by symptoms like paralysis, tumor formation, leukemia, and eye damage. Incubation period is months to years.

Etiology: Avian leucosis is caused by *Avian leucosis virus* (ALV). The ALV group contains both replication-competent and replication-defective viruses but defective viruses do not cause leukosis. ALV contains **10 subgroups,**

A to J on the basis of differences in envelope glycoproteins. ALVs are both endogenous (subgroup E) that occurs commonly in chickens, & exogenous. Only exogenous viruses cause avian leukosis. Subgroups A to E, and J viruses infect chickens. The other subgroup viruses occur in quail, partridges and pheasants. ALV subgroup A causes most outbreaks of avian leukosis that manifest as a lymphoid leukosis, **B cell lymphoma**, which is the most important and common neoplasm associated with the disease. Viruses of subgroup J have been associated with **myeloid leukosis in broilers.**

Occurrence: ALV infection is found worldwide and exist in virtually all chicken flocks except for some SPF (specific pathogen free) flocks from which it has been eradicated. Globally, the frequency of infection has been reduced in the primary breeding stocks of several commercial poultry breeding companies, & in recent years, due to the control program, ALV has become infrequent or absent in certain commercial flocks.

Hosts susceptible

ALVs occur in chickens, quail, partridges and pheasants worldwide and the disease is of immense economic importance to poutry farmers. Susceptibility varies considerably among different strains and types of stock - egg layers are generally more susceptible to lymphoid leukosis.

Transmission

Exogenous ALV is transmitted **vertically** or via close contact as the virus is present in feces and saliva. Vertical transmission occurs via hens with subclinical disease usually shedding virus or viral antigen into the albumen of eggs. Chickens infected at hatching shed virus through their entire lives. Horizontal transmission can occur by the fecal-oral route but is of secondary importance to vertical transmission. Chicks from infected eggs are persistently viremic & are the most important source of infection to the flock. Blood-sucking parasites act as potential vectors.

The causative viruses are rapidly inactivated at ambient temperature and on exposure to most disinfectants.

Pathogenesis

All ALV group viruses are **oncogenic, except subgroup** E. Development of neoplasia depends on genetics make up, the age and sex of the host. The **incubation period is variable from months to years.**

After infection the virus is disseminated to tissues throughout the body where it replicates. Within **B-cells,** the provirus induces neoplasia by integrating closely to the **host c-myc oncogene** causing stimulation of the cell to divide when the viral genes are being transcribed. In case of erythroblastosis, virus integration is near the c-erb B gene, with a similar outcome. Fast-transforming virus genome contains the **c-onc proto-oncogene.** Several copies of the c-onc gene causes over production of the oncoprotein, which stimulates cellular transformation. The oncoproteins produced act as hormones, growth factor receptors, transcription regulation factors, or kinases associated with cellular signaling.

Viruses of subgroups A through D & J are associated with a variety of neoplastic conditions in chickens, like lymphoid leukosis, erythroblastosis, myeloblastosis, myleocytoblastosis, osteopetrosis, nephroblastomas, hemangiomas, and sarcomas.

Clinical symptoms & lesions

Lymphoid leukosis is the most prevalent form of avian leukosis virus & reported in chickens at least 16 weeks of age and occurs more commonly in females. Clinical signs may be absent or birds may appear thrifty with pale combs. The abdomen may be enlarged due to massive tumor growth in the liver.

Osteopetrosis is a sporadic disease that occurs mainly in males in which the shafts of the long bones are thickened, often resulting in a stilted gait. Affected birds may be anemic and also have lesions of lymphoid leukosis.

Erythroblastosis is manifested in two forms, anemic or proliferative. The proliferative form is more common. Clinical signs are similar: chickens become depressed, emaciated, and dehydrated. Anemic form contains few circulating erythroblasts and chickens appear pale, as opposed to cyanotic with the proliferative form in which circulating erythroblasts are present in large numbers.

Myeloblastosisis similar clinically to erythroblastosis. There is an abnormal proliferation of myeloblasts resulting in severe leukemia.

Subclinical disease syndrome characterized by depressed egg production in the absence of tumour formation is more important economically than mortality from lymphoid leukosis.

Diagnosis

1. *Presumptive diagnosis*: Clinical symptoms, gross lesions & histopatological observations are indicatve of AL.
2. *Avian leucosis needs to be differentiated from MD & IBD*. Differential features include: nodular tumors in the bursa of Fabricius as opposed to diffuse enlargement with Marek's disease, intrafollicular cell proliferation in case of bursa of Fabricius as opposed to interfollicular cell proliferation

with Marek's disease. The cytologic appearance of lymphoid cells are uniformly **blast cells** with lymphoid leukosis but a mixture of **mature and immature pleomorphic cells with Marek's disease.**

Treatment & prevention: There is no treatment for ALV. Lymphoid leukosis appears to be controlled best by reduction and eventual eradication of the causative virus. Obtain chicks from breeder flocks free of the virus. Rear birds in isolation with adequate ventilation, follow good biosecurity and management procedures to prevent stress and control other diseases, and dispose of dead birds by composting, incineration or deep burial.

Vaccination: So far, vaccination for tumour prevention has not been promising. However, **recombinant vaccines have been developed that can induce antibodies in breeders to ensure protective maternal antibodies in chicks and these may be useful to assist with eradication** programs.

Rous Sarcoma

Rous sarcoma is a **spindle-cell sarcoma of fowls** which is transplantable, metastasizes & usually destroys the host bird within a short time, & is caused by the *Rous sarcoma virus*, which occurs in several serotypes and is transferable to rabbits, mice, rats, hamsters and primates as well as chickens. RSV was **discovered in 1911 by Peyton Rous & Rous was awarded the Novel prize for the** significance of his discovery in 1956. RSV has three genes: gag - encodes capsid proteins, pol - encodes reverse transcriptase &src - encodes a tyrosine kinase that attaches phosphate groups to the amino acid tyrosine in host cell proteins, & the env gene was lost during the recombination. The src gene is oncogene triggering uncontrolled mitosis of host cells, providing these cells for fresh infection.

Genus: *Betaretrovirus*

Jaagsiekte/ Ovine Pulmonary Adenocarcinoma

Jaagsiekte (JSRV) is **a contagious lung cancer in sheep called** Jaagsiekte, or **ovine pulmonary adenocarcinoma (OPA)**, which isa slowly progressing neoplastic lung disease of adult sheep being invariably fatal. The disease is characterized by clinical symptoms of **dispnea, respiratory distress on slight exercise, profuse watery pulmonary discharge, loud fluid sound on auscultation, prolonged clinical course, & progressive emaciation & almost fatal**. The disease was called "Jaagsiekte" based on Afrikans words for **Jaag= chase, and siecte= "sickness"** to describe the respiratory distress or animal becoming out of breath when being chased.

Etiology: Jaagsiekte/ovine pulmonary adenocarcinoma is caused by *Jaagsiekte sheep retrovirus* (JSRV). Both exogenous & endogenous form of JSRV viruses occur but only **exogenous virus is infectious.** Endogenous virus is present in the genomes of all sheep and goats, & sheep genome has about 27 copies of endogenous retroviruses (enJSRVs) that is highly related to JSRV. Endogenous JSRV has several roles in the evolution of the domestic sheep as they are able to block the JSRV replication, play a critical role in sheep conceptus, development and placental morphogenesis.

Occurrence

The disease has worldwide distribution except Australia & New Zealand.

Hosts susceptible

JSRV affects sheep & rarely goats.

Transmission

JSRV is transmitted through direct contact as **respiratory exudate** from the diseased sheep contains the virus, & aerosol inhalation spread between sheep. The virus spread is respiratory. In **endemic areas,** the majority of infected animals **never show clinical signs of infection,** but they are **shedding virus,** thus promoting introduction of the disease into previously unaffected flocks and new geographical areas.

Pathonenesis

JSRV is transmitted by the respiratory route, the virus infect **lung epithelia; also infect lymphocytes and myeloid cells.** The virus replicates in type II **pneumocytes in the alveolus & Clara cells in the terminal bronchioles which are transformed.** Expression of the JSRV envelope protein activates signaling cascades that promote cellular proliferation and malignant transformation of the cells. Initially, the tumour cells grow along the alveolar walls, but subsequently become **more invasive and metastasizing to the local lymph nodes.** Larger tumours may become necrotic and fibromatous at their centre. As the tumour grows, fluid production in the lung increases and promotes virus spread to other sheep. Adenomatous **ingrowth of alveolar epithelium occupies alveolar air space** causing anoxic anoxia. When the tumour reaches a large size, it interferes with lung function, & clinical signs appear. In **endemic areas,** the majority never shows clinical signs of infection, but they are shedding virus, thus spreading the disease into previously unaffected flocks and new geographical areas.

Clinical symptoms & lesions

Symptoms appear after an **incubation period of several months to 2 yrs.** The affected sheep are 3-4 years of age & have poor health, initially show occasional coughing, & panting after exercise. Later show dyspnea, respiratory distress, mouth breathing, weight loss, respiratory distress and fluid flowing from the nostrils when the head is lowered, moist rales are heard, & often only a few animals are infected in a herd. The course of the disease runs for months. Secondary bacterial infection, especially of pasteurellosis occurs. Affected animals die after 6 weeks to 4 months after the symptoms. Raising of the sheep's hindquarters whilst lowering the head (wheelbarrow test) often exaggerates the flow of clear fluid from the nostrils and can be a useful ancillary diagnostic test. The clinical signs in the earlier stages of the disease are not specific and there are currently no laboratory tests to support a diagnosis in the live animal.

Lesions include grossly increased lungs in size & weight, extensive neoplastic tissues, the affected areas are solid & raised , bronchial & medistinal lymph nodes are enlarged & hyperplastic. **Histologically,** alveolus is lined by cuboidal & columnar epithelia forming adenomatous ingrwoth of alveolar epithelium into alveolar space.

An important feature of JSRV infection is the **absence of any specific immune response** from the host. Probably the sheep are immunologically tolerant to JSRV antigens due to the expression of closely related **endogenous JSRV proteins in the fetal thymus during T lymphocyte development** and any JSRV-reactive T cells should be recognized as 'anti-self' and selectively removed. A second hypothesis is that tumor cells downregulate their Major Histocompatibility Class-I expression that might be the reason for the absence of any virus-specific Cytotoxic T Cell response (CTL).

Diagnosis

1. *Presumptive diagnosis:* By characteristic clinical symptoms, histological lesions in formalin fixed lung & bronchial lymph nodes are characteristics.
2. *Detection of the virus:* It is performed by ELISA test from lung exudate or washings.
3. *Detection of viral nucleic acid:* PCR test detects viral nucleic acid.

Treatment & prevention: No treatment exists. Regular inspection, culling of lean & breathless sheep on the onset of disease & culling progeny of the affected sheep is adopted. Keeping naïve younger sheep separate from older infected sheep helps reduce the incidence.

Mouse Mammary Tumor

Mouse mammary tumor virus (MMTV) causes mammary breast cancer, which is milk transmitted, formerly called as Bittner virus, or the **'milk factor'**. Dr. John Joseph Bittener established in 1936 the theory that a cancerous agent, or "milk factor", could be transmitted by cancerous mothers to young mice from a virus in their mother's milk. MMTV can be transferred either through an **exogenous (horizontally) or endogenous (vertical) routes.** If the virus is transferred exogenously, it is passed from the mother mouse to her pups through her milk via lymphocytes in the milk. Virus is contained as a DNA provirus integrated in the DNA of milk lymphocytes. The viruses infect **host immune cells-T cells**, become transported through the gastrointestinal tract to the Peyer's patches where they infect the new host's macrophages, and then to lymphocytes. Endogenous MMTV responds to **glucocorticoid hormones**, mostly progesterone, so when the mouse reaches puberty the virus begins to express its mRNA in the estrogen sensitive tissues. Hence, after puberty all mammary cells will contain the active retrovirus and begin to replicate in the genome and express viral mRNA is all new mammary tissue cells. The strongest hormone for virus production is the artificial cortisone dexamethasone. The role of mouse mammary tumor virus (MMTV) as a causative agent in human breast carcinogenesis has recently been the subject of interest, MMTV sequences has been detected in human breast cancer but not in healthy breast tissue. The virus, when transmitted exogenously, first infects cells of the immune systems, like T-cells which later carry the virus to the exocrine tissue in the mammary gland. The first step of development of breast cancer is characterized by the development of mammary hyperplasia, followed by the formation of hyperplastic alveolar nodules, which are not yet malignant, & some of these nodules can further develop in malignant tumors. The induction of the first malignant tumors caused by MMTV requires the presence of glucocorticoid hormones.

Genus: *Gammaretrovirus*

Feline Leukemia

Feline leukemia (FeLV) infects cats & causes **cancer of the blood cells (lymphocytes) leukemia.** FeLV can be transmitted between infected cats via saliva or nasal secretions, if not defeated by the animal's immune systems the virus can be lethal. The disease is characterized by varied signs: loss of appetite, poor coat condition, infections of the skin, bladder and respiratory tract, oral disease, seizers, lymphoadenopathy, skin lesions, fatigue, fever, weight loss, stomatitis, gingivitis, litter box avoidance, pancytopenia, poor grooming, reoccurring bacterial and viral illnesses, anemis, diarrhea, and jaundice.

Etiology: Feline leukemia is caused by *Feline leukemia virus* (FeLV). Four subgroups of FeLV exist: A; B; C, and T, but **only subgroup A** is transmissible between cats. The other subgroups arise *de novo* and as a result of recombination with an endogenous DNA feline sequence.

Occurrence

The disease occurs worldwide, & is a major, frequent malady of domestic cats, wild cats and jungle cats. Colostrum protect kittens for the first month of life but older kittens become susceptible with their susceptibility decreasing with age. It is estimated that only about 1 in 5 cats exposed at 10 weeks of age will develop persistent infection. Kittens of persistently infected queens usually become infected.

Hosts susceptible

Cats including wild cats are affected, & larger wild cat e.g. lynx, cheetah, and lions are also susceptible but FeLV is not transmissible to either humans or dogs. **Kittens under 4 months of age are susceptible to infection, but by 8 months are resistant to it.**

Transmission

Cats infected with FeLV act as focus of infection, such cats pass the virus through **saliva and & nasal secretions**, infect other cats via close contact, by biting another cat, through a litter box or food dish used by an infected cat, and from milk during nursing. Transmission takes place from an infected mother cat to her kittens, either before they are born *in utero* or while they are nursing.

Kittens can be born with FeV, having contracted it from their mother while in utero. Infection is far higher in city cats, stray or owned, than in rural cats: this is entirely due to contact the cats have with each other.

Pathogenesis

The disease has a wide range of effects. The cat can fight off the infection and become totally immune, can become a healthy carrier & never gets sick but can infect other cats, or the cat has beome immunocompromised. The development of lymphomas is a final stage of the disease. It is thought that virus protein induce lymphomas in cats.

Once the virus has entered the cat, there are **six phases** to a FeLV infection:

Phase one: The virus enters the cat through the pharynx where it infects the epithelial cells, the tonsil B-lymphocytes and macrophages. These white blood cells then pass to the lymph nodes and begin to replicate.

Phase two: The virus enters the blood stream and begins to distribute throughout the body.

Phase three: The lymphoid system becomes infected, with further virus distribution throughout the body.

Phase four: FeV can take control of body's immune system and cause viremia. During this phase the hemolymphatic system and intestines become infected.

If the cat's immune system does not fight off the virus, then it goes onto:

Phase five: The bone marrow becomes infected. **FeV will stay with the cat for the rest of its life**. In this phase, the virus replicates and is released four to seven days later in infected neutrophils, and sometimes lymphocytes, monocytes, and eosinophils.

Phase six: The cat's body is overwhelmed by infection and mucosal and glandular epithelial cells become infected. The virus replicates in epithelial tissues including salivary glands, oropharynx, stomach, esophagus, intestines, trachea, nasopharynx, renal tubules, bladder, pancreas, alveolar ducts, and sebaceous ducts from the muzzle.

Cats persistently infected may die within a few months or may remain asymptomatic for longer. The fatal diseases are leukemias, lymphomas, and non-regenerative anemia.

Neoplastic forms: About 20% of persistently infected cats develop one of the following lymphosarcoma forms: alimentary, multicentric, thymic, or lymphoid leukemia & the clinical signs vary with the different forms of tumors:

Alimentary form: Affected cats show signs of anorexia, vomiting and diarrhea. Abdominal masses involve the small intestine, cecum and colon.

Multicentric form: There are **generalized lymphoadenopathy, renal lymphosarcoma, splenomegaly, and hepatomegaly** usually seen in young cats.

Thymic form: The affected cats commonly show dysphagia, dyspnea, cyanosis may be present in advanced cases, & pleural fluid may contain neoplastic cells.

Lymphoid leukemic form: This form is seen when **bone marrow is involved, and transformed lymphocytes circulate in the blood**. Jaundice, fever, anemia and pallor of mucous membranes are seen. There is lymphadenopathy, splenomegaly and hepatomegaly are observed. The sick cats develop fever, anorexia and weakness are evident.

Myeloid leukemia: This form is seen in the **bone marrow** with secondary involvement in the liver, spleen and lymph nodes. Leukemia is named as per the precursor hematopoietic cells are affected, e.g., myelogenous leukemia, erythroleukemia, and lymphoblastic leukemia. There are signs of progressive anemia, recurring fever and weight loss.

Non-neoplastic forms

Immunosuppression: The immunosuppression **favours infections due to bacterial, fungal, protozoan, and viral agents.** Some of the symptoms: chronic recurring rhinitis and sinusitis, sores around claws, and peridontal disease are seen. Affected cats contract feline infectious peritonitis and *Haemobartonella felis* infection. In the the chronic infection, there is persistent fever with a progressive loss of weight and condition. FeLV infection may predispose to feline infectious anemia. A panleukopenia-like syndrome has been associated with FeLV infection. It has occurred in cats immunized against feline panleukopenia and is invariably fatal.

Reproductive Disorders: FeLV infection may cause **fetal death, abortion and infertility**. Fetal death is due to endometritis and placentitis, & about 75% of infected queens abort. Cats that survive to full term are persistently infected and the resulting kittens are weak and sickly.

Glomerulonephritis: Glomerulonephritis is seen in cats with persistent FeLV infection. It caused by the **deposition of immune complex** in the kidney which is an important cause of death in FeLV infection.

Diagnosis: Clinical samples for test include blood smears, tumors, bone marrow, serum, histopathologic examination of biopsies, bone marrow examinations, and cytology of thoracic and abdominal fluids.

Virus detection: Test for FeLV is the **ELISA,** while the **immunofluorescent antibody test (IFA)** is the recommended confirmatory test. **PCR test detects FeLV genome.** Commercial reagents are available to diagnostic laboratories for the ELISA and the IFA tests.

Treatment & prevention: Supportive therapy, chemotherapy and irradiation may prolong life in cats with neoplasia. Antiviral agents like human recombinant INF-α and AZT may delay the onset of clinical signs but are not curative.

Prevention includes inactivation by commonly used disinfectants as FeLV is labile and quickly loses its infectivity in the environment. The disease can be eradicated from the colonies by periodic serologic testing, the removal of positive cats, and disinfection of potentially contaminated areas, & new additions should be quarantined and tested before admission to the main colony. Cats in the main colony are retested at yearly intervals or less.

Vaccination: **Subunit and killed virus vaccines** are available and administered from **nine weeks of age** but these vaccines do not eliminate pre-existing infections. The vaccines don't interfere with tests for viral antigen. Non-adjuvanted **PUREVAX® FeLV (formerly EURIFEL V) Recombinant Leukemia Vaccine**-Merial is a non adjuvanted Canarypox vector vaccine administered with the VET JET™ transdermal vaccination system. Canarypoxvirus (ALVAC), the genome of which contains the env and gag genes and part of the pol gene of the subgroup A of the FeLV virus (strain vCP97). The vaccine is used SC for active immunization of cats of 8 weeks of age or older against feline leukaemia for the prevention of persistent viremia and clinical manifestations of the disease. The vaccine is effective against any oronasal FeLV challenge. The protection was shown to be solid against an oronasal challenge one year after the initial vaccination, and was effective against a very severe 'in-contact' challenge. It can also be used by transdermal vaccination system enhancing immune response through targeted antigen presentation. The vaccine stimulates both humoral and cell-mediated immune response. It needs lower volume dosage 0.25 ml into the skin of cat at nine weeks of age, another three weeks later, and annually thereafter. All vaccinated cats are protected from persistent FeLV infection in a challenge that infected 90% of the nonvaccinated controls.

Genus: *Deltaretrovirus*

Bovine Leukemia

Bovine leukemia **(BLV)** is a **B-cell leukemia called enzootic bovine leukosis** in adult cattle, & is characterized by **varied clinical signs, enlargement of superficial lymph nodes, a digestive form, a cardiac form, a nervous form, & a respiratory form.** Many cows remain in **preclinical form for years with** disease appearing in small no of these animals, 5-10% show **peracute case** & die suddenly with involvement of adrenal glands, rupture of abomasal ulcers or affected spleen, & **subacute to chronic (majority)** cases show loss of appetite, pallor & muscular weakness. BLV is an exogenous type C retrovirus that causes a benign mononucleosis-like disease in cattle, & only some of these animals later develop B-cell leukosis.

Etiology: Bovine leukemia is caused by *Bovine leukemia* virus (BLV). Only one antigenic type of BLV has been found, & only a small percentage of animals infected with BLV develop B cell lymphosarcoma. **Most infected animals develop a persistent lymphocytosis without any apparent clinical features.**

The virus produces **syncytia in cell cultures** and immune serum prevents syncytia formation. This is used as an assay for virus or antibody. **BLV** contains***gag, pol* and *env* genes, & also a X region located between the env and the 3' LTR.**

Occurrence

BLV occurrence of the disease in cattle is called leukosis, & was first reported by Leisering who described as early as in 1871 the presence of yellowish nodules in the enlarged spleen of a cow. BLV occurs worldwide with persistent infection, followed by persistent lymphocytosis. Some countries have controlled the disease by various means.

Hosts susceptible

Cattle are the only species infected, but sheep & goats can be infected experimentally. All breeds of cattle are susceptible, but cattle less than 2 years are rarely infected & **infection rate increases with age.**

Transmission

BLV transmission occurs through methods that transmit blood between animals, like gouge dehorning, vaccination and ear tagging with instruments, or needles that are not changed, rectal palpation with common sleeves, & via colostrum, milk, and in utero. Embryo transfer and artificial insemination are also a small means of spread. A small number of infections occur through common equipment and/or palpation sleeves, via blood feeding insects that transfer infected lymphocytes from one animal to the next. **Infection with BLV is life-long.** Under natural conditions the disease is transmitted **mainly by milk to the calf via infected lymphocytes in the milk.**

Pathogenesis

BLV affects B lymphocytes & causes persistent infection in some subpopulation of B lymphocytes by integrating its provirus DNA in host cell DNA. Cattle exposed to BLV go through 4 possible outcomes:

1. Some animals fail to become infected because of genetic resistance.
2. Some animals get infected & establish permanent infection & induce Abs production, & become latent carrier of infection.
3. Some cattle get infected, establish permanent infection, become seropositive & **develop persistent lymphocytosis**, which is a benign lymphoproliferative process.
4. Some infected, seropositive cases cause neoplastic transformation of the cells & develop **malignant tumours called lymphosarcoma.**

Clinical symptoms and lesions

Cattle any organ may be infected but most common organs are **abomasum, heart, visceral & peripheral lymph nodes, skin, reproductive tract** & others. Clinical signs are based on involvement of these organs.Tumors in abomasal wall cause impaired digestion & persistent diarrhea. When heart has tumours, cows can show signs of heart failure such as big jugular veins and brisket edema. When the spine is affected, cows can become progressively paralyzed, especially from the hind legs. **Cutaneous involvement** shows persistent intradermal thickening with neoplastic lymphocytes. Medistinal lymph nodes involvement causes **esophaseal obstruction.**

Diagnosis

Clinical samples for testing include serum & affected tissues.

Detection of viral antigen : Agar gel diffusion test detects 98% of the cases. Radioimmunoassay is used for individual cows testing. Serum & milk ELISA detects BLV in serum & milk, & is very sensitive test. PCR detects BLV in peripheral blood lymphocytes.

Tretment & prevention

There is no treatment or vaccine used against BLV. The control of BLV infection in a herd depends on detection of infected animals and their slaughter, culling or separation. The second option if infected animals are large is to keep them separately, & use every thing separately for them.

Genus: *Lentivirus*

Bovine Immunodeficiency

Bovine immunodeficiency (BIV)has been shown to be prevalent globally and variably associated with alterations in animal production, weight loss, secondary disease, diminished milk production and increased incidence of encephalitis. Although BIV induces **dysfunction of monocytes and neutrophils, BIV inoculated calves did not exhibit severe clinical symptoms**, and pathogenesis of BIV in cattle remains unclear. BIV is similar to Human immunodeficiency virus (HIV) and infects cattle. Mainly lymphocytes and monocytes/ macrophages are infected.

Etiology: Bovine immunodeficiency is caused by *Bovine immuno-deficiencyvirus* (BIV) in the genus *Lentivirus.*

Occurrence

BIVinfections have been shown to be prevalent globally. BIV in ten blood samples and one milk sample of cattle was detected **in India by Southern hybridization followed by PCR.** BIV was first reported by **Dr. Cameron Seger, a veterinarian of the Louisiana State University Agricultural Center, discovered BIV in 1966s** at the Southeast Louisiana Experiment Station at Franklinton, Louisiana. The cows showed with high white blood cell counts, referred to as persistent lymphocytosis (PL) which is associated with the development of bovine leukemia/lymphosarcoma. Van Der Maten & associates from USA in1972 identified BIV from a cow with persistent lymphocytosis, lymphoadenopathy, neuropathy & progressive emaciation.

Hosts susceptible

Cattle are susceptible to BIV.

Transmission

BIV is transmitted **via exchange of bodily fluids.** BIV infection is more prevalent in the southern United States and most prevalent in South America. Disease spread is also due to reuse of contaminated needles used in vaccinations, communal sharing of colostrum by calves and failure to completely sterilize instruments after invasive treatment.

Clinical symptoms & lesions

Leukocytosis and lymphadenopathy are associated with **early infection,** & the symptoms resemble those of AIDS in humans. BIV infections have been shown variably associated with alterations in animal production, weight loss, secondary bacterial infection, diminished milk production and increased incidence of encephalitis. Although, **BIV induces dysfunction of monocytes and neutrophils, overt clinical signs in seropositive cattle rarely appear** & experimentally BIV infected calves did not exhibit severe clinical symptoms. Thus, pathogenesis of BIV in cattle remains unclear. Even though the virus has not been linked to any specific disease condition in cattle, it certainly can aggravate certain illnesses in the animals, including **impairment of the immune system.**

Diagnosis

PCR assays targeting BIV env & pol sequences detects BIV -infected leukocytes in the blood and milk of BIV-seropositive cows, but did not adequately amplify Australian BIV sequences. PolTaqMan MGB assays showed 10-fold improved sensitivity to detect BIV over conventional PCR tests.

Treatment & prevention

Cell-associated bovine immunodeficiency virus (BIV) and cell-free BIV were subjected to increasing temperatures, including pasteurization; BIV was inactivated by heating to 47^{0}C for 30 min and by low- and high-temperature pasteurization conditions.

Equine Infectious Anemia

Equine infectious anemia (EIAV), also called as **swamp fever,** is a contagious, viral disease of horses that runs in 3 clinical forms: **acute, subacute & chronic forms** characterized by fever, depression, petechiae on mucous membrane & conjunctiva, & rarely severe epistaxis, ventral edema & death, but majority of sick horses recover. After varied period, **the disease recurs in recovered animals. In chronic form**, there are weight loss, anemia, ventral edema & debilitation leading to **death**.

Occurrence

The virus is endemic in the America, parts of Europe, the Middle East, Far East, Russia, and South Africa.

Hosts susceptible

EIA affects horses, ponies, donkey & mules. **Infected animals remain viremic throughout their life**. Recent research indicates that there are some breeds of horses with a tolerance to EIA.

Transmission

Like HIV, EIA can be transmitted through **blood, saliva, milk, and body secretions**. Transmission is mechanical through **biting flies**, such as the blood sucking horse fly and deer-fly- Haematophagus insects mainly *Tabanus* spp & *Stomoxys* spp on whose mouth parts the virus survives for only short period. The virus survives up to 4 hours in the carrier. **Iatrogenic** transmission occurs through contaminated surgical equipments, recycled needles and syringes, and bits can transmit the disease. **Mares** can transmit the disease to their foals **via the placenta**. The risk of transmitting the disease is greatest when an infected horse is ill, as the blood levels of the virus are then highest.Recent studies in Brazil on living wild horses have shown that in the Pantanal, about 30% of domesticated and about 5.5% of the wild horses are chronically infected with EIA. EIAV may also be transmitted between infected pregnant mares and unborn foals. About 10 percent of **foals born to infected mares are infected** with the virus. The virus may also be transmitted through natural service or breeding. Horses that are infected without showing detectable clinical signs are inapparent **carriers** of EIA.

Pathogenesis

EIAV replicates in in **macrophages, monocytes & Kupffer cells causing a cell-associated viremia** that disseminates the virus in the whole body & affect several organs. The infected animals develop antibodies that fail to eliminate EIAV. **The provirus remains integrated in the host-cell DNA as such horses become persistently infected.** During reverse transcription, frequent error in transcription occurs that causes mutation in glycoprotein resulting in more virulent strains. Such mutations cause febrile recurrent episodes & immune stimulation. Non neutralizing antibodies form **immune**

complexes that activate complement inducing fever, anemia, thrombocytopenia & glomerulonephritis. Haemolysis, erythrophagocytosis & reduced erythropoiesis result in anemia in chronic cases.

Clinical symptoms & lesions

Acute form: In the acute form, there is a sudden onset of the disease showing symptoms of high fever, anemia due to the breakdown of RBC, weakness, swelling of the lower abdomen and legs, weak pulse, and irregular heart beat. The horse may die suddenly.

Subacute: Disease progresses less severely & symptoms include recurrent fever, weight loss, an enlarged spleen, anemia, and swelling of the lower chest, abdominal wall, penile sheath, scrotum and legs.

Chronic form: In chronic form of the disease, horses tire easily and are unsuitable for work. Sick horses may have a recurrent fever and anemia, may relapse to the subacute or acute form even several years after the original attack.

EIA may cause **abortion** in pregnant mares **at any time during the pregnancy** if there is a relapse when the virus enters the blood. Most infected mares will abort, however some give birth to healthy foals. Foals are not necessarily infected.

A horse **may not show any symptoms, yet tests positive for EIA antibodies**. This horse can still pass on the disease. According to most veterinarians, horses diagnosed EIA positive are usually not showing any sign of sickness or disease.

Diagnosis

The **Coggins test**, which is a **agar immunodiffusion test**, is a very sensitive diagnostic test for EIAV developed by Dr. Leroy Coggins in the 1970s. Many countries require a negative Coggins test for inter-state travel. Most horses participating in shows, events or importation or in breeding farm require a negative Coggins test. A Coggins test should be done on an annual basis or every 6 months in case of increased travelling.

Treatment & prevention

Measures for positive horses include sending the horse to a recognized research facility, branding the horse and quarantining it at least 200 yards from other horses for the rest of its life, and euthanizing **the horse. It is suggested that the risks posed by infected horses, even if they are not showing any clinical signs, are enough to impose such stringent rules.** Syringes and needles should not be reused, & all horses that test positive should be reported as EIA-positive horses are infected for life.

Vaccination

A vaccine is used, called **Chinese live attenuated EIA vaccine,** developed in China and widely used there since 1983. Currently, EIA-positive horses throughout the world are being slaughtered or quarantined. This is a tragic, ineffective waste. However, the Chinese Live Attenuated EIA vaccine can prevent contracting the disease in horses. This vaccine offers new hope in developing a better understanding and treatment for retroviruses, including EIA and HIV. All vaccinated horses were asymptomatic and had a low level of virus replication (<10 copies ml^{-1}). The expression level of cytokines including gamma interferon, interleukin 2 and 12 in DLV immunized horses was 5-100-fold higher than that in non-vaccinated controls (n=4, P<0.01). After challenge with virulent LN strain, horses vaccinated with DLV showed lower viral loads (<10^3 copies ml^{-1}) with no temperature increase. High levels of EIAV-specific cytokines induced by the attenuated EIAV vaccine may contribute to the protective immune response against EIA disease.

Feline Immunodeficiency

Feline immunodeficiency (FIV) affects house cats worldwide and causes feline AIDS, characterized by 3 clinical forms: **acute, subclinical stage & chronic stages.** FIV is related to human immunodeficiency virus (HIV). FIV is the only non-primate lentivirus to cause an AIDS-like syndrome, but is **not fatal for cats,** as they can live healthily as carriers and transmit the disease for many years. A vaccine is available.

Etiology: Feline immunodeficiencyis caused by *Feline immunodeficiency virus* (FIV). Within FIV, 5 subtypes of FIV have been reported based on nucleotide sequence differences of env gene. Two subtypes of FIV- **FIV-O & FIV-P** have been detected with varying virulence.

Occurrence

FIV was first isolated in **1986 by Pedersen et al. in a colony of cats that had a high prevalence of opportunistic infections with degenerative conditions** but has since been identified as an endemic disease in domestic cat populations worldwide. FIV occurs in about 2.5% to 4.4% of cats worldwide and about 2.5% of cats in the USA are infected with FIV.

Hosts susceptible

FIV affects only **domestic house cats,** but related lentiviruses have been isolated from wild Felidae like **pumas & lions**. FIV prevalence is highest in cats **more than 6 yrs old**. FIV infects other feline species, and is endemic in some large wild cats, such as African lions, but these species do not exhibit symptoms, perhaps due to mutation that confers resistance.

Transmission

FIV is shed mainly in the **saliva,**& hence the virus is transmitted by **deep bite wounds and scratches**, where the infected cat's saliva enters the other cat's bloodstream, & **from pregnant females to their offspring in utero**. Adult cats having free roaming have the highest infection rate & non aggressive intimate contact spread the virus under natural condition.

Pathogenesis

FIV replicates in **CD^4 helper T lymphocytes, macrophases, astroccytes, microglial cells.** The infected cats remain **persistently viremic**. Viremia increases rapidly with peak in 7-8 weeks, & a **second peak of viremia is** seen at the terminal stage. CD^4 helper T lymphocytes are destroyed causing **progressive decline in cellular immunity** although humoral immunity is not affected. There are also reduced IL-2 production & response & impaired lymphogenesis. Simultaneous reduction in CD4 T lymphocytes, increased viremia, and appearance of varints with enhanced virulence induce development of immunodeficiency & opportunistic pathogens infection in such cats.

Clinical symptom & lesions

The disease occurs in three stages, **acute, suclinical stage & chronic stages.Acute stage** starts 1–2 months after transmission in which fever, depression, and generalized lymphoadenopathy are observed. **Subclinical Stage** starts 4 weeks to 10 months after transmission, in which symptoms of the disease decrease or disappear; however, **all cats remain viremic for life.** In the **chronic Stage**, cats succumb to chronic infections due to immunosuppression. Cats may show stomatitis, odontoclasia, periodontitis, gingivitis, rhinitis, conjunctivitis, pneumonia, enteritis & dermatitis in the later stages of infection. FIV positive cats are less prone to develop AIDS-like symptoms than HIV+ humans.

Diagnosis

Detection of viral antigen: PCR is used to detect provirus DNA.

Detection of antibody : ELISA detects Abs to FIV, & alternatively indirect immunofluorescence & immunoblotting are also very useful tests.

Treatment & prevention

Treatment includes use of antibiotics to control secondary infections.

Vaccination

Single strain vaccines proved efficacious against homologous FIV strains. A dual-subtype vaccine for FIV released in 2002 called Fel-O-Vax made it possible to immunize cats against more FIV strains. The vaccine has shown 100% effectiveness against two different subtype B FIV strains. Vaccination will cause cats to have positive results on FIV tests, making diagnosis more difficult.

Caprine Arthritis-Encephalitis

Caprine arthritis-encephalitis virus (CAEV) causes **polyarthritis** in adult animals, **encephalitis in kids between 2 and 6 months of age, a hard udder or mastitis, hypogalactia, chronic interstitial pneumonia, and progressive weight loss & infection resulting in a persistent, lifelong infection.** The CAE virus has a predilection to infect mononuclear cells, specifically tissue **macrophages of the lung, CNS, synovium, and mammary gland.**

Etiology: Caprine arthritis-encephalitis is caused by *Caprine arthritis-encephalitis virus* (CAEV).

Occurrence

This disease was first diagnosed in goats in 1974. Since that time, it has been diagnosed in North America, Europe, Africa, Arabia, Kenya, Peru, Australia, and New Zealand. Disease prevalence is highest where there is intensive dairy goat farming in confinement in countries like USA, France, Norway, Switzerland, and Canada.

Hosts susceptible

Dairy goats are susceptible.

Transmission

Viral transmission usually occurs **horizontally** through the ingestion of viral-infected **goat milk and/or goat colostrum.** Other sources of viral transmission include transmission***in utero***; contact with the vagina of an infected doe during parturition; via **saliva** or respiratory secretions; via contact with infected blood; viral contamination of milking equipment, needles, tattooing equipment; and breeding an infected animal with a non-infected animal.

Pathogenesis

Kids infected at **birth remains persistently infected for life** but only a few show clinical infection. CAE replicates in the **monocytes,** virus remains latent until the **monocytes mature into macrophages, which express & shed the virus.** The macrophages then disseminate the virus to other tissues such as mammary gland, choroid plexus, synovium, lung interstitium, and their associated draining lymph nodes. Clinical signs and lesions of CAE are associated with the viral replication in the infected macrophages. Active viral infection induces a **strong, but non-protective, humoral and cell mediated immune response.** The maternal antibodies passed in the colostrum are not protective for kids ingesting the colostrum. The neutralizing Abs does not arrest virus infection due to continual expression of antigenic variants. The immune complexes cause chronic inflammatory changes in tissues.

Recently it has been shown that the virus can develop a tropism for and replicate within **caprine oviduct epithelial cells (COEC)**, which are often utilized from untested slaughter house animals to aid *in vitro* fertilization techniques. COEC cells being highly susceptible to CAEV indicates that **embryo transfer may be a possible mode of transmission** for CAE.

Clinical symptoms and lesions

There are **five** major clinical forms associated with CAE: **arthritis, encephalitis, interstitial pneumonia, mastitis, and progressive weight loss.**

The **arthritic form** is the most common symptoms & is seen in mature goats (6 months and older), & arthritis tends to be chronic and progressive, with a sudden onset of lameness. Joints affected are: carpal joints, tarsal joints, stifle joints, fetlock joints, alantooccipital joint, and coxofemoral joints. All synovial membranes can be affected by CAE virus. Arthritic signs may be subtle or severe; subtle signs include stiffness, shifting leg lameness, decreased ambulation, weight loss, reluctance to rise, and abnormal posture after rising. More severe arthritic signs include acute swellings without pain upon palpation; joints that are drained of the fluid simply refill. Eventually these signs lead to a painful arthritis.

The **encephalitic form** affects **kids** between **2 and 6 months** of age showing incoordination and inappropriate placement of limbs while standing and walking. A gradual paresis and paralysis, commonly affecting the hind limbs and often progressing to the forelimbs, can occur. Lastly, the animal is unable to rise to a standing position. More commonly kids show **neurologic signs:** depression, nystagmus, abnormal pupillary response, blindness, head tilt, head tremor, dysphagia, torticollis, circling, and facial nerve deficits. Affected kids are afebrile.

Chronic interstitial pneumonia form shows initially, a deep chronic cough, & later, chronic dyspnea, weight loss, tachypnea, and abnormal lung sounds. Enlarged lymph nodes may contribute to some of the respiratory distress.

Mastitis form shows interstitial mastitis with distended udder from which milk cannot be expressed. The mastitis is mostly seen around parturition.

Chronic form shows progressive weight loss, which can occur with any of the other forms of the disease.

Diagnosis

Disease is diagnosed by various tests.

1. Clinical symptoms & lesions.
2. CSF shows increased mononuclear cell count & blood depicts reduced or inverted CD4: CD8 ratio.
3. Agar gel immunodiffusion test is very sensitive.

Treatment & prevention: There is no treatment that eliminates CAE virus or vaccine to prevent this disease. Prevention is based on maintaining a closed herd, & testing all animals for CAE every 6 months beginning at 6 months of age. Seropositive individuals should be segregated and culled. Kids born to seropositive does should be segregated from kids born to seronegative does. **Kids should only be fed heat-treated goat colostrum and heat-treated goat milk, heated at 56° C for one hour.** Seronegative animals should be milked first and the milking parlor should be disinfected after every milking. Seropositive and seronegative animals should not be bred to each other. Iatrogenic transmission of CAE virus should be avoided by using different instruments- needles, tattooing equipment, dehorning equipment, etc.

Visna/ Maedi

Visna virus (also called as Visna-Maedi virus, Maedi-Visna virus or ovine lentivirus) causes **encephalitis and chronic pneumonitis in sheep or ovine progressive pneumonia, or Montana sheep disease**. The disease is characterized by virus replication in mature macrophages, virus dissemination to various organs like lungs, mammary glands, joints and the brain, with **clinical signs of dyspnea, loss of weight, mastitis and arthritis, all related to the location of these lesions.** In these organs, the virus induces slowly progressing inflammatory lesions containing B and T lymphocytes.

VISNA is known as visna when found in the brain, and maedi when infecting the lungs. Life-long, persistent infections in sheep occur in the **lungs, lymph nodes, spleen, joimts, CNS, and mammary glands. Monocytes/ macrophages lineage are the target of Visna virus.**

Etiology: Visna/maedi is caused by *Visna/maedi virus* (VISNA). Phylogenetic analysis divides the viruses into four principal sequence groups, A to D. Sequence groups A and B are divided further into subtypes. Group A contains at least seven subtypes and group B at least two subtypes. To date, **subtypes A5 and A7, and groups C and D have been found only in goats. Subtypes A1 and A2 have been isolated only from sheep. Subtypes A3, A4, A6, B1 and B2 have been found in both species.** Recombination between a group A maedi-visna virus and a group B caprine arthritis-encephalitis virus has recently been demonstrated in goats infected with both viruses.

Occurrence

The disease was described in 1954 by Bjorn Sigurdsson in Iceland & was the first lentivirus to be isolated and characterized in 1957 by Sigurdsson. In Iceland "Maedi" means dyspnoea, and "visna" means "wasting" or "shrinking" of the spinal cord. The disease was introduced to Iceland following an import of Karakul sheep from Germany in 1933. Maedi-visna occurs in most sheep-raising countries other than Australia and New Zealand, & has been reported from most part of Europe, UK, USA, Canada, Peru, Kenya, South Africa, Israel, India, Myanmar and the southern regions of the former U.S.S.R.

Hosts susceptible

Maedi-visna **affects sheep and, to a lesser extent, goats.**The susceptibility of Maedi-Visna infection varies across sheep breeds; **coarse-wool breeds** apparently are more **susceptible** than fine-wool sheep. Breed susceptibility varies, **Texel, Border Leicester, and Finnish Landrace sheep are more susceptible** to disease than Columbia.

Transmission

Most animals become infected **early in life from infected colostrum or milk.** The virus also spread via close contact, probably by the respiratory route. Coinfection with Jaagsiekte virus increases visna titers in the respiratory tract, increasing contact transmission between sheep. Transmission has been reported from water contaminated with feces, but indirect spread is rare. Intrauterine spread is thought to be negligible or minor. VISNA **infects sheep or goats for life**, but viral burdens vary between individual animals. Both **asymptomatic and symptomatic animals can transmit this virus.**

Sheep can be a source of virus transmission to goats, and vice versa. The ingestion of contaminated colostrum or milk, or close contact between the two species in crowded barns has been suggested as a source of infection. Under experimental conditions, lambs that have nursed from infected goats can become persistently infected with the virus.

Pathogenesis

Viral replication occurs in the **monocyte/ macrophages in the infected tissues**, the majority of cells containing viral RNA do not produce infectious virus. The RNA genome integrates as provirus DNA into the infected cells. Virus disseminates to various organs like the **lungs, mammary glands, joints, lymph nodes, blood vessels and the brain.** After 2-8 weeks of virus replication, there occurs induction of immune response that fails to eliminate the virus. The virus replicates mainly in macrophages & pulmonary secretions & milk contain the infected macrophages & provide a source of infection to other susceptible animals. In these organs, the virus replicates in mature macrophages and induces slowly progressing inflammatory lesions containing B and T lymphocytes.. The persistence & virus replication in presence of antibodies lead to immune mediated lesions in various organs. In the lung there is gradual development of interstitial pneumonia, filling alveolar spaces. In the CNS, infiltration of lymphocytes occurs in the meninges & white matter. Similar infiltration occurs in the udder. The clinical signs of VISNA infection, i.e. dyspnea, loss of weight, mastitis and arthritis, are related to the location of these lesions.

Clinical symptoms and lesions

The **incubation period** for maedi is more than **two years,** & clinical signs appear when animals are 3 to 4r years old, the incubation period for visna is shorter, and symptoms are seen in sheep **as young as two years.**

Most VISNA infections are **asymptomatic**. The clinical signs are seen in several forms.

Maedi is the most common form in sheep, & show **wasting, progressive dyspnea and sometimes a dry cough**. Fever, bronchial exudates and depression are not usually seen. Maedi is lastly fatal; **death results from anoxia or secondary bacterial pneumonia.**

Visna occurs less frequently than maedi in sheep, but it is the more common form in goats. Visna initially show subtle neurologic signs such as hind-limb weakness, trembling of the lips or a head tilt, accompanied by loss of condition. The symptoms gradually progress to **ataxia, incoordination, muscle tremors, paresis and paraplegia**. Other neurological signs include blindness in rare cases. The clinical course can prolong for a year. Unattended animals usually die of inanition.

Slowly progressive arthritis is seen with severe lameness, or chronic indurative mastitis with decreased production of normal-appearing milk. Weight gain in lambs may be decreased due to low milk yields from dams with indurative mastitis.

Diagnosis

Infection with VISNA induces the formation of antibodies which can be detected by agar gel immunodiffusion, ELISA and the serum neutralization assay. Virus nucleic acid is detected by PCR assays, Southern blotting and *in situ* hybridization. PCR tests are used for rapid diagnosis.

Treatment & prevention

As **neither antiviral treatment nor vaccination** is available, diagnostic tests are the backbone of most of the schemes implemented to prevent the spread of the virus. Animals should be quarantined and tested before adding them to the herd; uninfected herds should also be kept away from contact with untested or seropositive herds. VISNA can be eradicated from a flock, or reduced in prevalence, by isolating lambs from seropositive dams immediately at birth & are raised on uninfected colostrum and pasteurized milk. The flock should also be tested frequently for MVV, and seronegative and seropositive sheep should be maintained separately.

□□□

Diagnosis

Infection with VISNA induces the formation of antibodies which can be detected by agar gel immunodiffusion, ELISA and the serum neutralization assay. Virus nucleic acid is detected by PCR assays, Southern blotting and in situ hybridization. PCR tests are used for rapid diagnosis.

Treatment & prevention

As neither antiviral treatment nor vaccination is available; diagnostic tests are the backbone of most of the schemes implemented to prevent the spread of the virus. Animals should be quarantined and tested before adding them to the herd; uninfected herds should also be kept away from contact with untested or seropositive herds. VISNA can be eradicated from a flock or reduced in prevalence, by isolating lambs from seropositive dams immediately at birth & are raised on uninfected colostrum and pasteurized milk. The flock should also be tested frequently for MVV, and seronegative and seropositive sheep should be maintained separately.

□□□

Chapter 33

Characteristics and Disease Caused by Group VII Hepadnaviruses (Family *Hepadnaviridae*:DNA-RT)

Contents

Characteristics of Hepadnaviruses

Hepadnaviruses (Hepar= liver, dna= DNA) of the family *Hepadnaviridae* are enveloped, spherical virions with a diameter of about 42 nm having an icosahedric capsid (T=4 capsid). Hepadnaviruses genome consists of **two uneven strands of DNA (partially ds & partially ss DNA, circular). (-) DNA strand is complete** & are 3-3.3 kb in size. **(+) DNA strand is** incomplete, is made of 1.7-2.8 kb. *Hepadnaviridae* has two recognized genera: Genus *Orthohepadnavirus*, type species: *Hepatitis B virus* & Genus *Avihepadnavirus*; type species: *Duck hepatitis virus.* Hepadnaviruses infect humans (the important hepatitis B virus), herons, ducks, woodchucks, squirrels & the virus has been recovered from other wild and domestic species such as geese, marsupials and orangutans. Hepadnaviruses are highly host specific & have a predilection for the liver and produce persistent infections.

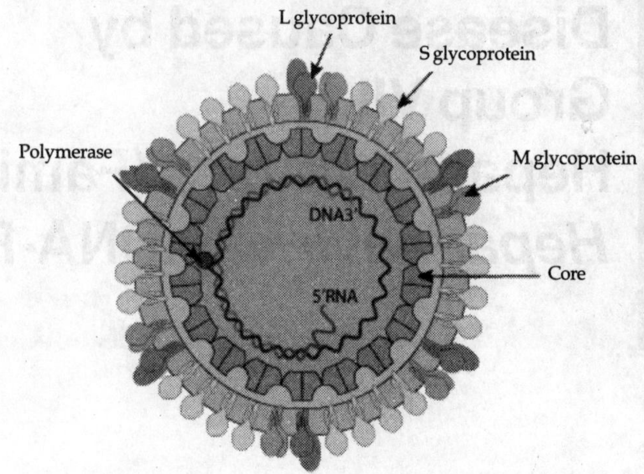

Figure 33.1 : Morphology of Hepadnavirus.

The Virus Genome Organization

Hepadnaviruses have very small genome & consists of **two uneven strands of DNA** (partially ds & partially ss DNA, circular). (-) DNA strand is complete & are 3-3.3 kb in size. (+) DNA strand is incomplete, & is made of 1.7-2.8 kb. Four main overlapping **open reading frames (ORFs)** include i. S or surface antige gene (includes Pre S) encodes the surface antigen HBs Ag. ii. P gene encodes the viral polymerase (P), iii. C or core protein gene (C/C2) encodes capsid proteins (HBcAg), & X gene encodes non-structural proteins whose .function and significance are poorly known. S gene transcribes 3 mRNAs surface antigens- pre S1, pre S2, and S (HBsAg).

C-ORF – encoding the core antigen and pre-core protein which are processed and secreted as HBcAg

S-ORF – codes for the surface antigen HBs Ag

P-ORF – encoding the viral polymerase

X ORF- encodes non structural proteins whose function is not fully understood

Hepadnaviruses fall in group VII ds DNA-RT, hence **replicate through an RNA intermediate**, which they transcribe back into cDNA using reverse transcriptase. The reverse transcriptase becomes covalently linked to a short 3- or 4-nucleotide primer. Most hepadnaviruses will only replicate in specific hosts, and this makes experiments using in vitro methods very difficult.

HBV is divided **into 8 genotypes, A to H differing in their nucleotide sequences & geographical distribution.**

Virus replication

Hepadnaviruses replicate in the cell nucleus. The virus binds to specific receptors on cells though major surface antigen, & the core particle enters the cell cytoplasm by unknown means. Then relaxed circular DNA (RC-DNA) is translocated to the nucleus. **In the nucleus the partially ds DNA is 'repaired' by the cell to form a** covalently closed complete circular DNA. It then undergoes **transcription by the host cell RNA polymerase II of the pregenomic RNA** (pgRNA) and subgenomic mRNAs, inducing synthesis of all the viral proteins by host cell ribosomes. Pregenomic RNA is encapsidated together with the P protein and reverse-transcribed inside the nucleocapsid in (-) DNA covalently linked to P protein. (+)DNA is synthesized from the (-) DNA template generating new cDNA. New RC-DNA is transported to the nucleus causing ds to covalently closed circular DNA amplification or alternatively, the RC-DNA containing nucleocapsids are enveloped and bud as virions. New virus particles acquire lipid from the endoplasmic reticulum of the host cell, and the genome is packaged within these particles, which then bud off from the cell. **Virus-infected cells translate the protein called as the virus surface antigen many times until there is too much protein to coat the virions formed.** These proteins then aggregate to form rod shapes, and it is this antigen, **known as the Australian or hepatitis B surface antigen, which is released from the cell and which leads to a very strong immune response from the host.**

Summary: The viruses replicate in the nucleus of hepatocytes > (-) DNA strand acts as a template > forms +RNA strand (full length) > +RNA is packaged into the viral core in the infected cell cytoplasm > viral reverse transcriptase copies ss (-) viral DNA strand from ss (+) RNA > + ssRNA is degraded > viral DNA pol II forms (+) DNA from (-) DNA template >± ds DNA is packaged into virion before full length +DNA is synthesized, thus (+) DNA remains incomplete.

Virus classification

Group; Group VII-Reverse transcribing dsDNA

Family: *Hepdnaviridae*

Genus1: *Orthohepadnavirus*, type species *Hepatitis B virus.* Other species within the genus include *Ground Squirrel Hepatitis B & Woodchuck Hepatitis B.*

Genus 2: *Avihepadnavirus*, type species: *Duck hepatitis virus.* Other species within the genus include *Heron hepatitis B virus* (HHBV), *Snow goose hepatitis*

B virus (SGHBV), *Ross Goose hepatitis B virus* (RGHBV) and *Stork hepatitis B virus* (SHBV).

Table 33.1 : Classification of the family *Hepadnaviridae* showing genera, species (Italized), serotypes & diseases caused by the members.

Genera	Species	Serotypes	Diseases caused
G1: *Orthohepad-navirus*	TS: *Hepatitis B virus*	HBV-A-H	**Hepatitis B virus** (HBV) infects the liver of humans, chimpanzees, gibbons, wooly monkeys and causes hepatitis. HBV is transmitted via exposure to infectious blood, body fluids containing blood, sexual contact, blood transfusion, reuse of infected needles & syringes and vertical transmission from mother to child. The CTL mediated host immune response & antigen- nonspecific inflam-matory cells cause both hepatocellular damage and viral clearance. **Acute infection leads to** acute viral hepatitis with ill-health, loss of appetite, nausea, vomiting, bodyache, mild fever, dark urine and then jaundice but gradually improves in most affected people. A few patients develop more severe liver disease, fulminant hepatic failure, and may die. The infection may be entirely asymptomatic. **Chronic infection** with HBV is either asymptomatic or chronic inflammation of the liver, chronic hepatitis leads to cirrhosis in several years & increases the incidence of hepatocellular carcinoma.
	Ground squirrel hepatitis virus	GSHV	*Ground squirrel hepatitis B virus* **(GSHBV)** rarely causes hepatitis or hepatocellular carcinoma. Disease occurs in squirrels in northern California - the Beechey squirrels. It is interesting that other breeds of squirrels are not susceptible or do not develop quite in the same progression.
	Woodchuk hepatitis virus	WHV	*Woodchuck hepatitis B virus* (WHBV) causes acute hepatitis & usually hepato-cellular carcinoma but not cirrhosis. Wood-chucks chronically infected with

			WHV develop progressively severe hepatitis and hepatocellular carcinoma, with similar lesions to that of HBV infection in humans.
	Wooly monkey hepatitis B virus	WMHBV	Asymptomatic Carrier State, hepatitis, hepatocellular carcinoma.
G 2: *Avihepadna-virus*	*Duck hepatitis B virus*	DHBV	*Duck hepatitis B virus* **(DHBV)** causes natural infection of Anas species ducks (not Muscovy ducks), acquired congenitally; produces chronic viremia but is not of economic importance.
	Heron hepatitis B virus	HHBV	
	Stork hepatitis B virus	STHBV	

Hepadnavirus Clinical Infections in Humans, Animal and Birds

Genus: Orthohepadnavirus

Hepatitis B virus **(HBV)** infects the liver of humans, chimpanzees, gibbons, wooly monkeys and causes hepatitis. The disease has caused epidemics in parts of Asia & Africa & is endemic in China. The virus is divided into **4 major serotypes-adr, adw, ayr, & ayw** based on envelop protein antigenic epitopes, and into **8 genotypes (A-H)** as per the nucleotide sequence variation of the genome.

Transmission

HBV is transmitted via exposure to infectious blood, body fluids containing blood, sexual contact, blood transfusion, reuse of infected needles & syringes, and vertical transmission from mother to child during childbirth. HBV can be transmitted between family members within households, possibly by contact of nonintact skin or mucous membrane with secretions or saliva containing HBV.

Pathogenesis

HBV interferes with the functions of the liver by replicating in liver cells, hepatocytes. HBV virions (DANE particle) bind to the host cell via the preS domain of the viral surface antigen, PreS and IgA receptors, & cellular receptors for HBV may also exist on extrahepatic cells. During HBV infection, the host immune response causes both hepatocellular damage and viral clearance. Virus-specific cytotoxic T lymphocytes (CTLs) contributes to most of the liver injury, CTLs eliminate HBV infection by killing infected cells and producing antiviral cytokines, which are then used to purge HBV from viable hepatocytes. Although liver damage is initiated and mediated by the CTLs, Ag- nonspecific inflammatory cells worsen CTL-induced immunopathology, and platelets activated at the site of infection may facilitate the accumulation of CTLs in the liver.

Acute infection with HBV causes acute viral hepatitis with ill-health, loss of appetite, nausea, vomiting, bodyache, mild fever, dark urine, and then jaundice lasting for a few weeks and then gradually improves in most affected people. A few patients may have more severe liver disease, fulminant hepatic failure, and may die as a result of it. The infection may be entirely asymptomatic and may go unrecognized.

Chronic infection with HBV is either asymptomatic or chronic inflammation of the liver; chronic hepatitis leads to cirrhosis in several years, & increases the incidence of hepatocellular carcinoma.

Genus : *Orthohepadnavirus*

Woodchuck hepatitis B virus **(WHBV)** causes acute hepatitis & usually hepatocellular carcinoma but not cirrhosis. Woodchucks chronically infected with WHV develop progressively severe hepatitis and hepatocellular carcinoma, with similar lesions to that of HBV **infection** in humans.

Ground squirrel hepatitis B virus **(GSHBV)** rarely causes hepatitis or hepatocellular carcinoma. Disease occurs in squirrels in northern California - the Beechey squirrels. It is interesting that other breeds of squirrels are not susceptible or do not develop quite in the same progression.

Genus : *Avihepadnavirus*

Duck hepatitis B virus (DHBV) causes natural infection of Anas species ducks (not Muscovy ducks), acquired congenitally; produces chronic viremia but is not of economic importance.

□□□

Chapter 34

Characteristics and Diseases Caused by Prion Proteins

Contents

Characteristics of Prions

Prions, collectively called **transmissible spongiform encephalopathies (TSE)** cause neurodegenerative diseases in humans & many animal species by forming aggregates extracellularly in CNS called **plaques or amyloid fibrils**, which disrupt the normal tissue structure, form holes or vacuoles in the neurons tissue giving spongy architecture, astrogliosis, absence of an inflammatory reaction & immune responses, very long incubation period (years), but after symptoms appear the disease progresses rapidly, leading to brain damage with clinical symptoms of behavioural or personality changes, weight loss, convulsion, dementia, ataxia and death. **Prion is used for several, unique group of neurodegenerative diseases, which induce spongiform degeneration in the grey matter of brain, & is fatal**, Prion diseases include **scrapie** of sheep & goat, **bovine spongiform encephalopathy (BSE), feline spongiform encephalopathy (FSE), transmissible mink encephalopathy** (TME), **chronic wasting dsease(CWD)** of White-tailed deer, elk mule &**exotic ungulate encephalopathy (EUE)** of nyalaoryx, & greater kudu, & human diseases- **Kuru & Creutzfeldt Jacob disease**.

The name **Prion** was coined in **1982 by Stanley B. Prusiner from** proteinaceous infection particle. Prusiner was awarded the Noble Prize in Physiology or Medicine in 1997 for his research into prions. While the infectious agent was named prion, the specific protein that the prion was composed of is also known as the **Prion Protein (PrP)**, though this protein occur both in infectious and non-infectious forms. The protein that prions are made of (PrP) is found throughout the body, even in healthy people and animals. However, PrP found in infectious material has a different structure and is **resistant to proteases**, the enzymes in the body that can normally break down proteins. **The normal form of the protein** is called **PrP^C** (C refers to 'cellular' or 'common' PrP), while the infectious form is called **PrP^{Sc}** (*Sc* refers to **srapie**, a prion disease occurring in sheep). **PrP^C** is structurally well-defined but **PrP^{Sc}** is certainly polydspers and defined at a relatively poor level. PrP can be induced to fold into other more-or-less well-defined isoforms in vitro, and their relationship to the form(s) that are pathogenic in vivo is not yet clear. **All known prion diseases affect the structure of the brain or other neural tissue and all are currently untreatable and universally fatal**. Prions are propagated by **transmitting a misfolded protein state**. When a prion enters a healthy organism, it induces existing, properly-folded proteins to convert into the disease-associated, prion form; the **prion acts as a template to guide the misfolding of more protein into**

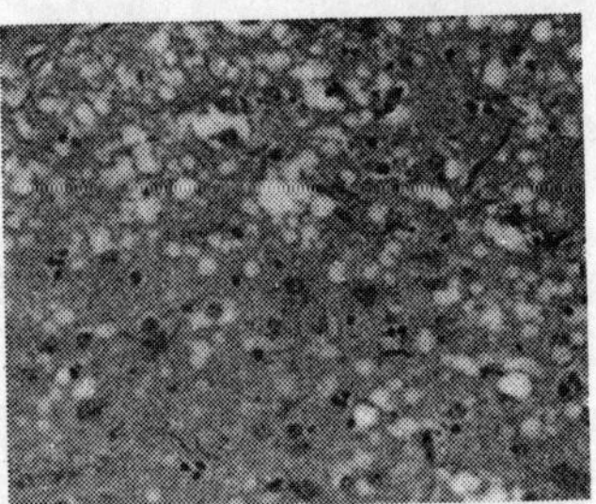

Microscopic "holes" are characteristicsin prion-affected tissue sections, causing the tissue to develop a "spongy" architecture.

prion form. These newly-formed prions can then go on to convert more prion proteins, thus triggers a chain reaction that produces large amounts of the prion form. **All known prions induce the formation of an amyloid fold**, in which the protein polymerises into an aggregate consisting of **tightly packed β sheets**. Amyloid aggregates are fibrils, growing at their ends, and replicating when breakage causes two growing ends to become four growing ends. The incubation perid of prion diseases is determined by the exponential growth associated with prion replication. Prions are proteinaceous particles derived from normal cell membrane glycoproteins, PrPc. They are unconventional because they **are devoid of nucleic acid, are non immunogenic, resistant to heat, chemical & irradiation & are stable at wide range of pH.**

PrP^C: The normal protein is called **PrP^C** (c= cellular), is a transmembrane glycoprotein normally found at the surface of certain cells, e.g., neural and hematopoietic stem cells, its **secondary structure is dominated by alpha helices**, is easily soluble, is easily digested by proteases, & is encoded by a gene called in humans ***PRNP* located on our chromosome 20.**

PrP^C has 209 amino acids (in humans), one disulfide bond, a molecular weight of 35-36 kDa and made of mainly α-helix structure. Several topological forms exist; one cell surface form anchored via glycoprotein and two transmembrane forms. The normal protein is not sedimentable; meaning it cannot be separated by centrifuging techniques.

PrP^C binds copper (II) ions with high affinity. The significance of this finding is not clear, but it presumably relates to PrP structure or function. PrP^C is readily digested by proteases K and can be liberated from the cell surface in vitro by the enzyme phosphoinositide phospholipase (PI-PLC), which cleaves the glycophosphatidylinositol (GPI) glycolipid anchor. PrP^C has been reported to play important roles in cell-cell adhesion, intracellular signaling *in vivo*, and may therefore be involved in cell-cell communication in the brain.

PrP^{Sc}: The abnormal, disease-producing protein is called PrP^{Sc} (Sc =scrapie), has the same amino acid sequence as the normal protein; that is, their primary structure is identical, but its **secondary structure is dominated by beta conformation**, is insoluble in all but the strongest solvents, & is highly resistant to digestion by proteases. **When PrP^{Sc} comes in contact with PrP^C**, it converts the PrP^C into more of PrP^{Sc}, even in the test tube. These molecules bind to each other forming aggregates. It is not yet clear if these aggregates are themselves the cause of the cell damage or are simply a side effect of the underlying disease process. PrP^{Sc} is the infectious isofom of **PrP^C**, is able to convert normal PrP^C proteins into the infectious isoform by changing their conformation, or shape; this, in turn, alters the way the proteins interconnect.

Although the exact 3D structure of PrP^{Sc} is not known, it has a higher proportion of β-sheet structure in place of the normal α-helix structure. **Aggregations of these abnormal isoforms form highly structured amyloid fibers**, which accumulate to form plaques. The end of each fiber acts as a template onto which free protein molecules may attach, allowing the fiber to grow. Only **PrP^{C}** molecules with an identical amino acid sequence to the infectious PrP^{Sc} are incorporated into the growing fiber.

Prion Diseases

Prion diseases are transmissible from host to host of a single species and, sometimes, even from one species to another (such as a laboratory animal), destroy brain tissue giving it a spongy appearance, & for these reasons, prion diseases are also called **transmissible spongiform encephalopathies** or **TSEs**. Before the victim dies of a TSE, the damage to the brain is reflected in such signs as loss of coordination and, in humans' dementia. **Injection of ground-up brain tissue from an animal or human patient with a prion disease into another animal transmits the disease**. This suggests that the disease is caused by an infectious agent such as a virus. But viruses have a genome and despite intense efforts, no evidence of a virus has ever been found in these brain extracts. In fact, treating the extracts with agents e.g., UV light that destroy DNA does not reduce their infectiousness. To date, the evidence indicates that the infectious agent in the TSEs is a protein.

It turns out that prions are molecules of a normal body protein that have **changed their three-dimensional configuration. Prions cause neurodegenerative disease by aggregating extracellularly within the CNS to form plaques known as amyloid, which disrupt the normal tissue structure**. This disruption is characterized by "holes" in the tissue with resultant spongy architecture due to the vacuole formation in the neurons. Other histological changes include astrogliosis and the absence of an inflammatory reaction. While the incubation period for prion diseases is generally quite long, once symptoms appear the disease progresses rapidly, leading to brain damage and death. Neurodegenerative symptoms can include **convulsions, dementia, ataxia (balance and coordination dysfunction), and behavioural or personality changes.**

All known prion diseases, collectively called *transmissible spongiform encephalopathies* (TSEs), **are untreatable and fatal**. A vaccine has been developed in mice, however, that may provide insight into providing a vaccine in humans to resist prion infections. Additionally, in 2006 scientists announced that they had genetically engineered cattle lacking a necessary gene for prion production, thus theoretically making them immune to BSE, building on research indicating that mice lacking normally occurring prion protein are resistant to infection by scrapie prion protein.

Many different mammalian species can be affected by prion diseases, as the prion protein (PrP) is very similar in all mammals. Due to small differences in PrP between different species, it is unusual for a prion disease to be transmitted from one species to another. The human prion disease variant Creutzfeldt-Jakob disease, however, is believed to be caused by a prion which typically infects cattle, causing Bovine spongiform encephalopathy and is transmitted through infected meat.

Various hypothesis

Protein hypothesis: Prior to the discovery of prions, it was thought that all pathogens used nuclei acid to direct their replication. The "protein hypothesis" states that a protein structure can replicate without the use of nucleic acid. This was initially controversial as it contradicts the so-called **"central dogma of molecular biology"**, which describes nucleic acid as the central form of replicative information.

Evidence in favor of a protein hypothesis includes:

No virus particles, bacteria, or fungi have been conclusively associated with prion diseases, although *Saccharomyces cerevisiae* has been known to be associated with infectious, yet non-lethal prions, such as Sup35p.

No nucleic acid has been conclusively associated with infectivity; agent is resistant to ultraviolet radiation, & induces no immune response to infection. PrP^{Sc} experimentally transmitted between one species and another results in PrP^{Sc} with the amino-acid sequence of the recipient species, suggesting that replication of the donor agent does not occur. Familial prion disease occurs in families with a mutation in the PrP gene, and mice with PrP mutations develop prion disease despite controlled conditions where transmission is prevented. Animals lacking PrP^{C} do not contract prion disease. Infectious prions can be formed *de novo* from purified non-infectious components, in the absence of gene-coding nucleic acids.

Genetic factors: A gene for the normal protein has been identified in humans called the **PRNP gene**. In all inherited cases of prion disease, there is a mutation in the *PRNP* gene. Many different *PRNP* mutations have been identified and it is thought that the mutations somehow make PrP^{C} more likely to change spontaneously into the abnormal PrP^{Sc} form. Although this discovery puts a hole in the general prion hypothesis, that prions can only aggregate proteins of identical amino acid make up. These mutations can occur throughout the gene. Some mutations involve expansion of the octapeptide repeat region at the N-terminal of PrP. Other mutations that have been identified as a cause of inherited prion disease occur at positions 102, 117 & 198 (GSS), 178, 200, 210 & 232 (CJD) and 178 (Fatal Familial Insomnia, FFI). The cause of prion disease can be sporadic, genetic, and infectious, or a combination of these factors. For example, in order to have scrapie, both an infectious agent and a susceptible genotype need to be present.

Multi-component hypothesis: In 2007, biochemist Surachai Supattapone and his colleagues at Dartmouth College produced purified infectious prions *de novo* from defined components (PrP^{C}, co-purified lipids, and a synthetic polyanionic molecule). These researchers also showed that the polyanionic molecule required for prion formation was selectively incorporated into high-affinity complexes with PrP molecules, leading them to hypothesize that infectious prions may be composed of multiple host components, including PrP, lipid, and polyanionic molecules, rather than PrP^{Sc} alone.

In 2010, Jiyan Ma and colleagues at The Ohio State University produced infectious prions from a recipe of bacterially expressed recombinant PrP, POPG phospholipid, and RNA, further supporting the multi-component hypothesis. This finding is in contrast to studies that found minimal infectious prions produced from recombinant PrP alone.

*Viral hypothesis:*The protein-only hypothesis has been criticized by those who feel that the simplest explanation of the evidence to date is viral. For more than a decade, Yale University neuropathologist Laura Manuelidis has been proposing that prion diseases are caused instead by an unidentified slow virus. In January 2007, she and her colleagues published an article reporting to have found a virus in 10%, or less, of their scrapie-infected cells in culture.

The virion hypothesis states that TSEs are caused by a replicable informational molecule (which is likely to be a nucleic acid) bound to PrP. Many TSEs, including scrapie and BSE, show strains with specific and distinct biological properties, a feature which supporters of the virion hypothesis feel is not explained by prions.

Evidence in favor of a viral hypothesis includes:

Strain variation: differences in prion infectivity, incubation, symptomology and progression among species resemble that seen between viruses, especially RNA.

The long incubation and rapid onset of symptoms resemble lentiviruses, such as HIV-induced AIDS. Viral-like particles that do not appear to be composed of PrP have been found in some of the cells of scrapie- or CJD-infected cell lines.

Recent studies propagating TSE infectivity in cell-free reactions and in purified component chemical reactions strongly suggest against TSE viral nature. More recently, using a similar defined recipe of multiple components (PrP, POPG lipid, RNA), Jiyan Ma and colleagues generated infectious prions from recombinant PrP expressed from *E. coli*, casting further doubt on the viral hypothesis.

Possible basis of species specificity of prions: A particular **PrP^{Sc}** can only convert **PrP^{C}** molecules of the same or at least similar primary structure. This requirement of "like-with-like" resides in a short sequence at the N-terminal of the protein (rather like an antibody epitope).

Yeasts engineered to form two types of prion form two types of "pure" aggregates within the cell. Even in the test tube, each type of prion finds and aggregates with others of its own type.

So the picture that emerges is that a molecule of **PrP^{Sc}** acts as a seed providing a template for converting **PrP^{C}** to more **PrP^{Sc}**. These interact with each other to form small soluble aggregates. These interact with each other to form large insoluble deposits.

Although only a small portion of the prion protein is responsible for its specificity, other parts of the molecule are needed for flipping the molecule from the alpha-helical to the beta conformation. All prion proteins contain tracts of repeated Gln-Asn residues which appear to be essential for the conversion process.

Transmission: It has been recognized that prion diseases can arise in three different ways: **acquired, familial, or sporadic**. It is often assumed that the diseased form directly interacts with the normal form to make it rearrange its structure. One idea, the "Protein X" hypothesis, is that an as-yet unidentified cellular protein (Protein X) enables the conversion of PrP^{C} to PrP^{Sc} by bringing a molecule of each of the two together into a complex.

Current research suggests that the primary method of infection in animals is **through ingestion**. It is thought that prions may be deposited in the environment through the **remains of dead animals and via urine, saliva, and other body fluids**. They may then linger in the soil by binding to clay and other minerals.

A University of Californian research team, led by Nobel prize winner Stanley Prusiner, has proven that infection can **occur from prions in manure**. Since manure is present in many areas surrounding water reservoirs, as well as used on many crop fields, it raises the **possibility of widespread transmission**. It was reported in January 2011 that researchers had discovered **prions spreading through airborne transmission on aerosol particles**, in an animal testing experiment focusing on scrapie infection in laboratory mice.

Preliminary evidence supporting the notion that prions can be transmitted through **use of urine-derived human menopausal gonadotrpin**, administered for the treatment of infertility, was published in 2011.

Pathogenesis of prion diseases: The unique feature of prion diseases is that they are **self-propagating and transmissible.** Once PrP^{TSE} is generated endogenously or introduced into the body from the environment, it converts normal PrP^{c} into abnormal ones. This conversion begins with the initial production of a **small polymer of misfolded prions, (a seed)**, perhaps no more than 28 molecules. This seed converts normal adjacent PrP^{c} into abnormal ones by an unknown mechanism. As more PrP^{TSE} polymers are produced, they, in turn, act as seeds, propagating the conversion of normal to abnormal prions. During the incubation period and active clinical phase of prion diseases, PrP^{TSE} is probably present (and can transmit the disease) in all tissues and body fluids, especially brain, nerves, and skeletal muscle. **Pathology develops only in the brain.** Initially, intracytoplasmic vacuoles appear in neurons. As the disease progresses, vacuolization becomes more pronounced and the cortical neuropil develops a spongy appearance, hence the term **spongiform encephalopathy**. In a process PrP^{Sc} has the ability to convert the normal prion protein, PrP^{C}, into more PrP^{Sc}. This abnormal protein builds up in the brain, forming clumps/ plaques that damage or destroys nerve cells. The loss of these cells creates microscopic sponge-like holes in the brain, which leads to the signs and symptoms of prion disease.

Sterilization: Infectious particles possessing nucleic acid are dependent upon it to direct their continued replication. Prions, however, are infectious by their effect on normal versions of the protein. **Sterilizing prions therefore involves the denaturation of the protein to a state where the molecule is no longer able to induce the abnormal folding of normal proteins.** Prions are generally quite resistant to proteases, heat, radiation, and formalin treatments, although their infectivity can be reduced by such treatments. Effective prion decontamination relies upon **protein hydrolysis or reduction or destruction of protein tertiary structure.** Examples include bleach, caustic soda, and strong acidic detergents such as LpH. 134°C (274°F) for 18 minutes in a pressurized steam autoclve may not be enough to deactivate the agent of disease. **Ozone sterilization** is currently being studied as a potential method for prion **denatures and deactivation.** Renaturation of a completely denatured prion to infectious status has not yet been achieved, however partially denatured prions can be renatured to an infective status under certain artificial conditions.

The WHO recommends any of the following three procedures for the sterilization of all heat-resistant surgical instruments to ensure that they are not contaminated with prions:

1. Immerse in a pan containing 1NNaOH and heat in a gravity-displacement autoclave at 121°C for 30 minutes; clean; rinse in water; and then perform routine sterilization processes.

2. Immerse in 1N NaOH or sodium hypochloride (20,000 parts per million available chlorine) for 1 hour; transfer instruments to water; heat in a gravity-displacement autoclave at 121°C for 1 hour; clean; and then perform routine sterilization processes.
3. Immerse in 1N NaOH or sodium hypochlorite (20,000 parts per million available chlorine) for 1 hour; remove and rinse in water, then transfer to an open pan and heat in a gravity-displacement (121°C) or in a porous-load (134°C) autoclave for 1 hour; clean; and then perform routine sterilization processes.

Evidence that prions are a "protein-only" phenomenon: A few molecules of a **PrP^{Sc}** form of the Sup35 protein, when introduced into yeast cells, convert the yeast cell's own Sup35 protein into prion aggregates. The resulting disease phenotype is then passed on to the cell's daughters. Yeast can be cured of their prion disease by increasing the activity of their chaperones. Presumably the chaperone helps maintain the folded state (with alpha helices) of the protein. When the gene for the glucocorticoid receptor is altered to include sequences coding for one part (domain) of the Sup35 protein, the resulting protein forms prions and produces an entirely new phenotype.

There are 4 types of prion diseases:

1. *Inherited prion diseases:* Include Creutzfeldt-Jacob disease (CJD), Gerstmann-Straussler-Scheinker disease (GSS), & Fatal familial insomnia (FFI)
2. *Infectious prion diseases:* Include scrapie, Kuru, bovine spongiform encephalopathy (BSE) or Mad cow disease,Creutzfeldt-Jacob disease (CJD), variant Creutzfeldt-Jacob disease (vCJD) & miscellaneous infectious prion diseases like feline spongiform encephalopathy (FSE) , Transmissible mink encephalopathy (TME) & chronic wasting disease (CWD) seen in North America in elk and mule deer in the Rocky Mountains of the U.S.
3. *Sporadic prion diseases:* Include **Creutzfeldt-Jacob disease** (CJD) and Familial fatal insomnis (FFI) that occasionally occur in people who have no family history of the disease and no known exposure to infectious prions. The cause of their disease is uncertain.
4. *Prions in Yeast:* Two proteins in yeast (*Saccharomyces cerevisiae*)- the Sup35 protein (Sup35p) and the Ure2 protein (Ure2p) are able to form prions, & they can exist either in a **PrP^{C}**-like form that is functional or in a **PrP^{Sc}**-like form that is not.

With all of these diseases, there is evidence that their amyloid-forming proteins, like PrP^{Sc}, **can act as a seed converting a correctly-folded protein**

into an incorrectly-folded one; have this effect spread from neuron to neuron in the brain. However, they do not seem to be able to be spread from person to person (unlike the TSEs). Perhaps this is because they are not so them. Furthermore, this binding blocks the ability of the proteasomes to process other proteins that are normal candidates for destruction. Because of the critical role of proteasomes in many cell functions, such as mitosis, it is easy to see why this action leads to death of the cell.

Transmissible spongiform encephalopathies of humans & animals

Table 34.1 : Diseases caused by prion proteins

Disease	Animal affected	Description
Scrapie	Sheep, goats	**Scrapie** is a non febrile, chronic, fatal, degenerative disease of sheep & goats characterized clinically by a long incubation period, pruritis, altered gait, involvement of CNS & convulsive collapse. Scrapie is caused by **prion protein, PrP^{Sc}** & is related to BSE or "mad cow disease, FSE and chronic wasting disease of deer. Scrapie has been known since the 18th century (1732) and does not appear to be transmissible to humans. The name scrapie is derived from the clinical signs of the condition, wherein affected animals scrape off their fleece against rocks, trees or fences. The disease apparently causes an itching sensation in the animals, lip-smacking, altered gaits, and convulsive collapse.
Bovine spongiform encephalopathy (BSE) or mad cow disease	Cattle	**Bovine spongiform encephalopathy (BSE)**, also called **mad-cow disease**, is a afebrile, subacute, fatal neurodegenerative disease in adult cattle of 4-5 years, all breeds being susceptible, causes a vacuolation of grey matter, neurophil & neuronal perikaya, neuronal spongy degeneration in the brain and gliosis with a long incubation period, 30 months to 8 years.
Transmissible mink encephalopathy (TME)	Mink	**Transmissible mink encephalopathy (TME)** is rare sporadic disease that affects the CNS of ranch-raised adult mink. Clinical signs include the

		characteristic behavioural changes such as confusion, loss of cleanliness, and aimless circling. Affected animals show signs of weight loss, matted fur, hind quarter ataxia and arching its tail over its back; seizures may rarely occur & at last stages, there are signs of drowsiness and unresponsiveness.
Feline spongiform encephalopathy (FSE)	Cat	**Feline spongiform encephalopathy (FSE)** is a disease that affects the brains and livers of domestic and captive feline. FSE is thought to be related to BSE. Lezmi S. et al. (2003), suggested that this infectious agent might be spread by both hematogenous & nervous pathways. Like BSE, this disease can take several years to develop. Probably the affected animals contract the disease by eating contaminated bovine meat. Ataxia was observed to last for about 8 weeks in the affected animals. The ultimate result is death of the infected animals.
Chronic wasting disease (CWD)	White-tailed deer, elk, mule, deer, moose	**Chronic wasting disease** (CWD) is a transmissible spongiform encephalopathy (TSE) of mule, deer, White-tailed deer, elk, & moose. To date, CWD has been found mainly in cervids (members of the deer family). First recognized as a **clinical "wasting" syndrome** in 1967 in mule deer in a wildlife research facility in northern Colarado, USA, it was identified as a TSE in 1978 and has spread to a dozen states and two Canadian provinces. CWD is manifested by **chronic weight loss leading to death.** There is no known relationship between CWD and any other TSE of animals or people.
Exotic ungulate encephalopathy (EUE)	Nyala, oryx, greater kudu	**Exotic ungulate encephalopathy is a** Transmissible spongiform encephalopathy (TSE), identified in infected organs of zoo animals like Nyala, Arabian & Scimitar oryx, greater kudu, gemsbok, the common eland, Ankole-Watusi cow & an American bison in UK.

		Transmission probably occurred via the consumption of feed supplemented with meat & bone meal, although some animals died after the British ban on ground offal in animal feed. All animals died during the 1990s, with the last death occurring in 1998.
Spongiform encephalopathy	Ostrich	Spongiform encephalopathy, but is has been shown to be transmissible.
Creutzfeldt–Jacob disease (CJD)	Humans	**Creutzfeldt-Jakob disease (CJD)** is a rare, degenerative, invariably fatal brain isorder, showing in the early stage symptoms of failing memory, behavioral changes, lack of coordination and visual disturbances. As the illness progresses, mental deterioration becomes pronounced and involuntary ovements, blindness, weakness of extremities, and coma may occur. CJD affects about one person in every one million people per year worldwide, usually appears in later life and runs a rapid course.
Variant Creutzfeldt -Jacob disease (vCJD)	Humans	Variant Creutzfeldt -Jacob disease **(vCJD)** human disorder appeared some years after the epidemic of BSE or Mad cow disease in UK through the cattle herds in Great Britain. Even though the cow and human *PRNP* genes differ at 30 codons, the sequence of their prions suggests that these patients (155 by 2005) acquired the disease from eating contaminated beef.
Familial Creutzfeldt -Jacob disease (fCJD)	Humans	**Familial Creutzfeldt -Jacob disease (fCJD)**: 10–15% of the cases are inherited; that is, the patient comes from a family in which the disease has appeared before. The disease is inherited as an autosomal **dominant**. The patients have inherited at least one copy of a mutated *PRNP* gene. Some of the most common mutations are: a change in codon 200 converting glutamic acid (E) at that position to

		lysine (K), designated "E200K", a change from aspartic acid (D) at position 178 in the protein to asparagine (D178N) when it is accompanied by a polymor phism in both *PRNP* genes that encodes valine at position 129.
Sporadic Creutzfeldt -Jacob disease (sCJD)	Humans	**Sporadic Creutzfeldt -Jacob diseases CJD** occurs in people who have no family history of the disease. Perhaps a spontaneous somatic mutation has occurred in one of the *PRNP* genes in a cell. Perhaps their normal PrP^{C} protein has spontaneously converted into the PrP^{Sc} form or perhaps the victims were simply unknowingly exposed to infectious prions, and sporadic prion diseases do not exist! All the cases are found in people with a susceptibility polymorphism in their *PRNP* gene.
Gerstmann-Straussrtar/Scheinker syndrome (GSS)	Humans	**Gerstmann-Straussrtar/ Scheinker syndrome (GSS)** is caused by the the inheritance of a *PRNP* gene with a mutations encoding most commonly: leucine instead of proline at position 102 (P102L) or valine instead of alanine at position 117 (A117V). Again, the disease is also strongly associated with homozygosity for a polymorphism at position 129 (both residues being methionine).
Fatal familial insomnia (FFI)	Humans	**Fatal familial insomnia (FFI)** people with this rare disorder have inherited a *PRNP* gene with asparagine instead of aspartic acid encoded at position 178 (D178N), & the susceptibility polymorphism of methionine at position 129 of the *PRNP* genes. Extracts from autopsied brains of FFI victims can transmit the disease to transgenic mice.
Kuru	Humans	**Kuru** was once found among the Fore tribe in Papua New Guinea whose rituals included eating the brain tissue of recently deceased members of the tribe. Since this practice was halted, the

disease has disappeared. Before then, the disease was studied by transmitting it to chimpanzees using injections of autopsied brain tissue from human victim.

Prion Diseases in Humans

Creutzfeldt-Jakob disease (CJD) is a rare, degenerative, invariably fatal brain disorder, showing in the early stage symptoms of failing memory, behavioral changes, lack of coordination and visual disturbances. As the illness progresses, mental deterioration becomes pronounced and involuntary movements, blindness, weakness of extremities, and coma may occur. CJD affects about one person in every one million people per year worldwide, usually appears in later life and runs a rapid course. Typically, onset of symptoms occurs about age 60, and about 90% die within 1 year. A number of humans have acquired CJD through accidental exposure to material contaminated with CJD prions. Grafts of duramater taken from patients with inherited CJD have transmitted the disease to more than 100 recipients. Corneal transplants have also inadvertently transmitted CJD.

Instruments used in brain surgery on patients with CJD have transmitted the disease to other patients. Two years after their supposed sterilization, these instruments remained infectious.

Over 100 people have acquired CJD from injections of human growth hormone (HGH) or human gonadotropins prepared from pooled pituitary glands that inadvertently included glands taken from humans with CJD. By 2009, the death toll among French children receiving contaminated HGH reached 116.

As both HGH and human gonadotropins are available through recombinant DNA technology, such infections need never recur.

Variant Creutzfeldt–Jacob disease(vCJD) human disorder appeared some years after the epidemic of BSE or Mad cow disease through the cattle herds in Great Britain. Even though the cow and human *PRNP* genes differ at 30 codons, the sequence of their prions suggests that these patients (155 by 2005) acquired the disease from eating contaminated beef. All the patients are homozygous for the susceptibility polymorphism of methionine at position 129. The BSE epidemic has waned, and slaughter techniques that allow cattle nervous tissue in beef for human consumption have been banned since 1989.

Familial Creutzfeldt –Jacob disease (fCJD): 10–15% of the cases are inherited; that is, the patient comes from a family in which the disease has appeared before. The disease is inherited as an autosomal **dominant**.

The patients have inherited at least one copy of a mutated *PRNP* gene. Some of the most common mutations are: a change in codon 200 converting glutamic acid (E) at that position to lysine (K), designated "E200K", a change from aspartic acid (D) at position 178 in the protein to asparagine (D178N) when it is accompanied by a polymorphism in both *PRNP* genes that encodes valine at position 129. When the polymorphism at codon 129 is Met on both genes, the D178N mutation produces Fatal familial insomnia, change from valine (V) at position 210 to isoleucine (V210I). Extracts of autopsied brain tissue from these patients can transmit the disease to apes (whose *PRNP* gene is probably almost identical to that of humans). Transgenic mice, which have been given a *Prnp* gene that contains part of the human sequence, contract the disease. These results lead to the important realization that prion diseases can only be transmitted to animals that already carry a *PRNP* gene with a sequence that is at least similar to the one that encoded the **PrP^{Sc}**. In fact, knockout mice with no *Prnp* genes at all cannot be infected by PrP^{Sc}.

Sporadic Creutzfeldt -Jacob disease sCJD occurs in people who have no family history of the disease. Perhaps a spontaneous somatic mutation has occurred in one of the *PRNP* genes in a cell. Perhaps their normal PrP^C protein has spontaneously converted into the PrP^{Sc} form. Or perhaps the victims were simply unknowingly exposed to infectious prions, and sporadic prion diseases do not exist! All the cases are found in people with a susceptibility polymorphism in their *PRNP* gene.

Gerstmann-Straussrtar/Scheinker syndrome (GSS) is caused by the inheritance of a *PRNP* gene with a mutations encoding most commonly: leucine instead of proline at position 102 (P102L) or valine instead of alanine at position 117 (A117V). Again, the disease is also strongly associated with homozygosity for a polymorphism at position 129 (both residues being methionine). Brain extracts from patients with GSS can transmit the disease to monkeys and apes, & to transgenic mice containing a portion of the human *PRNP* gene. Transgenic mice expressing the P102L gene develop the disease spontaneously.

Fatal familial insomnia (FFI) People with this rare disorder have inherited a *PRNP* gene with asparagine instead of aspartic acid encoded at position 178 (D178N), & the susceptibility polymorphism of methionine at position 129 of the *PRNP* genes. Extracts from autopsied brains of FFI victims can transmit the disease to transgenic mice.

Kuru was once found among the Fore tribe in Papua New Guinea whose rituals included eating the brain tissue of recently deceased members of the tribe. Since this practice was halted, the disease has disappeared. Before then, the disease was studied by transmitting it to chimpanzees using injections of autopsied brain tissue from human victim.

Prion Diseases in Animals

SCRAPIE

Scrapie is a non febrile, chronic, fatal, degenerative disease of sheep & goats characterized clinically by a **long incubation period, pruritis, altered gait, involvement of CNS & convulsive collapse.** The name scrapie is derived from the clinical signs of the condition, wherein affected animals scrape off their fleece against rocks, trees or fences. The disease apparently causes an itching sensation in the animals, lip-smacking, altered gaits, and convulsive collapse.

Etiology: Scrapie is caused by **prion protein, PrP^{Sc}** & is related to BSE or "mad cow disease, FSE and chronic wasting disease of deer. Scrapie has been known since the 18th century (1732) and does not appear to be transmissible to humans. There are > 15 strains of scrapie. The Nor98 form of scrapie was first reported from Norway in 1998. Since 2002, Nor98 and other atypical scrapie agents have been detected in a number of European countries. Nor98 was diagnosed for the first time in U.S. sheep in March 2007.

Occurrence

Scrapie is found worldwide, reported in Europe (including the United Kingdom), the Middle East, Japan, Canada, the United States, Kenya, South Africa, Columbia and parts of Asia but Australia and New Zealand have remained free of scrapie. Although outbreaks occurred in these two countries, the disease was eradicated by slaughtering the imported sheep and their flockmates soon after they were released from quarantine.

Hosts susceptible

Scrapie affects sheep, goats, and moufflon (*Ovis musimon*). Rats, mice, hamsters, monkeys and a variety of other laboratory and wild animals can be infected experimentally. The Nor98 form of scrapie has been reported in sheep and goats.

Transmission

Scrapie transmission is best understood in sheep. Infected animals **carry the scrapie prion for life**, and can transmit the agent even if they remain asymptomatic. Most animals become infected from their dam, either at or soon after birth. In genetically susceptible, infected ewes, prions may be found in the reproductive tract, including the **placenta,** during pregnancy. These ewes can produce either prion-positive or prion-negative placentas, depending on the genotype of the fetus. Neonatal animals become infected when they lick or ingest fetal membranes and fluids. In confined lambing areas, the disease can also spread to the offspring of uninfected sheep. Uninfected adult ewes may be infected from this source, although they are more resistant. Current evidence suggests that **transmission mainly occurs after birth.**

Transmission can also occur by direct contact between sheep. The scrapie agent has been detected in the **nervous system, salivary glands, tonsils, lymph nodes, nictitating membrane, spleen, distal ileum, proximal colon and muscles**. A recent report suggests that the scrapie agent persisted in a **sheep barn in Iceland for 16 years.** This prion has also been isolated from an experimentally contaminated soil sample after three years. **Transmission via contaminated fomites** such as knives is theoretically possible, and transmission has been reported in a contaminated **vaccine.**

Transmission has not been studied extensively **in goats.** Most infected goats have a history of contact with sheep, and are probably infected by contact with the placenta or nasal secretions. Experimental infections have been established in goats by feeding prion-containing fetal membranes, as well as by intracerebral or subcutaneous inoculation. Recent studies suggest that prions may be spread through **urine and persist in the environment for decades.**

Scrapie tends to persist in flocks and can also arise apparently spontaneously in flocks that have not previously had cases of the disease. This disease of sheep (and goats) was the first TSE to be studied. It seems to be transmitted from animal to animal in feed contaminated with nerve tissue. It can also be transmitted by injection of brain tissue.

Pathogenesis

After natural infection, PrP^{Sc} is firstly detected in **lymphoreticular system like spleen, tonsil, retropharyngeal & mesenteric lymph nodes** where replication occurs before invading nervous system. While in the lymph nodes, replication occurs in the **dendritic cells.** Following oral infection, it probably enters the **neural tissues** in the duodenum & ileum, PrP^{Sc} then spreads trough the fibres of autonomic nervous system to the **spinal cord & the medulla oblongata**. There occurs non inflammatory neuronal vacuolar degeneration of **grey matter, appearance of amyloid fibrils containing PrP^{Sc}**, & astroglyosis are associated with accumulation of PrP^{Sc} in the CNS. The PrP^{Sc} proteins are resistant to proteases & are not cleared from the brain by normal mechanism.

Clinical symptoms and lesions: **The incubation period is usually 2 to 5 years in sheep;** cases are rare in sheep less than a year old. Scrapie has been reported in 2 to 8 year old goats. The incubation period in experimentally infected goats is less than three years, with a range of 30 to 146 weeks

The symptoms of scrapie are **variable in sheep**, and influenced by the **strain of the prion, sheep's genotype and/or breed**. The first symptoms are usually behavioral changes: affected sheep tend to stand apart from the flock and may either trail or lead when the flock is driven. As the disease progresses, animals usually become hyperexcitable and have a high-stepping or unusual hopping gait and/or a fixed stare, with the head held high. Other symptoms may include **ataxia, incoordination, blindness, trembling, or convulsions when being handled.** Intense **pruritus** is common and may lead to rubbing, scraping or chewing. Scratching of the dorsum or pressure over the base of the tail may cause a characteristic nibbling response due to pruritus. **Loss of condition is common in the early stages**, and significant weight loss or emaciation may be seen later. The fleece may be dry and brittle. Drinking behavior and urination can also change, with affected animals drinking small quantities of water often. Most animals die two to six weeks after the onset of symptoms, but deaths may occur up to six months later.

In sheep with the **Nor98 variant**, incoordination and ataxia appear to be major symptoms. Pruritus seems to be minimal or uncommon, although it has been seen in some animals. Losses of body condition, anxiety, tremors, abnormal menace responses or a subdued mental status have been reported in some cases. Some cases of atypical scrapie have been found by routine surveillance in apparently healthy flocks at slaughter.

Variable clinical signs have been reported **in goats** with scrapie. In one case, the only symptoms were **listlessness, weight loss and premature cessation of lactation**. The clinical signs may also resemble scrapie in sheep, with behavioral changes such as irritability and loss of inquisitiveness, as well as hyperesthesia, incoordination, posture abnormalities, unusual alertness, restlessness, tremors, teeth grinding, salivation, impaired vision or regurgitation of rumen contents. Some goats have been reported to stamp and hold their heads down as if they are bothered by nonexistent flies. In late stages, animals may appear drowsy and have difficulty in rising. Pruritus is less common in goats than in sheep; if it occurs, it is typically less intense and often localized over the tailhead or withers. As in sheep, the disease is progressive, with prostration and death 1-6 months after the onset of symptoms.

Lesions: The carcass may be wasted or emaciated. No other gross lesions are found. The characteristic **histopathologic** lesions include neuronal vacuolation and non-inflammatory spongiform changes in the gray matter of the central nervous system (CNS). Astrocytosis and **amyloid plaques** may also be seen. These lesions are usually but not always bilaterally symmetrical.

Diagnosis: Scrapie is usually confirmed by detecting PrPSc in the CNS. Neuronal vacuolation and PrPSc accumulation typically occur in the brainstem at the level of the obex in sheep with the classical form of scrapie. In sheep with Nor98 scrapie, these abnormalities occur mainly in the cerebellar and cerebral cortices.

Treatment & prevention: There is no treatment for scrapie. Scrapie is a reportable disease in the United States. Risk of scrapie can be reduced by maintaining a closed flock or minimizing outside purchases of stock. If replacement animals must be added to the flock, they should be from flocks that are negative for this disease.

The use of scrapie-resistant genotypes also decreases the risk for the classical form of scrapie; however, atypical scrapie can occur in these animals, including those with highly resistant ARR/ARR genotypes. Goats usually become infected after contact with sheep. Goats should not be mixed with sheep of unknown scrapie status. Outside purchases of stock should be minimized.

Bovine Spongiform Encephalopathy (BSE)

Bovine spongiform encephalopathy (**BSE**), also called **mad-cow disease**, is a afebrile, subacute, fatal neurodegenerative disease in adult cattle of 4-5 years, all breeds being susceptible, causes a vacuolation of grey matter, neurophil & neuronal perikaya, neuronal spongy degeneration in the brain, and gliosis with a long incubation period, 30 months to 8 years.

Occurrrence

BSE started in UK, spread to Oman, Canada, Germany, Denmark, Belgium, Italy, France, Portugal, Switzerland & Ireland.

Transmission

Transmission occurred viacattle feed that contained brain tissue from sheep infected with scrapie. BSE also probably evolved from a spontaneous form of "mad cow disease" that has been seen occasionally in cattle for many centuries. Studies in 2008 suggest that mad cow disease also is caused by a **genetic mutation within a gene called Prion Protein Gene**. An epidemic of this disease began in Great Britain in 1985 and before it was controlled, some 800,000 cattle were sickened by it. Its origin appears to have been cattle feed that contained brain tissue from sheep infected with scrapie, and had been treated in a new way that no longer destroyed the infectiousness of the scrapie prions. The use of such food was banned in 1988 and after peaking in 1992, the epidemic declined quickly.

Transmissible Mink Encephalopathy (TME)

Transmissible mink encephalopathy (TME) is rare sporadic disease that affects the CNS of ranch-raised adult mink. Clinical signs include the characteristic behavioural changes such as confusion, loss of cleanliness, and aimless circling. Affected animals show signs of weight loss, matted fur, hind-quarter ataxia and arching its tail over its back; seizures may very rarely occur & at last stages signs of drowsiness and unresponsiveness.

Feline Spongiform Encephalopathy (FSE)

Feline spongiform encephalopathy (FSE) is a disease that affects the brains and livers of domestic and captive feline. FSE is thought to be related to BSE. Lezmi S. et al. (2003), suggested that this infectious agent might be spread by both hematogenous & nervous pathways. Like BSE, this disease can take several years to develop. Probably the affected animals contract the disease by eating contaminated bovine meat. Ataxia was observed to last for about 8 weeks in the affected animals. The ultimate result is death of the infected animals.

Chronic Wasting Disease (CWD)

Chronic wasting disease (CWD) is a transmissible spongiform encephalopathy (TSE) of mule, deer, White-tailed deer, elk, & moose. To date, CWD has been found mainly in cervids (members of the deer family). First recognized as a **clinical "wasting" syndrome in 1967** in mule deer in a wildlife research facility in northern Colorado, USA, it was identified as a TSE in 1978 and has spread to a dozen states and two Canadian provinces. CWD is manifested by **chronic weight loss leading to death**. There is no known relationship between CWD and any other TSE of animals or people.

Exotic Ungulate Encephalopathy (EUE)

Exotic ungulate encephalopathy (EUE) is a Transmissible spongiform encephalopathy (TSE), identified in infected organs of zoo animals like Nyala, Arabian & Scimitar oryx, greater kudu, gemsbok, the common eland, Ankole-Watusi cow & an American bison in UK. Transmission probably occurred via the consumption of feed supplemented with meat & bone meal, although some animals died after the British ban on ground offal in animal feed. All animals died during the 1990s, with the last death occurring in 1998.

□□□

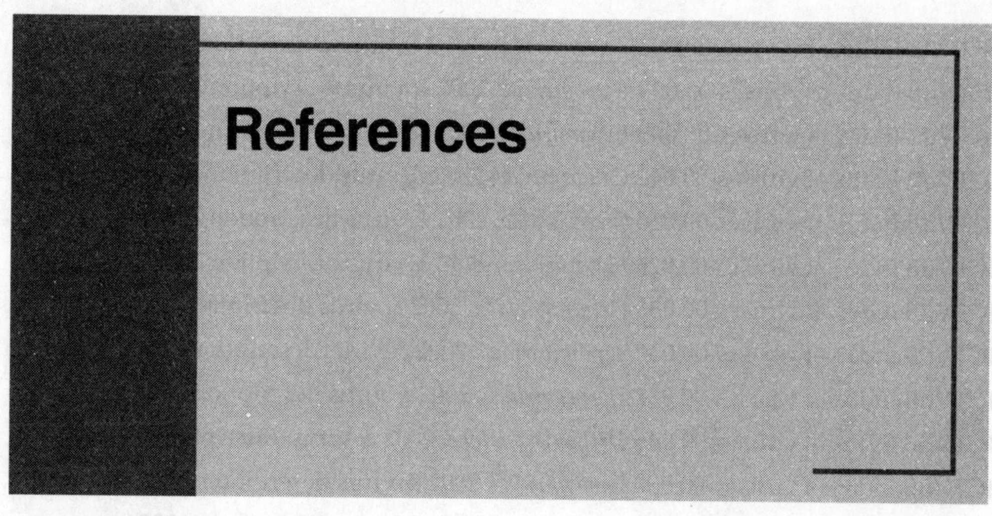

References

Internet references

Adenoviridae: From Wikipedia, the free encyclopedia, 2011

Arenaviridae: From Wikipedia, the free encyclopedia, 2011

Arteriaviridae: From Wikipedia, the free encyclopedia, 2011

Asfarviridae: From Wikipedia, the free encyclopedia, 2011

Astroviridae: From Wikipedia, the free encyclopedia, 2011

Birnaviridae: From Wikipedia, the free encyclopedia, 2011

Bornaviridae: From Wikipedia, the free encyclopedia, 2011

Bunyaviridae: From Wikipedia, the free encyclopedia, 2011

Caliciviridae: From Wikipedia, the free encyclopedia, 2011

Circoviridae: From Wikipedia, the free encyclopedia, 2011

Coronaviridae: From Wikipedia, the free encyclopedia, 2011

Filoviridae: From Wikipedia, the free encyclopedia, 2011

Flaviviridae: From Wikipedia, the free encyclopedia, 2011

Hepadnaviridae: From Wikipedia, the free encyclopedia, 2011

Herpesviridae: From Wikipedia, the free encyclopedia, 2011

ICTVdB description of Prions-90.001 *Hepdnaviridae*, 2002 & virus description 2006

ICTVdB Index of viruses-00.001 Adenoviridae, 2002 & virus description 2006

ICTVdB Index of viruses-00.002 *Asfarviridae*, 2002 & virus description 2006

ICTVdB Index of viruses-00.003 *Arenaviridae*, 2002 & virus description 2006

ICTVdB Index of viruses-00.003 *Bunyaviridae*, 2002 & virus description 2006
ICTVdB Index of viruses-00.005 *Astroviridae*, 2002 & virus description 2006
ICTVdB Index of viruses-00.009 *Birnaviridae*, 2002 & virus description 2006
ICTVdB Index of viruses-00.012 *Caliciviridae*, 2002 & virus description 2006
ICTVdB Index of viruses-00.016 *Circoviridae*, 2002 & virus description 2006
ICTVdB Index of viruses-00.026 *Flaviviridae*, 2002 & virus description 2006
ICTVdB Index of viruses-00.030 *Hepdnaviridae*, 2002 & virus description 2006
ICTVdB Index of viruses-00.030*Hepdnaviridae*, 2002 & virus description 2006
ICTVdB Index of viruses-00.031 *Herpesviridae*, 2002 & virus description 2006
ICTVdB Index of viruses-00.046 *Orthomxoviridae*, 2002 & virus description 2006
ICTVdB Index of viruses-00.050 *Parvoviridae*, 2002 & virus description 2006
ICTVdB Index of viruses-00.052 *Picornaviridae*, 2002 & virus description 2006
ICTVdB Index of viruses-00.058 *Poxviridae*, 2002 & virus description 2006
ICTVdB Index of viruses-00.060 *Reoviridae*, 2002 & virus description 2006
ICTVdB Index of viruses-00.061 *Retroviridae*, 2002 & virus description 2006
ICTVdB Index of viruses-00.073 *Togaviridae*, 2002 & virus description 2006
ICTVdB Index of viruses-00.099 *Papillomaviridae*, 2002 & virus description 2006
ICTVdB Index of viruses-00.099 *Polyomaviridae*, 2002 & virus description 2006
ICTVdB Index of viruses-01.025 *Filoviridae*, 2002 & virus description 2006
ICTVdB Index of viruses-01.025 *Filoviridae*, 2002 & virus description 2006
ICTVdB Index of viruses-01.048 *Parmyxoviridae*, 2002 & virus description 2006
ICTVdB Index of viruses-01.062 *Rhabdoviridae*, 2002 & virus description 2006
ICTVdB Index of viruses-01.081 *Bornaviridae*, 2002 & virus description 2006
ICTVdB Index of viruses-03.004 *Arteriviridae*, 2002 & virus description 2006
ICTVdB Index of viruses-03.019 *Coronaviridae*, 2002 & virus description 2006
Orthomyxoviridae: From Wikipedia, the free encyclopedia, 2011
Papillomaviridae: From Wikipedia, the free encyclopedia, 2011
Paramyxoviridae: From Wikipedia, the free encyclopedia, 2011
Parvoviridae: From Wikipedia, the free encyclopedia, 2011
Picornaviridae: From Wikipedia, the free encyclopedia, 2011
Polyomaaviridae: From Wikipedia, the free encyclopedia, 2011
Poxviridae: From Wikipedia, the free encyclopedia, 2011
Prion: From Wikipedia, the free encyclopedia, 2011
Reoviridae: From Wikipedia, the free encyclopedia, 2011

Retroviridae: From Wikipedia, the free encyclopedia, 2011

Rhabdoviridae: From Wikipedia, the free encyclopedia, 2011

Togaviridae: From Wikipedia, the free encyclopedia, 2011

ViralZone: *Arenaviridae 2011*

ViralZone: *Arteriviridae* 2011

ViralZone: *Astroviridae* 2011

ViralZone: *Birnaviridae* 2011

ViralZone: *Bornaviridae* 2011

ViralZone: *Bunyaviridae 2011*

ViralZone: *Caliciviridae* 2011

ViralZone: *Circoviridae* 2011

ViralZone: *Coronaviridae* 2011

ViralZone: *Filoviridae 2011*

ViralZone: *Flaviviridae* 2011

ViralZone: *Hepadnaviridae 2011*

ViralZone: *Herpesviridae* 2011

ViralZone: *Orthomyxoviridae* 2011

ViralZone: *Papillomaviridae* 2011

ViralZone: *Paramyxoviridae* 2011

ViralZone: *Parvoviridae* 2011

ViralZone: *Picornaviridae* 2011

ViralZone: *Polyomaviridae* 2011

ViralZone: *Poxviridae* 2011

ViralZone: *Reoviridae* 2011

ViralZone: *Retroviridae 2011*

ViralZone: *Rhabdoviridae* 2011

ViralZone: *Togaviridae* 2011

ViralZone:*Adenoviridae*, 2011

ViralZone:*Asfarviridae* 2011

Other references

Clinical Microbiology Review; 2007, 20(3): 489-510.

Current Science, 79(6): Sept. 25, 2000.

Federick A. Murphy, E. Paul J. Gibbs, Mavian C. Horiznek, M.J. Studdert Veterinary virology, 3rd edn. Academic Press.

Merck Veterinary Manual, 9th edn. 2008.

N. Agarwal, H. Korkaya and S. Jammel : How Viruses evade host responses International Centre for Genetic Engineering and Biotechnology, New Delhi.

N. James Maclachlan, Edward Dubovi : Fenner's Veterinary Virology Iredn. 2011, Elsevier/ Academic.

NT Meeusen, J. Walker, Andrew Peters, Paul-Pierre Pastoret and Gregers Jungersen : Current Status of Veterinary Vaccines.

Prion Diseases: Microbiology Bytes: Latest Updates, 2011

Prion Diseases; Centres for Disease Control & Prevention, 2011

Sharda SN, Adlakha S. Text Book of veterinary virology, 2009, IB DCO, Lucknow.

Surendran Mahalingam, Jayesh Meanger, Paul S. Foster and Brett A. Lidbury : The viral manipulation of the host cellular and immune environments to enhance propagation and survival : A focus on RNA viruses.

□□□

About the Author

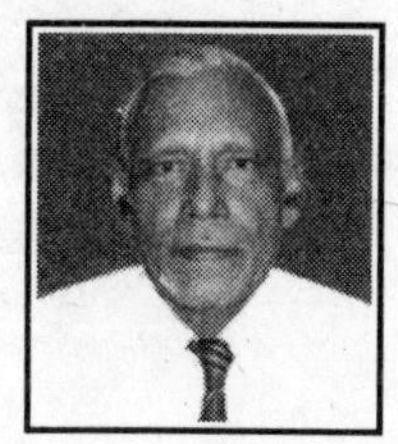

Dr. Chandra Bhushan Prasad, the author of the book, Veterinary Medical Virology was born in a village, Tope in Patna district on 6.7. 1938. He graduated (B. V. Sc. & A. H) from Bihar Veterinary College, Patna in 1960, & did M. V. Sc (Microbiology) from Mathura Veterinary College, UP in 1965. He obtained his Ph. D. degree in Virology in 1974 from Division of Virology, Central Drug Research Institute, Lucknow. He got FAO Fellowship & completed his FRVCS degree in 1972 from Royal Veterinary College, Stockholm (Sweden) under Dr Rubarth, the imminent pathologist. He pursued his research work at the National Institute of Bacteriology, Stockholm (Sweden) related to his dissertation research work in virology. He visited various Institutions in Sweden, Denmark, Helsinki (Finland), Norway & UK related to his research work. Under WHO/NICD training programme, he worked at NICD, Delhi in 1982.

He headed the dept of Veterinary Microbiology from 1974 to 1998 in the capacity of Assistant Professor, Associate Professor & University Professor cum Chief Scientist & Chairman. He was the Incharge of AICRP on Epidemiology of Foot-and-Mouth Disease, Patna Unit from 1978 to 1985 & visited all FMD Centers in India & participated in the deliberations of the Workshop on the Project. After his retirement in 1998, he taught Biochemistry, Biotechnology, Molecular Biology & Immunology at B. V. C., Patna, Sanjay Gandhi Institute of Dairy Technology, Patna & at Science College, Patna, the premiere college of Patna University at M. Sc. level. He was the subject matter expert of Bihar Public Service Commission, Bihar, Patna for the selection of Veterinary Officers & was the expert for selection of Professor at IVRI, Izatnagar, Agricultural University, Pantnagar & Central Agriculture University, Aizawl. He was the member of Management Board of ICAR Society for framing ICAR policy for four years. He is the life member of Infectious Diseases & Microbiologists of India & was on the Editorial Board of Indian Journal of Virology & other journals. He is credited with publication of more than 50 research papers & Lectures series in Veterinary Virology, Bacteriology, Immunology & Mycology.

About the Author

Dr. Chandra Bhushan Prasad, the author of the book Veterinary Medical Virology was born in Village Tope in Patna district on 6.7.1938. He graduated (B. V. Sc. & A. H) from Bihar Veterinary College, Patna in 1960 & did M. V. Sc (Microbiology) from Mathura Veterinary College, UP in 1965. He obtained his Ph. D. degree in Virology in 1974 from Division of Virology, Central Drug Research Institute, Lucknow. He got FAO Fellowship & completed his FRVCS degree in 1972 from Royal Veterinary College, Stockholm (Sweden) under Dr Rubarth, the imminent pathologist. He pursued his research work at the National Institute of Bacteriology, Stockholm (Sweden) related to his dissertation research work in virology. He visited various institutions in Sweden, Denmark, Helsinki (Finland), Norway & UK related to his research work. Under WHO/NICD training programme, he worked at NICD, Delhi in 1982.

He headed the dept of Veterinary Microbiology from 1974 to 1998 in the capacity of Assistant Professor, Associate Professor & University Professor cum Chief Scientist & Chairman. He was the Incharge of AICRP on Epidemiology of Foot-and-Mouth Disease, Patna Unit from 1978 to 1988 & visited all FMD centers in India & participated in the deliberations of the Workshop on the Project. After his retirement in 1998, he taught Biochemistry, Biotechnology, Molecular Biology & Immunology at B. V. C., Patna, Sanjay Gandhi Institute of Dairy Technology, Patna & at Science College, Patna, the premier college of Patna University at M.Sc level. He was the subject matter expert of Bihar Public Service Commission, Bihar, Patna for the selection of Veterinary Officers & was the expert for selection of Professor at IVRI, Izatnagar, Agricultural University, Pantnagar & Central Agriculture University, Aizawl. He was the member of Management Board of ICAR Society for framing ICAR policy for four years. He is the life member of Infectious Diseases & Microbiologists of India & was on the Editorial Board of Indian Journal of Virology & other journals. He is credited with publication of more than 50 research papers & Lectures series in Veterinary Virology, Bacteriology, Immunology & Mycology.